ANTEPARTAL AND INTRAPARTAL FETAL MONITORING

3rd Edition

By MICHELLE L. MURRAY, PhD, RNC

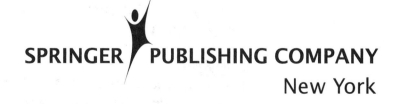

SPRINGER PUBLISHING COMPANY
New York

*"But many do not know that they do not know,
and many think they know when they know nothing."*

Balthasar Gracián
Originally written in 1637 in Spanish
Translated by Joseph Jacob
The Art of Worldly Wisdom
© 1993 Shambhala Publications, Inc.

Springer Publishing Company, LLC
11 West 42nd Street
New York, NY 10036
www.springerpub.com

Acquisitions Editor: James Costello
Production Editor: Rose Mary Piscitelli
Composition: International Graphic Services

07 08 09 10 / 5 4 3 2 1

Library of Congress Cataloging-in-Publication Data

Antepartal and intrapartal fetal monitoring / [edited] by Michelle L. Murray.–3rd ed.
    p. ; cm.
    Includes bibliographical references and index.
    ISBN 0-8261-3262-6
    1. Fetal monitoring. I. Murray, Michelle (Michelle L.)
    [DNLM: 1. Fetal Monitoring.   2. Heart Rate, Fetal.   WQ 209
A6271 2007]
RG628.A574 2007
618.3'2075--dc22

2006028397

Printed in the United States of America by Bang Printing

ANTEPARTAL AND INTRAPARTAL FETAL MONITORING
Third Edition

Michelle L. Murray, PhD, RNC
Author and Editor

Kenneth J. Moise, Jr., MD
Gary Joffe, MD
Sherrill L. Tillger, RN, MA
Contributing Editors

Contributions By:

Chapter 1
Penny Peterson, RNC, MSN
Corporate Sponsors

Chapter 2
Deborah J. Eganhouse, PhD, RNC
Sherrill L. Tillger, RN, MA
Jean Marie Yackey, RNC, MSN

Chapters 3 & 4
Tracey A. Kasnic, RNC, BSN, MBA

Chapter 5
Katherine W. O'Connell, RN, MN

Chapter 6
Linda Chagnon, RNC, MBA, MN
Julia M. B. Fine, PhD, RN
Joyce Vogler, DrPH, RN

Chapter 7
Kathy W. O'Connell, RN, MN

Chapter 8
Linda A. Petersen, RNC, BSN
Cheryl Wallerstedt, RNC, MS

Chapter 9
Carolyn L. Gegor, CNM, MS, RDMS

Chapter 10
Carolyn L. Gegor, CNM, MS, RDMS
Susan Nelson, RN

Preface

The dawn of a new era in treating the fetus as a patient arrived in 1958 when Dr. Edward Hon reported the capability to continuously assess the fetal heart rate by means of a fetal EKG monitor on the maternal abdomen. Commercial devices for bedside fetal heart rate monitoring were introduced in the late 1960s, and by the mid-1980s the great majority of laboring women in the United States underwent electronic fetal monitoring.

Our forefathers were so convinced that such surveillance would reduce the incidence of cerebral palsy and perinatal asphyxia that clinical trials were omitted before widespread implementation of fetal monitoring. Some 40 years later, we know this not to be the case. Clearly, a large percentage of perinatal asphyxia occurs prior to the onset of labor. Recent randomized trials have even questioned the validity of continuous electronic monitoring in any low-risk obstetrical patient. In addition, several authorities have concluded that monitoring has contributed to the disturbing rise in the rate of cesarean delivery.

Minimal advances have been achieved in monitoring techniques. Computer technology has brought us autocorrelation to improve our ability to assess fetal heart rate variability with external monitoring. Electronic sensors in specialized intrauterine pressure catheters with amnioinfusion ports have improved our capability to accurately assess intrauterine pressure and replace amniotic fluid volume in cases of variable decelerations. Yet in an era when space shuttle missions are so commonplace that they rarely receive prime time television coverage, we must still rely on the interaction between the fetal central nervous system and the fetal heart to establish in utero well-being. Perhaps the newest technology of fetal pulse oximetry, now in clinical trials, will aid us in accurately interpreting the fetal heart rate tracing. More likely, a continuous assessment of the fetal acid-base status will transform the art of evaluating fetal monitoring tracings into a true science.

Although the accurate interpretation of a fetal heart rate tracing is paramount to the care of the laboring patient, it remains one of the more difficult skills to master. One must learn to appreciate subtle changes in the baseline rate, short-term variability, and patterns of decelerations to determine that the tracing is nonreassuring. In her second edition of *Antepartal and Intrapartal Fetal Monitoring*, Michelle Murray, PhD, RNC, has provided us with an excellent tool to begin the process of understanding the basics as well as the more advanced aspects of fetal heart rate monitoring. The book has more than doubled in size since the publication of the first edition in 1988. Sections on maternal and fetal physiology have been added to describe the wealth of knowledge that has been acquired in these areas in the last decade. Dr. Murray has chosen to include a section on fetal pulse oximetry, a clear reflection of the contemporaneous nature of this book. Beginners will find this work extremely useful to master the endless patterns of fetal heart rate tracings. This book also deserves a special place on the front shelf of the seasoned practitioner as a useful reference text.

Kenneth J. Moise, Jr., MD
UpJohn Distinguished Professor of Obstetrics and Gynecology
Director, Division of Maternal-Fetal Medicine
University of North Carolina
Chapel Hill, North Carolina

Preface

In 1988, Michelle Murray's text, *Antepartal and Intrapartal Fetal Monitoring*, was published by the Nurses' Association of the American College of Obstetricians and Gynecologists (NAACOG). NAACOG is now known as the Association of Women's Health, Obstetric, and Neonatal Nurses (AWHONN). *Antepartal and Intrapartal Fetal Monitoring* has been referred to as "The Bible." It was updated in 1989, and has sold over 10,000 copies. In this new edition, Dr. Murray has expanded the depth and breadth of the original text. The second edition provides practitioners with the needed references and resources they need to provide quality care to women and their fetuses. It is a cutting edge resource for a practice-based discipline, with details and references that are specific and clear. In addition, the protocols and procedures found in the appendix are applicable to clinical practices that include fetal monitors.

The leadership role in fetal monitoring education for nurses came from AWHONN. AWHONN demonstrated their commitment to fetal monitoring by publishing the first edition of this text. AWHONN continues to take a leadership role in fetal monitoring education through their fetal monitoring courses and videotapes. AWHONN is to be commended in these endeavors.

Building on the traditions of AWHONN, Dr. Murray selected a broad base team of contributors and editors who represent every aspect of perinatal nursing and medicine from practice, research, business, industry, education, management, and academia. The educational preparation of this team is vast, representing the baccalaureate to the doctorate. All contributors have expertise in one or more aspects of fetal monitoring. Many are fetal monitoring instructors or instructor-trainers for AWHONN.

As with any book, there are people who help turn dreams into reality. One is Elaine Smiel who, during the pregnancy of her fourth child, undertook the task of typing this text. Indeed, it was a birthing process. Dr. Murray's sons, Sean and David, have been an inspiration and a grounding force for their mother. They have allowed her the opportunity to grow and create this new book for all of us to use in our practice settings. Most of all, this book is for you. To the nurses who care for mothers, babies, and families, may this text be the foundation for your excellence in practice, education, and research. To the physicians who read this text, our teamwork and common knowledge are an asset to the quality care families deserve.

Patricia Grant Higgins, PhD, RN
Professor of Parent-Child Nursing, retired
University of New Mexico Health Sciences Center
College of Nursing, Albuquerque, New Mexico
AWHONN Director-at-Large

Acknowledgments

The Decade of the 1970s

In the 1970s, when I became a labor and delivery staff nurse, the vast majority of nurses and physicians learned to use fetal monitors "on the job." A few books were available to help us learn basic fetal monitoring concepts. Journal articles started to appear that enhanced our understanding of the fetus. For example, the first case report on fetal seizures that included a fetal heart rate pattern was published in 1978 in the *American Journal of Obstetrics and Gynecology*.

The Decade of the 1980s

In 1980, I became an instructor in a 2 year associate degree program. My MSN was completed in May, 1981. The ADN curriculum included only $1/2$ hour on fetal monitoring concepts. Student nurses were rarely allowed to participate in the care of a woman during labor and delivery, other than to witness a delivery. Just as I had learned fetal monitoring, graduates of our program were expected to learn fetal monitoring "on the job."

   In 1984, I became the Ob/Gyn Nursing Education Coordinator for a 9 hospital system in New Mexico. I was tasked with developing a fetal monitoring education program for nurses. By 1986, I had taught 500 nurses fetal monitoring. The handout materials for that program grew into a book which later became the first edition of this text. The entire process of creating the first edition of *Antepartal and Intrapartal Fetal Monitoring* took 3 years. In 1985, I began my doctoral studies. *Antepartal and Intrapartal Fetal Monitoring* was published in 1988. I completed my doctoral studies in 1992.

The 1990s

Between 1986 and 1996, over 50,000 people from all 50 states and at least 7 foreign countries had attended my courses on fetal monitoring. The excellence of these courses is due, in part, to the dedicated staff at Professional Education Center in Chico, California. My participants have included student nurses, OB techs, licensed practical nurses, registered nurses, certified nurse midwives, residents, family practice physicians, obstetricians, chiefs of obstetrics, paralegals, insurance company employees, and lawyers. They have been my teachers and have generously shared their most interesting tracings and experiences with me. Many of their tracings are included in this text. I thank each and every one of them for their generous contributions and support.

   I wish to thank everyone who helped me finish the second edition, which was completed in 1 $1/2$ years. The reference librarians and employees at the New Mexico Health Sciences Center Library, especially Becca, Judy, and Tim, always maintained a pleasant attitude in spite of our pressures and deadlines. Whatever we needed, they helped us get. The quality of the reference lists reflects their excellence and the work of Elaine Smiel, who spent countless hours on the telephone with the librarians, or copying articles for me to read, or typing.

   My contributors are all very busy, talented, and dedicated people. Each offered as much support as they could so that this text could be revised. Some critiqued a chapter and made suggestions for additions. Others rewrote sections of the old edition. Some wrote sections of the new edition and even edited a chapter. Corporate sponsors offered support so that the text could be completed in as short a time as possible.

   It is with deep pride and intense love that I thank my sons, Sean and David, for their continued tolerance of my work to educate users of the fetal monitor. I wish to acknowledge my mother, Emma Sarah Angel Moise, who taught me, "If there's a will, there's a way." I had the will, I found the way. Now, Springer Publishing will help me reach more readers of this book. I am grateful for their dedication to excellence!

                                                                          Michelle L. Murray, PhD, RNC

Table of Contents

Contributors and Corporate Sponsors. iii

Preface iv

Acknowledgments vi

Chapter 1   Fetal and Maternal Monitoring Equipment 1

Chapter 2   The Baseline, Accelerations, and Decelerations. 59

Chapter 3   Intrinsic Factors that Affect the Fetal Heart Rate. 163

Chapter 4   Extrinsic Factors that Affect Oxygen Delivery and the FHR 197

Chapter 5   Acid-Base Balance 241

Chapter 6   Prediction and Prevention of Intrapartal Fetal Asphyxia 305

Chapter 7   Hemodynamic and Biochemical Fetal Monitoring 341

Chapter 8   Variations of the Fetal Heart Rate 391

Chapter 9   Antepartal Fetal Monitoring. 455

Chapter 10 Biophysical Fetal Assessment 489

Appendix   507

Index   517

1

Fetal and Maternal Monitoring Equipment

Advances in fetal monitor development have paralleled computer and ultrasound development. *First generation fetal monitors*, from the 1960s and 1970s, were equipped with ultrasound technology that poorly detected the fetal heart rate. In fact, 40 to 45 percent of the signals were missed which created gaps in the tracing (1). Experienced clinicians knew internal devices, such as the spiral electrode and intrauterine pressure catheter, provided better signal transmission than external devices such as the ultrasound transducer and tocotransducer.

A goal of the 1970s was to improve ultrasound (US) technology (2). Advanced microprocessors, wider beam US devices, and autocorrelation enhanced the signal to noise ratio resulting in a higher quality fetal heart rate (FHR) tracing. *Second generation monitors*, introduced in the 1980s, had this advanced technology (3-4). Their US signal loss was less than 20 percent in the less than 25 week gestation and less than 10 percent in the 25 or greater week gestation (5).

A goal of the 1980s was to reduce inconsistent tracing interpretations. Software programs were developed and tested in both antepartal and intrapartal settings (6-8). The goal of the next century is to improve these software programs, incorporating artificial intelligence so that management strategies can be recommended.

The value of electronic fetal monitors depends on the depth and breath of the user's knowledge of fetal and maternal physiology and technology. Chapter 2 examined fetal and maternal physiology related to regulation of the FHR. This chapter includes strengths and limitations of continuous electronic fetal monitoring (EFM), fetal monitor features, computer applications related to fetal monitoring,

external and internal monitoring devices, and the assessment and analysis of uterine activity (UA).

BENEFITS AND LIMITATIONS OF CONTINUOUS EFM

The application of a fetal monitor throughout labor with frequent evaluation of the FHR and UA pattern is known as continuous EFM. On the positive side, continuous EFM was associated with a decrease in fetal and neonatal death rates (0.05 percent vs. 0.43 percent) (9-13). However, controversy about the benefits of continuous EFM persist due to studies that found no relationship between EFM use and fetal death (14-17).

Continuous EFM has been associated with an increase in the cesarean section and post partum endometritis rates (9). However, EFM studies rarely examine other factors related to an abnormal FHR pattern or the decision to perform a cesarean section. Continuous EFM, in conjunction with fetal scalp pH sampling, was associated with a lower cesarean section rate than EFM use alone, but a higher cesarean section rate than intermittent auscultation (18). This finding implies scalp pH results support a decision to wait for a vaginal birth.

A fetus at high risk for intrapartal asphyxia, such as the intrauterine growth restricted (IUGR) fetus who has limited oxygen reserves, benefits the most from continuous surveillance. Benefits of continuous EFM must be weighed with its limitations (see Tables 1 and 2). Although there are more limitations than benefits, the impact of each point on the fetus, mother, and her support network should be considered.

Clinicians who overuse EFM may be fearful that labor increases the risk of fetal or neonatal neurologic injury. But, labor events are rarely the primary cause of cerebral palsy (12, 16, 19-22). Fear may precede "over monitoring," resulting in millions of monitor tracings for analysis by clinicians with differing educational backgrounds and interpretation skills. Thus, over monitoring may result in misinterpretation of FHR and UA patterns, conflicting interpretations, and unnecessary interventions (6-7).

Table 1: Benefits of Continuous EFM

1. Reliably identifies the healthy fetus (23-25).
2. Provides a means of antepartum fetal surveillance in high risk pregnancies (26).
3. Less labor intensive than auscultation (23).
4. External monitoring, like auscultation, is noninvasive.
5. Records FHR variability (23, 25).
6. Expedites twin and triplet monitoring.
7. Provides a continuous printout of the FHR and UA for evaluation by health care providers who may not be present at the bedside 100 percent of the time.
8. Enhances the woman's awareness of the onset of contractions so she can begin relaxation techniques (27-28).
9. Reassures women when they hear a normal FHR (27-28).
10. Less intrusive than auscultation with less interruption of maternal concentration than intermittent auscultation (27-28).
11. Preferred by obese women, high risk women, and women with a history of stillbirth (29).

Table 2: Limitations of Continuous EFM

1. EFM equipment is expensive (30).
2. The FHR pattern is not diagnostic, it does not *quantitate* hypoxia, and a hypoxic fetus may be missed (16, 23-26). Auscultation may also fail to identify a hypoxic fetus.
3. Fetal and maternal benefits are controversial (31-33).
4. May increase forceps and cesarean section deliveries (31-33).
5. Encourages other obstetric interventions (15, 31-33).
6. Subjective analysis of the tracing results in interpretation discrepancies and unnecessary operative interventions (6-7, 26).
7. Similar patterns of the FHR or UA have different causes.
8. Increased maternal or fetal risk of complications when internal monitoring devices are used, e.g., the spiral electrode (SE) may be dangerous in the very small preterm fetus (26, 34-35).
9. The tocotransducer (toco) may not detect contractions well in preterm, obese, or restless women (36-37).
10. The monitor medicalizes labor, may interfere with relaxation, and increases maternal immobility which may affect labor progress or precede weak and more painful contractions (26, 28, 30, 38).
11. Lack of knowledge of FHR and UA patterns may increase anxiety of the woman and her support network (28, 38).
12. Perpetuates the misconception that monitors replace nurses (28).
13. Places a barrier between the care giver and the laboring woman (28, 38).
14. The monitor can become the focal point in the room, distracting attention away from the laboring woman (28, 38).
15. The SE may transmit the maternal ECG (MECG) in a case of fetal demise. The maternal heart rate (MHR) will be printed on the tracing (39). The US may detect maternal aortic wall movement and the MHR will be printed. A failure to recognize the lack of a FHR may delay appropriate management.

EQUIPMENT: FETAL MONITOR FEATURES

Fetal monitors are capable of detecting, analyzing, and displaying fetal movement, the fetal ECG (FECG), and UA (40). Monitor features include:

1. *On/off recorder button:* Turns the paper recorder on or off.

2. *Paper and Paper tray:* Paper is heat sensitive with two distinct sections or channels. The top is referred to as the FHR channel and the bottom is the UA channel. Some monitors also record fetal movement in the UA channel. The FHR channel may be printed in 5 or 10 beats per minute (bpm) increments on the vertical scale. *USA scaled paper has 10 bpm increments* with 30 bpm per

centimeter (cm) on the vertical scale (30 to 240 bpm range). *European scaled paper is printed in 5 bpm increments* with 20 bpm/cm on the vertical scale, usually with a range of 50 to 210 bpm (2) (see Figure 1.1). Most monitors sold in the United States are preset for USA scaled paper. If European scaled paper is used, monitors can be adjusted to print on this paper. Once the monitor is set to print on European scaled paper, only European scaled paper should be used. Otherwise, if USA scaled paper is used, the FHR pattern would be misinterpreted. European scaled paper (5 bpm increments) widens the FHR baseline, and increases the height of accelerations and the depth of decelerations.

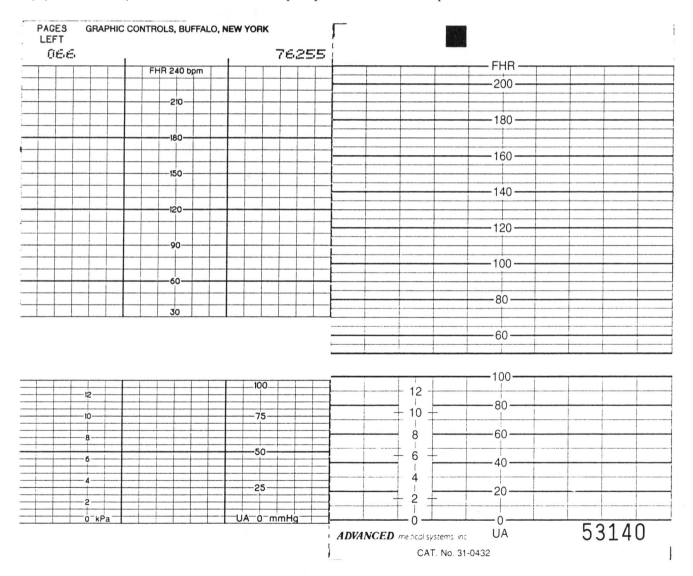

Figure 1.1 USA scaled paper on the left with 30 bpm/cm in the FHR channel. European scaled paper on the right with 20 bpm/cm. Note the uterine activity channel is similar, usually rising from 0 to 100 mm Hg in 5 to 10 mm Hg increments. Fetal monitor paper may be printed in 10 or 20 second increments. Uterine activity may be denoted in 0 to 13.3 kilopascal (kPa) units (1 kPa = 7.5 mm Hg). At 1, 2 or 3 cm/minute, both USA and European paper roll out of the fetal monitor at the same speed. At 3 cm/minute, 10 seconds = 0.5 cm, and 1 minute includes six 10 second boxes or three 20 second boxes. Paper may be printed with dark vertical lines 3 cm apart (1 minute) at 3 cm/minute speed.

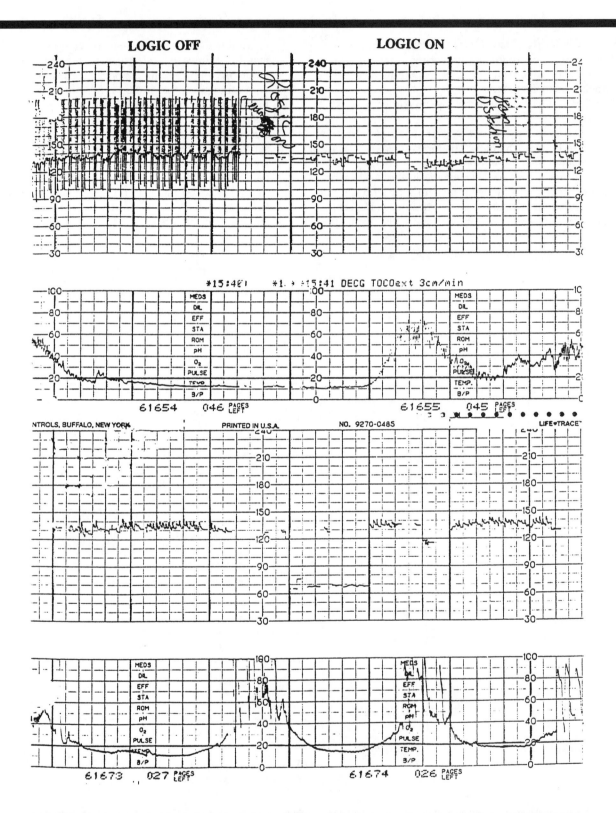

Figure 1.2: With a spiral electrode on the fetus and logic off, PVCs are represented by lines above and below the FHR baseline level. With logic on, PVC lines are deleted. The upward deflections reflect the rate calculated from the pulse interval between the normal R wave and the premature R wave. The downward deflections reflect the slower rate calculated using the pulse interval between the premature R wave and the R wave following a compensatory pause.

3. *Paper speed switch:* Fetal monitors may be set at 1, 2 or 3 cm/minute. *However, fetal monitors used in the USA <u>must</u> be set at 3 cm/minute.* Anything less would be below the national standard of practice (41). The standard may vary in other countries where paper speed may be 1, 2 or 3 cm/minute. The paper speed is often printed between the FHR and UA channels of the paper. The images at 1 or 2 cm/minute will be more compressed than those at 3 cm/minute and may be misinterpreted by people who are unfamiliar with the significance of those images.

4. *Printer:* Most fetal monitors have a heated thermal array printer, which is necessary when twins are monitored so that the FHR tracings can overlap. Some fetal monitors have thermal pens. The width of the printed dot (resolution) affects the accuracy of the printout when there are very small differences between consecutive calculated rates. Resolution is usually one bpm, but some monitors have a 1/2 bpm resolution. Date, time, monitoring mode,

and paper speed may be automatically printed at intervals on the paper. When the monitor is started, check the accuracy of this information.

5. *Logic or ECG artifact elimination switch:* Logic algorithms in the monitor software prevent the recording of extraneous noise and consecutive heart rates that are outside of pre-defined parameters. *It is best to leave logic off.* When the US is used, most second generation fetal monitors will not print consecutive rates that differ more than 25 bpm. When the SE is used and logic is ON, consecutive rates that differ more than 28 bpm will NOT be printed. When logic is OFF with SE use, all FHRs will be printed. Premature ventricular contractions will appear as long lines of similar length (see Figure 1.2).

6. *FECG plot:* Monitors that print the FECG on the paper have an ECG plot switch, not a logic switch. At the time of this writing, the AMS IM-76® and IM-77® (Advanced Medical

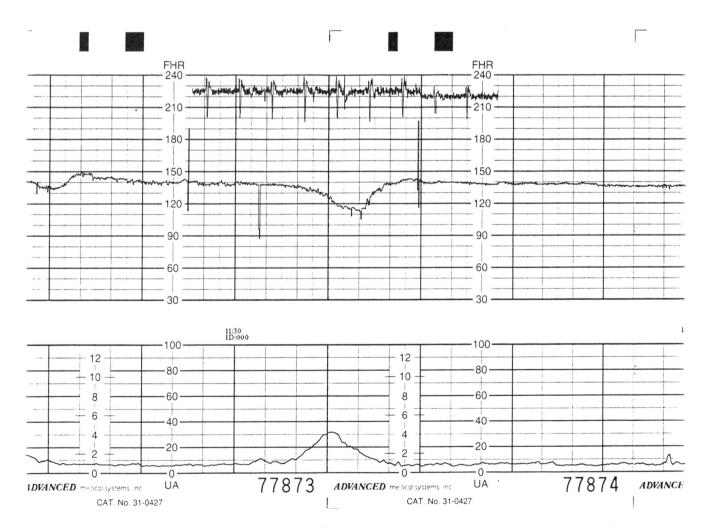

Figure 1.3: Fetal ECG printout automatically recorded at top of FHR channel if ECG plot is on (tracing provided by Advanced Medical Systems, Hamden, CT).

Systems, Hamden, CT) automatically plotted an FECG for 4 seconds at 25 mm/second on the top of the FHR channel if a SE were in use and the consecutive FHRs differed by more than 20 bpm (see Figure 1.3). This feature can be manually activated or deactivated. The Sonicaid Meridian® intrapartum fetal monitor (Oxford Instruments) also prints the FECG when the SE is used and the ECG plot is activated. Corometrics and Hewlett-Packard monitors do not print the FECG on the paper. To see the FECG, Corometrics monitors require a cable and ECG recorder.

7. *Test button:* Can be activated to check the internal circuitry of the monitor, the printer and paper feed. The digital displays of the FHR and UA are illuminated with a standard set of numbers. When the test button is pressed, the paper rolls out of the machine as the printer prints lines and/or words on the paper. The monitor circuitry can be tested with FHR and UA cables plugged in or out. When the monitor is first plugged in, it may run a self test. The monitor test may be manually activated.

8. *Uterine activity button:* Most monitors have a UA button to move the UA baseline to zero when an intrauterine pressure catheter (IUPC) is used. If a toco is used, this button or dial is used to return the UA baseline to a predetermined level such as 10 units.

9. *Fetal heart rate volume:* Used to increase or decrease the volume of the monitor's speaker.

10. *Loudspeaker:* The fetal monitor produces sounds. *These sounds are not actual heart sounds.* Therefore, it is inappropriate to inform women that the sound they hear is their baby's heart beat. If the transducer should slip and no sound is heard, she might think her baby is in jeopardy. Therefore, she needs to be informed that the sound is machine generated. Different sounds are produced by the Doppler shift when the US is used. If the sound is not manipulated by the equipment, the differences in the sounds reflected by different moving objects may be useful. Different sounds may also be heard when

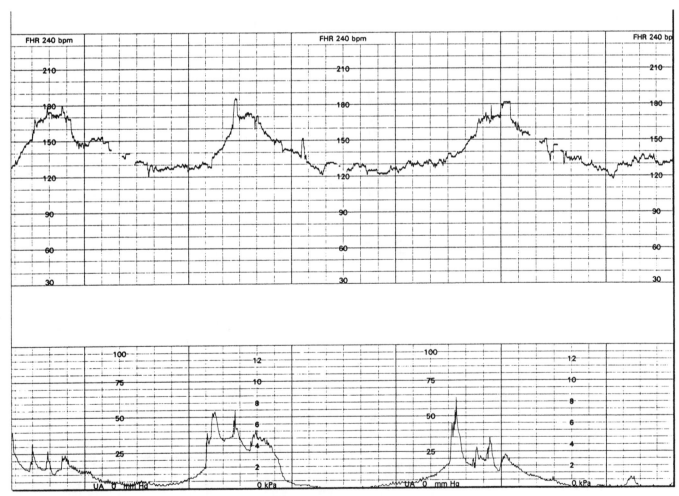

Figure 1.4: Maternal heart rate detected by ultrasound transducer during the second stage of labor. Suspect the fetus is not being recorded when there is a stable rate with uniform accelerations during times of maternal pain. This is entirely the MHR.

ANTEPARTAL AND INTRAPARTAL FETAL MONITORING

a hand-held Doppler is used. For example, cardiac wall motion produces a low *pulsing* sound, valve closure produces a *clicking* sound, umbilical or placental blood flow produces a *swishing* sound, and maternal arteries produce a *whispered rumble*. Since the actual heart sound is not heard, it is NOT appropriate to document "heart rate audible" when a fetal monitor is used. To hear the fetal heart beating (the ventricular rate), fetal heart sounds should be assessed by auscultation with a fetoscope or stethoscope. Fetal movement is not audible, but artificial sounds created by the monitor are often heard. However, rhythmic sounds in response to detected diaphragm movement may be heard when the fetus has hiccups.

11. *Automatic gain control:* Amplifies signals, increasing the signal to noise ratio which improves signal detection. The US placed over the maternal aorta detects maternal blood flow and aortic wall movement. Automatic gain control increases the strength of this weak signal and the MHR will be

recorded on the tracing. This has occurred in cases of fetal demise when an US or SE was used. For example, the weak MECG signal passes through the fetal body, is amplified by automatic gain control, and the MHR is printed.

Prior to application of the fetal monitor, the MHR should be assessed and a fetal movement history should be obtained. If there is a question regarding fetal life, the FHR should be determined. The FHR is best assessed by hearing the heart beat (fetoscope or stethoscope) or seeing it beat (real-time ultrasound). If a hand-held Doppler is used, the rate should be distinct from the MHR (7, 36, 42-43). If the maternal apical or radial pulse coincide with the rate printed on the tracing, the fetus is not being recorded (44-45).

Fetal death should be suspected if there is no fetal movement (FM), no fetal heart tones, the recorded baseline may be less than 100 bpm, uniform accelerations occur with contractions (the maternal pain response) (see Figure 1.4), and there is no acceleration following fetal scalp stimulation (45). In addition, the maternal heart rate

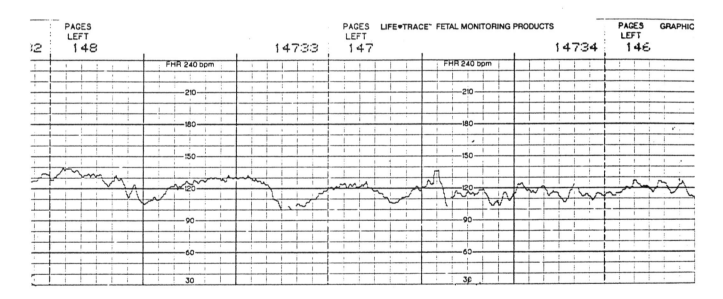

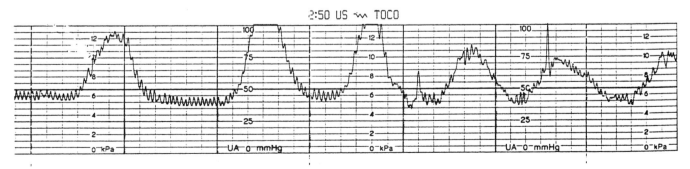

Figure 1.5: Maternal heart rate decelerations during contractions in a confirmed case of fetal demise.

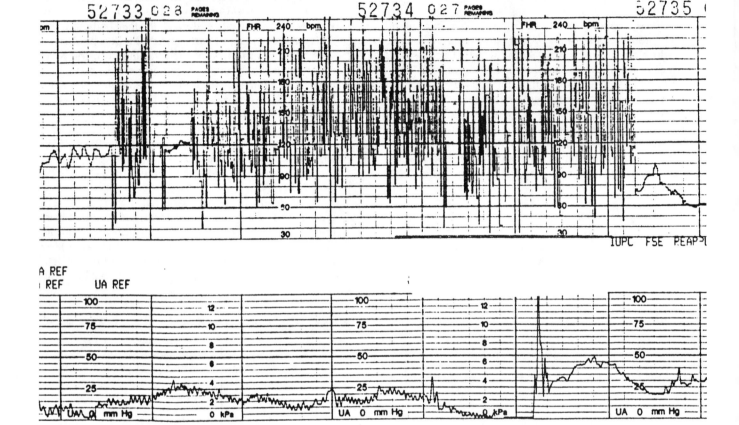

Figure 1.6: Artifact produced by signal loss or interference when the spiral electrode was in place. If artifact persists, it may be helpful to apply the ultrasound transducer and determine the cause of the artifact (see Table 5).

can decelerate, and may be mistaken for a FHR pattern (see Figure 1.5). Loss of the FHR signal, e.g., the US was over the maternal aorta, might create a small gap in the tracing, then MHR accelerations with a low baseline might be misinterpreted as FHR decelerations (46).

12. *Artifact:* When US is used, gaps and dots on the tracing may appear when the cardiac signal is undetected or too weak to be continuously recorded. When the SE is used, artifact includes *irregular lines with varying lengths,* unlike the regular lines of PVCs (see Figure 1.6). To improve signal transmission, the US transducer should be repositioned, coupling gel may be added or a SE may need to be applied. Signal interference when the SE wires bump the vaginal wall cause artifact. This "cervical interference" may also occur when the SE is first applied or the wires are touched during a vaginal examination.

13. *Monitor clock:* Clocks are battery-backed. If the printout reads "set time/date" when the monitor is plugged in and turned on, *backup batteries need replacement.* Reset the

clock if necessary, but consider replacing the back-up batteries as soon as possible. If each monitor's clock is reset to the nurse's watch, all the monitors will be set at different times. Then, events noted in the nurses' notes may not be timed to correspond with monitor times. This could create confusion as to the actual time of events. To avoid this confusion, it is better to set one's watch to the monitor then the monitor to one's watch.

14. *Monitoring ports:* Monitors may have two or three cardio ports. When only two cardio ports exist, one twin is monitored by US and the other by SE. If three cardio ports exist, twins may be simultaneously monitored by US. When the US and SE ports are used simultaneously, the US tracing is often darker than the SE tracing. When two US ports are used, the rate detected by US 2 often prints darker than the rate detected by US 1.

15. *Maternal ECG (MECG) cable:* The MHR may be calculated when the MECG is detected by a two lead or three lead ECG device adapted for the fetal monitor (see Figures 1.7

and 1.8). The MECG may be detected when a US or SE is in use in some monitors. In other monitors, the MECG can only be detected when an US is used as the MECG cable is inserted in the SE port. Dual maternal and fetal monitoring may be helpful when β-sympathomimetics, such as intravenous terbutaline, are administered or when a fetal demise is suspected. The MHR, not the MECG, and the FHR will be printed. In the case of fetal demise, the two rates will be nearly identical (47). When demise is suspected, the absence of fetal cardiac motion should be confirmed by real-time ultrasound.

Cross-channel verification™ (Hewlett-Packard M1350A®) helps identify maternal monitoring in the case of fetal demise or dual monitoring of one twin. Cross-channel verification triggers the printing of a question mark at the top of the FHR channel when more than one device, such as the MECG transducer, SE, or US detect a signal from the same source.

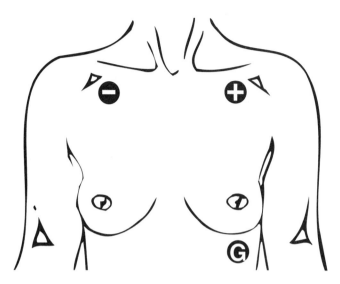

Figure 1.8: Suggested placement location for three lead maternal ECG cable. The electrodes are attached and the cable is plugged into the cardio or SE port on the fetal monitor. The two active electrodes may be placed anywhere on the upper thorax. The reference electrode (ground) should be at least 12 inches from the active electrodes.

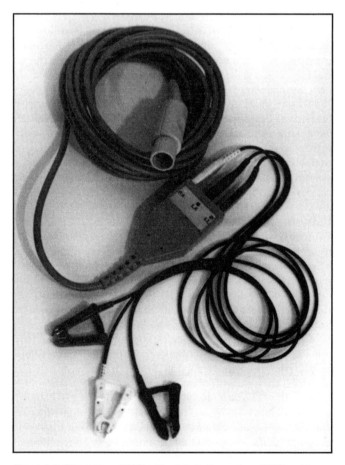

Figure 1.7: The maternal ECG cable detects the maternal ECG and transmits it to fetal monitor for analysis. The MHR will be printed on tracing. (Photographed by Barbara Gibson, Gibson Graphics, Albuquerque, NM)

16. *Twin baseline offset:* Some monitors print twin heart rates on two different numeric grids. Others have a baseline offset feature that adds 20 or 30 bpm to the twin monitored with US 1. Consult the manufacturer's guidelines for activation of this feature.

17. *Fetal Actocardiograph:* Some fetal monitors print fetal movement on the UA channel of the paper. For example, the Toitu Fetal Actocardiograph® detects and prints fetal movement as well as the FHR and UA (see book cover). Fetal movement is recorded as spikes at the bottom of the UA channel of the tracing. Dot marks also appear between the FHR and UA channels when FM speed exceeds a preset threshold.

18. *Data entry devices:* A keypad, keyboard, touch screen, light pen, or barcode reader have been used to enter comments on the tracing and in the nurses' notes. Entries appear between the FHR and UA channels on the fetal monitor paper.

19. *Peripheral equipment:* An automated noninvasive blood pressure cuff and SpO$_2$ monitor can be built in or connected via cables to the fetal monitor. After using these peripheral devices, blood pressure and SpO$_2$ should be printed on the strip. If they are not printed, additional hardware may need installation or adjustments, such as equalizing the baud rate of the fetal monitor and the peripheral equipment.

Fetal monitors can be connected by means of cables to computers for data storage. When a computer system is installed, the tracing and documentation may be stored on optical laser disks and the hard drive. Dual back-up disks are essential. As many as 10,000 records may be stored on a 20 megabyte hard drive (48). It is important to confirm the woman's tracing is actually stored as loose cable connections may result in storage of another woman's data. When tracings are stored on disk, all entries must be made using the data entry system as handwritten remarks are not stored.

Fetal monitors may store FHR and UA information. The AMS IM-77® (Advanced Medical Systems, Hamden, CT) stores approximately 60 minutes of strip data in its memory if the paper ends (out of paper memory™). Once new paper is placed in the paper tray, the stored information should be printed at a rapid rate until the strip catches up with the current data.

Data from fetal monitors may also be transmitted by a modem or telemetry (49). Modems utilize telephone lines to transmit data to a personal computer (PC) or a fax machine. Data can be stored for later transmission. For example, 100 minutes of stored data can be transferred in 10 minutes. Or, real-time data can be transmitted. Some receivers can accommodate multiple transmissions.

Telemetry is a wireless system that transmits data from one location to another. In 1979, telemetry was being created and was considered a promising line of development in 1987 (24, 50). A telemetry unit which transmits radio waves may be carried like a shoulder bag by the pregnant woman. Transducer cables are plugged into this unit. Its receiver is plugged into the back of the fetal monitor. Telemetry allows continuous recording of FHR and UA data when the woman is out of bed away from the monitor. In the future, fetal monitors may have different forms of telemetry. For example, Advanced Medical Systems (Hamden, CT) is seeking FDA approval for a fetal monitor with cableless toco and US transducers that transmit signals to the fetal monitor by electromagnetic waves.

COMPUTER APPLICATIONS IN OBSTETRICS

Initially, computers were used in hospitals for patient admissions, billing, and management reporting. The first computer systems designed for obstetrics were introduced in the mid-1980s. These systems were PC based and capable of transmission, archival and retrieval of maternal and fetal data. Electronic fetal monitor signals were captured, digitized, and stored within the computer's memory. The best computer systems can simultaneously record FHR and UA information and:
- display the tracing on a computer screen
- send it to another PC via modem
- print the tracing on a computer printer and
- store the information on a hard drive and laser optical disks.

Some computer systems are capable of:
- central display at the nurses' station
- remote display in hospital rooms, hallways, and lounges
- central and remote alarm systems
- electronic point-of-care charting
- interconnections to other biomedical devices such as a blood pressure monitor
- data retrieval and statistical report generation, and
- networking with other computer systems such as the "housewide" financial system.

Central and Remote Display Functions
Busy units may benefit from access to all fetal monitor tracings on one or more computer screens located at the nurses' station. The charge nurse's accountability expands as the number of displayed tracings increases.

Optical Disk Archiving
Storage of UA and FHR data on a computer disk should save space and time. Fetal monitor strips may be discarded and retrieval of tracings from the computer is faster than searching for microfilm in the medical records department. Some hospitals continue to microfilm the tracing prior to discard. This provides an exact copy of the tracing.

Computer-generated tracings are close facsimiles, not exact copies. In 1990, computerized systems were considered investigational and no final legal status of computer-archived tracings existed (51). Since 1990, however, they appear to have been accepted in medical malpractice cases.

To safeguard against loss or damage to one optical disk cartridge, dual optical disk storage should be installed. Computer systems can be installed with an electronically controlled security system to protect data from tampering or removal. Risk managers may prefer an optical disk storage system in which the strip is automatically archived and no strip review is allowed.

Point-of-Care Documentation
Computer systems have been designed to eliminate redundant charting. One entry can be sent to multiple places, a "single entry-multiple result" design. Documentation speed may be enhanced by use of a pen light and software with a Graphical User Interface (GUI) capable of point and click data entry. Data entry options may include a keyboard, mouse, trackball, touch screen, and light pen.

Computer software documentation programs should reflect expert clinician input and provide data entry options in all areas health care providers currently chart. For example, they should allow entries that reflect assessments such as the FHR baseline, short-term variability (STV), long-term variability (LTV), accelerations, decelerations, uterine contraction frequency, duration, intensity, peak intrauterine pressure (IUP), and relaxation or resting tone. The number of computers should be adequate to meet personnel needs and prevent documentation delays. Computer-generated documents should be easy to retrieve and read.

When changing from a paper documentation system to a computerized system, success depends on having enough computer workstations at each charting location. Success also requires the nurse manager's commitment to the change. User comfort with technology and a positive approach to change will increase acceptance of the new computerized system. Change requires a clear implementation plan and a quality assurance process that provides continuous feedback to staff. Everyone involved in the change should be *patient, persistent, and open-minded.* No other major changes should be competing for attention.

Data Retrieval: Reports and Statistics

The quantity and quality of retrieved data depends on the quantity and quality of data entered. If data entry is deficient, some say, "Garbage in, garbage out." Therefore, to ensure excellent reports, it is critical to determine who will enter data prior to purchase of a point-of-care charting module. Data entry tasks will be a major part of their job. Data may be collected for unit statistics, patient reports, and customizable reports. Reports that once took several days or weeks to generate can be generated in a few minutes. Some vendors do not offer a customizable report option.

Remote Access, Communications, and Networking

Data from the strip alone or the entire chart may be retrieved by midwives or physicians in their offices or homes or sent from community-based hospitals to tertiary centers. The physician or clinic may purchase a system by which the prenatal record is computerized and transmitted to labor and delivery or the antepartal unit via a modem.

Purchase of a Computer System

Many options are available for a comprehensive obstetrical information management system (see Figure 1.9). One or more of these options can be purchased. Some central display systems are not expandable. In other words, the central system "black box" technology is not upgradable or capable of being connected to other computer systems. Therefore, prior to purchase, costs and benefits as well as enhancement capabilities of each component of the system should be considered.

Prior to purchase, a computer system selection committee should perform a needs assessment. The committee should consist of the following people: the medical and nursing directors of perinatal services, antenatal and intrapartal unit nurse managers, clinical nurse specialists, the medical records department director, an information systems representative, and the risk manager. Issues to be discussed by the sales representative and this committee should include the computer system's ease of use, system flexibility, documentation capabilities, future software development plans, and configuration requirements to meet everyone's needs.

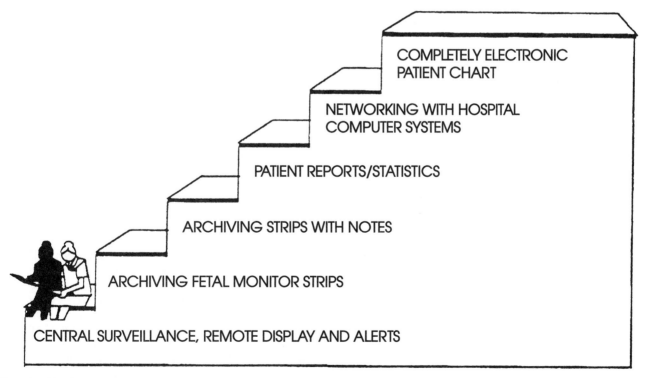

Figure 1.9: The steps to successful obstetrical information management (©1995 Peritronics Medical, Inc., reproduced with permission). **The bottom two steps are the basic requirements of an obstetric computer system.**

Prior to purchase of a computer system, the committee should answer the following questions:

1. Is a central display system critical?
2. Are remote display functions needed and if so, to what extent?
3. Is bed to bed surveillance needed?
4. Is an alert/alarm function needed and if so, is it customizable for each patient?
5. Is optical disk archiving a significant advantage or is the current EFM strip storage system adequate?
6. Is the system sold by a stable company who has been in business for some time?
7. Who will perform data entry?
8. Which data entry tasks would provide the greatest return on the investment?
9. What peripheral devices for data collection will be connected to the system?
10. Does the system support connection to different fetal monitors?
11. What data needs to be stored, reviewed, and retrieved?
12. Does the system support user-configurable report writing?
13. What technology standards does the system have?
14. Is the system's technology compatible with the hospital's strategic plan and future?
15. Does the system allow for growth and flexibility as future needs change?
16. Does the vendor have experience implementing a successful computerized documentation system?
17. Can you interview others who have succeeded in the areas you are interested in?
18. What support will be required to implement the system?
19. What support will be needed on an ongoing basis?
20. What support/training services does the company offer after installation?
21. Will the vendor provide training and support, and if so, at what cost?
22. What level of customization will be needed and who will be responsible for customization, the hospital or the vendor?
23. Will it be necessary to hire or train a full time specialist for internal support and training of the personnel who will use the computer system?

If all these issues are considered prior to purchase, computer systems should not be a source of frustration or disappointment. The budget should be adequate to cover the entire system required, including an adequate warranty provision and support services such as training of employees in the use of the system. Software may be very minimal and require extensive set-up and customization prior to use. Or, the data storage procedures will require tedious manual processes for backup and quality control. These indirect costs could be the burden of the obstetric department. Therefore, to avoid indirect costs, a realistic budget should be determined with the vendor prior to purchase.

Implementation of a Comprehensive OB Computer System

Changing to a computer-based documentation system from a paper system is a major event. The process may take more than a year. Adaptation to this change may be slow.

If the hospital wishes to change to bedside/point-of-care charting, staff may find it difficult to change if they are not accustomed to documenting at the bedside. Hospitals should look for a vendor that develops a long term partnership to work with the staff to facilitate this change.

Each component of the computer system should be implemented, evaluated, and deemed successful prior to installation of the next component. A quality assurance process should be in place to identify problems and areas for further training or system modifications. A forced or rapid change may create resentment or antagonism towards the process, and the project could fail. The department manager will need to be a coach and a leader with the patience to deal with minor and major obstacles in the change process. Commitment is required for success.

ANALYSIS OF THE FHR
Visual Analysis of the FHR Pattern

Agreement between nurses and physicians in the meaning of FHR and UA patterns is critical when the fetus is suffering from hypoxia, acidosis, or asphyxia or the woman has abnormal uterine activity as the result of a placental abruption or uterine rupture. *If the fetus is healthy, disagreements are of little consequence. However, if the fetus is not, disagreements may result in a treatment delay, fetal damage, fetal death, or maternal death.* Fortunately, nurses have a high rate of agreement in their interpretations of nonstress tests (NST) as reactive or nonreactive. Four hundred and twelve nurses agreed 84 to 98 percent of the time when they reviewed 5 NST strips (52). A failure to agree that the NST is nonreactive could precede inaction and fetal demise or the birth of a neonate with a significant risk for low Apgar scores, neonatal intensive care unit admission, or death (53). Physicians and nurses rarely experience total agreement with themselves when they take a second or third look at a tracing (intraobserver agreement) or when their interpretations are compared to each others' interpretations (interobserver agreement). Disagreements limit the predictive value of fetal monitoring and reflect different training and experiences (54-55).

Nurses and physicians may agree more often with their own interpretation than the interpretation of others (56). Some people agree with themselves less then they agree with others. For example, agreement with oneself occurred 22 percent of the time when obstetricians, perinatologists, and nurses took a second look at NST and labor strips. But, they agreed with each others' interpretation 42 to 55 percent of the time (57-58). Scoring systems may heighten agreement, but their use assumes the definitions and descriptions of FHR components are understood and accepted by the individuals using the system (59). One would think attendance by physicians and nurses at the same fetal monitoring educational seminars would heighten agreement. Yet, even when fetal monitoring education occurred within one hospital, differences in opinions persisted (56).

Even nurses and physicians, who considered themselves experts in fetal monitor strip interpretation, disagreed with each other's pattern interpretation. When 5 obstetricians reviewed 150 labor strips, all 5 only agreed on 44 of 150 tracings (29 percent) (60). When 8 nurse experts reviewed 45 FHR patterns, they only agreed on 25 of the 45 tracings (56 percent). Agreement was defined as consensus between 3 or more nurses. When 20 of 25 agreed upon tracings were randomly selected for review, the 8 nurse experts agreed 100 percent of the time on some, but not all, of the FHR pattern components. In one strip, there was only 54 percent agreement on the type of deceleration that was present (61-62). In Denmark, physician residents agreed the deceleration was a late deceleration or a variable deceleration less than 56 percent of the time (63).

Barriers to deceleration recognition include insufficient or erroneous recognition criteria or a limited mental image to compare with newly encountered examples (61). Recognition criteria help people see an image imbedded in a field. The field is the grid on the fetal monitor paper. The image may be the FHR baseline, STV, LTV, accelerations, or decelerations. A failure to learn appropriate recognition criteria could limit recognition skills.

Images in one's mind are called prototypes. Limited exposure to the various deceleration types and multiple examples of each type of deceleration limits the recognition of other decelerations in that category. Variable decelerations occur more often than late decelerations. Therefore, some late decelerations may not be recognized if there is limited prototype development. As more images are recognized, based on recognition criteria, prototypes become more abstract. A highly abstracted prototype increases image recognition.

Interpretation accuracy increases when the number of examples on a tracing increases and the number of people examining the tracing increases. For example, accuracy interpreting a 55 to 70 minute UA strip generated by a toco decreased when contractions lasted less than 40 seconds and were fewer than 4 per hour. One observer was only accurate in their assessment 70 percent of the time, 2 were accurate 82 percent of the time, and 3 were accurate 88 percent of the time (55).

Appropriate actions should be the response to accurate interpretation. Computer analysis of FHR data should diminish incorrect and inconsistent interpretations. But, clinical judgment will still be required to determine management strategies. The product of computer analysis is a summary of FHR and UA data, not a conclusion or plan of action. Many physicians have been working to refine software programs for FHR and UA pattern analysis. They believe FHR patterns are too complex for some users to interpret in a reliable, consistent or accurate way and that computer software increases the accuracy of FHR pattern analysis (40, 54, 64-66).

Computer Analysis of FHR Patterns

The fetal monitor transmits its data via a digital parallel port and cable to a PC for analysis (64). Software programs have been developed to identify components of the FHR pattern and UA. When a SE is on the fetus, the FECG is transmitted into the fetal monitor and transferred to the PC. R waves on the FECG waveform reflect the heart beat or systole. The computer determines a bpm rate based on one R to R or pulse interval. For example, if the pulse interval were ½ second or 500 milliseconds (msec), the minute rate would be 120 bpm.

The computer calculates STV by identifying the msec differences between two consecutive pulse intervals. LTV is calculated by adding 30 to 60 seconds of pulse intervals (67-68). The baseline rate is computed after 5 minutes of pulse intervals are analyzed (69). When a computer was used to analyze the FHR pattern, benefits included:

1. constant fetal surveillance
2. assistance in interpretation for inexperienced staff
3. multiple variables that set off an alarm
4. standardized interpretation
5. data storage, analysis, interpretation, recall, and display at any time and
6. data retrieval for research or legal purposes (48, 51, 69).

Researchers developed an experimental program with artificial intelligence that analyzed the FHR and UA patterns during antepartal testing and labor. The program made a diagnosis, prognosis, and recommended actions based on the findings, such as "repeat the test in standard conditions...". Prior to labor, the program was used to determine the Bishop's score and labor favorability. The program also predicted morbidity. During labor, the program evaluated FHR and UA patterns, and labor progress. Diagnoses were made as well as suggestions for management, such as a change in maternal position, fetal blood sampling, or maternal oxygen administration. The application of artificial intelligence techniques used in this program depended on data entry and the procedural and informational knowledge programmed into the software. While this type of program might be helpful to retrospectively evaluate antepartal tests or labor tracings and management, its applicability in a clinical setting may be hampered by a lack of data entry personnel and high speed computers. In addition, physicians did not always agree with the computer analysis of the tracing. Agreement between physician analysis and management and computer analysis and management varied between 71 to 85 percent (70).

Preliminary research in 1976 compared physician and computer analyses of tracings generated by a SE. There was 91 percent agreement between physician interpretation and computer analysis (69). Early problems with computer analysis included the lack of a precise formula to recognize contractions or to identify deceleration types. Plus, there were faulty alarms and a failure to evaluate some decelerations. The analysis of FHR data has challenged software developers (51). By 1990, software algorithms were more consistent in how the FHR was calculated but some researchers were still developing algorithms (64). Today, computer software analyzes the FHR and UA patterns *whether or not external (US and toco) or internal (IUPC and SE) devices are used.* Computer analysis of the FHR pattern generated by US yielded similar results as the computer analysis of the tracing generated by SE, except in the *measurement* of STV.

The Sonicaid system 8000® is a PC-based computer program that was developed in the United Kingdom to analyze the FHR and UA. Once analyzed, the following variables were printed:
- baseline or basal (BL) FHR
- variation of the baseline
- time spent in high variation (24 or more msec)
- time spent in low variation (less than 24 msec)
- fetal movement (FM) recorded by the woman or her nurse
- uterine contractions (UCs)
- accelerations that lasted more than 15 seconds and peaked 10 or more bpm above the baseline and
- decelerations dropping 10 or more bpm below the baseline lasting 1 or more minutes or dropping 20 bpm below the baseline lasting more than 30 seconds (1, 51).

This automated FHR and UA analysis works best with a near term fetus when the woman is not in labor. During labor, signal loss limits data acquisition. Software was programmed based on known changes in the FHR during different fetal behavioral states. A minimum of 45 minutes of monitoring is required if there are no episodes of high variation or accelerations (71).

Both LTV and STV are determined after each minute of pulse intervals is analyzed for a minimum of five minutes (48). The minimum and maximum pulse intervals determined during the five minutes become the bottom and top of the FHR baseline range.

Long-term variation is determined each minute by adding that minute's pulse interval differences. *The lower normal limit for LTV is 30 msec/minute (72-73). Twenty to 30 msec/minute is questionable. Less than 20 msec/minute is considered abnormal (72). "Decreased variation" best predicted acidemia, acidosis, and death in the post-term fetus (6, 74).* Nine of 10 fetuses with decreased variation during antepartal testing had "fetal distress" during labor. Seven of 12 with decreased variation during labor had acidemic cord artery pH values (74).

STV is calculated as the average pulse interval over a 1/16 minute (3.75 seconds) epoch. After each epoch, it was expected that the average pulse interval would vary slightly and create a small difference in each consecutive calculated rate. Fifty percent of consecutive rate differences were approximately 1 bpm when an abdominal FECG was used to calculate the FHR (75).

STV was determined with an US transducer in place. FHR patterns when an US is used to detect the FHR may look smoother than FHR patterns when a SE is used because autocorrelation averages pulse intervals over 0.5 to 1.2 seconds (3, 27, 76-79). Using US technology, *pulse interval differences for normoxic fetuses were 3 or more msec. A pulse interval difference of 4.17 msec creates one bpm change between consecutive rates. Pulse interval differences less than 2.6 msec were associated with acidemia, and less than 2 msec were associated with fetal death in less than 24 hours in 7 fetuses. Decelerations detected by computer analysis were also a warning of impending death (6).*

Bernardes and Pereira (65) hoped both visual and computer analysis would be complementary and enhance the detection of acidotic fetuses during labor. Unfortunately, labor was associated with FHR signal loss where no valid pulse intervals could be obtained for analysis (66). Signal loss was also more common in premature gestations and obese women (36).

Computer analysis of FHR patterns and FM yielded new data about variation, accelerations, and fetal behavior. For example, the average baseline FHR at 20 weeks was 149 bpm and 134 bpm at term (5). This indicates the vagus becomes more dominant as gestation advances. The baseline slowly drops between 24 and 30 weeks' gestation (68).

Low variation lasted up to 40 minutes near term and was often associated with a quiescent fetal sleep state (5, 68, 80). The amount of time spent in high variation increased as gestation progressed. The number of accelerations significantly increased between 20 to 41 weeks' gestation (5, 81-82). Thirteen percent of 20 to 30 week fetuses did not accelerate within a 60 minute observation period. "One big deceleration" occurred in 7 percent of fetuses 20 to 37 weeks' gestation. Between 30 and 41 weeks, fetal rest and activity episodes lengthened and became more distinct (5).

Visual and Computer Analysis
Visual interpretation of the FHR pattern is subjective and requires identification of the FHR baseline, its variability (STV and LTV), accelerations, decelerations, arrhythmias, and artifact. The UA pattern may be analyzed for frequency, duration, intensity, peak IUP, and relaxation or resting tone. Pattern analysis is coupled with clinical observations or tests to determine the meaning of the pattern.

Computer software programs that analyze tracings have been developed in countries such as the United Kingdom, Portugal, Italy, and the United States of America (26, 64, 83-84). Computer analysis of the FHR and UA is objective but limited as it does not factor in clinical observations (68, 73). Therefore, computer analysis is best used as an adjunct to clinical observations and decision making.

Visual analysis is *qualitative;* computer analysis is *quantitative* (85-86). Some felt the computer was "superior" in its analysis (87). Computer analysis is different than visual analysis. Therefore, comparing computer and visual analysis is synonymous with comparing apples to oranges. Therefore, any research that does so is open to criticism. It would be better to compare fetal outcomes, not tracing interpretations.

Humans and computers are similar in their ability to identify well fetuses who have normal birth outcomes (87). *Sometimes the computer was more sensitive than humans to abnormal findings,* but predicted well babies the same. For example, in a 1993 study, 93 percent of reactive tracings by visual analysis met the computer's requirements for reactive (88). The computer found 13 abnormal results that the reviewers felt were normal (73). This suggested visual analysis might miss an abnormal FHR pattern. On the other hand, the FHR pattern may have had low LTV and represented a fetus in a quiet sleep state rather than a hypoxic fetus.

Sometimes physicians were more sensitive than the computer to abnormal findings. When three physicians evaluated 148 NST strips, they found 17 to 19 were nonreactive. The computer found 14 were nonreactive. For the computer to identify the tracing as reactive, there had to be at least one FM or three accelerations and five of six minutes had to have high FHR variation and no large deceleration (72). The difference in "reactive" criteria partially explains different interpretations by the physicians and the computer.

Perinatal nurses and perinatologists reviewed NST strips, and for the most part they agreed with the computer's determination of the baseline rate (89). In another study, there was 82 percent agreement between visual and computer analysis of the baseline of 158 tracings, but less agreement with the number and duration of contractions, the number of accelerations, the number of decelerations, and the time between contractions and decelerations (83). Escarena (90) found physicians and the computer had poor agreement on STV. However, the computer used different criteria to assess STV than the physicians.

MONITOR START-UP and DISCONTINUANCE

Prior to using the electronic fetal monitor, inspect the power cord. If it is damaged, don't use it. Inspect the transducer cables for missing pins or loose wires. The lack of pins or loose wires may interrupt or diminish signal transmission. Damaged cables should not be used.

In case of an electrical outage, the fetal monitor should be disconnected from its power source until power is restored. However, even if a fetus were attached to a SE and the monitor were plugged in when power was restored, it is not possible that a

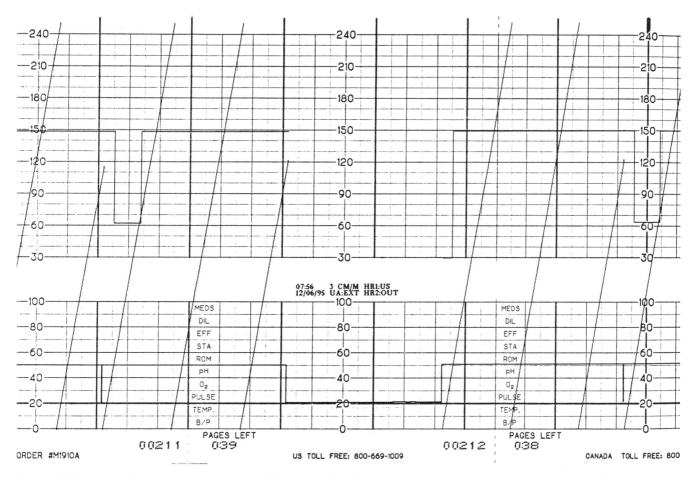

Figure 1.10: Some monitors run an automatic test of the electronic circuitry, printer, and paper feed. If a gap exists between the printed line and the paper grid line, the paper may need to be adjusted in the paper tray or the printer may need to be adjusted by a skilled technician.

power surge would override the surge protector in the fetal monitor, travel down the SE cable, through the SE wires to the fetus resulting in electrocution because the manufacturers have taken all precautions necessay to prevent direct current transfer to the fetus.

Equipment should be working properly prior to its use. When the monitor is plugged in, it may automatically go through an electronic test. A manual test of the fetal monitor circuitry could be performed at any time during monitor use by pressing the test button. Some monitors require transducers and the telemetry receiver be unplugged from the monitor when it is undergoing the initial self test. It is a good habit to test the monitor and its transducers prior to use. If a test strip is generated, it should remain part of the permanent medical record.

To test the connection between the fetal monitor and its component devices, e.g., the toco and the US, turn the monitor on after transducers are connected. If two ultrasounds are to be used for monitoring twins, plug in one US at a time. Press the test button. A digital readout on the fetal monitor FHR and UA screens should appear while the printer prints lines on the UA and FHR channels. An auditory signal should be heard at the same rate as that printed in the FHR channel. Examine the lines of the test pattern to ensure the printing is clear and consistent (see Figure 1.10). If there are gaps between the printed lines and the paper grid, reposition the paper in the paper tray and retest. If the gaps persist or the lines contain gaps or are too dark or too light, the monitor should be sent for printer repair or adjustment. Some monitors display an error message on the digital readout when equipment malfunctions. Peripheral devices, such as a barcode reader, may be tested using a barcode sheet.

A continuous line or squares printed on the paper indicates the paper end is approaching, often with less than 30 minutes remaining when a 3 cm/minute paper speed is used. If these lines are present prior to beginning monitoring, remove the old paper and add new paper to the tray.

THE TOCOTRANSDUCER: INDIRECT/EXTERNAL UTERINE MONITORING

The most common external monitoring devices are the uterine tocodynamometer or tocotransducer (toco) and the ultrasound transducer (US). "Toco" is similar to the Greek word "tokos" meaning childbirth. Uterine activity will be recorded on the lower portion of the tracing in the UA channel. Since this is an external device that rests on the abdomen, mm Hg or kPa units are not used in the analysis of the UA pattern. Instead, the waveform is examined for its shape.

The Tocodynamometer Mechanism

In the near term woman, the toco should be placed on the upper third of the abdomen. In the preterm gestation, it should be placed below the umbilicus (91). During a uterine contraction (UC), the uterus becomes more convex and rotates to the anterior abdominal wall. The traditional

guard-ring tocos contain a strain gauge in the form of a piston held in place by a metal ring. Pressure from the abdomen is exerted on the piston. The piston bends a metal strip which activates a Wheatstone bridge that converts mechanical energy to electrical energy for transmission into the fetal monitor (91). Another type of toco contains a pressure-sensitive piezoelectric computer chip connected to a Wheatstone bridge. Voltage transmitted from the Wheatstone bridge into the fetal monitor is amplified by automatic gain control prior to determination of the relative frequency, duration, intensity, and relaxation of contractions. A UA waveform will be printed on the tracing (92, 93).

Guard-ring tocos have been used for ambulatory preterm UA monitoring (94). Some home UA monitors store up to a week of UA data (95). Tocos used in the hospital may be insensitive to preterm UA. Other tocos may be set at different sensitivities for the preterm and term woman. If the tocotransducer is not highly sensitive, preterm labor contractions may not be recorded. To improve recognition of preterm UA, a highly sensitive toco should be used, and the feelings and complaints of women should be considered when the nurse or physician palpates the abdomen.

Some women complained they were in preterm labor, but were not contracting at all! Contractions appeared to be recorded on the paper, but they were created by the woman when she pressed on the toco or pushed out her abdomen (96). Woman-made UA patterns have UC waveforms that look more square then curved. Women who feign labor may have Munchausen Syndrome. In the case of suspected Munchausen Syndrome, a hand should be placed under the woman's lower back with another hand near the toco on the abdomen to prevent touching of the toco by the woman. UA is palpated while a psychosocial history is obtained. The tracing should be evaluated during the woman's sleep times. Women with Munchausen Syndrome cannot push the toco to register false contractions when they sleep.

Testing the Tocotransducer

To test the tocotransducer, plug the cable into its port on the fetal monitor, turn on the monitor, then press the toco's pressure-sensitive surface. Observe the digital readout on the monitor screen. The pressure should increase and be recorded at the top of the UA channel.

Setting the UA Baseline

Some tocos automatically set the UA baseline at zero, while others need to be manually set to a UA level of 10 units. As long as UA is recorded in the UA channel, and the beginning and end of the UA waveform are visible, the toco baseline can be placed at any level. Of course, it is preferable to see the entire UA waveform which is most common when the baseline is set near 10 units.

Analysis of UA

Contractions look like hills that last 30 or more seconds in the UA channel. Each contraction has an ascending limb, acme or peak, and descending limb or decrement reflecting the relative onset, peak, and offset of the contraction. When the toco is used, the recorded *waveform reflects pressure exerted by the abdomen in the area under the toco* which can be altered by the location of the toco, maternal activity such as turning to the side, or by adjusting the UA dial or button.

External UA monitoring with a toco provides qualitative not quantitative information. The assessment of UA by a toco was fairly reliable for UC frequency, less reliable for UC duration, and not reliable for peak pressures and resting tone (97). The recorded UC peaks depend upon the thickness of subcutaneous tissue, belt tightness, position of the toco on the abdomen, and maternal position.

Maternal position is an important assessment that should be recorded in the nurses' notes. A supine position might create supine hypotension and reduce uterine blood flow due to compression of the great vessels. The resulting uterine hypoxemia may precede weak, frequent contractions. A lateral position increases uterine blood flow, and may reduce UC frequency, but increase contraction duration and intensity (98).

When women bear down or hold their breath, their abdomen becomes distended and the contraction waveform extends past the actual contraction duration. This false duration may prevent some physicians and nurses from acknowledging the presence of late decelerations. While late decelerations return to the baseline after contractions end, when a toco is used, the exact end of a UC is unknown. Therefore, this recognition criteria for a late deceleration is the least significant when a toco is in place. Decelerations are identified first *by their shape, then by their timing* in relation to contractions. The timing alone does not determine the name given to the observed deceleration. If clarification of the deceleration pattern is needed, exact measurements of IUP can be obtained after an IUPC is inserted into the uterus (92-93).

Contractions are usually palpable and will be recorded prior to the woman's awareness of the onset of the contraction. The woman's coach can be instructed to identify the ascending limb of the contraction to help prepare the woman to cope with the contraction. *Recorded UA is relative when a toco is used*, therefore it is essential to palpate the woman's abdomen and listen to her subjective viewpoint to confirm UC duration, intensity, and relaxation. The uterus should be soft between contractions for at least 60 seconds. Women's subjective complaints, coupled with a review of the UA pattern, may suggest placental abruption. For example, contractions every 1 ½ to 2 minutes experienced by a restless and screaming woman who is requesting removal of transducer belts has been associated with abruption of the placenta.

EXTERNAL FHR MONITORING DEVICES

Four devices detect the FHR: the phonocardiotransducer, an abdominal wall electrocardiogram (indirect FECG), the ultrasound transducer, and the SE (direct FECG) (see Figure 1.11).

Phonocardiography

Phonocardiography was first used in 1908, and was available with the first clinically useful fetal monitor. However, it is rarely used in clinical practice. A microphone placed on the abdomen detects harmonic content of fetal heart sounds between 75 and 107 Hz. It also detects ambient noises. *Sound triggers a cardiotachometer for determination of the FHR.* Detection of heart sounds is hampered by excessive abdominal wall movement during contractions (99-100). Signal clarity is also affected by abdominal wall thickness, the quantity of amniotic fluid, and maternal and fetal position (2, 100). Because the actual beat of the heart during systole is determined, this device can be used to measure STV (2,99).

Abdominal Wall Fetal ECG (aFECG)

The fetal ECG (FECG) may be transmitted into the fetal monitor by a spiral electrode applied directly under the fetal skin. This is a direct ECG assessment and is abbreviated DECG. The FECG may also be detected by electrodes applied to the maternal abdomen, an indirect assessment of both the maternal and fetal ECGs. This indirect FECG assessment is abbreviated aFECG.

The first recorded aFECG occurred in 1906. Abdominal electrodes were placed over the uterine fundus and an electrode was placed in the vagina. This technique has been used to diagnose twins, fetal life, fetal position, and congenital heart defects (99). The technique is rarely used in clinical practice (101). Abdominal FECG electrodes may be noninvasive or invasive, i.e., three to six electrodes have been applied midline on the abdomen or three platinum electrodes have been inserted subcutaneously in the anterior abdominal wall (102-103). The FECG is analyzed by an abdominal electrocardiogram processor. The FHR can be calculated by a computer and printed on a computer screen.

The aFECG detects the FECG and MECG complexes and transmits them into the processor. The FECG is hidden in a sea of electrical noise. To extract the signal, a filter and averaging and subtraction of the MECG or substitution of the FECG have been used (2, 100, 104). The FECG is difficult to detect because it is often distorted and 2 to 10 times smaller than the MECG (99, 105-106). In addition, maternal skin has a high impedance, which diminishes signal detection (106).

When the MECG and FECG coincide, an averaging or substitution technique can be used to detect or replace the undetected FECG complex (107-108). If an averaging technique is used, an averaged MECG waveform is subtracted from the entire signal (109). This enables detection of all fetal QRS complexes, even if they coincide with MECG complexes. With pulse substitution, a FECG complex is entered when it should have occurred. This artificial signal reconstruction may lose any ectopic beats, such as premature ventricular contractions. Actual and substituted pulse intervals have been compared and were within 0 to 10 msec 98.5 percent of the time (101).

18

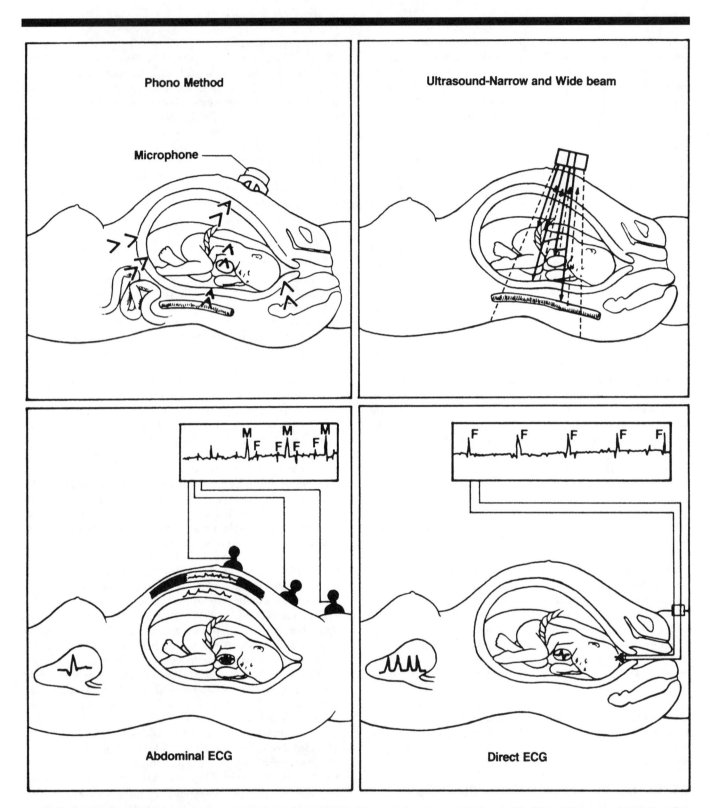

Figure 1.11: Techniques for fetal heart rate measurement. (Reproduced with permission of Marshall Klavan, MD: *Clinical Concepts of Fetal Heart Rate Monitoring*. Hewlett-Packard Company, 1977).

ANTEPARTAL AND INTRAPARTAL FETAL MONITORING

Automatic gain control constantly searches for a fetal signal to amplify. Automatic gain control increases in strength until it finds a signal and it shuts down when excessive electrical noise exists. In the absence of fetal life, it will amplify the MECG. Since R waves trigger the cardiotachometer, absence of a FECG would allow the MECG to trigger the cardiotachometer (97).

Once the FECG is detected and amplified, it is filtered and converted to a digital signal. The digital signal is filtered, and might be modified by averaging or substitution. Then, the refined ECG waveform is stored in memory, a rate is calculated, and the ECG may be plotted on ECG paper moving at 25 mm/second or the FECG and FHR may appear on a computer screen (101, 105-106, 110).

aFECG Reliability

In 1994, researchers reported as many as 35 percent of FECG signals were weak, not detected, or unsuitable for analysis (103). Signal strength varies with different electrodes and decreases during contractions and pushing. While phonocardiography provides a reliable signal to detect STV, aFECG may be less reliable due to signal averaging and/or substitution. When the FECG was substituted, STV was not exactly the same as when the FECG was transmitted by the SE. However, STV calculated by aFECG versus a SE was very similar (r = 0.83 ± 0.08). LTV was also similar between the aFECG and SE (r = 0.95 ± 0.02) (111). In spite of this limitation, STV calculated by aFECG predicted 12 of 17 cases of "fetal distress" (112). As technology advances, and software improves, it may be possible to use aFECG to detect STV during labor (78). Until then, the US and SE will continue to be the most common devices used to detect the FHR.

Gestational Age. Gestational age and position of the fetus, placenta, and woman decrease FECG transmission and result in a 35 percent or greater signal loss (99, 103). The FECG was detected only 50 to 80 percent of the time between 28 and 34 weeks' gestation, possibly due to the thick vernix caseosa on the fetus (1, 101). The best signals, and therefore the most accurate tracings, were obtained antepartally from fetuses 36 or more weeks' gestation who were in a cephalic presentation with electrodes placed midline above the symphysis pubis over the uterus and at the height of the uterine fundus (103,107).

Electrical Noise. The use of an aFECG during labor is nearly nonexistent, as an accurate, clear tracing is difficult to obtain (99, 107). The best results are obtained after epidural anesthesia (107). Maternal exertion during labor generates electromyographic interference or noise. In addition, electrical "noise" is created by the MECG, the abdominal muscles, the uterus, and equipment (100, 106).

Fetal and Maternal Position. Fetal postural changes alter the FECG configuration (99). The best FECG signal was obtained with the woman supine or at a 15 degree lateral tilt.

A dry cup electrode poorly transmitted the FECG signal; an electrode moistened with ECG paste was better (113).

T/QRS Ratio

In 1969, Dr. Edward Hon suggested changes in the P wave and ST segment duration in the FECG waveform might reflect asphyxia (99). Some believe the ST segment and T wave change prior to heart failure (114). To study FECG changes related to myocardial hypoxia and acidemia, researchers have developed equipment that analyzes the FECG, the ST segment, and the T/QRS ratio. The FECG is altered when the fetus becomes metabolically acidotic and the heart becomes depleted of glycogen and creatine-phosphate, plasma lactate, and epinephrine (from the adrenal glands) increase (103). As the *pH drops, the PR interval decreases and the pulse interval increases resulting in a decreased FHR.* The fetal *T/QRS ratio* is fairly stable during labor. With acidemia and a *drop in the pH,* the T wave increases and the T/QRS ratio increases.

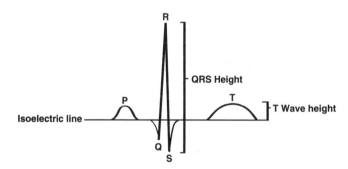

Figure 1.12: ECG schematic indicating T and QRS height used to calculate T/QRS ratio.

Researchers hoped the fetal T/QRS ratio could be used to rule out metabolic acidosis and reduce unnecessary cesarean sections or forceps without adversely affecting neonatal outcome (103). The STAN® fetal monitor (ST Analyzer, Cinventa AB, Sweden) is a conventional fetal monitor that plots the ST analysis alongside the FHR pattern. The STAN® monitor also prints a representation of an averaged FECG every two minutes on the fetal monitor paper. Advanced Medical Systems (Hamden, CT) monitors plot the ST segment or a FECG above the FHR pattern when the ECG plot is activated. In Figure 1.13, the tocotransducer is off (UA: out). The FHR is being monitored by a spiral electrode (HR1: ECG). The monitor has another cardio port (HR2: US) which is not in use.

Occasionally the S wave, not the R wave, becomes the counting trigger which creates a false high T/QRS ratio. A high T/QRS ratio is greater than 0.28 or 28 percent. In one study, a high T/QRS ratio predicted a low umbilical cord pH (< 7.12) twice as often as an abnormal FHR pattern (103). Conversely, a high T/QRS ratio detected fewer acidemic

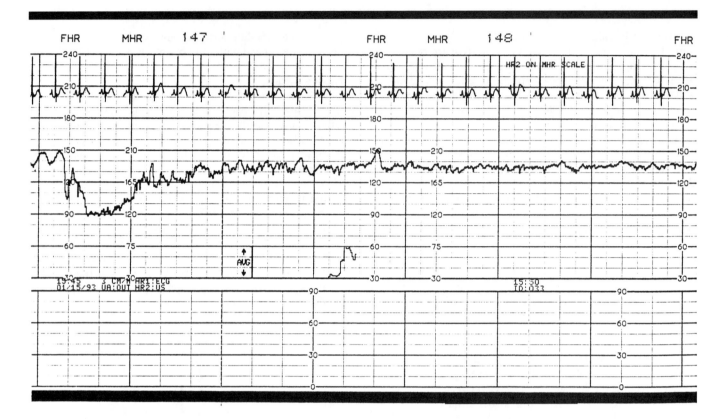

Figure 1.13: Segments of the fetal ECG (ST segments) are plotted above the FHR pattern. The dark line at the bottom of the paper indicates the end of paper is near.

fetuses than an abnormal FHR pattern (115). Others found no relationship between the T/QRS ratio and an abnormal FHR pattern (116). So far it appears that the relationship between the fetal ST waveform, T/QRS ratio, the FHR pattern, and Apgar scores is unclear (103). Additional prospective randomized controlled trials are needed before the T/QRS ratio becomes useful information in clinical practice.

THE ULTRASOUND TRANSDUCER: INDIRECT/EXTERNAL FHR and FM MONITORING

Ultrasound was created for submarine detection (117). Ultrasonography was first used in obstetrics in Scotland in the 1950s. By 1964, the first inexpensive Doppler instrument for detecting the human FHR was described (99). In 1968, fetal monitors with US transducers were available for purchase. US was used for over two decades when the first clinical study of obstetric ultrasound was published in 1980 (118). By 1987, US was used in as many as 40 percent of antenatal tests (117). Today, US use is common in antenatal and intrapartal settings.

Testing and Cleaning the Ultrasound Transducer

To test this component, plug the transducer cable into the monitor, turn on the power, and turn up the sound volume. Apply ultrasonic (coupling) gel or water to the transducer

face. Gently rub the transducer face in small circles, moving in a clockwise or counterclockwise direction. Where ever the transducer face is rubbed, static should be heard if the crystals inside the transducer are functioning. Another way to test the transducer is to hold it in one hand while moving the other hand toward and away from the transmitting surface. If the monitor produces a noise as the hand moves towards the transducer, the transducer is working.

Be gentle with US transducers to avoid damage of the delicate piezoelectric crystals inside (2). Usually, transducers and their cables should not be immersed in water. However, some manufacturers make immersible transducers. Transducers should be cleaned after use with a disinfectant solution, thoroughly rinsed with water, and dried with a clean cloth.

The Doppler Principle

Ultrasound devices, such as a hand-held Doppler, have one or more piezoelectric crystals inside which transmit high frequency US waves and receive reflected waves (see Figure 1.14). *Ultrasounds are motion detectors.* The Doppler Principle states that ultrahigh frequency sound wave echoes reflected from moving objects differ from those reflected from nonmoving objects. The difference in the frequency of the return waves is called the Doppler shift.

Ultrasound devices send US waves into the abdomen and

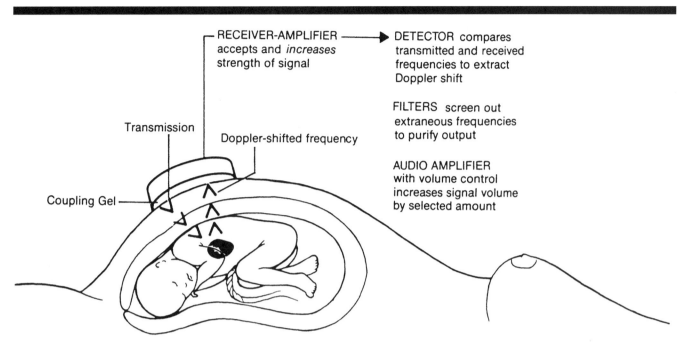

Figure 1.14: Continuous-wave ultrasound transducer devices simultaneously send and receive ultrasound waves. Hand-held Doppler devices may provide continuous or pulsed waves. Fetal monitors usually use pulsed-echo ultrasound technology.

uterus which are reflected back by moving objects, similar to a ping pong ball (US waves) and a ping pong paddle (moving object). The reflected beam may be increased or decreased in frequency based on the direction of motion. Movement perpendicular to and towards the face of the US transducer increases sound wave frequency. Movement away from the transducer decreases sound wave frequency (108).

"Moving objects" include maternal abdominal muscles, maternal blood flow through the aorta, the aortic wall, maternal bowel, fetal limbs, the umbilical cord, fetal atria and ventricles, and fetal heart valves (2-3). Movement that creates a signal for detection may not be from the fetus or the woman. A tracing has been generated when the US was unattached to the woman but was sitting on top of the fetal monitor. A tachycardic rate was recorded.

Since maternal aortic movement can reflect US waves which will be amplified and counted, the maternal pulse should be assessed and recorded prior to US application. The recorded rate should differ from the MHR. The MHR and fetal heart sounds or fetal movement should be confirmed and documented when the signal source of the tracing is unclear.

Confirmation of the FHR is also important when β-sympathomimetics are used for tocolysis or when fetal demise is suspected. (36-37, 44). To confirm fetal life, a *fetoscope or stethoscope should be used to hear fetal ventricular heart sounds,* or the fetus should be scanned by a real-time ultrasound to visualize cardiac motion. The MECG cable could be applied to distinguish the MHR from the

printed rate. A hand-held Doppler device could be used at the same time the MHR is assessed. The Doppler rate and the MHR should differ.

The US detects mechanical activity, *not electrical energy or sound.* Systole and diastole, with the respective valvular closures (closure of the mitral and tricuspid valves with systole and closure of the aortic and pulmonic valves with diastole), create two different frequencies of sound wave return. Fetal cardiac valve closure during systole sends US waves back into the transducer faster than any other cardiac motion. Therefore, mitral and tricuspid valve closure produces the greatest Doppler shift and a peak on the US waveform.

Once the raw US waveform is received, nonrandom events are filtered and extraneous random noise is canceled (see Figure 1.15). The FHR is determined by peak detection (uncorrelated) or autocorrelation. First generation monitors use peak detection. Second generation monitors use autocorrelation. When the rate is calculated, a dot representing the rate is printed on the fetal monitor paper. When the dots are connected, a FHR pattern develops.

Since the US indirectly assesses systole as a peak on a filtered and modified US waveform, and the SE directly assesses systole by identifying the R wave on the FECG, the FHR pattern generated by an US may be similar to the SE pattern, but not identical (37, 119). One monitor company has reported US measurement accuracy of 0.5%, meaning the US calculated rate will be 99.5 percent similar to the SE calculated rate (Toitu of America, Inc., Wayne, PA).

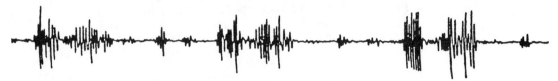

Figure 1.15: Illustration of raw ultrasound waveform received in fetal monitor prior to filtering (modified from Lewinsky, R. M., et al. (September/November 1992). Prediction of pregnancy outcome by combined analysis of the fetal electrocardiogram and systolic time intervals. *American Journal of Perinatology*, *9*(5/6), 349).

US Signal Transmission

To enhance signal transmission, the US transducer face should be at a right angle to the fetal heart. First generation monitors have a narrow beam US device, making FHR detection more difficult than the wide beam Dopplers of second generation monitors (120-121).

Like sonar of a ship or submarine, US waves travel best through water. Ultrasonic gel, such as Aquasonic gel® should be applied to the US transducer face to eliminate air between the transducer and the abdomen. Use of this coupling gel enhances US wave transmission. Lubifax®, K-Y Jelly®, or water can be used in lieu of coupling gel. When the woman is soaking in warm water during labor, she can arch her back to lift her abdomen out of the water for Doppler detection of the FHR.

Ultrasound Signal Reliability

US signal quality decreases when the transducer is not directly over the fetal heart. If a hand-held Doppler device is used, signal quality is affected by the pressure of the device on the maternal abdomen. The distance US waves travel limits their transmission and reception. For example, in obese women it was occasionally helpful to move the device to the lower abdomen, near the groin where there is less subcutaneous tissue, and point it upward toward the fetus. Sometimes, coupling gel may need to be added to the US transducer to enhance signal transmission. When twins are monitored, it is best to avoid directing US devices towards one another as incoming US waves may be detected and interpreted as fetal in origin. If the US beams are directed parallel to one another into the abdomen, sound wave interference is avoided.

Concerns: Ultrasound Energy (mW/cm²)

Unlike aFECG which is noninvasive, ultrasound waves enter tissue at ultrahigh speeds and exert a physical force or energy (106, 108, 117). *However, the energy emitted by fetal monitor ultrasound transducers or hand-held Dopplers is vastly below that used in animal research studies where tissue was destroyed.*

Second generation monitors have a pulsed Doppler US that emits as little as 1.5 mW/cm² of energy, with an average of 5 mW/cm² and a peak of 15 mW/cm². In general, fetal monitor US devices deliver less than 10 mW/cm². Pulsed-echo Doppler US devices alternate the emission of ultrasound waves with the reception of reflected waves and produce lower intensity US energy than continuous wave devices used in electronic fetal monitoring. This intermittent US emission exposes the fetus to less energy for shorter periods of time (122). For example, the Toitu Actocardiograph® pulsed Doppler delivers an US wave intensity *less than or equal to 1.5 mW/cm²*. Animal cells were disturbed or destroyed by energy at *100 mW/cm²* (123).

Fetal monitor US transducers contain seven to nine piezoelectric crystals. The pulsed-echo Doppler transducer has a wider beam than an array transducer, allowing its crystals to receive more sound wave transmissions (see Figures 1.16 and 1.17). The hand-held Doppler beam is narrow. Hand-held devices may emit a small, continuous US beam of low intensity, usually 5 to 12 mW/cm² of energy (124). Some hand-held Doppler devices are pulsed, waterproof, and have a digital display. Hand-held devices do not have internal logic to differentiate artifactual signals from fetal heart movement. In other words, the rate you hear when using a hand-held Doppler device may be from a maternal source. Therefore, *whenever a hand-held Doppler device is used the MHR should be assessed for a different rate than the Doppler generated rate.*

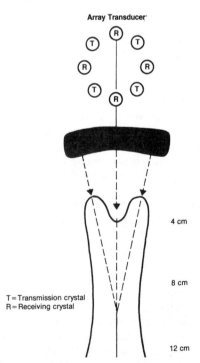

T = Transmission crystal
R = Receiving crystal

Figure 1.16: Array transducer with separate transmitting (T) and receiving (R) crystals.

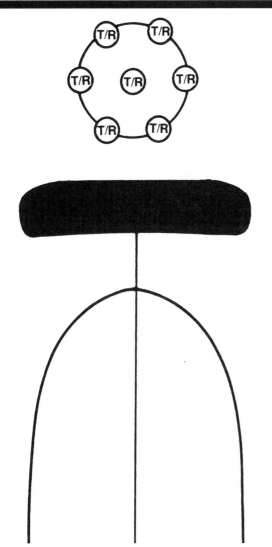

Figure 1.17: Pulsed-echo Doppler transducer. Every crystal is a transmitter and a receiver.

Health care providers and consumers are concerned about the potential hazardous effects of US waves. Human experiments using US during the antepartal period found no fetal damage (125). But, in animal cell studies with ultrahigh US energy levels and longer exposure times the following was discovered:
1. Damage to fetal animal cell DNA
2. Over-production of oxygen free radicals with gas formation (cavitation)
3. Significant increase in temperature with cell destruction
4. Cell lysis, inactivation, and/or modification of the its ultrastructure
5. Radiation force and disturbances in blood
6. Cell wall membrane alterations
7. Increased frequency of sister chromatid exchanges

8. Nucleoli fragmentation
9. Acoustic streaming of cytoplasm
10. Mitochondrial damage
11. Mitotic spindle disturbance
12. Increased frequency of giant cells
13. Abnormal eye pigmentation
14. Reduced litter size
15. Increase in skeletal abnormalities
16. Delay in nervous system maturation
17. Disturbance of bone marrow growth
18. Changes in contractility of muscles
19. Suppression of radioiodine uptake and
20. An effect on emotional behavior after birth (118, 124, 126).

Again, it is important to note that no significant biological effects were independently confirmed in human or mammalian tissue. Ultrasound exposures during fetal monitoring were less than 15 mW/cm². Cells were destroyed at levels at or near 100 mW/cm² (127).

Then and Now: Peak Detection and Autocorrelation
First generation monitors have an array, narrow beam US transducer and peak detection to calculate the FHR (2, 108). Peak detection measures the time between peaks of US waveforms to within 1 msec. These pulse intervals (peak to peak) are used to calculate an average pulse interval during 1/16 minute or 3.75 seconds (79). This averaged pulse interval creates greater variability in the tracing and made it look bumpier than it would with a SE in place.

Analysis of the US signal depends on the software capabilities in the fetal monitor (128). *First generation monitors were uncorrelated and poorly detected the FHR when the US was in use. They often tripled the actual STV and printed a rate within 10.9 bpm of the true rate* (37, 129-130). First generation monitors used "point trigger" technology to detect the tallest peaks of the raw US waveform, an estimate of systole. This was an uncorrelated technique where each peak was determined regardless of other ultrasound waveforms. Peak detection started with an inaccurate signal (the peak of the ultrasound waveform), then added a second distortion by averaging two to three consecutive heart beats (which were assumed to occur with each peak). When two consecutive heart beats were less than 5 msec apart, distortion was minimal. When there were large time differences between heart beats, the inaccuracies accumulated and created an exaggerated beat-to-beat variability (or STV) appearance in the FHR baseline.

Autocorrelation
Second generation monitors use autocorrelation which refines and smoothes the US waveform within the fetal monitor prior to calculation of the FHR. *Second generation monitors calculate the FHR within 2.5 bpm of the true rate* (129) (see Figure 1.18).

Autocorrelation significantly increases the fetal monitor's ability to detect the FHR. A high-speed data processor applies a complex, mathematically-intense formula to volumes of data derived from incoming US signals (130). Each incoming nonrandom US signal is amplified for detection. Random signals generated from motion of such things as maternal abdominal muscles or the intestines are cancelled. However, if the US is directed towards the maternal aorta or if the fetus has died, maternal aortic blood flow or wall movement would be amplified by automatic gain control and become the source of nonrandom signals. Since the calculated rate could be maternal, whenever the US is used, it is wise to compare the MHR with the printout at intervals throughout the monitoring period.

Once a nonrandom US signal is detected, the autocorrelation process begins. Incoming nonrandom US waveforms are compared with previous nonrandom waveforms while noise is continually canceled during 0.5 to 1.2 second epochs (77-79, 130). Within the computer's memory a pattern of refined Doppler waveforms is built (3) (see Figure 1.19).

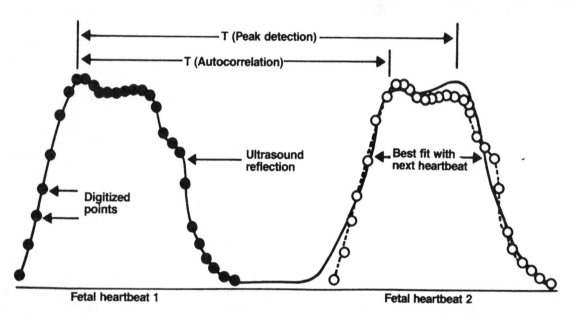

Autocorrelation vs. Peak Detection

Figure 1.18: Autocorrelation vs. peak detection: These two methods differ markedly in how they time heart beats. Peak detection builds in artificial variability because it can't pick up at a consistent point on the waveform. Doppler signal processing, with autocorrelation, yields a higher degree of accuracy and *permits evaluation of variability.* (Reproduced with permission of Patricia C. Wagner, et al. (Technology 1986). What's really new in EFM equipment? *Contemporary OB/GYN, 26* (special issue), 91-106, Medical Economics Company.).

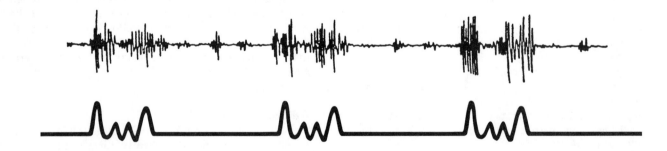

Figure 1.19: Illustration of raw US waveform above, autocorrelated waveform below. The peak of the autocorrelated wave corresponds with the greatest frequency of sound wave return. After 0.5 to 1.2 seconds are evaluated, the peaks trigger a cardiotachometer for calculation of the FHR (modified from Divon, M.Y., et al. (January 1, 1985). Correlation techniques in fetal monitoring. *American Journal of Obstetrics and Gynecology, 151*(1), 4).

The calculated rate is determined from analysis of the peaks of the nonrandom US waveforms that occurred during each 0.5 to 1.2 second epoch (79). The US-derived signal will only be printed if it falls within a predetermined bpm range. For example, when USA scaled paper is used, the Advanced Medical System IM-76®records FHRs between 50 and 210 bpm. The AMS IM-77® records FHRs between 50 and 216 bpm. The Toitu Actocardiograph® records 50 to 212 bpm. Corometrics monitors record FHRs between 50 to 210 bpm and the Hewlett-Packard M1350A® records FHRs between 50 to 240 bpm. Rates less than 50 bpm are not printed. Rates higher than 210 to 240 will not be printed (depending on the type of monitor). If European scaled paper is used, a line will be drawn at 210 bpm if the rate exceeds 210 bpm. Rates higher than 240 bpm are printed at half of the actual rate by most fetal monitors.

Even if the calculated rate fell within this predetermined range, the rate might not be printed if it was more than 14 bpm from the previous rate. For example, *in 1983, some fetal monitors programmed with autocorrelation only printed the new rate if it was less than or equal to a 14 bpm difference* (77). Research prior to 1983 found *the great majority of pulse intervals corresponded with consecutive rates that were within 15 bpm of one another* (131). If the first calculated rate was 120 bpm, and the next rate was 136 bpm, the second rate would not be printed as it fell out the 0 to 14 bpm range. If the next rate was 124 bpm, it would be printed. Therefore, gaps on the tracing when a US is used may suggest an arrhythmia such as premature ventricular contractions (PVCs) exists, as the calculated rate would be greater than a 14 bpm difference from the preceding rate (see Figure 1.20). By 1990, software had improved so that FHR differences of more than 14 bpm detected by US would be printed. Some monitors detect and print rate differences up to 25 bpm with the US and 28 bpm with the SE.

Short-term Variability and the US

The US-derived FHR pattern of first generation monitors often exaggerated fluctuations between calculated rates and was incapable of removing random noise from the US waveform. This contributed to a printout that was more bumpy than the true FHR baseline. Since the external baseline FHR was an exaggeration of the internal, SE-derived baseline, a flat (no LTV) and smooth (no STV) external baseline was even flatter and smoother when the SE was used. This lead some to say, *"If it looks bad on external, it's worse on internal."*

Since first generation monitors were inaccurate in their assessment of the FHR baseline, one never knew if the bumpy look corresponded with STV or not. Sometimes a bumpy external baseline was totally smooth when the SE was applied. Therefore, it was mandated that nurses *"Don't document STV when an external monitor is used"* (77, 132).

Extensive improvements in US technology, now found in second generation monitors, changed the thinking about external (US) and internal (SE) generated tracings. The new sayings are:

- "If it looks GOOD on external, it's probably GOOD on internal."
- "If it looks BAD on external (no STV), it may be better on internal."
- "If LTV and a reactive acceleration are present on external, metabolic acidosis is ruled out and STV is present."

STV has been measured and documented using US technology. In 1000 tracings analyzed by computer, STV averaged 7.78 msec, "medium" LTV averaged 42.4 msec (79). The US-derived FHR printout of autocorrelated fetal monitors is similar to the printout of a SE-derived FHR printout (130). *Therefore, the statement "Don't document STV when an external monitor is used" may not apply to autocorrelated fetal monitors under certain circumstances.*

Measurement and Documentation of STV

Second generation fetal monitors and some hand-held Doppler devices use autocorrelation. The International Federation of Obstetricians and Gynecologists met in November 1986 in Zurich to develop Guidelines for the Use of FHR Monitoring. They supported the notion that the US record "very closely" approached that of beat-to-beat variability (STV) generated from the SE (26).

When comparing tracings generated by an autocorrelated US signal and the SE, researchers found the US tracing was *a reasonable representation, virtually identical, with an accuracy close enough to the direct ECG* (46, 121). Based on these extensive improvements in US technology, *STV has been measured and documented by computer software during antepartal testing* (7, 37, 78-79, 129).

Some researchers found the *US printout had significantly less STV compared with the SE-derived FHR* (3, 31, 76-79). In other words, **"If it looks good on external, it probably is."** But, *until metabolic acidosis is ruled out* by a normal fetal scalp pH or the presence of LTV and a "reactive" acceleration, STV should NOT be documented as present because it can only be conceptualized as being present in a normoxic fetus who is not metabolically acidotic. *When the fetus is moving and LTV and a reactive acceleration are present, even when an US is used, the fetus is not metabolically acidotic and STV is conceptually present. In this case, health care providers have documented it as present, e.g., STV +.* If no accelerations are present within the 15 to 30 minutes being assessed, and there is concern that the fetus may be acidemic, a phonocardiotransducer, aFECG, or SE would need to be applied to more accurately *measure* STV. The latter device is the most common in clinical use today.

Halving and Doubling the Fetal Heart Rate

The FHR prints at half of its actual rate (halving) when the FHR is greater than 240 bpm (see Figure 1.21). US-derived rates between 240 and 300 bpm will not be printed by Hewlett-Packard Series 50® monitors, but the rate will be half-counted and printed if it exceeds 300 bpm. Sometimes the halved FHR pattern appears as a broken flat line on the tracing near 125 bpm when the actual rate is 250 bpm. FHRs

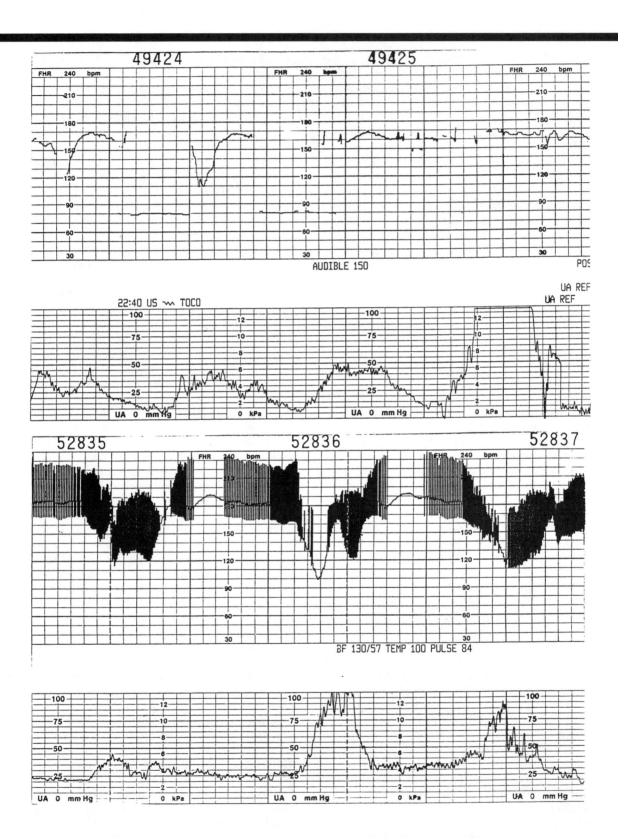

Figure 1.20: Ultrasound-derived FHR pattern on top, spiral electrode-derived FHR pattern on the bottom. With the ultrasound in place, the FHR difference between 2 or more consecutive 0.5 to 1.2 second periods was greater than 25 bpm and was not printed. When the spiral electrode was applied with logic off, PVC lines were evident. Neonatal Apgar scores were 8, 9, and 10 at 1, 5, and 10 minutes. Fetal arterial gases revealed hypoxia prior to birth.

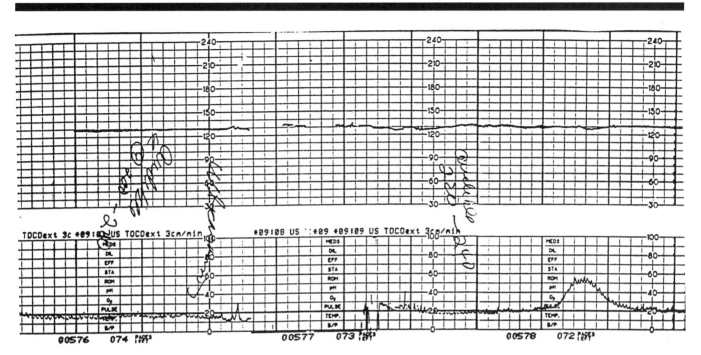

Figure 1.21: Most fetal monitors halve the fetal heart rate if it exceeds 240 bpm. When European scaled paper is used, a FHR above 210 but less than 240 will be printed as a line at 210 bpm. Over 240 bpm, the rate will be halved. An ultrasound and tocotransducer were in place.

above 240 bpm are usually associated with supraventricular tachycardia (SVT).

Fetal monitor software is programmed to ignore US signals for 250 to 280 msec after a nonrandom signal (representing the heart beat) is received. The time that incoming signals are ignored is called a "blanking" window or refractory window. The refractory window is 200 to 250 msec when a SE is used. Therefore, more signals will be counted when a SE is used than when the US is used. When the US is used and the heart contracts during the refractory window, heart movement will be ignored and the FHR may be calculated at half the actual rate (see Figure 1.22). Some second generation monitors accurately count the FHR to 300 bpm, whether or not the US or SE is used, e.g., Advanced Medical Systems and Hewlett-Packard. Even though the FHR is accurately counted, the paper scale ends and rates higher than 240 bpm will be printed at half their actual rate. In addition, Advanced Medical Systems monitors will put a dot at the 240 bpm line to indicate the printed rate is half the actual rate.

Because first generation fetal monitors had a longer refractory window than autocorrelated monitors, doubling and halving of the FHR occurred at rates below 80 bpm (doubling) and above 180 bpm (halving) (97, 133). But advances in fetal monitor software in second generation monitors allow accurate counting of the FHR to a low of 50 bpm. Second generation monitors will not double the FHR below 50 bpm but may double the MHR.

When the US of a first generation monitor is used and the FHR is slower than 80 bpm, the second signal from the same heart beat will be counted as a new heart beat. Second generation monitors may double the MHR when US signals due to aortic wall movement or aortic blood flow are equidistant.

Second Generation Monitors

With autocorrelated fetal monitors and the US, *the maternal heart rate (MHR) may be doubled* if the interval between peak US waveforms (reflective of aortic blood flow during systole and diastole) are symmetrical in their timing, and no FHR is detected. The two waveforms would be counted as two separate heart beats (see Figure 1.23). If it is suspected that the MHR is being recorded on the fetal monitor paper, the MHR and FHR should be assessed and compared with the printout. If fetal movement is present, locate the fetal spine using Leopold Maneuvers and place the US over it. If no FM is present, listen to the fetal heart sounds or visualize fetal cardiac motion with real-time ultrasound. A SE may need to be applied if continuous EFM is needed and the US was unable to detect fetal cardiac motion.

Fetal Movement Monitoring Using an US Transducer

Normally, fetuses stretch, roll, and move their trunk, limbs, and hands (134). They have clustered and isolated movements. They hiccup and have rapid eye movements (REM) (135). FM can be assessed by manual palpation, maternal perception, real-time ultrasound, spikes on the UA tracing when a toco is used, and by analysis of ultrasound frequencies (136-137). *Fetal movement (FM) is a sign of fetal well-being that rules out asphyxia* (138-139). Therefore, the presence of fetal movement should be documented. For example, the nurse might write, "FM noted by palpation."

REFRACTORY WINDOW: DOUBLING AND HALVING THE HEART RATE

S_1= first cardiac signal, usually synonymous with systole, S_2 = second cardiac signal, usually synonymous with diastole. RW = refractory window, RECEIVE = time nonrandom signal is detected and counted.

RW S_1	RECEIVE S_1	RW S_1	RECEIVE S_1	RW S_1	RECEIVE S_1	RW S_1	RECEIVE S_1

Cardiac signals are ignored during the refractory window resulting in a calculated rate that is half the actual rate. When the ultrasound is used, first generation monitors halve rates over 180 bpm. Some second generation monitors accurately count the fetal heart rate up to 300 bpm and print half the rate when it exceeds 240 bpm.

RW	RECEIVE S_1	RW	RECEIVE S_2	RW	RECEIVE S_1	RW	RECEIVE S_2

Fetal monitors double the maternal heart rate when ultrasound signals, due to aortic wall movement, are detected as nonrandom and equidistant. First generation monitors double rates less than 80 bpm when the ultrasound is used. Second generation monitors print accurately to 50 bpm. Doubling does NOT occur when a spiral electrode is used since each R wave of the ECG will be detected.

Figure 1.22: Doubling and halving the heart rate: Electronic logic inserts a "refractory window" (RW) following a detected heart beat when the ultrasound or spiral electrode are used (derived from Freeman, R.K., & Garite, T. J. (1981). *Fetal Heart Rate Monitoring.* Baltimore, MD: Williams and Wilkins, 47).

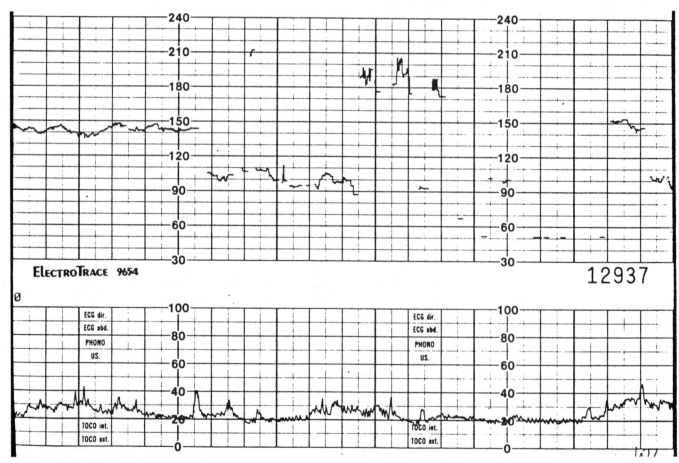

Figure 1.23: The maternal heart rate, in the 90s and 100s, doubled to the 180s to 200s for 5 to 10 seconds when the duration of systole and diastole US waveforms were similar. The tachometer counted aortic blood flow or movement as two separate heart beats. Gaps in the tracing are due to signal loss.

The absence of FM may indicate fetal demise. Women often know when their fetus is not adequately moving. If they were not prompted to go into the hospital, but showed up with the complaint of decreased FM, the fetus was usually dead (140).

Women perceive 4 to 8 fetal movements in 15 minutes when their fetus is 24 and 38 weeks' gestation (138). When examined by ultrasound, fetuses between 29 and 40 weeks' gestation moved once every 29 seconds, but only 16 percent of FM was perceived by the pregnant woman. Perhaps perception was low because movement had to last only one second to be counted (135).

Pregnant women were asked to determine how long it took for their fetus to move 10 times. Macrosomic fetuses moved 10 times in 14 to 18 minutes. IUGR fetuses moved 10 times in 12 to 16 minutes, and normal weight fetuses moved 10 times in 9 to 13 minutes (138). Therefore, one would *expect fetuses to move within 20 minutes of maternal observation.*

Since 98 percent of fetuses 24 to 27 weeks' gestation and *100 percent of fetuses 30 to 39 weeks' gestation move by the 75th minute of observation,* maternal perception of FM should occur within 1 1/2 hours (134). In fact, *one researcher felt that two hours should be the absolute maximum observation time for FM* (138).

Women perceive fetal movement when the fetus contacts the uterine wall. An anterior placenta decreased FM perception after the 28th week of gestation. Perception also depends on the woman's ability to concentrate (141). *Women most likely perceived FM if it lasted more than 20 seconds* (142). Baskett and Liston (139) reported that maternal perception of FM could be as high as 90 percent if awareness were heightened by showing the woman a real-time ultrasound of FM, and asking her to lie down versus sit or stand. Of 200 women queried about FM counting, 55 percent were reassured when they counted FM, 23 percent were worried, and a small percentage (17 percent) were neutral about FM counting (139). They were asked to count FM for 30 to 60 minutes once a day and were expected to perceive four or more fetal movements in an hour.

Processed US waveforms (using autocorrelation) can distinguish FM from the FHR. The ultrasound detects fetal spinal flexion-extension, trunk and limb movement, rolling, multiple, and isolated movements, and hiccups (143-144). However, US analysis cannot distinguish hand, mouth, breathing, and rapid eye movements (144-145).

The reflected US frequency is proportional to FM speed (145). The raw Doppler signal is analyzed by a band-pass filter. FM had US frequencies of 13 to 80 Hz lasting 200 or more msec (136). Fetal cardiac motion was associated with US frequencies greater than 150 to 220 Hz (143, 145). Maternal aortic motion greater than 200 Hz can be counted and recorded (3).

The Toitu Actocardiograph® uses a pulsed-echo Doppler ultrasound and autocorrelation to enhance FHR signal detection (77). High-frequency signals (due to cardiac valve closure) and low-frequency signals (due to FM) are identified

(78). The Hewlett-Packard M1350A® monitor also identifies FHR and FM, but does not print the movement of each twin like the Toitu monitor does. The Hewlett-Packard M1350A® records FM at the top of the UA channel as black bars lasting as long as FM lasts.

Fetuses move 0.4 to 4.8 cm per second. Their limbs move faster than their spine, which moves faster than rolling movements (145). The Toitu MT-320® monitor detected 88 percent of FM perceived by 27 women (142). The Toitu monitor detected 93 to 95.9 percent of all FM seen with real-time US. Using the US, FM detection was not affected by the placenta's location. Seven percent of spikes were false registrations due to maternal coughing, hiccups, abdominal wall movement, and movement of the US transducer (136, 144-145). False movement registrations or artifact can be decreased if the US is not moved or the woman is motionless (144). Since labor is accompanied by extensive maternal movement, more false FM registrations will be recorded than during antepartal testing.

The Toitu monitor records FM as spikes in the UA channel. The density of the spikes reflects the number of fetal movements. Spike amplitude reflects the speed of FM, i.e., *the taller the spike, the faster the movement* (146). A single or double spike was usually associated with an isolated limb movement. Spike clusters were usually associated with complex spinal movements, rolling, or sustained limb movements (145).

A benefit of actocardiography is the ease at which the relationship between FM and accelerations of the FHR can be examined. When twins were monitored, the Toitu monitor indicated each twin's heart rate (1 Dop and 2 Dop), and the corresponding activity of each twin (1 Act and 2 Act). Accelerations were defined by Baser (147) as an increase in the FHR of five bpm for any duration. Using this definition, accelerations were linked with FM 90 percent of the time in the third trimester in a sample of 166 women (147). A reactive acceleration (15 bpm above the baseline lasting 15 seconds at its base) ruled out metabolic acidosis. In the nonacidotic fetus, the majority of accelerations occurred near the time of FM (145). When accelerations were present in the oxygenated fetus, movement and "normal" variability of the FHR baseline were also present (143). Nonreactive NSTs had inadequate or absent accelerations and a 300 percent greater likelihood than reactive NSTs of no FM (141).

Fetuses evaluated by ultrasound had an average of 31 *gross body movements* per hour that lasted 10.6 to 11 seconds each (134). Fetuses moved most between 9 pm and 2 am at 38 to 40 weeks' gestation (102). Perhaps kick counts and NSTs should be performed after 9 pm, rather than during daylight hours. On the other hand, pregnant women need their sleep, so this is more ideal than practical.

It is a gross misconception that food causes fetuses, who may lack oxygen, to move and accelerate. *Fetuses moved more when maternal blood glucose levels were low. Meals, orange juice, and glucose had NO effect on gross body movements or the height or duration of accelerations in the 30 to 31 week, 34 to 35 week, or*

38 to 39 week old fetus (134, 148). *Therefore, in an attempt to stimulate FM or accelerations, the mother should **not** be fed.* She should not be given orange juice or any food until fetal well being is confirmed. After meals, the only change in fetal behavior was a significant increase in fetal breathing movements during the second and third hours after the meal and between 3 am and 7 am (102).

*The perceived lack of FM for **two or more hours** requires further evaluation* (138). *Reduced fetal movement may represent the effect of chronic fetal hypoxia* (149). Approximately half of 46 fetuses who were inactive for two or more hours were stillborn, tolerated labor poorly, or required resuscitation after birth (150). Fetal hypoxia was associated with fewer and smaller accelerations, decreased fetal swallowing, decreased lung fluid production, fewer breathing movement episodes, and decreased FM (149, 151-155). The gradual decrease in FM may take up to one week before death and is often associated with meconium and an abnormal FHR (155). As the fetus began to decompensate, accelerations and movement disassociated and occurred at different times (147). Then, there was an absence of fetal movement, and eventually there were spontaneous decelerations of the FHR. Therefore, the assessment of FM and accelerations over time may be valuable in the prevention of fetal acidosis, asphyxia, or death.

Fetal body movement should continue during pregnancy and even during labor (102). Barbiturates, narcotics, alcohol, valium, and nicotine may reduce the duration and number of FMs. FM also decreased when the fetus had a malformation such as hydrocephaly, gastroschisis, musculoskeletal deformities, and nonimmune hydrops. Nonimmune hydrops is associated with congestive heart failure (139, 156). FM decreases when there is a lack of amniotic fluid (oligohydramnios), partly due to hypoxia and partly due to the lack of a medium in which to move.

DIRECT/INTERNAL MONITORING TECHNIQUES: THE SPIRAL ELECTRODE (SE)

Very little additional clinical information will be gained by the application of a SE when compared with a consistent US-derived FHR pattern. Insertion of a SE requires the rupture of membranes and is an invasive procedure. The SE should be applied if:

1. continuous EFM is needed and
2. the US tracing is incomplete with multiple gaps and/or
3. accelerations and fetal movement have been absent for 75 minutes or more and/or
4. concern exists that the fetus may be developing metabolic acidosis and/or
5. there is an erratic tracing or
6. a suspected arrhythmia.

The arbitrary use of SEs should be avoided as the rupture of membranes for more than four hours was related to a significant increase in the transmission rate of the human

immunodeficiency virus (HIV) to the fetus (157). Until the HIV status is known for all laboring women, it is wise to assume they potentially have HIV. Since women who were HIV positive did not develop preeclampsia, one might think a woman with preeclampsia is more likely to be HIV negative (158). Preeclampsia is a high risk condition that requires increased fetal surveillance. Rupture of membranes for SE insertion would be wise if a continuous FHR is desired and a good US tracing cannot be obtained.

In 1963, Dr. Edward Hon created the predecessor of today's SE. The first electrode was not a spiral helix, but was an insulated clip similar to clips used in skin closure today (103). In 1967, Japanese doctors Kitahama and Sasaoka published the first description of the fetal SE. In 1972, Hon and his co-workers created a disposable SE (99).

Several types of electrodes have been used in the past, such as one with a clip, a suction cup, or a thin spiral wire (2). Spiral electrodes have a single or double helix (159). The double helix needed fewer replacements, whereas the clip electrode or the single helix electrode had to be replaced 20 to 38 percent of the time (160). There was no difference in the number of infections or scalp trauma when the clip electrode, single helix, or double helix were used. Three percent of the neonates developed scalp abscesses and three percent had minor infections. All wound infections were cured by the 10th day after birth (159).

The SE most in use today has two metallic surfaces that conduct an electrical current, a single helix and a reference electrode behind the white tip. In the past, electrode wires were composed of silver/silver chloride which raised the signal to noise ratio. Stainless steel electrodes are most common today because they are economical and the signal to noise ratio is sufficiently high (161). The spiral electrode is inserted through the fetal skin of the presenting part. The maternal lead or reference electrode should be in vaginal secretions. The US transducer should remain in place until the SE is attached to the fetus, electrode wires are attached to the leg plate, the leg plate is secured to the maternal leg, and a clear tracing is obtained. Then, the US should be removed.

Testing the DECG Cable Block/Leg Plate

Some fetal monitors have a ECG cable test capability. Consult the manufacturer's guidelines. For example, to test the cable of the Hewlett-Packard 8030A® or 8040A® monitors, the cable is plugged into the monitor and the end of the cable block is pressed against two protruding metal pins. The monitor is turned on and the digital readout reads 200 bpm and the audio speaker makes a sound at a 200 bpm rate. To test the cable block of the Hewlett-Packard M1350A®, an electrode must be in the fetus. The cable is plugged in and the electrode wires are removed from the leg plate. If "nop" appears in the digital display, the transducer cable is working correctly. With the wires out of the cable block, the test button is pressed and a rate of 200 bpm should appear on the digital display and should be recorded.

The Third Lead

Some monitors use a three-lead ECG set up. Only two leads are needed for the device to transmit signals into the fetal monitor. These leads include the fetal lead, attached to the green wire, and the maternal lead, attached to the red wire of the SE. Only one fetal and one maternal lead are needed for the SE to work. Two ECG complexes must enter the fetal monitor prior to calculating a heart rate.

A third lead is only needed when the reference electrode is in a dry pocket and is not transmitting the MECG into the fetal monitor. For this lead to work, conductive gel (ECG paste) may be applied to the leg under the leg plate. Conductive gel decreases surface tension on the skin and improves the contact between the leg plate and the skin. The leg plate will then become an active electrode and conduct the MECG signal. Some monitors use an ECG adhesive electrode that holds the green and red wires. For the system to work properly, the electrode pad must have complete contact with maternal skin. Therefore, the site is cleansed with alcohol and dried prior to application of the electrode pad. (21, 43, 162).

ECG paste serves no purpose with monitors that use a two-lead device, e.g., Hewlett-Packard. When a two-lead device is used, the leg plate or cable block simply holds the wires and transmits ECG signals back to the monitor. If the reference electrode is not in a wet pocket, a third lead can be established by applying an adhesive electrode to the maternal leg and attaching a red wire to it (single nonshielded lead with snap termination™). The red wire from the SE should be removed from the leg plate, and the new red wire should be inserted in its place. Then, the MECG will be conducted from the maternal le.g.

Application and Removal of the SE

The FECG is transmitted from the presenting part, which could be vertex or breech (see Figures 1.24 and 1.25). The SE is applied using sterile technique. After hand washing, usually only one hand is gloved (the one holding the SE). Once membranes are ruptured, the SE can be inserted by a physician, certified nurse midwife, or a staff nurse. The cervix should be at least 2 cm dilated, and the presenting part should be *accessible and identifiable*. When it is inserted, the single helix electrode is usually turned one-and-a-half *clockwise* rotations. The double helix need only be turned clockwise 180 degrees (103).

To remove the SE, slowly turn it *counterclockwise* while applying mild traction. Never pull the electrode from the fetal skin, cut the electrode, or try to reinsert it if it has fallen out.

Calculation of the FHR

When a SE is used, the FECG and MECG are transmitted into the fetal monitor. The direct ECG from the fetus is the stronger of the two signals and will be counted by the cardiotachometer (see Figure 1.26). The pulse intervals or R to R intervals are mapped out on a template in the computer's memory and then matched. Each dot on the tracing represents a newly calculated rate derived from dividing 60 seconds by the pulse interval. For example, if the pulse interval is 0.5 seconds, the calculated rate would be 60/0.5 or 600/5 or 120 bpm.

Consecutive rate changes, determined from consecutive pulse intervals, are plotted on moving fetal monitor graph paper. If the connected dots create a bumpy baseline, STV is present. *The SE is the most precise and reliable method used to*

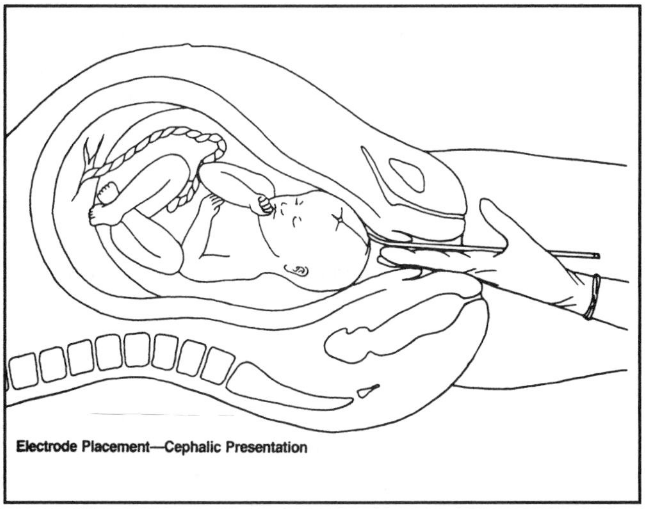

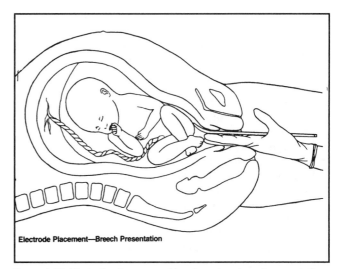

Figure 1.24: Electrode placement with fetus in a cephalic presentation. (Reproduced with permission of Marshall Klavan, MD: *Clinical Concepts of Fetal Heart Rate Monitoring*, Hewlett-Packard Company, 1977).

Figure 1.25: Electrode placement with a fetus in a breech presentation. (Reproduced with permission of Marshall Klavan, MD: *Clinical Concepts of Fetal Heart Rate Monitoring*, Hewlett-Packard Company, 1977).

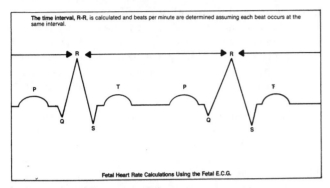

Figure 1.26: Fetal heart rate calculations using the fetal ECG. This illustration is based on the assumption that all beats occur at the same interval over a minute of time. The time interval between R waves on the fetal ECG is measured and the beats per minute rate is calculated, e.g., a pulse interval of 1 second will create a rate of 60 bpm.

measure STV (2, 26). Usually in cases of heart block, or when the pulse intervals do not change, STV is absent and the baseline is smooth (7, 43, 162).

When the SE is used, the Advanced Medical Systems (AMS) monitor plots a variability trend plot™ every ten minutes near the base of the FHR channel. The full variability trend graph is completed when 100 minutes of data has been received by the fetal monitor. The variability trend plot represents the combination of STV and LTV or variability in general. Variability will be plotted as average (AV), increased (↑) or decreased (↓).

Complications After SE Use
Although the SE precisely and reliably measures the FHR, the decision to perform an invasive procedure by applying the SE should be based on knowledge about its benefits and related complications. It should be applied to the scalp over a parietal bone or to the fetal buttocks. However, it should not be applied to the fetal face, fontanel, genitalia, or when there is placenta previa or a genital infection, such as active herpes lesions. The SE should not be used if there could be a transplacentally acquired coagulation defect, e.g., maternal thrombocytopenic purpura (163).

SE application is invasive and has been associated with several complications which include:
- finding a 7 cm electrode (it had been cut) imbedded in the uterus at the time of repeat cesarean section (164).
- scalp bruising, subcutaneous necrosis (103)
- scalp artery laceration (163)
- cephalhematoma with or without abscess (165)
- scalp abscess (166-168)
- septic scalp dermatitis (169)
- osteomyelitis (166, 170)
- meningitis, ventriculitis, hydrocephalus (171)
- E. coli sepsis and death of a 34 week premature baby (172)
- cerebrospinal fluid leaks

- injuries to the eyelids, e.g. lower eyelid attachment (173)
- injuries to the genitalia
- scalp alopecia at the site of the scar following an abscess and
- maternal endomyometritis (169).

Scalp Abscess. Scalp abscesses are usually diagnosed 1 to 14 days after birth, with the average being 3 days of age (171). Organisms isolated from scalp abscesses included Staphylococcus epidermidis, streptococcus, peptostreptococcus, peptococcus, bacteroides, and gonococci. The scalp may also become infected with the herpes simplex virus, although the source of the virus may be disputed, i.e., from maternal contact with the neonate versus vaginal contact during birth (171). Scalp abscesses may need to be incised and drained. Antibiotics will be given. In one case, the neonate had to be hospitalized for 11 days for treatment. In a case of a subperiosteal scalp abscess, E. coli was cultured. The baby developed an infected cephalhematoma, meningitis, ventriculitis, hydrocephalus, and seizures and was discharged from the hospital on the 54th day of hospitalization (167). In a case of osteomyelitis, there was a cephalhematoma that drained straw-colored fluid two to three days prior to admission. Staphalococcus epidermidis and a probable anaerobic sepsis were suspected. The hematoma was incised and drained and later debrided. Unfortunately, a craniotomy was needed for removal of a small portion of the right parietal bone and apex of the occipital bone and the adjacent portion of the left parietal bone. The infant spent 47 days in the hospital (169). Due to these rare (less than 1 percent risk) but potential infectious complications, the nursery staff should be informed about SE use and women should be taught the signs and symptoms of infection.

Endometritis. The incidence of maternal endomyometritis was related to the length of time the membranes had been ruptured, the number of vaginal examinations, the use of a SE, socioeconomic status, and the performance of a cesarean section. If the SE was in place nine or more hours, the risk of infection significantly increased. Clinic women had a higher risk (2.35 percent) of infection than private patients (0.1 percent). The most common causes of infection were Staphylococcus epidermidis and Bacteroides fragilis (169). Infection was markedly increased if a cesarean section was performed and any type of internal fetal monitoring was used. Even though maternal morbidity was related to the number of vaginal examinations in one study, it was not related to the duration of ruptured membranes or the number of vaginal examinations in another study (174). Cesarean section was the most significant factor contributing to febrile morbidity when it was compared with use of the clip electrode, spiral electrode, and the duration of ruptured membranes (163).

Human Immunodeficiency Virus (HIV) and Internal Monitoring
HIV is a RNA virus that infects cells with the CD4 antigen.

Cells with the CD4 antigen include lymphocytes, macrophages, the central nervous system, and the placenta. Acquired immunodeficiency syndrome (AIDS) is diagnosed when a person with HIV develops opportunistic infections, neoplasia, dementia encephalopathy and/or a wasting syndrome. People with AIDS often have a CD4 lymphocyte count below 200/mm³. Usually 6 to 12 weeks after exposure to HIV, seroconversion occurs and the woman is HIV positive. Seroconversion is confirmed when antibodies to HIV are found in serum (175).

In 1995, it was reported that 11 percent of the 315,000 people with AIDS in the United States were women. Sixty percent of these women were intravenous drug users or had male partners that used intravenous drugs. The majority of the remaining 40 percent had bisexual male partners (176). The majority of women and children with AIDS were black or Hispanic and not aware of any high risk behaviors (175). *It was projected that by the year 2000, there will be 10 million orphans and 10 million children with HIV in the world.*

Health care providers continue to be at risk for exposure to the HIV virus and other infectious diseases carried by blood and body secretions. They must balance the theoretic risk of HIV inoculation posed by invasive procedures against the benefits of those procedures (175). By December, 1994, the Center for Disease Control (CDC) in Atlanta, Georgia reported 42 cases, and 91 possible cases of occupational transmission of HIV. Of the 42 cases, 17 people now have AIDS or have died. Ninety percent of health care workers who had occupational transmission of HIV were exposed to blood. Others were exposed to a lab specimen or an unspecified fluid. Eighty-six percent had a hollow needle stick. Of those stuck by a needle, 1 in 250 to 300 seroconverted and now have the HIV virus. Obviously, needles must not be recapped and exposure to blood and body fluids must be avoided.

Health care providers have also contacted the herpes simplex virus, which caused herpes whitlow or herpes paronychia after the virus entered a cut in the skin or a newborn with the virus was handled (177). Hands should be washed before and after glove use because viruses and bacteria can enter the tiniest pinhole in a glove (178). Unused gloves have been found to be defective with perforations in 2 percent of 501 gloves. If a sterile vaginal examination (SVE) was done, 2.5 percent of gloves were perforated. If a SE was applied, 2.5 percent were perforated. But, the most exposure to maternal blood and body fluids (3.8 percent) was through the open cuff during a vaginal examination, especially when the hand was in a dependent position below the perineum (179). Naturally, if multiple vaginal examinations and invasive procedures are performed, there is heightened exposure to whatever virus or bacteria is lurking in the dark. Amstey (180) concluded that the risk outweighed the benefit for routine SE use.

Transmission of HIV from mother to fetus occurs during pregnancy, labor, and breastfeeding. White blood antigens, such as CD4, are low in women with HIV. Placentas vary in their impedance of the HIV-1 and virus. HIV-1 crosses the placenta in a concentration-dependent manner. In Kenya, as many as 31 percent of HIV infected women transmitted the virus to their fetus (181-182). Transmission rates were higher in developing countries (as high as 48 percent) and lower in industrial countries (as low as 13 percent) (182). Transmission rates increased if there was placental inflammation, such as chorioamnionitis with placental damage, a low maternal CD4 count, and/or a female fetus (182-183). It was theorized that the fetal female vagina provided a large area for viral entry. Neonates may have transplacentally acquired P24 antibodies in their plasma (181). However, the presence of HIV P24 antibodies in the neonate was not always associated with HIV transmission.

HIV may be transmitted vertically from the maternal vagina into the amniotic sac. Membranes must be ruptured to insert the SE or IUPC. If membranes are ruptured more than four hours, there is a dramatic increase in the rate of maternal to fetal transmission of HIV. Two hundred and seven HIV positive pregnant women participated in a study to examine the transmission rate of HIV to their fetus. Twenty four percent of their neonates had HIV (184). *If membranes were ruptured 4 or more hours, there was a 53 percent risk of neonatal infection with the virus. More than half of the neonates would become infected. But, if membranes were ruptured less than 4 hours, the risk of transmission decreased to 11.8 percent.*

A cesarean section for rupture of membranes for more than four hours may not be appropriate. Of 148 HIV seropositive women, there was a 29 percent HIV transmission rate when a scalp blood sample was obtained or a SE was applied versus a 25.6 percent HIV transmission when no invasive procedures were performed. This small increase in the rate of HIV transmission to the fetus prompted the recommendation that the arbitrary use of SEs be discouraged (157). *However, and perhaps more importantly, the arbitrary rupture of membranes should be discouraged, as well as the application of forceps, scalp pH sampling, and spiral electrode insertion.* In addition to in utero transfer of HIV, neonates may acquire HIV by a blood transfusion of HIV positive blood. There have been at least eight cases of HIV transmission to infants via blood transfusions (176).

Zidovudine, formerly called AZT or azidothymidine, decreases the rate of maternal-fetal HIV transmission. Oral zidovudine or Retrovir® may be given by mouth in a dose of 100 mg 5 times a day for 500 mg/day from the 14th to 34th week of gestation. This dose inhibited HIV from entering lymphocytes, monocytes, and placental cells, and prevented maternal-fetal transmission in 2/3 of cases. Zidovudine has also been administered intravenously during labor (185). Even if zidovudine were administered, HIV was still transmitted to the fetus, but at a lower rate. Prenatal oral AZT, IV AZT during labor, and oral AZT for the infant for 6 weeks has been recommended by the Centers for Disease Control. Even though some researchers have suggested large multicenter studies of maternal-fetal transmission of HIV are needed, they may never take place (186).

34

DIRECT/INTERNAL MONITORING TECHNIQUES: THE INTRAUTERINE PRESSURE CATHETER (IUPC)

In 1952, intrauterine pressure (IUP) monitoring was primitive and felt to be inferior to palpation (99). Almost forty years later, in 1990, the IUPC was thought by some to provide no advantage over the toco, even though the toco underestimated the true uterine pressure by as much as 10 to 40 percent (91, 187).

Since membranes must be ruptured prior to IUPC insertion, the decision to rupture membranes to insert an IUPC must be based on a "must know" situation (see HIV discussion). An IUPC is beneficial in obese women or when oxytocics are used in women with abnormal labor progress or a TOLAC on oxytocin, or the type of deceleration (early vs. late) is difficult to discern due to an unclear UA picture (34, 188-189). An IUPC must be inserted to administer an intrauterine infusion of normal saline or lactated Ringer's solution (amnioinfusion). Amnioinfusion cushions the umbilical cord and dilutes thick meconium (91-92).

An IUPC is *not required* when oxytocics are administered for induction or augmentation of labor. However, transducer belts may not fit around obese women who need close surveillance of the FHR and UA during induction. Therefore, insertion of an IUPC and/or SE may be required to meet the standard of practice, e.g., the FHR should be *closely monitored* when oxytocin is infusing (190-191). The IUPC should be used when it is *necessary* to better document contraction frequency, duration, intensity, and resting tone (34, 91-93, 189).

IUPC Insertion, Types, and Differences

The IUPC, or transcervical catheter, should be inserted by health care professionals in accordance with state practice acts, hospital policy, and after skill in the insertion technique has been demonstrated (see Figure 1.27). In some states, staff nurses may insert IUPCs. An IUPC may be inserted once membranes are ruptured and the cervix is 0.5 cm or more

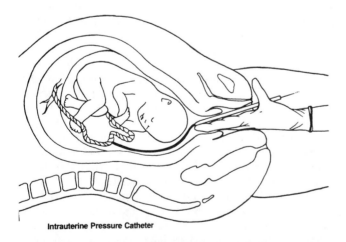

Intrauterine Pressure Catheter

Figure 1.27: The intrauterine pressure catheter (IUPC) is inserted using sterile technique. The catheter guide is placed just distal to the finger tip and the IUPC is advanced through the guide into the uterus.

ANTEPARTAL AND INTRAPARTAL FETAL MONITORING

dilated (192). However, insertion success is associated with the level of the woman's cooperation and a dilatation of more than one cm (193).

Insertion is contraindicated in the presence of uterine bleeding, uterine infection, and/or a low lying placenta with a risk of hemorrhage (26). Sterile technique is used and both hands are washed then gloved. Most IUPCs are inserted inside a guide tube. The IUPC may be passed into the uterus to a depth of 12 to 18 inches at clock positions of 6, 7, 8, or 12 (193). The IUPC should *never* be inserted against resistance. Once inserted, it is usually secured to the woman's leg with tape or a strap. Confirmation that the IUPC is in the uterus may be obtained if the woman coughs and a spike appears in the UA channel. Further confirmation is the appearance of the UC waveform.

Prior to insertion, single-lumen IUPCs should be flushed with normal saline or sterile water. The solution used to flush the catheter should be preservative-free. Preservatives, such as benzyl alcohol, have been associated with serious morbidity and mortality among very low birth weight infants, including intracranial hemorrhage (97, 165, 194-195).

Catheters may be fluid-filled or solid sensor-tipped. The first generation single-lumen fluid-filled IUPC may be attached to a sterile transducer dome on a nondisposable strain gauge or pressure transducer which is attached to a pole on the side of the fetal monitor. This type of strain gauge must be sterilized prior to use. After use, it must be disassembled, cleaned, dried, and resterilized as it is a potential source of nosocomial infection. Strain gauges that were only dried were positively cultured for pseudomonas, flavobacterium, Alcaligenes faecalis, and achromobacter (196). When a fluid-filled IUPC is used, artifact on the tracing is often due to maternal movement or catheter manipulation (193). Second-generation single-lumen catheters attach to a cable that contains a piezoelectric microchip and a Wheatstone bridge that senses pressure changes. The catheter must still be flushed with sterile saline or sterile water without preservatives prior to use and no air bubbles should be in the line. Air bubbles cause artifact.

Another type of fluid-filled IUPC is a closed system. When pressure is applied to this catheter, fluid pressure increases in the catheter and activates a sensor in the cable attached to the proximal end of the catheter. This catheter also has an amnioinfusion port (Lifetrace IUP 3000®, Graphic Controls, Buffalo, NY).

Solid sensor-tipped IUPCs have a micropressure transducer in their tip (193). The microtransducer changes its conductivity in proportion to the surrounding pressure (197) (see Figure 1.28). The transducer is a pressure-sensitive piezoelectric silicon chip and a Wheatstone Bridge strain gauge. Solid IUPCs usually have two lumens, one for amniotic fluid sampling and amnioinfusion and the other for IUP assessment. One such IUPC is the INTRAN Plus® (Utah Medical Products, Inc., Midvale, UT). Compared to fluid-filled systems, the set-up time for this catheter's insertion is substantially reduced.

35

Fetal and Maternal Monitoring Equipment

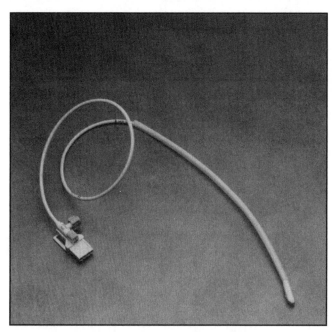

Figure 1.28: Intran Plus®. A pressure-sensitive piezoelectric silicon chip in the distal end senses a change in pressure at the catheter tip. (Photograph courtesy of Utah Medical Products, Inc., Midvale, UT)

Pressure Recordings

Researchers believed laws of hydrodynamics and muscle spheroids would apply to IUP measurements (197). Pascal's Law suggests IUP generated by a uterine contraction (UC) will be transmitted to a pressure transducer (193). However, IUP is affected by more than UCs. IUP is related to atmospheric pressure, hydrostatic pressure, elastic recoil of tissues within and around the uterus, and uterine contractions.

IUP = atmospheric pressure + hydrostatic pressure + elastic recoil + contractions
After zeroing, IUP = hydrostatic pressure + elastic recoil + contractions

Atmospheric pressure. Atmospheric pressure varies with the weather and adds to the IUP. This factor is removed by a "zeroing" process prior to monitoring UA. All IUPCs must be "zeroed" to negate atmospheric pressure (193). The INTRAN Plus® can be zeroed before or after insertion. After insertion, this device can be electronically zeroed by opening a sliding "door" (rezero switch) in the proximal end of the catheter near the cable. The UA level of the fetal monitor is set to zero when this "door" is open then the "door" is closed. Some solid IUPCs, such as INTRAN III®, are not equipped with a rezero capability. Therefore, these IUPCs can *only* be zeroed prior to insertion. Once the device package is open and it is attached to a cable that is plugged into the UA port, UA is set to zero and "0" appears on the digital readout and the IUPC waveform touches 0 mm Hg.

Traditional, single-lumen, fluid-filled IUPCs may be rezeroed or recalibrated any time after insertion because their pressure transducer is located outside of the uterus. To zero this device, the external strain gauge dome is opened to room air by turning a stopcock off to the IUPC and another stopcock off to the syringe used to flush the IUPC. The pressure sensitive transducer is now open to room air. The UA button is set to zero and "0" should appear on the FHR digital readout and the UA waveform should touch 0 mm Hg. Then the stopcocks are turned so that they are off to the syringe used to flush the catheter and off to room air. This leaves the IUPC open to transmit pressure to the strain gauge.

Another type of transducer-tipped IUPC necessitates the injection of one milliliter (ml) of air via a special port in the IUPC. Air inflates a little latex balloon over the pressure sensitive tip (Corometrics, Wallingford, CT). Once air surrounds the catheter tip, UA is set to zero. Air is then removed from the balloon by removing the one ml syringe from the port used to inject the air. This type of IUPC should never be used in a woman who has a latex allergy. Negating atmospheric pressure by zeroing creates IUP that is a reflection of hydrostatic, elastic recoil, and contraction pressures (198).

Hydrostatic pressure. The weight of amniotic fluid creates *hydrostatic pressure*. Hydrostatic pressure is related to the amniotic fluid index (AFI) and the quantity of amniotic fluid (199). One ml of amniotic fluid weighs 0.95 gm, supporting the saying *"a ml weighs a gram."*

Hydrostatic pressure is not equal throughout the uterus as the column of water varies in different quadrants (91). Each cm of fluid above the catheter tip adds 0.75 mm Hg (1 inch add 1.88 mm Hg) to the pressure reading (198, 200).

The pressure recorded from a fluid-filled catheter depends on the level of the tip of the catheter, air in the line, and the level of the pressure sensing transducer (strain gauge). To negate hydrostatic pressure, the tip of the fluid-filled catheter should be level with the external pressure sensitive strain gauge ("liquid level balancing"). Differences in the level of the strain gauge and the IUPC tip generate an offset error. If maternal position changes, the location of the fluid-filled IUPC also changes. Offset error is caused by an imbalance between the level of the catheter tip and the level of the strain gauge. If the catheter tip is lower than the external transducer, the recorded IUP is slightly lower than the actual pressure. Conversely, if the catheter tip is higher than the transducer, the recorded IUP is higher than the actual pressure (due to the weight of the water column in the catheter pressing on the transducer). If the transducer and catheter tip are at the same level, hydrostatic pressure is negated or zeroed out. If the IUPC were inserted at a position of 0600 (6:00 on a clock face or at the bottom of the uterus), with the woman supine there would be double the hydrostatic pressure as a catheter inserted at positions of 0300 or 0900 (with ½ the fluid above it) (198). Sometimes women change position and a different resting tone is recorded. This is due to the different amounts of amniotic fluid above the catheter tip which may increase or decrease resting tone 5 to 10 mm Hg (0.7 to 1.3 kPa) (91).

Offset error does not occur with solid IUPCs because the pressure-sensitive transducer is in the uterus detecting hydrostatic pressure (91-92). Pressure recorded by a sensor-tipped IUPC depends on the placement of the tip of the catheter and the height of the amniotic fluid above it. Some examples of sensor-tipped IUPCs are the Intran III® and Intran Plus (IUP 400)® from Utah Medical Products Inc. in Midvale, Utah (198).

Resting tone (tonus pressure). The resting tone or steady contraction of the uterine muscle is related to the normal *elastic recoil of tissues in and around the uterus* and contributes 7.5 to 15 mm Hg (1 to 2 kPa) to the IUP (91). If hydrostatic pressure is not part of the recorded IUP, resting tone would be approximately 7 to 15 mm Hg. However, hydrostatic pressure is usually a component of the recorded resting tone.

With fluid-filled IUPCs, normal resting tone ranges from 5 to 15 mm Hg. For example, during active labor resting tone was recorded at 10 mm Hg (200). In general, normal resting tone should be no greater than 25 mm Hg. Uterine resting tone appears as the straight, horizontal line between contractions and has been measured in cm H_2O (1 cm H_2O = 0.75 mm Hg) (200-201). Alvarez and Caldeyro-Barcia (201) found the following resting tones:

During pregnancy
    4-11 cm H_2O (3-8.25 mm Hg)
Last two weeks of pregnancy
    8-15 cm H_2O (6-11.25 mm Hg)
First and second stages of labor
    8-17 cm H_2O (6-12.75 mm Hg)
Third stage of labor (placental expulsion)
    5-10 cm H_2O (3.75-7.5 mm Hg).

Resting tone is derived from the hydrostatic pressure and elastic recoil of the uterus and surrounding tissues. It changes with maternal movement, and can increase during abruption and oxytocin administration (91). Normal resting tone depends on the type of IUPC used and the amount of amniotic fluid above the pressure transducer (hydrostatic pressure). It might have been suspected that pressures recorded by transducer-tipped IUPCs would be higher than pressures recorded by fluid-filled IUPCs due to the addition of hydrostatic pressure. However, pressures are reflective of the level of the transducer, a water column in fluid-filled systems, and whether the pressure transducer was inside or outside the uterus. In one study, the average *resting tone* measured by a fluid-filled catheter was 12.3 mm Hg, but with a sensor-tipped catheter it was 9.7 mm Hg when the woman was on her right side. On her left side, the fluid-filled catheter average resting tone was 10.1 mm Hg, and the sensor-tipped catheter was 7.4 mm Hg (Moise Jr., March 8, 1989 letter re: Intran I study). The fluid-filled transducer was

probably lower than the sensor tip of the solid IUPC, and the added weight of the column of water in the IUPC created higher pressures.

Contractions. Contractions of the uterus increase IUP (91, 198). *Uterine blood flow is significantly diminished when contraction pressures exceed 30 or more mm Hg.* The lowest uterine blood flow occurs at the contraction peak and recovers if there is no excessive uterine activity (98). During contractions, uterine blood flow (maternal) and umbilical artery blood flow (fetal) is uninterrupted before, during and after normal contractions (202). However, abnormally frequent, long, and/or strong contractions may diminish fetal oxygen delivery, requiring increased oxygen extraction by the fetus depleting oxygen reserves. Based on the relationship between UA and fetal oxygen delivery, *when the FHR is assessed, the UA should also be assessed and recorded.*

Laplace's Law states the pressure in a closed, fluid-filled sphere should be equal at all points within the sphere and should change in relation to sphere wall thickness and radius. Applying Laplace's Law to the uterus suggests *IUP should increase as the radius decreases*, i.e., the smaller the uterine size, the higher the pressure; and, IUP *should decrease as the radius increases*. However, the uterus is not a closed system. For example, in human and animal research the Law of Laplace did not apply (197, 203). When fluid was infused into the uterus of several sheep, the uterus became distended but there was *no change* in IUP (203). In another study of sheep and amnioinfusion, fetal vascular pressures decreased but pressure on maternal spiral arteries increased, *decreasing* blood flow to the placenta (204). Amnioinfusion to dilute thick meconium also *decreased* placental blood flow and preceded abnormal FHR patterns (205). If the FHR pattern deteriorates during amnioinfusion, the amnioinfusion should be discontinued, measures should be taken to improve maternal cardiac output and uterine oxygen delivery and the physician should be notified.

Pressure differences between fluid-filled and solid IUPCs. Fluid-filled and solid transducer-tipped IUPCs *should generate a similar UA activity waveform at slightly different pressures.* When the two catheters were used simultaneously, differences were found in the recorded resting tone and contraction peak pressures, but not the frequency and duration of contractions (see Figure 1.29) (91-92, 195, 206). Sometimes, peak IUPs were significantly higher with a sensor-tipped catheter than a fluid-filled catheter. Usually, the difference between the two types of IUPCs is 5 to 10 mm Hg (207).

With a fluid-filled catheter there should be no air in the line, otherwise the assessed UA would be inaccurate (2, 198). The position of the holes in the catheter affect the pressure reading (208). Sometimes these holes became clogged with vernix, blood, or meconium. A "flat top" on the UA waveform results from the catheter holes being plugged and the catheter should be flushed. Additional causes of artifact in the UA tracing may be caused by catheter "manipulation" or

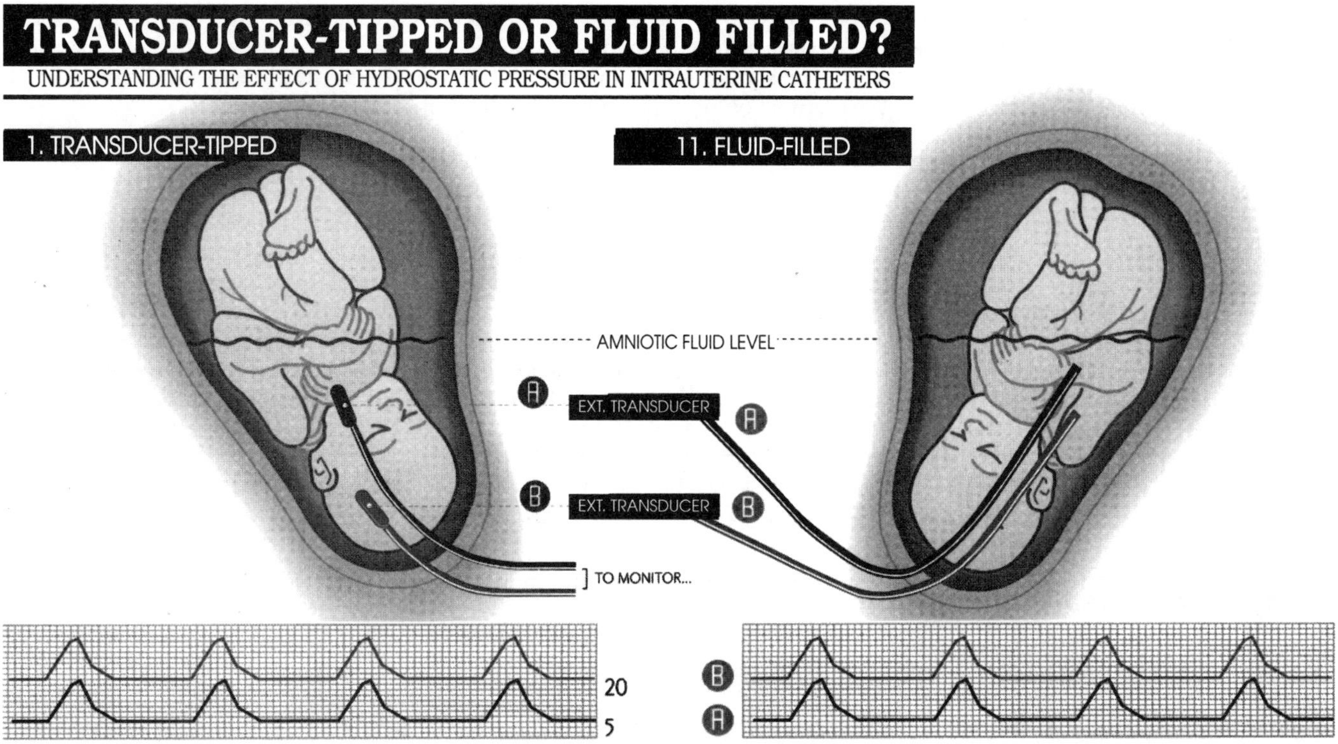

TRANSDUCER-TIPPED OR FLUID FILLED?

UNDERSTANDING THE EFFECT OF HYDROSTATIC PRESSURE IN INTRAUTERINE CATHETERS

Figure 1.29: Transducer-tipped IUPCs (on the left) detect hydrostatic pressure plus uterine resting tone and contraction pressure. If the catheter tip is near the top of the amniotic fluid column, recorded pressures will be less than if the catheter is near the bottom of the fluid column. Pressures detected by a fluid-filled IUPC depend on the level of the external pressure transducer in relation to the catheter tip. Theoretically, when the tip of the transducer-tipped IUPC is at the same level as the external transducer of the fluid-filled system, the tracings should register the same pressures. (Illustration provided by Utah Medical Products, Inc.)

a kink in the IUPC (193, 207). Fluid-filled IUPCs needed readjustments and had more unrecorded contractions and signal loss than solid IUPCs (207).

IUPC Complications

The use of an IUPC has potential but rare complications. One researcher reported problems occurred once in every 1400 uses (209). Some of these included:
a) perforation of placental vessels with minimal observed bleeding and fetal tachycardia
b) entanglement of the catheter with the umbilical cord and
c) uterine perforation (34)
d) perforation of a vessel on the fetal surface of the placenta (210).
e) perforation of a vessel in the amniotic sac with velamentous insertion of the cord, followed by fresh bright red vaginal bleeding, a single-lumen IUPC filled with blood, resulting in fetal demise (209)
f) entanglement with the umbilical cord resulting in variable decelerations two hours after IUPC insertion (209)
g) abruption (Moise Jr., March 8, 1989 letter)
h) water-borne contamination of reusable strain gauges (196) and
i) endometritis (192, 211).

Perforation. Signs of perforation of a fetal placental vessel included fresh vaginal bleeding, a soft nontender uterus, fetal tachycardia with "good" variability, and the absence of any contraction waveform on the monitor tracing (210). Uterine perforation may be asymptomatic (211). Or, the uterus may be hyperirritable (34). To avoid perforation, the IUPC should not be inserted against resistance *and the tip of the guide should not be inserted past the tip of the examining fingers or above the presenting part or past the internal cervical os* (173, 211). If resistance is felt, the IUPC should be repositioned and another attempt should be made at insertion (211).

Uterine perforation may be complicated by development of an intraperitoneal abscess. In one case, the catheter perforated the lower uterine segment and there was no UA waveform. When the woman performed a Valsalva maneuver, a spike was observed in the UA tracing. The catheter was withdrawn slightly and uterine contractions were then recorded. The woman delivered vaginally but complained of persistent right lower quadrant abdominal pain. Later, surgery revealed an abscess filled with several hundred ml of purulent material (212).

For suspected uterine perforation after IUPC insertion, the woman should be asked to perform a Valsalva maneuver. If a spike appears on in the UA channel, but there is no contraction waveform, suspect a uterine perforation.

Sometimes the woman feels some epigastric discomfort. At that point, the IUPC should be withdrawn. A physician who can manage complications such as uterine perforation should be immediately summoned to the bedside. The uterus should be monitored for hyperstimulation, while the fetus is monitored for signs of hypoxia. Following delivery, the woman should be monitored for signs and symptoms of infection. The hole in the uterus caused by the IUPC will heal without surgery.

Abruption. Abruption may be a complication of IUPC insertion, but it may also be related to cocaine use, preeclampsia, or infarctions of the placenta. To avoid abruption, it might be helpful to identify the location of the placenta, if a recent ultrasound report is available, prior to choosing the IUPC insertion point. A sign of abruption related to IUPC use is vaginal bleeding within 1 to 10 minutes after IUPC insertion (189).

Endometritis. The risk of infection related to IUPC use increases as the number of vaginal examinations increases, socioeconomic status decreases, and the duration of rupture of membranes increases (171). The chance the woman may develop endometritis significantly increases if membranes are ruptured more than 8 hours prior to delivery. Many times, the isolated pathogen is from the vagina. The authors recommend limited vaginal examinations and use of a toco prior to IUPC use to avoid rupture of membranes (213).

SOLVING EQUIPMENT PROBLEMS

Tables 3, 4, and 5 present common equipment problems, their possible causes, and possible solutions.

Table 3: The Ultrasound Transducer

PROBLEM	POSSIBLE CAUSE	POSSIBLE SOLUTION
Erratic printout with gaps in the tracing	• US not over fetal heart • Insufficient coupling gel • Loose belt • Very active fetus • Maternal movement • Maternal obesity	• Perform Leopold's maneuvers to locate the fetal back • Reposition US transducer over fetal back, perpendicular to the heart if possible • Reapply coupling gel and tighten belt • Encourage relaxation • Vary maternal position to see which results in the best signal transmission but avoid supine positioning
Doubling or halving the heart rate	• Maternal heart beat components, systole and diastole, counted as two beats (doubling) • Fetal arrhythmia with faster rate than top rate on the fetal monitoring paper (halving) • Old technology, first generation monitors were unable to count rates above 180 and below 80 due to their long refractory window (halving and doubling)	• Assess the maternal heart rate • Confirm fetal movement by palpation (confirm fetal life) • Auscultate the fetal heart rate with a fetoscope or stethoscope or • Compare the maternal heart rate with the fetal heart rate • Visualize the fetal heart beating with a real-time ultrasound • If the fetus is alive, see solutions for erratic printout
Burned tracing	• Bad paper feed • Overheated printer or thermal pen	• Examine paper feed • Refer to Biomedical Department for repair

Table 4: The Intrauterine Pressure Catheter (IUPC)

PROBLEM	POSSIBLE CAUSE	POSSIBLE SOLUTION
No contraction waveform	• IUPC fell out • IUPC is disconnected from monitor or poor cable/monitor connection • Uterine perforation, catheter in peritoneal cavity • Fetal vessel/placenta perforation • Fluid-filled system: catheter clogged • Solid IUPC with rezero feature: the rezero switch was left in the open (activated) position	• Check IUPC is in the uterus (examine marking on IUPC, should be near introitus) • Have woman perform a Valsalva maneuver, a spike indicates it's in the peritoneal cavity • If in the peritoneal cavity, pull IUPC out slightly, contraction waveform will be seen • Check connections between IUPC, cable, and monitor • Rezero IUPC transducer • Flush fluid-filled catheter • Replace IUPC if it is still needed and it fell out
Resting tone too low (less than 5 mm Hg) or Resting tone too high without apparent cause (greater than 25 mm Hg with uterus soft to palpation)	• IUPC malfunction • IUPC placement, e.g., entrapment between fetus and uterine wall may cause high pressure readings (or damped readings if a vacuum pocket forms at the tip) • Cable malfunction • Monitor malfunction	• Rezero IUPC transducer • Reposition catheter • If damped (less than 5 mm Hg) pressures continue, reposition by twisting catheter to reposition catheter tip • If pressures still continue below 5 mm Hg continue, replace IUPC • If high pressures continue in light of a soft uterus, pull back on IUPC to change its position • Discontinue oxytocin until the source of the high resting tone is determined
Straight line on tracing in UA channel	• IUPC fell out • Solid IUPC with rezero feature: the rezero switch was left in the open (activated) position • Loose connections between IUPC, cable, and/or fetal monitor • IUPC or cable is defective	• Tighten connections • Rezero IUPC • Close rezero switch • Change IUPC cable • Replace IUPC if needed
Artifact on contraction waveform or unusual, jagged tracing	• IUPC in dry area • IUPC defective	• Flush fluid-filled catheter • Pull back on IUPC • Replace IUPC if needed

Table 5: The Spiral Electrode (SE)

PROBLEM	POSSIBLE CAUSE	POSSIBLE SOLUTION
Gaps in the tracing	• Logic ON and fetal PVCs present • SE fell off presenting part or wire(s) fell out of leg plate/cable block • Faulty connection between cable and fetal monitor • Faulty cable block • Faulty SE • Reference (maternal) electrode in a dry area • Fetal demise	• Turn logic off • Check that SE wires are inserted in leg plate • Assess connection of SE to fetus by first gently pulling on SE and if not loose, confirm attachment by digital examination • Confirm fetal life (e.g., FM is palpated and/or fetal heart tones are heard by auscultation) • If SE is attached, test cable block (see manufacturer's guidelines for ECG cable test) • If SE is attached, and cable block is not malfunctioning: Set up a maternal lead by applying conductive gel to leg plate (3-lead device) or apply active electrode with single nonshielded lead with snap termination™(Hewlett-Packard) to leg. Replace SE red wire in leg plate with this wire. • Replace SE if it detached and is needed
Artifact on tracing	• Signal interruption, e.g., wires bumping against vaginal wall or SE in cervix • Malfunctioning SE (not conducting signals) • Loose connection between SE and leg plate • Reference electrode in dry area	• Reapply US transducer • Confirm fetal life • See "gaps in tracing" solutions

ASSESSMENT OF UTERINE ACTIVITY (UA)

Neither the American College of Obstetricians and Gynecologists (ACOG) nor the Association of Women's Health, Obstetric, and Neonatal Nurses (AWHONN) have formally endorsed a standard set of terms and definitions for interpretation of UA patterns. Clinicians in each facility should use consistent terms which have clearly defined meanings in order to "speak the same language" when communicating their interpretations of the FHR and UA tracings.

The terms chosen to describe UA in this chapter and the FHR pattern components in Chapter 5 were carefully selected after an extensive literature review and experience teaching fetal monitoring concepts to more than 50,000 nurses and physicians from all 50 states of the USA, two provinces of Canada, and 7 foreign countries.

Definition of UA Terms

Frequency: the time from the beginning of one contraction to the beginning of the next, some define it as the number of contractions over a period of time, e.g. 10 minutes (188). If the contractions are bell-shaped and not skewed, frequency may be timed from the peak of one contraction to the peak of the next contraction.

Duration: measured in seconds, it is the time from the beginning to the end of the contraction, some calculate a mean or average duration over a specified period of time (188).

Intensity: by palpation it is mild, moderate, or strong; by IUPC it is calculated as *the difference* between the peak pressure and the resting tone (peak minus tonus) (214). This difference (peak minus resting tone) is also known as the **amplitude or active pressure** (215).

Peak IUP: the acme of the contraction in mm Hg (or kPa) determined only when an IUPC is in place, also known as the **quality or strength** of the contraction (216-217)

Interval: the time from the end of one contraction to the beginning of the next, also known as the rest interval.

Resting Tone/Tonus/Baseline Tone/Mean Baseline Pressure/Relaxation: the intercontraction tension, the lowest intrauterine pressure found between contractions. By palpation, resting tone should be "soft between contractions" not "firm between contractions."

Hyperstimulation: also known as tachysystole or hypercontractility, abnormal contraction frequency (closer together than every two minutes) with the contraction interval less than 60 seconds. Hyperstimulation may or may not be accompanied by hypertonus.

Hypertonus: Abnormally high resting tone (above 30 mm Hg).

Oxytocin reaches a plateau or stable phase activity in each woman. Beyond that plateau, hypertonus can occur. When oxytocic agents are used, it is recommended that FHR and UA be recorded similarly to the standard for a high-risk woman in active labor, i.e., every 15 minutes (191).

To avoid hypertonus and hyperstimulation, oxytocin should be titrated until contraction frequency is 6 to 7 contractions per 15 minutes, rather than a certain peak IUP in mm Hg or kPas. *In at least one study, higher doses of oxytocin did not speed up labor.* For example, induction with 2.5 mU/minute increments every 30 minutes did not decrease the time to delivery when compared with 1.25 mU/minute increments. In fact, there was an increase in uterine hyperstimulation at the higher dose (218). The goal is to mimic spontaneous labor. In some cases, nulliparas may need 14 to 20 mU/minute to achieve this goal (219).

Montevideo Units (MVUs) were invented by physicians in Montevideo, Uruguay (214). Labor progress requires cervical effacement, dilatation, and descent of the fetus, regardless of UA. The Montevideo unit is used as a means to quantify contractions and determine their relationship to labor progress. If Montevideo units total 150 to 250, adequate labor progress should be anticipated (220-221).

Women who had normal labors had 66 to 340 MVUs with an average of 100 in early labor, 200 during the end of the first stage (10 cm), and 250 during the second stage (pushing). MVUs are higher when women ambulate (average 73.2 to 205.2) and lower when they are supine (79.6 to 175.6) (222). In normal labors, 250 MVUs were rarely surpassed (214). If MVUs are used to titrate oxytocin, they probably should be similar to those of women who had normal labor progress to avoid uterine hyperstimulation.

Some researchers believe MVUs are related to dilatation progress and can be used to evaluate labor progress (222). However, others found no relation between MVUs and labor progress. For example, women with hypocontractile labor had 21 to 313 MVUs (223). Since the MVU values for normal and hypocontractile labor were similar, Seitchik (223) felt MVUs could not be used to identify hypocontractility. However, MVUs might show a trend in UA when there is a failure to dilate.

Alexandria Units: Invented in 1967 by El Sahwi (221), Alexandria Units are not currently in widespread use. Alexandria units are calculated by determining the average intensity (average active pressure during 10 minutes) multiplied by the number of contractions in a 10 minute period (intensity x frequency) multiplied by the average duration of contractions in the same 10 minutes (intensity x frequency x duration).

Kilopascal Units (kPa): A unit of measurement of UA. 1 kPa = 7.5 mm Hg (192).

Active Pressure: peak IUP minus resting tone of that contraction (see intensity). The average active pressure during active labor was 37.6 mm Hg or 5.01 kPa (222).

Active Pressure Integral (API)/Uterine Activity Integral (UAI)/Active Pressure Area (APA)/Active Contraction Area (ACA): Invented by Steer in 1977 as the Active Pressure Integral (API), API is measured in kPa/time, and is related to MVUs (188, 222). API is calculated by adding each contraction's active pressure (in kPa) for a 15 minute period.

API is used to determine the **mean active pressure (API/time)**. The active pressure sum (API) is divided by 900 seconds (15 minutes) (91). A computer can be used to calculate API. API is reviewed to examine trends during labor. API increases as dilatation advances (222, 224). In a normal labor, API averaged 3390 per centimeter of dilatation. To ensure labor progress, some researchers suggested a goal of 1750 kPas/15 minutes in nulliparous women and 1500 kPas/15 minutes in multiparous women (221).

Oxytocin increases the API from an average of 1040 kPas/15 minutes to 1890 kPas/15 minutes or a mean active pressure of 0.58 to 1.05 kPa or 4.35 to 7.8 mm Hg (215). *The oxytocin dosage needed to achieve the*

75th percentile of UA in a normal labor was achieved at 8 or less mU/minute (224). When women were given oxytocin to induce labor, calculation of API was not related to the length of labor, mode of delivery, one and five minute Apgar scores, or cord arterial pH (219).

API/time (mean active pressure) was not superior to MVUs as a measure or predictor of dilatation (224). API, MVUs, and Alexandria Units poorly correlated with labor progress (215). Calculation of API along with the baseline pressure integral (BPI), mean active pressure (API/time), total duration of contractions, total number of contractions, and percent of contractions over time can be determined by a computer (188). More research is needed to clarify norms for these UA variables in normal labor before they will have clinical significance (225).

Documentation of UA

Contractions are displayed in the UA channel on the tracing. Contractions are usually bell-shaped with an ascending limb, peak or acme, and a descending limb. *Documentation of contractions may include frequency, duration, intensity, and relaxation* (226). When contractions are palpated, intensity may be recorded as mild, moderate, or strong. When an IUPC is used, the mm Hg or kPa of the peak intrauterine pressure (IUP) should be recorded, as well as the mm Hg or kPa of the resting tone. In the United States, mm Hg are documented. Calculation of intensity (amplitude or active pressure) is mostly done to determine MVUs.

Documentation should include the method of monitoring (227). More information can be obtained by a toco or IUPC than by palpation. The IUPC will record the onset of the contraction prior to the time it is palpated or perceived by the woman. The toco and palpation will detect the onset of the contraction prior to the woman's awareness (228).

The tracing is only one small, but important, part of the entire medical record. Although it was once thought that the tracing should be able to stand alone as evidence of labor events, thinking has changed (229). The tracing or strip provides limited evidence of events related to a woman's care and the standard of practice. The nurses' notes reflect assessments and observations, actions, fetal and maternal responses, and communications. Evidence of the standard of care provided should be found in the nurses' notes and need not be double-charted on the fetal monitor tracing. The nurses' notes should provide enough information about the UA and FHR patterns that *the tracing could be drawn if the strip were lost.*

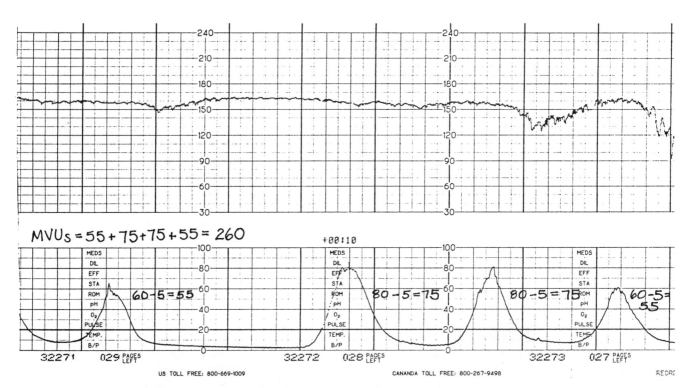

Figure 1.30: Calculation of MVUs. Subtract the resting tone from the peak IUP of each contraction to determine contraction intensity or active pressure. Then, add up the active pressure values of each contraction in a 10 minute period. This example includes 9 minutes at a paper speed of 3 cm/minute. In this example, an assumption was made that no additional contractions occurred in the minute preceeding or following the contractions. MVUs totaled 260. Labor progress would be expected.

Assessment of UA might be documented in the nurses' notes as follows:

Method of Assessment	Sample Documentation
Palpation:	UCs palpated q 3 min x 60 sec, strong, uterus soft between UCs.
Tocotransducer:	Toco, UCs q 3-3 ½ min x 60-80 sec, strong, uterus soft between UCs.
IUPC:	IUPC, UCs q 3-3 ½ min x 60-80 sec, ↑ 75-85 mm Hg, rest. tone 20-25 mm Hg. (The ↓ reflects the peak IUP).

Uterine Activity Pattern Deviations

Since palpation provides no permanent record of UA, it is important to record these UA assessments. Uterine activity should be confirmed when the contraction waveform is upside down (see Figure 1.31). This **uterine reversal pattern** occurs because the abdomen pulled away from the toco creating a negative pressure. This sometimes happens when a woman turns to her side or is obese. The toco should be moved to a position where the uterus pushes forward under the toco. The onset, peak, and offset of the UA waveform are visible, but they are upside down. Contraction frequency and duration can be timed from this pattern once the onset and offset of UA is confirmed by palpation.

Low amplitude, high frequency waves (LAHF waves) or uterine irritability often occurred 24 to 72 hours prior to the onset of preterm labor (230-231). A woman with a preterm gestation and LAHF waves should be evaluated for preterm labor. LAHF waves usually have a duration of less than 30 seconds, an interval of less than 15 seconds, and are occasionally felt by the woman. LAHF waves may be a uterine response to prostaglandin production stimulated by infection, such as a urinary tract infection (232). Occasionally, this pattern is associated with abruption of the placenta. When a woman presents preterm with LAHF waves, the physician should rule out preterm labor, infection, and abruption (see Figure 1.32).

Abnormal uterine activity. The shape, frequency, duration, and/or intensity of uterine contractions may reflect abnormal UA. The shape may be skewed, with a longer descending limb than ascending limb. The interval between contractions might be less than 60 seconds. Without a 60 second interval between contractions, the fetus might deplete

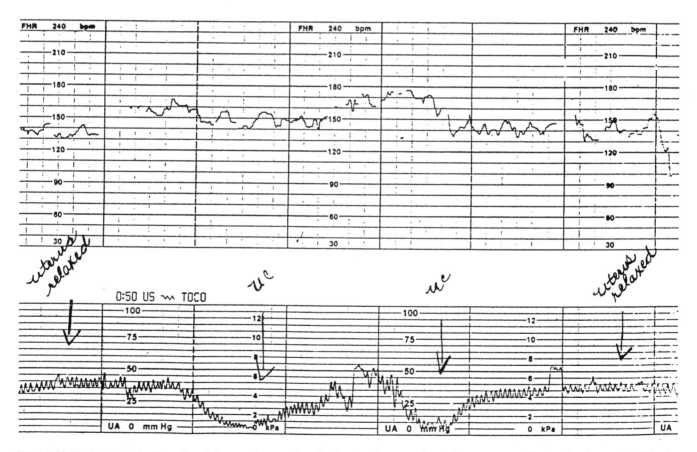

Figure 1.31: Uterine reversal pattern. The abdomen pulls away from the tocotransducer resulting in less pressure on the toco (tracing courtesy Columbus Hospital, Great Falls, MT).

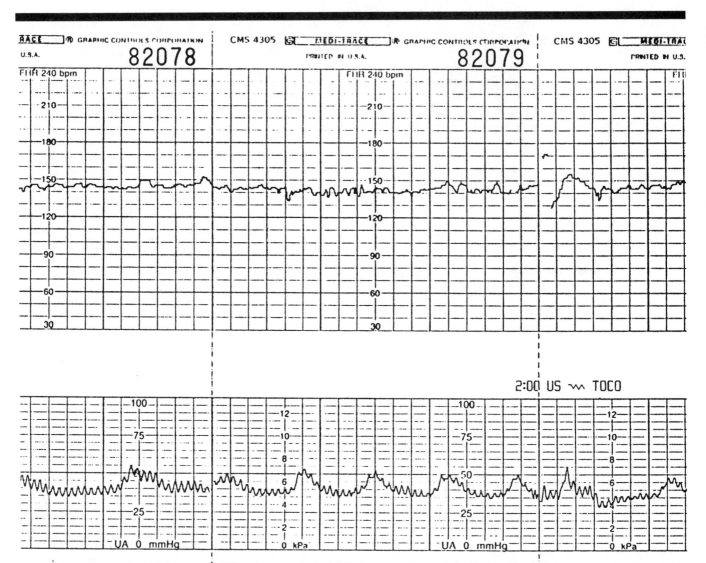

Figure 1.32: Low amplitude, high frequency (LAHF) waves or uterine irritability in response to prostaglandin formation. This is often seen as a precursor to preterm labor or in response to infection, such as a bladder infection. Occasionally, it is associated with abruption of the placenta.

its oxygen reserves. Contractions may last longer than 90 seconds and be strong with a peak IUP of 90 or more mm Hg. Long and strong contractions could limit entry of oxygen into the placenta which would deplete oxygen reserves.

Skewed Contractions. The contraction waveform is usually bell-shaped. Skewed contractions, seen when a toco is in place, may be a uterine response to an overdistended bladder. This has occurred after an epidural anesthetic was administered but the foley catheter had not yet been inserted. When a toco is in place, shewed contractions may occur during maternal apnea with abdominal distention after a contraction has ended (see Figure 1.33).

Increased Contraction Frequency (Short Contraction Interval): Polysystole, Tachysystole, Hyperstimulation, and Hypercontractility. Contractions are too frequent *when the*

interval between them is less than one minute and/or they occur closer together than every 2 minutes. Polysystole is a general term that includes all UC patterns where contraction frequency is less than every two minutes and contraction interval is less than 60 seconds (see Figure 1.34). Polysystole does not pose a threat to the fetus if uterine pressures are less than 30 mm Hg or contractions are very mild to palpation. However, oxygen reserves may become depleted if pressures exceed 30 mm Hg.

Polysystole exists when contractions occur in sets of two (doubling or coupling) or more with an interval less than 20 seconds. Doubled contractions usually posed little threat to the oxygen reserves of the fetus since the second contraction is always weaker than the first and there is an interval between sets of contractions of more than 60 seconds. But, when there are three contractions in a row (tripling), four in a row (quadrupling), or more than four in a row (hyperstimulation, hypercontractility, tachysystole), uterine resting tone typically rises and poses a threat to fetal oxygen reserves. The combination of too frequent contractions (hyperstimulation) with an inadequate resting tone (hypertonus) poses the greatest risk of fetal oxygen reserve depletion.

Doubling. In some locations, e.g., southern California, this pattern has been called "camel backs." In Montgomery, Alabama, the same pattern has been called "piggy backs." When doubling occurs, the first contraction is always longer and stronger than the second contraction (see Figure 1.35). The uterus rarely returns to the normal resting tone before the second contraction begins. The interval between the two contractions is usually less than 20 seconds. The interval between each set of contractions will be greater than 60 seconds.

Documentation of this pattern may be "Doubling q 4½ minutes x 40-80 sec, mild to moderate, uterus soft between UCs." In this example, the beginning of each set of contractions (frequency) is four and a half minutes apart. The second contraction lasts 40 seconds and the first lasts 80. The peak intensities are mild to moderate, and the uterus is at rest

between each set of contractions. Doubling or coupling has been observed when the fetus was in a malposition such as persistent occiput posterior (OP) or *persistent occiput transverse (OT)*.

Actions in response to doubling include discontinuing the oxytocin infusion and evaluating the pelvis and fetal position and size for fit. This pattern has been associated with cephalopelvic (fetopelvic) disproportion. If the fetus is not in a malposition, and the pelvis is found to be adequate for the fetus to descend and deliver vaginally, and oxytocin was infusing, and the FHR pattern demonstrated fetal well-being (reactive accelerations and no variable, late, or prolonged decelerations), the oxytocin infusion could be continued in order to establish a normal UA pattern. If the fetus has decelerations and oxytocin ordered to continue, the physician should be readily available to handle complications (190).

Hyperstimulation. This is a disorder of UC frequency with three names: hyperstimulation, hypercontractility, or tachysystole. The interval between contractions is less than one minute and contractions occur closer together than every

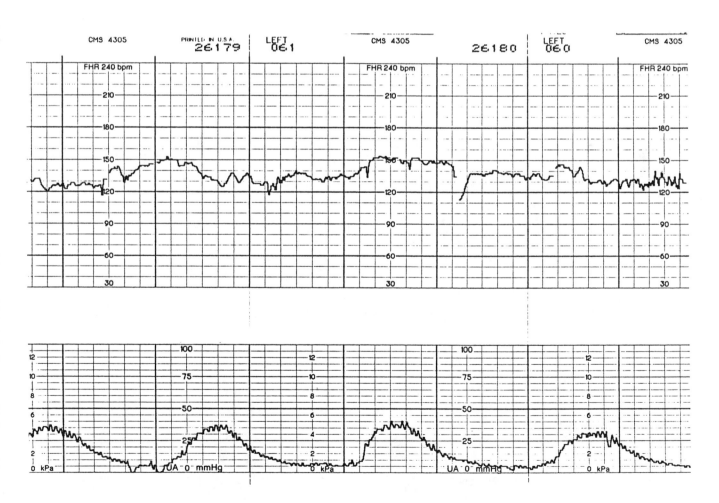

Figure 1.33: Skewed contractions with less than a 60 second interval. Intensity and relaxation of the uterus should be confirmed by palpation.

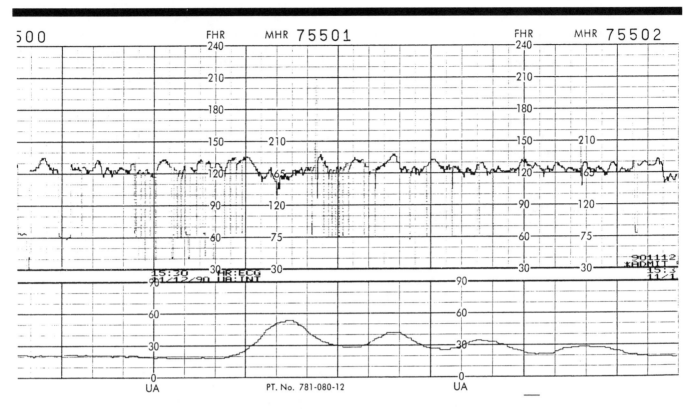

Figure 1.34: Polysystole with quadrupling. Also note artifact in the FHR record.

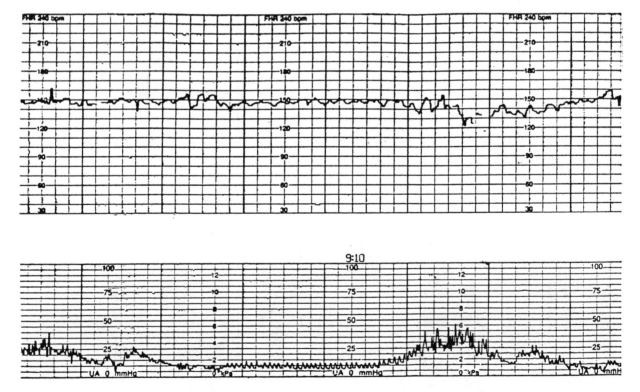

Figure 1.35: Doubling or coupling of uterine contractions.

two minutes (see Figure 1.36). The uterus may be contracting too frequently when the woman is dehydrated. In this case, she will be ketotic and have ketones in her urine. This pattern will in ineffective in dilating the cervix.

When the uterus is contracting too frequently (hyperstimulated) and the uterine resting tone is elevated above normal (hypertonus), the pattern is called *tachysystole with uterine hypertonus or hyperstimulation with uterine hypertonus.* Hyperstimulation with hypertonus is an abnormal response to oxytocin. It may also be a response to abruption, prostaglandin gel, or maternal hypoxia.

If an oxytocic drug, such as oxytocin, is infusing, it should be immediately discontinued. If oxytocin is ordered to be given, it should be withheld until the etiology of the hyperstimulation has been determined. If hyperstimulation continues, and the woman is not dehydrated, placenta abruption should be ruled out by the physician. The placenta can be abrupting even when the FHR pattern demonstrates no sign of fetal hypoxemia.

Increased Peak IUP, Duration, and/or Resting Tone.
Tetanic contractions are long and strong but not necessary close together. Tetanic contractions are strong to palpation or 90 or more mm Hg at their peak when an IUPC is in place. Tetanic contractions also last 90 or more seconds. Thus, some clinicians use a *"90 x 90"* rule to define a tetanic contraction

(see Figure 1.37). Tetanic contractions may precede birth! Therefore, a vaginal examination should be performed to assess dilatation and descent of the fetus. Tetanic contractions may *decrease* placental perfusion which would increase fetal oxygen extraction and deplete oxygen reserves. Tetanic contractions have occurred after exposure to cocaine. If cocaine addiction is suspected, a toxicology screen may be required.

Contractions may have an abnormally high resting tone. An elevated resting tone may be due to oxytocin or uterine overdistention, a complication of amnioinfusion. Oxytocin and/or the amnioinfusion should be immediately discontinued until resting tone is below 30 mm Hg. Hypertonus may be diminished by laternal positioning. Lateral positioning may also decrease contraction frequency and increase intercontraction relaxation (233). When hypertonus is noted, the fetus should be evaluated for signs of hypoxia. In response to fetal hypoxia or signs of stress, to diminish UA the physician may order a subcutaneous or intravenous injection of 0.125 to 0.25 mg of terbutaline to the woman.

CONCLUSION
Continuous EFM and internal FHR and UA monitoring has more limitations than benefits. Therefore, the decision to apply this technology requires an analysis of the potential risks and benefits and a "need to know."

Personal computers have been linked with fetal monitors

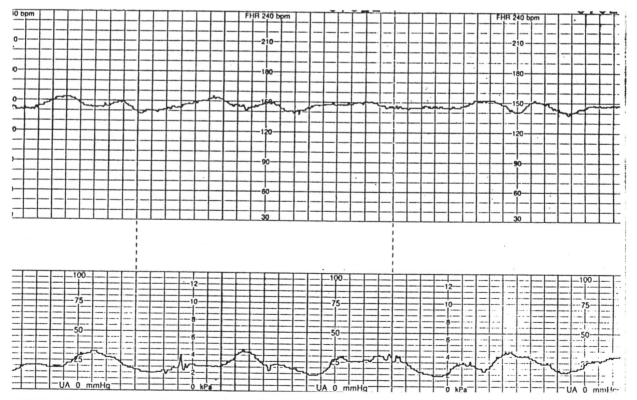

Figure 1.36: Hyperstimulation recorded with a tocotransducer in place. The placenta abrupted.

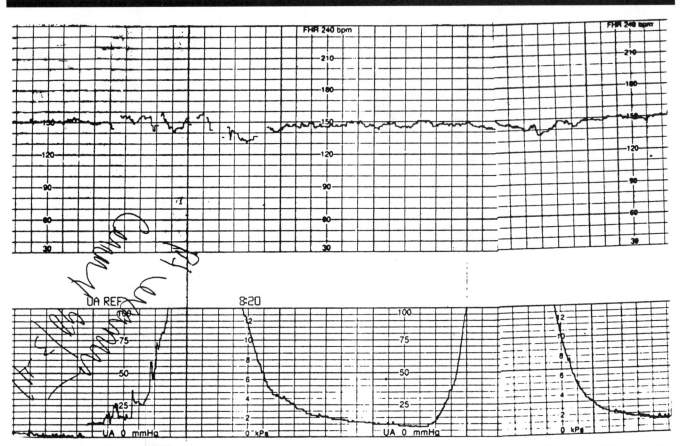

Figure 1.37: Tetanic contractions at 3 to 4 cm dilatation. The woman was a gravida 4, para 3, with a history of heroin abuse. She smoked 1/2 pack per day. Her admission blood pressure was 140/80, with a temperature of 99.2° F, a pulse of 90 bpm, and a respiratory rate of 20/minute. When membranes were artificially ruptured, thick meconium was noted. Approximately 4 1/2 hours after admission, she underwent a cesarean section. 17 minutes after delivery she had a cardiac arrest. She died 1 hour and 27 minutes after delivery. Her husband then admitted they had free-based heroin and crack cocaine the night prior to admission.

for tracing analysis, documentation, storage, retrieval, and communication via telephone modems. Computer analysis of FHR and UA patterns differs from physician analysis and was a helpful adjunct in some clinical situations (51).

Ultrasound technology has improved since the 1970s in its ability to detect the FHR signal. These improvements changed thinking about the ability of an external US to assess short-term variability. Short-term variability has been analyzed by computer and documented even when the US was used to determine the FHR.

Fluid-filled intrauterine pressure catheters and solid, transducer-tipped catheters may be used to assess intrauterine pressure. Intrauterine pressure variables have been identified which explain why these two types of IUPCs might register slightly different peak pressures and resting tones.

Fetal monitors are electronic machines filled with computer hardware and software. The devices attached to the machines may malfunction due to equipment failure, placement errors or loose connections. Sometimes the clinician can fix the problem, and other times, the monitor or its components must be repaired by a skilled technician.

The configuration of the contraction waveform may suggest the toco needs adjustment, or the women has Munchausen Syndrome, a risk of preterm labor, infection, cephalopelvic disproportion, dehydration, abruption, excessive oxytocin, uterine overdistention, cocaine addiction, or an impending birth. Analysis of UA provides a basis for interventions such as evaluation of the feto-pelvic relationship in the case of coupling, discontinuance of oxytocin in the case of hyperstimulation and/or hypertonus, an ultrasound to rule out abruption, discontinuance of an amnioinfusion related to hypertonus, a vaginal examination to rule out impending birth, or terbutaline administration to stop excessive UA.

Antepartal and intrapartal fetal monitoring technology has advanced over the last three decades and has created a "high tech" environment. It might be easier to focus on the machine and forget about the woman and her fetus. But, "high tech" can never replace "high touch" and caring. A listening ear, a soft touch, a gentle voice, and an empathetic word mean more to women and their families than the complex printout of a machine.

References

1. Dawes, G. S., Visser, G. H. A., Goodman, J. D. S., & Redman, C. W. G. (September 1, 1981). Numerical analysis of the human fetal heart rate: The quality of ultrasound records. American Journal of Obstetrics and Gynecology, 141(1), 43-52.

2. Serr, D. M. (April 1974). Methods for recording the continuous fetal heart rate and uterine contractions. Clinics in Obstetrics and Gynecology, 1(1), 169-190.

3. Divon, M. Y., Torres, F. P., Yeh, S-Y., & Paul, R. H. (January 1, 1985). Autocorrelation techniques in fetal monitoring. American Journal of Obstetrics and Gynecology, 151(1), 2-6.

4. Boehm, F. H., & Fields, L. M. (1984). Second generation EFM is waiting in the wings. Contemporary Obstetrics and Gynecology, 23, 179.

5. Snijders, R. J. M., McLaren, R., & Nicolaides, K. H. (1990). Computer-assisted analysis of fetal heart rate patterns at 20-40 weeks' gestation. Fetal Diagnosis and Therapy, 5(2), 70-83.

6. Dawes, G. S., Moulden, M., & Redman, C. W. G. (1991). The advantages of computerized fetal heart rate analysis. Journal of Perinatal Medicine, 19(1-2), 39-45.

7. Dawes, G. S. (March 1993). The fetal ECG: Accuracy of measurements. British Journal of Obstetrics and Gynaecology, 100(Suppl. 9), 15- 17.

8. Dawes, G. S., Lobb, M., Moulden, M., Redman, C. W. G., & Wheeler, T. (October 1992). Antenatal cardiotocogram quality and interpretation using computers. British Journal of Obstetrics and Gynaecology, 99, 791-797.

9. Amato, J. C. (September 1977). Fetal monitoring in a community hospital. A statistical analysis. Obstetrics & Gynecology, 50(3), 269-274.

10. Vintzileos, A. M., Antsaklis, A., Varvarigos, I., Papas, C., Sofatzis, I., & Montgomery, J. T. (June 1993). A randomized trial of intrapartum electronic fetal heart rate monitoring versus intermittent auscultation. Obstetrics & Gynecology, 81(6), 899-907.

11. Spencer, J. A. D. (1989). Intrapartum hypoxia, birth asphyxia and handicap. In J. A. D. Spencer (Ed.), Fetal monitoring: Physiology and techniques of antenatal and intrapartum assessment (pp. 228-232). Philadelphia: F. A. Davis.

12. Carter, B. S., Haverkamp, A. D., & Merenstein, G. B. (June 1993). The definition of acute perinatal asphyxia. Clinics In Perinatology, 20(2), 287-304.

13. Boylan, P. (March 1987). Intrapartum fetal monitoring. Bailliere's Clinical Obstetrics and Gynaecology, 1(1), 73-95.

14. Leveno, K. J., Cunningham, F. G., Nelson, S., Roark, M., Williams, M. L., Guzick, D. (September 1986). A prospective comparison of selective and universal electronic fetal monitoring in 34,995 pregnancies. New England Journal of Medicine, 315,615-619.

15. McCusker, J., Harris, D. R., & Hosmer, Jr., D. W. (September 1988). Association of electronic fetal monitoring during labor with cesarean section rate and with neonatal morbidity and mortality. American Journal of Public Health, 78(9), 1170-1174.

16. Shy, K. K., Luthy, D. A., Bennett, F. C., Whitfield, M., Larson, E. B., van Belle, G. (March 1, 1990). Effects of electronic fetal-heart-rate monitoring, as compared with periodic auscultation, on the neurologic development of premature infants. The New England Journal of Medicine, 322(9), 588-593.

17. Smith, C. V., Nguyen, H. N., Kovacs, B., McCart, D., Phelan, J. P., & Paul, R. H. (1987). Fetal death following antepartum fetal heart rate testing: A review of 65 cases. Obstetrics & Gynecology, 70(1), 18-20.

18. Prentice, A., & Lind, T. (December 12, 1987). Fetal heart rate monitoring during labour-too frequent intervention, too little benefit? The Lancet, 1375-1377.

19. Grant, A., Joy, M.-T., O'Brien, N., Hennessy, E., & MacDonald, D. (November 25, 1989). Cerebral palsy among children during the Dublin randomized trial of intrapartum monitoring. The Lancet(8674), 1233-1235.

20. Hoffmann, A. L., Hjortdal, J. O., Secher, N. J., & Weile, B. (March 12, 1990). The relationship between Apgar score, umbilical artery pH, and operative delivery for fetal distress in 2778 infants born at term. European Journal of Obstetrics, Gynecology and Reproductive Biology, 38, 97-101.

21. Kaiser, G. (May 1991). Do electronic fetal heart rate monitors improve delivery outcomes? Journal of the Florida Medical Association, 78(5), 303-307.

22. Nelson, K. B. (December 1989). Relationship of intrapartum and delivery room events to long-term neurologic outcome. Clinics in Perinatology, 16(4), 995-1007.

23. Anthony, M.Y., & Levene, M. I. (1990). An assessment of the benefits of intrapartum fetal monitoring. Developmental Medicine and Child Neurology, 32, 547-553.

24. Bossart, H., Jenkins, H. M. L., van Geijn, H. P., & Sureau, C. (February 1987). Fetal monitoring, present and future. European Journal of Obstetrics, Gynecology and Reproductive Biology, 24(2), 105-121.

25. Thacker, S. B. (1989). Effectiveness and safety of intrapartum fetal monitoring. In J. A. D. Spencer (Ed.), <u>Fetal monitoring: Physiology and techniques of antenatal and intrapartum assessment</u> (pp. 211-217) Philadelphia: F. A. Davis.

26. Guidelines for the use of fetal monitoring. (1987). <u>International Federation of Gynaecology & Obstetrics, 25,</u> 159-167.

27. Killien, M. G., & Shy, K. (March 1989). A randomized trial of electronic fetal monitoring in preterm labor: Mother's views. <u>Birth, 16</u>(1), 7-12.

28. Snydal, S. H. (September/October 1988). Responses of laboring women to fetal heart rate monitoring: A critical review of the literature. <u>Journal of Nurse-Midwifery, 33</u>(5), 208-216.

29. Snydal, S. H. (January/February 1988). Methods of fetal heart rate monitoring during labor: A selective review of the literature. <u>Journal of Nurse-Midwifery, 33</u>(1), 4-14.

30. Shearer, M. H. (Spring 1979). Auscultation is "acceptable" in low-risk women according to the National Institute of Child Health and Human Development task force. <u>Birth and the Family Journal, 6</u>(1), 3-6.

31. Carter, M. C. (1986). Advances in electronic fetal monitors - real or imaginary. <u>Journal of Perinatal Medicine, 14</u>(6), 405-410.

32. Sandmire, H. F. (December 1990). Whither electronic fetal monitoring? [Clinical Commentary]. <u>Obstetrics & Gynecology, 76</u>(6), 1130-1133.

33. Shy, K. K., Larson, E. B., & Luthy, D. A. (1987). Evaluating a new technology: The effectiveness of electronic fetal heart rate monitoring. <u>Annual Review of Public Health, 8,</u> 165-190.

34. Madanes, A. E., David, D., & Cetrulo, C. (March 1982). Major complications associated with intrauterine pressure monitoring. <u>Obstetrics and Gynecology, 59</u>(3), 389-391.

35. Sorokin, Y., Weintraub, Z., Rothschild, A., Iancu, T. C., & Abramovici, H. (November 1990). Cerebrospinal fluid leak in the neonate-complication of fetal scalp electrode monitoring. <u>Israel Journal of Medical Sciences, 26</u>(11), 633-635.

36. Dawes, G. S., Moulden, M. & Redman, C. W. G. (January 1991). Limitations of antenatal fetal heart rate monitors. <u>American Journal of Obstetrics and Gynecology, 162</u>(1), 170-173.

37. Docker, M. F. (March 1993). Doppler ultrasound monitoring technology. <u>British Journal of Obstetrics and Gynaecology, 100</u>(Suppl. 9), 18-20.

38. Simkin, P. (December 1986). Stress, pain, and catecholamines in labor: Part 2. Stress associated with childbirth events: A pilot survey of new mothers. <u>Birth, 13</u>(4), 234-240.

39. Gimovsky, M. L. (Ed.). (Summer 1988). Fetal heart rate monitoring casebook. <u>Journal of Perinatology, 8</u>(3), 276-281.

40. Redman, C. W. G. (March 1993). Communicating the significance of the fetal heart rate record to the user. <u>British Journal of Obstetrics and Gynecology, 100</u>(Suppl. 9), 24-27.

41. Tammelleo, A. (July 1986). Misuse of fetal monitor: Brain damage results. <u>The Regan Report on Nursing Law, 27</u>(2). Providence, RI: Medica Press.

42. Carter, M. C. (1993). Signal processing and display-cardiotocographs. <u>British Journal of Obstetrics and Gynaecology, 100</u>(Suppl. 9), 21-23.

43. Gray, J. (1989). A case of intrapartum fetal arrhythmia creating difficulties in cardiotocographic interpretation. <u>Australian and New Zealand Journal of Obstetrics and Gynaecology, 29</u>(3), 265-267.

44. Herbert, W. N. P., Stuart, N., & Butler, L. S. (July/August 1987). Electronic fetal heart rate monitoring with intrauterine fetal demise. <u>JOGNN</u> (4), 249-252.

45. Schneiderman, C. I., Waxman, B., & Goodman, C. J. (August 15, 1972). Maternal-fetal electrocardiogram conduction with intrapartum fetal death. <u>American Journal of Obstetrics and Gynecology, 113</u>(8), 1130-1133.

46. Amato, J. C. (December 15, 1983). Fetal heart rate monitoring. <u>American Journal of Obstetrics and Gynecology, 147</u>(8), 967-969.

47. Lackritz, R., Schiff, I., Gibson, M., & Safon, L. (March 1978). Decelerations on fetal electrocardiography with fetal demise. <u>Obstetrics & Gynecology, 51</u>(3), 367-368.

48. Dawes, G. S., Moulden, M., & Redman, C. W. G. (1991). System 8000: Computerized antenatal FHR analysis. <u>Journal of Perinatal Medicine, 19</u>(1-2), 47-51.

49. Bernardes, J. (December 1992). "Classic nonstress test" and "ambulatory stress test" in the assessment of umbilical cord compression [Letters]. <u>American Journal of Obstetrics and Gynecology, 167</u>(6), 1911.

50. Zuspan, F. P., Quilligan, E. J., & van Geijn, H. P. (December 1979). NICHD consensus development task force report: Predictors of intrapartum fetal distress -the role of electronic fetal monitoring. <u>The Journal of Pediatrics, 95</u>(6), 1026-1030.

51. Devoe, L. D. (April 1990). Computerized analysis of fetal heart rate. <u>The Female Patient, 15,</u> 41-47.

52. Chez, B. F., Skurnick, J. H., Chez, R. A., Verklan, M. T., Biggs, S., & Hage, M. L. (May/June 1990). Interpretations of nonstress tests by obstetric nurses. <u>JOGNN, 19</u>(3), 227-232.

53. Flynn, A. M., Kelly, J., Matthews, K., O'Conor, M., & Viegas, O. (June 1982). Predictive value of, and observer variability in, several ways of reporting antepartum cardiotocographs. <u>British Journal of Obstetrics and Gynecology, 89,</u> 434-440.

54. Steer, P. J. (February 1987). Fetal monitoring - present and future. <u>European Journal of Obstetrics and Gynecology, 24</u>(2), 112-117.

55. Scheerer, L. J., Campion, S., & Katz, M. (July 1990). Ambulatory tocodynamometry data interpretation: Evaluating variability and reliability. Obstetrics & Gynecology, 76(Suppl. 1), 67s-70s.

56. Lotgering, F. K., Wallenburg, H. C. S., & Schouten, H. J. A. (November 15, 1982). Interobserver and intraobserver variation in the assessment of antepartum and cardiotocograms. American Journal of Obstetrics and Gynecology, 144(6), 701-705.

57. Borgatta, L., Shrout, P. E., & Divon, M. Y. (September 1988). Reliability and reproducibility of nonstress test readings. American Journal of Obstetrics and Gynecology, 159(3), 554-558.

58. Nielsen, P. V., Stigsby, B., Nickelsen, C., & Nim, J. (1987). Intra- and inter-observer variability in the assessment of intrapartum cardiotocograms. Acta Obstetricia et Gynecologica Scandinavica, 66(5), 421-424.

59. Trimbos, J. B., & Keirse, M. J. N. C. (December 1978). Observed variability in assessment of antepartum cardiotocograms. British Journal of Obstetrics and Gynaecology, 85, 900-906.

60. Beaulieu, M.-D., Fabia, J., Leduc, B., Brisson, J., Bastide, A., Blouin, D. (August 1, 1982). The reproducibility of intrapartum cardiotocogram assessments. Canadian Medical Association Journal, 127(3), 214-216.

61. Murray, M. L. (1992). A comparison of fetal monitoring concept learning from a learner-controlled vs. teacher-controlled instructional strategy. (Doctoral Dissertation). Albuquerque, NM: University of New Mexico.

62. Murray, M. L., & Higgins, P. G. (February 1996). Computer versus lecture. Strategies for teaching fetal monitoring. Journal of Perinatology, 16(1), 15-19.

63. Lidegaard, O., Bottcher, L. M., & Weber, T. (January 1992). Description, evaluation and clinical decision making according to various fetal heart rate patterns. Inter-observer and regional variability. Acta Obstetricia et Gynecologica Scandinavica, 71(1), 48-53.

64. Bernardes, J., Moura, C., Marques de Sa, J. P., & Leite, L. P. (1991). The porto system for automated cardiotocographic signal analysis. Journal of Perinatal Medicine, 19(1-2), 61-65.

65. Bernardes, J., & Pereira, A. C. (April 1994). Automated methods of analyzing fetal heart rate tests: Already a good alternative to visual analysis? [Letters]. American Journal of Obstetrics and Gynecology, 170(4), 1207-1208.

66. Pello, L. C., Rosevear, S. K., Dawes, G. S., Moulden, M., & Redman, C. W. G. (October 1991). Computerized fetal heart rate analysis in labor. Obstetrics & Gynecology, 78(4), 602-610.

67. Organ, L. W., Hawrylyshyn, P. A., Goodwin, J. W., Milligan, J. E., & Bernstein, A. (January 1, 1978). Quantitative indices of short- and long-term heart rate variability. American Journal of Obstetrics and Gynecology, 130(1), 20-27.

68. Visser, G. H. A., Dawes, G. S., & Redman, C. W. G. (August 1981). Numerical analysis of the normal human antenatal fetal heart rate. British Journal of Obstetrics and Gynaecology, 88, 792-802.

69. Wade, M. E., Coleman, P. J., & White, S. C. (September 1976). A computerized fetal monitoring system. Obstetrics and Gynecology, 48(3), 287-291.

70. Alonso-Bentanzos, A., Moret-Bonillo, V., & Hernandez-Sande, C. (February 1991). Foetos: An expert system for fetal assessment. IEEE Transactions on Biomedical Engineering, 38(2), 199-211.

71. Dawes, G. S., & Redman, C. W. (December 1992). Automated analysis of the FHR: Evaluation? [Letters]. American Journal of Obstetrics and Gynecology, 167(6), 1912-1914.

72. Mantel, R., van Geijn, H. P., Ververs, A. P., & Copray, F. J. A. (July 1991). Automated analysis of near-term antepartum fetal heart rate in relation to fetal behavioral states: The Sonicaid system 8000. American Journal of Obstetrics and Gynecology, 165(1), 57-65.

73. Cheng, L. C., Gibb, D. M., Ajayi, R. A., & Soothill, P. W. (October 1992). A comparison between computerized (mean range) and clinical visual cardiotocographic assessment. British Journal of Obstetrics and Gynaecology, 99(10), 817-820.

74. Weiner, Z., Farmakides, G., Schulman, H., Kellner, L., & Maulik, D. (January 1994). Numeric analysis of FHR variation in post-term pregnancy. American Journal of Obstetrics and Gynecology, 170(1, Pt. 2), 397. SPO abstracts, #435.

75. Nageotte, M. P., Freeman, R. K., Freeman, A. G., & Dorchester, W. (March 1, 1983). Short-term variability assessment from abdominal electrocardiogram during the antepartum period. American Journal of Obstetrics and Gynecology, 145(5), 566-569.

76. Dawes, G. S., & Redman, C. W. G. (1985). Antenatal heart rate analysis at the bedside using a microprocessor. In W. Kunzel (Ed.), Fetal heart rate monitoring (pp. 63-65). Berlin: Springer-Verlag.

77. Lawson, G. W., Belcher, R., & Dawes, G. S. (1983). A comparison of ultrasound (with autocorrelation) and direct electrocardiogram fetal heart rate detector systems. American Journal of Obstetrics and Gynecology, 147(6), 721-722.

78. Fukushima, T., Flores, C. K. A., Hon, E. H., & Davidson, Jr., E. C. (November 15, 1985). Limitations of autocorrelation in fetal heart rate monitoring. American Journal of Obstetrics and Gynecology, 158(6), 685-692.

79. Dawes, G. S., Moulden, M., & Redman, C. W. G. (May 1990). Criteria for the design of fetal heart rate analysis systems. International Journal of Bio-medical Computing, 25(4), 287-294.

80.   Dawes, G. S., Houghton, C. R. S., & Redman, C. W. G. (April 1982). Baseline in human fetal heart-rate records. British Journal of Obstetrics and Gynaecology, 89, 270-275.

81.   Ribbert, L. S. M., Fidler, V., & Visser, G. H. A. (1991). Computer-assisted analysis of normal second trimester fetal heart rate patterns. Journal of Perinatal Medicine, 19, 53-59.

82.   Dawes, G. S., Houghton, C. R. S., Redman, C. W. G., & Visser, G. H. A. (April 1982). Pattern of the normal human fetal heart rate. British Journal of Obstetrics and Gynaecology, 89, 276-284.

83.   Arduini, D., & Rizzo, G. (May 1990). Quantitative analysis of fetal rate: Its application in antepartum clinical monitoring and behavioral pattern recognition. International Journal of Bio-medical Computing, 25(4), 247-252.

84.   Beksac, M. S., Karakas, U., Yalcin, S., Ozdemir, K., & Sanliturk, E. (1990). Computerized analysis of antepartum fetal heart rate tracings in normal pregnancies (version 88/2.29). European Journal of Obstetrics, Gynecology and Reproductive Biology, 37, 121-132.

85.   Larks, S. D., Webster, A., & Larks, G. G. (May 1, 1967). Quantitative studies in fetal electrocardiography. I. Prenatal prediction of the condition of the infant at birth (Apgar rating). American Journal of Obstetrics and Gynecology, 98(1), 52-55.

86.   Sureau, C. (February 1987). Fetal monitoring present and future - discussion. European Journal of Obstetrics, Gynecology and Reproductive Biology, 24(2), 119- 121.

87.   Abduljabbar, H. S. O., Ibrahim, Y., Elahi, T. F., Tawfiq, A. K., & Khoja, M. (1993). Use of the computer for interpretation of fetal heart tracings. International Journal of Gynecology and Obstetrics, 42, 251-254.

88.   Hiett, A. K., Devoe, L. D., Youssef, A., Gardner, P., & Black, M. (May 1993). A comparison of visual and automated methods of analyzing fetal heart rate tests. American Journal of Obstetrics and Gynecology, 168(5), 1517-1521.

89.   Gagnon, R., Campbell, M. K., & Hunse, C. (March 1993). A comparison between visual and computer analysis of antepartum fetal heart rate tracings. American Journal of Obstetrics and Gynecology, 168(3, Pt. 1), 842-847.

90.   Escarena, L., McKinney, R. D., & Depp, R. (November 1, 1979). Fetal baseline heart rate variability estimation. I. Comparison of clinical and stochastic quantification techniques. American Journal of Obstetrics and Gynecology, 135(5), 615-621.

91.   Steer, P. J. (March 1993). Standards in fetal monitoring-practical requirements for uterine activity measurement and recording. British Journal of Obstetrics and Gynaecology, 100(Suppl. 9), 32-36.

92.   Gibb, D. M. F. (March 1993). Measurement of uterine activity in labour-clinical aspects. British Journal of Obstetrics and Gynaecology, 100(Suppl. 9), 28-31.

93.   Hess, W. L., McCaul, J. F., Perry, K. G., Howard, P. R., & Morison, J. C. (July 1990). Correlation of uterine activity using the term guard monitor versus standard external tocodynamometry compared with the intrauterine pressure catheter. Obstetrics & Gynecology, 76(Suppl. 1), 52s-55s.

94.   Morrison, J. C., Martin, R. W., Johnson, C., & Hess, L. W. (July 1990). Characteristics of uterine activity in gestations less than 20 weeks. Obstetrics and Gynecology, 76(Suppl. 1), 605-625.

95.   Torok, M., Bota, J. L., & Gati, I. (November 1992). Contraction monitoring with a manager calculator. American Journal of Obstetrics and Gynecology, 167(5), 1389-1390.

96.   Goodlin, R. C. (September 15, 1985). Pregnant women with Munchausen syndrome. American Journal of Obstetrics and Gynecology, 153(2), 207-210.

97.   Hutson, J. M., & Petrie, R. H. (March 1986). Possible limitations of fetal monitoring. Clinical Obstetrics and Gynecology, 29(1), 104-113.

98.   Brotanek, V., Hendricks, C. H., & Yoshida, T. (April 15, 1969). Changes in uterine blood flow during uterine contractions. American Journal of Obstetrics and Gynecology, 103(8), 1108-1116.

99.   Goodlin, R. C. (February 1, 1979). History of fetal monitoring. American Journal of Obstetrics and Gynecology, 133(3), 323-352.

100. Tournaire, M., Sturbois, G., Zorn, J. R., Breart, G., & Sureau, C. (1980). Fetal monitoring before and during labor. In S. Aladjem, A. K. Brown, & C. Sureau (Eds.), Clinical perinatology. (pp. 331-361.) St. Louis: The C. V. Mosby Co.

101. Solum, T., Ingemarsson, I., Nygren, A. (1980). The accuracy of abdominal ECG for fetal electronic monitoring. Journal of Perinatal Medicine, 8(3), 142-149.

102. Carmichael, L., Campbell, K., & Patrick, J. (March 1, 1984). Fetal breathing, gross fetal body movements, and maternal and fetal heart rates before spontaneous labor at term. American Journal of Obstetrics and Gynecology, 148(5), 675-679.

103. Deans, A. C., & Steer, P. J. (January 1994). The use of fetal electrocardiogram in labour. British Journal of Obstetrics and Gynaecology, 101, 9-17.

104. Angel, E. S., Fox, H. E., & Titlebaum, E. L. (April 1979). Digital filtering and fetal heart rate variability. Computers & Biomedical Research, 12(2), 167- 180.

105. Frank, T. H., Blaumanis, O. R., Gibbs, R. K., & Wells, R. K. (October 1987). Adaptive filtering in ECG monitoring of the fetal heart rate. Journal of Electrocardiology, 20(Suppl.), 108-113.

106. Cicinelli, E., Bortone, A., Carbonara, I., Incampo, G., Bochicchio, M., Ventura, G. (April 1994). Improved equipment for abdominal fetal electrocardiogram recording: Description and clinical evaluation. International Journal of Bio-medical Computing, 35(3), 193-205.

107. Carter, M. C., Gunn, P., & Beard, R. W. (May 1980). Fetal heart rate monitoring using the abdominal fetal electrocardiogram. British Journal of Obstetrics and Gynaecology, 87, 396-401.

108. Lowensohn, R. I. (September/October 1976). Instrumentation for fetal heart rate monitoring. JOGNN,(Suppl.), 7s-10s.

109. Abboud, S., & Sadeh, D. (March 1990). Power spectrum analysis of fetal heart rate variability using the abdominal maternal electrocardiogram. Journal of Biomedical Engineering, 12(2), 161-164.

110. Cerutti, S., Baselli, G., Civardi, S., Ferrazzi, E., & Marconi, A. M. (1986). Variability analysis of fetal heart rate signals as obtained from abdominal electrocardiographic recordings. Journal of Perinatal Medicine, 14(6), 445-452.

111. Kariniemi, V., Hukkinen, K., Katila, T., Laine, H. (1979). Quantification of fetal heart rate variability by abdominal electrocardiography. Journal of Perinatal Medicine, 7(1).

112. Ammala, P., & Kariniemi, V. (1983). Short term variability of fetal heart rate during insulin-dependent diabetic pregnancies. Journal of Perinatal Medicine, 11(2), 97-102.

113. Kariniemi, V., Siimes, A., & Ammala, P. (1982). Antepartal analysis of fetal heart rate variability by abdominal electrocardiography. Journal of Perinatal Medicine, 10(2), 114-118.

114. Murphy, K. W., Russell, V., Johnson, P., & Valente, J. (January 1992). Clinical assessment of fetal electrocardiogram monitoring in labour. British Journal of Obstetrics and Gynecology, 99(1), 32-37.

115. Maclachlan, N. A., Spencer, J. A. D., Harding, K., & Arulkumaran, S. (1992). Fetal acidemia, the cardiotocogram and the T/QRS ratio of the fetal ECG in labour. British Journal of Obstetrics and Gynaecology, 99, 26-31.

116. Newbold, S., Wheeler, T., & Clewlow, F. (February 1991). Comparison of the T/QRS ratio of the fetal heart rate during labour and the relation of these variables to condition at delivery. British Journal of Obstetrics and Gynaecology, 98, 173-178.

117. Lewis, C., & Mocarski, V. (January/February 1987). Obstetric ultrasound: Application in a clinic setting. JOGNN, 16(1), 56-60.

118. Oakley, A. (March 1986). The history of ultrasonography in obstetrics. Birth, 13(1), 8-13.

119. Maulik, D. (December 1989). Biologic effects of ultrasound. Clinical Obstetrics and Gynecology, 32(4), 645-659.

120. Keirse, M. J., Trimbos, J. B., Mallens, T. E., & van der Heemst, M. (April 1981). Reliability of ultrasound as compared to direct fetal electrocardiography for antepartum cardiotography. British Journal of Obstetrics and Gynaecology, 88(4), 391-394.

121. Lauersen, N. H., Hochberg, H. M., George, M. E. D., Tegge, C. S., & Meighan, J. J. (February 1978). Technical aspects of ranged directional doppler: A new doppler method of fetal heart rate monitoring. Journal of Reproductive Medicine, 20(2), 77-83.

122. Wagner, P. C., Cabaniss, M. L., & Johnson, Jr., T. R. B. (1986). What's really new in EFM equipment [Special Issue]. Contemporary OB/GYN, 26, 91-106.

123. Bishop, E. H. (November 15, 1966). Obstetric uses of the ultrasonic motion sensor. American Journal of Obstetrics and Gynecology, 96, 863-867.

124. Taylor, K. J. W. (December 1990). A prudent approach to ultrasound imaging of the fetus and newborn. Birth, 17(4), 218-223.

125. Mole, R. (March 1986). Possible hazards of imaging and doppler ultrasound in obstetrics. Birth, 13(1), 29-38.

126. Bases, R. (1988). Commentary: The safety of diagnostic ultrasound [Letters]. British Journal of Obstetrics and Gynaecology, 95, 729-732.

127. Barnett, S. B., & Kossoff, G. (November 1983). A review of low intensity bioeffects and their relation to ß-mode ultrasonic imaging. Australasian Radiology, 27(3), 297-302.

128. Lawson, G., Dawes, G. S., & Redman, C. W. G. (August 1, 1982). A comparison of two fetal heart rate ultrasound detector systems. American Journal of Obstetrics and Gynecology, 143(7), 840-842.

129. Maulik, D. (December 1989). Basic principles of doppler ultrasound as applied in obstetrics. Clinical Obstetrics and Gynecology, 32(4), 628-644.

130. Boehm, F. H., Fields, L. M., Hutchison, J. M., Bowen, A. W., & Vaughn, W. K. (July 1986). The indirectly obtained fetal heart rate: Comparison of first- and second generation electronic fetal monitors. American Journal of Obstetrics and Gynecology, 155(1), 10-14.

131. Young, B. K., Weinstein, H. N., Hochberg, H. M., & George, M. E. (April 1978). Observations in perinatal heart rate monitoring. I. A quantitative method of describing baseline variability of the fetal heart rate. Journal of Reproductive Medicine, 20(4), 205-212.

132. Suidan, J. S., Young, B. K., Hochberg, H. M., & George, M. E. D. (July 1985). Observations on perinatal heart rate monitoring. II. Quantitative unreliability of dopper fetal heart rate variability. Journal of Reproductive Medicine, 30(7), 519-522.

133. Post, W. D., & Carson, G. D. (September 1, 1984). Masking of fetal supraventricular tachycardia by electronic monitoring artifact. Canadian Medical Association Journal, 131(5), 462-464.

134. Patrick, J., Campbell, K., Carmichael, L., Natale, R., & Richardson, B. (February 15, 1982). Patterns of gross fetal body movements over 24-hour observation intervals during the last 10 weeks of pregnancy. American Journal of Obstetrics and Gynecology, 142(4), 363-371.

135. Lowery, C. L., Russell, Jr., W. A., Wilson, J. D., Walls, R. C., & Murphy, P. (June 1995). Time-quantified fetal movement detection with two-transducer data fusion. American Journal of Obstetrics and Gynecology, 172(6), 1756-1764.

136. Schwobel, E., Fallenstein, F., Huch, R., Huch, A., & Rooth, G. (1987). Combined electronic fetal heart rate and fetal movement monitor-a preliminary report. Journal of Perinatal Medicine, 15, 179-184.

137. Stanco, L. M., Rabello, Y., Medearis, A. L., & Paul, R. H. (December 1993). Does doppler-detected fetal movement decrease the incidence of nonreactive nonstress tests? Obstetrics & Gynecology, 82(6), 999-1003.

138. Connors, G., Natale, R., & Nasello-Paterson, C. (February 1988). Maternally perceived fetal activity from twenty-four weeks' gestation to term in normal and at risk pregnancies. American Journal of Obstetrics and Gynecology, 158(2), 294-299.

139. Baskett, T. F., & Liston, R. M. (September 1989). Fetal movement monitoring: Clinical application. Clinics inPerinatology, 16(3), 613-625.

140. Weeks, J., Perlow, J., Asrat, T., & Towers, C. (January 1994). The significance of unsolicited patient complaints of decreased fetal movement. American Journal of Obstetrics and Gynecology, 170(1, Pt. 2), 319. SPO abstracts #151.

141. Hedriana, H. L., & Moore, T. R. (January 1994). Factors influencing maternal perception of fetal movement in the count-to-ten system. American Journal of Obstetrics and Gynecology, 170(1, Pt. 2), 319. SPO abstracts #153.

142. Johnson, T. R. B., Jordan, E. T., & Paine, L. L. (July 1990). Doppler recordings of fetal movement: II. Comparison with maternal perception. Obstetrics & Gynecology, 76(1), 42-43.

143. Devoe, L., Boehm, F., Paul, R., Frigoletto, F., Penso, C., Goldenberg, R. (February 1994). Clinical experience with the Hewlett-Packard M-1350A fetal monitor: Correlation of doppler-detected fetal body movements with fetal heart rate parameters and perinatal outcomes. American Journal of Obstetrics and Gynecology, 170(2), 650-655.

144. Melendez, T. D., Rayburn, W. F., & Smith C. V. (September 1992). Characterization of fetal body movement recorded by the Hewlett-Packard M-1350-A fetal monitor. American Journal of Obstetrics and Gynecology, 167(3), 700-702.

145. Besinger, R. E., Johnson, T. R. (August 1989). Doppler recording of fetal movement: Clinical correlation with real-time ultrasound. Obstetrics & Gynecology, 74(2), 277-280.

146. van Eyck, J., & Arabin, B. (April 1992). Acotocardiotocographic monitoring of triplets during vaginal delivery. American Journal of Obstetrics and Gynecology, 166(4), 1293-1294.

147. Baser, I., Johnson, T. R. B., & Paine, L. L. (July 1992). Coupling of fetal movement and fetal heart rate accelerations as an indicator of fetal health. Obstetrics & Gynecology, 80(1), 62-66.

148. Eglinton, G. S., Paul, R. H., Broussard, P. M., Wala, C.A., & Platt, L. D. (1984). Antepartum fetal heart rate testing. XI. Stimulation with orange juice. American Journal of Obstetrics and Gynecology, 150(1), 97-99.

149. Manning, F. A., Snijders, R., Harman, C. R., Nicolaides, K., Menticoglou, S., & Morrison, I. (October 1993). Fetal biophysical profile score. VI. Correlation with antepartum umbilical venous fetal pH. American Journal of Obstetrics and Gynecology, 69(4), 755-763.

150. Rayburn, W. F. (December 15, 1982). Clinical implications monitoring fetal activity. American Journal of Obstetrics and Gynecology, 144(8), 967-980.

151. Brace, R. A., Wlodek, M. E., Cook, M. L., & Harding, R. (September 1994). Swallowing of lung fluid and amniotic fluid by the ovine fetus under normoxic and hypoxic conditions. American Journal of Obstetrics and Gynecology, 171(3), 764-770.

152. Yoneyama, Y., Shin, S., Iwasaki, T., Power, G. G., & Araki, T. (September 1994). Relationship plasma adenosine concentration and breathing movements in growth-retarded fetuses. American Journal of Obstetrics and Gynecology, 171(3), 701-706.

153. Egerman, R. S., Bissonnette, J. M., & Hohimer, R. (October 1993). The effects of centrally administered adenosine on fetal heart rate accelerations. American Journal of Obstetrics and Gynecology, 169(4), 866-869.

154. Sadovsky, E., & Yaffe, H. (June 1973). Daily fetal movement recording and fetal prognosis. Obstetrics & Gynecology, 41(6), 845-850.

155. Mathews, D. D. (June 9, 1993). Fetal movements and fetal well being [Letters]. The Lancet, 1, 1315.

156. Goodman, J. D. S., Visser, F. G. A., & Dawes, G. S. (July 1984). Effects of maternal cigarette smoking on fetal trunk movements, fetal breathing movements and the fetal heart rate. British Journal of Obstetrics and Gynaecology, 91(7), 657-661.

157. Viscarello, R. R., Copperman, A. B., & DeGennaro, N. J. (March 1994). Is the risk of perinatal transmission of human immunodeficiency virus increased by the intrapartum use of spiral electrodes or fetal scalp pH sampling? American Journal Obstetrics and Gynecology, 170(3), 740-743.

158. Saade, G., Belfort, M., Vedernikov, Y., Hughes, H., Moise, Jr., K., & Suresh, M. (January 1994). The effect of lipid peroxides on isolated human umbilical arteries. American Journal of Obstetrics and Gynecology, 170(1, Pt. 2), 289, SPO Abstracts.

159. Calvert, J. P., & Newcombe, R. G. (February 16, 1980). Which fetal scalp electrode? [Letters]. The Lancet, 371.

160. Needs, L., Grant, A., Sleep, J., Ayers, S., & Henson, G. (April 1992). A randomized controlled trial to compare three types of fetal scalp electrode. British Journal of Obstetrics and Gynaecology, 99(4), 302-306.

161. Junge, H. D. (1973). A new disposable electrode model for clinical routine FHR monitoring. Journal of Perinatal Medicine, 1, 70-72.

162. Carter, M. C. (March 1993). Present-day performance qualities of cardiotocographs. British Journal of Obstetrics and Gynaecology, 100 (Suppl. 9), 10-14.

163. Ledger, W. J. (April 1978). Complications associated with invasive monitoring. Seminars in Perinatology, 2(2), 187-194.

164. Fernandez, C. M. (1983). Complications of fetal scalp electrodes: A case report. American Journal of Obstetrics and Gynecology, 145(7), 891.

165. Tutera, G., & Newman, R. L. (July 15, 1975). Fetal monitoring: Its effect on the perinatal mortality and cesarean section rates and its complications. American Journal of Obstetrics and Gynecology, 122(6), 750-754.

166. Overturf, G. D., & Balfour, G. (February 1975). Osteomyelitis and sepsis: Severe complications of fetal monitoring. Pediatrics, 55(2), 244-247.

167. Sola, A., Bednarek, F. J., Davidson, R., & Griffin, B. E. (November 1980). Meningitis, ventriculitis, and hydrocephalus: A complication of fetal monitoring. Obstetrics & Gynecology, 56(5), 663-665.

168. Okada, D. M., & Chow, A. W. (April 15, 1977). Neonatal scalp abscess following intrapartum fetal monitoring: Prospective comparison of two spiral electrodes. American Journal of Obstetrics and Gynecology, 127(8), 875-878.

169. Wagener, M. M., Rycheck, R. R., Yee, R. B., McVay, J. F., Buffenmyer, C. L., & Harger, J. H. (July 1984). Septic dermatitis of the neonatal scalp and maternal endomyometritis with intrapartum internal fetal monitoring. Pediatrics, 74(1), 81-85.

170. McGregor, J. A., & McFarren, T. (March 1989). Neonatal cranial osteomyelitis: A complication of fetal monitoring. Obstetrics & Gynecology, 73(3, Pt. 2), 490-492.

171. Mead, P. B. (1982). Maternal and fetal infection related to internal fetal monitoring. Perinatal Press, 127-129.

172. Turbeville, D. F., Heath, Jr., R. E., Bowen, Jr., F. W., & Killam, A. P. (June 15, 1975). Complications of fetal scalp electrodes: A case report. American Journal of Obstetrics and Gynecology, 122(4), 530-531.

173. Fernandez-Rocha, L., & Oullette, R. (August 15, 1976). Fetal bleeding: An unusual complication of fetal monitoring. American Journal of Obstetrics and Gynecology, 125(8), 1153-1155.

174. Hagen, D. (1975). Maternal febrile morbidity associated with fetal monitoring and cesarean section. Obstetrics & Gynecology, 46(3), 260-262.

175. Human immunodeficiency virus infections. (March 1992). Technical bulletin number 165, 1-11. Washington, DC: ACOG.

176. Zelewsky, M. G., & Birchfield, M. (February 1995). Women living with the human immunodeficiency virus: Home care needs. JOGNN, 24(2), 165-172 .

177. Jackson, M. M., & Rymer, T. E. (July/August 1995). Nurses: At special risk [Clinical issues]. JOGNN, 24(6), 533-540.

178. Mayhall, C. G., Simmons, B. P., & Hedrick, E. (July 1982). Guidelines for hand washing: When and how. Conversations in Infection Control, 3(4), 1-12.

179. Rhoton-Vlasak, A., & Duff, P. (February 1993). Glove perforations and blood contact associated with manipulation of the fetal scalp electrode. Obstetrics & Gynecology, 81(2), 224-226.

180. Amstey, M. S. (November 1982). Intrapartum inoculation of herpes simplex virus [Letters]. Obstetrics & Gynecology, 60(5), 669-670.

181. Bawdon, R. E., Gravell, M., Roberts, S., Hamilton, R., Dax, J., & Sever, J. (February 1995). Ex vivo human placental transfer of human immunodeficiency virus- 1 p24 antigen. American Journal of Obstetrics and Gynecology, 172(2, Pt. 1), 530-532.

182. Temmerman, M., Nyong'o, A. O., Bwayo, J., Fransen, K., Coppens, M., & Piot, P. (February 1995). Risk factors for mother-to-child transmission of human immunodeficiency virus-l infection. American Journal of Obstetrics and Gynecology, 172(2, Pt. 1), 700-705.

183. Collins, T. M., Saltzman, R. L., & Jordan, M. C. (1995). Viral infections. In Burrow, G. N., & Ferris, T. F., (Eds.), Medical complications during pregnancy. (4th ed.) (pp. 381-403). Philidelphia W. B. Sanders, Company.

184. Youchah, J., Minkoff, H., Landesman, S., Burns, D. N., Nugent, R., & Goedert, J. J. (January 1994). Longer duration of ruptured membranes in association with increased risk of vertical transmission of HIV infection. American Journal of Obstetrics and Gynecology, 170(1, Pt. 2), 415. SPO abstracts.

185. Zidovudine cuts rate of maternal transmission. (May 1994). American Journal of Nursing, 12.

186. Spence, M. R., & Harwell, T. (January 1995). Invasive fetal monitoring and human immunodeficiency virus transmission [Letters]. American Journal of Obstetrics and Gynecology, 172(1, Pt. 1), 243-244.

187. Chua, S., Kurup, A., Arulkumaran, S., & Ratman, S. S. (August 1990). Augmentation of labor: Does internal tocography result in better obstetric outcome than external tocography? Obstetrics & Gynecology, 76(2), 164-167.

188. Carter, M. C., & Steer, P. J. (March 1993). Working party on cardiotocograph technology - abstract, objectives and propositions. British Journal of Obstetrics and Gynaecology, 100(Suppl. 9), 1-3.

189. Sciscione, A. C., Manley, J. S., Pinizzotto, M. E., & Colmorgen, G. H. C. (January 1993). Placental abruption following placement of disposable intrauterine pressure transducer system. American Journal of Perinatology, 10(1), 21-23.

190. Standards for obstetric-gynecologic services (7th ed.). (1989). Washington, DC: ACOG.

191. Induction and augmentation of labor. (July 1991). Technical bulletin number 157. Washington, DC: ACOG.

192. Steer, P. J., Carter, M. C., Gordon, A. J., & Beard, R. W. (August 1978). The use of catheter-tip pressure transducers for the measurement of intrauterine pressure in labour-a significant advance. British Journal of Obstetrics and Gynaecology, 185(8), 561-566.

193. Strong, T. H., & Paul, R. H. (March 1989). Intrapartum uterine activity: Evaluation of an intrauterine pressure transducer. Obstetrics & Gynecology, 73(3, Pt. 1), 432-434.

194. Mead, P. B., Gallant, J. M., Hayward, R. G., & Hamel A. J. (June 19, 1986) ...And benzyl alcohol. Pediatric Alert, 11(13), 50.

195. Devoe, L. D., Smith, R. P., & Stoker, R. (August 1993). Intrauterine pressure catheter performance in an in vitro uterine model: A simulation of problems for intrapartum monitoring. Obstetrics & Gynecology, 82(2), 285-289.

196. Baker, O. (April 15, 1979). Water-borne contamination of intrauterine pressure transducers. American Journal of Obstetrics and Gynecology, 133, 923-924.

197. Csapo, A. (June 1970). The diagnostic significance of the intrauterine pressure. Obstetrical and Gynecological Survey, 402-435.

198. Stoker, R., & Wallace, D. (October 1, 1992). Intrauterine pressure monitoring, sales and marketing training. Midvale, UT: Utah Medical Products, Inc.

199. Merrill, D., & Weiner, C. (January 1994). Amniotic fluid pressure/volume relationship during human pregnancy. American Journal of Obstetrics and Gynecology, 170(1, Pt. 2), 342. SPO abstracts, #239.

200. Ross, M. G., & Walton, J. (1994). Artifactually elevated basal uterine tonus resulting from measurement of hydrostatic pressure by transducer-tipped intrauterine catheters. Journal of Perinatology, 14(5), 408-410.

201. Alvarez, H., & Caldeyro, R. (July 1950). Contractility of the human uterus recorded by new methods. Surgery, Gynecology, and Obstetrics, 91(1), 1-13.

202. Meizner, I., Levy, A., & Katz, M. (February/March 1993). Assessment of uterine and umbilical artery velocimetry during latent and active phases of normal labor. Israel Journal of Medical Sciences, 29(2-3), 82-85.

203. Shields, L. E., & Brace, R. A. (July 1994). Fetal vascular pressure responses to nonlabor uterine contractions: Dependence on amniotic fluid volume in the ovine fetus. American Journal of Obstetrics and Gynecology, 171(1), 84-89.

204. Flack, N. J., Bower, S., Sepulveda, W., Talbert, O. G., & Fisk, N. M. (January 1994). Changes in uterine artery blood flow in response to correction of amniotic fluid volume. American Journal of Obstetrics and Gynecology, 170(1, Pt. 2), 274. SPO abstracts.

205. Usta, I. M., Mercer, B. M., Aswad, N. K., & Sibai, B. M. (January 1994). The impact of amnioinfusion for meconium-stained amniotic fluid. American Journal of Obstetrics and Gynecology, 170(1, Pt. 2), 391. SPO abstracts.

206. Paul, M. J., & Smeltzer, J. S. (November 1991). Relationship of measured external tocodynamometry with measured internal uterine activity. American Journal of Perinatology, 8(6), 417-420.

207. Devoe, L. D., Gardner, P., Dear, C., & Searle, N. (October 1989). Monitoring intrauterine pressure during active labor. A prospective comparison of two methods. The Journal of Reproductive Medicine, 34(10), 811-814.

208. Odendaal, H. J., Neves Dos Santos, L. M., Henry, M. J., & Crawford, J. W. (March 1976). Experiments in the measurement of intrauterine pressure. British Journal of Obstetrics and Gynaecology, 83, 221-224.

209. Trudinger, B. J., & Pryse-Davies, J. (August 1978). Fetal hazards of the intrauterine pressure catheter: Five case reports. British Journal of Obstetrics and Gynaecology, 85, 567-572.

210. Nuttall, I. D. (August 1978). Perforation of a placental fetal vessel by an intrauterine pressure catheter. British Journal of Obstetrics and Gynaecology, 85, 573-574.

211. Chan, W. H., Paul, R. H., & Toews, J. (January 1973). Intrapartum fetal monitoring. Maternal and fetal morbidity and perinatal mortality. Obstetrics & Gynecology, 41(1), 7-13.

212. Haverkamp, A., Bowes, Jr., W. A. (July 1, 1971). Uterine perforation: A complication of continuous fetal monitoring. American Journal of Obstetrics and Gynecology, 110(5), 667-669.

213. Larsen, J. W., Goldkrand, J. W., Hanson, T. M., & Miller, C. R. (June 1974). Intrauterine infection on an obstetric service. Obstetrics & Gynecology, 43(6), 838-843.

214. Caldeyro-Barcia, R., Sica-Blanco, Y., Poseiro, J. J., Panizza, V. G., Mendez-Bauer, C., Fielitz, C., & Alvarez, H. (March 26, 1957). A quantitative study of the action of synthetic oxytocin on the pregnant human uterus. Journal of Pharmacology Experimental Therapy, 121, 18-31.

215. Jacobson, J. D., Gregerson, G. N., Dale, P. S., & Valenzuela, G. J. (November 1990). Real-time microcomputer-based analysis of spontaneous and augmented labor. Obstetrics & Gynecology, 76(5, Pt. 1), 755-758.

216. Drukker-Dauphinee, J. (October 1988). Ask the experts. [Newsletter]. NAACOG Newsletter, 15(10), 6, 8.

217. Reddi, K., Kambaran, S. R., Philpott, R. H., & Norman, R. J. (August 1988). Intrauterine pressure studies in multigravid patients in spontaneous labour: Effect of oxytocin augmentation in delayed first stage. <u>British Journal of Obstetrics and Gynaecology, 95,</u> 771-777.

218. Hourvitz, A., Seidman, D. S., Alcalay, M., Korach, J., Lusky, A., & Barkai, G. (January 1994). A prospective study of high- versus low-dose oxytocin for induction of labor. <u>American Journal of Obstetrics and Gynecology, 170</u>(1, Pt. 2), 285.

219. Arulkumaran, S., Ingemarsson, I., & Ratnam, S. S. (March 1987). Oxytocin titration to achieve preset active contraction area values does not improve the outcome of induced labour. <u>British Journal of Obstetrics and Gynaecology, 94,</u> 242-248.

220. Caldeyro-Barcia, R., & Alvarez, H. (1952). Abnormal uterine action in labor. <u>Journal of Obstetrics and Gynaecology of the British Empire, 59,</u> 646-656.

221. Phillips, G. F., & Calder, A. A. (March 1987). Units for the evaluation of uterine contractility. <u>British Journal of Obstetrics and Gynaecology, 94,</u> 236-241.

222. Steer, P. J., Carter, M. C., & Beard, R. W. (March 1984). Normal levels of active contraction area in spontaneous labour. <u>British Journal of Obstetrics and Gynaecology, 91,</u> 211-219.

223. Seitchik, J. (December 1, 1980). Measure of contraction strength in labor: Area and amplitude. <u>American Journal of Obstetrics and Gynecology, 138</u>(7, Pt. 1), 727-730.

224. Reddi, K., Kambaran, S. R., Philpott, R. H., & Norman, R. J. (August 1988). Intrauterine pressure studies in multigravid patients in spontaneous labour: Effect of oxytocin augmentation in delayed first stage. <u>British Journal of Obstetrics and Gynaecology, 95,</u> 771-777.

225. Miller, F. C., Yeh, S.-Y., Schifrin, B. S., Paul, R. H., & Hon, E. H. (February 15, 1976). Quantitation of uterine activity in 100 primiparous patients. <u>American Journal of Obstetrics and Gynecology, 124</u>(4), 398-405.

226. <u>Standards for the nursing care of women and newborns.</u> (4th ed.). (1991). Washington, DC: NAACOG.

227. Schmidt, J. (1987). Documenting EFM events. <u>Perinatal Press, 10</u>(6), 79-81.

228. Newman, R. B., Campbell, B. A., & Stramm, S. L. (December 1990). Objective tocodynamometry identifies labor onset earlier than subjective maternal perception. <u>Obstetrics & Gynecology, 76</u>(6), 1089-1092.

229. Chez, B. F., & Verklan, M. T. (1987). Documentation and electronic fetal monitoring: How, where, and what? <u>Journal of Perinatal and Neonatal Nursing, 1</u>(1), 22-28.

230. Martin, R. W., Gookin, K. S., Hill, W. C., Fleming, A. D., Knuppel, R. A., & Lake, M. F. (July 1990). Uterine activity compared with symptomatology in the detection of preterm labor. <u>Obstetrics & Gynecology, 76</u>(Suppl. 1), 19s-23s.

231. Garite, T. J., Bentley, D. L., Hamer, C. A., & Porto, M. L. (July 1990). Uterine activity characteristics in multiple gestations. <u>Obstetrics & Gynecology, 76</u>(Suppl. 1), 56s.

232. Romero, R., Sibai, B., Caritis, S., Paul, R., Depp, R., & Rosen, M. (October 1993). Antibiotic treatment of preterm labor with intact membranes: A multicenter, randomized, double-blinded, placebo-controlled trial. <u>American Journal of Obstetrics and Gynecology, 169</u>(4), 764-774.

233. LaCroix, G. E. (May 1, 1968). Monitoring labor by an external tokodynamometer. <u>American Journal of Obstetrics and Gynecology, 101</u>(1), 111-119.

Notes

2

The Baseline, Accelerations, and Decelerations

INTRODUCTION

The fetal heart rate is influenced by factors such as the fetus' gestational age, acid-base status, and medications (1). By evaluating the fetal heart rate (FHR) pattern, the influence of these variables may be evident. FHR patterns can be divided into three parts: the baseline, accelerations, and decelerations. In 1971, there was no *universally accepted* classification scheme for FHR pattern components (2). There continues to be a lack of consensus on labels, definitions, and recognition criteria which hinders communication and meaningful research on the etiology and efficacy of fetal monitoring (3-5). A consensus committee on fetal monitoring, composed of 17 physicians and 1 nurse, met between May 1995 and November 1996 at the National Institute of Child Health and Human Development (NICHD) to develop labels and definitions that could be consistently used in fetal monitoring research (5). Their 1997 publications indicted that the descriptions of concepts were not related to fetal physiology. Due to that limitiation, FHR pattern component labels, definitions, and recognition criteria used in this chapter were derived from a comprehensive review of medical and nursing literature spanning four decades. This chapter includes information on teaching and learning fetal monitoring concepts, *all* FHR pattern components, a discussion of amnioinfusion, FHR patterns of preterm fetuses and twins, and pattern classifications.

FETAL MONITORING CONCEPTS
Pattern Components

FHR pattern components are recognized after visual interpretation of images on moving graph paper. The plotted FHR is divided into the baseline (BL), accelerations (accels), and decelerations (decels). BL characteristics include the BL level, range or bandwidth, stability, and variability. Variability has two components: short-term variability (STV) and long-term variability (LTV). There are two types of accels and five types of decels. Accels may be spontaneous or uniform. Decels may be early, late, variable, prolonged, or spontaneous. Sometimes, the BL, accels, or decels cannot be distinguished due to the presence of artifact or an arrhythmia.

Perception

Decels are more readily seen than variability because the eye focuses on larger objects (6). To improve perception of small changes in the FHR, e.g., STV, a systematic analysis of the tracing is needed. A systematic analysis forces the eye to see all the parts of the tracing. Observed images are filtered by the brain. The filtered image and information associated with it are briefly stored in short-term memory which interacts with long-term memory where it is stored for the future (7).

Perception involves all the senses. It is continuous and is influenced by thoughts and feelings (8). Therefore, perception may be clouded by distracting thoughts or emotions. Decisions related to the tracing, such as the decision to perform a cesarean section, may be influenced by factors unrelated to the actual FHR pattern.

Concepts

A concept is a set of specific objects, symbols, or events which share certain characteristics. Concepts organize experiences (9). They are represented by names, labels, or symbols (10). Concepts are basic to thinking, they are tools of thought. Concepts help organize reality, interpret phenomena, solve problems, and help individuals respond to the physical world (10, 11). They promote effective communication (10). Failure to learn concepts, or disagreement on the presence or absence of that concept, may precede miscommunication or a communication failure.

Concept Labels

Labels and definitions connect concepts together and connect new concepts to the existing knowledge base (7, 12). The knowledge base can be divided into declarative knowledge or "knowing what" and procedural knowledge or "knowing how" to use concepts. Both types of knowledge are needed to recognize FHR pattern components, interpret the tracing, and respond appropriately to meet maternal and fetal needs (7). Declarative knowledge includes concept labels, definitions, and recognition criteria or critical attributes (13). Without declarative knowledge, a FHR pattern and its components will not be identified.

Procedural knowledge includes rules that tie two or more concepts together. For example, a rule of FHR monitoring is, "a hypoxic, but not metabolically acidotic, fetus may have late decelerations, accels, and STV." Once concept labels, definitions, recognition criteria, and rules are learned, images will be consistently recognized and communicated, and actions in response to the FHR pattern should be appropriate and timely.

Overgeneralizations and Undergeneralizations

Overgeneralizations, undergeneralizations, and misconceptions reflect a concept learning failure. Failure to discriminate a concept example from a nonexample reflects an overgeneralization, e.g., when early and variable decels are not distinguished, and are all called variable decels. To enhance discrimination skill and prevent overgeneralizations, recognition criteria should be used to evaluate the tracing.

Recognition criteria for decelerations includes the onset slope and duration, the lag time between the decel nadir and the contraction peak, and the usual shape of decels. To improve concept recognition, visualization and thinking time needs to increase (14). Unfortunately, in some obstetric settings processing time is very short, which increases the chance of recognition errors.

Undergeneralizations occur when a concept exists but is not identified. Either the clinician does not know the concept or recognition criteria are overly simplistic, limited, or erroneous. For example, accels may not be acknowledged if they are only defined as an increase in the FHR of 15 or more beats per minute (bpm) above the BL. Smaller accels will be ignored and undocumented. The failure to recognize small accels may mean there is no evidence of fetal well-being in the record. If the tracing is lost and it is alleged the fetus should have been delivered sooner due to a lack of well-being, the failure to document accels, even small ones, may make it difficult to defend nurses' and physicians' actions.

Recognition Criteria

Critical attributes are defining characteristics or distinctive features of a concept (15). In this chapter, critical attributes are called recognition criteria. Recognition criteria provide a basis for exclusion of concept nonexamples and identification of concept examples (9, 16).

Perception of discrete parts of a field is hindered when images are received in the brain with other information (17). To improve perception, images should be compared with recognition criteria (18). Irrelevant recognition criteria must be known in order to avoid recognition errors (19). For example, an irrelevant recognition criteria of a late decel *when a tocotransducer is used* is the FHR return to BL. When a spiral electrode and an intrauterine pressure catheter (IUPC) are in place, the FHR will return to the BL after the contraction ends. However, *a spiral electrode and IUPC are not needed to identify a late decel*. Instead, this recognition criteria must be considered irrelevant when a "toco" is in place. The "toco" does not accurately record the termination of the contraction. Therefore, relevant recognition criteria of a late decel when a "toco" is used include the:

- slope of descent (which is *always* gradual or slanted)
- duration from the onset of the decel to the nadir (30 or more seconds)
- lag time between the peak of the contraction and the nadir (18 or more seconds) and
- the similarity of shapes between consecutive decels, late decels are usually similar in shape for one to the next.

Principles and Rules: The Relationship Between Concepts

A principle or rule is a relationship between two or more concepts. A rule in fetal monitoring based on physiologic research is, *"variable or late decels often precede the disappearance of accels."* Rules provide guidelines for decisions (9, 11, 20). Rules that involve many steps and a decision tree are called deterministic rules. To acquire rules, learners must first know concept differences. They must also be skilled at identifying concepts in newly encountered FHR patterns (21).

Application of rules is a complex cognitive behavior (15). Novices of fetal monitoring are not prepared to use rules because they are still trying to identify one example of a concept at a time. With increased exposure to FHR patterns and clinical experience, rules can be learned and applied.

Misconceptions

A *misconception* occurs when an example of a concept and its nonexample are rejected or accepted based on irrelevant attributes or a lack of clear labels, definitions, or recognition criteria (22). For example, in 1969, the BL was defined as the FHR "determined *between* contractions or periodic FHR changes" (23-24). For years, nurses and physicians did not consider the FHR above contractions the BL, even though it was neither an accel or a decel. Thinking has now progressed.

The BL can exist anytime, but it does not include accels and decels. Whether or not the uterus is contracting does not determine if the BL exists or not.

Another misconception concerning the BL involves the time required to determine it. In 1977, Low, Pancham, and Worthington wrote that the BL was determined "in the interval between periodic FHR changes...for each 20 minute period" (25). There is no minimum time limit for determining a BL rate. In fact, a flat BL will be obvious in one minute!

Reactivity has been poorly and inconsistently defined in medical literature, promoting the creation of misconceptions. For example, O'Gureck, Roux, and Neuman (26) defined reactivity as a BL that fluctuates five or more bpm. Others thought reactivity was the presence of accels (27). Some thought accels were a function of FHR variability (28). Others said there was no reactivity unless accels peaked 15 bpm above the BL and lasted 15 seconds at their base. Based on these discrepancies, *reactivity should NOT be used in documentation* unless the term is clearly defined on the chart form or in a protocol known to all personnel at that facility. A "reactive" nonstress test (NST) or "reactive" acceleration have been clearly defined in the literature. A reactive accel peaks 15 bpm above the BL and lasts 15 seconds at its base. A reactive NST has two or more reactive accels within 20 minutes of monitoring.

Variability is a BL characteristic, not an accel or decel characteristic. Yet, in 1987, Moczko, Breborowicz, and Slomko suggested LTV included accels and decels (29). In 1990, Tortosa and Acién discussed "variability during decelerations" (30). These were anecdotal comments that were *not* based on research. When variability has been quantified using computer analysis, it has consistently been examined as a BL characteristic.

Names of decels proposed in the literature are confusing. For example, a *late/variable decel* implies the decel is a variable decel. Yet, a late/variable decel is actually a late decel that looks like a variable decel because of it's U or V shape. *Variable decels with a late component* are variable decels with a slow recovery and not late decels (31).

It is now time to standardize labels, definitions, and recognition criteria of fetal monitoring concepts. Unfortunately, unless all clinicians and researchers define concepts and their recognition criteria the same, misconceptions will continue to be perpetuated. *The perpetuation of imprecise terms delays concept acquisition and recognition, and may have serious maternal or fetal implications.*

Newly-invented words muddy the waters of fetal monitoring. They perpetuate misconceptions. For example, in an article written in 1990, several new terms were used which should *not* be adopted. The authors referred to variable decels as "Dip III or umbilical variable dips," "shoulders" (the common language) were "transitory ascents," and overshoots were considered accels (30). These terms and their definitions do not reflect existing terms and definitions. The creation of new terms prolongs the time until there will be universal acceptance of a common fetal monitoring language.

TEACHING AND LEARNING CONCEPTS
The FHR pattern will be an undifferentiated stimulus until concepts are learned (9, 11, 32). Teaching facilitates learning (33).

Instructor Responsibilities and Accountability
Instructors of fetal monitoring should have a comprehensive knowledge base which includes, but is not limited to:
- fetal monitoring equipment
- all the FHR pattern concepts
- fetal and maternal physiology
- appropriate actions in response to FHR and uterine activity patterns.

They need to have multiple examples of each concept they teach either on slides, overhead transparencies, or course handout materials. They should be prepared to present at least four examples of each concept.

Instructors of fetal monitoring are liable for the information they teach. They may convey their misconceptions to their pupils. These misconceptions will cause cognitive dissonance and learner frustration at a future learning experience with a more knowledgeable instructor. Therefore, it behooves all instructors of fetal monitoring to be experienced and well-versed in all aspects of fetal monitoring. Otherwise, it might be said, "the learner didn't learn because the teacher didn't teach" or "the learner learned it wrong because the teacher taught it wrong."

Learner Responsibilities and Characteristics
The learner has a responsibility to actively participate in the learning process. Fetal monitoring concept learning requires a mature mind, prototype formation, and discrimination skill (13). Gender is *not* related to concept attainment (13, 34). Since nurses and physicians are mature, a failure to learn concepts is often due to the teacher's failure to teach recognition criteria and rules or the learner's failure to learn (35).

An example of an important decel recognition rule is *"shape outweighs timing."* Both late and variable decels may have late timing, i.e., their nadir is past the contraction peak. However, variable decels often have a *jagged descent* and *usually* reach their nadir in *less than* 30 seconds. Late decels reach their nadir in 30 or more seconds. Variable decels *usually vary in shape* from one to the next. Late decels are *often similar in shape* from one to the next. Once the slope of onset, the jaggedness of the descent, and the overall shape of the decels are identified and compared, the lag time between the nadir and contraction peak becomes an irrelevant attribute.

Instructional Design
Fetal monitoring concept acquisition is promoted by instruction based on information processing theory not behavioristic theory. The information provided in this chapter on teaching and learning concepts is based on information processing theory. By designing instruction for concept acquisition, learners will form prototypes and develop a cognitive

structure consistent with the desired, learned performance (20, 36).

Prototype formation. A prototype is a mental image. For proper prototype development, the learner must first be exposed to the best example of the concept. Then, other examples may be presented. When prototypes are complete, there will be fewer recognition errors (12).

At least four examples of each concept should be presented for adequate prototype formation. Some learners will require fewer examples and others will require more to form a prototype (37). As the number of attributes on the display increases, the accuracy for recognizing any one particular attribute decreases (38). Therefore, learners should be given cues to help them attend to parts of the tracing. A laser pointer is helpful in focusing attention on parts of images projected on a screen.

Conceptual knowledge development. Once the initial prototype is formed, conceptual knowledge can be expanded by exposure to more *examples and nonexamples* of each concept. The instructor should describe and identify all the recognition criteria of each concept example (39). As more examples are presented, dimensions of new examples will be stored in memory, changing the prototype into a more abstract and comprehensive image. Expansion of the conceptual knowledge base depends on the number, sequence, and timing of exposure to examples. Reinforcement given to the learner's responses, and learner attention to relevant stimuli, impact prototype formation and concept acquisition (32).

Concept learning requires development of the ability to generalize and discriminate, which are classification skills. Classification skill requires storage of abstract prototypes and practice evaluating similar and different examples (35). If *prerequisite concepts* are not learned, or there are a *large number of relevant attributes* of the concept stored in memory, or there is a *high information load*, concept attainment will be delayed and difficult (32). An example of prerequisite knowledge is the paper scale and monitor features. Recognition of FHR pattern components is usually taught prior to physiology of each concept, as physiology may present a high information load.

Procedural knowledge development. Procedural knowledge is an intellectual skill of "knowing how" to use schema to solve problems (7, 12). In fetal monitoring, procedural knowledge exists when there is recognition of pattern components and an appropriate response to the pattern. Instructional design to promote procedural knowledge should include posing questions about new, divergent examples (7). Then, the learner could be asked what they would do in response to the pattern and the fetal or maternal physiology which prompted their choice of actions.

Learning to discriminate. Discrimination is a basic intellectual skill. It is the capability of making different responses to stimuli that differ in one or more physical dimensions (40). Intellectual ability of the learner and teaching methodology will determine how well concepts are learned (17). When concepts are learned, they will be responded to in an appropriate manner (9). For example, a response to late decels may include assessment of maternal blood pressure (BP). BP is not an appropriate assessment when variable decels are identified.

A taxonomy of uterine activity and FHR pattern components identifies the relationships between concepts and aids the discrimination process (see Tables 1 and 2). Discrimination between concepts is also enhanced when the learner is shown *coordinate concepts*, i.e., two examples of one concept are shown simultaneously. The instructor should highlight differences and similarities between coordinate examples (41). Discrimination ability is further enhanced when learners are exposed to *disordinate concepts*, i.e., examples of two different concepts that have similarities, e.g., early and late decels. The similarities and differences should be emphasized.

Evaluation of Learning

Learning is known by its outcome (9). To evaluate fetal monitoring concept learning, nurses and physicians may be shown tracings they have never seen before and asked to identify all the pattern components. Their responses may be verbalized or written. Learning could also be evaluated by comparing an actual tracing with documentation in the medical record. Contemporaneous observation of documentation at the bedside is another way to evaluate learning.

Documentation as a reflection of teaching and learning. It has been recommended that documentation include
- the method of monitoring
- the baseline
- short-term variability
- long-term variability
- accelerations
- decelerations and
- uterine activity (31).

It has also been suggested that documentation should be complete, accurate, objective, and free of bias (42). Documentation may not be complete due to the failure to identify a component of the FHR pattern. The failure to identify and document parts of the FHR pattern might be a result of a teaching failure, a learning failure, a lack of perception, or distractions during assessment of the tracing. In fact, documentation may be incomplete, inaccurate, subjective, and biased, especially when there is a lack of knowledge or lack of consensus on FHR pattern component definitions.

Table 1: Taxonomy of Uterine Activity Concepts

A. **UTERINE ACTIVITY (UA)**
   1. Low amplitude high frequency (LAHF) waves or uterine irritability
   2. Contraction
      a. Frequency
         1. tachysystole (hyperstimulation or hypercontractility)
         2. coupling (doubling, "camel backs,"* "piggy backs"*)
      b. Duration
         1. tetanic contraction
      c. Peak pressure (quality or strength)
      d. Intensity (peak pressure minus resting tone, amplitude, active pressure)
      e. Interval
      f. Resting tone (relaxation)
         1. hypertonus
      g. Other
         1. "picket fence"* or pushing pattern
         2. reversed or uterine reversal pattern
         3. skewed contractions

*Words that appear in quotes have been used in the clinical environment but are not usually used in documentation.

Table 2: Taxonomy of Fetal Heart Rate Pattern Concepts

A. **BASELINE (BL)**
   1. Level
      a. Normal
         1. Term and postterm: between 100 - 160 bpm
         2. Preterm: between 120 - 160 bpm
      b. Tachycardia: > 160 bpm for ≥ 10 minutes
         1. Moderate tachycardia: 161 - 180 bpm
         2. Marked tachycardia: ≥ 181 bpm
      c. Bradycardia
         1. Term and postterm: < 100 bpm for 10 minutes
         2. Preterm: < 120 bpm for ≥ 10 minutes
         3. End-stage bradycardia (second-stage bradycardia)
         4. Agonal Pattern
         5. Terminal bradycardia
   2. Rate
      a. Average level, e.g., 125 bpm
      b. Range, e.g., 120 - 130 bpm
   3. Stability
      a. Rising
      b. Falling
      c. Wandering
   4. Variation
      a. Short-term variation
      b. Long-term variation
   5. Variability
      a. Baseline variability
      b. Short-term variability (STV)
         1. Sawtooth Pattern (respiratory sinus arrhythmia)

    c. Long-term variability (LTV)
       1. cycles (oscillations, sine waves, cyclicity)
       2. amplitude (bandwidth)
       3. Saltatory Pattern
    d. Sinusoidal Pattern
       1. Benign
       2. Pathologic

B. ACCELERATIONS (Accels)
  1. Spontaneous
  2. Uniform (periodic)
  3. Lamba Pattern

C. DECELERATIONS (Decels)
  1. Early
  2. Late
    a. subtle
    b. reflex
    c. hypoxic myocardial failure
    d. late/variable
  3. Variable
    a. mild (< 30 seconds, no lower than 80 bpm)
    b. moderate (30 - 60 seconds, no lower than 70 bpm)
    c. severe (> 60 seconds, 70 bpm)
    d. typical (pure, classic)
       1. "shoulders" (primary and secondary acceleratory phases)
    e. atypical
       1. biphasic (W shape)
       2. slow return to baseline (late component)
       3. baseline returns to a lower level (after deceleration)
       4. overshoots
       5. smooth deceleration
       6. loss of primary shoulder/acceleratory phase
    f. Checkmark Pattern
  4. Prolonged
  5. Spontaneous

D. ARRHYTHMIA PATTERNS (see Chapter 8)

E. ARTIFACT (see Chapter 1)

SYSTEMATIC REVIEW

Human beings are information processors (43). To standardize how FHR patterns are processed, and to improve concept recognition, a systematic approach to FHR pattern review is recommended (3). A complete understanding of FHR and uterine activity concepts is required prior to performing a *complete* systematic review of the tracing. A systematic review includes determination of

1. *Uterine activity*, including uterine:
   - contraction frequency
   - duration
   - peak pressure or strength and
   - resting tone or relaxation
2. The *FHR pattern*, including:
   - baseline level, range, stability, and variability (STV and LTV)
   - accelerations
   - decelerations
   - arrhythmia and
   - artifact.

Once the components of the uterine activity and FHR patterns are identified, the FHR pattern is classified. Pattern classifications reflect where the fetus is believed to be on the acid-base continuum. Pattern classifications used in this text include reassuring, compensatory, nonreassuring, and ominous. Classifications influence the extent and timing of actions. If appropriate actions occur in a timely manner, the number of neonates born with acidemia should decrease (44). For example, if there is a nonreassuring pattern of late decels due to an abruption, and delivery is expedited, the fetus may be successfully resuscitated prior to permanent injury.

Documentation of the systematic review should be followed by documentation of *actions, communications*, including the person(s) notified and the general content of the conversation, and maternal and fetal *responses* to actions.

Identification of the Baseline

A decision rule provides cues to classify parts of the FHR pattern (45). For example, the rules to identify the BL are:

- The BL does not include accels or decels.
- The BL exists between accels and decels.

Identification of Accelerations and Decelerations

An accel is a transient increase in the FHR above the BL. A decel is a transient decrease in the FHR below the BL (46). Accels may be any height and duration as long as they are an obvious "bump" that could stand alone. Spontaneous accels usually peak 10 or more bpm above the middle of the BL and last 10 or more seconds at their base. Spontaneous accels vary in shape from one to the next. Uniform accels last 20 or more seconds, have a gradual onset, and are similar in shape from one to the next.

Decels vary in depth and duration. Early and late decels usually last as long as the contraction lasts. Prolonged decels last 2 to 10 minutes. But variable decels are not identified unless the drop in the FHR is at least 15 bpm and the decel lasts 15 or more seconds. Anything smaller is called a "dip." Spontaneous decels are usually accompanied by a lack of BL variability, decreased to absent fetal movement, and decreased amniotic fluid.

Identification of a Pattern

A pattern is a configuration of elements which are conceptually linked and visually assessed (47-48). Visualized images are compared to abstract images, i.e., prototypes in the mind (45). The FHR pattern is the combination of the BL, accels, and decels. A *pattern of decels* has been arbitrarily defined as the presence of five or more consecutive decels.

THE BASELINE (BL)

Label: baseline
Alternative labels: basal heart rate, baseline level
Definition: The FHR between and/or not including accels or decels (49 - 50).

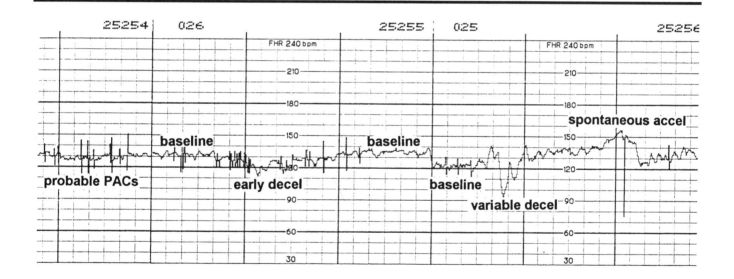

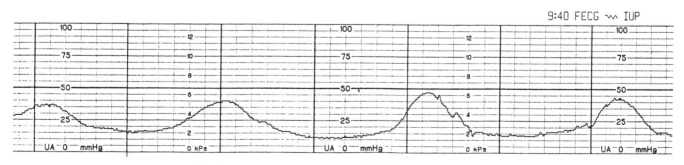

Figure 2.1: The baseline, accelerations, decelerations, arrhythmia, and artifact. The baseline fluctuates between 126 to 134 bpm and 130 to 140 bpm then shifts down to 120 to 128 bpm. The total baseline range (120 to 140) reflects normal modulation of the fetal heart rate. The small upward and downward deflections are most likely created by premature atrial contractions. The downward deflection in the last minute is called a "dropped beat" and usually represents a nonconducted premature atrial contraction or artifact.

Recognition Criteria:
- scan the FHR for a steady, stable area where *most* of the FHR is plotted.
- the BL may be determined in as little as one minute, especially if it is flat.
- the BL is often determined after 10 or more minutes of the tracing have been reviewed.

Cause(s)/Physiology of a Normal Baseline:
- sympathetic and parasympathetic nerve impulses (51).

Cause(s)/Physiology of an Abnormal Baseline:
- "decreased" variability, no accels, and variable or late decels are some of the features of an abnormal BL (27)
- arrhythmia
- abnormal central nervous system (CNS) function
- acid-base imbalance
- medications
- machine artifact.

Discussion

The BL is influenced by neural, humoral, and pharmacologic factors (52). Most term fetuses have a BL level between 110 and 160 bpm. However, many well-oxygenated term and postterm fetuses have a stable BL between 100 and 120 bpm (53). The BL level decreases as the fetal nervous system matures, the parasympathetic system becomes more dominant, and the heart enlarges. Between 11 and 20 weeks of gestation, the average BL was 162 bpm. It was 139 bpm between 31 and 40 weeks (50). Based on an extensive review of the literature, *the normal BL level is between*
100 - 160 bpm for term and postterm fetuses and
120 - 160 bpm for preterm fetuses.

Documentation of the Baseline

The BL may be documented as an average rate, e.g., 125 bpm,

or as a range, e.g., 120 - 130 bpm. If the baseline fluctuates, more than one BL could be recorded, e.g., 120 - 130 bpm, 125 -135 bpm. Or, the entire range of the BL could be documented with LTV, e.g., 120 - 135 bpm with average LTV. Average LTV is a cycle bandwidth of 6 to 10 bpm. If the tracing is lost, and the BL was recorded as one number, without recording LTV, the BL will be recreated from the nurse's notes as a flat line. If a range is recorded, even without LTV, the reader will be able to visualize the actual BL appearance.

Actions in Response to Any Abnormal FHR Pattern

It is a good habit to test the equipment prior to use. A stable, tachycardic rate could be recorded if the test button is stuck in the "in" position. In general, if any FHR pattern suggests an acid-base disturbance, high-risk factors (see list in appendix) and recent drug use should be assessed as possible causes of the pattern. Fetal well-being should be confirmed by assessment of
- fetal movement
- accels
- STV.

If there are no signs of fetal well-being, fetal acid-base status should be confirmed. If the fetus is thought to be hypoxic, actions should be implemented to enhance fetal oxygenation until the fetus is delivered or it is discovered that the abnormal pattern is not related to fetal oxygen deprivation (see Chapter 7 for actions to assess fetal acid-base status and to enhance fetal oxygenation). Health care providers should remain calm and explain their actions to the woman and her family. To gather more data, the spiral electrode and/or IUPC may be inserted. The physician or a skilled nurse may wish to ultrasound the fetus and intrauterine contents. The physician may request or perform an echocardiogram if an arrhythmia is suspected. Determination of maternal vital signs; cervical dilatation and effacement; fetal size,

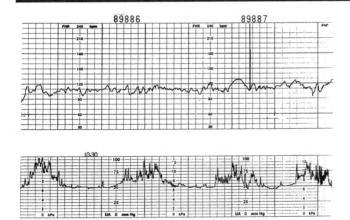

Figure 2.2: Baseline of a term fetus between 100 and 120 bpm. Note the presence of short-term variability, a small variable deceleration and a spontaneous acceleration. The upward deflection after the acceleration is probably artifact. The fetus delivered vaginally with Apgar scores of 8 and 9 at 1 and 5 minutes .

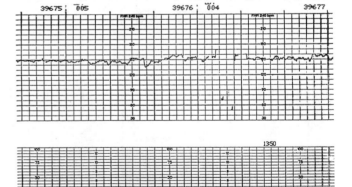

Figure 2.3: Baseline of a preterm fetus at 32 weeks of gestation. Note the stable baseline between 140 to 150 bpm and the acceleration prior to the gap in the tracing.

presentation, station, and position; uterine activity; complaints of pain; and, the color, amount, and odor of amniotic fluid (if membranes are ruptured) provide additional data that might explain the FHR pattern.

Tachycardia
Definitions:
- Tachycardia is a BL greater than 160 bpm for 10 or more minutes (49).
- Some have suggested tachycardia is a rate greater than 150 bpm (54).
- Moderate tachycardia is a BL level between 161 and 180 bpm.
- Marked tachycardia is a BL level of 181 bpm or more. Ten minutes is arbitrary, but is the common time minimum used to avoid labeling a long accel as tachycardia.

Recognition Criteria:
BL	greater than 160 bpm
STV	usually present but diminished due to sympathetic dominance
LTV	may be absent
ACCELS	may be absent
DECELS	may be absent

Classifications:
Tachycardia with spontaneous accels: compensatory or a tachyarrhythmia

Tachycardia with spontaneous accels and early decels: compensatory or a tachyarrhythmia

Tachycardia with variable decels, STV and LTV: compensatory, nonreassuring, or ominous depending on the depth of the decels, i.e., moderate and severe variable decels are associated with lower scalp pH values than mild variable decels (46)

Tachycardia with late decels: nonreassuring

Tachycardia with absent STV and LTV (a flat line): suspect machine artifact or an arrhythmia

Tachycardia (> 180 bpm) with no accels: ominous (55) or a tachyarrhythmia

Tachycardia, absent STV, absent LTV, variable or late decels: ominous.

Cause(s)/Physiology of Tachycardia
- increased sympathetic and/or decreased parasympathetic tone (56)
- sympathetic dominance may produce a sustained accel that is interpreted as tachycardia (57)
- tachyarrhythmia such as reentry supraventricular tachycardia or atrial ectopic tachycardia or junctional ectopic tachycardia (see Chapter 7) (58-59)
- hypoxia and/or acidosis with increased catecholamine levels possibly related to cigarette smoking (50, 60-65)
- amnionitis and/or sepsis (66-67)
- fetal anemia with a chemoreceptor-mediated sympathetic response (66)

- response to maternal catecholamines (anxiety), hyperthyroidism, or fever (66)
- response to drugs such as cocaine, amphetamines, terbutaline (68)
- partial umbilical cord occlusion (69)
- unknown cause (56).

Actions in Response to Tachycardia
In addition to actions in response to any abnormal FHR pattern, the nurse may wish to:

Assess recent drug use
- drugs which stimulate sympathetic nerves or are related to fetal hypoxia (70-71), e.g.,
  - over the counter medications
  - prescription medications
  - cigarettes
  - cocaine
  - amphetamines

Assess the maternal condition
- anxious?
- hyperthyroid?
- temperature and MHR (maternal tachycardia is related to chorioamnionitis and fetal sepsis)
- abdominal tenderness
- vaginal discharge (foul odor?)
- presence or absence of meconium
- white blood cell count

Assess the fetal condition:
- auscultate to confirm the rate if a tachyarrhythmia is suspected
- perform an ultrasound scan to examine fetal cardiac activity and possible hydrops

Act to:
- reduce maternal anxiety
- reduce maternal fever, e.g., provide a cool sponge bath, administer antipyretics
- determine fetal acid-base status
- if hypoxia is suspected: enhance fetal oxygenation, e.g., administer oxygen (O_2) at 8 to 10 liters per minutes by a tight-fitting face mask (72)

Communicate
- maternal assessments
- auscultated FHR
- actions
- FHR pattern and fetal movement
- fetal response to actions

The physician may choose to perform a cesarean section if:
- the fetus is near term with signs of congestive heart failure, e.g., hydrops or
- fetal well-being cannot be confirmed, e.g., the fetus does

not respond to acoustic stimulation or
- the scalp pH is less than 7.20.

Discussion

Tachycardia is a more favorable fetal finding than bradycardia (73). A rare cause of a tachycardic rate is a sustained accel which lasts 55 or more minutes. Accels of this duration occurred in only 1 in 10,000 fetuses (74). If the fetus is mildly tachycardic on admission to labor and delivery (160 to 170 bpm), it may be due to maternal catecholamines which entered fetal circulation. The FHR should steadily drop into the normal range within the first hour after admission as the woman calms down. However, other causes of tachycardia should not be ruled out just because the woman is anxious.

Tachycardia, absent STV, and absent LTV, with or without decels, is related to hypoxia and acidosis (58, 62). Tachycardic preterm fetuses, with absent to minimal LTV, and mild variable decels are likely to be acidotic (75). If the rate is tachycardic with STV and LTV, the fetus may be compensating for a mild hypoxic stress with catecholamine release and a

chemoreceptor/sympathetic nerve response. Therefore, the significance of the tachycardic rate depends on BL variability.

At a rate of 180 bpm, the fetal heart is beating at least 3 times a second. If the FHR is greater than 180 bpm with absent LTV, a tachyarrhythmia should be suspected. The lack of fetal movement suggests the fetus may be hydropic as well. Hydrops should be suspected when the woman complains of decreased fetal movement and/or the fundal height has grown more than 3 cm within a week. An ultrasound scan of the fetus will confirm hydrops. Eventually, myocardial fatigue and decompensation can occur. A BL greater than 180 bpm with absent STV is considered ominous partly because of the increased risk of fetal congestive heart failure, hydrops, and death.

Tachycardia is abnormal. The presence of tachycardia increases the risk of
- chorioamnionitis and sepsis
- meconium aspiration
- asphyxia

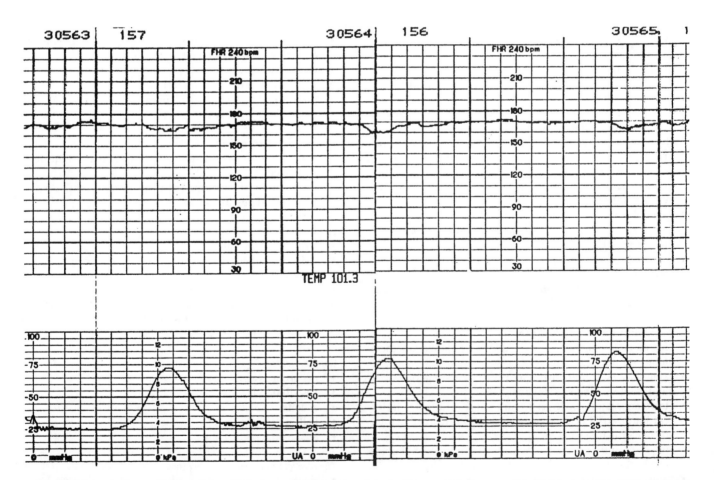

Figure 2.4: Tachycardia and early decelerations of a postdate fetus (41 5/7 weeks) of a 33 year old G_2P_0 woman admitted for induction. At 6 to 7 cm her temperature was 101.3° F and her pulse was 102 bpm. She was delivered by cesarean section 10 hours after rupture of the membranes. Meconium-stained amniotic fluid was noted. Apgar scores were 5 and 9 at 1 and 5 minutes.

- neonatal respiratory distress and
- neonatal pneumonia (50, 58, 76-78).

Chorioamnionitis. Fetal tachycardia may reflect a developing intrauterine infection. The intrauterine temperature is higher than the maternal temperature by 0.2 to 0.8° C. Sometimes, *the fetal temperature and FHR increase before maternal temperature increases* (50, 76). *Therefore,* **an afebrile woman may have chorioamnionitis.** A tachycardic BL with absent STV, has been associated with chorioamnionitis (58). In one study, only 17% of women whose fetus had tachycardia also had chorioamnionitis (77). In another study, 83% of women who were tachycardic had a neonate who was diagnosed with sepsis (78). Sixty-one percent of neonates (11 of 18) diagnosed with sepsis were *not* tachycardic (79). *Therefore, a fetal infection is associated with maternal tachycardia more than fetal tachycardia. Nurses should assess MHR and temperature at least every two hours after rupture of the membranes.* Abnormal vital signs should be reported to the certified nurse midwife and/or physician.

Fetal hypovolemia. Tachycardia may be a fetal compensatory response to a loss of blood with tissue hypoxia. Therefore, if there is a possibility of fetal blood loss, e.g., after maternal trauma, the physician should be notified immediately and actions should be directed at increasing fetal oxygenation.

Tachycardia and decelerations. Tachycardia with early decels was not related to a significant increase in catecholamines (80). However, tachycardia with variable decels was associated with fetal respiratory acidosis (66). Tachycardia and late decels may be a response to a placental abruption (50).

Bradycardia
Definitions:
- a BL less than 100 bpm in the term or postterm fetus (81).
- a BL less than 120 bpm in the preterm fetus.
- The duration that separates a prolonged decel from bradycardia has been arbitrarily determined to be 10 or more minutes. Therefore, a prolonged decel has a duration of 2 to 10 minutes. If the decel persists more than 10 minutes, it is labeled bradycardia.

Recognition Criteria:

BL	less than 100 bpm if term or postterm
	less than 120 bpm if preterm
STV	may be absent
LTV	may be absent
ACCELS	may be absent
DECELS	may be absent

Classifications:
Bradycardia > 90 bpm with or without accels, STV and LTV are present: compensatory

Bradycardia > 90 bpm, early decels, STV, and LTV: compensatory

Bradycardia > 80 bpm, variable decels, STV and LTV during second stage: compensatory

Bradycardia < 80 bpm preceded or followed by variable decels: nonreassuring

Bradycardia < 80 bpm, stable BL with absent STV and LTV: probable heart block

Bradycardia < 80 bpm, unstable BL, absent STV and LTV: ominous

Bradycardia, absent STV, absent LTV, late decels: ominous

Cause(s)/Physiology of Bradycardia in General:
- vagal response due to head compression and/or umbilical cord compression
- neurologic and/or myocardial depression, e.g., following umbilical cord prolapse
- medication side effect, e.g., Nubain® or β-blockers
- arrhythmia, e.g., complete heart block
- cord entanglement during external cephalic version procedure (82)
- central vagal stimulus during forceps application (83)
- fetal
  - hypothermia
  - hypothyroidism (58, 60)
  - panhypopituitarism (84).

The FHR was 90 to 120 bpm with "acceptable" LTV and no decels in a fetus with congenital panhypopituitarism (hypoplastic pituitary, thyroid, and adrenal glands), multiple anomalies of the heart and lungs, anemia, and IUGR (84).
- maternal
  - hypotension
  - hypoglycemia
  - hypothermia
- severe fetal acidosis (85)
- the MHR, not the FHR, is recorded.

Actions in Response to Bradycardia
In addition to actions in response to any abnormal FHR pattern,
Assess recent drug use that may contribute to an abruption or fetal decompensation:
- cocaine
- cigarettes

Assess the maternal condition:
- MHR and BP
  - a 3-lead ECG for the fetal monitor may be applied to compare the MHR with the printout
- labor progress
  - vaginal examination to rule out cord prolapse and identify cervical dilatation, effacement, and fetal presentation, station, and position, e.g., an occiput posterior (OP) position may be related to fetal bradycardia

If there is second-stage bradycardia and a decreasing rate or loss of variability, act to:
- limit maternal bearing-down efforts
- enhance fetal oxygenation, which may include:
  - encourage pushing with every other contraction
  - assist the woman in squatting or other upright position
  - encourage the woman to "moan" the baby out, rather than hold her breath
  - discontinue oxytocics
- the nurse
  - may obtain assistance to set up for delivery
  - may obtain assistance to assist with the vacuum extractor
  - should closely monitor and document the FHR
  - may obtain assistance to prepare for neonatal resuscitation.

If there is an agonal pattern or terminal bradycardia, act to:
- expedite delivery!

Measures to enhance fetal oxygenation will *not* improve the pattern (87).
- anticipate neonatal resuscitation (87)
- if at all possible, a physician who can manage neonatal complications should be present at delivery.

Communicate:
- maternal assessments
- actions
- FHR pattern
- fetal response to actions
- need for assistance, e.g., in calling personnel or setting up for delivery.

Discussion
In the past, all fetuses were grouped together, regardless of gestational age. Bradycardia in some references was defined as a BL less than 120 bpm for 1 to 2 minutes. In other publications, it was a rate less than 110 bpm or 120 bpm for 10 or more minutes. Moderate bradycardia was defined as a BL between 100 to 119 bpm. Marked bradycardia was a rate less than 100 bpm (88).

Term and postterm fetuses. The definition of bradycardia should be based on gestational age norms. It is clear that well-oxygenated term and postterm fetuses may have a BL between 100 and 120 bpm with accels, STV and LTV, especially in an occiput posterior (OP) or occiput transverse (OT) position (50, 58, 60, 89). The FHR decreases as the fetus matures (90). At term, sympathetic and parasympathetic nerves are almost equal in dominance. However, some term and postterm fetuses have a dominant vagus nerve. A rate near 100 bpm is normal because at birth a heart rate of 100 bpm receives 2 out of 2 possible Apgar points. Bradycardia in fetuses 38 or more weeks of gestation is a sustained rate *below* 100 bpm. An arbitrary time of 10 minutes has customarily been used to define "sustained."

Regional anesthesia and hypotension. "Reflex bradycardia" (due to the chemoreceptor-vagal reflex) following spinal or epidural anesthesia may be accompanied by fetal hypertension, hypoxia, or respiratory acidosis (91). If maternal hypotension is corrected and oxygen delivery is increased but the FHR remains bradycardic for 10 or more minutes, the fetus may become hypoxic due to decreased cardiac output and perfusion. Therefore, the physician should be notified of any bradycardic rate and maternal BP and the FHR should be closely monitored (see Chapter 6 for treatment of hypotension related to anesthesia).

End-stage Bradycardia
Alternative labels: second-stage bradycardia

Definition: A sustained BL drop of 15 to 30 bpm during the second-stage of labor.

Recognition Criteria:

BL	fluctuates, but usually > 80 and < 100 bpm
STV	present
LTV	may be marked
ACCELS	rare
DECELS	variable decels may be present prior to or during end-stage bradycardia

Classification of end-stage bradycardia:
Compensatory or nonreassuring

The classification depends on the FHR and the duration of the bradycardia. The presence of STV and accels suggest this is a compensatory vagal response. If the FHR *stays below 80 bpm* and/or there is a loss of variability, the FHR pattern becomes nonreassuring. Actions should be taken to improve fetal oxygenation and deliver the baby as safely and as soon as possible.

Discussion
During the second stage of labor, when the cervix is 10 cm dilated, it is common to see variable decels during bearing-down efforts. "Spikes" below the BL lasting less than 30 seconds often coincide with pushing efforts (92). End-stage bradycardia is common, occurring in as many as 91% of fetuses. *If end-stage bradycardia was preceded by a lack of accels, decreased variability, or late decels, the fetus was hypoxic (93).* If there was thick meconium in the amniotic fluid prior to the second stage of labor, there was an increased risk of decreased variability, late decels, bradycardia, and meconium aspiration syndrome (MAS) (94). Therefore, *it is important to be prepared to intervene to improve fetal oxygenation or expedite delivery if hypoxia exists prior to the second stage of labor.*

Hypoxia, acidosis, and decompensation. Marked LTV is a compensating response to hypoxia. To increase fetal oxygen delivery, woman should be encouraged to stop pushing with a few contractions or every other contraction while the fetal response is assessed (92). Efforts to increase fetal oxygenation, such as placing the woman in a squatting position, should also improve fetal O_2 delivery and expedite descent and birth.

Bradycardia or tachycardia during the second stage of labor were associated with a 20% risk of "acidosis" versus a 4% risk when there was a normal BL (95). Prolonged hypoxia may precede metabolic acidosis, failing circulation, sinus node depression, and terminal bradycardia (54, 56). At that point, measures to enhance fetal oxygenation will probably not help the fetus. The fetus must be delivered and resuscitated or terminal bradycardia will lead to fetal or neonatal death. Terminal bradycardia is classified as ominous (56).

"Terminal bradycardia" has occasionally been confused with "end-stage bradycardia." They are two different concepts at different ends of the acid-base continuum. Terminal bradycardia occurs near the end of life, a terminal event. The FHR is smooth near 60 bpm and falling. End-stage bradycardia, on the other hand, is chaotic and signals impending birth. Since there is torsion on the umbilical cord and compression of the fetal head, the neonate may have respiratory acidosis but not usually metabolic acidosis (96-97). These two concepts illustrate a rule in fetal monitoring, "chaos is good, smooth is bad."

Agonal Pattern
Definition: the FHR of a decompensating fetus with a surge of catecholamines.

BL	less than 100 bpm, often near 60 bpm, with upward and downward swings that last 20 or more seconds, often preceding terminal bradycardia
STV	absent
LTV	absent
ACCELS	absent
DECELS	absent
Classification:	ominous

Cause(s)/Physiology of Agonal Patterns:
- a surge of epinephrine and norepinephrine from the adrenal glands
- during fetal decompensation with complete cardiovascular collapse (87, 98)
- often as a result of cord prolapse (98).

Actions in Response to an Agonal Pattern:
- rule out umbilical cord prolapse (vaginal examination)
- if the umbilical cord is prolapsed, inflate the bladder if there is a delay to deliver (see Chapter 6)
- enhance fetal oxygenation, although these measures may not help the fetus or improve the FHR
- see actions for terminal bradycardia.

Terminal Bradycardia
Definition: the FHR of a decompensating fetus with sinus node depression.

BL	near 60 bpm and falling
STV	absent
LTV	absent
ACCELS	absent
DECELS	absent
Classification:	ominous

Cause(s)/Physiology of Terminal Bradycardia:
- fetal decompensation usually due to metabolic acidosis.

Actions in Response to Terminal Bradycardia:
- mobilize all available personnel
- set up for cesarean section if vaginal delivery is not imminent
- set up for neonatal resuscitation
- call stat:
  - "any available obstetrician" if the attending physician or surgeon is not in the hospital
  - anesthesia provider
  - neonatal resuscitation team, including a physician who can manage neonatal complications
- act to improve fetal oxygenation, although this may not change the FHR pattern
- prepare the woman for delivery, which may include minimal preparations for a cesarean section, e.g., a foley catheter
- ask family members to wait in the waiting room
- if personnel are available, a member of the health care team should stay with the family and explain events
- deliver the fetus as soon as the team is mobilized.

Stability of the Baseline
A well-oxygenated fetus should have STV, LTV, accels, and a BL level that fluctuates within a 25 bpm range (see Figure 2.1). The BL bandwidth should be less than 25 bpm in a well-oxygenated fetus, i.e., LTV will not be marked. Even though the BL shifts downward in Figure 2.1, it remains stable for forty seconds until the variable decel. The downward shift of the BL is probably a response to the vagal stimulus that created the variable decel.

Rising baseline. The BL may flatten and rise over a period of minutes or hours (see Figure 2.32). Accels may disappear. For example, a rising BL may begin in the 120s and be in the 130s within 30 minutes, the 140s in 1 hour, the 150s in another 30 minutes, until it becomes tachycardic. The rising BL is usually a fetal response to *infection* or *hypoxia* and is initially classified as compensatory (50, 99). The pattern becomes nonreassuring with the lack of accels and LTV (see Figure 5.9). A rising baseline is abnormal and the physician should be contacted to evaluate and/or deliver the fetus as soon as possible.

A review of previous NST strips could provide the fetus' normal BL level. To differentiate a rising BL from a prolonged accel, the rule is, "accels are rarely flat at the top." A rising BL is flat or nearly flat when it reaches 160 bpm. Fetuses with a prolonged accel have a fluctuating "top." In addition, fetuses with a rising BL reduce their movement. Fetuses with a long accel should be actively moving. Abdominal palpation may

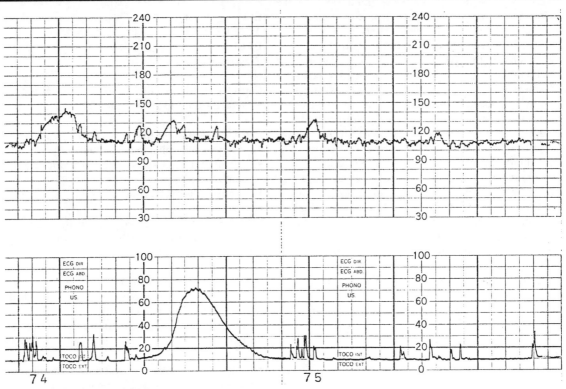

Figure 2.5: Formerly thought of as bradycardia, a baseline level between 100 and 120 bpm with short-term variability present, minimal (3 - 5 bpm) to average (6 - 10 bpm) long-term variability, and spontaneous accelerations in a well-oxygenated *term* fetus.

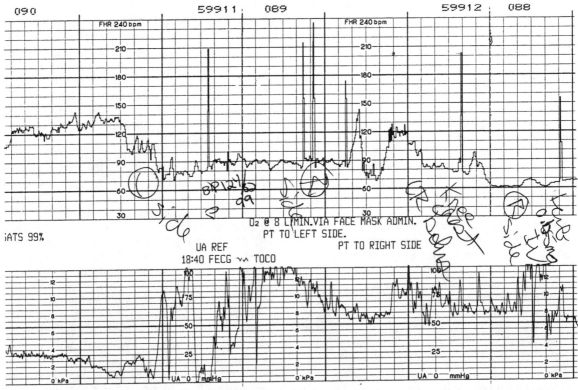

Figure 2.6: End-stage bradycardia at 10 cm dilatation and a +1 station. This 38^1/2 week fetus was delivered by vacuum extraction. Apgar scores were 8 and 9 at 1 and 5 minutes. Note the presence of short-term variability and a variable decel following the initial drop in the rate.

confirm fetal movement or the fetus may need to be scanned by ultrasound. Some fetuses remain in an active state for 20 or more minutes, delaying BL identification.

Falling baseline. The BL level *may abruptly or slowly drop.* This fall in the BL may be due to one of two mechanisms: a direct vagal response, e.g., the fetal head is compressed, or a response to hypoxia. The fetus needs to be immediately evaluated to determine the probable cause of the drop in the BL. A vaginal examination with palpation of the fetal head may suggest a tight fit. Labor progress should be reviewed.

Abruption may cause an *abrupt* drop in the BL. If an abruption is suspected, the physician should be called and measures to improve fetal oxygenation should be implemented.

A falling BL may be classified as compensatory or nonreassuring. If accels, STV, and LTV are present, the pattern is compensatory. If there are no accels and a loss of variability, and/or the BL continues to fall, the pattern is nonreassuring.

Wandering baseline. A smooth, meandering BL with absent STV and LTV is called a wandering BL or an unstable BL. A wandering BL is classified as ominous. For LTV to be present there needs to be at least 1 1/2 cycles per minute. The fetus may have a congenital defect or be metabolically acidotic. Measures to enhance fetal oxygenation should be instituted and delivery should be expedited.

BASELINE VARIABILITY

Short-term variability (STV) and long-term variability (LTV) were first described as separate concepts by Dr. Caldeyro-Barcia in 1966 (91). Visual inspection of the tracing and computer software have been used to quantify these two

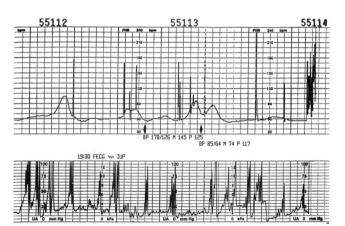

Figure 2.7: Agonal pattern of a 41 week fetus who had a vaginal birth with Apgar scores of 4 and 8 at 1 and 5 minutes. There were two loops of a tight nuchal cord.

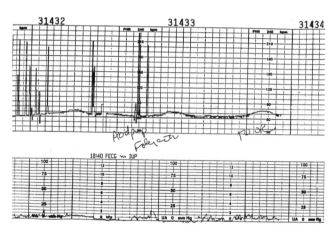

Figure 2.8: Terminal bradycardia of a 40 week fetus of a G_2P_1 with a history of cesarean section for failure to progress and a 9 lb 1 1/2 ounce fetus. The uterus ruptured. Apgar scores after the cesarean section were 2 and 7 at 1 and 5 minutes.

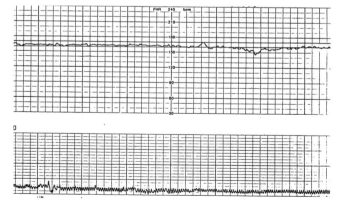

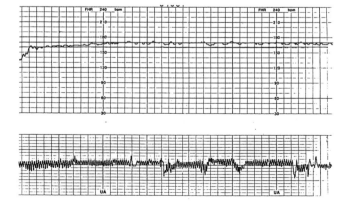

Figure 2.9: Rising baseline of a term fetus whose mother has chronic hypertension. Note the baseline on the left at 1430 is hugging 160 bpm. One hour later (on the right), the baseline is hugging 170 bpm. The ultrasound (biophysical profile) revealed a limp fetus with normal amniotic fluid volume and a score of 2 out of a possible 10. The fetus seized for over one hour after the ultrasound was completed and was stillborn at 1859. Placental cultures were negative, there was inflammation of the umbilical cord (funisitis). Permission for an autopsy was denied.

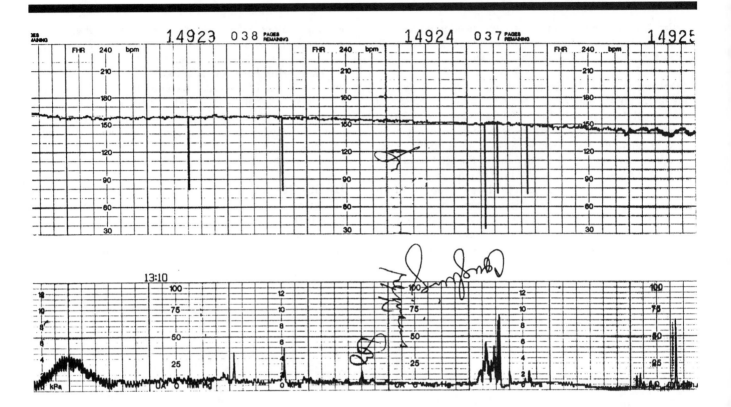

Figure 2.10: Falling baseline. At 40 weeks of gestation, a G_1P_0 woman with an uneventful, uncomplicated pregnancy was admitted after spontaneous rupture of the membranes, a dilatation of 1 to 2 cm, and a negative group B strep test. Induction of labor began at 0720 with insertion of a "mini-prostin" vaginal suppository. Pitocin was started at 1130 at 2 mU/minute to augment labor. This tracing was obtained at 1310, 3 minutes after terbutaline was given for uterine hyperstimulation and late decelerations. The fetus was delivered by cesarean section with Apgar scores of 7, 9, and 10 at 1, 5, and 10 minutes. There was "golden" vernix noted on the fetus, suggesting a release of meconium long before delivery.

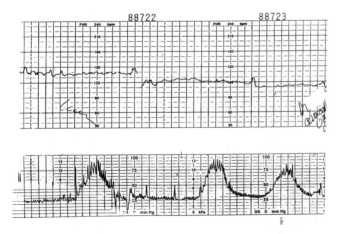

Figure 2.11: Abrupt fall in the baseline from the 130s to less than 120 bpm. The woman was delivered by cesarean section within 20 minutes. There was a complete abruption. The fetus was stillborn.

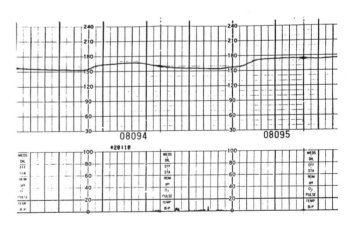

Figure 2.12: Wandering baseline of a fetus who had myasthenia gravis and was born "brain dead." The fetus expired at 7 days of age. See 2.18 for more of this fetus' tracing.

types of BL variability (100). In spite of clear differences between STV and LTV, some clinicians chose to not differentiate the two (101). Instead of documenting STV and LTV as separate concepts, they documented "variability."

Label: variability

Alternative labels: fluctuation, irregularity (50, 102)

Definitions:

- the FHR "around the BL" (103).
- the difference between the fastest and slowest FHR in one minute of the BL (104).

Recognition Criteria:

- variability is *present* when the BL is chaotic, irregular, and fluctuating (105-106)
- variability is *absent* when the BL is regular, nonchaotic, or smooth (105)

Cause(s)/Physiology of Baseline Variability:

- sympathovagal tone (push-pull effect) (46, 101, 107-109)
- rapid changes in the rate are vagal mediated (91)
- slow changes are sympathetic mediated (91)
- influenced by
  - neural impulses to and from the CNS
  - humoral substances such as catecholamines and arginine vasopressin and
  - drugs (106, 110-111)
- changes when a fetus has:
  - fetal breathing movements
  - sucking movements
  - mouthing movements
  - hiccups or a change in the
  - behavioral state (112).

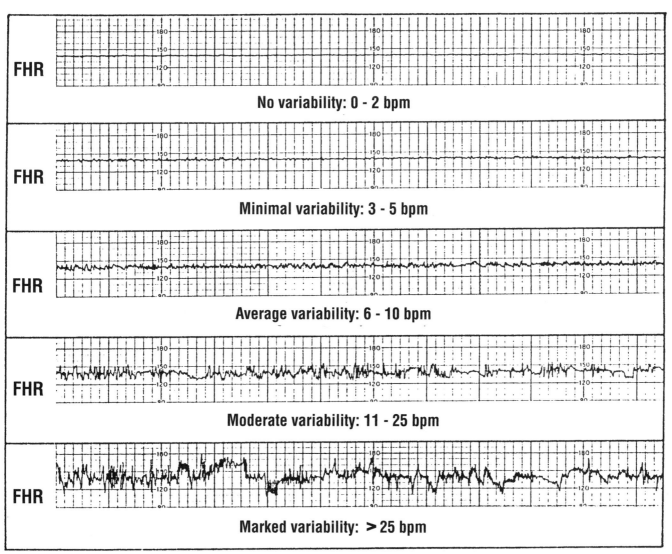

Figure 2.13: Variability, as a general concept, has been documented as absent, minimal, average, moderate, and marked based on the baseline bandwidth or range. The bandwidth is also used to classify long-term variability. (Reproduced with permission of Susan M. Tucker; *Fetal Monitoring and Fetal Assessment in High-Risk Pregnancy*, The C.V. Mosby Company, 1978.)

Discussion
Documentation of Variability

Unless variability as a general concept is defined in nursing protocol or on chart forms, other people reading the nurse's notes may not know if the nurse was referring to STV or LTV. The current practice is to separate the two when performing a systematic review of the tracing.

Words used to categorize variability vary in articles and texts. Three or more categories have been used to clas-sify BL variability as a general concept. *The classification of variability as a general concept is based on the BL bandwidth or range (see Table 3 and Figure 2.13). This is similar to the classification of LTV, which is also classified after determining the BL bandwidth.*

The three category system proposed in Table 3 did not include a category for "increased" or "saltatory" variability, and is therefore a limited system. A four-category system or a five-category system would be more complete. A drawback of a classification system that does not differentiate STV from LTV is that when variability (in general) is absent, it is assumed that both STV and LTV are absent. When variability is minimal to marked, it assumes STV is present. *Therefore, a pathologic sinusoidal pattern could not be classified by this system because pathologic sinusoidal patterns usually lack STV but have minimal to moderate LTV.*

Table 3: Classification of Variability (as a General Concept) (113)

CATEGORY	BL BANDWIDTH
Absent	< 3 bpm
Reduced	3 - 5 bpm
Normal	> 5 bpm

Visualization of variability. Variability, in general, is a "rough," irregular BL rather then a smooth BL (108). Variability is visible equally well on tracings generated by an ultrasound transducer or a spiral electrode (114). *Acute hypoxia increases variability and chronic hypoxia, with the accumulation of adenosine, decreases variability.*

Increased Variability

Catecholamine release, as a response to hypoxia, may increase variability (115-116). Maternal catecholamines may also increase fetal variability. Hypoxia may be the result of maternal hypotension following an epidural and Marcaine® administration. When variability decreases as a result of hypoxia, hyperoxygenation may increase variability. The presence of average to moderate variability implies the fetus is well-oxygenated with a mature nervous system. The fetus who becomes more active after scalp stimulation or electrode placement increases variability.

Term and postterm fetuses will have marked variability. The preterm fetus' nervous system is not mature enough to produce marked variability. This is helpful information if a woman presents with a history of no prenatal care and an unknown due date. The presence of marked variability suggests the fetus is term.

As the fetus matures, rapid eye movement (REM) sleep is accompanied by an increase in LTV and a decrease in STV. During nonREM sleep, LTV decreases and STV increases (117). Variability increases with increased parasympathetic activity. Parasympathetic activity increases as labor progresses and the fetal head descends into the pelvis or when the vacuum extractor is used (118). To summarize, variability may increase as a result of
- hypoxia
- catecholamines
- hyperoxygenation
- fetal stimulation
- normal maturation
- increased parasympathetic activity.

Actions in response to increased variability. No actions are required unless fetal hypoxia is suspected or birth appears imminent.

Decreased Variability

Decreased variability may reflect:
- normal fetal behavior
- a medication effect
- a response to hypoxia.

Atenolol (Tenormin®) decreases variability by suppressing sympathetic nerves, however, STV may increase due to β-blocking properties of this drug, which enhances the vagal influence on the FHR. Maternal medications, especially narcotics, depress the fetal CNS. After determining the probable cause of decreased variability, actions may include measures to increase fetal oxygen delivery. If the spiral electrode is contraindicated or cannot be applied, fetal acid-base status may be assessed by acoustic stimulation or scalp stimulation (see Chapter 7).

Absent Variability

The loss of variability may be caused by neural, humoral, or pharmacological mechanisms. *A flat line may be worse than a BL with decels*, particularly when the lack of variability is related to cerebellar hemorrhage or asphyxia (108). Variability will be absent when the fetus has complete heart block. Chronic hypoxia, with the accumulation of adenosine, may precede absent variability (119).

Actions in response to decreased or absent variability. Decreased variability is a sign of possible fetal jeopardy. However, *"good" variability should not be interpreted as reassuring unless accels are also present within the last 60 to 100 minutes of monitoring* (120). If the fetus is hypoxic, O_2 administration may increase variability (121). When variability is decreased or absent:

Assess recent maternal drug use:
- CNS depressants, e.g.,
  - alcohol
  - cigarettes (nicotine)
  - tranquilizers
  - narcotics
  - heroin or methadone

Assess the maternal condition:
- vital signs, hypotensive?

Assess the fetal condition:
- the time of the *last* accel
- color, amount, and odor of amniotic fluid

Act to:
- rule out metabolic acidosis, e.g., by using scalp stimulation to elicit an accel (122)

Communicate:
- maternal assessments
- actions
- FHR pattern and fetal movement
- fetal response to actions

The physician may choose to deliver the fetus by cesarean section if:
- fetal metabolic acidosis is suspected.

VARIATION VERSUS VARIABILITY

Variation is *not* the same as variability. Variation is only determined by computer software but variability may be determined by visual inspection. Variation is a *measure* of the difference between things. Variability is the quality of being different (123). Both variation and variability have been determined when an ultrasound transducer or spiral electrode were used to assess the FHR.

Variation and variability are characteristics of the BL, not characteristics of accels or decels (124). Variation and variability have been divided into short-term and long-term components. Short-term variation has also been called beat-to-beat variation (125-126). Short-term variability has been called beat-to-beat variability.

Just like variability, variation is nonlinear and chaotic (127). Variation is measured in milliseconds (msec). Variability is measured in bpm. Short-term variation is calculated by averaging the time between fetal heartbeats. The time between heartbeats is called the pulse interval. Pulse intervals over each 1/16th minute epoch (3.75 seconds) are calculated and averaged over a maximum of 64 minutes to determine short-term variation (123, 128). At 37 weeks of gestation, short-term variation was 9.5 ± 2.9 (SD) msec in 4188 tracings analyzed by the Oxford System 8000® software program. SD is the standard deviation. Thus, short-term variation was 6.6 to 12.8 *msec.*

Long-term variation is divided into high heart rate variation (HHRV) and low heart rate variation (LHRV). Both

HHRV and LHRV are calculated by adding the pulse interval *differences* for each minute of a five to six minute period (128). HHRV is usually greater than 32 msec and LHRV is less than 30 msec during the first 25 minutes of monitoring. If after 25 minutes there were no episodes of HHRV, the computer program automatically changed its parameters to greater than 24 msec for recognition of HHRV and less than 22 msec for LHRV.

Abnormal short-term variation and long-term variation. Just as STV is related to LTV, short-term variation is related to long-term variation. Short-term and long-term variation decrease when the fetus is IUGR, although not acidemic. Abnormally low variation may be due to direct myocardial hypoxic depression (129). Short-term variation less than 2.6 msec was associated with a low umbilical artery pH, low base excess, and an increased risk of intrauterine death. Long-term variation was low (19.4 to 21.l8 msec) in IUGR fetuses who had a low PaO_2, hypoglycemia, hyperalaninemia, increased lactic acid, and an increased level of amniotic fluid erythropoietin (129-130). *Short-term variation less than 2 msec was associated with fetal death within 24 hours* (128).

The computer calculations developed to reflect STV and LTV differ from the calculations for short-term variation and long-term variation. In 1973, Dr. Yeh proposed that STV and LTV could be determined by calculating the differential index (DI) (for STV) and the interval index (for LTV) (121). For example, the formula for the DI is $I_i - I_{i+1} \div I_i + I_{i+1}$ where previous intervals between R waves are $I_i - I_{i+1}$, and successive intervals between R waves are $I_i + I_{i+1}$ (131). The majority of current research uses software that calculates variation versus variability.

SHORT-TERM VARIABILITY (STV)

Alternative label: beat-to-beat variability (BTBV)
Definitions:
- BTBV is the fluctuation in pulse intervals measured in *msec* by a computer.
- BTBV determines STV.
- STV is the instantaneous, high-frequency, rhythmic fluctuations of the FHR, exclusive of accels or decels.
- STV is visualized as the *bpm* differences between consecutive FHRs.

Discussion
BTBV was used interchangeably with STV in documentation and research reports, even though they are technically different concepts. BTBV is the difference between time intervals between consecutive heartbeats and is created by rapidly oscillating vagal impulses (132-135). STV is calculated from BTBV and creates the "building blocks" of LTV (136-139). STV is superimposed on LTV (133). STV is strongly associated with LTV, i.e., if STV increases, LTV *usually* increases. If STV decreases, LTV *usually* decreases. STV consists of very *rapid fluctuations* of the FHR, LTV consists of *slow fluctuations or oscillations* of the FHR (140).

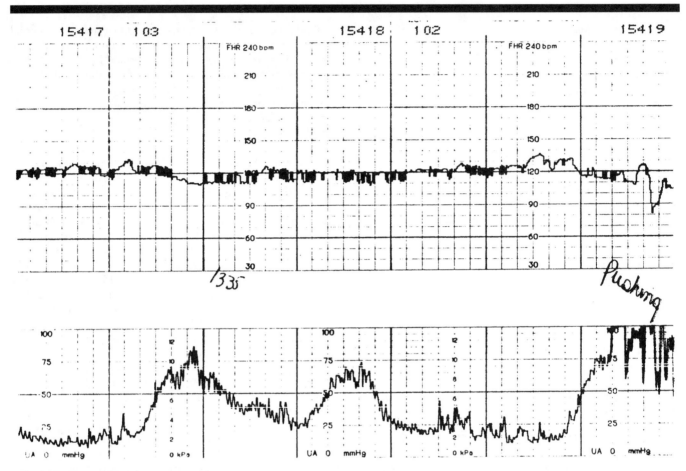

Figure 2.14: Short-term variability is determined from the interval between consecutive heartbeats. The calculated rates are plotted on moving fetal monitor paper. The calculated FHRs vary due to differences in the time between cardiac systoles (R waves or heartbeats). When short-term variability is present, the baseline will appear bumpy, rough, or grass-like. This is an example of STV with a "grass-like" appearance. Using computer analysis, these bpm changes (≥ 9 bpm) were classified as marked short-term variability (114). Short-term variability should be documented as "STV present" or "STV +."

Technically, BTBV cannot be visualized because it is calculated by a computer. The time between successive R waves is calculated. The bpm rate is determined based on the assumption that every heartbeat occurs at that interval for a full minute, e.g., if the R-R interval is $1/2$ second, the bpm rate will be 120 bpm (121).

Recognition Criteria of STV:
Present:
- STV is chaotic and nonlinear (106)
- the BL appears bumpy, rough, or grass-like

Absent:
- the BL appears smooth because pulse intervals are similar (101)

Cause(s)/Physiology of STV:
- *an intact, oxygenated vagus nerve* (141)
- moment-to-moment differences in *parasympathetic* cardiac regulatory activity (142)

- CNS function and cardiovascular reflexes (137, 143)
- fluctuates with fetal respiratory efforts (136)
- is affected by baroreceptors, chemoreceptors, catecholamines, and fetal behavior (132, 137, 144-145)
- STV increases in term and postterm hypoxic fetuses with increased sympathoadrenal activity (146)
- parasympatholytic drugs, e.g., atropine, decrease STV (147)
- hypoxia is related to decreased STV (117)
- therefore, the presence of STV is a sign of fetal well-being (106, 148-151).

Cause(s)/Physiology of Absent STV:
- STV decreases as the BL level increases due to sympathetic nerve dominance or as a result of
- depressed neurocirculatory control of the FHR (134, 152)
- STV decreases with medulla oblongata depression (152)
- the medulla oblongata is depressed
  - when acidosis develops, e.g., in the postterm acidotic fetus (153)

• when a CNS depressant drug, such as diazepam (Valium®) or a narcotic, is in the fetus
• but, magnesium sulfate ($MgSO_4$) may have no effect on STV, may increase it, or decrease it (132, 144-145, 154)
• during fetal quiet sleep (state 1F) or
• following maternal smoking (146, 152, 154-157)
• *severe acidemia* (118, 158)
• anencephaly (117)
• cerebellum and/or the bulbopontine respiratory center injury or hemorrhage (159-160)
• a fetus in a coma or a dying fetus lacks STV (152)
• there is no STV or LTV (the BL is flat) when there is fetal brain death, even with normal blood gases (161)
• infection, trauma, asphyxia, congenital vascular defects, and a blood dyscrasia such as thrombocytopenia have been associated with absent STV
• cocaine and fetal anoxia, often due to an abruption (160)

• STV was abolished by atropine or a vagotomy (in lambs) (117, 152).

Discussion

Abnormal brain anatomy may or may not affect STV. The FHR pattern of an anencephalic fetus depends on which brain tissue is missing. The BLs of 20 anencephalic fetuses were analyzed and found to be between 120 and 150 bpm. *If the medulla oblongata was present, the FHR pattern looked like that of a fetus with normal anatomy.* Decels were U-shaped. The lack of a medulla oblongata caused decels to be mostly V-shaped. The lack of accels was related to a damaged midbrain. In addition, STV was decreased (0.32 to 1.06 bpm versus 0.8 to 1.5 bpm in normal fetuses). LTV was decreased an average of 3.93 bpm in anencephalic fetuses versus normal fetuses (162).

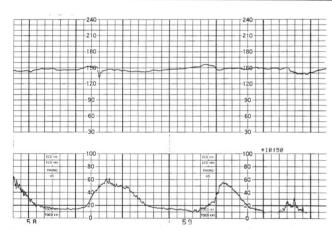

Figure 2.15: Absent short-term variability and absent long-term variability. This fetal heart rate was obtained with a spiral electrode.

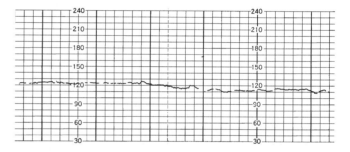

Figure 2.16: Absent short-term variability obtained when an ultrasound transducer was used to assess the fetal heart rate. The rule is, "if it looks bad on external, it's probably worse on internal." It is appropriate to document "0 STV, 0 LTV."

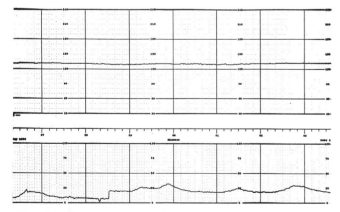

Figure 2.17: Absent short-term variability and long-term variability of a 27 week fetus. The woman is 41 years old, G_3P_2, with chronic hypertension and severe preeclampsia (superimposed preeclampsia) and no perceived fetal movement for 3 days. She admitted taking Valium® during the pregnancy for "stress" and "anxiety attacks." Apgar scores were 2, 6, and 7. The baby died 24 hours after birth.

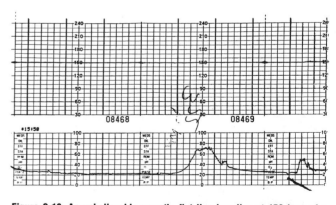

Figure 2.18: An unbelievable smooth, flat line baseline at 150 bpm of a term fetus of a G_2P_1 woman with a history of a neonatal death due to myasthenia gravis. The test button was *not* stuck in the "in" position. Myasthenia gravis is a muscle/nerve disturbance with a defect in the conduction of nerve impulses at the myoneural junction. The fetus was delivered vaginally with Apgar scores of 2 and 3 at 1 and 5 minutes. The "cord" pH was 7.38. The baby was "brain dead." The baby died a week later and was diagnosed at autopsy to have myasthenia gravis.

THE CONCEPT, MEASUREMENT, VISUALIZATION, AND DOCUMENTATION OF SHORT-TERM VARIABILITY

The Concept of Short-Term Variability

Variability is a BL characteristic, not an accel or decel characteristic. The presence of STV in an anatomically normal fetus reflects oxygenation of the brain, autonomic nervous system, and heart (163). There will be rapidly oscillating vagal impulses and a fetus who is *not* metabolically acidotic (106, 134, 141, 150).

If spontaneous accelerations are present, STV is present. Both the vagus and sympathetic nerves innervate the heart and receive their impulses from nerves in the medulla oblongata. Logically, both receive similar quantities of O_2. A "reactive" accel suggests the fetus is not metabolically acidotic. If the sympathetic nerves are not acidotic, the vagus nerve is not acidotic. *Therefore, when there is a chaotic BL, LTV is present, and at least one reactive accel (with a peak 15 bpm above the BL lasting 15 seconds at its base) is seen near the time of assessment of the FHR pattern,* **conceptually** *BTBV and STV are also present. STV may be conceptually present when an ultrasound transducer or a spiral electrode are used to assess the FHR.*

The Measurement of Short-term Variability

STV exists when BTBV exists. To measure BTBV, computer software and a spiral electrode or an abdominal fetal electrocardiogram (aFECG) are required (164). BTBV cannot be *measured* when a fetoscope or ultrasound transducer are used to assess the FHR (165-166). STV is created after consecutive FHRs are determined and printed on moving fetal monitor paper (167). *STV is* measured by *visualizing* the tracing and the digital display on the fetal monitor. If the digital display changes 0 to 1 bpm between consecutive FHRs, STV is absent. In one study, 28.7% of fetuses with STV less than 2.75 bpm had a "low" 1 minute Apgar score versus only 4.3% of fetuses who had STV greater than 2.75 bpm (168).

Table 4: The Normal Range of Short-term Variability

- 1.21 to 6.47 bpm (168)
- 3.50 to 5.71 bpm between contractions (169)
- 4.09 to 6.65 bpm between contractions (148)
- 4.82 to 8.10 bpm during contractions (148)
- 5.33 to 8.39 bpm during contractions (169)
- 3.92 to 8.50 bpm during fetal movement (148)
- 3 to 8 bpm (170)
- 5 to 8 bpm (149)
- 3 to 10 bpm (49, 109).
- less than 15 bpm (151).

In general, STV ranges between 3 to 8 bpm in well-oxygenated fetuses, but may be 2 to 10 bpm. *Researchers classified STV as "excessive" if it exceeded 11 bpm (54).* In one study, 50% of fetuses had consecutive FHRs that varied by only 1 bpm (28). In another study, 85% of fetuses who were 22 to 41 weeks of gestation had consecutive FHR differences of *5 bpm or less* (171). When STV increases, especially during contractions, the mechanism may be catecholamine release due to "mild hypoxia" plus increased vagal tone due to compression of the fetal head (169).

In 1985, Suidan and his colleagues analyzed the FHR using a computer and classified STV using five categories (see Table 5) (114). Young and his colleagues created four classifications of STV. STV was classified when 90% or more of all R-R intervals produced rates listed in Table 6 (151). Unlike Suidan (114), no category was described for STV where the bpm changes were 5 to 8 bpm.

Table 5: Short-term Variability Categories Based on Computer Analysis of Consecutive Heart Beats or Beat-to-Beat Variability (114)

Category for STV	Fluctuation in Beats Per Minute in the Calculated Fetal Heart Rate
Fixed	0 - 1
Minimal	1.1 - 1.5
Moderate	1.6 - 5.5
Increased	5.6 - 8.9
Marked	≥ 9

Table 6: Short-term Variability Categories Based on Computer Analysis of Consecutive Heart Beats or Beat-to-beat Variability (151)

Category for STV	Fluctuation in Beats Per Minute in the Calculated Fetal Heart Rate
Fixed	0 - 1
Minimal	1 - 2
Moderate	3 - 4
Marked	9 - 10

Misconceptions about the bpm range used to classify STV. In at least two publications, it was suggested that *STV, not LTV, should be classified as absent if consecutive FHRs changed 0 to 2 bpm, minimal if changes were 3 to 5 bpm, moderate if changes were 6 to 25 bpm, and marked if changes were greater than 25 bpm* (172-173). *While these STV categories agree with published research reports,* **the bpm ranges correspond with LTV and do not reflect STV research findings.** *STV never exceeds 15 bpm and rarely approaches 10 bpm. Using this system, marked STV will never be seen.* Therefore, nurses are encouraged to change their fetal monitoring course content, medical records forms, and protocol if they used this flawed system to categorize STV.

The Visualization of Short-term Variability
Technically, BTBV is never visualized by looking at a FHR printout, whether or not a spiral electrode or an ultrasound transducer are used. STV, on the other hand, is visualized as bpm differences between consecutive FHRs.

Measurement versus visualization of short-term variability. Kariniemi, Hukkinen, Katila, and Laine (131) compared STV measured when an aFECG was used to assess the FHR with human analysis of STV visualized from a printout generated from a spiral electrode (direct FECG). The relationship between the computer generated analysis and the visual analysis of STV was strong ($r = 0.83 \pm 0.8$). However, most researchers believe the human eye *cannot* discriminate the small bpm fluctuations in consecutive FHRs by examining a FHR tracing (107, 115, 174-175). To improve the assessment of STV, the tracing should be visually inspected and the digital display should be observed for several seconds. Of course, with retrospective tracing review, the digital display cannot be viewed. Then, the assessment of STV is a crude estimate based on visualization of the BL for one or more minutes. When STV is *present*, consecutive FHRs will vary and the BL has a bumpy, rough, or grass-like appearance (176). When STV is *absent*, the BL is smooth most of the time.

The Documentation of Short-term Variability
For more than 25 years, nurses were taught, "Don't chart STV when an external (ultrasound) is used." However, this rule does not differentiate BTBV from STV. Furthermore, this rule does not acknowledge the differences between the concept, measurement, visualization, and documentation of STV. This rule arose because *first generation* fetal monitors exaggerated FHR variability when an ultrasound transducer was used (177). Therefore, *visualization* of STV was totally inaccurate with these early fetal monitors. However, even if STV could not be visually assessed, it could have been *conceptually present and even documented as present.*

STV is present. Since the human eye cannot accurately see small differences in consecutive printed FHRs, it is reasonable and prudent for nurses and physicians to *document STV as present (STV+) or absent (0 STV or STV 0)* after scanning the BL. If a spiral electrode is used, a reactive accel need not be present to document STV as present. The BL just needs to appear bumpy, rough, or grass-like.

However, if an ultrasound transducer is in place, STV is conceptually present only when the BL is stable, chaotic (not flat), and a reactive accel is present. Nurses and physicians may choose to document STV as present when it is *conceptually* present. As long as there is evidence the fetus is not metabolically acidotic, documentation of STV as present is reasonable.

STV is absent. STV is absent when the BL is smooth or nearly smooth with consecutive FHR changes of *0 to 1 bpm*. The FHR BL will be flat or nearly flat, sinusoidal, or wandering. There will be no accels. There may be decels. STV may be documented as absent even when an ultrasound transducer is used to assess the FHR, because, "if it looks bad on external, it's worse on internal."

A two category system makes sense. A two category system for documentation of STV, i.e., it is present or absent, makes sense in that its presence is a sign of fetal well-being whether or not it is minimal or moderate. When only two categories are used to classify STV, nurses and physicians are more likely to agree on the assessment. Using two categories to classify and document STV is not new. In fact, during the last 14 years, several publications have supported a two category system (see Table 7). Other descriptions for STV and/or variability that are not clearly defined in the literature and are not recommended for use are: intermittent STV, decreased STV, diminished STV, reduced variability, and good variability (139, 177, 184).

If clinicians cannot accept a two category system, they should classify the BL according to the findings of researchers such as Suidan, Young, and their colleagues (see Figure 2.14 and Figures 2.19 to 2.21) (114, 151). In addition, they must look at the digital display before and after they inspect the BL since their eyes will not be able to distinguish between fixed and minimal STV. In some hospitals, the protocol requires inspection of the digital display for a minimum of 10 seconds and the lowest and highest FHR must be documented.

Table 7: Categories of Short-term Variability From Medical and Nursing Literature

YEAR	AUTHOR	STV CATEGORIES
1983	Parer (141)	absent or present
1988	Murray (179)	absent or present
1991	Bernardes (182)	absent or present
1993	AWHONN (183)	absent or present
1997	Murray	absent or present

When STV is Present but "Increased"

STV was considered to be "increased" when bpm differences in consecutive calculated rates were 5.6 to 8.9 bpm (114). STV was "excessive" if bpm differences were more than 11 bpm (54). STV will not exceed 15 bpm. If the fluctuation in consecutive FHRs is greater than 15 bpm, suspect an arrhythmia such as premature atrial contractions, and auscultate the FHR with a fetoscope. If there is no arrhythmia, increased or excessive STV suggests *the fetus is hypoxic* with increased vagal tone (61). STV may appear increased when there is a Sawtooth Pattern (185).

Actions in Response to "Increased" STV

Auscultate the FHR with a fetoscope if an arrhythmia is suspected
Apply a second generation fetal monitor
Assess recent drug use:
- regional anesthetics with possible maternal hypotension and fetal hypoxia

Assess the maternal condition:
- vital signs, hypotension?

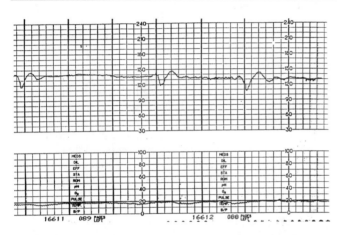

Figure 2.19: Fixed (absent) STV (0 - 1 bpm) of a 34 week fetus of a G_5P_3 woman who presented with abdominal pain and vaginal bleeding. The similar small V-shaped variable decelerations suggest the fetus was seizing or is beginning to seize. There is also a lack of long-term variability and accelerations making this an ominous tracing. An emergency cesarean section was performed. The Apgar scores were 3, 3, and 5 at 1, 5, and 10 minutes. The baby was seizing at birth.

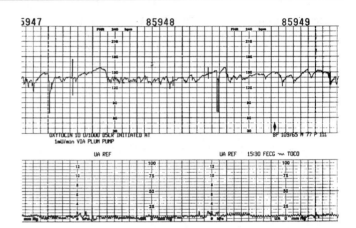

Figure 2.20: Minimal STV (1 - 2 bpm). STV creates the building blocks of LTV. LTV is average to moderate. There are spontaneous accelerations and an occasional dropped beat, which is most likely a baroreceptor/vagal response to an increase in fetal blood pressure during the acceleration. STV decreases when LTV increases during rapid eye movement (REM) fetal states (117). Fetuses have REM when they are active and accelerating in a 2F or 4F state.

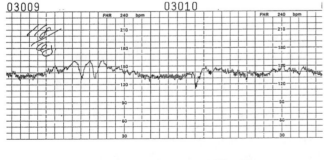

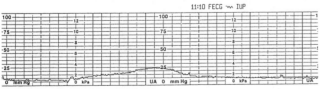

Figure 2.21: Moderate STV (1.6 - 5.5 bpm). The 39 4/7 week fetus of a G_3P_0 woman at 4 cm, 0 station. The fetus had a vaginal birth and Apgar scores of 4 and 8 at 1 and 5 minutes.

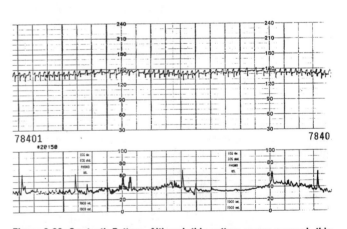

Figure 2.22: Sawtooth Pattern. Although this pattern seems unusual, this is a tracing of a normal fetus with a respiratory sinus arrhythmia. The fetus is 39 weeks. The G_2P_0 woman began prenatal care at 10 weeks of gestation and had an uncomplicated pregnancy. She is a nonsmoker, nondrug user now at 5 cm, -1 station. The vigorous female neonate delivered vaginally with Apgar scores of 8 and 9 at 1 and 5 minutes.

Assess the fetal condition:
- time and type of last accel
- color, amount, and odor of amniotic fluid (if hypoxia is suspected)

Act to:
- no action required unless hypoxia is suspected
- if hypoxia is suspected
  - change the maternal position
  - observe the pattern, if there are additional signs of hypoxia,
  - begin an IV bolus with a dextrose-free solution (unless contraindicated)
- if STV decreases to 2 to 5 bpm and/or accels return, return IV to its normal rate
- the return of STV to a normal range suggests the fetus recovered from hypoxia (144).
- if the pattern worsens, contact the certified nurse midwife and/or physician and

Communicate:
- maternal assessments
- actions
- FHR pattern
- time and type of last accel
- change in STV in response to actions.

Actions in Response to Absent STV and a Stable BL
When more than 10% of the entire tracing appears smooth, the incidence of a poor neonatal outcome increases (50). Therefore, if STV appears absent, when it was previously present, the entire tracing should be reviewed to determine the possible etiology of the change. In addition:
Rule out technical artifact:
- confirm the test button is not stuck in the "in" position

Assess recent drug use:
- CNS depressants

Assess the maternal condition:
- history of a seizure or other event that would deprive the fetus of oxygen
- vital signs (hypertension? preeclampsia?)
- uterine activity and labor progress (which may be important in determining the route and time of delivery)

Assess the fetal condition:
- obtain a fetal movement history
- determine current fetal movement, an ultrasound scan may be helpful

Act to:
- no actions are required if narcotic administration immediately preceded the loss of STV and/or LTV
- no actions are required if the fetus is in a 1F, quiescent state and there was an accel within the last 60 minutes

- stabilize the woman, e.g., if she has a history of eclampsia
- enhance fetal oxygenation if hypoxia, acidosis, or asphyxia are suspected

Communicate:
- *do not call the physician if the loss of variability is due to a narcotic or a fetal quiescent state*
- if concern exists about fetal acid-base balance:
  - describe maternal history, vital signs, and current condition
  - describe FHR pattern, time of last accel, fetal movement history, and fetal response to actions

The physician may choose to deliver the fetus by cesarean section if:
- the ultrasound confirms there is no lethal anomaly such as anencephaly
- there is no ultrasound evidence of fetal brain hemorrhage
- the fetus lacks tone (when examined by ultrasound)
- acid-base studies cannot be done at that facility, e.g., scalp blood pH.

A physician who can manage neonatal complications should be present at the time of delivery.

Actions in Response to Absent STV and an Unstable BL
The absence of STV may represent CNS depression from a lack of O_2, particularly when the smooth BL is not attributed to CNS depressant medication, fetal sleep, an arrhythmia, or a congenital brain or heart defect (91). Fetal death has frequently been preceded by a BL which lacks STV (58, 130). Therefore, actions in response to an unstable smooth BL should be directed at expediting delivery. If delivery is delayed because the operating team is not "in house," apply a spiral electrode if possible to maintain a continuous tracing. Enhance fetal oxygenation and evaluate fetal acid-base status (186-187).

Sawtooth Pattern
Alternative label: respiratory sinus arrhythmia

Definition: a BL with instantaneous, high-frequency, rhythmic FHR fluctuations that increase during inspiratory fetal breathing movements and decrease during expiratory fetal breathing movements.

Recognition Criteria:
- increase in the FHR during inspiratory movements (143, 188-189)
- decrease in the FHR during expiratory movements (143, 188-189)

Cause(s)/Physiology of a Sawtooth Pattern:
- a sign of fetal well-being (143)
- mediated primarily by the vagus nerve (188)
- suggests respiratory center, cardiovascular center, and CNS integrity (188)

- increased vagal tone during fetal breathing, decreased during fetal apnea (136, 190).

Actions in Response to a Sawtooth Pattern
- none, unless there are signs of O_2 deprivation, e.g., a rising BL, a loss of accels, variable or late decels.

LONG-TERM VARIABILITY (LTV)
Label: long-term variability
Definitions:
- irregular, crude sine waves which create a wavy appearance of the BL (134).
- oscillations of the FHR around an average level (133, 192).
- the sum of many small changes in the R-R interval and the calculated FHRs (151).

Recognition Criteria:
- LTV has two dimensions: cycles and amplitude (191-195)

Cause(s)/Physiology of LTV:
- primarily mediated by sympathetic nerves (136, 163)
- fluctuates with fetal BP, affected by baroreceptors and arginine vasopressin (136, 163).

Cycles
Cycles are the *horizontal* dimension of the BL and are counted during each minute of the BL. Although they are counted, the number of cycles is not usually documented. Cycle frequency is determined by counting the "zero-crossings" of the oscillations or cycles through an imaginary line drawn through the middle of the oscillations (3). When LTV is present *it is classified based on the amplitude, not the number, of cycles.* To be present, there must be at least $1^1/_2$ cycles per minute (cpm).

Label: cycles
Alternative labels: oscillations, sine waves, cyclicity, zero-crossings

Recognition Criteria:
- a BL characteristic
- does *NOT* include accels or decels
- consists of crude sine waves (193)
- oxygenated fetuses have 2 to 8 cpm (121)
- hypoxic or severely anemic fetuses may have as few as $1^1/_2$ cpm
- LTV is absent if there are fewer than $1^1/_2$ cpm

Discussion
Evaluation of LTV helps identify changes in the fetal behavioral state and the response to labor (194-195). During the first stage of labor, cpm increase. During the second stage of labor cpm decrease (see Table 8). In 1979, fewer than 3 cpm was considered "low" LTV, 3 to 6 cpm was "moderate" LTV, and more than 6 cpm was "high" LTV (196).

Table 8: Changes in the Cycles Per Minute of Long-term Variability During Labor (195)

Phase/Stage of Labor	Cycles Per Minute
Latent Phase	1 - 6
Active Phase	2 - 7
Second Stage	0 - 4

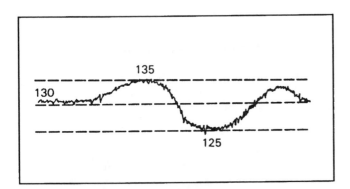

Figure 2.23: Long-term variability includes the oscillatory changes or cycles of the baseline over each minute. There are 1 1/2 cycles in this picture. (Reproduced with permission of Marshall Klavan, MD: *Clinical concepts of fetal heart rate monitoring.* Hewlett-Packard Company, 1977).

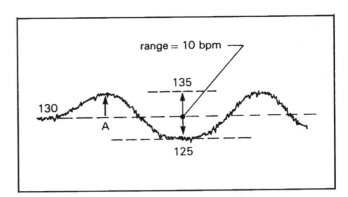

Figure 2.24: Cycle amplitude is calculated from the top to the bottom of *most* of the cycles. By estimating the range of the baseline over the course of each minute, long-term variability may be classified as absent, minimal (decreased), average (normal), moderate, and marked (saltatory). Documentation may include a combination of categories, e.g., "LTV absent to average." Some clinicians use a four category system to classify LTV. (Reproduced with permission of Marshall Klavan, MD: *Clinical concepts of fetal heart rate monitoring.* Hewlett-Packard, 1977).

Amplitude

Amplitude is the *vertical* dimension of the BL and refers to *the bandwidth or range* of **most** of the cycles of the BL. Amplitude of one cycle is measured as the bpm from the top to the bottom of the cycle (191). *If there are at least $1^1/2$ cpm, LTV is classified based on the bpm range or bandwidth (167).* Otherwise, if there are fewer than $1^1/2$ cpm or the BL appears flat and is within a 0 - 2 bpm range, LTV is classified as absent.

Label: amplitude
Alternative label: bandwidth, range

Definitions:
- the bpm between the top and bottom of *most* of the oscillations or cycles of the BL.

Recognition Criteria:
- determine the top of most of the cycles
- determine the bottom of most of the cycles
- calculate the bpm between these two levels, this is the bandwidth

Table 9: Categories of Long-term Variability
Proposed in 1973 by Saling, et al. (197)

CATEGORY	CYCLE BANDWIDTH (bpm)
Minimal	0 - 2
Decreased	3 - 5
Moderate	6 - 10
Increased	11 - 25
Marked	> 25

Table 10: Categories of Long-term Variability
Proposed in 1979 by Krebs, et al. (196)

CATEGORY	CYCLE BANDWIDTH (bpm)
Silent	< 3
Narrowed	3 - 5
Undulating	6 - 25
Saltatory	> 25

Table 11: Categories of Long-term Variability
from 1988 to the Present (27, 179, 183)

CATEGORY	BANDWIDTH (bpm)	ABBREVIATIONS
Absent	0 - 2	LTV 0
Minimal*	3 - 5	LTV min, LTV ↓
Average*	6 - 25	LTV av or LTV mod
Marked*	> 25	LTV marked, LTV ↑

*Minimal LTV has also been called "decreased" LTV. Average LTV may be subdivided into average LTV (6 - 10 bpm) and moderate LTV (11 - 25 bpm). Marked LTV has been called a saltatory pattern or "increased" LTV.

Within a 15 to 30 minute period of observation, LTV might include all of these categories. Yet, the BL may only be documented as an average rate, e.g., 125 bpm. The BL may be documented as several ranges if the BL changes during the assessment period, e.g., BL 120 - 130 bpm, 115 - 155 bpm. In this case, LTV might also be documented as "LTV av to marked." LTV has also been classified with fewer than four categories, e.g., absent, decreased, and normal (99). This three category system does not account for marked LTV. All clinicians working in the same setting need to know the definitions and recognition criteria of LTV, so that documentation is consistent, comprehensive, and understood.

Absent Long-term Variability
Alternative labels: fixed BL, flat BL, silent BL
Recognition Criteria:
- < $1^1/2$ cpm or
- a BL with a bandwidth of 0 to 2 bpm or
- a flat line

Cause(s)/Physiology of Absent LTV:
- machine artifact: test button is stuck in the "in" position
- fetal 1F quiescent state that may last 93 minutes (198-199)
- medications, e.g., CNS depressants
- hypoxia due to placental insufficiency (73)
- severe fetal anemia, e.g., as a result of a fetal viral infection
- arrhythmia such as supraventricular tachycardia or complete heart block
- fetal brain death or decerebration (161, 200)
- congenital brain anomaly, e.g., anencephaly, or heart anomaly or conduction defect (58, 61, 162, 201-202)
- cardiovascular lesions or chromosomal aberration, often accompanied by bradycardia and variable decels (201)
- cerebral ischemia and isoelectric electroencephalogram (200, 203)
- a late sign of deterioration of the IUGR fetus (204)
- fetuses who seized as newborns had absent LTV (205)
- *bradycardia and absent LTV, not related to an arrhythmia, suggests impending intrauterine death, e.g., terminal bradycardia (73).*

Actions in Response to *Absent* LTV
A flat BL during antepartal tests was associated with lower birth weights, prematurity, lower Apgar scores at 5 minutes of age, IUGR, and an increased risk for intrauterine fetal demise (199). Therefore, absent LTV is nonreassuring until the etiology is determined. In addition to actions in response to any abnormal FHR pattern:
Rule out machine artifact:
- is the test button stuck in the "in" position?

Assess recent drug use:
- CNS depressants
- cigarettes (nicotine)
- cocaine (drugs that contribute to fetal anoxia)

Assess the maternal condition:
- vital signs: infection?

Assess the fetal condition:
- fetal movement history, e.g., has the fetus moved in the last 100 minutes?
- history of IUGR
- ultrasound reports: oligohydramnios?
- color, amount, and odor of amniotic fluid: oligohydramnios? infection?

If the fetus is not in a 1F, quiescent state, act to:
- enhance fetal oxygenation
- the pattern will remain unchanged or not improve if the fetus already has CNS damage

Communicate if the fetus is not suspected to be in a 1F, quiescent state:
- maternal assessments and actions
- fetal movement history
- FHR pattern and response to actions

The physician may choose to deliver the fetus by cesarean section if:
- the ultrasound confirms the lack of a lethal anomaly and/or brain hemorrhage.

A physician who can manage neonatal complications should be present at the time of delivery.

Causes(s)/Physiology of *Minimal* LTV (3 - 5 bpm)
Alternative Label: decreased LTV
Minimal LTV may be present when the fetus has:
- a temperature elevation (tachycardia will be present too)
- hypovolemia, hypoxia, or acidosis (tachycardia may be present too)
- a CNS depressant medication "on board"
- moved into a quiescent (1F) state (58)

Cause(s)/Physiology of *Average* LTV (6 - 10 bpm):
- neural integrity

Cause(s)/Physiology of *Moderate* LTV (11 - 25 bpm):
- 4 F fetal behavioral state
- application of the vacuum extractor (may also see marked LTV)
- maternal ephedrine to correct hypotension (may also see marked LTV).
- mild hypoxia increases LTV 9 to 14 bpm (in lambs) (61, 206)

Marked LTV
Alternative Label: Saltatory Pattern
Saltar means "to jump" in Spanish. Therefore, saltatory describes a BL that is highly chaotic and "jumps" up and down multiple times each minute.

Definition: A pattern of excessive LTV with a bandwidth of more than 25 bpm and a frequency of at least 6 cpm.

Recognition Criteria:
- usually very chaotic in appearance
- previously normal BL
- may be preceded by variable decels
- cycle amplitude > 25 bpm for at least 1 minute
- cycle frequency > 6 cpm for at least 1 minute (207)

Cause(s)/Physiology of Marked LTV:
- if noted when an ultrasound transducer is used, may be caused by a fetal dysrhythmia such as premature ventricular contractions
- rare in preterm fetuses (98)
- high incidence in postterm fetuses, possibly due to neurologic maturation (98)
- usually a compensatory response to a hypoxic event, e.g., umbilical cord compression or uterine hyperstimulation (56, 163, 207)
- may follow ephedrine administration (207)
- may be observed during the second stage of labor, especially with use of the vacuum extractor (207).

Actions in Response to Marked LTV
In addition to actions in response to any abnormal FHR pattern:
Assess recent drug use:
- regional anesthetic?

Assess the maternal condition:
- BP, hypotension?
- vaginal examination: impending birth?

Assess the fetal condition:
- auscultate the FHR with a fetoscope, if irregular, apply a spiral electrode
- STV present?
- color, amount, and odor of amniotic fluid, meconium?

Act to:
- increase maternal BP if hypotensive
- enhance fetal oxygenation

Communicate:
- maternal assessments and actions
- request ephedrine administration if it is needed
- FHR pattern and fetal response to actions.

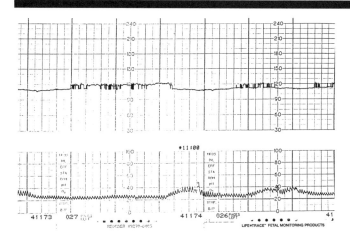

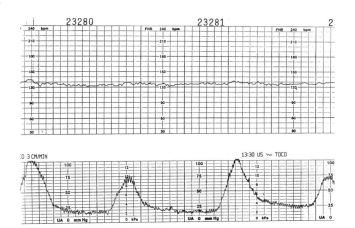

Figure 2.25: Absent LTV (0 - 2 bpm), present STV. Note STV is intermittently present and "marked" (≥ 9 bpm) suggesting an increased vagal response. The fetal monitor was changed and produced a similar printout. The physician was "concerned about cephalopelvic disproportion." Pressure on the fetal head and/or hypoxia may be related to the fetal heart rate pattern. The fetus was delivered by cesarean section with Apgar scores of 8 and 8 at 1 and 5 minutes.

Figure 2.26: Minimal LTV (3 - 5 bpm) in a term fetus of a G_2P_1 low-risk woman who delivered vaginally with Apgar scores of 8 and 9 at 1 and 5 minutes.

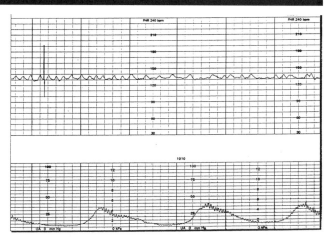

Figure 2.27: Average LTV (6 - 25 bpm in a 4-category system, 6 - 11 bpm in a 5-category system). This fetal heart rate and uterine activity information was stored on an optical disk then retrieved to produce this high-quality printout.

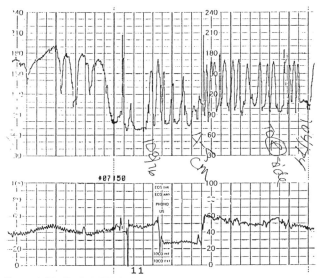

Figure 2.28: Marked LTV (> 25 bpm) and decelerations in a fetus of a multigravida woman at 4 to 5 cm dilatation with a history of a prior cesarean section for cephalopelvic disproportion. Apgar scores at 1 and 5 minutes were 7 and 8. There were two loops of nuchal cord and a "cord pH" of 7.20. The previous baseline was 120 to 130 bpm when the woman presented in labor at 3 cm 5 hours prior to this tracing.

If the FHR pattern returns to "normal" after acting to improve fetal oxygen delivery, no additional measures are required. Expect a good neonatal outcome (207). A very unusual, nonchaotic, nonreassuring pattern of marked LTV appears in Figure 2.29. In this case, the physician's immediate presence at the bedside should be requested. Acid-base evaluation and/or expeditious delivery is recommended.

Documentation of LTV

In the United States, LTV is classified and documented based on the bandwidth of most of the cycles, i.e., the vertical dimension. *LTV* is documented as *absent* if:

* the bandwidth is 0 to 2 bpm or
* there are fewer than $1^1/_2$ cpm and
* the BL is not sinusoidal.

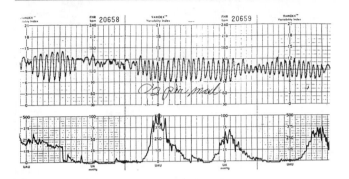

Figure 2.29: When LTV looks bizarre, fetal acid-base status should be evaluated. Although there appeared to be STV at times, the fetus was born with Apgar scores of 0 and 1 at 1 and 5 minutes.

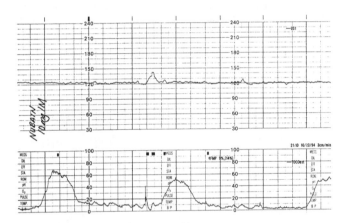

Figure 2.30: Minimal long-term variability (3 - 5 bpm) with spontaneous acceleration. Nubain® 10 mg was given IM at 2104. A benign sinusoidal pattern began 13 minutes later and persisted 2 hours. (See Figure 2.31).

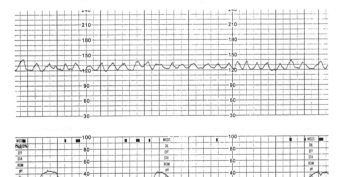

Figure 2.31 The small black rectangles at the top of the uterine activity channel represent fetal movement (Hewlett-Packard® monitor). Fetuses with a benign sinusoidal pattern are usually moving. Fetuses who have a pathologic sinusoidal pattern decrease their movement.

LTV is present if :
- the bandwidth is 3 or more bpm and
- there are at least $1^1/2$ cpm.

When LTV is present, it is best to classify it then document the classification. Classifications categories for LTV have been previously discussed. It is important to classify and document LTV when the average BL rate is documented, e.g., 125 bpm. If the BL range is documented, e.g., 130 - 140 bpm, LTV may not be documented, unless it varies in and around that BL range, e.g., minimal to moderate.

SINUSOIDAL PATTERNS

A cycle of the BL is also called a sine wave. A series of sine waves with a *similar*, but not always identical, duration and amplitude produces a sinusoidal BL or a sinusoidal pattern. There are two types of sinusoidal patterns: benign and pathologic. Benign sinusoidal patterns may have accels and decels. Pathologic sinusoidal patterns never have accels. In other words, "pathological sinusoidal patterns are bad, benign sinusoidal patterns are good."

Benign sinusoidal patterns require no treatment and precede fetal life. The key finding that differentiates the two types of sinusoidal patterns are accels. Accels are present before and after a benign sinusoidal pattern. When accels are present, fetal movement is usually palpable.

Pathologic sinusoidal patterns are associated with fetal anemia, hypoxia, and acidosis (208). Fetuses who have a pathologic sinusoidal pattern are always nonreactive (209). Pathologic sinusoidal patterns that go untreated can precede fetal decompensation and death. The fetus may have diminished movement or no movement, depending on the severity of the anemia and/or acid-base disturbance.

Benign (Physiologic) Sinusoidal Pattern
Alternative label: pseudosinusoidal pattern
Recognition Criteria:

BL	usually a normal level
STV	present
LTV	usually minimal (3 - 5 bpm) to moderate (11 - 25 bpm)
	rarely $1^1/2$ to 2 cpm, usually 4 or more cpm
ACCELS	present before and after sinusoidal BL
DECELS	may be present
DURATION	short-lived: may begin as early as 5 to 10 minutes after narcotic administration and last up to 47 minutes to 4 hours. The longer duration is associated with IV meperidine (Demerol®) (210-211).

Cause(s)/Physiology of a Benign Sinusoidal Pattern:
- mechanism in human fetuses is not clear (212)
- related to high-voltage sleep on the fetal lamb electrocorticogram (ECoG) (213)

- following administration of maternal narcotics:
  - meperidine (Demerol®)
  - Demerol and promethazine (Phenergan®)
  - butorphanol (Stadol®)
  - nalbuphine (Nubain®)
  - Nubain® and Phenergan® and in the past
  - alphaprodine (Nisentil®), a synthetic narcotic available prior to September, 1981 (26, 58, 210-212, 214-217).
- fetal sucking or mouthing with 1.7 to 2.2 cpm (218-219)
- clusters of fetal breathing movements (220)
- CNS malformations: reported in a 26 week fetus with hydraencephaly (66)
- gastroschisis with a hematocrit of 65% (221).

Actions in Response to a Benign Sinusoidal Pattern
- no specific responses are needed (212)
- document signs of fetal well-being that occurred prior to and after the pattern, e.g., fetal movement, accels, and/or STV. The nurse's note may read, "0 STV, 0 LTV s/p narcotic." "s/p" stands for status post or after.

Discussion
Benign sinusoidal patterns are uncommon and usually have a limited duration (50). Actual fetal sucking movements are rare, but mouthing movements are common. Sucking involves synchronized activity of the neck and buccal muscle groups versus movement of the mouth (219). Only 3.2% of fetuses whose mother received 50 mg of Demerol® and 25 mg of Phenergan® IV had a benign sinusoidal pattern (210). If the admission FHR pattern is sinusoidal, it may be difficult to distinguish a benign from a pathologic pattern. *If the fetus was actively moving just prior to fetal monitoring, the pattern is most likely benign. If acoustic or scalp stimulation produce an accel, the pattern definitely is benign.*

Pathologic Sinusoidal Pattern
Alternative label: true pseudosinusoidal pattern

Recognition Criteria:
BL	110 - 180 bpm, may be unstable sinusoidal BL may be intermittent may be tachycardic, rarely bradycardic
STV	decreased if hypoxic, absent if metabolically acidotic or asphyxiated
LTV	1^1/$_2$ to 5 cpm with an amplitude of 5 to 40 bpm some cycles "hang" below the BL like a "V" cycles are followed by a flat BL, e.g., 6 minute of cycles, 4 minutes of flat BL, 2 minutes with decelerations as the fetus deteriorates
ACCELS	none
DECELS	variable or late, never early decels
DURATION	often intermittent and followed by a flat BL or bradycardia when the fetus decompensates (222). Fetal movement will be significantly decreased if the fetus is hypoxic and anemic.

Fetal movement will be absent if the fetus is asphyxiated. *If fetal movement is palpable after measures to enhance fetal oxygenation have begun, the fetus is most likely anemic and hypoxic and not asphyxiated. Fetal movement may be the only sign of fetal well-being.*

Cause(s)/Physiology of a Pathologic Sinusoidal Pattern:
- *hypoxia, metabolic acidosis, and/or asphyxia* (50, 223-226)
- possible cord compression, hypoxia, and/or infection (229).
- preeclampsia, abruption, or amnionitis, probably related to hypoxia (51, 230)

Tissue **hypoxia** and the release of **arginine vasopressin** (AVP) could produce a sinusoidal pattern (226-227). AVP is secreted by the pituitary gland in response to hypoxia, hypotension, and hypernatremia to increase blood flow to the brain and heart (134). The loss of efferent vagal tone in the presence of AVP in fetal lambs produced a sinusoidal pattern (213, 221, 228).

Katz, Wilson, and Young (230) found 3 to 5 cpm with an amplitude of 5 to 40 bpm for a minimum of 10 minutes in anemic and hypoxic fetuses. They reported two cases of sinusoidal patterns: one in a preeclamptic woman who had a partial abruption, another in a woman whose fetus had "variable decels with a late component" due to an occult cord prolapse.

- severe fetal anemia (with hypoxia), possibly associated with:
  - maternal Rh isoimmunization and transplacental transfer of red blood cell (RBC) antibodies such as anti-C, anti-c, anti-D, anti-Kell, anti-E, anti-e, anti-MNS, anti Fy (Duffy), and anti-JK. Anti-D is the most immunogenic (231-232)
  - approximately 1/1000 live births has Rh D hemolytic disease of the newborn (232)
  - fetomaternal hemorrhage (transfusion), which occurs in 1 in 800 to 1 in 6000 live births and may precede fetal hydrops, seizures, and death (233-234)
  - transplacental transfer of anti-M antibodies which cause mild fetal hemolytic disease (235-236)
  - twin-twin transfusion (237-238)
  - fetal hemorrhage.

Fetal hemorrhage occurred as the result of an injury suffered during a motor vehicle accident. The anemic fetus was tachycardic (BL 170 to 180 bpm) with a sinusoidal BL. Cordocentesis revealed a fetal hematocrit of 17%. Intrauterine transfusion consisted of 70 ml of packed, washed, irradiated, cytomegalovirus-negative, O negative RBCs. Daily nonstress tests were done, as well as ultrasounds for fetal growth and movement (biophysical profile). The fetus recovered and the woman was discharged on the sixth hospital day (239). Other causes of fetal anemia are:

- umbilical vein thrombosis not related to intrauterine transfusion (233)
- cytomegalovirus (240)
- human parvovirus (B19) (HPV-B19).

Fifth's Disease

Pregnant women who have parvovirus may not have a "slapped cheek" facial rash. However, there may be a rash on their trunk and extremities with a lace-like (reticulated) pattern (241). Women may also have fever, malaise, swollen glands, myalgia, arthritis, pruritus, and upper respiratory symptoms (241-242). HPV-B19 virus infects the bone marrow and arrests RBC production and causes liver dysfunction (243). If the woman is exposed to parvovirus early in her pregnancy, she has an increased risk of abortion. Parvovirus is also associated with a small for gestational age (SGA) neonate and a fetus with aplastic anemia, thrombocytopenia, congestive heart failure, hydrops, and death (242, 244-246). There is no treatment or vaccine for this infection (243). Fetuses with parvovirus have a flat, not a sinusoidal, BL (see Figures 2.32 and 2.33) (244, 247).

Actions in Response to a Pathologic Sinusoidal Pattern

Rule out a benign sinusoidal pattern:
Assess recent self-administered drugs:
- narcotics?

Assess the fetal condition:
- recently active?
- accelerates with acoustic stimulation?
- ultrasound to confirm fetal well-being, e.g., sucking movements or clusters of breathing movements

If it is a pathologic sinusoidal pattern:
Assess maternal and fetal risk factors for anemia and/or hypoxia:
- maternal blood type, Rh negative?
- preeclampsia, abruption, infection?

- history of trauma?
- history of procedures, e.g., cordocentesis?
- twins?

Assess the maternal condition:
- vital signs, infection?
- urine color

Women may have an *immune reaction* from a fetomaternal transfusion of blood (248). In fact, they may suffer from *anaphylaxis, acute renal failure, and/or disseminated intravascular coagulopathy* if there is a large fetomaternal blood transfusion (209). Hoag (233) reported a case of a woman who had rust-colored urine without urgency, frequency, or dysuria. During a nipple stimulation contraction stress test, the FHR pattern was sinusoidal with late decels. The pale baby had a thin, empty cord and a hematocrit of 16%. The Kleihauer-Betke test suggested 185 ml of fetal blood had entered maternal circulation.

Assess the fetal condition:
- fetal movement is often decreased but not yet absent in the anemic fetus with a sinusoidal pattern (233)
- color, amount, and odor of amniotic fluid (infection? meconium?)

Act to:
- confirm fetal-acid base status, e.g., the fetus will *not* accel after acoustic stimulation
- enhance fetal oxygenation

Communicate:
- maternal condition and high-risk factors, if any, related to fetal anemia or hypoxia
- Sinusoidal Pattern and actions
- request the physician's immediate presence

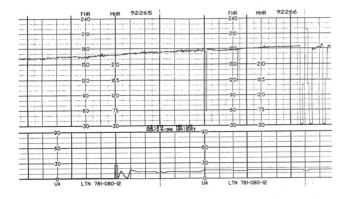

Figure 2.32: Tachycardic, rising baseline of a 27 week fetus who was diagnosed with parvovirus. Note the absence of accelerations, short-term variability, and long-term variability. The downward deflections are artifact. The baseline rose to 180 beats per minute.

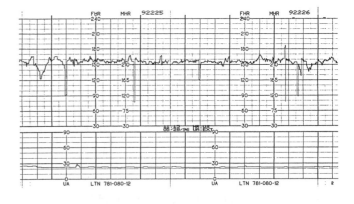

Figure 2.33: Fetal heart rate pattern of the same fetus in Figure 2.32 four days after an intrauterine transfusion. Note the baseline dropped to 150 - 160 bpm (a normal range for a 27 week fetus) with long-term variability, a spontaneous acceleration, and small variable decelerations.

If the fetus is term or near term, delivery should be expedited to avoid further fetal blood loss or deterioration of the acid-base status:

- prior to a decision to deliver by cesarean section, the physician may wish to determine the fetal scalp capillary pH and the hematocrit (58)
- prepare for neonatal resuscitation
- a physician that can manage neonatal complications, such as hypovolemic shock, should be present at the time of delivery

If the fetus is preterm, the physician may:

- obtain additional information about the woman's history and risk factors
- order a Kleihauer-Betke stain to detect fetal RBCs in maternal blood (233).
- perform an amniocentesis to
  - examine amniotic fluid optical density (to assess for bilirubin, a byproduct of RBC destruction)
  - culture the fluid for a virus (249-250)
- ultrasound the fetus to determine the presence of hydrops and to determine amniotic fluid volume
- obtain Doppler ultrasound studies of the middle cerebral artery or inferior vena cava
- transfuse the fetus.

Oligohydramnios/polyhydramnios may be present in twin pregnancies suspected to have twin-twin transfusion. Nonimmune hydrops may be due to hypoproteinemia, anemia, and/or cardiac failure (251).

Blood velocity in the middle cerebral artery increases during systole in the anemic fetus (252-254). The pre-load index (based on inferior vena cava studies) and the fetal hematocrit were 87% predictive of fetal anemia (255). Umbilical artery pressure was not affected by fetal anemia (256).

Intrauterine transfusion. Percutaneous umbilical cord blood sampling and determination of maternal Rh and antibody titers provides information to decide the need for transfusion. Blood for transfusion will usually be O negative, leukocyte-poor, washed adult RBCs (238). Fetuses will receive a transfusion based on a:

- hematocrit less than 30%, a diagnostic criteria for fetal anemia (257-258) and an
- elevated reticulocyte count and mean corpuscular volume (259).

If the cause of fetal anemia, confirmed by a Kleihauer-Betke test, is fetomaternal hemorrhage, women may donate their own blood for fetal intrauterine transfusion (258). Intrauterine transfusion requires collaboration between physicians, nurses, blood bank personnel, the woman, and her family. A genetic counselor may become part of the team. If an autologous transfusion is desired, the dietician should also be part of this collaborative team.

When a pregnant woman donates her own blood for fetal transfusion, she will need to increase her intake of vitamin C, iron, folic acid, cobalamin (B$_{12}$), pyridoxine (B$_6$), copper, zinc, and protein. Her hemoglobin should remain above 11 gm/dl (258).

The nurse will often interpret or clarify the medical plan of care and provide psychological support to the woman and her family prior to the day of the intrauterine transfusion. The nurse may assist with ultrasound guidance during the procedure, place fetal blood in labeled tubes for a complete blood count (CBC) and differential, blood type and antibody screen, direct and indirect Coombs test, and karyotype. The nurse will notify the physician of test results. After the procedure, the nurse or physician should review symptoms of anemia with the woman, e.g., fatigue, irritability, and a loss of a sense of well-being (257-258).

Prior to the transfusion, the fetus is given a drug to cause temporary paralysis (260). During the procedure, Doppler velocimetry of the umbilical vein and artery may be used to monitor the effects of the transfusion (261). The transfusion of blood into the umbilical vein is performed under ultrasound guidance. Within 24 hours following the transfusion, fetal hemodynamic values and the FHR should return to normal (262).

Success of the intrauterine transfusion. A continuous sinusoidal pattern after fetal transfusion suggests an unsuccessful transfusion (224). A transient sinusoidal pattern after fetal transfusion suggests a compensating fetus (225). Resolution or absence of the sinusoidal pattern after transfusion reflects a successful transfusion (224).

Prior to and after an intrauterine transfusion, the nurse will monitor the fetus and uterine activity. Electronic fetal monitoring is used prior to and after intrauterine transfusion to assess uterine activity, the effect of tocolytics on the uterus, and the FHR pattern. Preparations should be made prior to the intrauterine transfusion to deliver the fetus by cesarean section if necessary. Prior to the procedure, the nurse should assess maternal:

- anxiety or fear
- knowledge regarding the procedure

After the procedure, the nurse should assess:

- pain
- puncture sites (258).

The physician should be notified of the need for analgesics. Pressure with a sterile 4 x 4 gauze may be applied to the needle puncture site to stop bleeding.

Complications of intrauterine transfusion include bleeding from the puncture site, *fetal bradycardia*, chorioamnionitis, rupture of membranes, and umbilical vessel thrombosis (263). Therefore, maternal temperature and heart rate should be monitored after the procedure. The lack of uterine activity and rupture of membranes should be documented. The woman is usually discharged within 24 hours of the procedure. Following the procedure, the woman may return twice a week for a nonstress test and ultrasound examination (biophysical profile). Each week thereafter, she may have Doppler blood flow studies and ultrasounds to determine fetal growth. She should take her temperature twice a day and be asked to report an elevation of 100° F or more, cramps, vaginal discharge or leaking, abdominal pain, and decreased fetal movement (257).

Discussion

Previous reports of sinusoidal patterns provided limited recognition criteria which might lead to undergeneralizations and the failure to recognize a pathologic sinusoidal BL. For example, a sinusoidal pattern *was* described as a regular, smooth, undulating, sine wave pattern with no areas of normal variability, a relatively fixed periodicity or oscillations, and a duration of 2 to 10 minutes. In addition, the following recognition criteria were described:

BL	stable between 120 and 160 bpm with
STV	fixed (absent) STV and
LTV	uniform LTV, 2 to 8 cpm with a range of 5 to 40 bpm
ACCELS	no spontaneous accels
DECELS	not discussed in these reports (58, 215, 223, 264)

These criteria are actually misleading because severely anemic fetuses have had:
- an unstable, sinusoidal BL
- a sinusoidal BL less than 120 bpm
- a sinusoidal BL greater than 160 bpm

- $1^1/2$ cpm
- cycles that were *not* uniform, i.e., some cycles may appear to hang lower than others
- STV that was present but diminished in the hypoxic, nonacidotic fetus
- and a duration of 5 or more hours.

When nurses and physicians are looking for the "perfect" sinusoidal pattern within a normal BL range, they will miss other pathologic sinusoidal patterns. Pathologic sinusoidal patterns may have decels. Some believe if the baby can still decelerate, the fetus is more likely to be hypoxic and not yet acidotic.

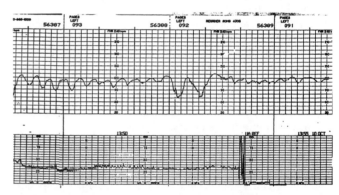

Figure 2.35: A rare pathologic sinusoidal pattern below 120 bpm with biphasic variable decelerations in a 30 week fetus of a 35 year old, G_3P_2 woman with severe preeclampsia who abrupted (BP 180/100, 4+ proteinuria). The fetus weighed 2 lb 12 oz and had Apgar scores of 7 and 8 at 1 and 5 minutes. A pathologic sinusoidal pattern is related to fetal hypoxia.

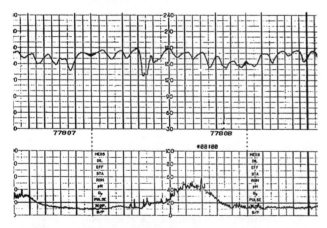

Figure 2.34: Unstable sinusoidal baseline with variable decelerations in a $33^1/2$ week fetus whose mother had premature rupture of the membranes, a history of a low-lying placenta, and vaginal bleeding. The fetus was delivered by cesarean section with Apgar scores of 8 and 9 by the physician and 6 and 8 by the nurse. The person with the infant at 1 and 5 minutes should declare the Apgar scores.

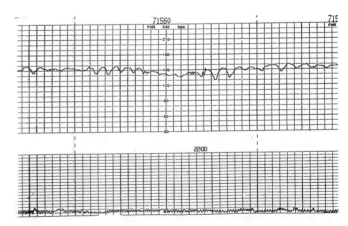

Figure 2.36: Sinusoidal pattern with cycles that are not uniform and an unstable baseline. The G_5P_3 woman at 35 weeks of gestation reported *decreased fetal movement*. The nonstress test was *nonreactive*. The plan was to "observe the patient throughout the night." A biophysical profile was scheduled for the following morning. The fetus decompensated at 5 am and was delivered stillborn by cesarean section before 6 am.

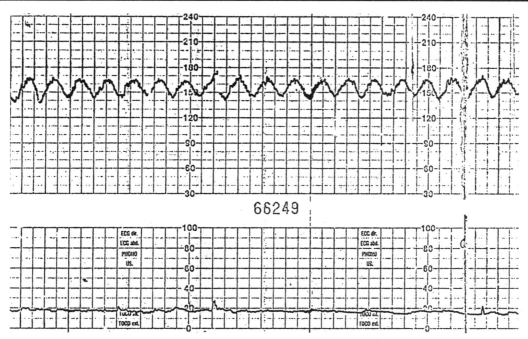

Figure 2.37: A sinusoidal pattern of a fetus of a G_1P_0 woman at term who presented for labor evaluation. She was 1 cm dilated and was sent home. She returned the next day with a fetal demise. The bumpy look of the baseline is technological artifact. An ultrasound transducer was used to assess the fetal heart rate.

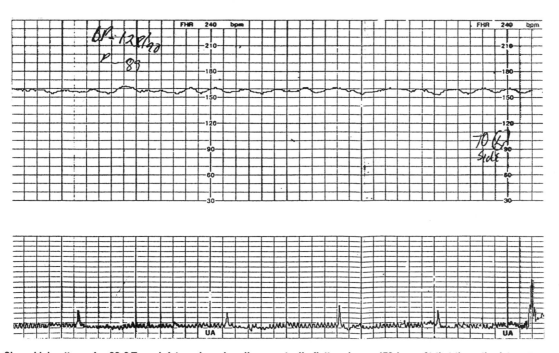

Figure 2.38: Sinusoidal pattern of a 36 3/7 week fetus whose baseline eventually flattened near 172 bpm. At that time, the fetus was unresponsive to acoustic stimulation. An anemic baby was delivered by cesarean section, with Apgar scores of 6 and 9 at 1 and 5 minutes and a hemoglobin of 4.5 gm/dl. The etiology of the fetomaternal bleed was not reported, but the woman presented with a headache, epigastric pain, and decreased fetal movement. Preeclampsia was ruled out. When the woman was turned to her side, given an intravenous bolus of lactated Ringer's solution, and hyperoxygenated with 10 liters per minute by face mask, 5 fetal movements were palpated by the nurse within a 10 minute period beginning 15 minutes after intrauterine resuscitation measures were instituted. This reflected a hypoxic fetus versus an asphyxiated fetus. An asphyxiated fetus doesn't move.

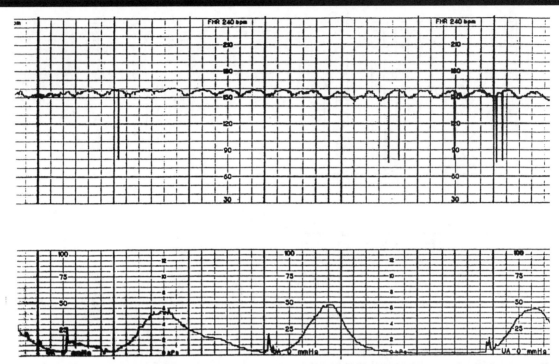

Figure 2.39: Sinusoidal pattern of an asphyxiated fetus. The G_2P_0 woman who had a benign pregnancy course had thick meconium when membranes were ruptured. An amnioinfusion was ordered. After forceps were applied, a compound presentation was discovered. A cesarean section was performed. The severely depressed neonate required intubation, chest compressions, and ventilator support. The umbilical artery gases were: pH 6.82, PO_2 22 mm Hg, PCO_2 107.9, base excess -18.1 mEq/L. The neonate seized on the second day of life and was later diagnosed with cerebral palsy. The infant died at 17 months of age.

AVP and Pathologic Sinusoidal Patterns

As late as 1989, the cause of a pathologic sinusoidal pattern was "unclear" (208). Then, in 1993 and 1994, Drs. Ninomiya, McMahan, Murata, Wakatsuki, Masaoka, Porto, and Tyner reported fetal lambs, who had a complete or partial vagal blockade due to a vagotomy or atropine administration, were given IV arginine vasopressin (AVP) and they developed a persistent sinusoidal pattern (213, 228). In human fetuses, AVP increases in the presence of hypoxia. Hypoxia may result from fetal anemia. If vagal tone remains, there will be STV, although it may be significantly diminished (189).

Given the results of Ninomiya and his colleagues, and the pathophysiology of the pattern proposed by Young, Katz, and Wilson in 1980 (226), and Modanlou and his colleagues in 1982 (223), a pathologic sinusoidal pattern appears to have the following pathophysiology:

Fetal Hypoxia
▼
Release of Arginine Vasopressin (AVP)
▼
Tissue Hypoxia in Medulla Oblongata
▼
Cardiac Regulatory Nerves Depressed
▼
Vagus and Sympathetic Nerves Depressed
▼
Fetal Heart Rate Regulated by AVP → Blood Pressure Rhythmically Fluctuates → Affecting Baroreceptors → Stimulating
    Sympathetic Nerves to create a
▼
Pathologic Sinusoidal Pattern

Figure 2.40: Proposed pathophysiology of a pathologic sinusoidal pattern.

Table 12: Benign versus Pathologic Sinusoidal Pattern Features

	BENIGN SINUSOIDAL	PATHOLOGIC SINUSOIDAL
CAUSE	high-voltage brain activity with sucking, mouthing, narcotics	loss of vagal tone, AVP as response to anemia and/or hypoxia, acidosis, and asphyxia
SINUSOIDAL BL	will not persist	may be followed by absent LTV, possibly unstable BL, decels
ACCELS	before and after pattern	*none*
STV	present	diminished or absent
LTV	average to moderate, *never marked*	minimal to moderate, *rarely marked*
FETAL MOVEMENT	moving	*decreased or absent movement*
ACTIONS	none	evaluate for hypoxia, anemia, treat for hypoxia and/or anemia
PROGNOSIS	expect healthy neonate	expect neonate requiring resuscitation and other treatment, e.g., for anemia

Documentation Of A Sinusoidal Pattern

A Benign Sinusoidal Pattern is not usually acknowledged in the nurse's notes. Instead, documentation may be, "STV present, average LTV with rhythmic undulations s/p narcotic administration." If a pathologic sinusoidal pattern is present, document "sinusoidal BL," "sinusoidal pattern," or the BL range, stability, STV, and LTV indicating "with regular undulations." For example, after seeing a pathologic sinusoidal pattern the nurse might write, "stable BL, 130 to 140 bpm, 0 accels, 0 STV, LTV average with regular undulations and intermittent flat areas." Also document decels. It is clearly more efficient to document "sinusoidal pattern" when describing the BL.

ACCELERATIONS (Accels)

Definition of an Acceleration in General:
- transient increase in the FHR above the BL (46).

In 1987, an accel was defined as *an increase in the FHR over the BL for 10 seconds to 2 minutes* (103). Unfortunately, this definition does not differentiate uniform from spontaneous accels. Only spontaneous accels may last longer than 2 minutes.

Recognition Criteria:
- a "bump" that could stand alone
- usually peaks at 10 or more bpm above the middle of the BL and
- lasts longer than 10 seconds at its base

Cause(s)/Physiology of Accelerations:
- increase in β-adrenergic (sympathetic) activity (99)
- less commonly, blockade of parasympathetic tone (99)
- accels often occur when the fetus is moving (265)
- accels *are associated with* fetal movement and not caused by fetal movement
- accels reflect fetal well-being (50)

- "extremely" premature fetuses are less likely to accel following movement than term or postterm fetuses (266).
- accel height, number, and duration decrease in IUGR fetuses due to hypoxia and adenosine (52, 267)
- accels may be absent due to
  - a medication such as atenolol (Tenormin®), a β-blocker
  - hypoxia, adenosine accumulation, and/or metabolic acidosis
  - neurologic or cardiac defect
  - brain death.

Actions in Response to a Lack of Accelerations

If the BL is sinusoidal, see Actions in Response to a Sinusoidal Pattern. If the BL is *not* sinusoidal and there have been no accels during a *40 minute period* of monitoring:

Assess recent drug use:
- CNS depressants, e.g., a narcotic
- β-blockers, e.g., atenolol (Tenormin®)

Assess the maternal condition:
- vital signs, infection?

Assess the fetal condition:
- determine when the fetus was last perceived by the woman to be moving
- palpate fetal movement or
- ultrasound the fetus and observe movement
- apply a spiral electrode and assess STV
- color, amount, and odor of amniotic fluid, infection? meconium?

Act to:
- confirm fetal acid-base status
- enhance fetal oxygenation if hypoxia is suspected

Communicate:
- fetal movement information

- time since last accel
- the FHR pattern
- FHR response to actions

The physician may choose to deliver the fetus by cesarean section if
- STV is absent
- the ultrasound examination reveals a limp fetus or
- the scalp pH is less than 7.20.

Discussion

A nonreactive nonstress test should be communicated to the physician after *40* minutes of monitoring (268). In other words, the NST should end after 40 minutes of monitoring. If it was nonreactive, the physician may request an ultrasound examination of the fetus (see Chapter 9). Some physicians prefer a contraction stress test after a nonreactive NST (see Chapter 8).

The rule that the physician should be notified of a nonreactive NST after 40 minutes of monitoring may not apply to the tracing generated during labor. It is known that the FHR may not accel during periods of fetal "sleep" (state 1F) which could last up to 100 minutes (269). However, it would be unwise to wait 100 minutes to report the lack of accels to the physician, especially if there are other signs of hypoxia such as meconium or a flat BL. *During labor, report the FHR if the fetus has not accelerated within the last 60 minutes and/or concern exists about acid-base status.*

Accels, in the presence of STV and LTV, indicate an intact nervous system. Accel *duration* is calculated from the time the FHR leaves the BL until it returns to the BL. The amplitude or height of the accel is usually calculated as the bpm from an imaginary line drawn through the middle of the BL to the top of the accel.

Misconceptions about accelerations. Some clinicians and researchers have adopted a definition of an accel that requires it to peak 15 bpm above the BL to be recognized. This definition is limited. Accels exist that do not attain this arbitrary height (270). For example, preterm fetuses may produce small accels that do not meet the 15 x 15 criteria (48). Their FHR pattern might be nonreactive but "appropriate for gestational age" versus "not appropriate for gestational age."

Only "reactive" accels should be defined by their height or duration, i.e., they peak at least 15 bpm above the BL and last 15 seconds at their base (268). During a nonstress test, when there are 2 reactive accels during 20 minutes of monitoring, the FHR is classified as *reactive* (268).

Accelerations during labor. It was reported that 95.5% of accels occurred during contractions (271). However, researchers did not specify whether the accels were uniform or spontaneous. *A tracing that remains nonreactive for 60 minutes is associated with fetal hypoxemia, acidemia, and low birth weight* (272). Accels often occur between contractions. Therefore, the 1975 definition of an accel as *an increase in the FHR in response to uterine contractions* is limited (273).

Uniform accels may occur *in response to* uterine contraction pressure on the umbilical cord, followed by a chemoreceptor, baroreceptor, sympathetic nerve response. Spontaneous accels may coincidentally occur during contractions in response to a sensory stimulus that precedes motor and sympathetic nerve impulses.

Both types of accels may occur during or between contractions. Therefore, timing words such as "periodic" and "nonperiodic" do not help identify the type of accel. To differentiate the two types of accels, it is best to **look at their shape, not their timing** *in relation to contractions.*

SPONTANEOUS ACCELERATIONS
(Spont Accels)

Alternative labels: sporadic accelerations, variable accelerations, nonperiodic accelerations, omega pattern (Ω) (180, 274).

These alternative labels are not commonly used in clinical practice and are not recommended for use.

Definition: An abrupt transient increase in the FHR with an abrupt return to the BL.

Recognition Criteria:

ONSET	abrupt, usually to the peak in less than 20 seconds, sometimes with a jagged slope
AMPLITUDE (PEAK)	varies from one to the next
OFFSET	usually abrupt return to BL, FHR may dip below the BL before or after the accel creating a Lambda pattern (λ) (274)
DURATION	usually varies from one to the next
SHAPE	if the tracing is *turned upside down*, spontaneous accels often look like variable decels due to their varying shapes
BL	usually greater than 100 bpm but may be lower
STV	present
LTV	usually present before and after the accel
DECELS	may be present

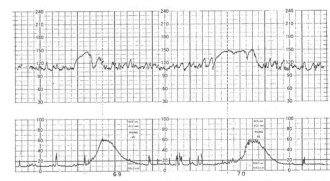

Figure 2.41: Spontaneous accelerations of a term fetus. The baseline is between 100 and 120 bpm. Short-term variability is present. Long-term variability is moderate (11 - 25 bpm). Look at the accelerations upside down. They vary in shape.

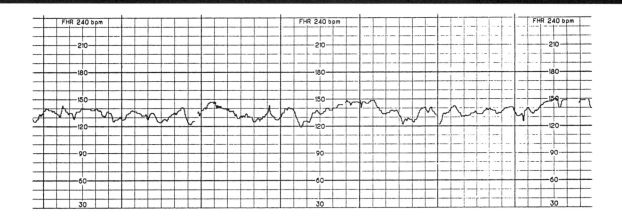

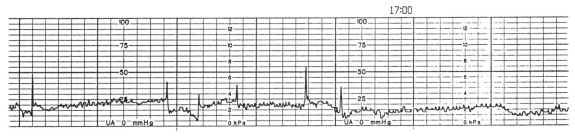

Figure 2.42: Spontaneous accelerations and moderate long-term variability (6 - 25 bpm) of a preterm fetus at 27 weeks of gestation. The woman was discharged after treatment for dehydration.

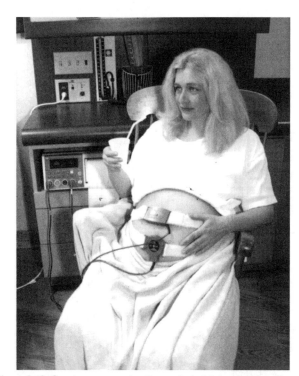

Figure 2.43: Spontaneous accelerations rule in fetal well-being. To maintain fetal oxygenation, the woman should be positioned off of her back in a position of comfort which may include an upright position in a rocking chair. (Photograph by Barbara Gibson, Albuquerque, NM courtesy of Lovelace Medical Center, Albuquerque, NM).

Cause(s)/Physiology of Spontaneous Accelerations:
- sympathetic nerve stimulus (274)
- found in 99.8% of tracings of well fetuses (55)
- *in association with* fetal movement, not caused by fetal movement
- suggesting coordination within the CNS (275)
- nerve cells associated with motor function and cells associated with cardiovascular function are anatomically in close proximity (276)
- accels may occur independent of fetal movement.

Discussion

The autonomic nervous system is thought to be mature by 30 weeks of gestation (277). However, the FHR can accel as early as 16 weeks after conception (269). Spontaneous accels are usually associated with fetal movement, whether or not the movement is palpable or perceived by the woman. Fetal movement may appear as a "spike" in the uterine activity pattern recorded when a tocotransducer is used.

Usually one to three seconds prior to a spontaneous accel, the fetus begins to move. Fetal movement is usually perceived by the woman after 20 seconds. Women may perceive as few as 16% or many as 96.7% of all fetal movements (278-279). The appearance of spontaneous accels in association with movement is a sign of fetal well-being.

A hypothyroid fetus may fail to produce reactive accels. Hypoxic fetuses also decrease the frequency, amplitude, and duration of accels. They reduce their activity

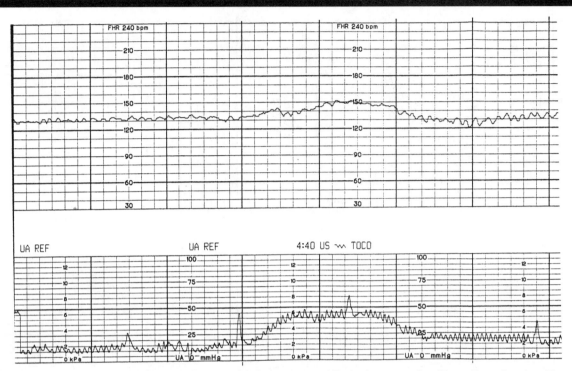

Figure 2.44: Uniform acceleration. The presence of a uniform acceleration suggests umbilical vein compression. Change the maternal position and observe the fetal response. The baseline is stable at 130 to 135 bpm prior to the acceleration. The subtle late deceleration following the uniform acceleration is most likely a response to the contraction which lasted 130 seconds causing a significant drop in the fetal PaO_2. A variable deceleration occurred 8 minutes after the uniform acceleration. Late decelerations never recurred.

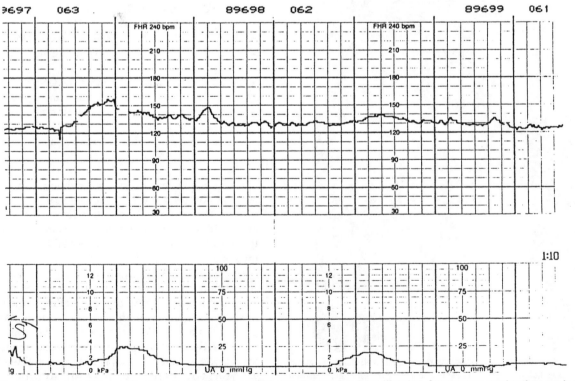

Figure 2.45: Spontaneous and uniform accelerations in a breech fetus, which was diagnosed at 7 cm dilatation. Spontaneous accelerations are in the minutes between 89697 and 89698. A definite uniform acceleration is in the minute after "062." The acceleration under "063" is a little jagged at the top, which suggests it is a spontaneous acceleration.

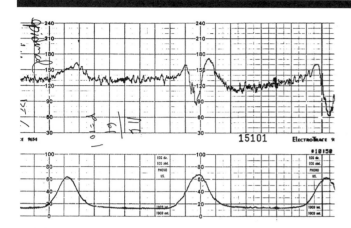

Figure 2.46: Uniform acceleration followed by mixed variable deceleration/late deceleration. If you cover the variable deceleration with your finger, you can imagine a uniform acceleration. The reflex late deceleration was most likely a result of a drop in maternal blood pressure from 136/61 to 116//61 after her epidural was redosed. The presence of short-term variability and accelerations that are at least 15 bpm high and 15 seconds at their base rule out fetal metabolic acidosis.

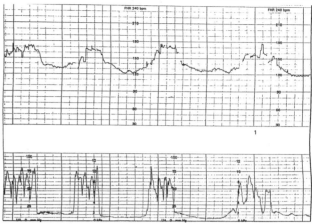

Figure 2.47: Uniform accelerations of the maternal heart rate in response to pain during pushing efforts. The Apgar scores were 5 and 9 at 1 and 5 minutes and there was meconium-stained amniotic fluid at the time of vaginal birth. Fetuses, prior to birth usually decelerate not accelerate due to a vagal response resulting from head and cord compression.

(280). *Perceived fetal inactivity and the lack of accels for two or more hours suggests fetal compromise and increases the risk of stillbirth, poor tolerance of labor, and the need for neonatal resuscitation* (202).

UNIFORM ACCELERATIONS

Alternative labels: periodic accelerations, pure accelerations, late accelerations (141, 281-282).

The most common alternative label is periodic accelerations. Pure accelerations and late accelerations are confusing terms and are not recommended for use.

Definitions:
- transient increase of the FHR in response to stimulation of chemoreceptors and baroreceptors when the umbilical cord is mildly compressed.
- accels with a gradual onset and usually a gradual offset or return to BL.

Recognition Criteria:

ONSET	gradual, reaches the peak in 20 or more seconds
AMPLITUDE (PEAK)	similar from one uniform accel to the next
OFFSET	usually a gradual return to BL
DURATION	similar, but not necessarily the same, from one to the next
USUAL SHAPE	similar to contractions (49), usually with one "hump" to confirm their similar shapes: copy the tracing onto a transparency and lay the transparency on the tracing, moving accels over one another...they are similar in shape!
ALTERNATE SHAPE	may have two humps (184)

BL	greater than 100 bpm
STV	may be absent
LTV	may be absent
DECELS	usually variable decels follow two or more uniform accels when they are due to umbilical cord compression and not the MHR response to pain

Cause(s)/Physiology of Uniform Accelerations:
- partial umbilical cord occlusion (60-61, 283)
- baroreceptor and chemoreceptor-induced sympathetic increase in the FHR (184)
- sympathetic stimulation greater than vagal stimulation (49, 141)
- when the umbilical cord is mildly compressed, there is a small decrease in fetal BP and PaO_2 with an increase in the FHR of 16 to 19 bpm (284-285)
- some uniform accels have an amplitude greater than 19 bpm
- normoxic fetus who has become hypoxemic or hypoxic from umbilical vein compression (55, 149, 274, 281, 284, 286-288)
- the term breech fetus during transition (7 to 10 cm dilatation), probably due to cord compression when the fetus is being pushed into the pelvis during contractions
- may be a precursor to variable decels (60-61, 289).
- indicative of an intact, responsive nervous system when STV and LTV are also present
- *may be the MHR*, especially if the fetus is dead and the woman is in pain (86, 290-291).

Actions in Response to Uniform Accelerations
Review previous ultrasound reports:
- possibility of IUGR? oligohydramnios?

Estimate fetal size, possibly small?
- by palpation
- by measuring the fundal height

Assess fetal movement
- fetuses move less when there is oligohydramnios versus a normal fluid volume

Rule out a breech presentation:
- Leopold's maneuvers (282)
- vaginal examination to assess presenting part

Rule out recording of the MHR and her pain response:
- assess MHR, it should differ from the printout
- if in doubt, apply the 3-lead ECG and plug into the fetal monitor and/or
- auscultate the fetus
- position the ultrasound transducer over the fetus' back or apply a spiral electrode

If the printout is not related to a fetus in a breech presentation or the MHR, but is due to mild cord compression, the only initial action is to change the maternal position and note the fetal response.
- consider other actions to improve fetal oxygenation if the pattern worsens

Since cord compression is the probable etiology of uniform accels, other actions may include:
- rupture of the membranes to assess color, amount, and odor of the fluid
- amnioinfusion

Communicate:
- findings, e.g., a breech presentation, fetal movement
- FHR pattern and response to actions
- concern about possible oligohydramnios
- abnormal amniotic fluid findings

Expedite delivery if :
- the MHR is being recorded, e.g., during pushing in the second stage of labor,
- the ultrasound has been repositioned over the fetal back or the spiral electrode has been applied and
- the FHR which *was* present is no longer transmitted.

Discussion

The MHR often increases due to pain during contractions. To rule out MHR as a cause of uniform accels, palpate her pulse while observing the printout and digital readout of the fetal monitor. Both the ultrasound and spiral electrode may transmit the MHR in the case of a fetal demise (86).

With umbilical vein occlusion, there is decreased blood return to the fetal heart, decreased cardiac output, hypotension, and stimulation of baroreceptors and chemoreceptors (61). Uniform accels are an appropriate neurologic response

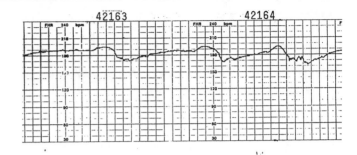

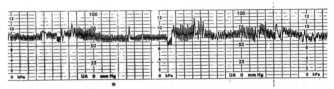

Figure 2.48: An overgeneralization will cause the clinician to mistake this ominous pattern for uniform accelerations. The baseline is near 190 bpm with absent short-term variability and absent long-term variability. The baseline is flat due to adenosine accumulation as a result of asphyxia. The increase in the fetal heart rate is most likely due to a surge of catecholamines, and the decrease in the fetal heart rate is probably due to myocardial failure. This tracing should be documented as "BL 190, 0 STV, 0 LTV, FHR ↑ 195 bpm, ↓ 170 bpm."

to mild hypoxia. As the cord becomes progressively more compressed during labor, uniform accels may disappear and variable decels will appear. Unlike uniform accels which are a response to umbilical vein compression, variable decels occur in response to compression of the umbilical vein and arteries.

If the uniform accels are thought to be due to mild umbilical cord compression, maternal repositioning may alleviate cord compression by changing the relationship between the cord, fetus, and uterus. Uniform accels have also been observed when the fetus is breech, especially near the end of the first stage of labor. The etiology of uniform accels when the fetus is breech is purely speculative and thought to be due to umbilical cord compression, particularly during strong contractions.

Compression of the umbilical vein decreases fetal PaO_2 and BP, which activates chemoreceptors and baroreceptors. A message travels to the medulla oblongata cardioregulatory nerves. The sympathetic nerves, more so than the vagus, are stimulated to increase the FHR (184). This is the same physiology as the "shoulders" on a variable decel. With greater cord compression, variable decels will appear.

Uniform accels described as a "blunt sympathetic response" may be associated with hypoxemia and acidemia (55). *They warn of impending umbilical cord complications* (284). They are often present when there is oligohydramnios. Clinicians who do not know this concept may miss an opportunity to diagnose oligohydramnios. For example, *if uniform accels, not spontaneous accels, appear during a nonstress test, they may be the first hint the cord is vulnerable due to the lack of amniotic fluid. Therefore, uniform accels should trigger thoughts and actions related to a vulnerable umbilical cord.*

Depending on the effect of acidemia on the FHR, STV and LTV may be present or absent. If there is tachycardia, absent STV, absent LTV, and a blunt increase in the FHR resembling an accel, the transient increase in the rate should not be documented as an accel because it is most likely a catecholamine response to hypoxia (see Figure 2.48). Measures should be taken to improve fetal O_2 delivery and the physician should be requested to promptly come to the bedside for expeditious delivery, which may be by cesarean section. The lack of accels, STV, and LTV plus the tachycardic BL makes this an ominous pattern.

LAMBDA PATTERN (λ)

Definition: a transient increase in the FHR preceded and/or followed by a dip in the FHR.

Recognition Criteria:
- a spontaneous or uniform accel with
- a dip in the FHR below the BL level before and/or after the accel

Cause(s)/Physiology of a Lambda Pattern:
- believed to be a baroreceptor/vagal response to a BP shift
- 10 to 20 second dips in the FHR are common between 20 to 30 weeks of gestation, and may be seen after fetal movement (292-294)
- may even occur in fetuses prior to 20 weeks' gestation
- the sympathetic and parasympathetic nervous system modulate FHR changes in response to BP fluctuations (135)
- often noted early in labor
- no association with decels
- no increased risk of adverse neonatal outcomes (274, 295).

Actions in Response to a Lambda Pattern:
- no specific actions are required.

Discussion

A potential problem is overgeneralization of a Lambda pattern, thinking variable or late decels exist (295). Lambda patterns are common, yet they are not commonly documented. One reason "Lambda pattern" may not be documented is that some clinicians do not know what a Lambda pattern is. In addition, it is a benign, innocuous pattern which requires no special actions.

Stimuli for accels and decels are different. Accels follow activation of the sympathetic nervous system. Dips in the FHR follow activation of the vagus nerve. Note that there is an abrupt drop in the FHR which descends to a level below the BL. Variable decels often have a similar abrupt drop because in both cases, the Lambda pattern and variable decels, the vagus is activated to decrease the FHR.

Timor-Tritsch and his colleagues (296) found that accels were followed by brief dips in 66.7% of fetuses. These dips (which the authors called decels) were of small amplitude, usually less than the amplitude of the accel, and were more prominent in early gestations. It was theorized that these brief "dips" which follow accels may be caused by stimulation of the vagus nerve by carotid baroreceptors. The presence of accels, followed by small, brief dips is indicative of an intact nervous system and responsive heart.

Differentiating a Lambda Pattern From an Accel/Decel Combination

The clinician is challenged to differentiate a Lambda pattern from accels that immediately precede an early, variable, or late decel. The significance of these combination accel/decel patterns depends on the presence or absence of STV, the BL rate, and pertinent clinical observations.

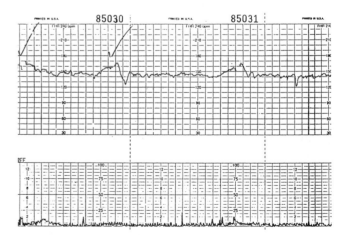

Figure 2.50: Lambda pattern of a uniform acceleration with a dip (see below 85030) during a nonstress test. This is a reactive nonstress test but it also suggests there is a vulnerable umbilical cord. It is possible there is oligohydramnios. The woman should move into several different positions. If there are no variable decelerations she may be discharged. If there are two or more variable decelerations, an ultrasound should be done to establish fetal well-being, the umbilical cord's position, and amniotic fluid volume.

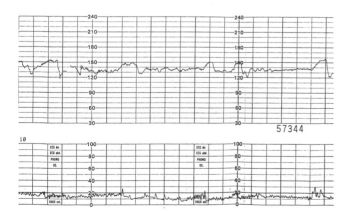

Figure 2.49: A Lambda pattern is an acceleration with a "dip." The baseline is higher than 130 bpm. Note the dips below 130 bpm in 4 out of 5 accelerations. Apgar scores were 8 and 9 at 1 and 5 minutes.

PERIODIC AND NONPERIODIC CHANGES

"Periodic" and "nonperiodic" are descriptive terms that were used to illustrate the time accels and decels occurred in relation to contractions. If accels or decels occurred in relation to a contraction, they were periodic changes. If accels and decels occurred without any relation to uterine activity, or between contractions, they were called nonperiodic changes.

Avoid the Use of "Periodic" and "Nonperiodic" When Describing Accelerations

Spontaneous accels are a response to a stimulus, which may be direct pressure of a contraction on the fetus. However, it does not make sense to call spontaneous accels that occur with contractions "periodic spontaneous accels." Alternatively, it is not necessary to call spontaneous accels that occur between contractions "nonperiodic spontaneous accels." It is best to simply label the accel as a spontaneous accel because it is not physiologically significant if a spontaneous accel occurs with or between contractions. Spontaneous accels may be documented as "spont accels."

Uniform accels are a response to mild umbilical cord compression. The alternative name for uniform accels is periodic accels. In 1975, when they were originally named, they were called periodic accels because they were noted to occur with contractions (281). If periodic accels occur during contractions, their name makes sense. However, periodic or uniform accels may also occur when the cord is compressed between contractions, especially if there is oligohydramnios. They then become nonperiodic periodic accels or nonperiodic uniform accels. To avoid confusion, nurses and physicians are encouraged to adopt the label uniform accels instead of periodic accels.

Periodic decelerations. Periodic decels are classified on the basis of their shape or waveform and their timing in relation to the onset, peak, and offset of the contraction. The three types of periodic decels are: early decels, late decels, and variable decels. Periodic decelerations occur in response to contractions and

- direct pressure on the head, which creates **early decels**
- umbilical cord compression and head compression which creates **variable decels** and/or
- hypoxia, usually due to uteroplacental insufficiency, which creates **late decels** (58).

Sometimes during the second stage of labor, late decelerations occur which may be partly caused by umbilical cord compression and variable decels may be due to fetal head compression and cord compression.

Early, variable, and late decels may occur separately or immediately follow one another. A mixed deceleration pattern is a periodic decel pattern that combines two of the three types of periodic decels. For example, there may be an early, late decel combination or a variable, late decel combination.

Nonperiodic decelerations. Nonperiodic decels are classified on the basis of their shape. Variable, prolonged, and spontaneous decels are the three types of nonperiodic decels. They are not related to uterine activity. Nonperiodic variable decels most commonly occur when the cord is compressed between contractions, often associated with oligohydramnios or an umbilical cord prolapse. A FHR pattern of nonperiodic variable decels, bradycardia, and absent variability has been associated with congenital neurologic and/or cardiac defects (201). In fact, the fetus with that type of pattern may be seizing, which is rare, and is called a Checkmark Pattern.

Table 13: Taxonomy of Periodic and Nonperiodic Decelerations

PERIODIC CHANGES	NONPERIODIC CHANGES

• Early deceleration(s)
 • Late deceleration(s)
 • Variable deceleration(s)
	
	 • Variable decelerations
	   • due to umbilical cord compression
	   • Checkmark Pattern (fetal seizures)
	 • Prolonged deceleration(s)
	 • Spontaneous deceleration(s)

EARLY DECELERATIONS

Alternative label (old and not recommended for use): Type I dip(s) (24)

Definition: periodic deceleration(s) due to intense fetal head compression.

Recognition Criteria:

ONSET	gradual, descent usually begins shortly after onset of the contraction may begin as late as 20 seconds after the contraction begins (pressure must be high enough to create a vagal response) may reach the nadir in 10 seconds, usually reaches the nadir in 30 or more seconds
PEAK TO NADIR	
LAG TIME	nadir is *usually* ≤ 18 seconds after the contraction peak (29)
OFFSET	gradual, with return to BL shortly after the contraction ends
DEPTH	usually drop is not > 25 bpm, but may be greater with substantial head compression
DURATION	usually same duration as the contraction, but may be up to 10 seconds less, e.g., if the contraction lasted 60 seconds, the early decel may last 50 to 60 seconds

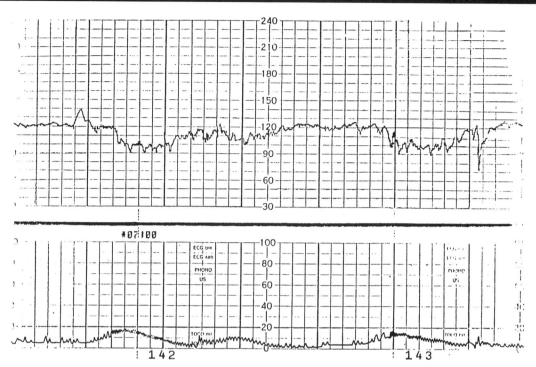

Figure 2.51: Early decelerations of a term fetus who was delivered by cesarean section due to a diagnosis of cephalopelvic disproportion. Short-term variability and long-term variability are present. The fetus is not hypoxic but has a vagal response due to increased intracranial pressure. Note the spontaneous acceleration in the first minute.

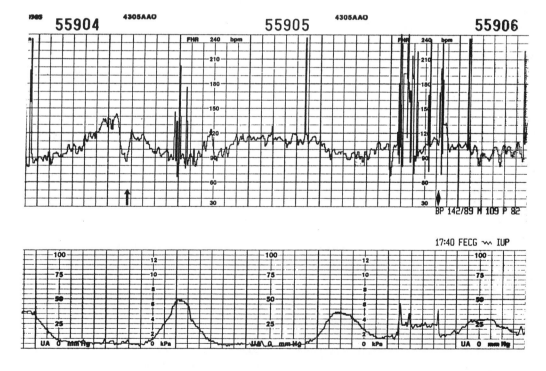

Figure 2.52: Early decelerations of a term IUGR fetus with oligohydramnios at 5 cm, -1 to -2. The arrow mark denotes perceived fetal movement. About 20 seconds before the arrow, the "shoulder" of the variable deceleration begins. Women perceive fetal movement after it lasts at least 20 seconds. When the fetus moved, the cord was mildly compressed, and the "shoulder" reflects that. A 5 lb 3 ounce fetus was delivered by cesarean section for failure to descend with Apgar scores of 8 and 9 at 1 and 5 minutes. Oligohydramnios increases the risk of an asynclitic presentation and failure to descend.

SHAPE	similar from one decel to the next, curvilinear like a smile, saucer or spoon; if the decel were cut in half, each half would be a mirror image
BL	stable, usually greater than 90 bpm
STV	usually present
LTV	usually present
ACCELS	usually present

Rules of Recognition:
- "If it has a "shoulder" it is not an early decel, it is a blunt variable decel."
- If after palpating the fetal head during a vaginal examination it is high, and/or it is not swollen (no caput), and/or there is no molding, and/or the cervix is not close to 4 cm or more dilated, it is not an early. It is probably a "blunt" variable decel (both early decels and variable decels are a response to vagal stimulation).
- calculate the duration of the contraction and duration of the decel, they should be within 10 seconds of each other.

Significance of Early Decelerations
- previously considered benign (196)
- not necessarily innocuous (297)
- significance depends on severity of in utero head compression and the risk of trauma related to a vaginal birth, e.g., subarachnoid hemorrhage
- usually first seen when the woman is 4 to 7 cm dilated, but may be present between 7 and 10 cm
- associated with cephalopelvic disproportion (CPD)
- part of a reassuring (nonhypoxic) FHR pattern when there are no signs of hypoxia, acidosis, or asphyxia, such as the absence of accels in the last 60 minutes.

Cause(s)/Physiology of Early Decelerations:
- not seen during the antepartal period due to the lack of significant fetal head compression
- a "squeeze" on the fetal head and possible carotid arteries with
- a transient decrease in cerebral blood flow but stable transcutaneous scalp PO_2 (298-300)
- creating a vagal stimulus, with the possible release of meconium (50, 299, 301)
- in lambs, decels occurred after pressure exceeded 200 mm Hg on the fetal head (298, 302)
- pressure on the fetal head may be 200% higher than the intrauterine pressure (IUP) prior to rupture of membranes (298-299)
- pressure on the fetal head exceeds 400% of the IUP after rupture of membranes (298-299)
- depending on the fit of the head in the pelvis, the "squeeze" can become excessive (302)
- deformation of the fetal head with increased intracranial pressure can occur (299)
- because CPD often manifests as an arrest of active labor, early decels are often seen during active labor between 4 and 7 cm dilatation, especially in primigravida women

- the physician must distinguish between CPD and inefficient uterine activity prior to making a decision to deliver the fetus by a cesarean section
- uterine activity when CPD is present is no different than uterine hypocontractility, therefore uterine activity alone does not predict CPD (303-304)
- if fetal descent or cervical dilatation cease when there are adequate contractions, CPD is diagnosed (303)
- to determine if there are adequate contractions, an IUPC is usually inserted and an oxytocic may be administered. When an oxytocic is administered, the fetus should be closely monitored.

Classifications:
- Early decels with normal BL level, STV, LTV, and accels: reassuring, the fetus is nonhypoxic. Concern should exist regarding the possibility of CPD and the potential for an intracranial bleed.
- Early decels, variable decels, BL > 100 bpm, STV present, average LTV: compensatory
- Early decels, tachycardia, and "poor" STV: nonreassuring, implies impending acidosis (125).

Actions in Response to Early Decelerations
Assess the maternal condition:
- review prenatal records: pelvic dimensions? height? weight gain?
- gestational diabetes?

Assess fetal size:
- *estimate* fetal weight by palpation of the abdomen and uterus, ultrasound reports regarding fetal size?
- a large baby in a small bony pelvis increases the risk of CPD (303)

Determine fetal/pelvic fit:
- in the past, x-ray pelvimetry was justified to diagnose CPD (305)
- now, clinical pelvimetry, estimation of fetal weight, and evaluation of labor progress are used to determine the risk of CPD (306)
- plot a labor curve

  Abnormal labor increases the probability of CPD as 50% of women who had an arrest of labor had CPD (303).

- assess fetal station (relationship of the skull bone, not caput, to the ischial spines) (307)
- assess cervical swelling, caput, molding, and fetal position (307)

If the fetal head is *not* engaged or there is a persistent occipitoposterior (OP) position, a cesarean section may be the best route of delivery (306). A swollen cervix suggests a tight fit. A persistent OP position suggests a tight fit.

Deliver by cesarean section if CPD is diagnosed (308).

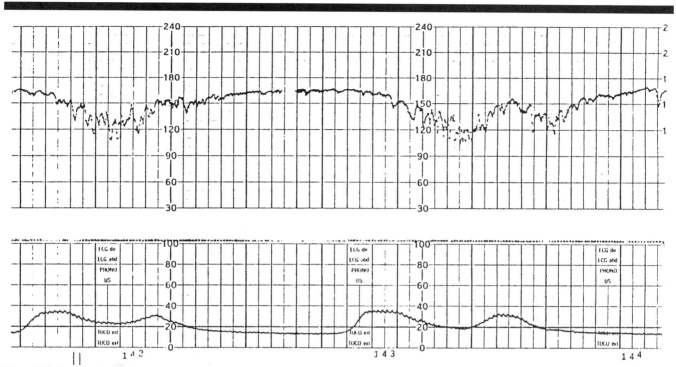

Figure 2.53: Late decelerations represent the fetal response to hypoxia caused by uteroplacental insufficiency. The baseline is 160 to 165 bpm with minimal long-term variability. There are no accelerations to rule out metabolic acidosis. Note coupling or doubling of uterine contractions. (Contributed by Micki Cabaniss, MD, FACOG).

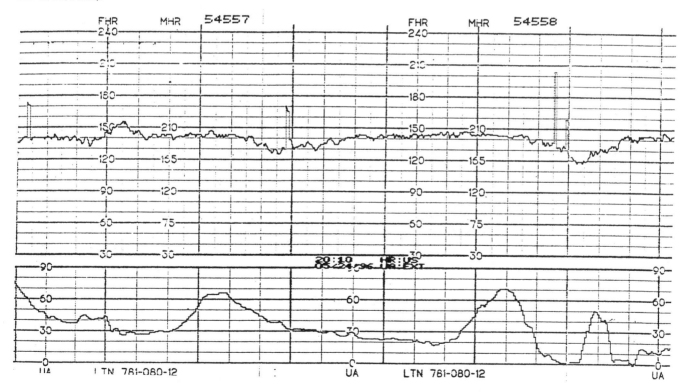

Figure 2.54: Late decelerations may be seen in the presence of STV and accelerations. This is the FHR pattern of a 41 week fetus of a G_1P_0 nonsmoker, non-drug user who was admitted at 3 cm/90%/-2 at 0830. It is now 2010. Membranes were ruptured 5 minutes later to reveal thick meconium. An amnioinfusion was performed. The fetus was delivered by cesarean section at 0230. Prior to delivery, the woman was completely dilated with a +2 station. There were moderate and severe variable decelerations and the baseline was tachycardic. Apgar scores were 1, 1, and 4 at 1, 5, and 10 minutes. The fetus was intubated.

LATE DECELERATIONS
Alternative label (old and not recommended for use): Type II dip(s) (24, 309)

Definitions:

- periodic deceleration(s) due to uteroplacental insufficiency
- transient decrease or slowing in the FHR in response to contractions and hypoxia (104, 133)
- isolated late decel, i.e., one late decel can occur, especially if the woman has only one contraction (310)
- a pattern of late decels is five or more consecutive late decels (311).

Recognition Rules and Criteria:
- late decels do not occur in the absence of contractions
- "if there is a "shoulder," it is not a late decel."
- if it looks like a late decel but contractions are not recorded:
  - palpate the abdomen for contractions (mark the onset and offset on the paper)
  - reposition the tocotransducer
  - "rezero" the IUPC or insert an IUPC
  - rule out uterine rupture (even with uterine rupture, contractions should be recorded)

ONSET	descent of the FHR begins after the contraction begins and reaches the nadir in ≥ 10 seconds
PEAK TO NADIR	
LAG TIME	lag time > 18 seconds (25, 29)
OFFSET	may be abrupt after late decels that decrease > 50 bpm below the BL, if IUPC and spiral electrode (SE) are used, FHR will be back to BL after the contraction ends, *IUPC and SE are not required to identify a late decel*
DEPTH	nadir may reach 60 bpm (312)

SHAPE	usually similar from one to another
BL	may be bradycardic, tachycardic, or in a normal range
STV	present, will become absent as fetal acid-base status deteriorates
LTV	present, will become absent as fetal acid-base status deteriorates
ACCELS	may be present in the nonacidotic fetus, e.g., in response to maternal hypotension

Significance
- fetal compensatory response to hypoxia from uteroplacental insufficiency
- the deeper the late decel, the lower the pH (119)
- repetitive late decels have been labeled "fetal distress" (105, 205)
- significance of pattern depends on presence or absence of accels and STV.

Prognosis
- good if accels are present
- poor if there are no accels, absent LTV, and diminished or absent STV.

Classification
- late decels with accels and STV present: compensatory
- late decels with no accels and STV present: nonreassuring
- late decels with tachycardia and absent STV: ominous (2)
- late decels with no accels, absent to minimal LTV, diminished or absent STV: ominous (310).

Cause(s)/Physiology of Late Decelerations
- two mechanisms: direct SA node depression (vagal response) and myocardial depression (58, 287)
- a vagal reflex in the nonacidotic hypoxic fetus (56)

Fetal well-being (nonhypoxic)	→	Accelerations and fetal movement
▼		▼
Hypoxia (PaO$_2$) *Chemoreceptor, baroreceptor, vagal response*	→	*Late decelerations*
▼		▼
Adenosine accumulation	→	Loss of accelerations, LTV and STV decrease
▼		▼
Metabolic acidosis and risk of asphyxia *Direct myocardial depression*	→	Absent LTV and STV
		▼
		BL rises or falls
		▼
		Bradycardia, absent LTV and STV
		▼
		Fetal Death

Figure 2.55: The continuum as the fetus deteriorates due to uteroplacental insufficiency. Late decelerations are often the first sign of fetal hypoxia. Note two mechanisms for late decelerations: a vagal response and direct myocardial depression (64, 90, 175, 314, 317, 320, 328-329).

- an occasional, single late decel may occur in the presence of normal BL variability, and may be associated with changes in the fetal behavioral state ("sleep lates") or fetal breathing movements (294, 273, 313)
- initially, late decels reflect a chemoreceptor, baroreceptor, vagal response to hypoxia (314-315)
- *hypoxia,* with a fetal PaO_2 less than 17 to 19 mm Hg in humans, 19 mm Hg in rhesus and java monkeys and baboons, and less than 10 to 30 mm Hg in fetal sheep (58, 90, 99, 287, 310)
- late decels were a fetal response to a massive chronic feto-maternal hemorrhage with an estimated total fetal blood loss (over time) of 700 ml (322)
- when STV and LTV are absent, late decels are due to direct hypoxic myocardial depression (314)
- which has been confirmed with umbilical artery systolic/diastolic (S/D) ratios consistent with fetal hypertension and hypoxic myocardial depression (323)
- hypoxia and late decels were also associated with
  - maternal hypotension and hypertension (324-326)
  - uterine hypertonus, oxytocin use, and abruption (324)
  - maternal drug use, e.g., a nasal decongestant with oxymetazoline (70)
- in lambs, maternal hyperoxygenation was more effective when there was decreased uterine blood flow (late decels) versus decreased umbilical blood flow (variable decels) (327).

FOUR TYPES OF LATE DECELERATIONS

Late decelerations have been classified based on their shape, depth, and the presence or absence of STV. There are four classifications for late decels: subtle, reflex, hypoxic myocardial failure, and late/variables. These classifications are not recommended for documentation. Instead, documenting "late decels" should be sufficient, since they all represent a fetal hypoxic response. It is important to include the rest of the systematic review, i.e., BL rate, STV, LTV, accels, and uterine activity when documenting the FHR pattern.

Subtle Late Decelerations

Definition: Shallow late decels with a gradual onset and offset.

ONSET   gradual, descent of the FHR begins after the contraction begins and reaches the nadir in ≥ 30 seconds

PEAK TO NADIR

LAG TIME	> 18 seconds (25, 29)
OFFSET	gradual or slanted appearance
DEPTH	usually no more than a 10 bpm drop in the FHR
SHAPE	shallow like a bowl, saucer, or spoon
BL	usually above 100 bpm, often tachycardic
STV	absent or present
LTV	usually absent to minimal (3 - 5 bpm)
ACCELS	usually none

A misconception about subtle late decels is that they are "worse" than obvious late decels (330). The presence of accels and STV determines the significance of the pattern, not the depth of the decel(s). For example, if subtle late decels are present and there is tachycardia and absent STV the fetus is often acidotic (see Figure 2.56). In that case, a pattern of subtle late decels would be worse than a pattern of deeper lates with STV and accels present.

Reflex Late Decelerations

Alternative label: "good" lates

Definition: Late decels with a stable BL and STV present.

ONSET   gradual, descent of the FHR begins after the contraction begins and reaches the nadir in ≥ 10 seconds

PEAK TO NADIR

LAG TIME	> 18 seconds (25, 29)
OFFSET	varies, may be gradual or abrupt
DEPTH	varies, may be shallow or deep
SHAPE	varies, may be shaped like a spoon or a box
BL	any level
STV	**always present**
LTV	minimal (3 - 5 bpm) to moderate (11 - 25 bpm)
ACCELS	may be present

Discussion

Parer (331) suggested there were two types of late decel patterns: those with STV and those without STV. When the FHR pattern has been normal and an acute hypoxic event occurs, such as maternal hypotension or the beginning of a placental abruption, late decels may be the first sign of a problem. STV is still present, signifying adequate fetal compensation and maintenance of cerebral O_2 intake (see Figure 2.57). The fetus is stressed but has not decompensated. Actions should be taken to increase fetal oxygenation. The physician should be notified of all assessments, e.g., hypotension, vaginal bleeding, or abdominal pain, the FHR pattern, actions, and fetal and maternal responses to actions. Delivery may be expedited, especially if actions do not alleviate the late decel pattern or if STV decreases.

Hypoxic Myocardial Failure Late Decelerations

Alternative label: "bad" lates

Definition: Late decels with a gradual onset and offset, absent LTV, and diminished or absent STV.

ONSET   gradual, descent of the FHR begins after the contraction begins and reaches the nadir in ≥ 10 seconds

PEAK TO NADIR

LAG TIME	> 18 seconds (25, 29)
OFFSET	**always gradual or slanted**
DEPTH	varies, may be shallow or deep
SHAPE	like a bowl or flattened "U," sometimes a "V"
BL	may be tachycardic
STV	**diminished or absent**
LTV	absent
ACCELS	absent

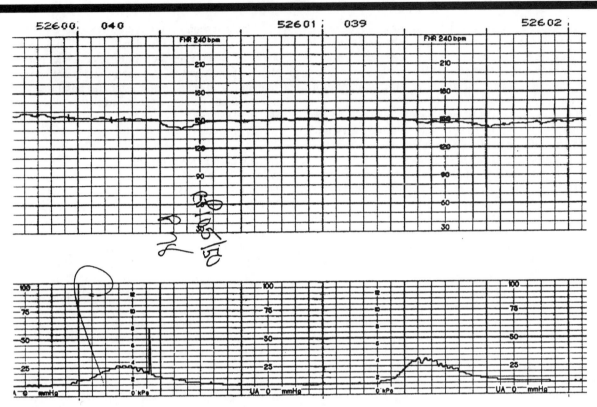

Figure 2.56: Subtle late decelerations. A G_2P_1 woman at term who smokes $1^1/2$ packs per day presented at 4 cm for a trial of labor. She delivered an 8 lb 6 ounce female (VBAC) at 2128 (more than 3 hours after this tracing). Her temperature was 100.3⁰ F at 2030 and there was clear amniotic fluid. Apgar scores were 1, 6, and 9 at 1, 5, and 10 minutes. Meconium was noted at delivery. The baby had a "prolonged stay" in the special care nursery.

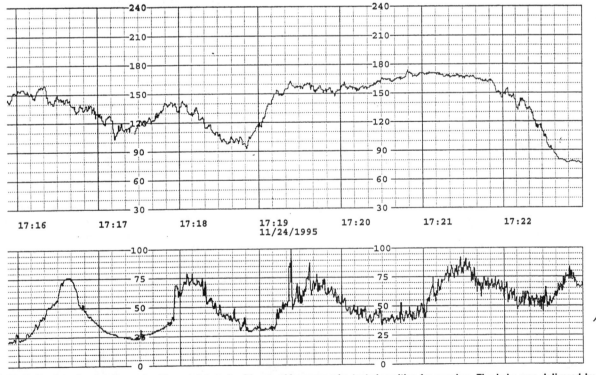

Figure 2.57: Reflex late decelerations of a 35 week fetus of a 27 year old woman who tested positive for cocaine. The baby was delivered by vacuum extraction with Apgar scores of 3, 5, and 8 at 1, 5, and 10 minutes. Note uterine hyperstimulation.

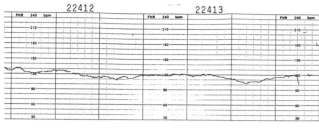

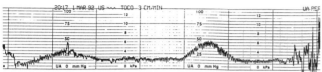

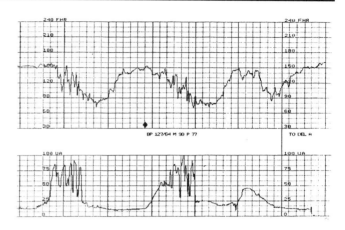

Figure 2.58: Hypoxic myocardial failure late decelerations *are ominous and require expeditious delivery to avoid fetal and neonatal morbidity and mortality.* A woman who was 39^1/2 weeks pregnant presented to labor and delivery with ruptured membranes x 4 days and 1 cm dilatation. She was given a pitocin augmentation. Bradycardia developed. The 8 lb 13^1/2 ounce baby was delivered by low forceps but was stillborn. Cord blood cultures were negative.

Figure 2.59: Two late/variable decelerations of a 39 week fetus of a G_2P_1 single 32 year old woman who admitted to alcohol abuse and smoking 12 packs of cigarettes a week. The baby was delivered by low forceps with Apgar scores of 5, 8, and 9. The placenta was stained with meconium. The cord pH values were 7.22 (artery) and 7.26 (vein). Based on her history, both cord compression and uteroplacental insufficiency could contribute to the creation of this pattern.

Discussion

Parer (331) describes this pattern as "late decelerations with virtually absent FHR variability" (see Figure 2.58). This pattern reflects myocardial failure and decreased cerebral oxygenation. Scalp blood pH will be abnormally low and the fetus should be delivered without hesitation, unless, of course, delivery by cesarean section would jeopardize the life of the woman, e.g., she has a coagulopathy.

Late/Variable Decelerations

Alternative label: severe late decels

Definition: Deep late decels with a gradual onset and usually an abrupt offset.

Recognition Criteria:

ONSET	gradual, reaching the nadir in ≥ 30 seconds
PEAK TO NADIR	
LAG TIME	> 18 seconds (25, 29)
OFFSET	**usually abrupt**
DEPTH	deep, > 50 bpm, may drop to 60 bpm (312)
SHAPE	U or V shape, never a W shape
BL	will become bradycardic if intervention is delayed
STV	present or absent
LTV	usually absent to minimal (3 - 5 bpm)
ACCELS	absent

Discussion

If decels meet the recognition criteria of late decels, they should be documented as late decels. Late/variable decels are recorded as late decels in the notes, even though cord compression may be related to the FHR pattern, e.g., during the second stage with pushing efforts. Cord compression is suspected when the descent is jagged (see Figure 2.59) versus smooth. Smooth late/variable decels are usually found in fetuses of women who have severe preeclampsia. Look at the BL to decide the significance of the pattern. If there is STV, the reflex late/variable decels are aggressively treated. If there is absent STV, the hypoxic myocardial failure late/variable decels should prompt delivery of the fetus.

Actions in Response to Late Decelerations

In addition to actions in response to any abnormal FHR pattern:

Determine the probable etiology of uteroplacental insufficiency and fetal hypoxia:

- the woman
  - assess vital signs, hypotensive? tachycardic?
  - urine toxicology screen if illicit drug use is suspected (70-71, 332)
- her uterus
  - hyperstimulation as a result of an oxytocic? abruption?
  - uterine rupture?
- the placenta
  - inspect color, amount, and odor of amniotic fluid, meconium?
  - vaginal bleeding, pain, abruption?

Act to:

- increase fetal oxygenation, including administration of 8 to 10 liters of O_2 per minute via a tight-fitting face mask (319)
- remove or wash out prostaglandin gel, e.g., the open end of IV tubing which is attached to a bag of normal saline

or lactated Ringer's solution may be inserted into the vagina. Then, the IV flow rate is increased. The tubing acts like a small hose and washes out the vagina. Clinicians have also used a Fleet's enema® or wet 4 x 4 gauze to remove prostaglandin gel.

- maintain a continuous tracing, which may include adjustment of the ultrasound transducer, tocotransducer, application of a spiral electrode, or insertion of an IUPC (62)

Communicate:
- maternal assessments and actions
- FHR pattern, including presence or absence of accels and STV
- fetal response to actions

The physician may choose to deliver the fetus by cesarean section if:
- STV is absent or
- fetal well-being cannot be confirmed, i.e., scalp pH studies indicate a pH less than 7.20 or
- the fetus does not respond to efforts to improve oxygen delivery and the FHR pattern worsens
- an abruption is diagnosed and vaginal birth is not imminent

After delivery:
- umbilical cord or placental gases may be obtained
- the placenta may be sent to pathology for analysis.

Discussion
In 1970, it was believed that the persistence of late decels was an indication for delivery (89). In 1987 and 1988, it was felt that if late decels persisted following measures to maximize fetal oxygenation, preparations should be made for expeditious delivery (324, 333-334). In 1988, a time frame between initiation of actions and delivery was suggested, i.e., *"Late decelerations not responsive to O$_2$, IV fluids, and positional changes should be treated aggressively with delivery within 1 hour of their occurrence...if a patient is followed conservatively, i.e., labor is allowed to continue, a full acid-base profile of the fetus should be readily available"* (335, p. 281).

A review of maternal high-risk conditions, and an assessment of maternal habits, such as smoking and illicit drug use, will prepare clinicians for the possibility of late decels. Late decels are usually a response to hypoxia. Therefore, late decels are a call for action, but not necessarily a cesarean section. When there is a pattern of late decels (five or more), women should be hyperoxygenated (see Chapter 7 for other actions that improve fetal oxygen delivery).

Common characteristics of late deceleration patterns.
All late decels have a gradual onset, reaching their nadir in 30 or more seconds. All late decels have a lag time of 18 or more seconds between the peak of the contraction and the nadir of the decel. But, late decels may be present with or without STV. Some late decels are shallow, others are deep. If a tocotransducer is used, the FHR return to BL is an irrele-

vant recognition criteria since the end of the contraction is not clear with a "toco" in place. *A spiral electrode and/or IUPC are not necessary to identify and document late decels if the onset to nadir, lag time, and shape of the decel meet recognition criteria.*

There are two mechanisms that cause late decels: a vagal response and direct myocardial depression. In animal experiments, the vagal component of late decels was abolished by atropine administration. But, if metabolic acidosis was present, late decels still appeared.

There are four classifications or "types" of late decels: subtle, reflex, hypoxic myocardial failure, and late/variables. Late decels are usually curvilinear, but some may look "boxy," like a U, or like a V. If the BL has STV, the late decel pattern is a reflex late decel pattern. Reflex late decel patterns often contain accels. If there is no STV, the pattern is called hypoxic myocardial failure lates. There may be subtle reflex lates or late/variable reflex lates. Conversely, there may be subtle hypoxic myocardial failure lates or late/variable hypoxic myocardial failure lates. All are documented as "late decels" with the rest of the systematic review.

All late decel patterns should prompt immediate action to improve fetal oxygenation to treat hypoxia and prevent metabolic acidosis (336). Signs of fetal well-being, such as STV and spontaneous accels should be documented (50). A reflex late decel pattern is usually caused by an acute event, such as maternal hypotension. When reflex lates are noted, BP and MHR should be assessed. If the FHR pattern improves and late decels disappear, the O$_2$ mask may be removed, the IV infusion may be returned to its normal rate, and oxytocin administration may be resumed. Usually oxytocin is restarted at half the mU/minute that existed when the infusion was discontinued.

Hypoxic myocardial failure late decels, with the absence of STV and LTV, require expeditious delivery. The lack of STV and back-to-back late decels suggests an abruption. Measures to maximize fetal oxygenation should be instituted and the physician and operating team should be paged to come to the unit stat. Preparations should also be made for neonatal resuscitation. If possible, a physician who can manage neonatal complications should be present at the birth. An example of appropriate nursing documentation under these circumstances might be:

date/time   "late decels, 0 STV, 0 LTV, 0 accels, uterine hyperstim, no vag. bleeding, c/o intense abd pain, pit dc'd, to L side, IV bolus LR, O$_2$ 10 LPM, Dr. — notified of FHR and maternal pain, requested to come to L & D stat. CRNA — called. NBN notified of impending birth, pedi requested. Nurse's signature."

The abbreviations in this note represent the following words:

decels	decelerations
STV	short-term variability
LTV	long-term variability
accels	accelerations
hyperstim	hyperstimulation

vag.	vaginal
c/o	complains of
abd	abdominal
pit	pitocin
dc'd	discontinued
L	left
IV	intravenous
LR	lactated Ringer's solution
O_2	oxygen
LPM	liters per minute (or liters per mask)
Dr.	doctor
FHR	fetal heart rate
L & D	labor and delivery
CRNA	certified registered nurse anesthetist
NBN	newborn nursery
pedi	pediatrician.

(See appendix for additional abbreviations).

VARIABLE DECELERATIONS

Definitions:
• transient decrease in the FHR with a U, V, or W shape.
• decels lasting at least 15 seconds, decreasing 15 or more bpm with a U, V, or W shape.

Recognition Criteria:

ONSET	abrupt, may be a jagged slope to nadir usually in less than 30 seconds
DEPTH	varies
NADIR	If periodic: over contraction peak, if nonperiodic, after contraction peak or between contractions
OFFSET	usually abrupt, a slow recovery (> 30 seconds) suggests myocardial depression
SHAPE	U, V, or W

Shoulders
Alternative labels:
• primary and secondary acceleratory phases of the deceleration pattern
• compensatory acceleratory phases

Recognition Criteria:
• will precede and/or follow a variable decel if the umbilical vein is compressed
• usually increases ≤ 20 bpm x ≤ 20 seconds

Cause(s)/Physiology:
• mild cord compression
• umbilical vein occlusion causing
• "mild" hypoxia and hypotension
• chemoreceptor and baroreceptor activation
• sympathetic nerve stimulus.

Discussion
A shoulder is not an accel. It is an acceleratory phase of the deceleration pattern. It should not be documented as an accel. "Shoulders" are a compensatory sign and indicate an intact fetal CNS. "Variable decels with shoulders" are descriptive, commonly used words, which may be documented. Otherwise, documentation might include cumbersome language such as, "variable decels with primary and secondary acceleratory phases." When the variable decel is *preceded and followed* by a shoulder, it has been called a classic, pure, or typical variable deceleration.

Overshoots
Alternative label: rebound accel (62)
This alternative label should be avoided in documentation as it is poorly defined in the literature and may confuse the reader. *An overshoot is not an accel.* An overshoot is "attached" to the variable decel and is part of a variable decel pattern.

Definitions:
• a rebound increase in the FHR following a variable decel.
• "a shoulder with epinephrine on board."

Recognition Criteria:
• immediately following a variable decel the FHR
  • rises 20 or more bpm above the BL or
  • rises above the BL for more than 20 seconds.

Cause(s)/Physiology:
• *significant* hypoxemia or hypoxia (337-338)
• activated adrenal glands (337)
• catecholamine release (264, 289, 338).

Discussion
The variable appearance of variable decels is due to differences in the intensity of cord compression (336, 339). When the umbilical cord was compressed, a "low" fetal pH was associated with:
• a rising BL
• tachycardia
• a decrease in BL variability and/or
• recurrent overshoots (62)

Overshoots are a nonreassuring sign (289). The physician should be notified of the FHR pattern, particularly when STV is absent and/or the BL is rising. Measures to improve fetal oxygenation are required.

Cause(s)/Physiology of Variable Decelerations
• fetal head compression, cord compression, or seizures
• most commonly associated with umbilical cord compression due to oligohydramnios, loss of amniotic fluid after rupture of membranes, or cord malposition (165, 324, 340-341)
• head compression and cord compression during the second stage of labor (336, 342)
• cord compression occurs in 1/3rd to 50% of all labors (61, 288, 340)

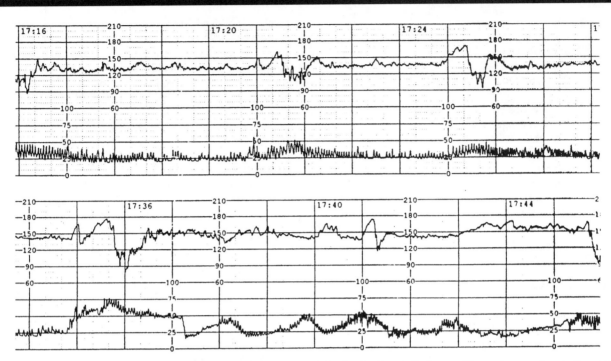

Figure 2.60: Variable decelerations with "shoulders" in a 41 week fetus. The variable decelerations in the top panel have primary and secondary acceleratory phases or shoulders. The variable decelerations in the bottom panel only have primary shoulders. There was a "very short cord." Delivery was by cesarean section. Apgar scores were 8 and 9 at 1 and 5 minutes.

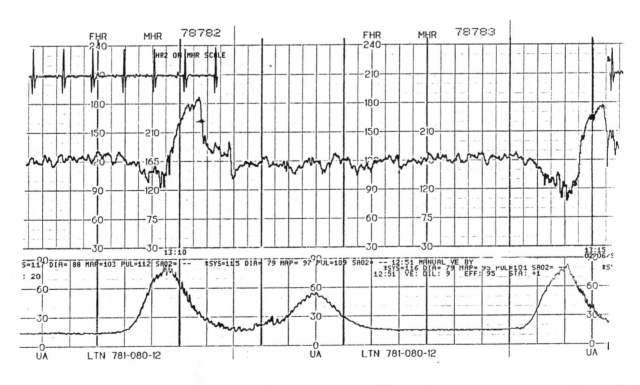

Figure 2.61: Variable decelerations with overshoots. Some overshoots "shoot up" and are more than 20 bpm above the baseline. Others "shoot out" and last more than 20 seconds. The 37 week fetus of a low-risk G_2P_1 woman had two loops of nuchal cord. The baby was delivered by low forceps with Apgar scores of 9 and 9 at 1 and 5 minutes. Although overshoots are part of a nonreassuring pattern because they reflect fetal compensation for hypoxia, the presence of short-term variability suggests the fetus is not metabolically acidotic and has adequate cerebral perfusion.

- a decrease in transcutaneous PO_2 and PaO_2, increase in PCO_2, decrease in pH, and activation of chemoreceptors and baroreceptors following cord compression (300, 316, 343-346)
- vagotomy (of fetal lambs) abolished variable decels (336)
- a mechanical obstruction of the umbilical cord may cause an abrupt increase in placental resistance, a halt in placental perfusion, and blood moving forward and backward in the umbilical arteries (339)
- after cord compression ceases, the FHR should begin to return to the BL in 8 to 27 seconds and be at the BL level in 3 to 17 seconds, therefore, the offset of most variable decels is abrupt (345)
- uncorrected variable decels have been associated with fetal metabolic acidosis and low Apgar scores (203)
- cord length may be related to variable decels, i.e., a short cord, 32 to 35 cm or less (12.8 to 14 inches), pulled flat when stretched as the fetus descended was related to variable decels in 63% of labors versus 37% of labors with a normal cord length (347-348)
- a long cord, 80 to 100 cm (32 to 40 inches), was related to cord accidents, inadequate descent, variable decels in 87% of labors (vs. 35% with a normal cord length) (348)
- a long umbilical cord may be related to W-shaped (biphasic) decels when loops of cord are compressed in more than one location in sequence, i.e., the cord is compressed and the FHR falls, then it recovers, but the cord is compressed somewhere else, and the FHR falls again (347)
- a true knot in the cord causes variable decels (348) the incidence of a true knot: none if short cord, 1% if normal length, 3% if long cord (348)
- a nuchal cord causes variable decels the incidence of a nuchal cord: 14% if short cord, 23% if normal length, 53% if long cord (348-349)
- if after acoustic stimulation there is an accel/decel combination, there is probably a nuchal cord (350)
- cord compression may also be associated with a truncal cord, cord around a body part such as the ankles or shoulder, a straight cord, thin cord, or two-vessel cord
- cord prolapse: none if short cord, 0.4% if normal length, 6% if long cord (348)
- an entangled cord increases the risk of meconium release, "abnormal" FHR patterns, operative vaginal delivery, and "mild" umbilical artery acidosis (349)
- entangled cords usually form after 35 weeks of gestation when the cord is 4/5ths as long as the fetus (351)
- entangled cords may resolve in utero prior to birth (351)
- the fetus grasps its cord: acoustic stimulation caused the fetus to drop the cord then fetal hiccups began (352)
- uterine rupture with extrusion of the fetus and cord into the abdomen
- acute inflammation of the umbilical cord with vasoconstriction (353)

- variable decels with a nadir below 60 bpm have been associated with a *vagal arrest* or *temporary asystole* (a transient sinus arrest or temporary cardiac arrest) in fetal animals (354). The FHR returns to the BL when cord compression was relieved (see figure 2.77).
- in the absence of cord prolapse, sudden death during an episode of variable decels is rare (62).

CLASSIFICATION OF VARIABLE DECELERATIONS

Differences in the depth and duration of variable decels have been used in the past to classify variable decels as mild, moderate, and severe (23, 337). If these words are used in documentation to identify decels, hospital protocol or the chart form should describe recognition criteria so that everyone pictures the same decels in their minds when they read the notes. If these criteria are not readily available or documented, it is better to document the duration and depth of variable decels. The time from the nadir to the BL (the recovery time) is rarely documented. When it is slow, e.g., longer than *30* seconds, it may be documented as "recovery to BL x — seconds."

Mild Variable Decelerations
Recognition Criteria:
DURATION   < 30 seconds
NADIR/DEPTH any depth, but not < 70 to 80 bpm

Moderate Variable Decelerations
Recognition Criteria:
DURATION   30 to 60 seconds
NADIR/DEPTH not less than 70 bpm

Severe Variable Decelerations
Recognition Criteria:
DURATION   > 60 seconds
NADIR/DEPTH < 70 bpm when baseline is not tachycardic.

Umbilical cord compression causes fetal hypoxemia (56). As long as tissue O_2 reserves exist, fetal hypoxemia will not progress to tissue hypoxia, acidemia, or acidosis. In fetal lambs, variable decels became deeper and wider during hypoxia and high-voltage electrocortical activity (355). The depth of the variable decel indirectly reflects the degree of fetal hypertension and hypoxia (356). Fetal O_2 reserves become depleted when the FHR is *less than 80 bpm*. Severe variable decels (> 60 seconds and < 70 bpm) were associated with a fetal scalp pH less than 7.20 (105, 153). At the nadir of severe variable decels, there may be a transient vagal arrest or transient complete atrioventricular block which suggests *complete occlusion* of the blood vessels in the umbilical cord. When pressure on the umbilical cord is released, there is a prompt increase in fetal PaO_2, SaO_2, and a prompt decrease in $PaCO_2$ (354).

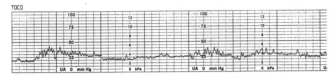

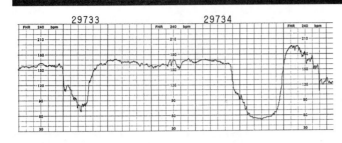

Figure 2.62: Moderate variable deceleration followed by a severe variable deceleration in the fetal heart rate of a term fetus in a G_1P_0 woman who smokes 1/2 pack per day, is 5 ft 4 inches tall, weighs 235 lbs, and has a blood pressure at the time of this pattern of 170/90. A cesarean section was performed for failure to progress. Apgar scores were 6, 9, and 9 at 1, 5, and 10 minutes. Note the overshoot after the severe variable deceleration indicating the fetus has released catecholamines as a compensatory response to hypoxia.

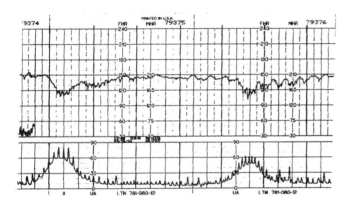

Figure 2.63: Atypical variable decelerations with a "late component." The first deceleration is a better example of this concept than the second deceleration. The fetus delivered vaginally with Apgar scores of 9 and 9 at 1 and 5 minutes.

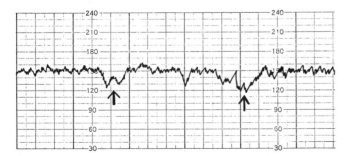

Figure 2.64: Atypical biphasic variable decelerations (above arrows) in a simulated tracing.

TYPICAL VERSUS ATYPICAL VARIABLE DECELERATIONS

Typical Variable Deceleration(s)

Definition: Variable decel(s) with primary and secondary "shoulders."

Alternative labels for typical variable decelerations: classic variable decelerations, pure variable decelerations

ONSET	abrupt drop in the FHR, may be jagged descent, usually reaching the nadir in less than 30 seconds
NADIR/	
LAG TIME	may occur during or after the contraction peak
OFFSET	abrupt
DEPTH	usually nadir $\geq$ 80 bpm
SHAPE	**primary and secondary acceleratory phases ("shoulders") are present**

Discussion

Pure or typical variable decels have a primary "shoulder," rapid deceleration to the nadir, rapid return to BL, and a secondary "shoulder." Adverse neonatal outcomes are uncommon (337).

Atypical Variable Deceleration(s)

Definition: Variable decel(s) that are missing a "shoulder," have a W shape or smooth appearance and/or an overshoot, and do not meet offset criteria for a typical variable decel.

ONSET	abrupt drop in the FHR, may be jagged descent, usually reaching the nadir in less than 30 seconds
NADIR/	
LAG TIME	may occur during or after the contraction peak
OFFSET	may be slow or have a "late component"
DEPTH	any depth
SHAPE	W shape (biphasic) or smooth deceleration or missing one or both shoulders, may have an overshoot
BL	may be at a lower level after the deceleration
STV	may be absent
LTV	may be absent
ACCELS	may be absent

Discussion

A variable decel that begins to recover then flattens out then returns to BL is a variable decel with a "late component"(see Figure 2.63). The late component is *not* a late decel. It is part of the recovery of the FHR. When a variable decel is followed by a late decel, the FHR will reach the BL between the two decels and a mixed decel pattern will exist. A variable decel with a late component is just one decel.

When *atypical* variable decels occurred *during the last 30 minutes of labor*, fetal PO_2 was less than 15 mm Hg. This occurred in 19% of 1,996 labors (337). Atypical variable decels are identified based on their shape. They may have a slow return to BL, be smooth, lack a "shoulder," have an overshoot,

Atypical Variable Decelerations

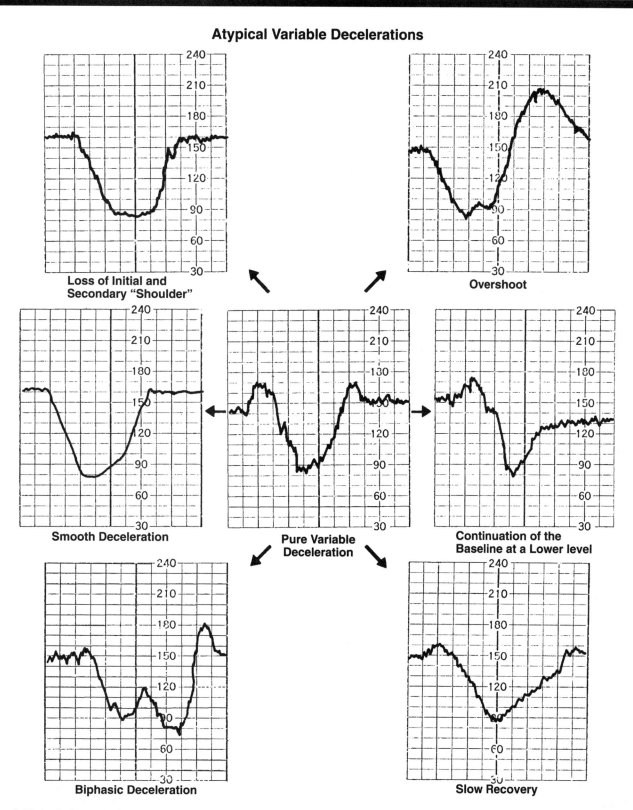

Loss of Initial and Secondary "Shoulder"

Overshoot

Smooth Deceleration

Pure Variable Deceleration

Continuation of the Baseline at a Lower level

Biphasic Deceleration

Slow Recovery

Figure 2.65: Atypical variable decelerations. (Reproduced with permission of the C. V. Mosby Company from Krebs, H. B., Petres, R. E., & Dunn, L. J. (February 1, 1983). Intrapartum fetal heart rate monitoring. VIII. Atypical variable decelerations. *American Journal of Obstetrics and Gynecology, 145*(3), 298). Labels have been modified to conform with this text.

have a BL that returns to a lower level following the decel, have a "late component," or have a W shape. Apgar scores at 1 and 5 minutes were associated with the
- duration of the variable decel
- number of atypical features and
- presence or absence of variability.

The depth and duration of variable decels were less significant in predicting Apgar scores or fetal scalp pH than the presence or absence of BL variability. The incidence of low Apgar scores increased as variability decreased, especially in combination with tachycardia or bradycardia and an increase in the number of atypical features or the duration of the variable decels. *Smooth decels predicted the highest incidence of low one and five minute Apgar scores.* The loss of the initial shoulder, a slow return to BL, and biphasic decels, were the most common findings (337).

Biphasic variable decelerations. Variable decels, which look like a "W" are called biphasic decels (see Figure 2.64). In one study, biphasic variable decels were defined as "2 or more variable decels dropping at least *10* bpm which occur in rapid succession with only a transient return to BL between the 2 decels." The same researchers suggested that W-shaped decels were related to a nuchal cord and an Apgar score less than 7 at 5 minutes (357). However, nuchal cords are common. They are found in up to 25% of all deliveries (358). Nuchal cords may also be associated with other decel shapes and higher Apgar scores. Therefore, it should not be assumed that the presence of biphasic variable decels predicts the presence of a nuchal cord.

Actions in Response to Variable Decelerations
There is a continuum in the fetal response to cord compression ranging from
- uniform accels to
- typical variable decels (with shoulders) to
- atypical variable decels
- a loss of variability and
- bradycardia (359-360).

The nursing response will depend on where the fetus is on this continuum. Since hypercapnia increases the risk of fetal gasping and MAS, when meconium is noted in the amniotic fluid all possible actions should be undertaken to prevent more intense cord compression (361).

In addition to actions in response to any abnormal FHR pattern,
Determine the etiology of variable decels:
- umbilical cord compression?
- fetal head compression?
- fetal seizures?
- ultrasound to confirm fetal seizure activity (see Checkmark Pattern)

Actions reflect the suspected etiology:
If cord compression is suspected, actions *may* include all or part of the following:
- review ultrasound reports, e.g., a straight cord? oligohydramnios? twins?
- change maternal position
- vaginal examination to rule out an umbilical cord prolapse
- IV bolus with a dextrose-free solution
- hyperoxygenate if variable decel nadirs are < 80 bpm
- hyperoxygenation during the second stage of labor does not improve umbilical artery gases if they are in a normal range (362)
- amnioinfusion
- discontinue oxytocics
- bladder inflation (for umbilical cord prolapse)(see Chapter 6)

If head compression is suspected:
- perform a vaginal examination to
  - determine labor progress: second stage?
  - ascertain compression on the fetal head: caput? molding?

If variable decels are deepening (< 80 bpm) and lengthening (≥ 60 seconds):
- maintain a continuous tracing
- apply a spiral electrode and/or insert an IUPC
- prepare for neonatal resuscitation (363)

Communicate:
- maternal assessments
- actions

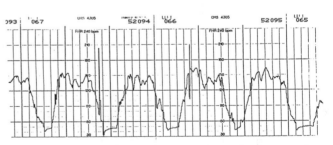
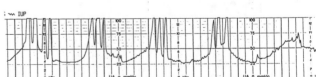

Figure 2.66: Documentation of moderate variable decelerations may be "var. decels x 40 - 45 seconds ↓ 35 - 45 bpm, prompt recovery, STV+, LTV moderate." Note the woman is pushing. These are second-stage variable decelerations and are a combination of umbilical cord torsion (there was a tight nuchal cord) and fetal head compression. The vigorous baby was born within less than 5 minutes of this tracing. Apgar scores were 8 and 8 at 1 and 5 minutes.

- FHR pattern
- fetal response to actions

The physician may choose to deliver the fetus by cesarean section if:
- fetal well-being cannot be confirmed, e.g., the fetus does not respond to acoustic stimulation, scalp stimulation, or the spiral electrode test (see Chapter 6)
- scalp pH values falls below 7.20
- the umbilical cord prolapsed.

After delivery:
- measure and document the umbilical cord length if it looks short or long
- document cord position and appearance, e.g., "tight true knot," "cord over shoulder and around the waist in seatbelt fashion," "thin, two-vessel cord."

Documentation of Variable Decelerations

Early and late decels have clear physiologic implications: early decels are *not* related to hypoxia, late decels are related to hypoxia. Because of their clear significance, it is common to document "early decels" and "late decels" in addition to the rest of the systematic review.

Since variable decels vary in configuration, duration, and depth, it is more common to use abbreviations to document a range of durations and depths. For example, if protocol define mild, moderate, and severe variable decel attributes, the nurse may record, "mod to sev var decels." If these criteria are not defined in institution protocol or on chart forms, the duration and depth of variable decels should be described. For example, one variable decel might be documented as "var decel x 25 sec ↓ 90 bpm." If more than one variable decel is present, the range of durations and depths may be recorded, e.g., "var decels x 30 - 45 sec, ↓ 80 - 90 bpm." If the recovery to the BL takes more than 30 seconds, it would be considered an abnormal recovery and may be documented, e.g., "var decels x 75 - 100 sec, ↓ 60 - 70 bpm, with return to BL x 30 - 40 seconds." Nurses and physicians should collaborate on nomenclature and abbreviations that should be used in institutional documentation (364).

AMNIOINFUSION

Definition: controlled intrauterine instillation of sterile normal saline or lactated Ringer's solution.

Intrapartal amnioinfusion was first described by Miyazaki and Taylor in 1983. IV fluid was infused into the uterus through an IUPC for the treatment of recurrent variable decels during the first stage of labor (365). Additionally, it has been done to dilute thick meconium.

Requirements Prior to Intrapartal Amnioinfusion
- vaginal examination to rule out an umbilical cord prolapse and to determine dilatation and presentation
- rupture of membranes, which increases the risk of cord compression (366)
- insertion of an IUPC and possibly a spiral electrode (367).

Indications
Transcervical Amnioinfusion (During Labor):
- oligohydramnios, with an amniotic fluid index (AFI) of 5 cm or less (368-369)
- premature rupture of the membranes (369-371)
- dilution of thick, particulate meconium (372-373)
- repetitive variable decels or prolonged decels during the first stage of labor (368, 374)
- instillation of antibiotics after rupture of membranes (375).

Transabdominal Amnioinfusion (Prior to Labor):
- diagnostic amnioinfusion, e.g., to aid in the ultrasonographic diagnosis of a fetus with bilateral renal agenesis (Potter's syndrome) (376-377)
- 250 ml was infused over 20 minutes via a 22 gauge needle under ultrasound guidance (378).

Type of Fluid for Amnioinfusion
- sterile normal saline (370)
- sterile lactated Ringer's solution (379)
- a sterile solution that contained dextrose has *only* been used under experimental conditions and is not recommended for use. A dextrose solution was infused into the uterus of 18 women under experimental conditions, and it did not affect neonatal glucose levels (380). In another report, 200 ml of 5% glucose was infused into the uterus (transabdominal amnioinfusion) for marked oligohydramnios, IUGR, and bilateral renal agenesis (381). A dextrose solution heightens the risk of intrauterine infection.

Amount of Fluid Infused
Transabdominal (Antepartal) Amnioinfusion:
- 200 to 500 ml (382)

Transcervical (Intrapartal) Amnioinfusion:
- 10 to 20 ml/hour for premature rupture of the membranes (PROM) when immediate delivery is not desirable and there is oligohydramnios from continuous leakage of amniotic fluid (371)
- 250 to 800 ml initial bolus over 15 to 60 minutes (359, 367, 369)
- average initial bolus was 600 ml, followed by a continuous infusion of 180 ml (383)
- Miyazaki (367) recommended that there should never be an infusion of more than 800 ml at any one time
- Wenstrom and Parsons (372) instilled 1000 ml of normal saline over 20 to 40 minutes
- 250 ml increased the AFI an average of 4 to 5.8 cm if it was ≤ 5 cm prior to the amnioinfusion (369, 384)
- the initial bolus should be decreased 25 to 30% if the fetus is less than 32 weeks' gestation (385)
- initial bolus may be followed by
  - ultrasound evaluation (367)
  - continuous amnioinfusion at 60 to 180 ml/hour (367, 383)
  - another 250 ml bolus (367).

118

Some researchers believe the persistence of variable decels after instillation of 800 ml is an indication that amnioinfusion will not improve the FHR pattern (374).

Ultrasound Prior to the Initial Bolus

Amnioinfusion is more successful in decreasing the number of variable decels when the AFI is 8 cm or less prior to amnioinfusion (386). Therefore, many physicians perform an ultrasound before amnioinfusion begins. The deepest vertical cord-free pocket in each of the four uterine quadrants is measured and added to calculate the AFI. If the AFI was less than 5 cm, 500 ml of warmed saline was instilled. If the AFI was 5 to 10 cm, 250 ml of warmed saline were infused (387). Some titrate the amnioinfusion, with the help of serial AFIs, to maintain the AFI at 8 or more cm throughout labor (388).

Contraindications
- placenta previa
- a need to avoid amniotomy, e.g., in a preterm gestation
- "distress" (378)
- vaginal bleeding, especially if an abruption is suspected (378)
- tachycardia ≥ 180 bpm
- late decels and absent variability
- a nonvertex presentation (378, 389).

Oligohydramnios is a sign of insufficient placental function (96). If oligohydramnios is associated with signs of abruption or fetal metabolic acidosis, amnioinfusion should be discontinued or not started and the fetus should be expeditiously delivered.

Benefits
Transabdominal Amnioinfusion:
For diagnostic purposes:
- aids visualization of the fetus
- enables the practitioner to define the cause of oligohydramnios (390)

For oligohydramnios:
- in 16 women with oligohydramnios and transabdominal amnioinfusion, there were no cesarean sections, no "cord" pH values less than 7.20, and no 5 minute Apgar scores less than 7. In 15 women who had oligohydramnios but did *not* have an amnioinfusion, there were 2 cesarean sections, 3 babies with "cord" pH values less than 7.20, and 1 with an Apgar score less than 7 at 5 minutes of age (378)
- indicated in term women *with oligohydramnios* whose cervical Bishop's score is 6 or less (unripe cervix) with a singleton pregnancy and vertex presentation, a reactive NST, estimated fetal weight by ultrasound of 2500 or more gm, and *intact membranes.* There were as many spontaneous vaginal births in the transabdominal amnioinfused group as the group without amnioinfu-

sion. However, there were fewer "abnormal" patterns during labor and fewer cesarean sections for "fetal distress" in the amnioinfused group (391).

Transcervical Amnioinfusion:
- fewer variable decels during the first stage of labor (359, 368, 370, 392)
- decreased incidence of end-stage bradycardia (359)
- higher one minute Apgar scores (372)
- fewer forceps deliveries (372)
- fewer cesarean sections for "fetal distress" (359, 372, 383, 393)
- higher umbilical artery pH than if no amnioinfusion was provided (393-394)
- when there was PROM prior to 35 weeks of gestation, umbilical vein and artery pH values were higher when women were amnioinfused (358)
- when thick meconium was present, umbilical artery pH was significantly *higher* in the amnioinfused group (395)
- decreased incidence of meconium below the vocal cords, e.g., 4.2% in the amnioinfused group versus 62.1% if there was no amnioinfusion or 18.2% if amnioinfused and 29.1% if not (372, 383, 395-397, 394-398)
- fewer babies with MAS, e.g., 2.1% versus 13.8% (359, 372, 396, 399)
- decreased incidence of neonatal respiratory distress and resuscitation (359, 394)
- in women with oligohydramnios: fewer maternal and neonatal hospital days (400)
- amnioinfusion of normal saline did not affect neonatal electrolytes (359, 401).

Limitations
Most prospective, randomized controlled studies of amnioinfusion were performed with term fetuses. Therefore, data is limited on the effects of fluid warming on preterm fetuses or the use of an IV pump versus gravity flow. In pregnancies near term or term, warming the fluid and an IV pump offered no additional benefits (383).

Transabdominal Amnioinfusion:
- when there was oligohydramnios, amnioinfusion altered uteroplacental perfusion and increased the resistance index and pulsatility index in the uterine artery but did not affect the incidence of fetal breathing movements (402-403)
- "severe" chorioamnionitis in 4 of 22 women (18.18%) (382)
- "clinical" chorioamnionitis in 2 of 89 women (2.25%) (404)

Transcervical Amnioinfusion:
Mixed scalp blood pH and blood gas findings:
- no difference or improvement in fetal scalp pH, even though there were fewer "abnormal" FHR patterns, between the amnioinfused group and women who did

not receive an amnioinfusion (372, 405)
- no significant difference in umbilical cord blood gases in the amnioinfused group versus women who did not have an amnioinfusion (359, 406)
- doesn't abolish variable decels during the second stage of labor as decels reflect a vagal stimulus from fetal head compression (336)
- no decrease in MAS (383)

In a 1994 study of 440 women who were amnioinfused due to thick meconium, and 497 who were not, there were fewer neonatal deaths but *no statistically significant decrease in the incidence of MAS* (407).
- following a historical review of medical records at a large medical institution, there was no decrease in the incidence of MAS after instituting amnioinfusion compared to the incidence of MAS prior to the use of amnioinfusion (408).

Complications of Amnioinfusion
- *chorioamnionitis*
The presence of meconium significantly increases the risk of infection (409-410). *When membranes are ruptured, the maternal temperature and heart rate should be assessed at least every two hours.*

- *uterine hypertonus*
During amnioinfusion, resting tone increases (367, 411). For example, 55 to 500 ml of normal saline increased resting tone an average of 4.7 mm Hg. *Assess and record uterine resting tone and the FHR at least every half hour* during an amnioinfusion. Hypertonus with or without fetal bradycardia suggests overdistention (389, 412-414).

- *uterine overdistention (iatrogenic hydramnios)*
Overdistention was related to iatrogenic polyhydramnios and umbilical cord prolapse (383, 412, 415). Amniotic fluid pressure was significantly increased when the deepest pocket of amniotic fluid was greater than 15 cm, but it was normal when the pocket was less than 15 cm (416). To prevent overdistention, *intrauterine intake and output should be determined.* Intake may be recorded every hour. Output will be recorded when the underpad is changed. The underpad may be weighed and the weight of a dry underpad should be deducted from the weight of the wet underpad. One ml of fluid weighs approximately 1 gram.

- *maternal cardiac or respiratory compromise*
Maternal distress may be the result of an acute increase in intrauterine volume (410, 417). The overexpanded uterus may apply pressure against the diaphragm. *Maternal comfort should be assessed* during the amnioinfusion. Any complaint of shortness of breath, hypotension, or tachycardia should be followed by immediate discontinuation of the amnioinfusion and assessment of MHR, BP, and respiratory rate. The

certified nurse midwife or physician should be asked to evaluate the woman.

- *fetal bradycardia*
Fetal bradycardia may occur with the *rapid infusion of* cool, room temperature fluid. Fetal bradycardia may also be the result of maternal distress. For example, uterine hypertonus, with a resting tone of greater than 50 mm Hg, occurred when more than 4300 ml was infused into the uterus. The FHR dropped to 70 bpm. The FHR recovered after 900 ml was removed from the uterus (389). To remove fluid from the uterus, the physician may apply pressure to the presenting part to lift it up. This procedure should be performed by a physician with cesarean section privileges in case the umbilical cord prolapses.

Nursing actions in response to fetal bradycardia during an amnioinfusion include:
- discontinuation of the amnioinfusion and, if applicable, the oxytocic infusion
- lateral or an upright position
- a vaginal examination to confirm the lack of an umbilical cord prolapse
- an IV bolus with a dextrose-free solution
- hyperoxygenation with a tight-fitting face mask at 8 to 10 liters per minute
- determination of uterine resting tone
- assessment of maternal BP if hypotension is suspected
- evaluation of intrauterine intake and output
- notification of the certified nurse midwife and/or physician of assessments, actions, and maternal and fetal responses.

Trial of Labor After Cesarean (TOLAC) and Amnioinfusion
Amnioinfusion does not increase the risk of uterine rupture but it does decrease the chance of a successful vaginal birth after a cesarean section (VBAC). Strong and his colleagues (418) amnioinfused 122 women who were undergoing a trial of labor. Only 58.2% delivered vaginally. One woman's uterine scar separated. Cook, Roy, and Spinnato (419) found an *increased rate of endomyometritis* (12.5% versus 1.9%) in women undergoing amnioinfusion during a TOLAC compared to women who were not amnioinfused. Women were *also less likely to have a VBAC* if they received an amnioinfusion (70.5% VBAC rate versus 86.7% if there was no amnioinfusion). Six of the 146 women who were undergoing a TOLAC and who received an amnioinfusion had a uterine scar separation (4.1%). But this was not statistically different than scar separation in women who did not have an amnioinfusion. Therefore, although uterine rupture should always be a concern in a woman undergoing a TOLAC, *the rate of uterine rupture was not greater in these women than women undergoing a trial of labor who did not have an amnioinfusion* (387). It is not clear why amnioinfusion would decrease the chance of delivering vaginally. Perhaps, it is related

to dysfunctional labor due to intrauterine infection or the need to perform a cesarean section for fetal signs of infection.

Uterine Rupture is Not a Risk of Intrapartal Amnioinfusion
It was thought that amnioinfusion might increase the risk of uterine rupture (410). However, the rate of uterine rupture did not increase in women undergoing a TOLAC (418-419). The risk of uterine rupture only increased if amnioinfusion included instillation of prostaglandins or hypertonic saline for midtrimester abortion (420).

Amnioinfusion and Amniotic Fluid Embolism
Amniotic fluid embolism (AFE) occurred in women who received an amnioinfusion. While some have speculated possible reasons for the AFE, no conclusions regarding the role of IV pumps in this complication could be made based on a meta-analysis of 14 prospective studies (383).

AFE has less "lethality" when amniotic fluid has a low particulate concentration and lacks meconium. During the first trimester, amniotic fluid lacks protein and particulate matter and consists of approximately 50 ml (421). Therefore, it comes as no surprise that there have been no cases of AFE reported during the first trimester.

Women who were 13 or more weeks pregnant have had an AFE. They had to have had *disruption of the membranes, open uterine or cervical blood vessels, and a pressure gradient to drive fluid into their circulation* (422-423). Stromme and Fromke (424) reported a case of AFE following uterine evacuation for a missed abortion.

Between 26 and 40 weeks of gestation, AFE has occurred:
- prior to labor due to cord entanglement and abruption with a marginal tear of the membranes (425)
- during hypertonic saline-induced abortion (426)
- after preterm PROM (427)
- within two minutes of insertion of an IUPC
- during delivery of the baby's head through the abdomen (428)
- after vaginal birth before delivery of the placenta (429)
- during a cesarean section as the baby was being delivered (428)
- 7 hours after a cesarean section (430) and
- after a cesarean hysterectomy for placenta previa with placenta accreta (431).

AFE has never been reported on the day following delivery.

AFE in the United States occurs in 1 in 20,000 to 30,000 live births (432). In Sweden, AFE occurred in 1 in 83,000 live births (433). One could speculate that AFE may be related to differences in obstetric practice between the United States and Sweden, differences in women or their amniotic fluid content, differences in criteria used to diagnose AFE, or differences in data collection techniques. Clark, Hankins, Dudley, Dildy, and Porter (434) reviewed 46 cases of AFE that occurred in the United States and found the following:

- no definitive predisposing factors
- 70% occurred during labor
- 69% had clear amniotic fluid
- 67% had a male fetus
- 61% maternal and fetal mortality
- 41% had a history of a drug allergy
- 30% of women seized
- 27% had dyspnea
- 17% had fetal bradycardia
- 13% were related to the insertion of an IUPC near the time of onset of symptoms
- 13% had hypotension
- 12% had intact membranes
- 1 woman had sepsis
- 1 woman had an unrecognized uterine rupture
- 1 woman became cyanotic.

Amniotic fluid contains fetal squamous cells, mucin, and lanugo. During pregnancy, fetal squamous cells routinely enter the venous circulation of pregnant women. These substances have been found in blood obtained from women who did not have an AFE (421). AFE does not occur until whole amniotic fluid-derived humoral substances, such as leukotrienes, enter maternal circulation which probably triggers a massive immune response (421, 427, 435-437).

Signs and symptoms of AFE include:
- nausea and vomiting
- abdominal cramps or pain
- anxiety
- tachypnea
- dyspnea
- light-headedness
- hypotension
- shock
- cyanosis
- unresponsiveness
- a grand mal seizure
- cardiopulmonary collapse (cardiac arrest) and
- disseminated intravascular coagulopathy (DIC) (427, 430, 438-440).

A convulsion suggests emboli entered cerebral vessels causing hypoxia. Emboli in pulmonary vessels limit the effectiveness of tracheal intubation and ventilation (428). DIC, the result of a severe hemodynamic disturbance, occurs in approximately 40% of women who have an AFE. Hemorrhage, a complication of DIC, further compromises tissue oxygenation. Histamine, bradykinin, cytokines, prostaglandins, leukotrienes, and thromboxane have been implicated in the pathophysiology of AFE (434). Bradykinin is related to vasodilation and hypotension. Prostaglandins cause uterine hyperstimulation and hypertonus. Leukotrienes and vasoactive substances with thromboplastin-like properties found in amniotic fluid probably trigger DIC (440). Collagen in amniotic fluid may activate platelets (431).

The Phases of AFE

AFE occurs in two phases that are *clinically identical to anaphylaxis* and pulmonary arteriolar spasm (441). AFE presents like "shock lung" syndrome (431). It happens without forewarning. There is no test for hypersensitivity to amniotic fluid.

Phase I. During phase I, pulmonary capillary wedge pressure and pulmonary artery pressure increase due to increased pulmonary vascular resistance and pulmonary hypertension. Right ventricular failure occurs with decreased blood flow to the lungs. The clinician will note

- tachypnea
- tachycardia
- uterine hyperstimulation and hypertonus
- fetal bradycardia and
- possibly a maternal seizure. All this can occur within 17 minutes or less.

Phase II. During phase II, there is left ventricular failure with a decrease in left ventricular stroke volume (442). The clinician observes

- hypotension and
- cardiorespiratory collapse.

Because emboli are in pulmonary vessels, immediate intubation, hyperventilation, and cardiopulmonary resuscitation (CPR) may not improve maternal oxygenation. In fact, SpO_2 will be near 80% in spite of all efforts to raise it. DIC and hemorrhage further compromise oxygenation.

Modified response to AFE. Isolated, fatal DIC in pregnant women who did not have hypotension, hypoxia, or other events or disease processes associated with AFE may be a *forme fruste* of AFE. In 8 women (1 with triplets, 2 with twins, and 5 with singletons), acute hemorrhage in the postpartum period (7/8) and intrapartal period (1/8) occurred. Six of the 8 exsanguinated and died despite appropriate management. In 3 of the 4 women who were autopsied, evidence of an AFE was found (443). AFE is confirmed during autopsy when fetal epithelial squames and lanugo are found in blood vessels in the cervix (after hysterectomy) or capillaries of the woman's lungs. Pulmonary edema will also be evident (441, 444-445).

Factors Associated with AFE

Researchers have been interested in factors associated with AFE.

Oxytocin. Some believe oxytocics are *not* related to AFE and that evidence that vigorous labor or hypertonic contractions are associated with AFE is based on anecdotal reports (434, 442). However, the possible contribution of oxytocics to the occurrence of AFE cannot be ignored.

For example, in Singapore between 1983 and 1992, 10 women died of AFE. Three (30%) had a labor induction or augmentation, 5 had an emergency cesarean section, and 3 of the 10 had a uterine rupture (440). AFE has occurred following induction with prostaglandins and Syntocinon® (an oxytocic) (446). In Sweden between 1951 and 1980, 38 women had a fatal AFE. Twenty (52.6%) received oxytocin during labor (433). In Sweden, AFE was also *related to*:

- polyhydramnios
- placental abruption
- *hypertonic labor*
- rupture of the birth canal
- macrosomia and
- fundal pressure (433).

Table 14: Case Reports of Amniotic Fluid Embolism Associated with Amnioinfusion

Researcher	Solution	IV Pump?	Meconium	Other Information
Maher (449) (2 confirmed cases)	NS 750 ml given over 1.5 hrs	*yes*	*yes*	*Rapid labor*, bradycardia, and hypotension 3 hrs after start of amnioinfusion and 12 minutes after *epidural* fentanyl, maternal death.
	NS	*yes* 125 ml/hr total 1800 ml	*yes*	*102° F, epidural* prior to cesarean for failure to progress, seizure, maternal death.
Dibble (421) (2 cases of *possible* AFE)	NS 600 ml given over 45 min.	no mention	no	Preterm labor, *38° C* 1 hr. after starting amnioinfusion, woman became dyspneic, cyanotic, and survived.
	NS 800 ml per hr	no mention	did not say	34 years old, 50 minutes after starting amnioinfusion developed dyspnea, hypotension, tachycardia, and survived.

NS = normal saline

AFE is usually lethal due to refractory cardiopulmonary arrest and its sequelae. Sixty-one to 86% of women and 50 to 61% of their fetuses die (434-435). AFE accounts for 10 to 20% of maternal deaths (447). Maternal deaths in Japan between 1964 and 1980 were reviewed. Most women died from hemorrhage. Of 16 women whose deaths were related to drugs such as oxytocin, 6 had an AFE (37.5%), 3 had a uterine rupture, and 2 had a cervical laceration. The remaining 5 deaths were unresolved as to the cause (448). Therefore, while the use of oxytocin may not "cause" an AFE, it is no doubt a dangerous drug that may increase the risk of maternal or fetal demise, especially if it is misused.

Other factors *related to* AFE are:
- preterm labor and maternal fever (38.5º C rectal temperature) (430)
- rupture of membranes (429)
- advanced maternal age (which was not defined) (422, 435)
- multiparity (422, 429, 435)
- a large fetus (422 , 433)
- a "short," tumultuous labor (422)
- fetal demise (435) and
- meconium (435).

Maternal fever is associated with infection. Rupture of membranes increases the risk of an intrauterine infection. Infection is associated with an increase in leukotrienes. Leukotrienes have been implicated in the pathogenesis of AFE. Multiparous women have an increased risk of spontaneous uterine rupture. Uterine rupture has been associated with AFE (440). It is not clear how a large fetus might be related to AFE, however, if the large fetus was a male, there is an association with AFE (434). When the fetus dies in utero, tissue thromboplastins may be released which can trigger DIC.

Meconium, Amnioinfusion, and Amniotic Fluid Embolism
Meconium is particulate. The presence of particulate matter in amniotic fluid heightens the risk of AFE (421). There have been at least 2 women who died from AFE which developed during an amnioinfusion for thick meconium. Normal saline was pumped into the uterus and both women had an epidural. One woman had a fever (see Table 14) (414, 449).

Nursing Response to a Suspected Amniotic Fluid Embolism
The goals of management of the woman who may have an AFE are to
- optimize maternal and fetal perfusion and oxygenation
- maximize maternal cardiac output and BP and
- deliver a live fetus.

If DIC occurs, an additional goal is to correct the coagulopathy (422, 435, 439).

In response to a suspected AFE, the nurse should
- discontinue the amnioinfusion, if applicable
- discontinue or remove any uterine stimulants, e.g., prostaglandin gel
- activate the emergency medical system, e.g., call a code blue
- notify the operating team, obstetrician(s), and neonatal team stat
- bring emergency equipment to the bedside
- apply a pulse oximeter and cardiac monitor
- assist the respiratory therapist, CRNA, or anesthesiologist with maternal intubation and provide O_2 (423, 435)
- assess vital signs, report abnormal findings
- clear the room of all unnecessary persons, beds, and equipment
- someone should stay with the family to explain events
- if an IV line is not in place, begin two IV lines if possible, using large bore catheters, infuse lactated Ringer's solution or normal saline as ordered
- observe for vaginal bleeding and blood which fails to clot
- notify the blood bank of the potential need for blood and blood products
- be prepared to infuse blood and blood products (429)
- transport the woman to the operating room
- assist the physician as requested
- document times, assessments, actions, personnel involved, and maternal and fetal responses.

Should the IV Fluid Used in Amnioinfusion be Warm?
It was believed that a rapid amnioinfusion of a cold solution could cause fetal bradycardia (412). However, warming fluid did not offer any added benefits when women were near term, term, or postterm (383, 392). In the original 1983 report on amnioinfusion by Miyazaki and Taylor, room temperature normal saline was instilled in the uterus (374, 385). In 1985, Miyazaki and Nevarez reported the use of room temperature normal saline which resolved 51% of the variable decels in the amnioinfused group and only 4.2% of the variable decels in the noninfused group (385). Thomas and Nageotte (385) reported amnioinfusion of normal saline at 10 ml/minute for 60 minutes then a continuous infusion of 3 ml/minute for the treatment of PPROM. No mention was made as to whether or not the fluid was warmed. However, at 3 ml/minute, even with room temperature fluid, fetal bradycardia is highly unlikely.

Prospective, randomized, controlled studies are needed to determine the risks and benefits of warm and room temperature fluid. Smith, Jr. and Snider (450) advocated the use of fluid warmed to body temperature. Warmed saline has been used in women who were not in labor and who were undergoing genetic amniocentesis due to "severe" oligohydramnios (451). Warmed saline has also been instilled during labor (387). In one report, fluid for amnioinfusion was warmed by a blanket warmer (413)!

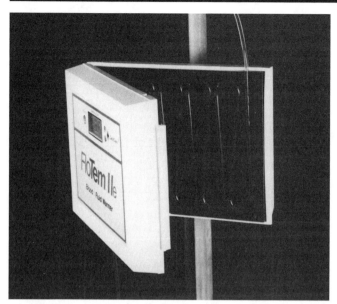

Figure 2.67: The Flo Tem IIe® was an easy to use fluid warmer that attached to an IV pole. A continuously warmed solution was provided during amnioinfusion. (Photograph courtesy of DataChem, Inc. Indianapolis, IN).

About That Blanket Warmer

A blanket warmer was made to warm blankets under steamed heat and bottles of sterile saline and water used in the operating room during cesarean sections. It was not made to warm IV fluid bags! Most blanket warmers don't have a thermometer in them. And, if they do, they are warming blankets to near 120°F! *IV fluid for amnioinfusion should NEVER be stored in the blanket warmer as blanket warmers are usually hotter than the manufacturers' recommendations for storage of IV fluid, i.e., 104° to 115° F* (personal communication from Abbott, November 14, 1994 and Baxter, November 11, 1994).

Dry heat warmers, with a calibrated thermometer, may be used for warming IV fluid bags. They were designed specifically for that purpose. *If IV bags are placed in a dry heat warmer, they should be labeled with the date and time. Heated IV bags stored for 14 or more days must be discarded as the contents of the solution may change.* **IV bags should NEVER be placed in a microwave oven** (personal communication from Abbott, November 14, 1994 and Baxter, November 11, 1994). *Hot fluid may scorch the fetus.* If a blood warmer or infusion warmer are not available, it is safer to use room temperature fluid than the extremely overheated fluid from a blanket warmer or a microwave oven.

A blood/infusion warmer, such as the Flo Tem IIe® (DataChem, Inc. Indianapolis, IN), or a blood warmer, are the only acceptable devices for continuous amnioinfusion of warmed saline or lactated Ringer's solution (see Figure 2.67) (389). The Flo Tem IIe® mounts on an IV pole with a "C" clamp and has aluminum plates with grooves for long IV tubing.

The plates heat to 40° C and can warm saline or blood to 33° C or more if the infusion is at a rate less than 50 ml per minute (452). Even if an infusion/blood warmer is used, if the infusion is very slow, fluid will cool to room temperature between the warming unit and the woman (453). Radiant heat loss occurs between the warming unit and the IUPC as the tubing is exposed to room air. If the tubing is insulated or short, fluid entering the IUPC will be closer to the temperature of the warming unit. Therefore, to realize the maximal benefit of a warming device, tubing should be as short as possible between the warming unit and the IUPC. A rapid infusion carries more heat than a slow infusion, and insulated tubing delivers warmer fluid than exposed tubing (453-454).

Medical and Nursing Responsibilities During Amnioinfusion

The woman should be informed of the risks and benefits of this procedure by her midwife or physician (389). While the midwife or physician are talking to the woman, the nurse can set up the IV bag and tubing. Continuous electronic fetal monitoring is essential. If a continuous ultrasound-derived tracing cannot be maintained, the spiral electrode should be inserted. Vigilant nursing care is required when a woman is receiving an amnioinfusion.

In general, the nurse should:
- monitor maternal comfort
- change the underpad as needed
- provide perineal care
- assess vital signs
  - temperature every two hours
  - BP, MHR, and respiratory rate at least once an hour
- assess uterine activity
- assess the FHR
- record intrauterine intake and output.

It has been recommended that uterine intake and output be assessed and recorded every hour (395). However, if concern exists at any time that fluid is only infusing into the uterus and not flowing out of the uterus, the amnioinfusion should be discontinued and the underpad should be weighed to determine amniotic fluid loss. The weight of a dry linen protector is subtracted from the weight of the wet linen protector.

During the amnioinfusion, uterine resting tone should be documented every 30 minutes. If it is greater than 25 mm Hg, the amnioinfusion may be discontinued until resting tone returns to 25 mm Hg or less (385). Nursing documentation should include the time the IUPC was inserted and by whom, the time the amnioinfusion began and/or was discontinued, the solution used, the rate of infusion, the bolus amount and continuous infusion rate, devices used to regulate and/or warm the solution, maternal and fetal assessments, maternal comfort and care, position changes, intrauterine intake and output,

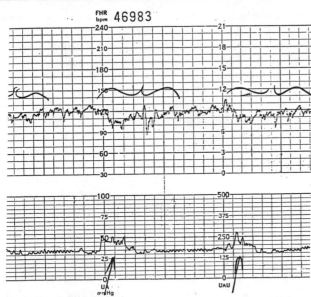

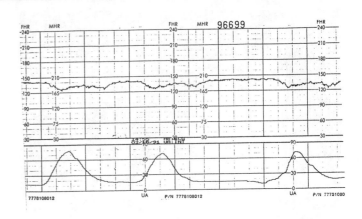

Figure 2.68: Mixed deceleration pattern of early and variable decelerations over first contraction in a postterm fetus with oligohydramnios who was delivered by cesarean section for cephalopelvic disproportion after over 6 hours at 5 cm/0 station. The baby had a cephalhematoma, subdural hemorrhage, normal blood gases, and was later diagnosed with cerebral palsy.

Figure 2.69: Mixed deceleration pattern of early and late decelerations. If the fetus is hypoxic and adenosine levels are high, the decelerations that look like early decelerations could, in fact, be caused by umbilical cord compression. If the vaginal examination does not confirm fetal caput and molding (signs of head compression), these are "blunt" variable decelerations. Fetal acid-base status should be determined. STV is absent or nearly absent. LTV is absent, suggesting hypoxia and possible metabolic acidosis.

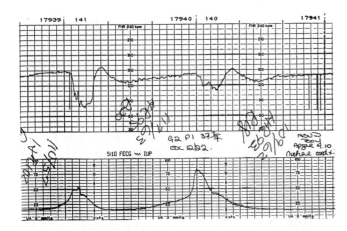

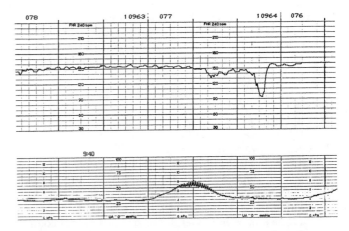

Figure 2.70: Mixed deceleration pattern of variable and late decelerations. This is NOT a variable deceleration with a "late component." There are two mechanisms for this pattern: cord compression and uteroplacental insufficiency. Actions should be directed at relief of both to avoid worsening hypoxia and metabolic acidosis.

Figure 2.71: A rare mixed deceleration pattern of late and variable decelerations. However, the late deceleration does not meet strict onset recognition criteria. Suspect oligohydramnios when there are signs of uteroplacental insufficiency (late decelerations) and cord compression (variable decelerations). An ultrasound scan to determine amniotic fluid volume, fetal size and well-being may be helpful in determining the cause of this pattern. During labor, membranes should be ruptured to assess for the presence of fluid and/or meconium.

application of the spiral electrode (if applicable), interventions, and communications.

MIXED DECELERATION PATTERNS

Alternative labels: combination deceleration pattern, combined deceleration pattern (273)

Recognition Criteria:
- early decel immediately followed by a late decel
- variable decel immediately followed by a late decel
- late decel immediately followed by a variable decel
- any decel immediately followed by a prolonged decel

Actions in Response to Mixed Decelerations
The response to the pattern will depend on the BL level, STV, LTV, and the type of decels present. Consider the physiologic basis for the pattern prior to intervening.

Discussion
Occasionally head compression or cord compression or cord compression and uteroplacental insufficiency may occur at a similar point in time. Interventions should be based on the types of decels identified. Assess and record signs of fetal well-being, such as accels, STV, and fetal movement. The physician should be notified of the FHR pattern, actions, and the fetal response to actions.

NONPERIODIC DECELERATIONS
CHECKMARK PATTERN
Definition: FHR pattern produced when the fetus is seizing.

Recognition Criteria:

BL	usually between 100 and 170 bpm, usually stable, but may be unstable and/or preceded or followed by a flat BL (181, 455)
STV	**absent**
LTV	**usually absent**, may look wavy and not "normal" in appearance
ACCELS	**absent**
DECELS	nonperiodic, repetitive variable decels that are similar in shape
Duration	usually 10 to 25 seconds
Depth	10 - 35 bpm
Shape	similar in shape, depth, and duration from one to the next
	mostly V-shaped, rarely U-shaped, never W-shaped
	may or may not be preceded by a 5 second "bump" or followed by a 10 - 20 second "bump"
	if "checkmarks" last l0 seconds, the BL is usually tachycardic and flat
	if BL is tachycardic, there is usually no "bump" before and/or after the decel
Nadir	every 30 to 75 seconds (nadir to nadir), although, "checkmark" (decel) every 20 seconds has been reported (181)

Significance	the cord is NOT compressed, the fetus is seizing
Classification	ominous
Incidence	rare (456), ratio of fetal seizures to live births is unknown

Cause(s)/Physiology of Fetal Seizures:
- abnormal neuronal electrical discharges due to
- an altered neuron environment
- intermittent bursts of high-frequency electrical discharges
- brain dysfunction or damage (181, 336)
- found in a fetus with a brain anomaly, e.g., hydraencephaly (456)
- a result of "severe" fetal hypoxia following four maternal eclamptic seizures, cardiorespiratory arrest, and pulmonary edema (455)
- a result of ischemia, acidosis, and/or asphyxia with CNS damage (lambs) (458-459)
- following a skull fracture and brain trauma as a result of a motor vehicle accident
- related to a structural or metabolic CNS abnormality (460)
- as a result of cocaine with marked cerebral hypoxia (in lambs) (461)
- due to fetal pyridoxine (B_6) deficiency or dependency, a rare congenital metabolic disturbance that exclusively affects the CNS (258, 462)
  - B_6 is found in pork, veal, lamb, glandular meats, milk, eggs, potatoes, oatmeal, wheat germ, bananas, cabbage, and carrots and is a mediator of protein metabolism and formation of essential brain chemicals
  - pyridoxine changes to pyridoxalphosphate and is a coenzyme in biochemical reactions
  - pyridoxalphosphate is needed to change glutamic acid to other byproducts
  - maternal treatment with 110 mg/day of B_6 stopped intrauterine fetal convulsions in the 5th and 7th months of pregnancy in 3 women (462)
- seizures were more common in female than male rats and may be hormonally dependent (463)
- unknown reasons (456)
- in neonates, seizures have been related to asphyxia, intracranial hemorrhage, metabolic abnormalities, CNS trauma, cerebral cortex malformations, congenital infections, and drug withdrawal (460).

Actions in Response to a Checkmark Pattern
- immediately notify the woman's physician
- initiate measures to increase fetal oxygenation, which may or may not be needed but nonetheless are appropriate as it is impossible to determine which seizures are due to anoxia and which are not
- prior to a cesarean section, the physician may elect to ultrasound the fetus to confirm seizure activity and rule out a lethal anomaly
- a physician who can manage neonatal seizures should be present at delivery.

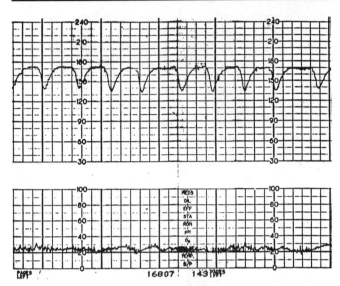

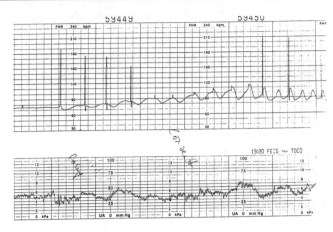

Figure 2.72: Checkmark Pattern of a fetus seizing in utero in a woman with pancreatitis. Pancreatitis occurs in approximately 1 in 3000 pregnant women and is related to gallbladder or biliary tract disease, gallstones, gallbladder sludge, and/or a thickened gallbladder wall. In nonpregnant women, pancreatitis is often due to alcoholism. Pregnant women who have pancreatitis need a bowel rest, IV hydration, antibiotics, and analgesics (457). The woman was unstable and could not be delivered by cesarean section. The fetus died prior to delivery. The cause of fetal seizures was not reported.

Figure 2.73: Brain anoxia causes seizures but may only be a transient asphyxial insult that causes no permanent injury. This is a Checkmark Pattern of a 40 4/7 week fetus who was seizing while recovering from terminal bradycardia. The previous pattern was stable and reassuring or compensatory, with spontaneous accelerations, a baseline of 120 to 135, and some variable decelerations. The sudden onset of terminal bradycardia suggests a cord prolapse. The fetal heart rate recovered to 120 to 150 with absent long-term variability and present short-term variability prior to the cesarean section. The neonatologist was present at the birth and the Apgar scores were 7 and 9 at 1 and 5 minutes. Umbilical "cord" gases were: pH 7.18, PO_2 37 mm Hg, PCO_2 38 mm Hg, and base excess -14 mEq/L. The high PO_2 suggests these are umbilical venous gases. The neonate was discharged with a normal acid-base status and no abnormalities.

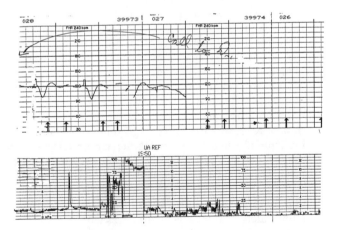

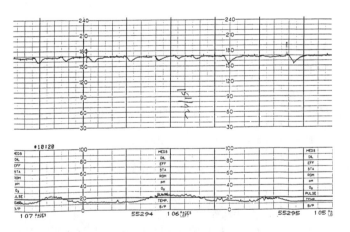

Figure 2.74: Checkmark Pattern of a 38 week fetus whose mother was G_1P_0 admitted for induction due to preeclampsia. She was asked to mark fetal movement (see arrows). These marks of fetal movement strongly suggest human fetuses, like seizing fetal lambs, also have jerking movements of the head and extremities between the "checkmarks" and the seizing movements repeat ever 20 to 30 seconds (460, 464, 467).

Figure 2.75: A tachycardic Checkmark Pattern. For an unknown reason, when the baseline approaches 170 bpm there are no "bumps" before or after the "checkmarks." The G_6P_4 39 year old woman at 39 6/7 weeks gestation reported fetal hiccup-type movements since 3:30 am. This tracing was obtained near 10:20 am. She had a fever one week prior to this admission. The fetus stopped seizing at 10:54 am and had a totally flat line at 170 bpm. The "brain dead" 8 lb 13 ounce baby was delivered by cesarean section with Apgar scores of 2, 5, and 6 at 1, 5, and 6 minutes and subsequently died. The autopsy report was not available.

Discussion

This pattern is caused by the changing FHR during fetal seizure activity. Seizure activity can last a few minutes to several hours. The fetus may never seize as a newborn if resuscitation is prompt and effective. Blood gases may be normal, especially if a structural abnormality is responsible for seizure activity.

Fetal seizures may consist of regular, very intense movements at the rate of two movements each second or single twitches several times a minute (462). Women report the fetus is "fluttering" or "hiccuping," especially when they have been pregnant before and hiccups are the only thing they can relate to (464). The fetus will have rapid, repetitive, episodic jerking movements (456).

Diagnostic tests for fetal seizures may delay delivery and their need must be carefully considered prior to their use. They have included a fetal electroencephalogram (EEG), real-time ultrasound, and toxicology screen for cocaine (456, 460-461, 465-466). During real-time ultrasound, the fetus may have recurrent jerking motions of its head, arms, and legs for 5 to 10 seconds, which repeat every 20 to 30 seconds for 3 or more minutes, then no fetal movement for 5 to 10 minutes (460, 464, 467).

The *neonatal* EEG may reveal intermittent electrical discharges (468). The neonate may have symmetrical, myoclonic twitchings followed by tonic convulsions for 5 seconds each. Seizing fetal lambs had rapid, deep fetal breathing movements or gasping-like movements synchronous with the "checkmark" decels. They also had tachycardia or bradycardia. *The deceleration occurred before or between seizure episodes* (459, 469).

If fetal seizures occur during the second trimester or early in the third trimester, a fetal pyridoxine deficiency is a possible cause of the seizures (462). If seizures are diagnosed in labor, there may be no time to investigate the possible cause, especially if the cause is anoxia. A delay to deliver may result in a fetal demise. Cord blood gases may be normal (181). Some seizing fetuses had severe retardation at 17 months of age and the etiology of seizures was never found (467).

DIFFERENTIATING SEIZURES, HICCUPS, AND CORD COMPRESSION

Fetal Hiccups Versus Seizures

Fetal hiccups occur in 1 in 50 fetuses, and are considered "normal." They appear at a similar time of the day and may persist after birth. Hiccups are not associated with morbidity or mortality and can be confirmed by real-time ultrasound. Hiccups are felt as abrupt, repetitive fetal movements or they may be felt as irregular, jerky fetal movements. Expect the FHR pattern to be reassuring, possibly with little dots (artifact) during the hiccuping episodes, and possibly with 2 to 20 second "dips" in the FHR. *Accels will be present.* A Checkmark Pattern lacks accels (470).

Differentiating a Checkmark Pattern Due to Seizures From Variable Decelerations Due to Umbilical Cord Compression

The "W" shape will help differentiate between a Checkmark Pattern and a variable decel pattern due to cord compression. If a W (biphasic) decel is observed, the cord is compressed.

Seizures are CNS mediated and produce similar decels. Variable decels, due to umbilical cord compression, vary in duration, depth, and shape (471).

Look for accelerations. In addition, there are no accels during fetal seizure activity, but there may be uniform accels when the cord is mildly compressed or spontaneous accels may occur following scalp stimulation or acoustic stimulation.

PROLONGED DECELERATION(S)

Definition: A nonperiodic deceleration of the FHR that lasts 2 to 10 minutes.

Recognition Criteria:

ONSET	acute, steep, abrupt drop
DEPTH	≥ 30 bpm from the BL level (264)
OFFSET	gradual recovery (163)
DURATION	≥ 2 minutes but ≤ 10 minutes, if > 10 minutes it is classified as bradycardia (264, 472).

Classification:

One prolonged decel: compensatory, especially if it is a response to maternal hypotension.

Two or more prolonged decels: nonreassuring, consider cord entanglement or prolapse.

Rebound tachycardia following a prolonged deceleration has been considered ominous (264).

Cause(s)/Physiology of Prolonged Decelerations:

Anesthesia
- hypotension following epidural anesthesia (473-474)
- possibly direct fetal effect or vasoconstriction or a change in uterine tone following epidural anesthesia with 2% lignocaine with adrenaline or bupivacaine (Marcaine®) with adrenaline (474)
- paracervical block with possible direct fetal effect (475-477)

Umbilical cord compression
- partial or complete umbilical cord compression (345)
- umbilical cord vessel spasm, e.g., during intrauterine transfusion
- hypoxia-chemoreceptor-vagal reflex (264, 478)
- prolapsed umbilical cord

Uterine activity
- hyperstimulation and/or hypertonus
- uterine rupture

Other
- maternal voiding (possibly due to a supine position and hypotension while on a bedpan) (58)
- vaginal examinations with pressure on the fetal fontanel

Actions in Response to a Prolonged Deceleration
Determine etiology of the prolonged decel:
- maternal hypotension?
- umbilical cord compression, prolapse?
- excessive uterine activity?
- direct anesthetic response?

Note the time of onset of the decel in relation to regional or paracervical anesthetic administration. The prolonged decel may be a direct anesthetic response if it occurs within 7 to 8 minutes of the epidural anesthesia test dose.

Assess the maternal condition:
- BP and MHR
- pain
- vaginal bleeding: uterine rupture? abruption? vasa previa?

Assess the fetal condition:
- signs of well-being: accels? STV present?
- meconium?

Act to:
- enhance fetal oxygenation
- increase maternal BP if hypotensive: ephedrine may be needed

- rule out a prolapsed cord (vaginal examination)
- rule out uterine rupture, i.e., the fetus may have an ascending station
- if hyperstimulation is related to the pattern: discontinue oxytocics and/or remove the prostaglandin gel, insert, or tablet
- administer a tocolytic if ordered by the physician (324, 333, 479)

Communicate:
- maternal assessments
- actions
- FHR pattern before and after the prolonged decel

The physician may choose to perform a cesarean section if:
- a cord prolapse is diagnosed and/or
- a uterine rupture is diagnosed and/or
- the FHR becomes bradycardic in spite of actions to enhance oxygen delivery.

Discussion
A prolonged decel may occur as the result of a central vagal stimulus or hypoxia, with activation of the chemoreceptors, baroreceptors, and vagus nerve (282, 480). Prolonged decels, following "caine" anesthetic administration, may be a response to an increase in contraction frequency, resting tone, and hypoxia. These decels lasted an average of 6 minutes after a paracervical injection with 100 mg of mepivacaine, and 2 to 4 minutes after low dose bupivacaine (476-477). The physician's decision to wait and observe the tracing is weighed against the decision to perform a cesarean delivery of an infant whose CNS depression may be due to the effects of a "caine" medication. Delivery of an infant who is

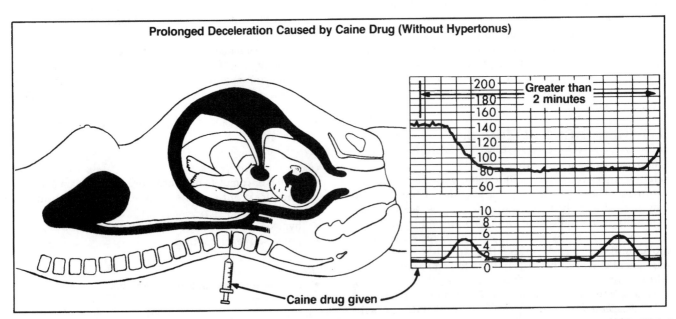

Figure 2.76: Prolonged deceleration caused by a "caine" drug (without uterine hypertonus). (Reproduced with permission of Marshall Klavan, MD: *Clinical concepts of fetal heart rate monitoring.* **Hewlett-Packard Company, 1977).**

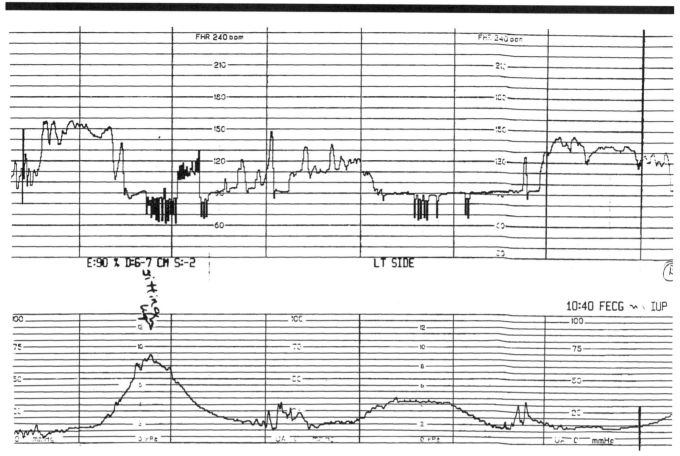

Figure 2.77: Prolonged deceleration following a variable deceleration in a 40 3/7 week fetus. The G_4P_3 woman had a history of 3 vaginal births. The fetus was delivered vaginally with Apgar scores of 8 and 9 at 1 and 5 minutes. Note the downward deflections (transient vagal arrest or sinus arrest) during the prolonged decel suggesting complete occlusion of the umbilical cord.

depressed from a "caine" medication may be followed by cardiovascular collapse and a very difficult resuscitation. Patience is needed, especially when the prolonged deceleration was preceded by a stable BL, STV, and accels. Within 8 to 25 minutes, the FHR should return to BL as the drug is excreted.

Prolonged decels may also be a response to hypoxia caused by maternal hypotension, hemorrhage, seizures, uterine hyperstimulation and/or hypertonus, and umbilical cord compression (58, 480). When hypoxia is present, variability may decrease and accels may disappear (475, 477). Even with a drop in fetal pH, recovery was complete following actions to improve maternal BP, decrease uterine activity, and increase fetal oxygenation. Prolongation of the decel over 10 minutes, creating bradycardia, was associated with PR interval shortening due to sinoatrial node depression and hypoxia (476).

SPONTANEOUS DECELERATIONS

Definition: nonperiodic smooth decels due to hypoxia and myocardial depression, usually observed in the antepartal period.

Recognition Criteria:

ONSET	gradual
DEPTH	varies, usually falls < 20 bpm
OFFSET	gradual
SHAPE	often a smooth decel, occasionally resembling a subtle late decel
BL	≥ 120 bpm
STV	absent
LTV	absent to minimal (3 - 5 bpm)
ACCELS	none

Significance abnormally high placental vascular resistance or placental dysfunction with fetal compromise from hypoxia, the fetus may already be acidotic (481).

Classification ominous

Cause(s)/Physiology of Spontaneous Decelerations:
- increased placental vascular resistance (481)
- abnormal umbilical artery S/D ratio (481)
- absent umbilical artery end-diastolic velocity (481).

- associated with IUGR (482)
- associated with fetal infection and hypoxia
- preceded by uncoupled accels and movements, indicative of fetal compromise (483)
- precedes fetal death (482)
- expect to resuscitate the neonate
- the return of middle cerebral artery flow velocity to a normal level is a harbinger of fetal jeopardy (481).

Accelerations

Fewer accelerations, smaller in size

Decreased fetal movement

Decoupling of accelerations and fetal movement
(i.e., there is no relationship between the two)

No accelerations or fetal movement

Decreased LTV and STV

Spontaneous decelerations

Figure 2.78: The continuum from oxygenated to compromised with the production of spontaneous decelerations (484).

Actions in Response to Spontaneous Decelerations:
In addition to actions in response to any abnormal FHR pattern:
Assess recent drug use:
- CNS depressants
- antihypertensives

This pattern is a sign of fetal compromise that often occurs in hypertensive women.

Review prenatal records:
- is this the fetus' normal BL level?
- ultrasound reports: IUGR? oligohydramnios?
- results of antepartal tests

Assess the maternal condition:
- vital signs
- signs of infection?
- signs of abruption?

Assess the fetal condition:
- fetal movement history
- movement palpable?
- when was the last accel?
- BL rising? any variability?
- amniotic fluid volume (oligohydramnios?)
- estimate fetal size, measure fundal height, or ultrasound: small baby? IUGR? tone?

Act to:
- enhance fetal oxygenation (see actions in Chapter 6)
- **keep the woman NPO** (nothing by mouth) until the physician evaluates the fetus

Communicate:
- pertinent maternal history
- maternal assessments
- actions
- pertinent fetal history
- fetal response to actions

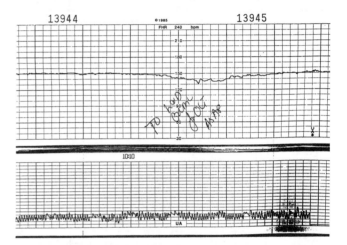

Figure 2.79: Spontaneous deceleration during a nonstress test of a 36 week fetus. The woman was a G$_3$P$_1$ insulin-dependent gestational diabetic (Class A$_2$) with labile blood pressures and proteinuria. She reported decreased fetal movement during the last 48 hours. A cesarean was performed with Apgar scores were 4, 6, and 7 at 1, 5, and 10 minutes.

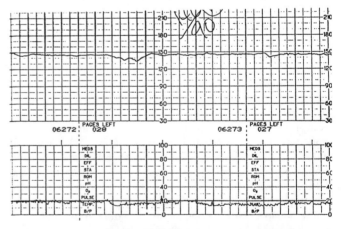

Figure 2.80: Spontaneous decelerations of an intrauterine growth restricted (IUGR) 33^1/$_2$ week fetus whose mother had blood pressures ranging from 146/90 to 160/100. An ultrasound scan revealed "severe" oligohydramnios. The fetus was delivered by cesarean section with Apgar scores of 1, 3, and 5 at 1, 5, and 10 minutes. An abruption was found at the time of delivery.

Document:
- the systematic review, e.g., "BL 120 - 122 bpm, 0 LTV, 0 STV, 0 accels, spont. decels x 2."
- communication time, person(s) spoken to, content of conversation

The physician may choose to deliver the fetus by cesarean section if:
- after 40 minutes of monitoring, the FHR pattern is nonreactive and
- the ultrasound examination reveals:
  - oligohydramnios and/or
  - absent fetal tone and/or
  - an abruption

Nurses should collaborate with physicians to decide who will call the:
- CRNA or anesthesiologist
- assistant surgeon
- physician who can manage neonatal complications to request their presence at the delivery.

Nurses witness signing of the consent form, call the OR team, and prepare the woman for surgery. The physician should discuss the plan of care with the woman and her family.

MONITORING THE PRETERM FETUS
FHR pattern characteristics of the preterm fetus have only recently been identified. Preterm fetuses differ from term and postterm fetuses in their normal BL range, accel amplitude, and behavioral state duration (485). As the fetus matures:
- the BL level decreases 1 bpm per week beginning at 16 weeks of gestation
- the BL level stabilizes (becomes fairly constant) between 30 to 40 weeks of gestation
- LTV and the BL bandwidth increase
- STV increases
- the number of accels increases
- the time between accels decreases
- the number of "reactive" NSTs increases

Specifically,
- at 20 to 30 weeks, only 13% of fetuses did not have an accel in 60 minutes of monitoring
- at ≤ 22 weeks, decels and asystole for ≤ 10 seconds occur
- at ≥ 23 weeks, rest-activity cycles begin
- between 20 and 30 weeks, 10 to 20 second dips are more common than accels
- by 24 to 26 weeks, prolonged (2 to 4 minute) decels disappear
- between 24 and 32 weeks, fetal breathing movements increase and the number of gross body movements decrease
- between 24 and 32 weeks, 20% of accels are not related to fetal movement, 30% of fetal movements are not related to accels

- between 24 and 32 weeks, a prolonged absence of fetal movement is rare
- by 27 weeks, rest/activity episodes can be distinguished by high and low variation changes
- by 36 weeks, it is easy to distinguish 4 behavioral states (269, 277, 293, 486-492).

Variation, Fetal Movement, and Betamethasone Administration
Fetal biophysical parameters decrease following betamethasone which is given to increase fetal lung maturity. Mulder (493) found *a significant decrease in FHR variation following betamethasone administration*, possibly mediated by centrally located glucocorticoid receptors. *Fetal movement also decreased.* Fetal breathing time, fetal breathing movements, limb and gross body movements decreased 48 hours after betamethasone (12 mg) was administered. Accels slightly decreased in their frequency and amplitude (from a maximum of 9 to a maximum of 6 during 30 minutes of observation). *Biophysical profile parameters returned to normal within 96 hours after drug administration (494).*

Baseline Level
As the fetus matures, the BL decreases, STV and LTV increase, the number and amplitude of accels increase, and behavioral state changes, indirectly reflected in changes in the FHR pattern, become more evident (52, 269, 294, 486). "Immature" fetuses have less STV than term fetuses (155). They do not produce *marked* LTV (207). The FHR averages 85 bpm between 4.5 and 7 weeks of gestation (495). The FHR rises until the 16th week, then it drops 1 bpm each week as the parasympathetic nervous system matures (269).

In the first and second trimesters, FHR patterns are related to inherent myocardial rhythmicity. By the third trimester, considerable autonomic control is demonstrated by the presence of STV and LTV (110). The autonomic nervous system matures about 30 weeks of gestation (277). As term approaches, the sympathetic and parasympathetic nerves are almost equal in dominance.

Baseline Variability
"Normal" variability predicted a nonacidemic umbilical artery pH in 24 of 29 fetuses who were 27.4 to 32.4 weeks of gestation. "Decreased" variability predicted an umbilical artery pH less than 7.20 in 5 of 7 fetuses (496).

Accelerations
Fetuses at 16 weeks of gestation accelerate (292). By 24 weeks of gestation, some preterm fetuses accel while moving (497). Between 25 and 28 weeks of gestation, 92% of fetuses had two or more accels that peaked *10* or more bpm in a 15 minute period of monitoring (498). A common finding prior to 30 weeks of gestation was small accels, with an amplitude of 10 bpm and a duration of 10 or more seconds. Preterm fetuses increase the number of accels and range of BL variability during maternal hyperoxygenation (497).

Nonstress testing. Using 15 x 15 criteria, fetuses at 23 to 27 weeks of gestation were reactive only 16.7% of the time. Between 28 and 32 weeks of gestation they were reactive only 65.6% of the time. *Preterm fetuses between 33 and 37 weeks' gestation have "reactive" accels 90.6% of the time* (266). Depending on their gestational age and ability to hear, preterm fetuses accelerated in response to acoustic stimulation 46% of the time, but 70% of term fetuses responded (499).

Ware and Devoe (52) urged different norms be developed for interpretation of the NST for fetuses who are less than 32 weeks' gestation. Perhaps the "reactive" criteria for fetuses less than 32 weeks of gestation should be 2 10 x 10 or 10 x 15 accels in 20 minutes. Before NST criteria change, results from prospective, randomized, controlled studies must be examined. Until then, the antepartal FHR prior to 32 weeks of gestation may be described in the notes as "FHR appropriate for gestational age" or "FHR not appropriate for gestational age."

Accelerations Versus Decelerations

At 20 weeks of gestation, accels were as frequent as decels (487). However, "decels" in the FHR, were actually "dips" because most of the reported "decels" were only 10 to 20 seconds in duration (293). Decels that lasted 2 to 4 minutes were also common *prior to* 20 weeks of gestation (488). Very immature fetuses (up to 22 weeks of gestation) had decels and even asystole lasting up to 10 seconds (292). Schifrin (294) found fetal movement often preceded small "decels" instead of accels.

When to Begin Monitoring

The rule for monitoring any baby is, "you must be willing to act on the information you receive." In addition, knowledge of normal preterm FHR patterns and behavior is essential so that the tracing is not misinterpreted. *The "age of viability" appears to be between 23 and 24 weeks of gestation.* "Extremely preterm" fetuses are 23 to 24 weeks of gestation. Prior to 23 weeks of gestation, electronic fetal monitoring is not usually considered appropriate. At a gestation of 23 weeks or less, approximately 1/3rd of fetuses survived, but only 30% were "normal" at 18 months of age. By 24 to 25 weeks, 47 to 48% survived. At 26 or more weeks, 72% survived. Steroids, to mature the fetal lungs, increased the *overall survival rate* from 38% to 68% (500-501). Based on these findings, fetuses less than 24 weeks of gestation are rarely monitored in some settings (502). For example, at the Baylor College of Medicine, researchers found only 8% of babies born at 23 weeks of gestation were discharged home without a major handicap, but 39% of babies born at or after 24 weeks were discharged without a major handicap. Therefore, they chose to develop an aggressive management plan for fetuses at 23.9 or more weeks of gestation (503).

Can the FHR Pattern Predict Intraventricular Hemorrhage?

A prenatal event, such as a maternal seizure, may contribute to the development of a fetal intraventricular hemorrhage (IVH) (504). Decreased fetal movement and intrapartal hypoxia and asphyxia were associated with IVH (505). Yet, *there is no specific FHR pattern predictive of IVH (472).*

Preterm fetuses lack the ability to autoregulate cerebral blood flow and are susceptible to blood vessel rupture when blood is redistributed during hypoxia (505). A cesarean section does not influence the incidence of a large IVH unless it is performed prior to the onset of labor (506). Therefore, *to prevent IVH in preterm fetuses, it is essential that at the earliest indication of hypoxic stress, interventions to maximize fetal oxygenation and minimize hypoxia should be implemented* (507).

Preterm Response to Hypoxia

Baseline changes. If a preterm fetus, 24 to 26 weeks of gestation, has tachycardia or bradycardia in the hour prior to delivery, neonatal death is predicted. Tachycardia and the loss of variability preceded poor neonatal outcomes (508). Severely anemic preterm fetuses may have a sinusoidal pattern (181).

Variable decelerations. Vagal responses in the immature fetus are decreased, therefore decels are highly significant and "more ominous" than decels in term babies (508). Because of the immature vagus, bradycardia is ominous.

Preterm and low birth weight infants poorly tolerate cord compression compared to term fetuses (509). Yet, some extremely preterm fetuses with cord compression do remarkably well. For example, a $23^{1}/_{2}$ week fetus who weighed 630 grams had "deep" variable decels and was delivered with normal blood gases and Apgar scores of 3 and 7 at 1 and 5 minutes. The baby survived without major complications. Another baby, delivered at 23 weeks of gestation, had normal blood gases and Apgar scores of 4 and 7 at 1 and 5 minutes, and also survived without major complications (510). If recurrent variable decels are not ameliorated with position change, discontinuation of oxytocin, hydration and hyperoxygenation, amnioinfusion may be helpful (358). Severe variable decels in fetuses less than 32 weeks of gestation were related to a significant increase in nucleated red blood cells. Some fetuses with severe variable decels had chronic vasculitis of the umbilical cord (511). Acidotic preterm fetuses were tachycardic with decreased variability and "relatively benign" variable decels (75). Transient tachycardia may be a sympathoadrenal response to hypoxia (512).

Late decelerations. *FHR patterns, such as late decels, that suggest compromise in the term fetus are also reliable markers of compromise in the preterm fetus* (110). Zanini, Paul, and Huey Jr. (513) considered late decels *ominous* in preterm fetuses, as significantly more preterm fetuses who had late decels were acidemic than preterm fetuses who had variable decels. Acidemic preterm fetuses who died had no accels, overall BL variability less than 5 bpm, and late decels (52). Preterm fetuses who were 27.9 to 31.8 weeks of gestation who lacked accels and had late decels or "pronounced" variable decels

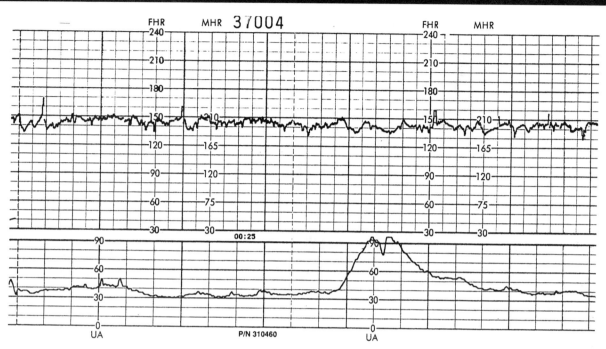

Figure 2.81: A well-oxygenated preterm fetus at 27 weeks of gestation in a G_1P_0 woman in "threatened preterm labor." The cervix was closed. Contractions ceased after tocolytics were administered.

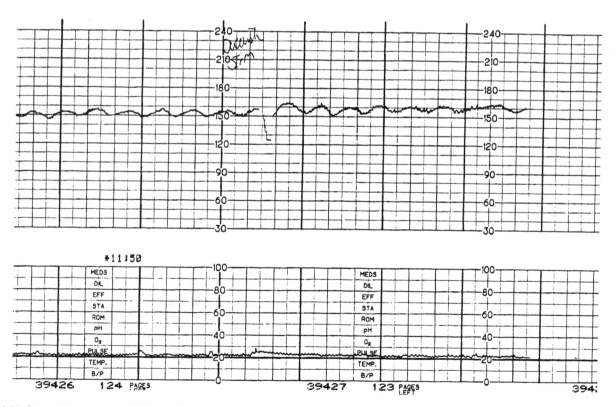

Figure 2.82: Sinusoidal pattern of a 33 5/7 week fetus whose mother had gestational diabetes and was delivered by cesarean section. The Apgar scores were 7 and 8 at 1 and 5 minutes. The baby weighed 4 lb 9 ounces and had a hemoglobin and hematocrit of 2.6 gm/dl and 9.2%, and was transfused with 50 cc of packed red blood cells. Note the failure of the fetus to respond to acoustic stimulation.

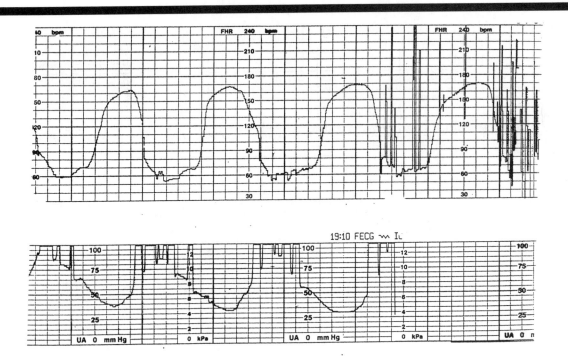

Figure 2.83: Preterm fetus with severe variable decelerations. This 31 2/7 week fetus of a G_2P_1 woman, who smokes a pack a day and who had a previous cesarean section, had a reactive nonstress test in the physician's office prior to admission for preterm labor. She was 4 to 5 cm/50%/-1/vertex with a positive group B streptococcus screen and a negative toxicology screen. The baby delivered vaginally (VBAC) with Apgar scores of 5 and 5 at 1 and 5 minutes. Umbilical artery gases were: pH 7.203, PO_2 18 mm Hg, PCO_2 56.4 mm Hg, and base excess -6 mEq/L. Umbilical vein gases were: pH 7.265, PO_2 21 mm Hg, PCO_2 47.2 mm Hg, and base excess -5 mEq/L.

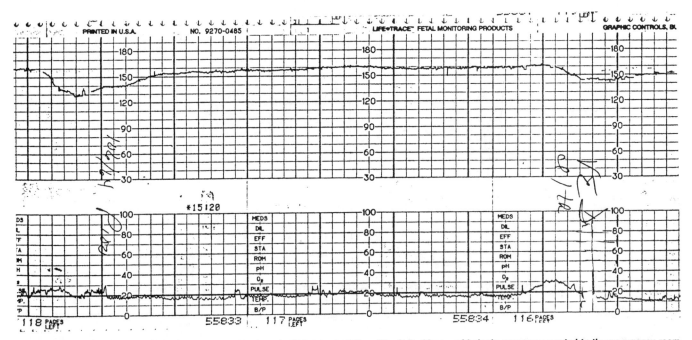

Figure 2.84: Preterm fetus with late decelerations. The fetus is 32 weeks gestation. The G_1P_0 20 year old single woman presented to the emergency room. She was traveling in a car with her boyfriend when she felt a gush of fluid and saw it was blood. The cervix was 1 cm dilated and the fetus was breech. The primary cesarean section revealed a bicornuate uterus, an abruption, and a neonate with Apgar scores of 2, 2, and 5 at 1, 5, and 10 minutes.

had an increased risk of asphyxia (507). Therefore, just like term fetuses, accels rule in well-being.

Preterm fetuses, less than 29 weeks of gestation, *with absent umbilical artery end-diastolic velocity* were slower to develop late decels than older fetuses. Only 10% of fetuses, who were less than 29 weeks' gestation with absent end-diastolic umbilical artery velocity had late decels 7 days later. However, 60.7% of fetuses who were 29 or more weeks' gestation had late decels within 7 days (514). Some preterm fetuses will not even demonstrate clinical signs of hypoxia, e.g., tachycardia, late decels, and loss of variability, for many hours until the moments preceding death. In addition, stressed preterm fetuses rarely pass meconium (98). Preterm fetuses produce a smaller quantity of catecholamines than term fetuses (64, 515).

MONITORING TWINS

With increasing use of ovulation-inducing agents, the number of twins and triplets increased in the United States between 1978 and 1988 by 33% and 101% respectively (516). Multiple gestation is associated with an increased risk of preterm birth, premature rupture of membranes, intrauterine fetal demise (IUFD), polyhydramnios, IUGR, abruption, and preeclampsia (517-520). Fewer fetal deaths occurred if twins weighed 2800 to 3700 grams and were delivered at 36 to 39 weeks of gestation (521-524). If women gained 1.5 pounds or more each week after the 20th week of gestation, their fetuses weighed 2500 or more grams (525). Compared to singletons who had an IUFD ratio of 6.6/1000 live births, twins had a 24.9/1000 IUFD ratio (526). In a review of 41 years of medical records, Saacks, Thorp, and Hendricks (519) found 23% of twins had a birth weight discordancy of 20% or more. If one twin was small for gestational age (SGA), the other twin, who was appropriate for gestational age (AGA), was smaller than two AGA twins of a similar gestational age (527). Discordant twins need heightened fetal surveillance (528).

Monozygotic (identical) twins. Monozygotic twins with one placenta and one sac have a 200 to 300% higher morbidity and mortality rate than dizygotic (fraternal) twins due to circulatory connections in the placenta, twin-to-twin transfusion with growth differences or discordance, cord entanglement, and intrauterine hypoxia (527, 529-531). *Discordance is the most significant predictor of fetal hypoxia when there are multiple fetuses.*

Identical twins may also have a shared, monochorionic placenta but two sacs. A monochorionic placenta may have vessel anastomoses that promote twin-to-twin transfusion. Using intrauterine laser surgery, perinatologists were able to occlude these vessels prior to 25 weeks of gestation and prolong pregnancies until an average of 32.3 weeks of gestation (532). If twin-twin transfusion is diagnosed, cordocentesis and Doppler velocimetry may be helpful to determine each fetus' hematocrit and hemodynamic state (533).

Dizygotic (fraternal) twins. Seventy-five percent of twins are dizygotic, with two placentae and two sacs (534). Antepartal tests, such as the NST, are common during pregnancies with multiple fetuses (535). Antepartal electronic fetal monitors may have two ultrasound transducers to monitor twins simultaneously. But, if two separate fetal monitors are used, it is imperative to compare the printouts to make sure that both twins are actually being monitored (534, 536).

Who is A and Who is B?

When the first NST is performed, the nurse should determine which twin will be named "A" and which will be "B." The BL rate for each twin should be recorded, preferably on the outside of the prenatal record or in a prominent place on the inside of the record. In addition to each twin's FHR BL, the position of the baby in the uterus should be documented. Then, during a future NST, and in light of the fact the FHR drops 1 bpm per week, it should be easy to relocate A and B based on the FHR, not position in the uterus. If A and B have nearly identical BLs, it may be impossible to keep A as A and B as B. At the time of birth, the twin who is delivered first is "first twin," and the other baby is "second twin" (537). The note in the medical record could be written as, "First twin (B), second twin (A)" or vice versa. Once the first twin is delivered, there is no time limit on delivery of the second twin as long as there is no clinical indication for delivery (538). In vertex/vertex twins, two hours passed between the birth of the first twin and the second twin without a negative effect (539). Other physicians found a delay of 15 or more minutes increased the need for a cesarean delivery of the second twin (540). If possible, a spiral electrode is usually applied to the second twin for continuous monitoring prior to a vaginal birth. The nurse should have Piper forceps available for vaginal delivery of the second twin who is breech. Real-time ultrasound images of the second twin may be obtained after birth of the first twin (531). Twins are usually delivered by cesarean section if the presenting twin is breech or the second twin's estimated weight is less than 1800 grams (538, 541). By keeping A as A and B as B, if a retrospective review of the medical records and tracings is required, the history and progress of twin A and twin B are easily distinguished. Document on the tracing "twin A" and "twin B" from time to time, e.g., every half hour, so that any one who reviews the tracing will readily know who was who. Care of women who have twins should also include:

- a 1:1 nurse:woman ratio
- frequent position changes, avoid a supine position
- confirmation that each twin is being monitored (the printouts should vary)
- if two fetal monitors are used, the clocks should be set to identical times
- if at all possible, two tocotransducers should be used when two monitors are used so that uterine activity is recorded on both tracings (try to use only two belts with

two transducers on each belt)

- if bradycardia is noted, the MHR should be confirmed and documented and the ultrasound transducer should be adjusted to record the FHR
- document the location of the twins and their FHRs
- report nonreactive or abnormal patterns as soon as possible to the physician
- institute measures to increase fetal oxygenation as needed
- at delivery have "two of everything" (534).

Multiple Gestation: Fetal Movements/Kick Counts

Fetal growth and well-being during multiple gestation is often monitored beginning at 28 weeks after conception (530). The pregnant woman may be asked to count fetal movements. If more than one fetus is moving, kick counts should be higher than in singleton pregnancies. Thirty-three women with twins, 6 with triplets, 1 with quadruplets, and 1 with quintuplets were asked to monitor fetal movement for 30 minutes 3 times a day. At 20 weeks' gestation, twins averaged 200 "kicks." At 32 weeks, a maximum of 575 "kicks" were recorded. Then, there was a gradual decline in the number of movements to an average of 282 at 40 weeks of gestation (120). If there are 282 movements in 90 minutes, fetuses move at least 3 times a minute. It would be reasonable to ask women who have turns to count fetal movement twice a day and call if 10 movements have not been felt within 60 minutes. However, each facility will need to establish a protocol for fetal movement assessment. When fetal movement of twins was observed with an ultrasound, 24 to 26% of fetal gross body movements were simultaneous and 49% of fetal breathing movements were simultaneous (542).

The Baseline

During NSTs of IUGR twins, "reduced" BL variability, the absence of accels, and the presence of late decels was associated with lower Apgar scores at 1 minute and more neonatal morbidity than twins who had variability, accels, and no late decels (543).

Accelerations

Synchrony. The fetus on the right side moves for longer periods of time and has longer episodes of breathing movements (544). Twins accelerate together about 57 to 58% of the time (545-546). Synchrony, the occurrence of accels within 15 seconds of each other, emerges as early as 27 weeks of gestation (545, 547-548). A reactive NST was 96.2% predictive of a twin's ability to tolerate labor within 1 week of the test (531, 549). If the tracing was nonreactive, a biophysical profile was helpful in identifying fetal compromise. A biophysical profile score of 7 or less (out of a possible 12) suggested fetal compromise (550).

Characteristics of synchronous twin tracings include similar frequency and timing of accels, similar baseline oscillations, and similar periodic decels. Synchrony may be related to placenta location, fetal weight, or vibration (542, 545-547). Synchrony can make it more difficult to obtain clear tracings of both fetuses when simultaneous monitoring is done, unless the fetal monitor distinguishes between the twins, e.g., Toitu® monitors, or has two FHR grids for plotting the FHRs. When 33 to 37 week gestation twins were acoustically stimulated, there were simultaneous or synchronous accels and fetal movement 100% of the time (546). Acoustic stimulation will make asynchronous FHRs synchronous (534).

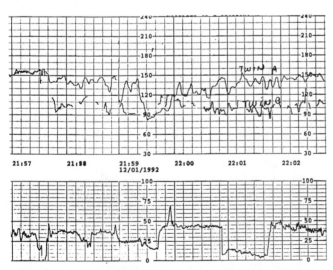

Figure 2.85: Labeling twin A and B on the tracing makes it easier for the person reviewing the FHR patterns to keep them clear in their mind.

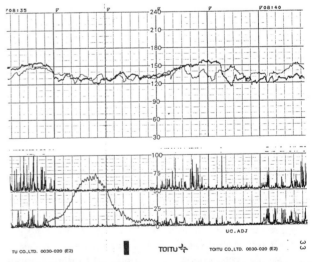

Figure 2.86: Synchronous fetal heart rates. Note the large uniform accelerations, the lack of fetal movement during the contraction, and the uniform acceleration in one twin (the darker tracing) when the other twin had spontaneous accelerations. (Tracing courtesy of Toitu of America, Wayne, PA).

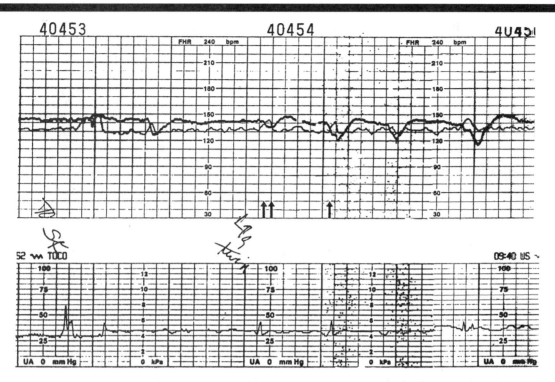

Figure 2.87: Asynchronous twin fetal heart rates at 36 1/2 weeks of gestation. One fetus was reactive and the other was nonreactive with a Checkmark Pattern (seizing). Unfortunately, the woman was discharged from the hospital and returned 4 days later. The fetus who was seizing had died. At delivery it was discovered that the umbilical cord was wrapped tightly around the baby's neck (nuchal cord x 3).

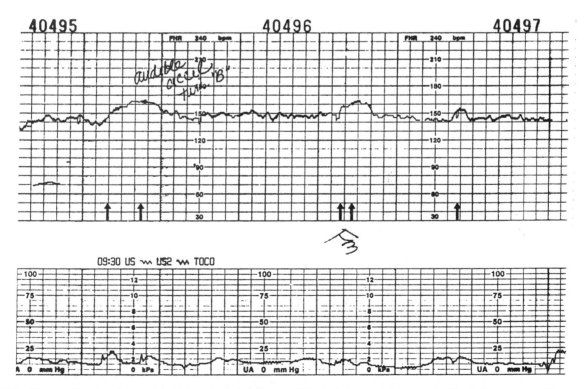

Figure 2.88: Double recording of surviving twin's fetal heart rate (see Figure 2.87). The baby was delivered vaginally with Apgar scores of 9 and 9 at 1 and 5 minutes.

Asynchronous accelerations. Asynchronous twin tracings may also occur and are most important during antepartal testing when one test is reactive and the other is nonreactive. Additional surveillance methods such as a biophysical profile, may help clarify the status of the nonreactive twin. When asynchrony occurs abruptly, e.g., the onset of bradycardia, it is imperative to assess the MHR and the FHRs (534). In some cases (see Figure 5.87), asynchrony may indicate a pathologic condition (548).

THE CONTINUUM OF FETAL WELFARE
The concept of a continuum of fetal welfare is clinically important because it represents the fetus as an adaptable, dynamic organism who is capable of recovery from most hypoxic stress when intervention is prompt and appropriate. FHR patterns help the clinician place the fetus on this continuum. For example, spontaneous accels and STV are signs of an adequate fetal O_2 reserve (287). Late decels, severe or atypical variable decels, and a loss of variability reflect a low O_2 reserve (316). Several umbrella terms have been suggested to categorize FHR patterns within this continuum. For example, intrapartal FHR patterns have been categorized as reassuring, normal, suspicious, questionable, suboptimal, fetal stress, threatening, warning, compensatory, decelerative, nonreassuring, pathological, fetal distress, terminal, and ominous (1-2, 133, 364, 508, 551-554). In July, 1995, ACOG (72) separated FHR patterns into only two categories: reassuring and nonreassuring. Reassuring implied a fetus with "normal O_2 and acid-base status." Nonreassuring patterns were nonspecific and had factors other than hypoxia as their cause. "Fetal distress" has been applied to many abnormal patterns, with different acid-base values (72).

Categorization of the FHR pattern is not based on the emotional state of the caregiver. In fact, they may feel "nonreassured" when there is a reassuring pattern. Categorization of the FHR pattern should reflect where the fetus is believed to be on the "continuum of fetal welfare." Categorization of the FHR pattern is a mental exercise that influences the speed and extent of interventions. It is best to avoid documentation of these categories in the medical record since they may not be agreed upon by other nurses and physicians. Categorization of the FHR pattern is NOT a diagnosis since electronic fetal monitoring is not a diagnostic technique. Physicians and nurses have been known to disagree on the classification of the FHR pattern or the FHR pattern components, but they should agree on the probable physiology, i.e., is the fetus hypoxic or not (555)?

Based on terms suggested by AWHONN (183) and an extensive review of the literature, the continuum of fetal welfare has been divided into four categories in this text: reassuring, compensatory, nonreassuring, and ominous. A well-oxygenated fetus with a *reassuring FHR pattern* should be able to compensate for a decrease in O_2 delivery during contractions. If a hypoxic insult, such as umbilical cord compression or uteroplacental insufficiency occurs, the

previously normoxic fetus (with a reassuring pattern) should develop a FHR pattern indicative of a *compensatory response* to hypoxia. If hypoxia persists, the fetus may quickly deteriorate and demonstrate a *nonreassuring or even an ominous pattern*. A nonreassuring pattern often precedes the birth of an acidemic newborn (556). However, a nonreassuring pattern may also precede the birth of a newborn who has high Apgar scores and normal umbilical cord blood gases (557). In fact, an abnormal tracing alone has been found to only predict an umbilical artery pH less then 7.17 25% of the time (558). An ominous pattern precedes neonatal resuscitation and may precede fetal or neonatal death.

Reassuring FHR Patterns
The *nonhypoxic* fetus has a reassuring pattern. A reassuring pattern is usually preceded by the presence of STV and spontaneous accels and followed by the birth of a responsive, oxygenated neonate. Reassuring patterns have the following recognition criteria:

BL	normal level, neither bradycardic nor tachycardic
STV	present
LTV	may be absent at times, e.g., during fetal quiescence (1F)
ACCELS	spontaneous
DECELS	possibly early decels
Patterns	Sawtooth Pattern, Benign Sinusoidal Pattern, Lambda Pattern

Discussion
The fetus with a reassuring pattern has normal blood gases and absolutely no hypoxic stress. However, the fetal head may be compressed to produce early decels. Some people consider mild variable decels to be part of a reassuring pattern if the BL level is stable, STV and LTV are normal, the decels have an abrupt onset and offset, and there are spontaneous accels.

Compensatory FHR Patterns
The fetus *compensating for hypoxia*, hypovolemia, hypotension, and/or hypertension will demonstrate characteristic changes in the FHR pattern. Interventions should be directed at improving fetal oxygenation and diminishing or removing the suspected cause of hypoxia. Compensatory patterns have the following recognition criteria:

BL	normal level or tachycardia with spontaneous accels or bradycardia with spontaneous accels
STV	present
LTV	usually minimal (3 - 5 bpm) to moderate (11 - 25 bpm), may be marked with STV present
ACCELS	spontaneous or uniform if uniform accels only, BL must be a normal level
DECELS	early decels with tachycardia or bradycardia

mild variable decels (not a Checkmark Pattern)
reflex late decels with "normal" BL variability and possibly accels
only one prolonged decel with an identifiable cause, e.g., maternal hypotension.

Patterns   Saltatory Pattern

Discussion

Tachycardia alone is not usually associated with acidosis (23). The presence of a "reactive" spontaneous accel when there is a tachycardic BL confirms the lack of metabolic acidosis. However, concern about fetal infection or a fetal arrhythmia should be expressed to the physician when tachycardia exists. Late decels with BL STV and accels (reflex late decels) have preceded the birth of nonacidotic neonates (122). The presence of accels and STV suggest metabolic acidosis has not yet occurred. If more than one compensatory sign is seen, e.g., a tachycardic BL and variable decels, the fetus may be becoming progressively more hypoxic, increasing the risk of metabolic acidosis. Measures to elicit an accel, such as scalp stimulation, will confirm the fetus is not yet metabolically acidotic. If an accel is not evident and hypoxia is not relieved, respiratory and/or metabolic acidosis and fetal decompensation may occur and the FHR pattern becomes nonreassuring.

Nonreassuring Patterns

Nonreassuring patterns reflect the deteriorating fetal status due to *hypoxia and the continuing depletion of O_2 reserves which increase the fetal risk of metabolic acidosis*. Fetuses with nonreassuring patterns need prompt attention. *If meconium is in the amniotic fluid, particularly during the second stage of labor, the risk for an abnormal Apgar score and low cord pH doubles (559).* Interventions to prevent further hypoxia and to maximize fetal oxygenation are needed. In some cases, interventions may be taken to identify the fetal acid-base status. Consequently, fetal scalp sampling or stimulation may be helpful to rule out metabolic acidosis. Nonreassuring patterns have the following recognition criteria:

BL   may be tachycardic or bradycardic
STV   may be absent, usually present until the fetus is metabolically acidotic
LTV   usually absent to minimal (3 - 5 bpm), may be marked (> 25 bpm)
ACCELS   **none**
DECELS   early decels with tachycardia, no accels, and absent LTV
variable decels and/or
late decels and/or
2 or more prolonged decels or
spontaneous decels or
a mixed variable and late decel pattern
Other   overshoots
Patterns   Pathologic Sinusoidal Pattern

Discussion

Variability decreases as the fetus becomes progressively more hypoxic (129). Fetal movement also decreases. Tachycardia, "poor" variability, and "significant" variable decels or late decels were associated with abnormally low fetal SpO_2 levels (2, 560). "Intermittent" late decels, "decreased" variability, and tachycardia for more than 30 minutes have been classified as "suspicious" and representative of "fetal distress" (472). Boylan (113) considered marked tachycardia, moderate tachycardia with reduced variability, moderate bradycardia with reduced variability, moderate variable decels, and a normal BL level with minimal variability "suspicious." Words such as reduced and minimal were never defined. Overshoots are an exaggerated sympathoadrenal gland response to hypoxia. When a nonreassuring pattern is seen, it is important to determine

* maternal vital signs
* complaints of pain or discomfort
* amniotic fluid color, amount, and odor
* any vaginal bleeding
* maternal subjective complaints, e.g., could she be abrupting?
* vaginal examination findings to decide the best time and route of delivery.

Interventions should be individualized. Actions should be explained. Maternal anxiety should not be heightened. Delivery decisions will depend on the fetal gestational age, duration of the pattern, estimated time to vaginal birth, predicted ease of delivery, presence of other risk factors, and the response of the fetus to measures used to optimize fetal oxygenation, including amnioinfusion.

In 1995, ACOG (72) had several recommendations when a persistently nonreassuring FHR pattern occurs during labor:

* determine the etiology of the pattern (when possible)
* act to correct the pattern, e.g., improve fetal oxygenation
* if the pattern continues in spite of corrective measures, obtain a scalp pH
* determine if and when operative intervention is warranted.

Ominous Patterns

Persistent, uncorrectable fetal bradycardia, e.g., terminal bradycardia, and repetitive severe variable decels, repetitive late decels, "blunt" decels, or prolonged decels have all been classified as ominous (95, 472). However, the FHR pattern is not really ominous unless the fetus has absolutely no variability and has *metabolic acidosis or asphyxia*. Ominous patterns are associated with fetal death, poor neonatal outcomes, and neonatal death. They *require delivery as soon as possible and neonatal resuscitation*. If at all possible, a physician who is skilled in neonatal intubation and the management of neonatal complications should be present in the delivery room at the time of birth. Recognition criteria of ominous patterns include:

BL   may be any level
STV   **absent**
LTV   absent or absent to minimal (3-5 bpm)

ACCELS   none
DECELS   variable decels with or without overshoots
          late decels
          prolonged decels
          spontaneous decels
PATTERNS Silent Pattern (flat line), Checkmark Pattern,
          Agonal Pattern, wandering baseline

Actions in Response to an Ominous Pattern
- determine the probable etiology
  - which may require an ultrasound scan to rule out a fetal defect, brain death, or seizures
- act to increase fetal oxygenation
- vaginal examination to determine the best route of delivery and to rule out an umbilical cord prolapse
- bladder inflation if a cord prolapse is found (see Chapter 6)
- immediate notification of the physician
- delivery as soon as possible
- neonatal resuscitation
- a physician skilled in neonatal intubation and management of neonatal complications should be present at the birth if at all possible.

Discussion
Late decels with absent BL variability (hypoxic myocardial failure lates) and severe variable decels preceded the delivery of acidotic neonates (23, 119). Usually, the more prolonged the pattern of late decels is, the more severe the acidosis is (146). As variability decreases, so does the pH (119). The drop in pH may be due to respiratory or metabolic acidosis or both. The lowest fetal pH values were found when late decels were associated with "diminished" variability and tachycardia (122). In other words, a combination of FHR changes associated with hypoxia such as absent to minimal LTV, absent STV, tachycardia or bradycardia, and late decels, predicted more cases of acidosis. Cibils (98) found preterm, term, and postterm fetuses who had a flat (fixed) tachycardic BL and variable or late decels often developed bradycardia, an Agonal Pattern, then died. Sometimes, the Agonal Pattern

was associated with an umbilical cord prolapse or meconium. Cibils (98) also found preterm fetuses do not always show clinical signs of severe hypoxic stress for many hours, until the very moment of death, and they rarely pass meconium. However, severely stressed term fetuses consistently passed meconium.

CONCLUSION
Competence in using fetal monitors and interpreting the data they produce is one small part of the many responsibilities and roles of nurses and physicians who care for women and their fetus(s) during the antepartal and intrapartal periods. Although it is "one part," the significance of this part should not be minimized because incorrect interpretation can result in maternal or fetal damage or death. The ability to accurately interpret the monitor tracing requires intense study of electronic monitoring technology, fetal physiology, and the fetal heart rate patterns produced in response to hemodynamic changes in the woman or her fetus. A fetal heart rate pattern may be divided into a baseline, accelerations, and decelerations. It may also contain an arrhythmia or artifact. Two types of accelerations and five types of decelerations may be identified, as well as patterns such as a Sawtooth Pattern, Saltatory Pattern, Lambda Pattern, Sinusoidal Pattern, Agonal Pattern, and Checkmark Pattern. Labels, definitions, recognition criteria, physiology, and actions in response to each of these concepts were presented. Once a systematic review of the baseline, accelerations, and decelerations is completed, the pattern may be classified as reassuring, compensatory, nonreassuring, or ominous. Categorization of the pattern precedes actions and determines the speed at which actions should be implemented and reported to the physician. If all nurses and physicians in the same facility agree with fetal heart rate pattern and uterine activity terms, definitions, recognition criteria, and their physiologic basis, actions in response to the FHR pattern should be consistent. A common knowledge base should facilitate communication and optimize fetal and neonatal outcomes.

References

1.   Cibils, L. A. (April 1996). On intrapartum fetal monitoring. <u>American Journal of Obstetrics and Gynecology, 174</u>(4), 1382-1389.

2.   Beard, R. W., Filshie, G. M., Knight, C. A., & Roberts, G. M. (October 1971). The significance of the changes in the continuous fetal heart rate in the first stage of labour. <u>Journal of Obstetrics and Gynaecology of the British Commonwealth, 78</u>(10), 865-881.

3.   Trimbos, J. B., Keirse, M. J. N. C. (December 1978). Observer variability in assessment of antepartum cardiotocograms. <u>British Journal of Obstetrics & Gynaecology, 85,</u> 900-906.

4.   Afriat, C. I., Simpson, K. R., Chez, B. F., & Miller, L. A. (December 1994). Electronic fetal monitoring competency—To validate or not to validate: The opinions of experts. <u>Journal of Perinatal Nursing, 8</u>(3), 1-16.

5.   Electronic fetal heart rate and monitoring: Research guidelines for interpretation. National Institute of Child Health and Human Development research and planning workshop. (1997). <u>JOGNN,</u> 26(6), 635-640.

6.   Pello, L. C., Dawes, G. S., Smith, J., & Redman, C. W. G. (November 1988). Screening of the fetal heart rate in early labour. <u>British Journal of Obstetrics and Gynaecology, 95,</u> 1128-1136.

7.   Tennyson, R. D. (February 26-March 1, 1987). Computer-based enhancements for the improvement of learning. In M. R. Simonson <u>". . . Mere vehicles. . .": Discussion of what the research says by those who are doing the saying.</u> Symposium conducted at the annual meeting of the association for Educational Communication and Technology, Atlanta, GA.

8.   Murphy, G., & Hochberg, J. (1951). Perceptual development: Some tentative hypothesis. <u>Psychological Review, 58,</u> 332-349.

9.   Gagné, R. M. (1970). Discrimination; Concrete concept learning. <u>The conditions of learning</u> (2nd ed., pp. 155-188). New York, NY: Holt, Rinehart, and Winston, Inc.

10.   McKinney, C. W. (January 1985). A comparison of the effects of a definition, examples, and nonexamples on student acquisition of the concept of "transfer propaganda." <u>Social Education, 49</u>(1), 66, 68-70.

11.   Klausmeier, H. J., & Sipple, T. S. (1980). <u>Learning and teaching concepts: A strategy for testing applications of theory.</u> New York, NY: Academic Press.

12.   Tennyson, R. D., & Cocchiarella, M. J. (1986). An empirically based instructional design theory for teaching concepts. <u>Review of Educational Research, 56</u>(1), 40-71.

13.   Jassal, R. S., & Tennyson, R. D. (1981/1982). Application of concept learning research in the design of instructional systems. <u>International Journal of Instructional Media, 9</u>(3), 185-205.

14.   Mewhort, D. J. K., Merikle, P. M., & Bryden, M. P. (1969). On the transfer from iconic to short-term memory. <u>Journal of Experimental Psychology, 81</u>(1), 89-94.

15.   Tennyson, R. D., & Tennyson, C. L. (1975). Rule acquisition design strategy variables: Degree of instance divergence, sequence, and instance analysis. <u>Journal of Educational Psychology, 67</u>(6), 852-859.

16.   Markle, S. M., & Tiemann, P. W. (1970). <u>Really understanding concepts: Or infrumious pursuit of the jabberwock.</u> Champaign, IL: Stipes Publishing Company.

17.   Ostrow, C. L. (April 1986). The interaction of cognitive style, teaching methodology and cumulative GPA in baccalaureate nursing students. <u>Journal of Nursing Education, 25</u>(4), 148-155.

18.   Park, O. (Spring 1984). Example comparison strategy versus attribute identification strategy in concept learning. <u>American Educational Research Journal, 21</u>(1), 145-162.

19.   Tennyson, R. D. (1973). Effect of negative instances in concept acquisition using a verbal-learning task. <u>Journal of Educational Psychology, 64</u>(2), 247-260.

20.   Merrill, M. D. (1987). The new component design theory: Instructional design for courseware authoring. <u>Instructional Science, 16</u>(1), 19-34.

21.   Haygood, R. C., & Bourne, Jr., L. E. (1965). Attribute- and rule-learning aspects of conceptual behavior. <u>Psychological Review, 72,</u> 175-195.

22.   Woolley, F. R., & Tennyson, R. D. (April 1972). Conceptual model of classification behavior. <u>Educational Technology, 12,</u> 37-39.

23.   Kubli, F. W., Hon, E. H., Khazin, A. F., & Takemura, H. (August 15, 1969). Observations on heart rate and pH in the human fetus during labor. <u>American Journal of Obstetrics and Gynecology, 104</u>(8), 1190-1206.

24.   Wood, C., Newman, W., Lumley, J., & Hammond, J. (November 15, 1969). Classification of fetal heart rate in relation to fetal scalp blood measurements and Apgar score. <u>American Journal of Obstetrics and Gynecology, 105</u>(6), 942-948.

25. Low, J. A., Pancham, S. R., & Worthington, D. N. (April 1, 1977). Intrapartum fetal heart rate profiles with and without asphyxia. American Journal of Obstetrics and Gynecology, 127(7), 729-737.

26. O'Gureck, J. E., Roux, J. F., & Neuman, M. R. (September 1972). A practical classification of fetal heart rate patterns. Obstetrics & Gynecology, 49(3), 356-361.

27. Sarno, Jr. A. P., Phelan, J. P., & Ahn, M. O. (March 1990). Relationship of early intrapartum fetal heart rate patterns to subsequent patterns and fetal outcome. Journal of Reproductive Medicine, 35(3), 239-242.

28. Nageotte, M. P., Freeman, R. K., Freeman, A. G., & Dorchester, W. (March 1, 1983). Short-term variability assessment from abdominal electrocardiogram during the antepartum period. American Journal of Obstetrics and Gynecology, 145(5), 566-569.

29. Moczko, J. A., Breborowicz, G., & Slomko, Z. (1987). A comparative study of usefulness of quantitative parameters in the description of cardiotocogram records. Medical Informatics, 12(3), 231-238.

30. Tortosa, M. N., & Acien, P. (1990). Evaluation of variable decelerations of fetal heart rate with the deceleration index: Influence of associated abnormal parameters and their relation to the state and evolution of the newborn. European Journal of Obstetrics, Gynecology, and Reproductive Biology , 34(3), 235-245.

31. Schmidt, J. (1987). Documenting EFM events. Perinatal Press, 10(6), 79-81.

32. Carroll, J. B. (1964). Words, meanings and concepts. Harvard Educational Review, 34, 178-202.

33. Murphy, D., & Kember, D. (August 1990). Alternative new directions for instructional design. Educational Technology, 42-47.

34. Clark, D. C. (June 1971). Teaching concepts in the classroom: A set of teaching prescriptions derived from experimental research [Monograph]. Journal of Educational Psychology, 62(3), 253-278.

35. Tennyson, R. D., Youngers, J., & Suebsonthi, P. (1983). Concept learning by children using instructional presentation forms for prototype formation and classification-skill development. Journal of Educational Psychology, 75(2), 280-291.

36. Tennyson, R. D., & Park, S. I. (June 1984). Process learning time as an adaptive design variable in concept learning using computer-based instruction. Journal of Educational Psychology, 76(3), 452-465.

37. Tennyson, R. D., & Rothen, W. (1977). Pretask and on-task adaptive design strategies for selecting number of instances in concept acquisition. Journal of Educational Psychology, 69(5), 586-592.

38. Miller, G. A. (March 1956). The magical number seven, plus or minus two: Some limits on our capacity for processing information. The Psychological Review, 63(2), 81-97.

39. Tennyson, R. D., Steve, M. W., & Boutwell, R. C. (1975). Instance sequence and analysis of instance attribute representation in concept acquisition. Journal of Educational Psychology, 67(6), 821-827.

40. Gagné, R. M., Briggs, L. J., & Wager, W. W. (1988). Principles of instructional design (3rd ed., pp. 57-58, 252-253). New York, NY: Holt, Rinehart, and Winston, Inc.

41. Tennyson, C. L., Tennyson, R. D., & Rothen, W. (1980). Content structure and instructional control content structure and instructional control strategies as design variables in concept acquisition. Journal of Educational Psychology, 72(4), 499-505.

42. Chez, B. F., & Verklan, M. T. (1987). Documentation and electronic fetal monitoring: How, where, and what? Journal of Perinatal and Neonatal Nursing, 1(1), 22-28.

43. Irwin, H. J. (April 1978). ESP and the human information processing system. The Journal of the American Society for Psychical Research, 72(2), 111-126.

44. Sandmire, H. F., De Mott, R. K. (April 1, 1996). Intrapartum fetal heart rate assessment: Which method is superior? American Journal of Obstetrics and Gynecology, 174(4), 1395.

45. Reed, S. K. (1972). Pattern recognition and categorization. Cognitive Psychology, 3, 382-407.

46. Tainish, Jr., R. E. (Winter 1990). Fetal heart rate monitoring. International Anesthesiology Clinics, 28(1), 30-32.

47. Strauss, S. S., & Clarke, B. A. (Spring 1992). Decision-making patterns in adolescent mothers. IMAGE: Journal of Nursing Scholarship, 24(1), 69-74.

48. Lawson, G. W., Dawes, C. S., & Redman, C. (June 1984). Analysis of fetal heart rate on-line at 32 weeks gestation. British Journal of Obstetrics and Gynaecology, 91(6), 542-550.

49. Hon, E. H. (1975). An introduction to fetal heart rate monitoring (2nd ed.). Publisher not listed on document.

50. Tournaire, M., Sturbois, G., Zorn, J. R., Breart, G., & Sureau, C. (1980). Fetal monitoring before and during labor: In S. Aladjem, A. K. Brown, & C. Sureau. (Eds.), Clinical perinatology (pp. 331-361). St. Louis, Toronto, London: The C. V. Mosby Company.

51. Bailey, D., Flynn, A. M., & Kelly, J. (July 1980). Antepartum fetal heart-rate monitoring in multiple pregnancy. British Journal of Obstetrics and Gynaecology, 87, 561-564.

52. Ware, D. J., & Devoe, L. D. (December 1994). The nonstress test reassessment of the "gold standard." Clinics in Perinatology, 21(4), 779-797.

53.   Steer, P. J. (February 1987). Fetal monitoring-present and future. <u>European Journal of Obstetrics , Gynaecology, and Reproductive Biology, 24</u>(2), 112-117.

54.   Rey, H. R., James, L. S., & Wiele, R. V. (November/December 1979). Optimized search for parameters useful in the interpretation of fetal heart rate data. <u>Medical Instrumentation, 13</u>(6), 337-343.

55.   Krebs, H. B., Petres, R. E., Dunn, L. J., & Smith, P. J. (February 1, 1982). Intrapartum fetal heart rate monitoring. VI. Prognostic significance of accelerations. <u>American Journal of Obstetrics and Gynecology, 142</u>(3), 297-305.

56.   Martin, C. B., & Gingerich, B. (September/October 1976). Factors affecting the fetal heart rate: Genesis of FHR patterns. <u>JOGNN, 5</u>(5, Suppl.), 16s-25s, 30s-40s.

57.   Emory, E. K., & Noonan, J. R. (August 1984). Fetal cardiac responding: A correlate of birth weight and neonatal behavior. <u>Child Development, 55</u>(4), 1651-1657.

58.   Gimovsky, M. L., & Caritis, S. N. (June 1982). Diagnosis and management of hypoxic fetal heart rate patterns. <u>Clinics in Perinatology, 9</u>(2), 313-324.

59.   Knudson, J. M., Kleinman, C. S., Copel, J. A., & Rosenfeld, L. E. (1994). Ectopic atrial tachycardia in utero. <u>Obstetrics & Gynecology, 84</u>(4), 686-689.

60.   Yunek, M. J., & Lojek, R. M. (December 1978). Fetal and maternal monitoring: Intrapartal fetal monitoring. <u>American Journal of Nursing, 78</u>(12), 2102-2109.

61.   Freeman, R. K., & Garite, T. J. (1981). <u>Fetal heart rate monitoring.</u> Baltimore, MD: Williams and Wilkins.

62.   Schifrin, B. S., Weissman, H., & Wiley, J. (June 1985). Electronic fetal monitoring and obstetrical malpractice. <u>Law, Medicine, and Health Care, 13</u>(3), 100-104.

63.   Ritchie, K. (October 1980). The fetal response to changes in the composition of maternal inspired air in human pregnancy. <u>Seminars in Perinatology, 4</u>(4), 295-299.

64.   Lagercrantz, H., & Bistoletti, P. (August 1977). Catecholamine release in the newborn infant at birth. <u>Pediatric Resuscitation, 11</u>(8), 889-893.

65.   Benson, R. C., Shubeck, F., Deutschberger, J., Weiss, W., & Berendes, H. (August 1968). Fetal heart rate as a predictor of fetal distress. A report from the collaborative project. <u>Obstetrics & Gynecology, 32</u>(2), 259-266.

66.   Gimovsky, M. L., & Bruce, S. L. (March 1986). Aspects of FHR tracings as warning signals. <u>Clinical Obstetrics and Gynecology, 29</u>(1), 51-63.

67. Youchah, J., Chazotte, C., & Cohen, W. R. (July 1989). Heart rate patterns and fetal sepsis. <u>American Journal of Perinatology, 6</u>(3), 356-359.

68.   Rana, J., Ebert, G. A., & Kappy, K. A. (April 1995). Adverse perinatal outcome in patients with an abnormal umbilical coiling index. <u>Obstretrics & Gynecology, 85</u>(4), 573-577.

69.   Matsuda, Y., Patrick, J., Carmichael, L., Fraher, L., & Richardson, B. (May 1994). Recovery of the ovine fetus from sustained hypoxia: Effects on endocrine, cardiovascular, and biophysical activity. <u>American Journal of Obstetrics and Gynecology, 170</u>(5, Pt.1), 1433-1441.

70.   Baxi, L. V., Gindoff, P. R., Pregenzer, G. J., & Parras, M. K. (December 1, 1985). Fetal heart rate changes following maternal administration of a nasal decongestant. <u>American Journal of Obstetrics and Gynecology, 153,</u> 799-800.

71.   Rosevear, S. K., & Hope, P. L. (April 1989). Favourable neonatal outcome following maternal paracetamol overdose and severe fetal distress. Case report. <u>British Journal of Obstetrics and Gynaecology, 96,</u> 491-493.

72.   Fetal heart rate patterns: Monitoring, interpretation, and management. (July 1995). <u>Technical bulletin number 207.</u> Washington, DC: ACOG.

73.   Hammacher, K., Huter, K. A., Bokelmann, J., & Werners, P. H. (1968). Foetal heart frequency and perinatal condition of the foetus and newborn. <u>Gynaecologia, 166,</u> 349-360.

74.   Dawes, G. S., Moulden, M., & Redman, C. W. G. (October 1995). Computerized analysis of antepartum fetal heart rate. <u>American Journal of Obstetrics and Gynecology, 175</u>(4), 1353-1354.

75.   Westgren, M., Holmquist, P., Svenningsen, N. W., & Ingemarsson, I. (July 1982). Intrapartum fetal monitoring in preterm deliveries: Prospective study. <u>Obstetrics & Gynecology, 60</u>(1), 99-106.

76.   Macaulay, J. H., Randall, N. R., Bond, K., & Steer, P. J. (March 1992). Continuous monitoring of fetal temperature by noninvasive probe and its relationship to maternal temperature, fetal heart rate, and cord arterial oxygen and pH. <u>Obstetrics & Gynecology, 79</u>(3), 469-474.

77.   Hager, W. D., & Pauly, T. H. (August 1985). Fetal tachycardia as an indicator of maternal and neonatal morbidity. <u>Obstetrics & Gynecology, 66</u>(2), 191-194.

78.   Youchah, J., Chazotte, C., & Cohen, W. R. (July 1989). Heart rate patterns and fetal sepsis. <u>Journal of Perinatology, 6</u>(3), 356-359.

79.   Day, D., Ugol, J. H., French, J. I., Haverkamp, A., Wall, R. E., & McGregor, J. A. (January 1992). Fetal monitoring in perinatal sepsis. <u>American Journal of Perinatology, 9</u>(1), 28-33.

80.   Cooper, R. L., & Goldenberg, R. L. (May/June 1990). Catecholamine secretion in fetal adaptation to stress. <u>JOGNN, 19</u>(3), 223-226.

81.   Lilien, A. A. (1970). Term intrapartum fetal death. <u>American Journal of Obstetrics and Gynecology, 107</u>(4), 595-603.

82. Phelan, J. P., Stine, L. E., Mueller, E., McCart, D., & Yeh, S. (July 15, 1984). Observations of fetal heart rate characteristics related to external cephalic version and tocolysis. <u>American Journal of Obstetrics and Gynecology, 149</u>(6), 405-410.

83. Persianinov, L. S. (1973). The effect of normal and abnormal labour on the foetus. <u>Acta Obstetricia et Gynecologica Scandinavica, 52</u>(1), 29-36.

84. Marsh, T. D., Lagrew, D. C., Cook, L. N., & Lavery, J. P. (April 1987). Unexplained fetal baseline bradycardia in congenital panhypopituitarism. <u>American Journal of Obstetrics and Gynecology, 156</u>(4), 977-979.

85. Roberts, J. E. (November/December 1989). Managing fetal bradycardia during second stage of labor. <u>MCN, 14,</u> 394-398.

86. Herbert, W. N. P., Stuart, N. N., & Butler, L. S. (July/August 1987). Electronic fetal heart rate monitoring with intrauterine fetal demise...need to distinguish maternal and fetal heart rate. <u>JOGNN, 16</u>(4), 249-252.

87. Block, B. S., Schlafer, D. H., Wentworth, R. A., Kreitzer, L. A., & Nathanielsz, P. W. (May 1990). Intrauterine asphyxia and the breakdown of physiologic circulatory compensation in fetal sheep. <u>American Journal of Obstetrics and Gynecology, 162</u>(5), 1325-1331.

88. Young, B. K., & Weinstein, H. M. (September 15, 1976). Moderate fetal bradycardia. <u>American Journal of Obstetrics and Gynecology, 126</u>(2), 271-275.

89. Wood, E. C. (November 1970). Studies of the human fetus during normal and abnormal labor. <u>International Journal of Gynaecology and Obstetrics, 8</u>(6, Pt. 2), 856-871.

90. Lavery, J. P. (December 1982). Nonstress fetal heart rate testing. <u>Clinical Obstetrics and Gynecology, 25</u>(4), 689-704.

91. Goodlin, R. C. (February 1, 1979). History of fetal monitoring. <u>American Journal of Obstetrics and Gynecology, 133</u>(3), 323-352.

92. Roberts, J., & Goodlin, R. (November/December 1987). Approaches to second stage labor bradycardia. <u>JOGNN, 16</u>(6), 438.

93. Krebs, H. B., Petres, R. E., & Dunn, L. J. (June 15, 1981). Intrapartum fetal heart rate monitoring V. Fetal heart rate patterns in the second stage of labor. <u>American Journal of Obstetrics and Gynecology, 140</u>(4), 435-439.

94. Morel, M., Mikhail, M. S., Stoessel, R., Anyaegbunam, A. (January 1993). Fetal heart rate (FHR) patterns associated with meconium aspiration. <u>American Journal of Obstetrics and Gynecology, 168</u>(1, Pt. 2), 343. SPO abstracts #159.

95. Gilstrap, III, L. C., Hauth, J. C., Schiano, S., & Connor, K. D. (May 1984). Neonatal acidosis and method of delivery. <u>Obstetrics & Gynecology, 63</u>(5), 681-685.

96. Vorherr, H. (September 1, 1975). Placental insufficiency in relation to postterm pregnancy and fetal postmaturity. <u>American Journal of Obstetrics and Gynecology, 123</u>(1), 67-102.

97. Fruchter, O. (June 1993). Variable decelerations during the second stage of labor. <u>American Journal of Obstetrics and Gynecology, 168</u>(6, Pt. 1), 1892-1893.

98. Cibils, L. A. (December 15, 1977). Clinical significance of fetal heart rate patterns during labor. <u>American Journal of Obstetrics and Gynecology, 129</u>(8), 833-843.

99. Low, J. A., Cox, M. J., Karchmar, E. J., McGrath, M. J., Pancham, S. R., & Piercy, W. N. (February 1, 1981). The prediction of intrapartum fetal metabolic acidosis by fetal heart rate monitoring. <u>American Journal of Obstetrics and Gynecology, 139</u>(3), 299-305.

100. Organ, L. W., Hawrylyshyn, P. A., Goodwin, J. W., Milligan, J. E., & Bernstein, A. (January 1, 1978). Quantitative indices of short and long-term heart rate variability. <u>American Journal of Obstetrics and Gynecology, 130</u>(1), 20-27.

101. Tucker, S. M. (1978). <u>Fetal monitoring and fetal assessment in high-risk pregnancy.</u> St. Louis, MO: The C. V. Mosby Company.

102. Roemer, V. M., Holzhauser, B., & Heinzl, S. (1979). The evaluation and significance of intrapartum FHR-oscillation patterns. <u>Journal of Perinatal Medicine, 7</u>(1), 46-52.

103. Donker, D. K., van Geijn, H. P., Derom, R., & Duisterhout, J. S. (1987). Processing and results of a pilot study on interventions based upon cardiotocographic recordings. In K. Dalton, & R. D. S. Fawdry (Eds.), <u>The computer in obstetrics and gynaecology</u> (pp. 159-165). Oxford, England: IRL Press.

104. McCune, G. S., Doig, J., & Ridley, W. (August 1983). Antepartum non-stress cardiotocography in 'high risk' pregnancies. <u>British Journal of Obstetrics and Gynaecology, 90</u>(8), 697-704.

105. Pincus, S. M., & Viscarello, R. R. (February 1992). Approximate entropy: A regularity measure for fetal heart rate analysis. <u>Obstetrics & Gynecology, 79</u>(2), 249-255.

106. Chaffin, D. G., Goldberg, C. C., & Reed, K. L. (November 1991). The dimension of chaos in the fetal heart rate. <u>American Journal of Obstetrics and Gynecology, 165</u>(5, Pt. 1), 1425-1429.

107. Oppenheimer, L. W., & Lewinsky, R. M. (September 1994). Power spectral analysis of fetal heart rate review. <u>Baillieres Clinical Obstetrics and Gynaecology, 8</u>(3), 643-661.

108. Martin, G. R., & Ruckman, R. N. (January/February 1990). Fetal echocardiography: A large clinical experience and follow-up. <u>Journal of the American Society of Echocardiography, 3</u>(1), 4-8.

109. Gabbe, S. G., Niebyl, J. R., & Simpson, J. L. (Eds.) (1991). <u>Obstetrics normal and problem pregnancies</u> (2nd ed.). NY: Churchill Livingstone.

110. Lagrew, D. C. (December 1987). Fetal evaluation in early gestational ages. <u>Clinical Obstetrics and Gynecology, 30</u>(4), 992-998.

111. Dalton, K. J., Dawes, G. S., & Patrick, J. E. (June 15, 1983). The autonomic nervous system and fetal heart rate variability. American Journal of Obstetrics and Gynecology, 146(4), 456-462.

112. Dawes, G. S., & Redman, C. W. G. (December 1992). Automated analysis of the FHR: Evaluation? American Journal of Obstetrics and Gynecology, 167(6), 1912-1916.

113. Boylan, P. (March 1987). Intrapartum fetal monitoring. Bailliere's Clinical and Gynaecology, 1(1), 73-95.

114. Suidan, J. S., Young, B. K., Hochberg, H. M., & George, M. E. (July 1985). Observations of perinatal heart rate monitoring. II. Quantitive unreliability of doppler fetal heart rate variability. Journal of Reproductive Medicine, 30(7), 519-522.

115. Steyn, D. W., & Odendaal, H. J. (November 1994). Fetal heart rate variability prior to delivery in women with severe hypertension who developed placental abruption. British Journal of Obstetrics and Gynaecology, 101, 1005-1006.

116. Parer, J. T., Dijkstra, H. R., Vredebregt, P. P. M., Harris, J. L., Krueger, T. R., & Reuss, M. L. (1980). Increased fetal heart rate variability with acute hypoxia in chronically instrumented sheep. European Journal of Obstetrics, Gynaecology, and Reproductive Biology, 10(6), 393-399.

117. van Ravenswaaij-Arts, C. M. A., Kollee, L. A. A., Hopman, J. C. W., Stoelinga, G. B. A., & van Geijn, H. P. (March 15, 1993). Heart rate variability. Annals of Internal Medicine, 118(6), 436-446.

118. Huey, Jr., J. R., Paul, R. H., Hadjiev, A. A., Jilek, J., & Hon, E. H. (July 15, 1979). Fetal heart rate variability: An approach to automated assessment. American Journal of Obstetrics and Gynecology, 134(6), 691-695.

119. Paul, R. H., Suidan, A. K., Yeh, S-Y., Schifrin, B. S., & Hon, E. H. (September 15, 1975). Clinical fetal monitoring. VII. The evaluation and significance of intrapartum baseline FHR variability. American Journal of Obstetrics and Gynecology, 123(2), 206-210.

120. Samueloff, A., Evron, S., & Sadovsky, E. (August 1, 1983). Fetal movements in multiple pregnancy. American Journal of Obstetrics and Gynecology, 146(7), 789-792.

121. Angel, E. S., Fox, H. E., & Titlebaum, E. L. (April 1979). Digital filtering and fetal heart rate variability. Computer & Biomedical Research, 12(2), 167-180.

122. Clark, S., Gimovsky, M. L., & Miller, F. C. (February 1, 1984). The scalp stimulation test: A clinical alternative to fetal scalp blood sampling. American Journal of Obstetrics and Gynecology, 148(3), 274-277.

123. Dawes, G. S. (July 1995). Beat-to-beat variation. American Journal of Obstetrics and Gynecology, 173(1), 349-351.

124. Dawes, G. S., Visser, G. H. A., Goodman, J. D. S., & Redman, C. W. G. (September 1, 1981). Numerical analysis of the human fetal heart rate: The quality of ultrasound records. American Journal of Obstetrics and Gynecology, 141(1), 43-52.

125. Anthony, M. Y., & Levene, M. I. (1990). An assessment of the benefits of intrapartum fetal monitoring for low-risk full-term fetus. Developmental Medicine and Child Neurology, 32, 547-553.

126. Lawson, G. W., Belcher, R., Dawes, G. S., & Redman, C. W. G. (November 15, 1983). A comparison of ultrasound (with autocorrelation) and direct electrocardiogram fetal heart rate detector systems. American Journal of Obstetrics and Gynecology, 147(6), 721-722.

127. Breborowicz, G., Moczko, J., & Gadzinowski, J. (1988). Quantification of the fetal heart rate variability by spectral analysis in growth-retarded fetuses. Gynecologic & Obstetric Investigation, 25(3), 186-191.

128. Dawes, G. S., Moulden, M., & Redman, C. W. G. (1991). The advantages of computerized fetal heart rate analysis. Journal of Perinatal Medicine, 19(1-2), 39-45.

129. Smith, J. H., Arnand, K. J. S., Cotes, P. M., Dawes, G. S., Harkness, R. A., & Howlett, T. A. (October 1988). Antenatal fetal heart rate variation in relation to the respiratory and metabolic status of the compromised human fetus. British Journal of Obstetrics and Gynaecology, 95, 980-989.

130. Street, P., Dawes, G. S., Moulden, M., & Redman, C. W. G. (September 1991). Short-term variation in abnormal antenatal fetal heart rate records. American Journal of Obstetrics and Gynecology, 165(3), 515-523.

131. Kariniemi, V., Hukkinen, K., Katila, L., & Laine, H. (1979). Quantification of fetal heart rate variability by abdominal electrocardiography. Journal of Perinatal Medicine, 7(1), 27-32.

132. deHaan, J. (1985). Short- and long-term variability in fetal heart rate pattern and its relation to basal heart frequency. In W. Kunzel (Ed.), Fetal heart rate monitoring. Clinical practice and pathophysiology (pp. 191-202). Berlin: Springer-Verlag.

133. Guidelines for the use of fetal monitoring. (1987). International Federation of Gynaecology & Obstetrics, 25, 159-167.

134. Arnold-Aldea, S. A., & Parer, J. T. (1990). Fetal cardiovascular physiology. In R. D. Eden & F. H. Boehm (Eds.), Assessment and care of the fetus: Physiological, clinical and medicolegal principles (pp. 29-41). Norwalk, CT: Appleton & Lange.

135. Akselrod, S., Gordon, D., Ubel, F. A., Shannon, D. C., Barger, A. C., & Cohen, R. J. (July 10, 1981). Power spectrum analysis of heart rate fluctuation: A quantitive probe of beat-to-beat cardiovascular control. Science, 213, 220-222.

136. Groome, L. J., Mooney, D. M., Bentz, L. S., & Wilson, J. D. (January 1994). Vagal tone in normal term fetuses during quiet sleep. American Journal of Obstetrics and Gynecology, 170(1, Pt. 2), 303. SPO abstracts #88.

137. Abboud, S., & Sadeh, D. (March 1990). Power spectrum analysis of fetal heart rate variability using the abdominal maternal electrocardiogram. Journal of Biomedical Engineering, 12(2), 161-164.

138. Visser, G. H. A., Dawes, G. S., & Redman, C. W. G. (August 1981). Numerical analysis of the normal human antenatal fetal heart rate. British Journal of Obstetrics and Gynaecology, 88, 792-802.

139. Bell, P. (May 1978). Heart rate variability in health and disease: A study of adult men. Doctoral dissertation. New Haven, CT: Yale University

140. Roemer, V. M., Heinzl, S., Peters, F. D., Mietzner, S., Ruhl, G., & Heering, P. (June 1979). Oscillation-frequency and baseline fetal heart rate in the last 30 minutes or labour. British Journal of Obstetrics and Gynaecology, 86, 472-479.

141. Parer, J. T. (1983). Handbook of fetal heart monitoring. Philadelphia, PA: W. B. Sanders Company.

142. Low, J. A., Cox, M. J., Karchmar, E. J., McGrath, M. J., Pancham, S. R., & Piercy, W. N. (February 1, 1981). The effect of maternal, labor, and fetal factors upon fetal heart rate during the intrapartum period. American Journal of Obstetrics and Gynecology, 139(3), 306-310.

143. Brown, J. S., Gee, H., Olah, K. S., Docker, M. F., & Taylor, E. W. (May 1992). A new technique for the identification of respiratory sinus arrhythmia in utero. Journal of Biomedical Engineering, 14(3), 263-267.

144. Dawes, G. S., Visser, G. H. A., Goodman, J. D., & Levine, D. H. (July 1, 1981). Numerical analysis of the human fetal heart rate: Modulation by breathing and movement. American Journal of Obstetrics and Gynecology, 140(5), 535-544.

145. van Geijn, H. P., Jongsma, H. W., deHaan, J., Eskes, T. K., & Precht, H. F. (April 15, 1980). Heart rate as an indicator of the behavioral state. Studies in the newborn and prospects for fetal heart rate monitoring. American Journal of Obstetrics and Gynecology, 136(8), 1061-1066.

146. Bistoletti, P., Lagercrantz, H., & Lunell, N. O. (January 1983). Fetal plasma catecholamine concentrations and fetal heart-rate variability during first stage of labour. British Journal of Obstetrics and Gynaecology, 90, 11-15.

147. Ayromlooi, J., Tobias, M., & Berg, P. (December 1980). The effects of scopolamine and ancillary analgesic upon the fetal heart rate recording. Journal of Reproductive Medicine, 25(6), 323-326.

148. Zimmer, E. Z., Divon, M. Y., & Vadasz, A. (1988). Fetal heart rate beat-to-beat variability in uncomplicated labor. Gynecologic & Obstetric Investigation, 25(2), 80-82.

149. The role of fetal monitoring today. (February 15, 1986). Patient Care, 91-93, 96-97, 100, 102, 107-108, 111, 114.

150. Frank, T. H., Blaumanis, O. R., Chen, S. H., Petrie, R. H., Gibbs, R. K., & Wells, R. L. (1992). Noninvasive fetal ECG mode fetal heart rate monitoring by adaptive digital filtering. Journal of Perinatal Medicine, 20(2), 93-100.

151. Young, B. K., Weinstein, H. N., Hochberg, H. M., & George, M. E. D. (April 1978). Observations in perinatal heart rate monitoring. I. A quantitative method of describing baseline variability of the fetal heart rate. Journal of Reproductive Medicine, 20(4), 205-212.

152. Hon, E. H., & Yeh, S. Y. (October/November 1969). Electronic evaluation of fetal heart rate X. The fetal arrhythmia index. Medical Research Engineering, 8(5), 14-19.

153. Shaw, K., & Clark, S. L. (December 1988). Reliability of intrapartum fetal heart rate monitoring in the postterm fetus with meconium passage. Obstetrics & Gynecology, 72(6), 886-889.

154. Atkinson, M. W., Belfort, M. A., Saade, G. R., & Moise, Jr., K. J. (June 1994). The relation between magnesium sulfate therapy and fetal heart rate variability. Obstetrics & Gynecology, 83(6), 967-970.

155. Yeh, S-Y., Forsythe, A., & Hon, E. H. (March 1973). Quantification of fetal heart beat-to-beat interval differences. Obstetrics & Gynecology, 41(3), 355-363.

156. Goodman, J. D. S., Visser, F. G. A., & Dawes, G. S. (July 1984). Effects of maternal cigarette smoking on fetal trunk movements, fetal breathing movements and the fetal heart rate. British Journal of Obstetrics and Gynaecology, 91(7), 657-661.

157. Eriksen, P. S., Gennser, G., Lindvall, R., & Nilsson, K. (1984). Acute effects of maternal smoking on fetal heart beat intervals. Acta Obstetricia et Gynecologica Scandinavica, 63, 385-390.

158. deHaan, J., et al. (1979). Pathophysiological mechanisms underlying fetal heart rate patterns. In O. Thalhammer, et al. (Eds.). Perinatale Medizin (p. 200). Stuttgart: Thieme.

159. ennett, R. J., Daily, W. J., Tarby, T. J., & Manwaring, K. H. (June 1990). Prenatal diagnosis of intracerebellular hemorrhage: Case report. American Journal of Obstetrics and Gynecology, 162(6), 1472-1475.

160. Hadi, H. A., Finley, J., Mallette, J. Q., & Strickland, D. (May 1994). Prenatal diagnosis of cerebellar hemorrhage: Medicolegal implications. American Journal of Obstetrics and Gynecology, 170(5, Pt. 1), 1392-1395.

161. Nijhuis, J. G., Kruyt, N., & Van Wijck, J. A. M. (February 1988). Fetal brain death. Two case reports. British Journal of Obstetrics and Gynaecology, 95, 197-200.

162. Terao, T., Kawashima, Y., Noto, H., Inamoto, Y., Lin, T. Y., Sumimoto, K., & Maeda, M. (May 15, 1984). Neurological control of fetal heart rate in 20 cases of anencephalic fetuses. American Journal of Obstetrics and Gynecology, 149(2), 201-208.

163. Fields, L. M., Haire, M. F., & Troiano, N. H. (1985). Current concepts in fetal monitoring. Litton Datamedix.

164. Frank, T. H., Blaumanis, O. R., Gibbs, R. K., & Wells, R. K. (October 1987). Adaptive filtering in ECG monitoring of the fetal heart rate. Journal of Electrocardiology, 20(Suppl.), 108-113.

165. Lawrence, L. (Winter 1992/1993). Fetal heart monitoring with a fetoscope. Midwifery Today, 24, 30-37.

166. Frank, T. H., Blaumanis, O. R., Chen, S. H., Petrie, R. H., Gibbs, R. K., Wells, R. L. (1992). Noninvasive fetal ECG mode fetal heart rate monitoring by adaptive digital filtering. Journal of Perinatal Medicine, 20(2), 93-100.

167. Solum, T., Ingemarsson, I., & Nygren, A. (1980). The accuracy of abdominal ECG for fetal electronic monitoring. Journal of Perinatal Medicine, 8(3), 142-149.

168. Maulik, D., Saini, V., & Zigrossi, S. T. (1983). Clinical significance of short-term variability computed from heart-rate waveforms. Journal of Perinatal Medicine, 11(5), 243-248.

169. Divon, M. Y., Platt, L. D., Muskat, Y., Sarna, Z., & Paldi, E. (January 1986). Quantification of changes in fetal heart rate and beat-to-beat variability during labor. American Journal of Perinatology, 3(1), 63.

170. Petrie, R. H. (1991). Intrapartum fetal evaluation. In S. G. Gabbe, J. R. Niebyl, J. R., & J. L. Simpson (Eds.), Obstetrics normal and problem pregnancies (2nd ed., pp. 457-491). NY: Churchill Livingstone.

171. Kariniemi, V., Siimes, A., & Ammala, P. (1982). Antepartal analysis of fetal heart rate variability by abdominal electrocardiography. Journal of Perinatal Medicine, 10(2), 114-118.

172. Harvey, C. J. (March/April 1989). Interpreting the electronic fetal monitor: Strategies for management. Journal of Nurse-Midwifery, 34(2), 75-84.

173. Daddario, J. B. (December 1992). Fetal surveillance in the intensive care unit: Understanding electronic fetal monitoring. Critical Care Nursing Clinics of North America, 4(4), 711-719.

174. Weiner, Z., Farmakides, G., Schulman, H., Kellner, L., Plancher, S., & Maulik, D. (October 1994). Computerized analysis of fetal heart rate variation in postterm pregnancy: Prediction of intrapartum fetal distress and fetal acidosis. American Journal of Obstetrics and Gynecology, 171(4), 1132-1138.

175. Gagnon, R., Campbell, M. K., & Hunse, C. (March 1993). A comparison between visual and computer analysis of antepartum fetal heart rate tracings. American Journal of Obstetrics and Gynecology, 168(3, Pt. 3), 842-847.

176. Knopf, K., Parer, J. T., Espinoza, M. I., Horton, J. I., Gunn, A. J., & Williams, C. E. (December 1991). Comparison of mathematical indices of fetal heart rate variability with visual assessment in the human and sheep. Journal of Developmental Physiology, 16(6), 367-372.

177. Sampson, M. B., Mudaliar, N. A., & Lele, A. S. (May 1980). Fetal heart rate variability as an indicator of fetal status. Postgraduate Medicine, 67(5), 207-210, 213-215.

178. Arduini, D., & Rizzo, G. (May 1990). Quantitative analysis of fetal rate: Its application in antepartum clinical monitoring and behavioural pattern recognition. International Journal of Bio-Medical Computing, 25(4), 247-252.

179. Murray, M. (1988). Antepartal and intrapartal fetal monitoring (pp. 192-193). Washington, DC: AWHONN.

180. Afriat, C. I. (1989). Electronic fetal monitoring. Rockville, MD: Aspen Publishers, Inc.

181. Freeman, R. K., Garite, T. J., & Nageotte, M. P. (1991). Fetal heart rate monitoring (2nd ed.). Baltimore, MD: Williams & Wilkins.

182. Bernardes, J., Mourd, C., Marques de Sa, J. P., & Leite, L. P. (1991). The porto system for automated cardiotocographic signal analysis. Journal of Perinatal Medicine, 19(1-2), 61-65.

183. Fetal heart monitoring. Principles & practices. (December 1993). Washington, DC: AWHONN.

184. Cabaniss, M. L. (1993). Fetal monitoring interpretation. Philadelphia, PA: J. B. Lippincott Company.

185. Divon, M. Y., Zimmer, E. Z., Platt, L. D., & Paldi, E. (1985). Human fetal breathing: Associated changes in heart rate and beat-to-beat variability. American Journal of Obstetrics and Gynecology, 151(3), 403-406.

186. Reed, N. N., Mohajer, M. P., & James, D. K. (September 1994). Plymouth randomized control trial of cardiotocogram only versus ST waveform plus cardiotocogram for intrapartum monitoring in 2400 cases. American Journal of Obstetrics and Gynecology, 171(3), 867-868.

187. Westgate, J., Harris, M., Curnow, J. S., & Greene, K. R. (November 1993). Plymouth randomized trial of carditocogram only versus ST waveform plus carditocogram for intrapartum monitoring in 2400 cases. American Journal of Obstetrics and Gynecology, 169(5), 1151-1160.

188. Donchin, Y., Caton, D., & Porges, S. W. (April 15, 1984). Spectral analysis of fetal heart rate in sheep: The occurrence of respiratory sinus arrhythmia. American Journal of Obstetrics and Gynecology, 148(8), 1130-1135.

189. Dalton, K. J., Dawes, G.S., & Patrick, J. E. (February 15, 1977). Diurnal, respiratory, and other rhythms of fetal heart rate in lambs. American Journal of Obstetrics and Gynecology, 127(4), 414-424.

190. Ohno, Y., Tsuji, M., Fujibayashi, H., Tomioka, M., Yamamoto, T., & Okada, H. (June 1986). Assessment of fetal heart rate variability with abdominal fetal electrocardiogram: Changes during fetal breathing movement. Asia-Oceania Journal of Obstetrics and Gynaecology, 12(2), 301-304.

191. Glanze, W. D., Anderson, K. N., & Anderson, L. E. (Eds.). (1990). Mosby's medical, nursing, and allied health dictionary (3rd ed.). St. Louis, MO: The C. V. Mosby Company.

192. Arabin, B., Lorenz, U., Ruttgers, H., & Kubli, F. (July 1988). Course and predictive value of fetal heart rate parameters. American Journal of Perinatology, 5(3), 272-277.

193. Shariati, M. A., & Dripps, J. H., Shariati, H., & Boddy, K. (1993). Linear time series analysis of long term fetal heart rate variability patterns. Biomedical Sciences Instrumentations, 29, 161-168.

194. Visser, G. H., Mulder, E. J., Stevenson, H., & Verweij, R. (September 1993). Heart rate variation during fetal behavioural states 1 and 2. Early Human Development, 34(1-2), 21-28.

195. Petrikovsky, B. M., Vintzileos, A. M., & Nochimson, D. J. (July 1989). Heart rate cyclicity during labor in healthy term fetuses. American Journal of Perinatology, 6(3), 289-291.

196. Krebs, H. B., Petres, R. E., Dunn, L. J., Jordaan, H. V. F., & Segreti, A. (April 1, 1979). Intrapartum fetal heart rate monitoring. I. Classification and prognosis of fetal heart rate patterns. American Journal of Obstetrics and Gynecology, 133(7), 762-772.

197. Saling, E. Z., & Dudenhausen, J. W. (1973). The present situation of clinical monitoring of the fetus during labor. Journal of Perinatal Medicine, 1, 75-103.

198. Spencer, J. A., & Johnson, P. (April 1986). Fetal heart rate variability changes and fetal behavioural cycles during labour. British Journal of Obstetrics and Gynaecology, 93(4), 314-321.

199. Odendaal, H. J. (May 19, 1990). More perinatal deaths associated with poor long-term variability during antenatal fetal heart-rate monitoring. South African Medical Journal, 77(10), 506-508.

200. Nijhuis, J. G., Crevels, A. J., & Van Dongen, P. W. J. (1990). Fetal brain death: The definition of a fetal heart rate pattern and its clinical consequences. Obstetrical and Gynecological Survey, 45(4), 229-232.

201. Biale, Y., Brawer-Ostrovsky, Y., & Insler, V. (January 1985). Fetal heart rate tracings in fetuses with congenital malformations. The Journal of Reproductive Medicine, 30(1), 43-47.

202. Rayburn, W. F. (December 15, 1982). Clinical implications from monitoring fetal activity. American Journal of Obstetrics and Gynecology, 144(8), 967-980.

203. Van der Moer, P. E., Gerretsen, M. D., &Visser, G. H. A. (January 1985). Fixed fetal heart rate pattern after intrauterine accidental decerebration. Obstetrics & Gynecology, 65(1), 125-127.

204. Snijders, R. J. M., Ribbert, L. S. M., Visser, G. H. A., & Mulder, E. J. H. (January 1992). Numeric analysis of heart rate variation in intrauterine growth-retarded fetuses: A longitudinal study. American Journal of Obstetrics and Gynecology, 166(1, Pt. 1), 22-27.

205. Keegan, Jr., K. A., Waffarn, F., & Quilligan, E. J. (December 1, 1985). Obstetric characteristics and fetal heart rate patterns of infants who convulse during the newborn period. American Journal of Obstetrics and Gynecology, 153(7), 732-737.

206. Parer, J. T. (1980). The effect of acute maternal hypoxia on fetal oxygenation and the umbilical circulation in the sheep. European Journal of Obstetrics, Gynecology, and Reproductive Biology, 10(2), 125-136.

207. O'Brien-Abel, N. E., & Benedetti, T. J. (1992). Saltatory fetal heart rate pattern. Journal of Perinatology, 12(1), 13-17.

208. Olah, K. S., Gee, H., & Taylor, E. W. (May 1989). The aetiology and clinical significance of the sinusoidal fetal heart-rate pattern; two case reports. European Journal of Obstetrics, Gynecology, and Reproductive Biology, 31(2), 189-193.

209. O'Grady, J. P., Joseph, J. F., & Gimovsky, M. L. (September/October 1993). Fetal heart rate monitoring casebook. Sinusoidal FHR pattern. Journal of Perinatology, 13(5), 405-409.

210. Busacca, M., Gementi, P., Ciralli, I., & Vignali, M. (1982). Sinusoidal fetal heart rate associated with maternal administration of meperidine and promethazine in labor. Journal of Perinatal Medicine, 10, 215-218.

211. Epstein, H., Waxman, A., Gleicher, N., & Lauersen, N. H. (June 1982). Meperidine-induced sinusoidal fetal heart rate pattern and reversal with naloxone. Obstetrics & Gynecology, 59(Suppl., 6), 22s-25s.

212. Hatjis, C. G., & Meis, P. J. (March 1986). Sinusoidal fetal heart rate pattern associated with butorphanol administration. Obstetrics & Gynecology, 67(3), 377-380.

213. Ninomiya, Y., Murata, Y., Wakatsuki, A., Masaoka, N., Porto, M., & Tyner, J. G. (May 1994). Experimentally induced intermittent sinusoidal heart rate pattern and sleep cycle in fetal lambs. American Journal of Obstetrics and Gynecology, 170(5, Pt. 1), 1421-1424.

214. Veren, D., Boehm, F. H., & Killam, A. P. (July 1982). The clinical significance of a sinusoidal fetal heart rate pattern associated with alphaprodine administration. Journal of Reproductive Medicine, 27(7), 411-414.

215. Funk, M., & Buerkle, L. (July/August 1986). Intrauterine treatment of fetal tachycardia. JOGNN, 15(4), 298-305.

216. Whatever happened to nisentil? (October 1981). The APRS Federal Monitor, 4(7), 4.

217. Spielman, F. J. (September 1987). Systemic analgesics during labor. Clinical Obstetrics and Gynecology, 30(3), 495-503.

218. van Woerden, E. E., van Geijn, H. P., Swartjes, J. M., Caron, F. J. M., Brons, J. T. J., & Arts, N. F. T. (1988). Fetal heart rhythms during behavioural state 1F. European Journal of Obstetrics, Gynecology, and Reproductive Biology, 28, 29-38.

219. Nijhuis, J. G., Staisch, K. J., Martin, Jr., C. B., & Prechtl, H. F. R. (1984). Case reports. A sinusoidal-like fetal heart-rate pattern in association with fetal sucking—report of 2 cases. European Journal of Obstetrics, Gynecology, and Reproductive Biology, 16, 353-358.

220. Sherer, D. M., D'Amico, M. L., Arnold, C., Ron, M., & Abramowicz, J. S. (July 1993). Physiology of isolated long-term variability of the fetal heart rate. <u>American Journal of Obstetrics and Gynecology, 169</u>(1), 113-115.

221. Elliott, J. P., Castro, R. J., & O'Keeffe, D. F. (July 1, 1988). Sinusoidal fetal heart rate associated with gastroschisis. <u>American Journal of Perinatology, 5</u>(3), 295-296.

222. Breart, G., Goupil, F., Legrand, H., Vaquier, J., Rochart, F., & Milliez, J. (February 1981). Antepartum fetal heart rate monitoring. I. A semi-quantitative evaluation of the 'non-stressed' fetal heart rate. <u>European Journal of Obstetrics, Gynecology, and Reproductive Biology, 11</u>(4), 227-237.

223. Modanlou, H. D., & Freeman, R. K. (April 15, 1982). Sinusoidal fetal heart rate pattern: Its definition and clinical significance. <u>American Journal of Obstetrics and Gynecology, 142</u>(8), 1033-1038.

224. Lowe, T. W., Leveno, K. J., Quirk, J. G., Santos-Ramos, R., & Williams, M. L. (September 1984). Sinusoidal fetal heart rate pattern after intrauterine transfusion. <u>Obstetrics & Gynecology, 64</u>(3, Suppl.), 21s-25s.

225. Mueller-Heubach, E., Caritis, S. N., & Edelstone, D. I. (July 1978). Sinusoidal fetal heart rate following intrauterine fetal transfusion. <u>Obstetrics & Gynecology, 52</u>(1, Suppl.), 43s-46s.

226. Young, B. K., Katz, M., & Wilson, S. T. (March 1, 1980). Sinusoidal fetal heart rate. <u>American Journal of Obstetrics and Gynecology, 136</u>(5), 587-597.

227. Baskett, T. F., & Koh, K. S. (September 1974). Sinusoidal fetal heart pattern. A sign of fetal hypoxia. <u>Obstetrics & Gynecology, 44</u>(3), 379-382.

228. Ninomiya, Y., McMahan, P. C., Murata, Y., Wakatsuki, A., Masaoka, N., & Porto, M. (February 1993). Intermittent sinusoidal heart rate pattern in vagotomized fetal lambs. <u>American Journal of Obstetrics and Gynecology, 168</u>(2), 731-735.

229. Kigawa, J., Makio, A., Torii, Y., Narita, K., & Aoki, S. (September 1986). Sinusoidal fetal heart rate pattern in twin pregnancies. <u>Asia-Oceania Journal Obstetrics and Gynaecology, 12</u>(3), 347-352.

230. Katz, M., Wilson, S. J., & Young, B. K. (March 1, 1980). Sinusoidal fetal heart rate. II. Continuous tissue pH studies. <u>American Journal of Obstetrics and Gynecology, 136</u>(5), 594-596.

231. Geifman-Holtzman, O., Kosmas, E., & Wojtowycz, M. (January 1996). Female sensitization with antibodies known to cause hemolytic disease. <u>American Journal of Obstetrics and Gynecology, 174</u>(1, Pt. 2), 446. SPO abstracts #499.

232. Geifman-Holtzman, O., Bernstein, I. M., Berry, S. M., Holtzman, E. J., Vadnais, T. J., & DeMarie, M. A. (March 1996). Fetal RhD genotyping in fetal cells flow sorted from maternal blood. <u>American Journal of Obstetrics and Gynecology, 174</u>(3), 818-822.

233. Hoag, R. W. (June 1986). Fetomaternal hemorrhage associated with umbilical vein thrombosis. Case report. <u>American Journal of Obstetrics and Gynecology, 154</u>(6), 1271-1274.

234. Westover, T. (January 1995). Neonatal outcome after spontaneous massive fetomaternal hemorrhage. <u>American Journal of Obstetrics and Gynecology, 172</u>(1, Pt. 2), 370. SPO abstracts #404.

235. Goodrum, L., Saade, G., Belfort, M., Knudsen, L., Carpenter, R., & Moise Jr., K. (January 1994). The effect of intrauterine transfusions on fetal serum bilirubin in red cell alloimmunization. <u>American Journal of Obstetrics and Gynecology, 170</u>(1, Pt. 2), 400. SPO abstracts #448.

236. Boyle, J., Rose, R., DeYoung, A., Kennedy, M., Waheed, A., & O'Shaughnessy, R. (January 1996). Management and outcome of anti-M isoimmunization. <u>American Journal of Obstetrics and Gynecology, 174</u>(1, Pt. 2), 488. SPO abstracts #659.

237. Ryan, G., Barrett, J. F. R., Mantay, E., Mullen, B., Farine, D., & Morrow, R. J. (January 1994). Misleading tests in the diagnosis of twin-twin transfusion syndrome (TTTS). <u>American Journal of Obstetrics and Gynecology, 170</u>(1, Pt. 2), 399. SPO abstracts #445.

238. Bruner, J., & Rosemond, R. (January 1993). Twin-to-twin transfusion syndrome: A subset of the twin oligohydramnios/polyhydramnios sequence (tops). <u>American Journal of Obstetrics and Gynecology, 168</u>(1, Pt. 2), 360. SPO abstracts #224.

239. Del Valle, G. O., Joffe, G. M., Izquierdo, L. A., Smith, J. F., Kasnic, T., & Gibson, G. J. (January 1992). Acute postraumatic fetal anemia treated with fetal intravascular transfusion. <u>American Journal Obstetrics and Gynecology, 166</u>(1, Pt. 1), 127-129.

240. Gimovsky, M. L. (Spring 1987). Fetal heart rate monitoring casebook. <u>Journal of Perinatology, 7</u>(2), 161-163.

241. Mead, P. B. (September 1989). Parvovirus B19 infection and pregnancy. <u>Contemporary OB/GYN,</u> 56-70.

242. Helstrom, K. K. (February 1990). Fifth disease and pregnancy: What the childbirth educator should know. <u>International Journal of Childbirth Education,</u> 29-30.

243. Finch, C. M. (July/August 1995). Human parvovirus B19 in pregnancy. <u>JOGNN, 24</u>(6), 495-498.

244. Thorsen, P., Jensen, I. P., Jensen, C. F., Jeune, B., Moller, B. R., & Vestergaard, B. F. (January 1996). An epidemic of parvovirus B19 in a population of 3600 pregnant women. A study of demographic risk factors. <u>American Journal of Obstetrics and Gynecology, 174</u>(1, Pt. 2), 403. SPO abstracts #336.

245. Jordan, J. A. (January 1996). Identification of human parvovirus B19 infection in idiopathic nonimmune hydrops fetalis. <u>American Journal of Obstetrics and Gynecology, 174</u>(1, Pt. 1), 37-42.

246. Strodtbeck, F. (September 1995). Viral infections of the newborn. <u>JOGNN, 24</u>(7), 659-667.

247. Shilletto, N., Barrett, J. F. R., Allen, L., Ryan, G., Morrow, R. J., & Farine, D. (January 1996). Human parvovirus B19 related hydrops and elevated fetal creatine kinase. <u>American Journal of Obstetrics and Gynecology, 174</u>(1, Pt. 2), 403. SPO abstracts #335.

248. Management of isoimmunization in pregnancy. (October 1990). <u>Technical bulletin number 148</u>. Washington, DC: ACOG.

249. MacGregor, S. N., Silver, R. K., Gupta, A., Ragin, A., King, G., & Perkins, J. (January 1995). Prediction of fetal anemia in red blood cell isoimmunization not receiving in utero transfusion using serial maternal antibody titers. <u>American Journal of Obstetrics and Gynecology, 172</u>(1, Pt. 2), 336. SPO abstracts #276.

250. Hutchison, C., Lyon, E., Varner, M., & Ward, K. (January 1995). Perinatal parvovirus diagnosis by nested polymerase chain reaction. <u>American Journal of Obstetrics and Gynecology, 172</u>(1, Pt. 2), 306. SPO abstracts #162.

251. Johnson, P., Sharland, G., Allan, L. D., Tynan, M. J., & Maxwell, D. J. (November 1992). Umbilical venous pressure in nonimmune hydrops fetalis: Correlation will cardiac size. <u>American Journal of Obstetrics and Gynecology, 167</u>(5), 1309-1313.

252. Mari, G., Rahman, F., Olofsson, P., Hamdi, A., Arefi, L., & Ammar, M. A. (January 1996). Acute increase of fetal hematocrit and doppler flow velocity of the middle cerebral artery. <u>American Journal of Obstetrics and Gynecology, 174</u>(1, Pt. 2), 458. SPO abstracts #545.

253. Mari, G., Ludomirsky, A., Abuhamad, A., Adrignola, A., Jones, D., & Copel, J. A. (January 1994). Doppler ultrasound in the management of the pregnancy complicated by fetal anemia II. <u>American Journal of Obstetrics and Gynecology, 170</u>(1, Pt. 2), 401. SPO abstracts #452.

254. Mari, G., Adrignolo, A., Abuhamad, A., Moise, K. J., Kirshon, B., & Copel, J. A. (January 1993). Doppler ultrasound in the management of the pregnancy complicated by fetal anemia. <u>American Journal of Obstetrics and Gynecology, 168</u>(1, Pt. 2), 318. SPO abstracts #70.

255. Lysikiewicz, A., Bracero, L. A., & Tejani, N. (January 1993). Fetal preload index predicts fetal hematocrit. <u>American Journal of Obstetrics and Gynecology, 168</u>(1, Pt. 2), 356. SPO abstracts #209.

256. Moise Jr., K. J., Saade, G., Goodrum, L., Belfort, M., & Carpenter, R. J. (January 1994). The effect of advancing gestational age on fetal arterial pressure. <u>American Journal of Obstetrics and Gynecology, 170</u>(1, Pt. 2), 286. SPO abstracts #50.

257. Dunn, P. A., Weiner, S., & Ludomirski, A. (September/October 1988). Percutaneous umbilical blood sampling. <u>JOGNN, 17</u>(5), 308-313.

258. Sala, D. J., Moise, Jr., K. J., Weber, V. E., & Cordella-Simon, L. (September/October 1992). Maternal blood donation for intrauterine transfusion. <u>JOGNN, 21</u>(5), 365-374.

259. Uckele, J. C., Berry, S. M., Bottoms, S. F., Puder, K. S., Dombroski, M. P., & Cotton, D. B. (January 1994). Fetal mean corpuscular volumes and reticulocyte counts predict need for intrauterine transfusion in Rh isoimmunized pregnancies. <u>American Journal of Obstetrics and Gynecology, 170</u>(1, Pt. 2), 399. SPO abstracts #444.

260. Stek, A., Fisher, B., Baker, S., & Clark, K. (January 1994). Cardiovascular responses to methamphetamine in fetal sheep. <u>American Journal of Obstetrics and Gynecology, 170</u>(1, Pt. 2), 269. SPO abstracts #12.

261. Rotmensch, S., Liberati, M., Luo, J-S., & Hobbins, J. C. (November 1992). Monitoring of intravascular fetal transfusions with doppler velocimetry. <u>American Journal of Obstetrics and Gynecology, 167</u>(5), 1314-1316.

262. Macphail, S., & Morrow, R. (January 1994). The fetal hemodynamic response to in-utero transfusion - an ovine model. <u>American Journal of Obstetrics and Gynecology, 170</u>(1, Pt. 2), 310. SPO abstracts #116.

263. Ludomirsky, A. (January 1993). Intrauterine fetal blood sampling-A multicenter registry, evaluation of 7462 procedures between 1987-1991. <u>American Journal of Obstetrics and Gynecology, 168</u>(1, Pt. 2), 318. SPO abstracts #69.

264. Schneider, E. P., & Tropper, P. J. (March 1986). The variable deceleration, prolonged deceleration, and sinusoidal fetal heart rate. <u>Clinical Obstetrics and Gynecology, 29</u>(1), 64-72.

265. Johnson, T. R. B., Besinger, R. E., & Thomas, R. L. (May 1988). New clues to fetal behavior and well-being. <u>Contemporary OB/GYN, 31</u>(5), 108-123.

266. Smith, C. V., Phelan, J. P., & Paul, R. H. (December 1, 1985). A prospective analysis of the influence of gestational age on the baseline fetal heart rate reactivity in low-risk population. <u>American Journal of Obstetrics and Gynecology, 153</u>(7), 780-782.

267. Ferrazzi, E., Bellotti, M., Barbera, A., Flisi, L., Bozzetti, P., & Pardi, G. (January 1994). Peak velocity of the outflow tract of the aorta and heart rate characteristics in growth retarded fetuses. <u>American Journal of Obstetrics and Gynecology, 170</u>(1, Pt. 2), 304. SPO abstracts #94.

268. Antepartum fetal surveillance. (January 1994). <u>Technical bulletin number 188.</u> Washington, DC: ACOG.

269. Pillai, M., & James, D. (January 1990). Behavioural states in normal mature human fetuses. <u>Archives of Disease in Childhood, 65</u>(1 Spec No.), 39-43.

270. Patrick, J., Carmichael, L., Chess, L., Probert, C., & Staples, C. (January 15, 1985). The distribution of accelerations of the human fetal heart rate at 38 to 40 weeks' gestational age. <u>American Journal of Obstetrics and Gynecology, 151</u>(2), 283-287.

271. Freeman, R. (Speaker). (1979). <u>Fetal monitoring: Policy, protocol, pitfalls. #327. The network for continuing medical education (videotape).</u> 15 Columbus Circle, New York 10023.

272. Pello, L. C., Rosevear, S. K., Dawes, G. S., Moulden, M., & Redman, C. W. (October 1991). Computerized fetal heart rate analysis in labor. <u>Obstetrics & Gynecology, 78</u>(4), 602-640.

273. Fetal heart rate monitoring. Guidelines for monitoring, terminology, and instrumentation. (June 1975). Technical bulletin number 32. Washington, DC: ACOG.

274. Aladjem, S., Rest, J., & Stojanovic, J. (July 1977). Fetal heart rate responses to fetal movements. British Journal of Obstetrics and Gynaecology, 84(7), 487-491.

275. Baser, I., Johnson, T. R. B., & Paine, L. L. (July 1992). Coupling of fetal movement and fetal heart rate accelerations as an indicator of fetal health. Obstetrics & Gynecology, 80(1), 62-66.

276. Sadovsky, E., Rabinowitz, R., Freeman, A., & Yarkoni, S. (May 15, 1984). The relationship between fetal heart rate accelerations, fetal movements, and uterine contractions. American Journal of Obstetrics and Gynecology, 149(2), 187-189.

277. Gagnon, R., Campbell, K., Hunse, C., & Patrick, J. (September 1987). Patterns of human fetal heart rate accelerations from 26 weeks to term. American Journal of Obstetrics and Gynecology, 157(3), 743-748.

278. Johnson, T. R., Jordan, E. T., & Paine, L. L. (July 1990). Doppler recordings of fetal movement: II. Comparison with maternal perception. Obstetrics & Gynecology, 76(1), 42-43.

279. Thomas, R. L., Johnson, T. R., Besinger, R. E., Rafkin, D., Treanor, C., & Strobino, D. (July 1989). Preterm and term fetal cardiac and movement responses to vibratory acoustic stimulation. American Journal of Obstetrics and Gynecology, 161(1), 141-145.

280. Baskett, T. F., & Liston, R. M. (September 1989). Fetal movement monitoring: Clinical application. Clinics in Perinatology, 16(3), 613-625.

281. Lee, C. Y., Di Loreto, P. C., & O'Lane, J. M. (February 1975). A study of fetal heart rate acceleration patterns. Obstetrics & Gynecology, 45(2), 142-146.

282. Klavan, M., Laver, A. T., & Boscola, M. (1977). Clinical concepts of fetal heart rate monitoring. Massachusetts: Hewlett-Packard Company.

283. Oxorn-Foote, H. (1986). Human labor & birth (5th ed.). Norwalk, CT: Appleton-Century-Crofts.

284. James, L. S., Yeh, M-N., Morishima, H. O., Daniel, S. S., Caritis, S. N., Niemann, W. H., & Indyk, L. (September 15, 1976). Umbilical vein occlusion and transient acceleration of the fetal heart rate. Experimental observations in subhuman primates. American Journal of Obstetrics and Gynecology, 126(2), 276-283.

285. Cerutti, S., Baselli, G., Civardi, S., Ferrazzi, E., Marconi, A. M., & Pagani, M. (1986). Variability analysis of fetal heart rate signals as obtained from abdominal electrocardiographic recordings. Journal of Perinatal Medicine, 14(6), 445-452.

286. Janulis, D. M. (1989). Primer on electronic fetal monitoring. Personal injury review, 175-214. New York, NY: Matthew Bender.

287. Krebs, H. B., Jordaan, H. V. F., Petres, R. E., Dunn, L. J., & Segreti, A. (April 1, 1979). II. Multifactorial analysis of intrapartum fetal heart rate tracings. American Journal of Obstetrics and Gynecology, 133(7), 773-780.

288. Goldkrand, J. W., & Speichinger, J. P. (May 15, 1975). "Mixed cord compression," fetal heart rate pattern, and its relation to abnormal cord position. American Journal of Obstetrics and Gynecology, 122(2), 144-150.

289. Weingold, A. B., Yonekura, M. L., & O'Kiefe, J. (September 15, 1980). Nonstress testing. American Journal of Obstetrics and Gynecology, 138(2), 195-202.

290. Schneiderman, C. I., Waxman, B., & Goodman, C. J. (August 15, 1972). Maternal-fetal ECG conduction with intrapartum fetal death. American Journal of Obstetrics and Gynecology, 113(8), 1130-1133.

291. Amato, J. C. (December 15, 1983). Fetal heart rate monitoring. American Journal of Obstetrics and Gynecology, 147(8), 967-969.

292. Pillai, M., & James, D. (November 1990). The development of fetal heart rate patterns during normal pregnancy. Obstetrics & Gynecology, 76(5, Pt. 1), 812-816.

293. Sorokin, Y., Bottoms, S. F., Dierker, Jr., L. J., & Rosen, M. G. (August 15, 1982). The clustering of fetal heart rate changes and fetal movements in pregnancies between 20 and 30 weeks of gestation. American Journal of Obstetrics and Gynecology, 143(8), 952-957.

294. Schifrin, B. S., & Clement, D. (1990). Why fetal monitoring remains a good idea. Contemporary OB/GYN, 35, 70-86.

295. Brubaker, K., & Garite, T. J. (December 1988). The lambda fetal heart rate pattern: An assessment of its significance in the intrapartum period. Obstetrics & Gynecology, 72(6), 881-885.

296. Timor-Tritsch, I. E., Dierker, L. J., Zador, I., Hertz, R. H., & Rosen, M. G. (June 1, 1978). Fetal movements associated with fetal heart rate accelerations and decelerations. American Journal of Obstetrics and Gynecology, 131(3), 276-280.

297. O'Gureck, J. E., Roux, J. F., & Neuman, M. R. (September 1972). Neonatal depression and fetal heart rate patterns during labor. Obstetrics & Gynecology, 40(3), 347-355.

298. O'Brien, W. F., Davis, S. E., Grissom, M. P., Eng, R. R., & Golden, S. M. (April 1984). Effect of cephalic pressure on fetal cerebral blood flow. American Journal of Obstetrics and Gynecology, 1(3), 223-226.

299. Mann, L., Carmichael, A., & Duchin, S. (May 1972). The effect of head compression on FHR, brain metabolism and function. Obstetrics & Gynecology, 39(5), 721-726.

300. Okane, M., Shigemitsu, S., Inaba, J., Koresawa, M., Kubo, T., & Iwasaki, H. (1989). Non-invasive continuous fetal transcutaneous pO_2 and pCO_2 monitoring during labor. Journal of Perinatal Medicine, 17(6), 399-410.

301. Richey, S. D., Ramin, S. M., Bawdon, R. E., Roberts, S. W., Dax, J., & Roberts, J. (April 1995). Markers of acute and chronic asphyxia in infants with meconium-stained amniotic fluid. <u>American Journal of Obstetrics and Gynecology, 172</u>(4, Pt. 1), 1212-1215.

302. Kelly, J. V. (March 1, 1963). Compression of the fetal brain. <u>American Journal of Obstetrics and Gynecology, 85</u>(5), 687-694.

303. Anderson, N. (September 1983). X-ray pelvimetry: Helpful or harmful? <u>The Journal of Family Practice, 17</u>(3), 405-412.

304. Seitchik, J., & Chatkoff, M. L. (1977). Intrauterine pressure wave form characteristics of successful and failed first stage labor. <u>Gynecologic Investigation, 8,</u> 246-253.

305. Mandry, J., Grandjean, H., Reme, J. M., Pastor, J., Levade, C., & Pontonnier, G. (July 1983). Assessment of the predictive value of x-ray pelvimetry and biparietal diameter in cephalopelvic disproportion. <u>European Journal of Obstetrics, Gynaecology, and Reproductive Biology, 15</u>(3), 173-179.

306. Yamazaki, H., Uchida, K., & Eng, D. (September 1, 1983). A mathematical approach to problems of cephalopelvic disproportion at the pelvic inlet. <u>American Journal of Obstetrics and Gynecology, 147</u>(1), 25-37.

307. Obstetric forceps. (August 1989). <u>Committee opinion no. 71.</u> Washington, DC: ACOG.

308. Silbar, E. L. (May 1986). Factors related to the increasing cesarean section rates for cephalopelvic disproportion. <u>American Journal of Obstetrics and Gynecology, 154</u>(5), 1095-1098.

309. Myers, R. E. (May 1, 1975). Maternal psychological stress and fetal asphyxia: A study in the monkey. <u>American Journal of Obstetrics and Gynecology, 122</u>(1), 47-59.

310. Willcourt, R. J., King, J. C., Indyk, L., & Queenan, J. T. (August 1, 1981). The relationship of fetal heart rate patterns to the fetal transcutaneous PO_2. <u>American Journal of Obstetrics and Gynecology, 140</u>(7), 760-769.

311. Thomas, G. (February 1975). The aetiology, characteristics and diagnostic relevance of late deceleration patterns in routine obstetric practice. <u>British Journal of Obstetrics and Gynaecology, 82,</u> 121-125.

312. van Geijn, H. P., Copray, F. J. A., Donkers, D. K., & Bos, M. H. (December 1991). Diagnosis and management of intrapartum fetal distress. <u>European Journal of Obstetrics, Gynecology and Reproductive Biology, 42</u>(Suppl.), s63-s72.

313. Mulder, E. J. H., & Visser, G.H. A. (1987). Braxton-Hicks contractions and motor behavior in the near-term human fetus. <u>American Journal of Obstetrics and Gynecology, 156,</u> 543.

314. Parer, J. T., Krueger, T. R., & Harris, J. L. (February 15, 1980). Fetal oxygen consumption and mechanisms of heart rate response during artificially produced late decelerations of fetal heart rate in sheep. <u>American Journal of Obstetrics and Gynecology, 136</u>(4), 478-482.

315. Takemura, H. (1973). Pathophysiological classification of perinatal depressions and cybernetics in obstetrics—a working hypothesis for a model of life. <u>Journal of Perinatal Medicine, 1,</u> 24-35.

316. Krebs, H. B., Petres, R. E., Dunn, L. J., & Segretti, A. (September 15, 1980). Intrapartum fetal heart rate monitoring. IV. Observations on elective and nonelective fetal heart rate monitoring. <u>American Journal of Obstetrics and Gynecology, 138</u>(2), 213-219.

317. Bekedam, D. J., Visser, G. H. A., Mulder, E. J. H., Poelmann-Weesjes, G. (1987). Heart rate variation and movement incidence in growth-retarded fetuses: The significance of antenatal late heart rate decelerations. <u>American Journal of Obstetrics and Gynecology, 157,</u> 126-133.

318. Van Hook, J., Harvey, C., Anderson, G., Shailer, T., & Troyer, L. (January 1995). Increases in human fetal hemoglobin oxygen saturation during late fetal heart rate decelerations as a response to intrauterine stress. <u>American Journal of Obstetrics and Gynecology, 172</u>(1, Pt. 2), 365. SPO abstracts #383.

319. Morishima, H. O., Daniel, S. S., Richards, R. T., & James, L. S. (October 1, 1975). The effect of increased maternal PaO_2 upon the fetus duing labor. <u>American Journal of Obstetrics and Gynecology, 123</u>(3), 257-264.

320. James, L. S., Morishima, H. O., Daniel, S. S., Bowe, E. T., Cohen, H., & Niemann, W. H. (July 1, 1972). Mechanism of late deceleration of the fetal heart rate. <u>American Journal of Obstetrics and Gynecology, 113</u>(5), 578-582.

321. Aldrich, C. J., D'Antona, D., Spencer, J. A., Wyatt, J. S., Peebles, D. M., & Delpy, D. T. (January 1995). Late fetal heart decelerations and changes in cerebral oxygenation during the first stage of labour. <u>British Journal of Obstetrics & Gynaecology, 102</u>(1), 9-13.

322. Willis, C., & Foreman, Jr., C. S. (March 1988). Chronic massive fetomaternal hemorrhage: A case report. <u>Obstetrics & Gynecology, 71</u>(3, Pt. 2), 459-461.

323. Damron, D. P., Chaffin, D. G., Anderson, C. F., & Reed, K. L. (January 1994). Umbilical arterial velocity ratios and venous pulsations in fetuses with late decelerations. <u>American Journal of Obstetrics and Gynecology, 170</u>(1, Pt. 2), 402. SPO abstracts #459.

324. Sarno, Jr., A. P., & Phelan, J. P. (July 1988). Intrauterine resuscitation of the fetus. <u>Contemporary OB/GYN, 32</u>(1), 143-145, 149-152.

325. Schifrin, B. S. (April 1972). Fetal heart rate patterns following epidural anaesthesia and oxytocin infusion during labour. <u>Journal of Obstetrics and Gynaecology of the British Commonwealth, 79,</u> 332-339.

326. Trudinger, B. J., Wu, Z., Song, J., & Rowlands, S. (January 1996). Placental insufficiency is characterized by platelet activation in fetus and mother. <u>American Journal of Obstetrics and Gynecology, 174</u>(1, Pt. 2), 391. SPO abstracts #295.

327. Paulick, R. P., Meyers, R. L., & Rudolph, A. M. (July 1992). Effect of maternal oxygen administration on fetal oxygenation during graded reduction of umbilical or uterine blood flow in fetal sheep. <u>American Journal of Obstetrics and Gynecology, 167</u>(1), 233-239.

328. Murata, Y., Martin, Jr., C. B., Ikenoue, T., Hashimoto, T., Taira, S., & Sagawa, T. (September 15, 1982). Fetal heart rate accelerations and late decelerations during the course of intrauterine death in chronically catherized rhesus monkeys. American Journal of Obstetrics and Gynecology, 144(2), 218-223.

329. Harris, J. L., Krueger, T. R., & Parer, J. T. (November 1, 1982). Mechanisms of late decelerations of the fetal heart rate during hypoxia. American Journal of Obstetrics and Gynecology, 144(5), 491-496.

330. Afriat, C. I. (March 1983). The nurse's role in fetal resuscitation. Perinatology/Neonatology, 7(3), 29-30, 32.

331. Parer, J. T. (1985). Fetal hemodynamic responses to reduced uterine blood flow in the sheep fetus. In W. Kunzel (Ed.), Fetal heart rate monitoring. Clinical practice and pathophysiology (pp. 82-93). Berlin: Springer-Verlag.

332. Silva, P. D., Miller, K. D., Madden, J., & Keegan, K. A. (1987). Abnormal fetal heart rate pattern associated with severe intrapartum maternal ethanol intoxication. A case report. Journal of Reproductive Medicine, 32(2), 144-146.

333. Mendez-Bauer, C., Shekarloo, A., Cook, V., & Freese, U. (1987). Treatment of acute intrapartum fetal distress by 2-sympathomimetics. American Journal of Obstetrics and Gynecology, 156(3), 638-642.

334. Patriarco, M. S., Viechnicki, B. M., Hutchinson, T. A., Klasko, S. K., & Yeh, S-Y. (August 1987). A study on intrauterine fetal resuscitation with terbutaline. American Journal of Obstetrics and Gynecology, 157(2), 384-387.

335. Gimovsky, M. L. (Summer 1988). Fetal heart rate monitoring casebook. Journal of Perinatology, 8(3), 276-281.

336. Ball, R. H., & Parer, J. T. (June 1992). The physiologic mechanisms of variable decelerations. American Journal of Obstetrics and Gynecology, 166(6, Pt. 1), 1683-1689.

337. Krebs, H. B., Petres, R.E., & Dunn, L. J. (February 1, 1983). Intrapartum fetal heart rate monitoring. VIII. Atypical variable decelerations. American Journal of Obstetrics and Gynecology, 145(3), 297-305.

338. Goodlin, R. C., & Lowe, E. W. (January 1974). A functional umbilical cord occlusion heart rate pattern. The significance of overshoot. Obstetrics & Gynecology, 43(1), 22-30.

339. Weiss, E., Hitschold, T., & Berle, P. (February 1991). Umbilical artery blood flow velocity waveforms during variable decelerations of the fetal heart rate. American Journal of Obstetrics and Gynecology, 164(2), 534-540.

340. Gaziano, E. P. (October 1, 1979). A study of variable decelerations in association with other heart rate patterns during monitored labor. American Journal of Obstetrics and Gynecology, 135(3), 360-363.

341. Premature rupture of membranes. (April 1988). Technical bulletin number 115. Washington, DC: ACOG.

342. Chung, F., & Hon, E. H. (June 1959). The electronic evaluation of fetal heart rate: I. With pressure on the fetal skull. Obstetrics & Gynecology, 13(6), 633-640.

343. Richardson, B., Carmichael, L., Homan, J., & Johnston, L. (January 1996). Cerebral metabolism in the ovine fetus during heart rate decelerations with umbilical cord compression. American Journal of Obstetrics and Gynecology, 174(1, Pt. 2), 378. SPO abstracts #243.

344. Itskovitz, J., La Gamma, E. F., & Rudolph, A. M. (October 1983). Heart rate and blood pressure responses to umbilical cord compression in fetal lambs with special reference to the mechanism of variable decelerations. American Journal of Obstetrics and Gynecology, 147(4), 451-457.

345. Lee, S. T., & Hon, E. H. (November 1963). Fetal hemodynamic response to umbilical cord compression. Obstetrics & Gynecology, 22(5), 553-562.

346. Bergmans, M., Stevens, G., Keunen, H., & Hasaart, T. (January 1996). Transcutaneous and arterial carbon dioxide tension during intermittent umbilical cord occlusion in lambs. American Journal of Obstetrics and Gynecology, 174(1, Pt. 2), 335. SPO abstracts #77.

347. Welt, S. I. (March 1984). The fetal heart rate W-sign. Obstetrics & Gynecology, 63(3), 405-408.

348. Rayburn, W. F., Beynen, & Brinkman, D. L. (April 1981). Umbilical cord length and intrapartum complications. Obstetrics & Gynecology, 57(4), 450-452.

349. Larson, J. D., Rayburn, W. F., Crosby, S., & Thurnau, G. R. (October 1995). Multiple nuchal cord entanglements and intrapartum complications. American Journal of Obstetrics and Gynecology, 173(4), 1228-1231.

350. Anyaegbunam, A., Ditchik, A., Stoessel, R., & Mikhail, M. S. (January 1993). Vibroacoustic stimulation (VAS) of the fetus entering second stage of labor. American Journal of Obstetrics and Gynecology, 168(1, Pt. 2), 343. SPO abstracts #161.

351. Collins, J. H., Collins, C. L., Weckwerth, S. R., & De Angelis, L. (1995). Nuchal cords: Timing of prenatal diagnosis and duration. American Journal of Obstetrics and Gynecology, 173, 768.

352. Petrikovsky, B. (March 1995). Fetal grasping of the umbilical cord [Letters]. American Journal of Obstetrics and Gynecology, 172(3), 1071.

353. Spong, C. Y., Salafia, C. M., Sherer, D. M., Ghidini, A., & Minior, V. K. (January 1996). Severe fetal heart rate variable decelerations are associated with umbilical vasculitis/histologic amnionitis in preterm infants. American Journal of Obstetrics and Gynecology, 174(1, Pt. 2), 490. SPO abstracts #667.

354. Yeh, M-N., Morishima, H. O., Niemann, W. H., & James, L. S. (April 1, 1975). Myocardial conduction defects in association with compression of the umbilical cord. American Journal of Obstetrics and Gynecology, 121(7), 951-957.

355. Murata, Y., Quilligan, E. J., Ninomiya, Y., Wakatsuki, A., Masaoka, N., & Oka, S. (February 1994). Variable fetal heart rate decelerations and electrocortical activities. American Journal of Obstetrics and Gynecology, 170(2), 689-692.

356. Edelstone, D. I. (July 1984). Fetal compensatory responses to reduced oxygen delivery. Seminars in Perinatology, 8(3), 184-191.

357. Simmons, J. N., Rufleth, P., & Lewis, P. E. (February 1985). Identification of nuchal cords during nonstress testing. The Journal of Reproductive Medicine, 30(2), 97-100.

358. Goodlin, R. C. (December 1986). Mechanism of amnioinfusion [Letters]. American Journal of Obstetrics and Gynecology, 155(6), 1359-1360.

359. Puder, K. S., Sorokin, Y., Bottoms, S. F., Hallak, M., & Cotton, D. B. (December 1994). Amnioinfusion: Does the choice of solution adversely affect neonatal electrolyte balance? Obstetrics & Gynecology, 84(6), 956-959.

360. Patil, N., Damle, P. S., & Sangamnerkar, A. V. (March 1982). Application of heart rate variability analysis to detect foetal distress. Indian Journal of Medical Research, 75, 366-371.

361. Ramin, K., Leveno, K., Kelly, M., & Carmody, T. (January 1994). Observations concerning the pathophysiology of meconium aspiration syndrome. American Journal of Obstetrics and Gynecology, 170(1, Pt. 2), 312. SPO abstracts #124.

362. Thorp, J. A., Trobough, T., Evans, R., Hendricks, J., & Yeast, J. D. (1994). Oxygen administration in the second stage of labor and cord blood co-oximetry. American Journal of Obstetrics and Gynecology, 170(1, Pt. 2), 305. SPO abstracts #98.

363. Singquefield, G. (January/February 1985). Midwifery management of end-stage decelerations. Journal of Nurse-Midwifery, 30(1), 49-52.

364. Eganhouse, D. J. (January/February 1991). Electronic fetal monitoring education and quality assurance. JOGNN, 20,(1), 16-22.

365. Burchfield, D. J. (February 1995). Amnioinfusion-A method to reduce the need for neonatal resuscitation. Intermountain West NRP News, 2(1), 1.

366. Mercer, B. M., McNanley, T., O'Brien, J., Randal, L., & Sibai, B. M. (October 1995). Early versus late amniotomy for labor induction: A randomized trial. American Journal of Obstetrics and Gynecology, 173(4), 1321-1325.

367. Miyazaki, F. S. (1987). 18 serial amnioinfusions for relief of cord compressions. In J. T. Queenan, & J. C. Hobbins (Eds.), Protocols for high-risk pregnancies (2nd ed., pp. 100-103). Oradell, NJ: Medical Economics Books.

368. Miyazaki, F. S., & Nevarez, F. (October 1, 1985). Saline amnioinfusion for relief of repetitive variable decelerations: A prospective randomized study. American Journal of Obstetrics and Gynecology, 153(3), 301-306.

369. Strong, Jr., T. H., Hetzler, G., & Paul, R. H. (March 1990). Amniotic fluid volume increase after amnioinfusion of a fixed volume. American Journal of Obstetrics and Gynecology, 162(3), 746-748.

370. Nageotte, M. P., Freeman, R. K., Garite, T. J., & Dorchester, W. (1985). Prophylactic intrapartum amnioinfusion in patients with preterm premature rupture of membranes. American Journal of Obstetrics and Gynecology, 153(5), 557-562.

371. Imanaka, M., Ogita, S., & Sugawa, T. (July 1989). Saline solution amnioinfusion for oligohydramnios after premature rupture of the membranes. A preliminary report. American Journal of Obstetrics and Gynecology, 161(1), 102-106.

372. Wenstrom, K. D., & Parsons, M. T. (April 1989). The prevention of meconium aspiration in labor using amnioinfusion. Obstetrics & Gynecology, 73(4), 647-651.

373. Cooper Nellist, K. (September 1, 1993). Questions meconium aspiration syndrome etiology. Ob Gyn News, 1, 35.

374. Miyazaki, F. S., & Taylor, N. A. (July 15, 1983). Saline amnioinfusion for relief of variable or prolonged decelerations. A preliminary report. American Journal of Obstetrics and Gynecology, 146(6), 670-678.

375. Ogita, S., Imanaka, M., Matsumoto, M., Oka, T., & Sugawa, T. (January 1988). Transcervical amnioinfusion of antibiotics: A basic study for managing premature rupture of membranes. American Journal of Obstetrics and Gynecology, 158(1), 23-27.

376. Wolfe, H. M., Dombrowski, M. P., Zador, I. E., Treadwell, M. C., & Sokol, R. J. (January 1993). Amniotic fluid volume: A major determinant of fetal visualization. American Journal of Obstetrics and Gynecology, 168(1, Pt. 2), 350. SPO abstracts #184.

377. Sherer, D. M., McAndrew, J. A., Liberto, L., & Woods, Jr., J. R. (January 1992). Recurring bilateral renal agenesis diagnosed by ultrasound with the aid of amnioinfusion at 18 weeks' gestation. American Journal of Perinatology, 9(1), 49-51.

378. Busowski, J., Pendergraft, J. S., Parsons, M., & O'Brien, W. (January 1995). Transabdominal amnioinfusion prior to induction of labor. American Journal of Obstetrics and Gynecology, 172(1, Pt. 2), 287. SPO abstracts #87.

379. Blakemore, K., Pressman, E., McGowan, K., Rossiter, J., Crino, J., & Callan, N. (January 1993). Amniolyte: A physiologic solution for artificial amniotic fluid. American Journal of Obstetrics and Gynecology, 168(1, Pt. 2), 353. SPO abstracts #194.

380. Pressman, E., & Blakemore, K. (January 1996). A prospectively randomized trial of two solutions for intrapartum amnioinfusion: Effects on fetal electrolytes, osmolality and acid-base status. American Journal of Obstetrics and Gynecology, 174(1, Pt. 2), 387. SPO abstracts #280.

381. van den Wijngaard, J. A., Pijpers, L., Reuss, A., & Wladimiroff, J. W. (1987). Effect of amnioinfusion on the umbilical doppler flow velocity waveform: A case report. Fetal Therapy, 2(1), 27-30.

382. Pryde, P. G., Isada, N. B., Johnson, M. P., Romero, R., Reichler, A., & Evans, M. I. (January 1994). Prenatal diagnostic amnioinfusion: Does oligohydramnios predispose to infection? American Journal of Obstetrics and Gynecology, 170(1, Pt. 2), 401. SPO abstracts #451.

383. Glantz, J. C., & Letteney, D. L. (January 1996). Pumps and warmers during amnioinfusion: Is either necessary? Obstetrics & Gynecology, 87(1), 150-155.

384. Chauhan, S. P. (November 1991). Amniotic fluid index before and after amnioinfusion of a fixed volume of normal saline. Journal of Reproductive Medicine, 36(11), 801-802.

385. Thomas, S. J., & Nageotte, M. P. (June 1993). Amniotic fluid during labor and delivery. Seminars in Perinatology, 17(3), 210-219.

386. Spong, C. Y., McKindsey, F., & Ross, M. G. (January 1996). Amniotic fluid index (AFI) predicts the relief of variable decelerations following amnioinfusion bolus. American Journal of Obstetrics and Gynecology, 174(1, Pt. 2), 480. SPO abstracts #626.

387. Ouzounian, J. G., Miller, D. A., & Paul, R. H. (February 1996). Amnioinfusion in women with previous cesarean births: A preliminary report. American Journal of Obstetrics and Gynecology, 174(2), 783-786.

388. Strong, Jr., T. H., Hetzler, G., Sarno, A. P., & Paul, R. H. (June 1990). Prophylactic intrapartum amnioinfusion: A randomized clinical trial. American Journal of Obstetrics and Gynecology, 162(6), 1370-1374.

389. Haubrich, K. L. (July/August 1990). Amnioinfusion: A technique for the relief of variable deceleration. JOGNN, 19(4), 299-303.

390. Stringer, M., Librizzi, R., & Weiner, S. (June 1990). Management of midtrimester oligohydramnios: A case for amnioinfusion. Journal of Perinatology, 10(2), 143-145.

391. Vergani, P., Ceruti, P., Strobelt, N., Locatelli, A., D'Oria, P., Mariani, S., & Ghidini, A. (January 1996). Transabdominal amnioinfusion in oligo-hydramnios at term with intact membranes prior to induction of labor: A randomized clinical trial. American Journal of Obstetrics and Gynecology, 174(1, Pt. 2), 490. SPO abstracts #668.

392. Nageotte, M. P., Bertucci, L., Towers, C. V., Lagrew, D. L., & Modanlou, H. (May 1991). Prophylactic amnioinfusion in pregnancies complicated by oligohydramnios: A prospective study. Obstetrics & Gynecology, 77(5), 677-680.

393. Schrimmer, D. B., Macri, C. J., & Paul, R. H. (October 1991). Prophylactic amnioinfusion as a treatment for oligohydramnios in laboring patients: A prospective, randomized trial. American Journal of Obstetrics and Gynecology, 165(4, Pt. 1), 972-975.

394. Sadovsky, Y., Amon, E., Bade, M. E., & Petrie, R. H. (September 1989). Prophylactic amnioinfusion during labor complicated by meconium: A preliminary report. American Journal of Obstetrics and Gynecology, 161(3), 613-617.

395. Cialone, P. R., Sherer, D. M., Ryan, R. M., Sinkin, R. A., & Abramowicz, J. J. (March 1994). Amnioinfusion during labor complicated by particulate meconium-stained amniotic fluid decreases neonatal morbidity. American Journal of Obstetrics and Gynecology, 170(3), 842-849.

396. Cialone, P. R., Abramowicz, J. S., Ryan, R. M., Sinkin, R. A., & Sherer, D. M. (January 1993). Markedly significant decrease in neonatal morbidity associated with amnioinfusion for labor complicated by particulate meconium. American Journal of Obstetrics and Gynecology, 168(1, Pt. 2), 319. SPO abstracts #75.

397. Eriksen, N. L., Hostetter, M., & Parisi, V. M. (October 1994). Prophylactic amnioinfusion in pregnancies complicated by thick meconium. American Journal of Obstetrics and Gynecology, 171(4), 1026-1030.

398. Uhing, M. R., Bhat, R., Philobos, M., & Raju, T. N. K. (January 1993). Value of amnioinfusion in reducing meconium aspiration syndrome. American Journal of Perinatology, 10(1), 43-45.

399. Wu, B. T., Sun, L. J., & Tang, L. Y. (March 1991). Intrapartum amnioinfusion for replacement of meconium-stained amniotic fluid to prevent meconium aspiration syndrome. Chinese Medical Journal-Peking, 104(3), 221-224.

400. Chauhan, S. P., & Morrison, J. C. (March 1993). Questions on prophylactic amnioinfusion as a treatment for oligohydramnios [Letters]. American Journal of Obstetrics and Gynecology, 168(3, Pt. 1), 1006-1007.

401. Nageotte, M. P., Bertucci, L., Towers, C. V., Lagrew, D. C., & Mondanlou, H. (January 23-27, 1990). Prophylactic amnioinfusion in pregnancies complicated by oligohydramnios or thick meconium: A prospective study (abstract #68). Presented at the tenth annual meeting of the Society of Perinatal Obstetricians, Houston, TX.

402. Bower, S. J., Flack, N. J., Sepulveda, W., Talbert, D. G., & Fisk, N. M. (August 1995). Uterine artery blood flow response to correction of amni-otic fluid volume. American Journal of Obstetrics and Gynecology 173(2), 502-507.

403. Fisk, N. M., Talbert, D. G., Nicolini, U., Vaughan, J., & Rodeck, C. H. (June 1992). Fetal breathing movements in oligohydramnios are not increased by amnioinfusion. British Journal of Obstetrics & Gynaecology, 99(6), 464-468.

404. Fisk, N. M., Ronderos-Dumit, D., Soliani, A., Nicolini, U., Vaughan, J., & Rodeck, C. H. (August 1991). Diagnostic and therapeutic transabdominal amnioinfusion in oligohydramnios. Obstetrics & Gynecology, 78(2), 270-278.

405. Blackstone, J., Young, B. K., Bautista, J., Ordorica, S., & Hoskins, I. A. (January 1994). Does amnioinfusion affect fetal acid-base status? American Journal of Obstetrics and Gynecology, 170(1, Pt. 2), 398. SPO abstracts #441.

406. MacGregor, S. N., Banzhaf, W. C., Silver, R. K., & Depp, R. (January 1991). A prospective, randomized evaluation of intrapartum amnioinfusion. Fetal acid-base status and cesarean delivery. Journal of Reproductive Medicine, 36(1), 69-73.

407. Usta, I. M., Mercer, B. M., Aswood, N. K., & Sibai, B. M. (January 1994). The impact of a policy of amnioinfusion for meconium-stained amniotic fluid. American Journal of Obstetrics and Gynecology, 170(1, Pt. 2), 391. SPO abstracts #422.

408. Sigman, R. (January 1996). Does the availability of amnioinfusion reduce the incidence of meconium aspiration syndrome (MAS)? <u>American Journal of Obstetrics and Gynecology, 174</u>(1, Pt. 2), 359. SPO abstracts #176.

409. Spong, C. Y., Ogundipe, O. A., & Ross, M. G. (January 1994). Prophylactic amnioinfusion for meconium stained amniotic fluid. <u>American Journal of Obstetrics and Gynecology, 170</u>(1, Pt. 2), 285. SPO abstracts #46.

410. Wenstrom, K. D., Andrews, W. W., & Maher, J. E. (January 1994). Prevalence, protocols, and complications associated with amnioinfusion. <u>American Journal of Obstetrics and Gynecology, 170</u>(1, Pt. 2), 341. SPO abstracts #235.

411. Posner, M. D., Ballagh, S. A., & Paul, R. H. (September 1990). The effect of amnioinfusion on uterine pressure and activity: A preliminary report. <u>American Journal of Obstetrics and Gynecology, 163</u>(3), 813-818.

412. Knorr, L. J. (September/October 1989). Relieving fetal distress with amnioinfusion. <u>MCN, 14,</u> 346-350.

413. Galvan, B. J., Van Mullem, C., & Broekhuizen, F. F. (May/June 1989). Using amnioinfusion for the relief of repetitive variable decelerations during labor. <u>JOGNN, 18</u>(8), 222-229.

414. Wallerstedt, C., Higgins, P., Kasnic, T., & Curet, L. B. (September 1994). Amnioinfusion: An update. <u>JOGNN, 23</u>(7), 573-578.

415. Tabor, B. L., & Maier, J. A. (January 1987). Polyhydramnios and elevated intrauterine pressure during amnioinfusion. <u>American Journal of Obstetrics and Gynecology, 156</u>(1), 130-131.

416. Fisk, N. M., Tannirandorn, Y., Nicolini, U., Talbert, D. G., & Rodeck, C. H. (August 1990). Amniotic pressure in disorders of amniotic fluid volume. <u>Obstetrics & Gynecology, 76</u>(2), 210-214.

417. Sorensen, T., Sobeck, J., & Benedetti, T. (November 1991). Intrauterine pressure in acute iatrogenic hydramnios. <u>Obstetrics & Gynecology, 78</u>(5, Pt. 2), 917-919.

418. Strong, Jr., T. H., Vega, J. S., O'Shaughnessy, M. J., Feldman, D. B., & Koemptgen, J. G. (May 1992). Amnioinfusion among women attempting vaginal birth after cesarean delivery. <u>Obstetrics & Gynecology, 79</u>(5, Pt. 1), 673-674.

419. Cook, V., Roy, W., & Spinnato, J. A. (January 1994). Amnioinfusion and vaginal birth after cesarean section. <u>American Journal of Obstetrics and Gynecology, 170</u>(1, Pt. 2) . SPO abstracts #379.

420. Hagay, Z. J., Leiberman, J. R., Picard, R., & Katz, M. (November 1989). Uterine rupture complicating midtrimester abortion. A report of two cases. <u>Journal of Reproductive Medicine, 34</u>(11), 912-916.

421. Dibble, L. A., & Elliott, J. P. (September/October 1992). Possible amniotic fluid embolism associated with amnioinfusion. <u>Journal of Maternal-Fetal Medicine, 1</u>(5), 263-266.

422. Sprung, J., Cheng, E. Y., Patel, S., & Kampine, J. P. (May/June 1992). Understanding and management of amniotic fluid embolism. <u>Journal of Clinical Anesthesia, 4</u>(3), 235-240.

423. Hardin, L., Fox, L. S., & O'Quinn, A. G. (August 1991). Amniotic fluid embolism. <u>Southern Medical Journal, 84</u>(8), 1046-1048.

424. Stromme, W. B., & Fromke, V. L. (July 1978). Amniotic fluid embolism and disseminated intravascular coagulation after evacuation of missed abortion. <u>Obstetrics & Gynecology, 52</u>(Suppl., 1), 76s-80s.

425. Corridan, M., Kendall, E. D., & Begg, J. D. (November 1980). Cord entanglement causing premature placental separation and amniotic fluid embolism. Case report. <u>British Journal of Obstetrics and Gynaecology, 87</u>(11), 935-940.

426. Mirchandani, H. G., Mirchandani, I. H., & Parikh, S. R. (March 1988). Hypernatremia due to amniotic fluid embolism during a saline-induced abortion. <u>American Journal of Forensic Medicine & Pathology, 9</u>(1), 48-50.

427. Benson, M. D. (September 1993). Nonfatal amniotic fluid embolism. Three possible cases and a new clinical definition. <u>Archives of Family Medicine, 2</u>(9), 989-994.

428. Noble, W. H., & St. Amand, J. (October 1993). Amniotic fluid embolus. <u>Canadian Journal of Anaesthesia, 40</u>(10), 971-980.

429. Chung, A. F., & Merkatz, I. R. (December 1973). Survival following amniotic fluid embolism with early heparinization. <u>Obstetrics & Gynecology, 42</u>(6), 809-812.

430. Dolyniuk, M., Orfei, E., Vania, H., Karlman, R., & Tomich, P., (March 1983). Rapid diagnosis of amniotic fluid embolism. <u>Obstetrics & Gynecology, 61</u>(3, Suppl.), 28s-30s.

431. Hammerschmidt, D. E., Ogburn, P. L., & Williams, J. E. (December 1984). Amniotic fluid activates complement. A role in amniotic fluid embolism syndrome? <u>Journal of Laboratory & Clinical Medicine, 104</u>(6), 901-907.

432. Arnone, B. (March/April 1989). Amniotic fluid embolism: A case report. <u>Journal of Nurse-Midwifery, 34</u>(2), 92-94.

433. Hogberg, U., & Joelsson, I. (1985). Amniotic fluid embolism in Sweden. <u>Gynecologic & Obstetric Investigation, 20</u>(3), 130-137.

434. Clark, S. L., Hankins, G. D. V., Dudley, D. A., Dildy, G. A., & Porter, T. F. (April 1995). Amniotic fluid embolism: Analysis of the national registry. <u>American Journal Obstetrics and Gynecology, 172</u>(4, Pt. 1), 1158-1169.

435. Sisson, M. C. (December 1992). Amniotic fluid embolism. <u>Critical Care Nursing Clinics of North America, 4</u>(4), 667-673.

436. Kobayashi, H., Ohi, H., & Terao, T. (March 1993). A simple, noninvasive, sensitive method for diagnosis of amniotic fluid embolism by monoclonal antibody TKH-2 that recognizes NeuAc 2-6GalNAc. <u>American Journal of Obstetrics and Gynecology, 168</u>(3, Pt. 1), 848-853.

437. Azegami, M., & Mori, N. (November 1986). Amniotic fluid embolism and leukotrienes. <u>American Journal of Obstetrics and Gynecology, 155</u>(5), 1119-1124.

438. Davies, M. G., & Harrison, J. C. (May 20-June 2, 1992). Amniotic fluid embolism: Maternal mortality revisited. <u>British Journal of Hospital Medicine, 47</u>(10), 775-776.

439. Johnson, T. R. B., Abbasi, I. A., & Urso, P. J. (July 1987). Fetal heart rate patterns associated with amniotic fluid embolism. <u>American Journal of Perinatology, 4</u>(3), 187-190.

440. Lau, G., & Chui, P. P. (April 1994). Amniotic fluid embolism: A review of 10 fatal cases. <u>Singapore Medical Journal, 35</u>(2), 180-183.

441. Mulder, J. L. (June 15, 1985). Amniotic fluid embolism: An overview and case report. <u>American Journal of Obstetrics and Gynecology, 152</u>(4), 430-435.

442. Clark, S. L. (October 1991). Amniotic fluid embolism. <u>Critical Care Clinics, 7</u>(4), 877-882.

443. Porter, T. F., Clark, S. L., Dildy, G. A., Hankins, G. D. V. (January 1996). Isolated disseminated intravascular coagulation and amniotic fluid embolism. <u>American Journal of Obstetrics and Gynecology, 174</u>(1, Pt.2), 486. SPO abstracts #650.

444. Cheung, A. N., & Luk, S. C. (1994). The importance of extensive sampling and examination of cervix in suspected cases of amniotic fluid embolism. <u>Archives of Gynecology & Obstetrics, 255</u>(2), 101-105.

445. Masson, R. G., & Ruggieri, J. (December 1985). Pulmonary microvascular cytology. A new diagnostic application of the pulmonary artery catheter. <u>Chest, 88</u>(6), 908-914.

446. Roungsipragarn, R., & Herabutya, Y. (January 1993). Amniotic fluid embolism: A case report. <u>Journal of the Medical Association of Thailand, 76</u>(Suppl., 1), 105-107.

447. Masson, R. G. (December 1992). Amniotic fluid embolism. <u>Clinics in Chest Medicine, 13</u>(4), 657-665.

448. Shinagawa, S., Katagiri, S., Noro, S., & Nishihira, M. (February 1983). An autopsy study of 306 cases of maternal death in Japan. <u>Nippon Sanka Fujinka Gakkai Zasshi - Acta Obsetrica et Gynaecologica Japonica, 35</u>(2), 194-200.

449. Maher, J. E., Wenstrom, K. D., Hauth, J. C., & Meis, P. J. (May 1994). Amniotic fluid embolism after saline amnioinfusion: Two cases and review of the literature. <u>Obstetrics & Gynecology, 83</u>(5, Pt. 2), 851-854.

450. Smith, Jr., J. S., & Snider, M. T. (March 1989). An improved technique for rapid infusion of warmed fluid using a level 1™ fluid warmer. <u>Surgery, Gynecology and Obstetrics, 168,</u> 273-274.

451. Quetel, T. A., Mejides, A. A., Salman, F. A., & Torres-Rodriguez, M. M. (August 1992). Amnioinfusion: An aid in the ultrasonographic evaluation of severe oligohydramnios in pregnancy. <u>American Journal of Obstetrics and Gynecology, 167</u>(2), 333-336.

452. Uhl, L., Pacini, D., & Kruskall, M. S. (November 1992). A comparative study of blood warmer performance. <u>Anesthesiology, 77</u>(5), 1022-1028.

453. Presson, Jr., R. G., Bezruczko, A. P., Hillier, S. C., & McNiece, W. L. (May 1993). Evaluation of a new fluid warmer effective at low to moderate flow rates. <u>Anesthesiology, 78</u>(5), 974-980.

454. Faries, G., Johnston, C., Pruitt, K. M., & Plouff, R. T. (November 1, 1991). Temperature relationship to distance and flow rate of warmed IV fluids. <u>Annals of Emergency Medicine, 20</u>(11), 1198-1200.

455. Cruikshank, D. P. (January 1, 1978). An unusual fetal heart rate pattern. <u>American Journal of Obstetrics and Gynecology, 130</u>(1), 101-102.

456. Landy, H. J., Khoury, A. N., & Heyl, P. S. (August 1989). Antenatal ultrasonographic diagnosis of fetal seizure activity. <u>American Journal of Obstetrics and Gynecology, 161</u>(2), 308.

457. Ramin, K. D., Ramin, S. M., Richey, S. D., & Cunningham, F. G. (July 1995). Acute pancreatitis in pregnancy. <u>American Journal of Obstetrics and Gynecology, 173</u>(1), 187-191.

458. Ball, R. H., Espinoza, M. I., Parer, J. T., Alon, E., Vertommen, J., & Johnson, J. (January 1994). Regional blood flow in asphyxiated fetuses with seizures. <u>American Journal of Obstetrics and Gynecology, 170</u>(1, Pt. 1), 156-161.

459. Doi, S., Murata, Y., Quilligan, E. J., Nagata, N., Ikeda, T., & Park, S. (January 1996). Effects of fetal seizure activities on fetal heart rate, blood pressure and breathing movements in fetal lambs. <u>American Journal of Obstetrics and Gynecology, 174</u>(1, Pt. 2), 380. SPO abstracts #251.

460. Conover, W. B., Yarwood, R. L., Peacock, M. D., & Thomas, B. A. (October 1986). Antenatal diagnosis of fetal seizure activity with use of real-time ultrasound. <u>American Journal of Obstetrics and Gynecology, 155</u>(4), 846-847.

461. Peters, A. J. M., Abrams, R. M., Burchfield, D. J., & Gilmore, R. L. (November/December 1992). Seizures in a fetal lamb after cocaine exposure: A case report. <u>Epilepsia, 33</u>(6), 1001-1004.

462. Bejsovec, M. I. R., Kulenda, Z., & Ponca, E. (April 1967). Familial intrauterine convulsions in pyridoxine dependency. <u>Archives of Disease in Childhood, 42</u>(222), 201-207.

463. Standley, C. A., Irtenkauf, S. M., Mason, B. A., & Cotton, D. B. (January 1995). Differential regulation of seizure activity in the hippocampus of male and female rats. <u>American Journal of Obstetrics and Gynecology, 172</u>(1, Pt. 2), 316. SPO abstracts #194.

464. Williamson, D. A. J. (December 12, 1968). Fits in utero, followed by infantile myoclonic twitchings. <u>Proceedings of the Royal Society of Medicine, 61</u>(12), 1255-1256.

465. Sokol, R. J., Rosen, M. G., Borgstedt, A. D., Lawrence, R. A., & Steinbrecher, M. (August 1974). Abnormal electrical activity of the fetal brain and seizures of the infant. <u>American Journal of Diseases of Children, 127</u>(4), 477-483.

466. Young, S. L., Vosper, H. J., & Phillips, S. A. (1992). Cocaine: Its effect on maternal and child health. <u>Pharmacotherapy, 12</u>(1), 2-17.

467. Shimizu, T., Nagai, T., Nishimura, R., Amano, H., Ihara, Y., & Yomura, W. (June 1991). Does fetal seizure activity mean a poor outcome? A case report. <u>Journal of Reproductive Medicine, 36</u>(6), 453-454.

468. Maouris, P. G. (October 1987). Spontaneous fetal seizures in utero [Correspondence]. <u>American Journal of Obstetrics and Gynecology, 157</u>(4, Pt. 1), 1009-1010.

469. Nagata, N., Murata, Y., Fujimori, K., Hirano, T., Doi, S., & Matsuura, M. (January 1995). Heart rate changes associated with abnormal breathing movements in fetuses prior to death. <u>American Journal of Obstetrics and Gynecology, 172</u>(1, Pt. 2), 322. SPO abstracts #219.

470. Miller, F. C., Gonzales, F., Mueller, E., & McCart, D. (August 1983). Case reports. Fetal hiccups: An associated fetal heart rate pattern. <u>Obstetrics & Gynecology, 62</u>(2), 253-255.

471. Goodlin, R. C., & Haesslein, A. C. (December 15, 1977). Fetal reacting bradycardia. <u>American Journal of Obstetrics and Gynecology, 129</u>(8), 845-856.

472. Rayburn, W. F., Johnson, M. Z., Hoffman, K. L., Donn, S. M., & Nelson, Jr., R. M. (April 1987). Intrapartum fetal heart patterns and neonatal intraventricular hemorrhage. <u>American Journal of Perinatology, 4</u>(2), 98-101.

473. Mills, P., Moreno, R., & Loy, G. (January 1993). Predictability of brachial blood pressure changes for fetal heart rate decelerations following epidural anesthesia. <u>American Journal of Obstetrics and Gynecology, 168</u>(1, Pt. 2), 438. SPO abstracts #518.

474. Stavrou, C., Hofmeyr, G. J., & Boezaart, A. P. (January 20, 1990). Prolonged fetal bradycardia during epidural analgesia. Incidence, timing and significance. <u>South African Medical Journal, 77</u>(2), 66-68.

475. Puolakka, J., Jouppila, R., Jouppila, P., & Puukka, M. (1984). Maternal and fetal effects of low-dosage bupivacaine paracervical block. <u>Journal of Perinatal Medicine, 12</u>, 75-84.

476. Freeman, R. K., Gutierrez, N. A., Ray, M. L., Stovall, D., Paul, R. K., & Hon, E. H. (July 1, 1972). Fetal cardiac response to paracervical block anesthesia. Part I. <u>American Journal of Obstetrics and Gynecology, 113</u>(5), 583-591.

477. Achiron, R., Rojansky, N., & Zakut, H. (1987). Fetal heart rate and uterine activity following paracervical block. <u>Clinical Experiments in Obstetrics and Gynecology, 14</u>(1), 52-56.

478. Fujimori, K., Endo, C., Kin, S., Funata, Y., Araki, T., & Sato, A. (August 1994). Endocrinologic and biophysical responses to prolonged (24-hour) hypoxemia in fetal goats. <u>American Journal of Obstetrics and Gynecology, 171</u>(2), 470-477.

479. Lipshitz, J., Shaver, D. C., & Anderson, G. D. (November 1980). Hexoprenaline tocolysis for intrapartum fetal distress and acidosis. <u>Journal of Reproductive Medicine, 31</u>(11), 1023-1026.

480. Leveno, K. J., Quirk, J. G., Cunningham, F. G., Nelson, S. D., Santos-Ramos, R., & Toofanian, A. (November 1, 1984). Prolonged pregnancy. I. Observations concerning the causes of fetal distress. <u>American Journal of Obstetrics and Gynecology, 150</u>(5, Pt. 1), 465-473.

481. Forouzan, I. (January 1995). Hemodynamic changes in fetuses with absent end-diastolic velocity in umbilical artery. <u>American Journal of Obstetrics and Gynecology, 172</u>(1, Pt. 1), 244.

482. Sfameni, S. F., Cole, M., McBain, J., & Heath, P. (August 1986). The significance of cardiotocographic monitoring in pregnancy complicated by intrauterine growth retardation and prematurity. <u>Australian & New Zealand Journal of Obstetrics and Gynaecology, 26</u>(3), 185-192.

483. Devoe, L., Boehm, F., Paul, R., Frigoletto, F., Penso, C., & Goldenberg, R. (February 1994). Clinical experience with the Hewlett-Packard M-1350A fetal monitor: Correlation of doppler-detected fetal body movements with fetal heart rate parameters and perinatal outcome. <u>American Journal of Obstetrics and Gynecology, 170</u>(2), 650-655.

484. Fetal movement profile (May 1991). Germany: Hewlett-Packard.

485. Eganhouse, D. J., & Burnside, S. M. (September/October 1992). Nursing assessment and responsibilities in monitoring the preterm pregnancy. <u>JOGNN, 21</u>(5), 355-363.

486. Castillo, R. A., Devoe, L. D., Arthur, M., Searle, N., Metheny, W. P., & Ruedrich, D. A. (January 1989). The preterm nonstress test: Effects of gestational age and length of study. <u>American Journal of Obstetrics and Gynecology, 160</u>(1), 172-175.

487. Swartjes, J. M., van Geijn, H. P., Mantel, R., & Shoemaker, H. C. (January 1992). Quantitated fetal heart rhythm at 20, 32 and 38 weeks of gestation and dependence on rest-activity patterns. <u>Early Human Development, 28</u>(1), 27-36.

488. Visser, G. H. A. (May 1984). Antenatal cardiotocography in the evaluation of fetal well-being. <u>Australian and New Zealand Journal of Obstetrics & Gynaecology, 24</u>(2), 80-85.

489. Wakatsuki, A., Kutty, K. K., Murata, Y., Ninomiya, Y., & Masaoka, N. (1992). Control of baseline heart rate in the fetal lambs. <u>Journal of Maternal-Fetal Medicine, 1</u>, 20-23.

490. Ikuo, S., Akio, I., Taro, T., (June/July 1992). Longitudinal measurements of fetal heart rate (FHR) monitoring in second trimester. Early Human Development, 29(1-3), 251-257.

491. Natale, R., Nasello-Paterson, C., & Turliuk, R. (January 15, 1985). Longitudinal measurements of fetal breathing, body movements, heart rate, and heart rate accelerations and decelerations at 24 to 32 weeks of gestation. American Journal of Obstetrics and Gynecology, 151(2), 256-263.

492. Snijders, R. J. M., McLaren, R., & Nicolaides, K. H. (1990). Computer-assisted analysis of fetal heart rate patterns at 20-40 weeks' gestation. Fetal Diagnosis and Therapy, 5(2), 79-83.

493. Mulder, E. J., Derks, J. B., Zonneveld, M. F., Bruinse, H. W., & Visser, G. H. (January 1994). Transient reduction in fetal activity and heart rate variation after maternal betamethasone administration. Early Human Development, 36(1), 49-60.

494. Rotmensch, S., Liberati, M., Sahavi, Z., Lev, S., Efrat, Z., & Kobo, M. (January 1996). Suppression of fetal biophysical activity and false diagnosis of asphyxia following antenatal steroid administration. American Journal of Obstetrics and Gynecology, 174(1, Pt. 2), 336. SPO abstracts #83.

495. May, D. A., & Sturtevant, N. V. (October 1991). Embryonal heart rate as a predictor of pregnancy outcome: A prospective analysis. Journal of Ultrasound in Medicine, 10(10), 591-593.

496. Bowes, Jr., W. A., Gabre, S. G., & Bowes, C. (August 1, 1980). Fetal heart rate monitoring in premature infants weighing 1,500 grams or less. American Journal of Obstetrics and Gynecology, 137(7), 791-796.

497. Bartnicki, J., & Saling, E. (May 1994). The influence of maternal oxygen administration on the fetus. International Federation of Gynecology and Obstetrics, 45, 87-95.

498. Guinn, D. A., Kimberlin, D. F., Wigton, T. R., Socol, M. L., & Frederiksen, M. C. (January 1995). Fetal heart rate characteristics at 25-28 weeks. American Journal of Obstetrics and Gynecology, 172(1, Pt. 2), 341. SPO abstracts #294.

499. Thomas, R. L. (July 1989). Preterm-term fetal cardiac and movement responses to vibratory acoustic stimulation. American Journal of Obstetrics and Gynecology, 161(1), 141-145.

500. Amon, E., Steigerwald, J., & Winn, H. (January 1995). Obstetric factors associated with survival of the borderline viable liveborn infant (500-750 gm.). American Journal of Obstetrics and Gynecology, 172(1, Pt. 2), 418. SPO abstracts #579.

501. LeFebvre, F., Glorieux, J., & St. Laurent-Gagnon, T. (March 1996). Neonatal survival and disability rate at age 18 months for infants born between 23 and 28 weeks of gestation. American Journal of Obstetrics and Gynecology, 174(3), 833-838.

502. Whyte, H. E., Fitzhardinge, P. M., Shennan, A. T., Lennox, K., & Lacy, J. (July 1993). Extreme immaturity: Outcome of 568 pregnancies of 23-26 weeks' gestation. Obstetrics & Gynecology, 82(1), 1-7.

503. Kramer, W., Saade, G., Goodrum, L., Montgomery, L., Belfort, M., & Moise, Jr., K. (January 1995). Neonatal outcome after aggressive perinatal management of the very premature infant. American Journal of Obstetrics and Gynecology, 172(1, Pt. 2), 417. SPO abstracts #574.

504. Minkoff, H., Schaffer, R. M., Delke, I., & Grunebaum, A. N. (March 1985). Diagnosis of intracranial hemorrhage in utero after a maternal seizure. Obstetrics & Gynecology, 65(3, Suppl.), 22s-24s.

505. Bowes, Jr., W. A. (September 1988). Clinical management of preterm delivery. Clinical Obstetrics & Gynecology, 31(3), 652-660.

506. Johnson, D., Shew, S., Dougherty, G., Moore, T., & Bejar, R. (January 1993). The contribution of delivery route and labor to the development of large intraventricular hemorrhages (IVH) in preterm infants. American Journal of Obstetrics and Gynecology, 168(1, Pt. 2), 366. SPO abstracts #249.

507. Westgren, L. M. R., Malcus, P., & Svenningsen, N. W. (April 1986). Intrauterine asphyxia and long-term outcome in preterm fetuses. Obstetrics & Gynecology, 67(4), 512-516.

508. Burrus, D. R., O'Shea, Jr., T. M., Veille, J-C., & Mueller-Heubach, E. (October 1994). The predictive value of intrapartum fetal heart rate abnormalities in the extremely premature infant. American Journal of Obstetrics and Gynecology, 171(4), 1128-1132.

509. Nageotte, M. P. (1986). Amnioinfusion. Perinatal Outreach Program, (6), 14. (Memorial Medical Center of Long Beach; Women's Hospital, 2801 Atlantic Avenue, Long Beach, California 90801-1428).

510. Vintzileos, A. M., Campbell, W. A., Dreiss, R. J., Neckles, S., & Nochimson, D. J. (March 15, 1985). Intrapartum fetal heart rate monitoring of the extremely premature fetus. American Journal of Obstetrics and Gynecology, 151(6), 744-751.

511. Salafia, C. M., Spong, C. Y., Minior, V. K., & Sherer, D. M. (January 1996). The combination of severe fetal heart rate variable decelerations and decreased variability are associated with elevated initial nRBC values in preterm newborns. American Journal of Obstetrics and Gynecology, 174(1, Pt. 2), 490. SPO abstracts #666.

512. Assali, W. S., Brinkman, III, C. R., Woods, Jr., J. R., Dandavine, A., & Nuwayhid, B. (December 1, 1977). Development of neurohumoral control of fetal, neonatal, and develop cardiovascular function. American Journal of Obstetrics and Gynecology, 129(7), 740-759.

513. Zanini, B., Paul, R. H., & Huey, J. R. (January 1, 1980). Intrapartum fetal heart rate: Correlation with scalp pH in the preterm fetus. American Journal of Obstetrics and Gynecology, 136(1), 43-47.

514. Arduini, D., Rizzo, G., & Romanini, C. (January 1993). The development of abnormal heart rate patterns after absent end-diastolic velocity in umbilical artery: Analysis of risk factors. American Journal of Obstetrics and Gynecology, 168(1, Pt. 1), 43-54.

515. Simkin, P. (December 1986). Stress, pain, and catecholamines in labor: Part 1. A review. Birth, 13(4), 227-233.

516. Van Eyck, J., & Arabin, B. (April 1992). Actocardiotocographic monitoring of triplets during vaginal delivery. American Journal of Obstetrics and Gynecology, 166(4), 1293-1294.

517. Kurzel, R. B., Kovacs, B. W., Goodwin, T. M., Gazit, G., & Evertson, L. R. (January 1995). Delivery of previable twins: When to attempt delay of delivery of the second twin. American Journal of Obstetrics and Gynecology, 172(1, Pt. 2), 413. SPO abstracts #558.

518. Daw, E. (1988). Continuous foetal heart rate monitoring of twins during labor. Clinical and Experimental Obstetrics and Gynecology, 15(4), 151-153.

519. Saacks, C. B., Thorp, Jr., J. M., & Hendricks, C. H. (August 1995). Cohort study of twinning in an academic health center: Changes in management and outcome over forty years. American Journal of Obstetrics and Gynecology, 173(2), 432-439.

520. Buekens, P., & Wilcox, A. (March 1993). Why do small twins have a lower mortality rate than small singletons? American Journal of Obstetrics and Gynecology, 168(3, Pt. 1), 937-941.

521. Luke, B. (January 1996). Reducing fetal deaths in multiple births: Optimal birth weights and gestational age. American Journal of Obstetrics and Gynecology, 174(1, Pt. 2), 347.

522. Chien, E., & Loy, G. (January 1995). Timing of delivery in twin gestation. American Journal of Obstetrics and Gynecology, 172(1, Pt. 2), 292. SPO abstracts #106.

523. Stone, J., Lapinski, R., Alvarez, M., & Lockwood, C. (January 1995). Are twins ≥ 38 weeks gestation "postdates"? American Journal of Obstetrics and Gynecology, 172(1, Pt. 2), 276. SPO abstracts #60.

524. Luke, B., Minogue, J., Witter, F. R., Keith, L. G., & Johnson, T. R. B. (September 1993). The ideal twin pregnancy: Patterns of weight gain, discordancy, and length of gestation. American Journal of Obstetrics and Gynecology, 169(3), 588-597.

525. Lantz, M. E., Chez, R. A., Porter, K. B., & Rodriguez, A. (January 1995). Maternal weight gain patterns during twin pregnancy and birth-weight outcome. American Journal of Obstetrics and Gynecology, 172(1, Pt. 2), 413. SPO abstracts #560.

526. Peaceman, A. M., Bonebrake, J., Garcia, P. M., & Wall, S. (January 1996). Risk of fetal death by gestational age in twin and singleton pregnancies. American Journal of Obstetrics and Gynecology, 174(1, Pt. 2), 346. SPO abstracts #122.

527. Barnhard, Y., & Divon, M. Y. (January 1993). Abnormal fetal growth in twin gestation. American Journal of Obstetrics and Gynecology, 168(1, Pt. 2), 438. SPO abstracts #515.

528. Schwartz, D., Goyert, G., Daoud, Y., Wright, D., Zazula, P., & Copes, J. (January 1993). Evaluation of twin discordance by second and third trimester ultrasound. American Journal of Obstetrics and Gynecology, 168(1, Pt. 2), 351. SPO abstracts #187.

529. Belfort, M. A., Moise, Jr., K. J., Kirshon, B., & Saade, G. (February 1993). The use of color flow doppler ultrasonography to diagnose umbilical cord entanglement in monoamniotic twin gestations. American Journal of Obstetrics and Gynecology, 168(2), 601-604.

530. Newton, E. R. (January 1986). Antepartum care in multiple gestation. Seminars in Perinatology, 10(11), 19-29.

531. Multiple gestation. (1989). Technical bulletin number 131. Washington, DC: ACOG.

532. De Lia, J., Kuhlmann, R., Harstad, T., & Cruikshank, D. (January 1993). Twin-twin transfusion syndrome treated by fetoscopic neodymium: Yag laser occlusion of chorioangiopagus. American Journal Obstetrics and Gynecology, 168(1, Pt. 2), 308. SPO abstracts #50.

533. Dickinson, J. E., Newnham, J. P., & Phillips, J. M. (January 1994). Concordance in umbilical artery doppler velocimetry is an indicator of successful therapy in twin-twin transfusion syndrome. American Journal of Obstetrics and Gynecology, 170(1, Pt. 2), 402. SPO abstracts #457.

534. Eganhouse, D. J. (January/February 1992). Fetal monitoring of twins. JOGNN, 21(1), 17-27.

535. Kim, E. S., Croom, C. S., & Devoe, L. D. (January 1994). Determination of fetal well-being in twin gestation by doppler velocimetry, nonstress testing, and sonographic growth. American Journal of Obstetrics and Gynecology, 170(1, Pt. 2), 320. SPO abstracts #155.

536. Gimovsky, M. L., Loredo, S., Wohlmuth, C., & Romero, B. (Fall 1988). Fetal heart rate monitoring casebook. Journal of Perinatology, 8(4), 379-386.

537. Fishman, A., Grubb, D. K., & Kovacs, B. W. (March 1993). Vaginal delivery of the nonvertex second twin. American Journal of Obstetrics and Gynecology, 168(3, Pt. 1), 861-864.

538. Warenski, J. C., & Kochenour, N. K. (December 1989). Intrapartum management of twin gestation. Clinics in Perinatology, 16(4), 889-897.

539. Gandhi, J., Wang, K., & Yeh, S. (January 1993). Second stage labor pattern for second twin. American Journal of Obstetrics and Gynecology, 168(1, Pt. 2), 365. SPO abstracts #243.

540. Thomas, S. J., Keegan, Jr., K. A., & Morgan, M. A. (January 1993). The delivery time interval of twins and the incidence of fetal distress in the second twin. American Journal of Obstetrics and Gynecology,168(1, Pt. 2), 438. SPO abstracts #516.

541. DiGiovanni, L., Shipp, T., & Rudman, C. (January 1993). Twins: Effect of delivery method on neonatal outcome when one or both fetuses is noncephalic. American Journal of Obstetrics and Gynecology,168(1, Pt. 2), 438. SPO abstracts #517.

542. Zimmer, E. Z., & Goldstein, I. (March 1991). The occurrence of simultaneous fetal heart rate accelerations in twins during nonstress testing. Obstetrics & Gynecology, 77(3), 491-492.

543. Lenstrup, C. (1984). Predictive value of antepartum non-stress test in multiple pregnancies. <u>Acta Obstetricia et Gynecologica Scandinavica,</u> <u>63</u>(7), 597-601.

544. Zimmer, E. Z., Goldstein, I., & Alglay, S. (1988). Simultaneous recording of fetal breathing movements and body movements in twin pregnancy. <u>Journal of Perinatal Medicine, 16</u>(2), 109-112.

545. Sherer, D. M., Nawrocki, M. N., Peco, N. E., Metlay, L. A., & Woods, Jr., J. R. (November 1990). The occurrence of simultaneous fetal heart rate accelerations in twins during nonstress testing. <u>Obstetrics & Gynecology, 76</u>(5, Pt. 1), 817-821.

546. Sherer, D. M., Abramowicz, J. S., D'Amico, M. L., Caverly, C. B., & Woods, Jr., J. R. (April 1991). Fetal vibratory acoustic stimulation in twin gestations with simultaneous fetal heart rate monitoring. <u>American Journal of Obstetrics and Gynecology, 164</u>(4), 1104-1106.

547. Devoe, L. D., & Azor, H. (October 1981). Simultaneous nonstress fetal heart rate testing in twin pregnancy. <u>Obstetrics & Gynecology, 58</u>(4), 450-455.

548. Gallagher, M. W., Costigan, K., & Johnson, T. R. B. (1992). Fetal heart rate accelerations, fetal movement, and fetal behavior patterns in twin gestations. <u>American Journal of Obstetrics and Gynecology, 167</u>(4, Pt. 1), 1140-1144.

549. Blake, G. D., Knuppel, R. A., Ingardia, C. J., Lake, M., Aumann, G., & Hanson, M. (1984). Evaluation of nonstress fetal heart rate testing in multiple gestations. <u>Obstetrics & Gynecology, 63,</u> 528-532.

550. Lodiero, J. G., Vintzileos, A. M., Feinstein, S. J., Campbell, W. A., & Nochimson, D. J. (1986). Fetal biophysical profile in twin gestations. <u>Obstetrics & Gynecology, 67,</u> 824-827.

551. Schneider, E., Schulman, H., Farmakides, G., & Paksima, S. (1991). Comparison of the interpretation of antepartum fetal heart rate tracings between a computer program and experts. <u>Journal of Maternal-Fetal Investigation, 1,</u> 205-208.

552. Lumley, J. (1988). Does continuous intrapartum fetal monitoring predict long-term neurological disorders? <u>Paediatric and Perinatal Epidemiology, 2,</u> 299-307.

553. Lotgering, F. K., Wallenburg, H. C. S., & Schouten, H. J. (November 15, 1982). Interobserver and intraobserver variation in the assessment of antepartum cardiotocograms. <u>American Journal of Obstetrics and Gynecology, 144</u>(6), 701-705.

554. Dellinger, E., & Boehm, F. (January 1995). Diagnosing fetal stress and distress: A practical classification system. <u>American Journal of Obstetrics and Gynecology, 172</u>(1, Pt. 2), 366. SPO abstracts #390.

555. Cohen, A. B., Klapholz, H., & Thompson, M. S. (1982). Electronic fetal monitoring and clinical practice. A survey of obstetric opinion. <u>Medical Decision Making, 2</u>(1), 79-95.

556. Fleischer, A., Schulman, H., Jagani, N., Mitchell, J., & Randolph, G. (September 1, 1982). The development of fetal acidosis in the presence of an abnormal feta heart rate tracing. I. The average for gestational age fetus. <u>American Journal of Obstetrics and Gynecology, 144</u>(1), 55-60.

557. Clark, S. L., & Paul, R. H. (October 1986). Fetal heart rate monitoring patterns. <u>American Journal of Obstetrics and Gynecology, 15</u>(4), 916.

558. Bossart, H., Jenkins, H. M. L., van Geijn, H. P., & Sureau, C. (February 1987). Fetal monitoring, present and future. <u>European Journal of Obstetrics, Gynecology, and Reproductive Biology, 24</u>(2), 105-121.

559. Berkus, M., Samueloff, A., Xenakis, E., Field, N., & Langer, O. (January 1993). Meconium-stained amniotic fluid: What's reassuring? <u>American Journal of Obstetrics and Gynecology, 168</u>(1, Pt. 2), 343. SPO abstracts #160.

560. Katz, M., Petrick, T., Richichi, K., & Belluomini, J. (January 1993). Oxygen saturation (SaO$_2$) monitoring in the presence of non-reassuring fetal heart rate (FHR) patterns. <u>American Journal of Obstetrics and Gynecology, 168</u>(1, Pt. 2), 341. SPO abstracts #153.

Notes

3

Intrinsic Factors that Affect the Fetal Heart Rate

INTRODUCTION

The fetal heart rate (FHR) reflects *conduction* of an impulse from the brainstem to autonomic nerves to the heart and the state of fetal oxygenation. Skilled clinicians *identify maternal, placental, umbilical cord, and fetal factors that might limit fetal oxygen (O$_2$) delivery. They react to the probable physiology causing the tracing, not the images on the paper.* This chapter presents intrinsic neurohumoral factors that directly and indirectly influence the FHR. The fetal compensatory response to hypoxia is also discussed.

FHR CONTROL MECHANISMS

The primary factors that regulate the FHR are the medulla oblongata in the brainstem, the autonomic nervous system, baroreceptors, and chemoreceptors. Secondary, intrinsic humoral or endocrine factors that affect the FHR, blood composition and volume, blood vessel diameter, cardiac contractility, and amniotic fluid composition include substances released from the hypothalamus, pituitary gland, adrenal glands, adipose tissue, pancreas, kidneys, intestines, liver, spleen, bone marrow, and heart. When O$_2$ delivery decreases by more than 50 percent, neurohumoral mechanisms are activated as a compensatory, adaptive response to maintain fetal homeostasis (1).

The Brainstem

Nerves in the medulla oblongata control the autonomic nervous system. The cardioregulatory nerves include the *cardioaccelerator* nerves which stimulate efferent sympathetic nerves to the heart and blood vessels, and the *cardiodecelerator* or cardioinhibitory nerves, from the parasympathetic center in the brainstem, which stimulates the vagus. The vagus is the 10th cranial nerve. It innervates the heart's sinoatrial (SA) and atrioventricular (AV) nodes.

A normal FHR pattern reflects an intact, oxygenated brainstem, autonomic nervous system, and heart. The fetus may have an abnormal brain yet still have a normal FHR pattern if the brainstem, nerves, and heart respond to activation of the cardioregulatory nerves. *Only a brainstem is required to have a normal FHR pattern.* The fetus may lack part of its brain or may not even have a head, just a neck and a brainstem. As tragic as this sounds, these type of defects exist. For example, anencephalic fetuses often have "normal" FHR patterns (see Figure 3.1). Therefore, it is important to avoid saying, "the fetus looks healthy" when the pattern is reviewed. "Healthy" can be interpreted as physically normal. It is far better to say, "this looks good to me" when reviewing the FHR pattern, or "the fetus appears to be well-oxygenated."

Brain damage that has occurred prior to labor may be suggested by the FHR pattern. For example, a fetus with a massive cerebellar hemorrhage had a smooth, flat FHR baseline and was moving less than normal. Fetal cerebral hemorrhage may be caused by trauma, asphyxia, infection, a congenital vascular defect, a blood dyscrasia with platelet dysfunction, maternal ingestion of drugs that cause platelet dysfunction such as aspirin, and/or thrombocytopenia (2).

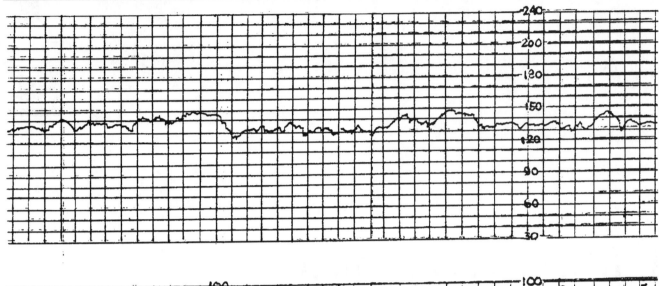

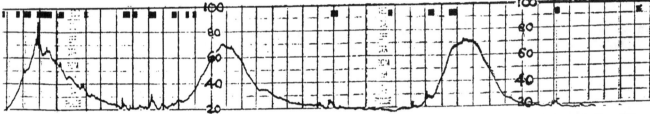

Figure 3.1: The normal heart rate pattern of an anencephalic fetus. The 33 year old woman refused α-fetoprotein studies. She had a gut feeling at 29 weeks' gestation that something was wrong. An ultrasound revealed an anencephalic fetus. She delivered vaginally at 42 weeks' gestation. The neonate was stillborn following severe shoulder dystocia.

Fetal breathing movements and FHR short-term variability. In the well-oxygenated fetus, changes in fetal behavior accompany changes in the FHR (3). The brainstem contains motor nerves that regulate fetal movement, respiratory nerves that regulate fetal breathing movements (FBM), and autonomic nerves that regulate the FHR. FBM are controlled by several centers or groups of neurons in the brainstem. The bulbopontine respiratory center is in the posterior fossa, close to the cerebellum, and plays the fundamental role in the control of FBM (2).

Stimuli that activate motor nerves or respiratory nerves precede gross body movements (GBM) and FBM. FBM are associated with an increase in short-term variability (STV). STV is determined by calculating the beats per minute (bpm) rate from the interval between two consecutive heart beats (3-5). When the bpm rates are plotted on moving fetal monitor paper, a bumpy FHR baseline appears when STV is present.

GBM are associated with changes in the FHR. However, movement *does not cause* a change in the FHR. The stimulus for GBM also precedes a sympathetic nerve stimulus and acceleration of the FHR. The neurologic mechanisms that tie GBM and FBM to the FHR may include afferent messages to the brainstem from mechanoreceptors (4).

Mechanoreceptors are sensory nerves found in the skin, deep tissues, ears (for hearing), arteries (chemoreceptors and baroreceptors), in and on the surface of the medulla oblongata

in the brainstem, and in the hypothalamus (chemoreceptors). There are chemoreceptors for taste, smell, and osmolality. Osmolality is the osmotic pressure of a solution which can be measured in osmols or milliosmols per kilogram of water (mmol/kg) (6).

Hypothalamic chemoreceptors are sensitive to changes in blood glucose, amino acids, and fatty acids (6). The association between GBM, FBM and the FHR reflects the broad stimulation of brainstem centers from mechanoreceptors and higher levels of the brain, such as the cerebral cortex motor center.

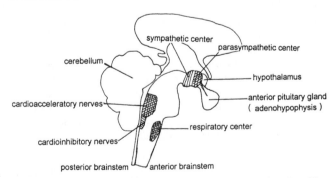

Figure 3.2: Autonomic control centers of the brainstem are in close proximity to one another. Nerves that regulate the heart rate and blood vessel diameter are near the hypothalamus, pituitary gland, motor nerve and respiratory nerve centers (modified from Guyton, A. C., *Textbook of medical physiology.* 7th ed. Philadelphia, PA: W. B. Saunders Company).

Respiratory sinus arrhythmia. Fetal breathing movements are seen with real-time ultrasound as chest wall and abdominal movements. The vagus and respiratory nerves interact. If FBM are observed, the FHR may increase with inspiratory movements and decrease with expiratory movements. The change in the FHR with FBM is called a

respiratory sinus arrhythmia (RSA) (7). The vagus, which innervates the SA node of the heart (the cardiac "pacemaker") is responsible for creating the RSA (8). Researchers noted that FBM and fluctuations in the R-R or beat-to-beat interval and fluctuations in the bpm rate occurred at the same time (9). This is due to an increase in SA node firing during inspiration

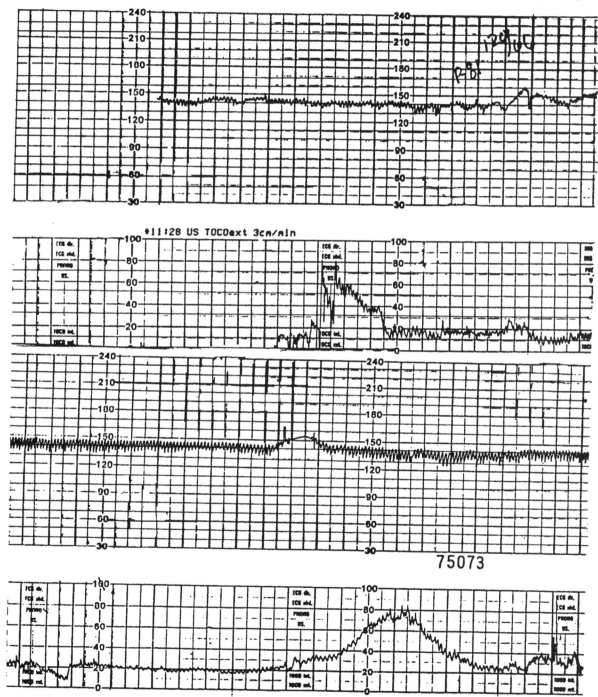

Figure 3.3: Sawtooth pattern reflective of a respiratory sinus arrhythmia created during low voltage, fast electrocortical activity and vagal influences on the sinoatrial node and the FHR. Maternal risk factors included a history of a miscarriage and tobacco use (she smoked 1/2 to 1 pack of cigarettes each day). Apgar scores were 8, 9, and 10 at 1, 5, and 10 minutes.

and a decrease in impulse generation during expiration.

Changes in brain activity modulate the brainstem and efferent vagal impulses to the heart and SA node (8-9). Afferent impulses from the pulmonary stretch reflex (a mechanoreceptor reflex), and/or respiratory centers in the brainstem, and/or baroreceptors that respond to changes in thoracic blood pressure with respiratory efforts, may contribute to changes in vagal tone (9).

FBM is associated with low voltage, fast electrocortical activity of the brain (3, 10). *The lack of FBM is associated with high voltage, slow activity in the brain* (11). In the presence of FBM and low voltage, fast electrocortical activity, the FHR pattern *resembles teeth on a saw and is called a "sawtooth" pattern* (see Figure 3.3). It is believed this pattern represents *a fetal RSA and an intact central nervous system. Therefore, a sawtooth pattern is a "good" finding.* A RSA and a sawtooth pattern may appear and disappear throughout the monitoring period. When RSA is absent, "normal" baseline variability should reappear (12).

Clustered FBM and long-term variability. A cluster of FBM or rhythmic sucking or mouthing movements have been associated with the acceleratory phase of the FHR baseline cycles or long-term variability (LTV) (see Figure 3.4). When FBM were clustered, the FHR baseline had 3 to 5 cycles/minute with a range from top to bottom (baseline amplitude) of 5 to 20 bpm. The cycles appeared to be smooth and sinusoidal-like and *not* associated with any fetal pathology.

Therefore, it has been called a physiological or benign sinusoidal pattern versus a pathological sinusoidal pattern. Pathological sinusoidal patterns are associated with fetal anemia, hypoxia, and/or asphyxia (13-14).

Fetal movement and accelerations. The relationship between motor nerves and sympathetic nerves in the oxygenated brainstem often results in fetal movement (FM) prior to an increase or acceleration in the FHR. For example, 20 to 22 week fetuses accelerated after 62.4 percent of FM (15). Using ultrasound observation and observer and maternal perception of FM, researchers noted that fetuses 24 to 41 weeks' gestation with 1 to 3 seconds of perceived FM did not accelerate 1.8 percent of the time, accelerated 31.5 percent of the time, and accelerated then "decelerated" for approximately 10 seconds 66.7 percent of the time. The acceleration/ "deceleration" combination is called a Lambda pattern. When FM was perceived to last 3 or more seconds, an acceleration followed FM 99.8 percent of the time. The lag time between perception of FM and the acceleration averaged 1.3 seconds (16).

Timor-Tritsch (15) found 28 to 30 week fetuses accelerated after 81.8 percent of FM (15). In another study, 28 to 42 week fetuses accelerated 10 bpm after 3 seconds of perceived FM. Accelerations followed FM 99.8 percent of the time. The lag time between FM perception and the acceleration was 1.3 seconds (17). As gestation advances, the number and height of accelerations increases (15, 17).

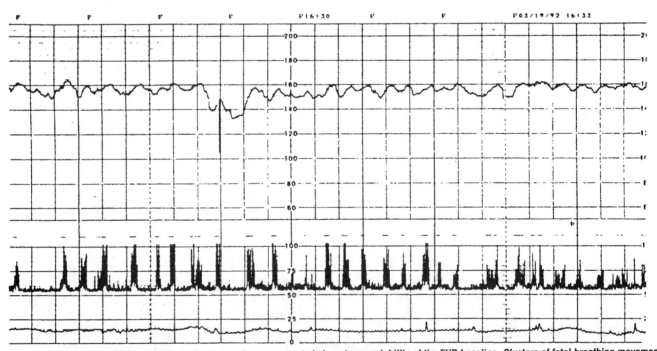

Figure 3.4: The movement of the FHR above and below the average rate is long-term variability of the FHR baseline. Clusters of fetal breathing movements in a 39 week, 6 day old fetus are associated with this physiological sinusoidal pattern. During each acceleratory phase of the baseline is a cluster of fetal breathing movements which were confirmed by real-time ultrasound. A Toitu Actocardiograph MT-430 monitor was used. The spikes in the uterine activity channel represent fetal movement (reproduced with permission of Mosby-Year Book, Inc. from Sherer, D. M., et al. (July 1993). Physiology of isolated long-term variability of the fetal heart rate. *American Journal of Obstetrics and Gynecology, 169*(1), 113-115).

Fetal movement and decelerations. FHR "decelerations" are common prior to 30 weeks' gestation. Prior to 30 weeks' gestation, approximately 97 percent of FHR changes are "decelerations" not accelerations (15, 17). The "deceleration" often consists of an abrupt drop in the FHR of about 40 bpm with a return to baseline within 10 seconds (17). These "decelerations" should be called "dips" to avoid confusion with the five types of decelerations: early, late, variable, prolonged, and spontaneous. Some clinicians have called dips "carrots." Of course, one would never document "dips" or "carrots" in their notes.

Preterm fetuses "dip" more than term fetuses. During mid-pregnancy some "dips" last 20 to 30 seconds and are 50 to 70 bpm at their lowest point or nadir. Decelerations even lasted 90 seconds and were followed by a compensatory sinus tachycardia lasting 1 to 2 minutes (18).

Between 20 to 30 weeks' gestation, "dips" in the FHR were associated with fetal swallowing, defecation, increased central nervous system pressure, startles, cord compression, apnea, and hypoxemia (17). "Dips" in the FHR have also been observed following large respiratory movements that created a negative lung pressure of 10 mm Hg or more. Researchers speculated the decrease in the FHR was probably a result of activation of stretch receptors, the brainstem, and the vagus (3). A vagal reflex may also be preceded by *compression of the fetal head or umbilical cord, hypoxia, or a blood pressure change.*

Fetal behavioral cycles. Fetal behavioral changes are accompanied by changes in FHR variability and acceleration frequency (19). However, fetal behavior was not related to a change in the average FHR baseline level. Fetuses startle, stretch, retroflex their head, flex and extend their spine, rotate their trunk, have regular and irregular breathing movements, move their jaw with regular and irregular mouthing movements, have rapid eye movements (REM) and slow eye movements (SEM), hiccup, yawn, suck, and swallow (3, 20). Fetuses swallow lung and amniotic fluid. Of the total fluid swallowed by the fetal lamb, about 18 percent was lung fluid and 82 percent was amniotic fluid. If the fetal PaO_2 decreased, lung fluid production decreased (21).

Lung fluid first appears in the embryo and increases in volume as gestation advances. Lung fluid is needed for normal lung and alveoli development. A deficiency of lung fluid could result in lung hypoplasia. Fetuses with renal agenesis (Potter's Syndrome) and laryngeal atresia have a deficiency of fluid in their lungs and they develop hypoplastic lungs (21).

Fetal rest and activity cycles begin to appear after 23 weeks' gestation. By 33 weeks' gestation, distinct behavioral states were identified by real-time ultrasound (22). They include 1F, 2F, 3F, and 4F. The F stands for fetal. These four fetal states correspond with neonatal states 1 to 4. By the 36th week of gestation, each fetal behavioral state should be easily identified by ultrasound evaluation (20). Table 1 summarizes the behavioral states, fetal behavior, and FHR pattern

Table 1: Fetal Behavioral States and Corresponding FHR Characteristics

STATE		BEHAVIOR	FHR CHARACTERISTICS
1F	Quiescence/ Quiet Sleep	absent eye movement regular FBM regular mouthing movements brief gross body movements occasional startle	stable FHR absent to minimal LTV (0-5 bpm range) **isolated accelerations** with movement
2F	Active Sleep	REM and SEM frequent gross body movements stretch of arms and legs retroflexion irregular FBM irregular mouthing movements	wider FHR baseline than 1F **frequent accelerations** with movement
3F	Quiet Awake	REM and SEM no gross body movements irregular mouthing movements	stable FHR baseline, wider than 1F **no accelerations**
4F	Active Awake	continuous eye movement vigorous, continual body movement irregular FBM and mouthing movements	unstable FHR **large, long-lasting accelerations** coalescence of accelerations/tachycardic rate

As the fetus ages, time spent in 1F increases to a maximum of 40 minutes at 38 to 40 weeks' gestation (20, 22). To determine if a fetus lacks O_2 or is simply in a 1F state, an auditory stimulus can be applied with a device that emits a loud sound, preferably over 90 decibels (see Figure 3.5).

characteristics that occur during each behavioral state.

Fetuses in a 1F state have fewer FBM and less baseline variability than fetuses in state 2F. Fetuses in 2F have frequent bursts of somatic activity. Fetuses in 3F have baseline variability that is similar to, but slightly less than, variability of fetuses in 2F. Fetuses in state 3F do not accelerate (23-24). Fetuses in 4F often accelerate and sustain a tachycardic rate, with is not tachycardia per se, but rather a prolonged acceleration (See figure 3.5) (22). Some fetuses in 4F have multiple accelerations rather than a coalescence of accelerations and a tachycardic rate (see Figure 3.6). They are well-oxygenated fetuses who may accelerate for more than one hour. Palpation of FM will confirm fetal well-being when this type of acceleratory pattern is observed.

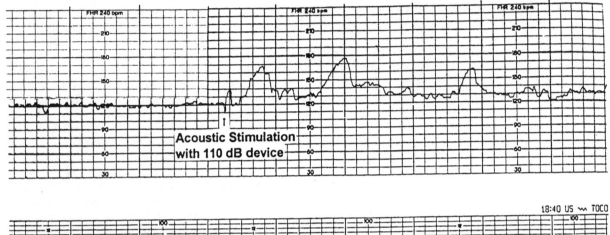
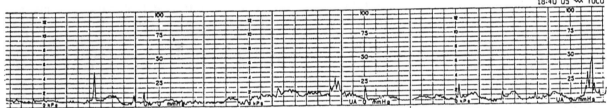

Figure 3.5: FHR pattern representative of 1F quiescent fetal behavioral state and 4F state following acoustic stimulation with a 110 decibel device.

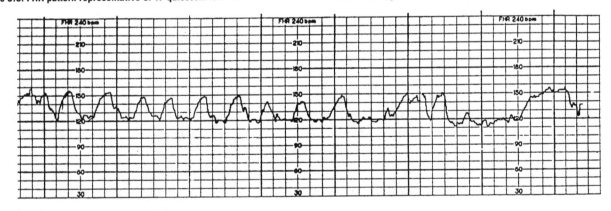
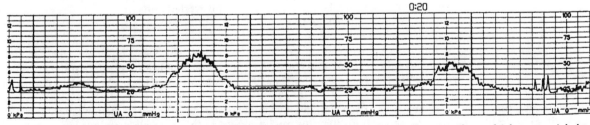

Figure 3.6: Multiple accelerations in the fetal heart rate, probably due to the fetus being in a 4F state. Expect continuous fetal movement during this time. Palpate the maternal abdomen to feel for fetal movement. The pattern reflects fetal well-being.

Table 2: Fetal EEG Patterns and Their Association with Fetal Behavior and the FHR

High voltage, slow activity
- nonREM sleep (10)
- no FBM (11)
- associated with higher levels of arginine vasopressin (26)

Low voltage, fast activity
- present 53 percent of the time if fetal SaO_2 was greater than 60% (27)
- rapid, irregular FBM (3, 10)
- fetal swallowing (28)
- increased short-term variability (3, 26)

Decreased incidence of low voltage, fast activity:
- hypoxemia (in human fetuses) (25)
- hypoxemia and metabolic acidosis (in lambs) (27)
- fewer accelerations (26-27)
- increased adenosine in the brainstem (27)

The Fetal Electroencephalogram (FEEG)

From the preceding discussion, it is clear that fetal electrocortical and biophysical activities are related. Researchers have examined FEEGs which are technically difficult to obtain. Two platinum pin electrodes are inserted into the fetal vertex after rupture of membranes. They are held in place by suction cups. A single channel FEEG is printed on a strip chart at 30 mm/second (25). Two distinct FEEG patterns have been identified: high voltage slow and low voltage fast (see Table 2).

During labor, transient FEEG changes occurred during contraction-induced hypoxemia. However, *there were no FEEG changes due to head compression* (10, 25). When the umbilical cord was compressed, causing a drop in fetal O_2 levels, there was a decrease in both high and low voltage electrocortical states (19, 25). If fetal hemoglobin O_2 saturation (SaO_2) decreased 30 to 60 percent, there was a marginal decrease in low voltage electrocortical activity. If SaO_2 was reduced to less than 30 percent, low voltage activity occurred only 35 percent of the time (versus a norm of 53 percent). Decreased low voltage activity was associated with metabolic acidosis in fetal lambs (27). Asphyxiated lambs, with a pH less than or equal to 7.00, had a pronounced decrease in brain neurological activity. High voltage activity was replaced with isoelectric activity or no activity (periodic tracing). Researchers felt the fetus should be able to recover from an acute asphyxial insult if the pH is greater than 7.00 (19). They found persistent low voltage activity was a grave prognostic sign (25). In another study, women were asked to breathe supplemental O_2 which increased the FEEG voltage within two minutes of initiation of O_2 therapy (10). Two assumptions can be made based on these research findings: *supplemental O_2 reaches the fetus when the FEEG improves and the fetus that increases its FEEG voltage probably had a pH of 7.00 or higher.*

An abnormal FEEG preceded abnormal neonatal neurological development and seizures. Abnormal FEEGs had persistent sharp wave activity, prolonged low voltage activity, or a periodic tracing. Some abnormal FEEGs consisted of high voltage, slow waves and bursts of sharp waves (hypsarrhythmia). Hypsarrhythmia is associated with mental deficit and early death, often by the age of three years. Other abnormal FEEGs had sharp waves, small bursts of spikes, and slowing. Sharp waves are repetitive spikes with the same polarity, higher in amplitude than the surrounding FEEG of short duration that occur during times of FEEG silence (25).

Hypoxia and Fetal Movement (FM)

The lack of adequate O_2 to meet tissue oxidative metabolic needs triggers chemoreceptors and sets off a chain of events to regulate the FHR, redistribute blood, and decrease FM (29). A decrease in FM may also occur in well-oxygenated fetuses when they move into a 1F state (30). Clinicians are challenged to distinguish the hypoxic, nonmoving fetus from the well-oxygenated, nonmoving fetus.

The Autonomic Nervous System

The autonomic nervous system is composed of *parasympathetic and sympathetic nerves* which originate in the brainstem and innervate cardiac muscle, smooth muscle, organs, and glands. The autonomic nervous system influences the FHR in a nonlinear, chaotic manner creating fluctuations in the FHR that are similar to fluctuations in the adult heart rate (31- 32). Therefore, chaos is normal whereas a fixed FHR suggests denervation of the autonomic nervous system (33). Clinicians who understand this know when they examine the FHR baseline, *"Chaos is good, smooth and flat is bad"* (34).

The Parasympathetic Nervous System: The Vagus

The parasympathetic nervous system has many nerve branches including the 10th cranial nerve or the vagus. Vagal nerve fibers, called vagi, appear in the fetal heart at 8 weeks' gestation, prior to the appearance of sympathetic nerves. Sympathetic nerves are found mainly in the heart muscle and first appear about 12 weeks' gestation (35).

The human heart begins to contract 22 days after conception. Cholinesterase-positive nerve cells appear in the heart ventricles even before vagi (35). The embryonic heart rate is related to its survival. *If at 4.5 to 7.3 weeks the embyro's heart rate was 85 bpm or higher, the embryo, no more than 1 centimeter long, was more likely to survive.* Surviving embryos increased their heart rate as gestation advanced. Their rate at 5 to 6 weeks was 90 to 110 bpm. At 7 weeks, their average heart rate was 128 bpm (36).

The right vagal branch innervates the sinoatrial (SA) node and the left vagal branch innervates the atrioventricular (AV) node. Vagal nerve endings secrete acetylcholine. Nerves that secrete acetylcholine are called cholinergic nerves. Acetylcholine inhibits SA nodal activity as early as the 10th week of life. Acetylcholine inhibits the SA node by creating an influx of sodium and an outward flow of potassium from the node which blocks calcium from entering the node (35).

Low voltage, fast electrocortical activity is associated with more vagal tone than sympathetic tone. High voltage, slow electrocortical activity is associated with more sympathetic tone than vagal tone. Sympathetic tone is stronger than vagal

tone early in gestation, therefore the baseline FHR is higher in younger fetuses than older fetuses (37). From an average rate near 162 bpm between 11 to 20 weeks' gestation, the FHR decreases to an average of 140 bpm at term (33, 38). This decline often begins at the 16th week but may begin as early as 12 weeks' gestation (see Figure 3.7) (22, 38-41). Pillai (22) and his colleagues found the *FHR baseline decreased 1 bpm per week of gestation from the 16th week on* and that accelerations began to appear at 16 weeks' gestation. Some researchers have found the FHR stabilizes after 35 weeks' gestation (39).

Vagal and sympathetic tone increases with age. As the fetus grows the heart becomes less sensitive to the sympathetic neurotransmitter norepinephrine and the catecholamines epinephrine and norepinephrine. At the same time, the vagus is maturing and vagal tone is increasing. The decline in FHR has also been attributed to a decrease in sympathetic tone, cardioacceleratory drive, and metabolic needs and an increase in cardiac mass and cardiac work (11, 37, 41-42).

Some term and post-term fetuses have a baseline FHR between 100 and 120 bpm as a result of normal neurologic maturation and changing metabolic needs. In these babies, a rate that might be considered bradycardic in some textbooks is normal. Table 3 summarizes research findings related to the FHR and increasing gestational age:

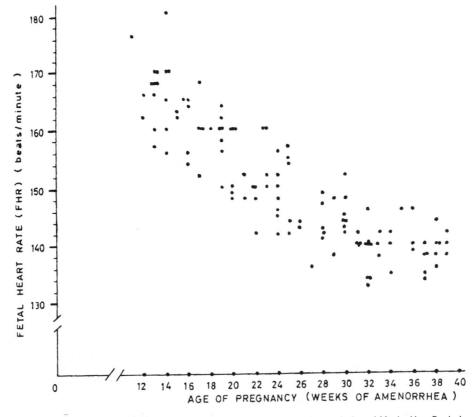

Figure 3.7: FHR average values from early pregnancy until term in 24 cases (reproduced with permission of Mosby-Year Book, Inc. from Ibarra-Polo, A. A., Guiloff, F. E., & Gomez-Rogers, C. (July 1972). Fetal heart rate throughout pregnancy. *American Journal of Obstetrics and Gynecology, 113*(6), 814-818.).

Table 3: The Average FHR Decreases as Gestational Age Increases

Gestational Age (weeks)	Average FHR (bpm)
11 to 20	161.8 (38)
20	155 (33)
21 to 30	147.5 (38)
26 to 28	143.1-145.7 (43)
31 to 35	139.3 (38)
38 to 42	140 (33)

Textbooks have defined fetal tachycardia as a baseline FHR above 160 bpm for 10 or more minutes. Although preterm fetuses have a higher average FHR than term fetuses, *only the extremely immature fetus, less than 20 weeks' gestation, will have a baseline greater than 160 bpm. Therefore, it is a myth that premies are tachycardic.* Clinicians who believe preterm fetuses are tachycardic may delay investigation into the cause of the elevated FHR.

Tonic and Oscillatory Effects of the Vagus

Tonic effect. The vagus exerts two effects on the FHR, one tonic and the other oscillatory. The tonic effect slows the FHR as the fetus matures and creates decelerations or bradycardia. For example, with application of a vacuum extractor or forceps and traction, the FHR decelerated or became bradycardic (44-49). The mechanism for the deceleration or bradycardia was thought to be compression of the dura and a direct vagal stimulus (49). The fetal head can also be compressed by the pelvis, uterus, cervix, perineum, or the clinician's hand pressing on a fontanel (46-50). Pressure on a fontanel causes an average drop in the FHR of 31 bpm (anterior fontanel) or 20 bpm (posterior fontanel) (47). With pressures of 50 mm Hg on the fetal lamb's head, blood pressure and FHR increased, then a deceleration appeared (50). Decelerations elicited by direct fontanel pressure were preceded by a small increase in the FHR. Decelerations elicited by direct fontanel pressure varied in shape (variable decelerations) and were not gradual in onset or offset. Decelerations in fetal lambs did not occur following a vagotomy (45).

Head compression. It is believed the mechanism of the deceleration during head compression is:

Pressure on the fetal skull and dura (45)
▼
Increased intracranial pressure with
Compression of cerebral vessels (47-48) and
Possible compression of carotid vessels (45)
▼
Increased cerebral vascular resistance (50) and
Possible increased carotid artery resistance (45)
▼
Decreased blood flow to the cerebral cortex and brainstem (46, 48)
Decreased venous return from the brain (50)

Decreased arterial flow to the brain (45)
Transient cerebral ischemia (48)
▼
Increased aortic blood pressure and
Increased right ventricular systolic pressure (50)
▼
Activation of chemoreceptors and baroreceptors
▼
Afferent signals to cardioregulatory nerves in the brainstem
▼
Efferent vagal and sympathetic impulses
▼
Slight increase in the FHR and fetal blood pressure *may* occur with appearance of a primary acceleratory phase or "shoulder" (46, 50) [sympathetic response]
▼
Variable deceleration or early deceleration [vagal response]

The shape of the deceleration during compression of the fetal skull may be classified as an early deceleration or a variable deceleration (see examples in Chapter 2). Both types of decelerations have been produced by fetal head compression. For example, five seconds of abdominal pressure applied close to the fetal head produced a vagal response and a variable deceleration (51). During the deceleration there is an increase in right atrial diastolic filling which augments cerebral blood flow (49). Therefore, *decelerations that accompany head compression have been considered a compensatory response to decreased cerebral oxygenation.* "Head compression" decelerations are well tolerated if they do not fall to a rate less than 80 bpm and head compression is not severe enough to cause intracranial bleeding. At a FHR near 60 bpm, fetal cardiac output and umbilical blood flow cannot be maintained (45). Fortunately, the deceleration from head compression usually lasts less than 1 minute, rarely reaches 60 bpm, and is rarely severe enough to cause intracranial bleeding.

Some believe pressure on the presenting fetal head is 2 ½ times higher than intrauterine pressure (IUP). Pressure on the fetal head increases when membranes are ruptured and the fetus descends into the pelvis (48). During the first stage of labor, contractions that create a peak IUP of 40 to 80 mm Hg exert 11 to 22 pounds (lbs) of pressure on the fetus. When the woman is 10 centimeters (cm) dilated she begins the second stage of labor. This is considered the most dangerous time for the fetus and is divided into two phases. The first phase of the second stage is the latent resting phase when the woman has no urge to push because the fetus is not yet pressing on perineal nerves. Pressure on the perineal nerves elicits Ferguson's reflex and an urge to bear down. The second phase of the second stage is the active pushing phase with descent and rotation of the fetal head and the sensation of a need to bear down (52).

During the second stage of labor, with maternal pushing

efforts, IUP peak pressures can reach 120 mm Hg and exert a force of 33 lbs. A Valsalva maneuver can exert a force of 30 lbs. Fundal pressure can exert a force of 15 to 20 lbs, and forceps can exert a force as high as 50 lbs with maximal traction (48-49). If the mother is using closed glottal pushing (Valsalva maneuver), and fundal pressure is applied while forceps are being pulled with maximal traction, the fetal head could be pressed with a force of 100 lbs!

If fetal head compression is unusually severe, brain damage can occur. The brain is covered by the dura and calvaria or skull. The dura fixes the brain to the skull and supports blood vessels. The dura also has thickened bands of connective tissue called "stress bands." These bands are stretched when the fetal head is compressed during labor. The bands may tear and even lacerate veins resulting in a subdural hemorrhage, brain damage, and cerebral palsy. A cephalhematoma may appear as well. The cephalhematoma develops on the side of the head that was pressed against the sacral prominence of the maternal spine. If the fetus turns in utero, two cephalhematomas may appear. A subdural hemorrhage could also result from a fetal skull fracture as a result of domestic violence, a motor vehicle accident, or excessive pressure during a forceps extraction (49).

Oscillatory effect. The oscillatory effect exerted by the vagus nerve causes the time interval between two consecutive heart beats to vary (53-54). This beat-to-beat interval is also called the R to R interval or the pulse interval. Pulse interval differences create small differences between consecutive calculated FHRs. These different rates, when plotted on moving fetal monitor paper, create a bumpy appearance in the FHR baseline. This bumpy appearance is called short-term variability (STV). The presence of STV reflects an intact, nonacidotic vagus nerve (55).

Atropine and scopolamine. Parasympatetolytic drugs, such as atropine and scopolamine, block the effect of acetylcholine and increase the FHR 20 bpm while decreasing STV approximately 65 percent (11, 56). Atropine prolongs high voltage FEEG activity and decreases FBM 30 to 40 percent in the fetal lamb (11).

Metabolic acidosis and asphyxia decrease or obliterate STV (57). In lambs, a vagotomy obliterated STV (58). In the past, atropine was given to women in an attempt to reverse decelerations or bradycardia. However, atropine did not abolish deceleration patterns nor improve fetal outcomes (59). Scopolamine was given in the past to induce "twilight sleep." Fortunately, the practice of modern obstetrics encourages women to be awake during labor and birth (60). When decelerations, bradycardia, or diminished or absent STV exist, clinicians take action to *remove the insult* that is probably causing the change in the FHR. If O_2 deprivation is causing the pattern, they then act to *increase fetal O_2 delivery*.

The Sympathetic Nervous System

At 6 weeks' gestation, the embryo begins to show signs of sympathetic nervous system development. Paraganglia outside of the heart produce norepinephrine and epinephrine (61). By 7 weeks' gestation, organs are formed and the embryo becomes a fetus (62). By 9 weeks' gestation, receptors sensitive to the catecholamines norepinephrine and epinephrine appear in the heart. When these receptors are activated, the FHR and myocardial contractile strength increase (35). Catecholamines regulate the cardiovascular system in the embryo and fetus prior to the development of sympathetic nerves (33).

Paraganglia continue to produce catecholamines and modulate sympathetic-like cardiac activity until the 12th to 13th week of gestation (35, 63). At that time, sympathetic nerve fibers appear near the sinoatrial node and in the ventricular musculature. By 13 to 14 weeks, the fetus is 10 to 11.9 cm long and the heart can produce positive and negative inotropic effects or increase and decrease myocardial contractility. The maximum positive effect occurred 15 seconds after sympathetic nerve stimulation (35). By 16 weeks' gestation, accelerations in the FHR appear (22). By 38 weeks, sympathetic nerve endings are widely distributed in the myocardium (39).

Norepinephrine is the primary neurotransmitter of sympathetic nerves, although some sympathetic nerves secrete acetylcholine (6, 64). Norepinephrine is also called noradrenaline (6). Nerves that secrete norepinephrine are adrenergic nerves (33).

There are two types of adrenergic receptors, alpha (α)-receptors and beta (β)-receptors. *Relatively speaking, cardiac α-receptor dominance decreases and α-receptor-mediated blood vessel tone increases as gestation advances* (33). Cardiac α-receptors slow the FHR (65). Blood vessel α-receptors cause vasoconstriction which increases systemic blood pressure. Stimulation of β_2-receptors causes vasodilation of renal and mesenteric vessels. Norepinephrine also exerts a strong vasodilator effect on blood vessels that supply the brain, heart, and adrenal glands (6, 33).

β_1-adrenergic receptors in the heart are activated by norepinephrine from sympathetic nerves but they can also be activated by norepinephrine and epinephrine from the adrenal medullae. Norepinephrine from the adrenal glands mostly excites α-receptors, and slightly excites β-receptors. Epinephrine from the adrenal medullae equally excites both types of receptors (6). The activation of β_1-receptors increases the FHR and the vigor of cardiac contractions (6, 33, 35, 53). *Thus, sympathetic nerves and catecholamines increase the FHR baseline or create accelerations or tachycardia.*

Beta blockers. Beta blockers are sympathetolytic drugs administered to clients to treat hypertension, thyroid, or cardiac disease (66). They have chronotropic effects that affect the heart rate, and inotropic effects that affect the heart muscle (67). β-blockers block the action of norepinephrine on the heart and blood vessels and also enter the placenta and fetus. When the action of norepinephrine is blocked, cardiac contractile strength diminishes, blood vessels dilate, and the

FHR will not accelerate, even though the fetus moves and is well (68). *Therefore, when the woman is taking a β -blocker, a non-stress test would be an inappropriate fetal surveillance technique to assess fetal well-being since the height and duration of accelerations is used to determine test results.* A contraction stress test and/or an ultrasound examination (biophysical profile) would be better tests for women who use β-blockers.

Propranolol (Inderal®) is a β-blocker that is rarely used in pregnancy due to fetal and neonatal adverse effects. Maternal Inderal use was associated with a lower than expected FHR in the presence of fetal hypoxia because vagal nerve responses were unopposed by β-adrenergic stimulation. Inderal does not change baseline variability (11, 67). Other examples of β-blockers include labetalol (Trandate® or Normodyne®) and atenolol (Tenormin®).

Long-term Variability:
Vagal and Sympathetic Influences

Long-term variability (LTV) is a FHR baseline characteristic with two features: cycles and bandwidth. In the well-oxygenated fetus, LTV appears to be created by both the vagus and sympathetic nerves (31, 54, 69).

Cycles. LTV is present when the FHR moves above and below an average baseline rate. When LTV is present, the baseline has crude sine waves called cycles (33). In a well-oxygenated fetus, the FHR baseline has two or more cycles per minute (see Figure 3.8) (54).

Bandwidth. The distance in bpm from the top of the cycles to the bottom of the cycles is called the bandwidth. Prior to 28 weeks' gestation, LTV bandwidth did not vary between fetal rest and activity states. However, as the well-oxygenated fetus matures, the baseline bandwidth increases to a maximum of 12 bpm at 30 weeks' gestation. The minimum bandwidth was 4 to 6 bpm and was observed after 36 weeks' gestation (22).

Benign versus Pathological Sinusoidal Patterns

Benign sinusoidal patterns correspond with clusters of FBM, rhythmic fetal mouthing or sucking, and nonREM sleep (58). Pathological sinusoidal patterns are related to severe fetal anemia and/or acidosis and asphyxia with absent vagal tone and increased arginine vasopressin (AVP). Fetal lambs were vagotomized and given intravenous AVP

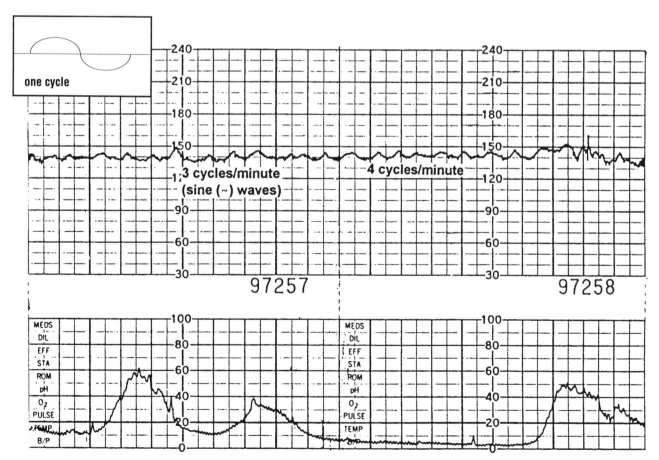

Figure 3.8: Illustration of one cycle or sine wave and cycles/minute of an actual FHR baseline. The baseline FHR of a well-oxygenated fetus has two or more cycles per minute of long-term variability (LTV) plus small, instantaneous fluctuations ("bumps") of short-term variability (STV).

which created high voltage FEEG changes and a sinusoidal pattern (26, 58, 70-71). The sinusoidal pattern persisted when there was high blood AVP, complete vagal blockade, and no low voltage FEEG activity (26).

True or pathological sinusoidal patterns are associated with seriously deteriorating fetuses who are anemic or asphyxiated and who have decreased to no autonomic control of the FHR (26, 58). AVP, released from the posterior pituitary gland when fetal tissues are O_2 deprived, probably causes the sinusoidal pattern when there is a loss of vagal and sympathetic control of the FHR. Examples of true sinusoidal patterns appear in Chapter 5.

Baroreceptors and Chemoreceptors

Control of the cardiovascular system is complex and includes afferent feedback to the brainstem from specialized mechanoreceptors called baroreceptors and chemoreceptors. They are the scouts in the fetal environment that send messages back to the brainstem to increase or decrease the

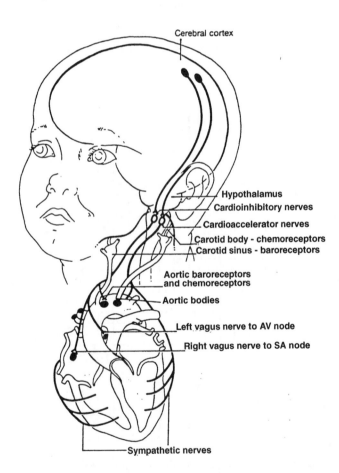

Figure 3.9: Chemoreceptors in carotid bodies send messages via Hering's nerves to glossopharyngeal nerves to the brainstem's cardioregulatory nerves. Baroreceptors send messages from the aorta via the vagus to the brainstem and from carotid sinuses via Hering's nerves to glossopharyngeal nerves to the brainstem's cardioregulatory nerves (modified and reproduced with permission of The C. V. Mosby Company from Tucker, S. M. (1978). *Fetal monitoring and fetal assessment in high-risk pregnancy.*).

FHR. Baro- and chemoreceptors help maintain fetal homeostasis by *indirectly* altering the FHR, atrioventricular conduction, contractility of the heart, and peripheral vascular resistance (6, 53). Activation of chemoreceptors may precede an increase in LTV (marked LTV or a saltatory pattern) when the fetus is hypoxic (33, 42, 45, 53, 72).

Baroreceptors. *Baroreceptors are blood pressure sensitive.* They are also called stretch receptors or pressor receptors. Baroreceptors are free nerve endings in carotid sinuses at the junction of the internal and external carotid arteries and in the wall of the aorta and walls of major arteries (33, 39, 53). Afferent signals from baroreceptors are transmitted from the aortic arch by vagus nerves to the medulla oblongata. Baroreceptors in the carotid sinus transmit signals to the medulla oblongata through Hering's nerves and glossopharyngeal nerves (6).

The FHR and blood pressure (BP) rise and fall together. Baroreceptors can send a message to the brainstem to increase or decrease the FHR in response to a decrease or increase in the BP. They are sensitive to changes in fetal BP because they sense changes in arterial wall diameter. An increase in blood volume may increase BP, which would stretch and activate the baroreceptors to send a message to the brainstem and vagus to decrease the FHR. If the fetus loses blood, arterial diameter may decrease and baroreceptors will send a message to the brainstem and sympathetic nerves to increase the FHR.

Chemoreceptors. *Chemoreceptors are chemistry sensitive. Chemoreceptors that affect the FHR are sensitive to the hydrogen, oxygen, and carbon dioxide (CO_2) concentration in cerebrospinal fluid and blood, specifically, pH, PaO_2, and $PaCO_2$.* Central chemoreceptors, sensitive to cerebrospinal fluid pH, are in the medulla oblongata near the fourth ventricle. Peripheral chemoreceptors are in the carotid and aortic bodies (6, 33, 39, 53).

A change in cerebrospinal fluid pH and plasma pH, PaO_2, and $PaCO_2$ initiates a chemoreceptor response. PCO_2 and pH have an inverse linear relationship. When PCO_2 increases pH decreases (73). Peripheral chemoreceptor activation requires blood circulation. Therefore, if vasoconstriction decreases blood flow, chemoreceptor sensitivity may decrease (74).

Peripheral chemoreceptor messages travel from the carotid or aortic bodies via nerve fibers in Hering's nerves to glossopharyngeal nerves into the brainstem. An efferent sympathetic stimulus will elevate the FHR and blood pressure in order to deliver more O_2 to tissues and remove CO_2 and hydrogen ions from tissues (6). A chemoreceptor-mediated efferent vagal stimulus will slow the FHR and decrease blood pressure. If a deceleration or bradycardia appears, the vagally-mediated decrease in the FHR occurred with a simultaneous sympathetic stimulus. However, the sympathetic response was less intense than the vagal response (45). The chemoreceptor response is considered a compensatory, adaptive response to maintain fetal homeostasis.

Umbilical Cord Compression and Activation of Baro- and Chemoreceptors.

The umbilical cord contains three vessels: one vein and two arteries. The vein delivers blood and O_2 to the fetus. The arteries deliver blood and CO_2 to the placenta.

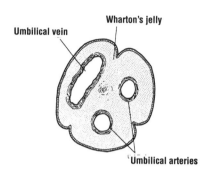

Figure 3.10: Cross section of umbilical cord. The arteries have thick walls. The vein has a thinner wall and a larger lumen than the arteries (reproduced with permission of The C. V. Mosby Company from Korones, S. B. (1981). *High-risk newborn infants. The basis for intensive nursing care.* 3rd ed.).

Vein compression. Baro- and chemoreceptors are activated when the umbilical cord is mildly compressed. Since the vein is thin and soft walled, it is compressed prior to compression of the thick-walled arteries. This curtails blood and O_2 delivery to the fetus. Since the arteries are patent, blood leaves the fetal body to the placenta. Blood

pressure may drop causing a mild hypotension since blood leaves the fetal body but does not reenter. In addition, O_2 delivery decreases which creates a state of hypoxemia. The change in blood pressure activates baroreceptors. The change in O_2 activates chemoreceptors. The brainstem and sympathetic nerves respond to create a uniform acceleration or acceleratory phase of the variable deceleration pattern ("shoulder"). Examples of *uniform accelerations and "shoulders"* appear in Chapter 2. The increase in the FHR is a protective mechanism that increases blood flow to the brain (53).

Vein and artery compression. When umbilical cord vessels are at least 75 percent occluded, neither blood nor O_2 reaches the fetus and CO_2 accumulates in fetal blood. Arterial diameter increases because blood cannot leave the fetal body. Baroreceptors are activated. When PaO_2 falls below a "critical level," chemoreceptors are activated.

Compression of the umbilical vein and arteries results in a decrease in the FHR. The decrease may appear as a *variable deceleration or bradycardia.* If the cause of O_2 deprivation is decreased uteroplacental blood flow or decreased placental O_2 transfer to fetal circulation, a late deceleration occurs (see Figure 3.11). Examples of variable and late decelerations and bradycardia appear in Chapter 2.

Baroreceptors and the Lambda Pattern
Blood pressure is FHR dependent. When the FHR increases, BP increases. When the FHR decreases, BP decreases. The FHR

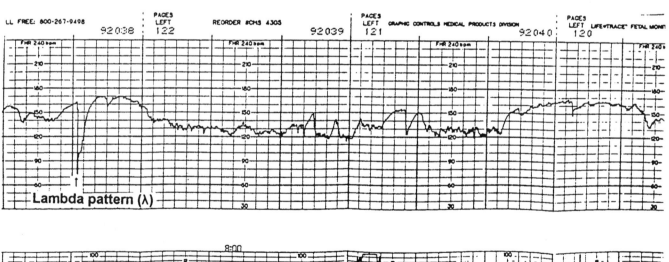

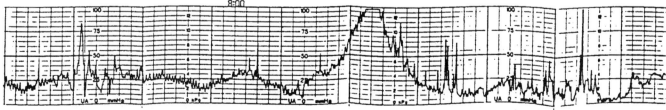

Figure 3.11: Lambda pattern is an acceleration/dip combination. It is innocuous and is not consistently related to any type of deceleration pattern.

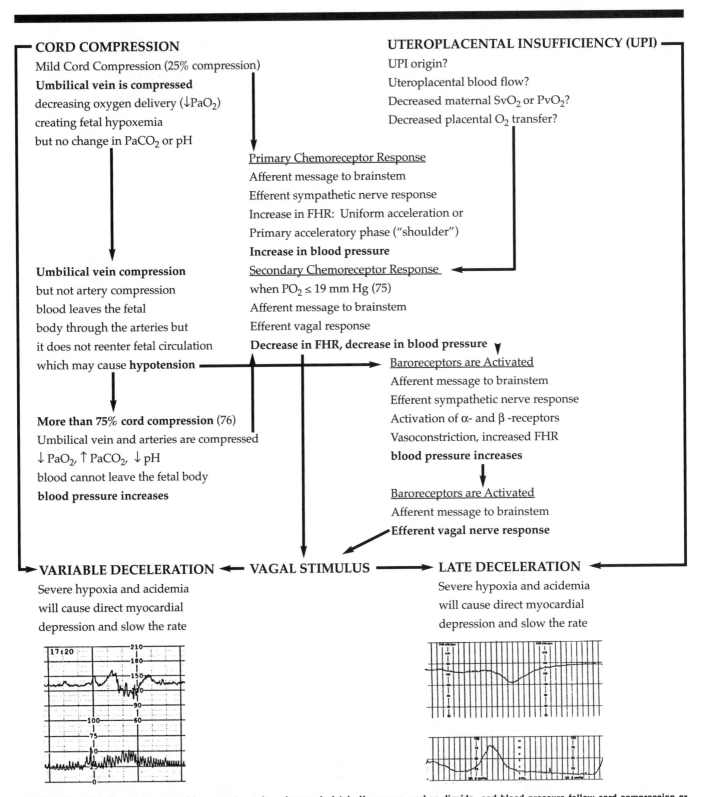

CORD COMPRESSION

Mild Cord Compression (25% compression)

Umbilical vein is compressed

decreasing oxygen delivery ($\downarrow PaO_2$)

creating fetal hypoxemia

but no change in $PaCO_2$ or pH

Umbilical vein compression

but not artery compression

blood leaves the fetal

body through the arteries but

it does not reenter fetal circulation

which may cause **hypotension**

More than 75% cord compression (76)

Umbilical vein and arteries are compressed

$\downarrow PaO_2$, $\uparrow PaCO_2$, $\downarrow$ pH

blood cannot leave the fetal body

blood pressure increases

UTEROPLACENTAL INSUFFICIENCY (UPI)

UPI origin?

Uteroplacental blood flow?

Decreased maternal SvO_2 or PvO_2?

Decreased placental O_2 transfer?

Primary Chemoreceptor Response

Afferent message to brainstem

Efferent sympathetic nerve response

Increase in FHR: Uniform acceleration or

Primary acceleratory phase ("shoulder")

Increase in blood pressure

Secondary Chemoreceptor Response

when $PO_2 \leq 19$ mm Hg (75)

Afferent message to brainstem

Efferent vagal response

Decrease in FHR, decrease in blood pressure

Baroreceptors are Activated

Afferent message to brainstem

Efferent sympathetic nerve response

Activation of α- and β-receptors

Vasoconstriction, increased FHR

blood pressure increases

Baroreceptors are Activated

Afferent message to brainstem

Efferent vagal nerve response

VARIABLE DECELERATION ← VAGAL STIMULUS → LATE DECELERATION

Severe hypoxia and acidemia will cause direct myocardial depression and slow the rate

Severe hypoxia and acidemia will cause direct myocardial depression and slow the rate

Figure 3.12: Activation of chemo- and baroreceptors when changes in fetal pH, oxygen, carbon dioxide, and blood pressure follow cord compression or uteroplacental insufficiency (76). In the human fetus, the critical PaO_2 when chemoreceptors precede an efferent vagal stimulus appears to be 17 to 19 mm Hg (75-77). Normally PaO_2 is 20 to 30 mm Hg (78). The baroreceptor-vagal reflex can override the chemoreceptor-sympathetic-β-adrenergic response (79). If total cord occlusion occurs, the fetus will become bradycardic due to hypoxemia, hypertension, and activation of the chemo- and baroreceptors (76). Bradycardia may also be a response to direct myocardial depression.

often accelerates after FM. If, during movement, the umbilical cord is pulled, cord vessels may spasm which would result in an increase in fetal systemic resistance and BP, activating baroreceptors and the vagus (80).

The acceleration following fetal movement may be immediately preceded or followed by a "dip" in the FHR. An acceleration followed by a dip is called a *Lambda pattern*, after the Greek letter lambda (λ). The "dip" in the FHR may consist of a 10 to 40 bpm decrease which may take as long as 30 seconds to return to the previous baseline level.

Lambda patterns are innocuous. *A Lambda pattern reflects a baroreceptor response to elevated BP. It always includes a FHR acceleration and is not related to any deceleration pattern* (see Figure 3.12) (80-81).

Table 4: Primary Intrinsic Factors That Regulate The Fetal Heart Rate

FACTOR	LOCATION	ACTION	EFFECT
1. Cerebral cortex	Brain	Stimulates lower brain centers, contains motor nerves	Affects FHR, variability, and movement
2. Medulla oblongata	Brainstem	Cardioregulation Maintains balance between cardioacceleration and cardiodeceleration nerves Mediates vasomotor center which regulates blood vessel diameter	Stimulates vagal and sympathetic nerves
3. The Vagus	Originates in medulla oblongata, branches innervate SA and AV nodes of the heart	Oscillatory and tonic actions Nerve endings secrete acetylcholine (cholinergic)	Creates short-term variability, decelerations, and bradycardia
4. Sympathetic Nerves	Originate in medulla oblongata, branches are widely distributed in heart muscle (myocardium)	Nerve endings primarily secrete norepinephrine (adrenergic); some secrete acetylcholine	Increase the FHR, cardiac output, cardiac contractility, change blood vessel diameter
5. Chemoreceptors (chemistry sensitive)	Central: in and on surface of medulla oblongata Peripheral: in aortic and carotid bodies	Send afferent messages to the brainstem Triggered by decrease in O_2 and pH or increase in CO_2	Increase or decrease the FHR
6. Baroreceptors (blood pressure sensitive) also called stretch receptors or pressor receptors	Carotid sinuses and aorta	Send afferent messages to the brainstem Triggered by a change in blood vessel diameter	Increase or decrease the FHR

COMPENSATORY MECHANISMS
Homeostasis
Homeostasis is the "relative constancy in the internal environment of the body" (82-83). When the fetus is stressed by deficient O_2 delivery, automatic mechanisms respond to maintain tissue oxidative metabolism. There may be a decrease in REM, FBM, GBM, and electrocortical activity. FHR changes usually occur (27). The hypothalamus, pituitary gland, sympathetic nerves, adrenal glands, kidneys, intestines, pancreas, liver, spleen, bone marrow, blood vessels, and heart will secrete substances into the blood stream to redistribute blood flow to vital organs, to increase intravascular volume and oxygen-carrying capacity of blood, and to increase the concentration of glucose for anaerobic metabolism (33, 84).

The Hypothalamic-Pituitary-Adrenal Axis
Changes in fetal pH, PaO_2, and $PaCO_2$ trigger chemoreceptors that activate the hypothalamic-pituitary-adrenal axis and the sympathoadrenal medullary system to maintain fetal homeostasis. The hypothalamus regulates endocrine activities (6). A decrease in plasma volume or an increase in plasma osmolality triggers the release of AVP from the posterior pituitary gland. Hypoxia triggers the release of adrenocorticotropic releasing hormone (ACTH) from the anterior pituitary gland or adenohypophysis (6, 64). ACTH is also produced by the placenta (85). In addition to ACTH, the adenohypophysis secretes β-endorphin, a hormone with an opiate effect on the nervous system, and β-lipotropin, a hormone which may stimulate the adrenal cortex to release aldosterone. β-endorphin is also found in the hypothalamus (6).

Endorphins. Endorphins are neuropeptides composed of amino acids. Another name for endorphins is opioids (33, 86). The specific action of endorphins in the human fetus during hypoxia remains to be elucidated. Perhaps endorphins decrease central nervous system activity and FM which conserves O_2.

ACTH. When fetal PaO_2 *acutely* falls 12 to 28 percent below control values (in fetal lambs), ACTH and cortisol levels increase. If fetal PaO_2 stays 25 percent below normal for more than 24 hours, ACTH and cortisol levels eventually return to near normal levels (87). ACTH and catecholamines stimulate the adrenal cortex to release cortisol and aldosterone. The high level of cortisol provides feedback to the pituitary to decrease ACTH release (88).

Arginine vasopressin (AVP). AVP is formed in the hypothalamus but transported to the posterior pituitary gland where it is stored and secreted into the blood (6). In animal experiments, AVP release was triggered by hypertonic saline, furosemide (Lasix®), hemorrhage, and hypoxia (89). AVP acts on the kidneys and blood vessels. In normoxic fetal lambs, AVP is nearly undetectable. However, AVP plasma concentration increases if the fetal lamb becomes hypoxic, hypotensive, or hyponatremic (64, 90).

Kidneys control water and electrolyte balance (91). AVP is the primary determinant of renal free water absorption and is known as antidiuretic hormone. In the kidneys, AVP is a membrane-active hormone that increases distal renal tubule and collecting duct epithelial cell permeability. When water absorption increases, intravascular volume and BP increase (92).

AVP directly affects blood vessel diameter. AVP is a potent vasopressor that helps restore cardiovascular homeostasis (29). AVP may also increase placental vascular resistance (33, 64). An increase in AVP has been associated with a decrease in FBM in fetal goats. If hypoxemia was prolonged, fetal goat AVP peaked after 6 hours then normalized after 24 hours (88).

The Adrenal Cortex
Cortisol. Hypoxemia triggers chemoreceptors and the hypothalamus to send a message to the adenohypophysis to secrete ACTH. ACTH activates adenylate cyclase which stimulates the adrenal cortex to release cortisol (93). Cortisol is a steroid needed for gluconeogenesis, protein and fat mobilization, and lysosome stabilization (6, 64, 93-94). Lysosomes are an intracellular digestive system that help cells digest and remove unwanted substances (6).

When hypoxemia in goat fetuses was prolonged, cortisol levels peaked after two hours and remained elevated (88). In addition to hypoxemia, cortisol levels are related to cytokines such as transforming growth factor-β and tissue necrotic factor-α (TNF-α) (94). Cytokines are found in cells. Cytokines activate the immune system. The source of TNF-α may be trophoblast cells, T cells, thymocytes, B cells, natural killer cells, amniotic membrane, or decidua cells. TNF-α stimulates cortisol and endothelium-derived relaxing factor (EDRF) production. EDRF is also known as nitric oxide and is a potent vasodilator and brain neurotransmitter (95-96).

EDRF stimulates AVP release (96). The following illustrates the relationship between ACTH, cortisol, EDRF, and AVP:

$$\text{Hypothalamus} \rightarrow \text{adenohypophysis} \rightarrow \text{ACTH} + \text{TNF-}\alpha \rightarrow$$
$$\text{cortisol} \rightarrow \uparrow \text{EDRF} \rightarrow \uparrow \text{AVP}$$
$$\text{vasodilation} \quad \uparrow\text{intravascular volume}$$

Aldosterone. In addition to cortisol, the adrenal cortex releases aldosterone. Aldosterone is a steroid hormone that regulates intravascular sodium and potassium. In the adult, aldosterone acts on sweat glands, salivary glands, intestines, and renal tubules to reabsorb sodium chloride (salt) and excrete potassium and bicarbonate (6). Retention of sodium chloride increases intravascular fluid retention. Both AVP and aldosterone precede an increase in intravascular water which increases intravascular volume.

The Heart

Atrial natriuretic peptide factor (ANP), natriuresis and diuresis. ANP is a peptide hormone synthesized, stored, and secreted by atrial cardiocytes in the walls of the two atria (6, 89). ANP plays a role in regulation of intravascular volume. It is secreted when there is an increase in intravascular volume, hemoconcentration, an increase in right atrial pressure due to an acute increase in venous return, or a decrease in fetal SaO_2, PaO_2, or pH (6, 28, 89). ANP has a vasodilator effect which reduces blood pressure (89).

ANP stimulates urinary sodium excretion or natriuresis. Even though sodium is lost in the urine, plasma sodium may be normal but potassium will be elevated (28). If ANP is significantly elevated, there will be significant sodium loss and vasodilation (6).

Rh isoimmunization and ANP. Rh D (Rho) positive fetuses, who are exposed to Rh D antibodies from maternal serum, may become swollen or edematous. Swelling of their subcutaneous tissue is called hydrops. ANP was almost 200 percent higher than normal in hydropic, anemic fetuses. Nonhydropic, fetuses had normal ANP values. After an intrauterine blood transfusion to treat anemia, fetuses that were hydropic increased serum ANP (due to hemoconcentration) which then decreased over the next few weeks. As the ANP level decreased, fetal hydrops decreased (89). Researchers did not elaborate on the reason for this relationship between ANP and hydrops. Perhaps, hypoxia, as a result of severe hemolytic anemia, increased vascular wall permeability which created hydrops. The loss of intravascular fluid to extravascular spaces caused hemoconcentration which increased ANP production.

ANP, EDRF, and AVP. Diuresis and sodium excretion (naturiesis) is related to the increase in ANP, EDRF, and AVP. Diuresis is also related to cAMP, prostaglandin E_2 (PGE_2), renal blood flow, and the glomerular filtration rate (28, 97). During 24 hours of fetal lamb hypoxemia, PGE_2 levels increased in the last 12 hours and appeared to be related to the level of AVP. PGE_2 was also associated with a decrease in cAMP production.

Fetal diuresis helps the fetus excrete the "acid load," such as lactate, which is produced from anaerobic glucose metabolism. During the first 24 hours of hypoxia, fetal lambs increased their urine output from an average of 256 (milliliters) ml to 614 ml. They also decreased swallowing of lung and amniotic fluid (28). Therefore, *amniotic fluid volume may be normal in the first 24 hours of hypoxia.* If hypoxia is prolonged more than 24 hours, the risk of intrauterine growth restriction (IUGR) and oligohydramnios increases.

Blood Vessels

Prostaglandins. The fetus produces prostaglandins from arachidonic acid found in different cell membranes. For example, arachidonic acid from endothelial blood vessel cells is acted on by the enzyme cyclooxygenase to produce prostaglandin I_2 (prostacyclin) which is a vasodilator that also decreases platelet adhesiveness (33).

PGE_2 is produced by endothelial cells, the placenta, the amnion, and the endometrium (64, 89). PGI_2 and PGE_2 are released from blood vessels as a result of an increase in arterial pulse pressure and shear force following an intrauterine blood transfusion to treat fetal anemia (89).

The levels of PGE_2 and prostaglandin F increase during fetal hypoxemia. PGE_2 may activate the adrenal cortex to increase plasma cortisol when the adrenal glands are immature and unresponsive to ACTH (89). Vasodilation from PGI_2 and PGE_2 may improve O_2 delivery to vital organs (98).

The Kidneys

Renin-angiotensin. Renin is a proteolytic enzyme that is produced by and stored in kidneys in the juxtaglomerular apparatus that surrounds each arteriole as it enters a glomerulus (82). Renin is an enzyme that catalyzes the change of angiotensinogen to angiotensin, a strong vasopressor. Renin and angiotensin help retain salt and water and prevent large blood pressure changes which maintains stability of the cardiovascular system (6, 56). In the fetus, hypoxemia appears to have little effect on the fetal renin-angiotensin system (33, 90).

The Sympathoadrenal Medullary System

The sympathoadrenal medullary system consists of paraganglia, the sympathetic nerves, and the adrenal medullae. This system controls circulation and matures throughout gestation (65). A surge of epinephrine and norepinephrine enters the fetal blood stream in response to deficient tissue oxygenation, a low pH, or cooling (63, 91, 99).

The Adrenal Medullae

The adrenal medullae produce epinephrine and norepinephrine, hormones known as amines or catecholamines (33). The fetus produces more catecholamines per kilogram (kg) than the adult (65). Catecholamines bind with β_1- and β_2-receptors on target organs. In the heart, norepinephrine and epinephrine bind with β_1-receptors to increase the heart rate and myocardial contractility (6, 35, 53). In blood vessels, catecholamines bind with α-receptors and β-receptors. Activation of β_2-receptors causes vasodilation; activation of α-receptors causes vasoconstriction (6).

Sympathetic nerves, in response to a chemoreceptor-brainstem stimulus, cause the adrenal medullae to secrete catecholamines (100). There is an inverse relationship between fetal pH and PaO_2 and the levels of catecholamines. *As fetal blood pH and PaO_2 fall, catecholamines increase* (39). More epinephrine is released from the adrenal medullae than norepinephrine. Approximately 75 percent is epinephrine and 25 percent is norepinephrine (6). Catecholamine release is a fetal protective mechanism against asphyxia and is responsible for blood being shunted to the brain, heart, adrenals, and placenta and away from the rest of the body (88, 100). Placenta catechol-o-methyl transferase and monoamine oxidase rapidly degrade catecholamines (63, 99).

Serotonin. Serotonin, dopamine, norepinephrine, and epinephrine are amines, neurotransmitters, and hormones that act on blood vessels. *Serotonin* is derived from the amino acid tryptophan. Tryptophan is derived from niacin, a water-soluble B vitamin. Sources of niacin and tryptophan include poultry, fish, liver, kidney, eggs, seeds, nuts, peanut butter, brewer's yeast, grains, wheat germ, and legumes.

In the brainstem, serotonin is secreted by nerve cells and acts as an inhibitor of pain pathways. An increase in serotonin may decrease fetal movement. In blood vessels, serotonin is released from platelets and acts as a potent vasoconstrictor (6, 82).

Niacin → Tryptophan → Serotonin → pain inhibitor (brainstem)
↓
vasoconstrictor (blood vessels)

Dopamine. Dopamine is a sympathomimetic catecholamine. It is secreted by nerves in the brainstem and is found in terminal nerve endings where it is converted to norepinephrine. In the adrenal medullae, through a process called methylation, norepinephrine becomes epinephrine (6, 82).

Tyrosine → DOPA (an amino acid) → Dopamine →
Norepinephrine → Epinephrine

THE METABOLIC AND CIRCULATORY FETAL RESPONSE TO HYPOXIA

In addition to activation of the hypothalamic-pituitary-adrenal axis and the sympathoadrenal medullary system, the fetus increases glucose production and redistributes blood so that the vital organs can continue to function (101).

The Pancreas, Liver, and Adipose Tissue

Acetylcholine and norepinephrine from sympathetic nerves stimulate α- and β-adrenergic receptors in the intestines, pancreas, liver, and adipose tissue (66). As a result, insulin and glucagon are secreted by the pancreas, glucose is secreted by the liver, and free fatty acids are secreted by adipose tissue. The intestines release glucagon (6, 66, 102).

The pancreas, insulin, and glucagon. The pancreas and intestines store glucagon (93). Glucagon is needed to break down liver glycogen (glycogenolysis) and to increase glucose production by the liver (gluconeogenesis) (6). The pancreas also stores insulin. *Insulin is needed for fetal and placental tissue glucose and amino acid uptake and lipid synthesis* (93).

Catecholamines activate β_2-receptors in the pancreas which releases glucagon and insulin into the bloodstream (93, 103). Glucagon release can stimulate a 50 percent increase in plasma glucose (103). The increase in glucose is accompanied by an increase in cortisol and insulin (6, 93, 104-106). Cortisol enhances glucose storage. A decrease in glucose, alanine, arginine, and pyruvate decreases the concentration of plasma glucagon. An increase in glucose, alanine, and pyruvate increases plasma glucagon (93).

The liver. The liver stores glucose as glycogen and creates glucose from amino acids (gluconeogenesis) or the breakdown of glycogen (glycogenolysis).

Glucose. Glucose reaches the fetus after being transported through the microvillous plasma membrane of placental villi. Vesicles in the villi take in glucose from maternal blood and transport it to fetal blood. Glucose also stays within placental cells (107-108).

The fetus receives a continuous supply of glucose via the placenta and stores it in its brain, heart, skeletal muscle, liver, and adipose tissue (101, 109). The fetal liver also stores lactate, glycerol, and amino acids. When there is a need for supplemental fetal glucose, e.g., in the case of hypoglycemia or hypoxia, catecholamines, glucagon, and cortisol stimulate hepatic production of glucose (103).

There is an association between the level of glucose, O_2, and tissue growth. D-glucose is the major fetal metabolic fuel which is consumed during oxidative (aerobic) metabolism (101, 110). It sustains 50 to 70 percent of oxidative metabolism in fetal lambs (101). *A chronic decrease in O_2 has been associated with fetal IUGR.*

During oxidative metabolism in red blood cells (RBCs), glucose becomes CO_2, water (H_2O), lactate, and adenosine triphosphate (ATP). ATP is an enzyme and an energy source. The fetus produces approximately 0.6 μl of CO_2 per minute (111).

Glucose $\Rightarrow CO_2 + H_2O$ + Lactate + ATP
(Oxidative Metabolism)

Gluconeogenesis. The fetus derives approximately 25 percent of its energy requirements from the degradation of amino acids (glucose sustains up to 70 percent of energy requirements). Amino acids are the nitrogenous building blocks of proteins and glucose (112). ^{14}C-alanine, an amino acid, is converted to ^{14}C-glucose in the liver when the fetus is hypoglycemic. Glucose is created in the liver with the help of glucose-6-phosphatase, phosphoenolpyruvate carboxykinase (PEP), and aminotransferases. Aminotransferases degrade amino acids. Cortisol enhances aminotransferase synthesis. Catecholamines and glucagon induce enzymes to break down amino acids and glucose (93).

Glycogenolysis. The rate glycogen is broken down into glucose depends on plasma O_2 and glucose levels (93). *When O_2 content decreases by 65 percent, activation of β_2-receptors in the liver by sympathetic nerves and epinephrine stimulates anaerobic glycogenolysis where glycogen is converted to glucose and lactate* (93, 113).

Adipose tissue, lipolysis, and free fatty acids. Catecholamines and sympathetic nerves activate β_1-receptors in adipocytes causing lipolysis and nonshivering thermogenesis (99). Lipolysis of white and brown fat increases fetal body temperature which decreases the bond between O_2 and hemoglobin (Hb) and frees O_2 for tissue use (66). Lipolysis also provides glycerol, a gluconeogenesis substrate, and free fatty acid, an energy source for gluconeogenesis (103).

Anaerobic Metabolism

Anaerobic metabolism occurs when the fetus is hypoxemic (114). Plasma growth hormone and glucose levels increase as a fetal compensatory response to fetal hypoxia and/or hypoglycemia (93, 99, 103). Catecholamines stimulate energy creation from the metabolism of fat and glycogen (115). If hypoxia and/or hypoglycemia are prolonged, glycogen stores will eventually be depleted (109).

The fetus cannot continue glucose oxidative metabolism when O_2 levels are reduced by 65 percent (107-108). At that point, the major sources of energy during anaerobic metabolism become glycogen, creatine-phosphate, and ATP. Creatine is needed for brain energy (116). ATP is formed in cell mitochondria and supplies energy for cellular function. Anaerobic glucose metabolism produces lactate and pyruvate (118-119). If there is nerve damage in the brain, N-acetyl compounds, such as N-acetylaspartate and choline, will be found. Choline is produced by metabolism of lipids. Researchers used proton magnetic resonance spectroscopy of human fetal brains to determine these chemical changes. More research is needed in this area (116).

During anaerobic metabolism, energy rich phosphates, such as creatine-phosphate and ATP are depleted. Byproducts of ATP metabolism are adenosine diphosphate, adenosine monophosphate, and adenosine. Cells are permeable to adenosine so some is lost into circulating blood. Adenosine is a vasodilator (6).

Once there is marked depletion of liver glycogen, brain cell glycogen is depleted first, then creatine-phosphate, and lastly ATP will be depleted at which point the cell dies (6). Depletion of ATP was related to fetal bradycardia with atrioventricular block in guinea pig fetuses (109). Eventually, fetal tissue will reach a "critical level" where O_2 consumption decreases and the fetus can no longer adjust its cardiac output and cardiovascular system to prevent the development of metabolic acidosis (107-108, 119).

Metabolic acidosis and lactate. Lactate is a salt or ester of lactic acid (107). L-lactate and pyruvate are byproducts of glycogen and glucose *anaerobic* metabolism (107-108, 117). Fetal lactate levels are stable during normoxic conditions (119). Normally, lactate is not used as a metabolic substrate, is partially consumed by the placenta, and some is transferred to maternal circulation by facilitated transport (108, 119). During hypoxia, the fetus may increase plasma lactate 200 percent (93). The enzyme lactate dehydrogenase (LDH), found in all body tissues and RBCs, catalyzes the oxidation of L-lactate to pyruvate (107, 120).

Lactic acid. When lactate is hydrolyzed in plasma, hydrogen ions (H^+) are released and lactic acid is formed.

The accumulation of H^+ lowers blood pH. *The accumulation of pyruvate, lactate, lactic acid, and H^+ are measures of the magnitude and duration of O_2 deprivation and the extent of anaerobic metabolism* (114, 117, 120).

Lactic acid levels increased when fetal lamb SaO_2 was less than 40 percent and fetal guinea pig O_2 was less than 25 percent (27, 121). In response to excess H^+ ions (an acid), bicarbonate (HCO_3^-), a base, is depleted (117-118). The decrease in the quantity of base, measured as a decrease in base excess or an increase in base deficit, is proportional to the increase in lactic acid (121). *A significant decrease in base excess or increase in base deficit indirectly reflects abnormally high levels of lactic acid and H^+ in the blood.* When blood gas values are reviewed, metabolic acidosis is reflected by an abnormal decrease in base excess and pH.

Due to redistribution of oxygenated blood to the vital organs (the brain, heart, and adrenal glands), cells of the body produce lactic acid prior to cells of the fetal brain, heart, and adrenal glands. Therefore, a low fetal scalp pH might not reflect the actual pH in the fetal brain (122).

Lactic acid is excreted in fetal urine or transferred to maternal circulation by the placenta. *It takes a long time for lactic acid to clear fetal circulation. When fetal lamb SaO_2 was greater than 60 percent* (a normal value), 2.2 percent of lactic acid per minute was oxidized or converted to pyruvic acid and glucose and 2.2 percent per minute was transferred across the placenta. Thus, only 4.4 percent of lactic acid will leave the fetal circulation per minute at a normal SaO_2 of 60 percent. At that rate, *it would take approximately 14 minutes to remove all the lactic acid* (121). Since it takes so long to clear lactic acid from the fetal circulation, lactic acid is often elevated at the time of birth (123). The following diagram illustrates anaerobic metabolism:

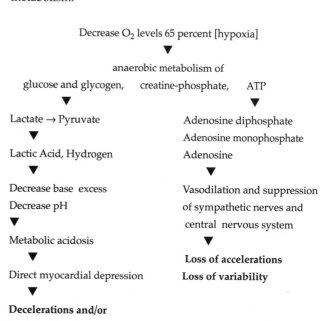

Decrease O_2 levels 65 percent [hypoxia]
▼
anaerobic metabolism of
glucose and glycogen,   creatine-phosphate,   ATP
▼   ▼
Lactate → Pyruvate   Adenosine diphosphate
▼   Adenosine monophosphate
Lactic Acid, Hydrogen   Adenosine
▼   ▼
Decrease base excess   Vasodilation and suppression
Decrease pH   of sympathetic nerves and
▼   central nervous system
Metabolic acidosis   ▼
▼   **Loss of accelerations**
Direct myocardial depression **Loss of variability**
▼
Decelerations and/or
Bradycardia

Table 5: Secondary Intrinsic Factors that Affect the FHR (Homeostatic Factors)

FACTOR	LOCATION	ACTION	EFFECT
1. Chemoreceptors	Hypothalamus	Regulates anterior pituitary and endocrine activities	Stimulates production of glucose, amino acids, free fatty acids (FFA) FFA stimulate heat production which increases release of O_2 from hemoglobin for cell use
2. Endorphins	Anterior Pituitary (Adenohypophysis)	Opiate effect on the nervous system Brain has opiate receptors	Possibly related to reduction in breathing and body movements
3. ACTH	Anterior Pituitary	Stimulates adrenal cortex	Release of cortisol
4. AVP	Posterior Pituitary	In kidneys On blood vessels	Water absorption Vasoconstriction Cyclic BP, FHR changes
5. Aldosterone	Adrenal cortex	Acts on renal tubules, sweat glands, salivary glands, intestines	Decreases sodium loss, increases water retention, increases intravascular volume, decreases blood viscosity
6. Cortisol	Adrenal cortex	Stimulates EDRF and AVP production or release	Vasodilation Increases intravascular volume Enhances glucose storage
7. Norepinephrine Epinephrine (Catecholamines)	Adrenal medullae	Sympathetic nerve receptors are activated	Increases heart rate, cardiac output, cardiac contractility, vasodilation to vital organs, vasoconstriction to less vital organs
8. Renin-angiotensin	Kidneys	Converts angiotensinogen to angiotensin	Retention of salt and water
9. Prostaglandins I_2 (Prostacyclin) and E_2 (PGE$_2$)	Produced from cell arachidonic acid in blood vessels	Affect blood vessel diameter and platelet adhesiveness	Vasodilation

Fetal Circulation and the Redistribution of Blood

Streaming. Fetal circulatory patterns differ considerably from those of the adult. Blood returning to the fetus through the umbilical vein passes through the ductus venosus into the inferior vena cava where it flows preferentially through the foramen ovale (an anatomic shunt between the atria) and into the left atrium (89). Streaming refers to the presence of two distinct streams of relatively unmixed blood in the fetal inferior vena cava. One stream is the oxygen-rich blood from the placenta and umbilical vein. The other stream is the systemic venous deoxygenated blood from the fetus' lower body. Some mixing of the two streams occurs in the inferior vena cava.

Anatomic Shunts. The *ductus venosus* shunts blood from the umbilical vein to the inferior vena cava. Blood from the inferior vena cava and superior vena cava enter the right atrium of the fetal heart. Blood from the right atrium enters the left atrium of the heart via the *foramen ovale*, an anatomic shunt. Blood also enters the right ventricle through the tricuspid valve (125). Most of the blood from the right ventricle bypasses the lungs and enters the ascending aorta through the *ductus arteriosus*, another anatomic shunt.

The placenta, not the lungs, is the fetal respiratory organ. Very little blood from the right ventricle enters the pulmonary artery (124). Instead, most of the right ventricular blood goes to the lower body, via the ductus arteriosus and aorta, and to

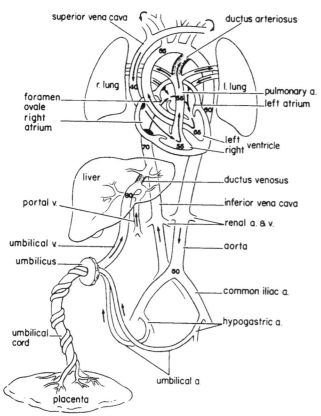

Figure 3.13: Illustration of fetal circulation. The numbers represent approximate values of the percentage of saturation of hemoglobin with oxygen. Anatomic shunts are like small doors that open when blood pushes against them. They include the ductus venosus, foramen ovale, and ductus arteriosus. These shunts help distribute oxygenated blood throughout the fetal body. Anatomic shunts normally close promptly after birth (modified and reproduced with permission from the W. B. Saunders Company from Parer, J. T. (1983). *Handbook of fetal heart rate monitoring.*).

the placenta. In fact, 40 percent of cardiac output goes to the placenta. Blood from the left atrium enters the left ventricle through the mitral valve. Most of the left ventricular blood goes into the ascending aorta to the fetal head and upper body (see Figure 3.13) (125, 126).

Fetal blood in the placenta releases CO_2 and picks up O_2. Then, most of the O_2 travels on Hb in the umbilical vein as oxyhemoglobin ($S_{uv}O_2$) and a small percentage of unbound O_2 travels in the plasma ($P_{uv}O_2$).

Shunting of blood to vital organs. The dive reflex causes the redistribution of blood to the heart, brain, and adrenal glands (vital organs) and away from arms, legs, and internal organs such as the liver, spleen, and pancreas (127). Fetal shunting, as a response to hypoxia, is similar to the dive reflex. Cardiac output is maintained and circulatory patterns change to preferentially divert or shunt oxygenated umbilical vein blood through the fetal liver and the ductus venosus to

the right side of the heart through the foramen ovale to the left side of the heart for distribution to coronary arteries, the brain, and adrenal glands (117, 122, 128-129). Blood vessels to the brain, heart, and adrenal glands dilate but blood vessels to other tissues constrict.

Human fetal O_2 consumption is 7 to 10 ml/min/kg, almost double adult O_2 consumption (130). During acute hypoxia of fetal lambs, blood flow to the heart and adrenal glands increased 135 and 156 percent (122). Blood flow to the heart may increase as much as 300 percent (73). *Blood flow to the brainstem, pons, medulla, and subcortical areas increased. Blood flow decreased to the cerebellum and cerebral cortex which increases their susceptibility to ischemic damage.* For example, when the umbilical cord was compressed 10 minutes, fetal lambs suffered from hippocampal damage (131). The hippocampus is the most medial portion of the temporal lobe cortex that folds underneath the brain and upward into the lower surface of the lateral ventricle (6). *O_2 consumption was maintained* (101, 122).

Because of selective shunting, blood flow to less vital organs diminishes due to vasoconstriction. Vasoconstriction increases systemic BP and may elicit a baroreceptor-vagal response and a decrease in the FHR (115, 132). *Acute and chronic hypoxia* cause blood flow to decrease to nonvital tissues such as the lungs, kidneys, intestines, skin, muscles, spleen, and skeleton (101, 132-133). Blood flow to the placenta is maintained or slightly decreases (33, 122). If hypoxia is prolonged, the fetus decreases lung fluid production and urine (due to shunting of blood away from the fetal kidneys) which creates oligohydramnios. *Oligohydramnios is a chronic hypoxia marker.* The mechanism causing oligohydramnios is often:

Uteroplacental insufficiency due to an increase in uteroplacental vascular resistance
▼
Decrease in fetal PaO_2
▼
Chemoreceptor-Brainstem-Sympathomedullary Stimulus
▼
Vasoconstriction—increased fetal pulmonary and systemic vascular resistance
▼
Increased right afterload, decreased lung perfusion
▼
Decreased lung fluid production
+
Increased right afterload, decreased umbilical cord perfusion
▼
Decreased end diastolic umbilical artery velocity
+
Increased left afterload
▼
Decreased renal perfusion
▼
Decreased urinary output
▼
Oligohydramnios

If hypoxia is prolonged or chronic, cardiac output may decrease and there will be no change in blood flow to the brain or heart. The slight decrease in cardiac output is primarily due to the decrease in right ventricular output. Since chronic hypoxia can result in chronic shunting of oxygenated blood and nutrients away from the fetal body, the fetus may develop *asymmetrical intrauterine growth restriction (IUGR) (122). Thus, IUGR and oligohydramnios are chronic hypoxia markers.*

CONCLUSION

Cardioregulatory nerves in the brainstem control the fetal heart rate. Afferent stimuli to the brainstem may influence cardio-regulatory nerves. Efferent nerves to muscles control fetal movement. Efferent vagal and sympathetic nerve impulses control the fetal heart rate. Fetal behavioral states are related to electrocortical activity, fetal movement, and the fetal heart rate. Fetal breathing movements are related to cyclical changes in the fetal heart rate and a respiratory sinus arrhythmia. Compression of the fetal head causes early and variable decelerations.

When homeostatic balance is altered by decreased oxygen delivery to the fetus and/or a change in fetal blood pressure, afferent impulses to the brainstem from chemoreceptors and/or baroreceptors initiate a neurohumoral compensatory response. An increase in fetal blood pressure when the fetal heart rate accelerates may activate baroreceptors, the brainstem, and the vagus to slow the rate creating a Lambda pattern.

If oxygen delivery to the fetus decreases, the neuro-humoral response includes activation of the *hypothalamic-pituitary-adrenal axis* and the *sympathoadrenal medullary system.* As a result, adrenocorticotropic releasing hormone (ACTH), arginine vasopressin (AVP), cortisol, norepinephrine, epinephrine, aldosterone, atrial natriuretic peptide factor (ANP), prostaglandins, renin, and endorphins are released. In addition, the intestines, pancreas, liver, and adipose tissue release substances such as glucagon, glucose, and free fatty acids into the blood stream. Fetal body temperature increases causing a right shift in the oxygen-hemoglobin dissociation curve. Oxygen is more readily released to tissues to meet oxidative metabolic needs.

Lactic acid will be produced as a byproduct of anaerobic glucose metabolism. ATP will be metabolized and adenosine will be its byproduct. If hypoxia is prolonged, the kidneys, spleen, and liver will release erythropoietin and eventually nucleated red blood cells will be synthesized to increase the blood's oxygen-carrying capacity. The fetal heart rate pattern is analyzed to determine the fetal response to oxygen deprivation.

References

1.	Carter, A. M. (1989). Factors affecting gas transfer across the placenta and the oxygen supply to the fetus. <u>Journal of Developmental Physiology, 12</u>(6), 305-322.

2.	Hadi, H. A., Finley, J., Mallette, J. Q., & Strickland, D. (May 1994). Prenatal diagnosis of cerebellar hemorrhage: Medicolegal implications. <u>American Journal of Obstetrics and Gynecology, 170</u>(5, Pt. 1), 1392-1395.

3.	Dalton, K. J., Dawes, G. S., & Patrick, J. E. (February 15, 1977). Diurnal, respiratory, and other rhythms of fetal heart rate in lambs. <u>American Journal of Obstetrics and Gynecology, 127</u>(4), 414-424.

4.	Campogrande, M., Alemanno, M. G., Viora, E., & Bussolino, S. (1982). FHR short and long-term variability associated with fetal breathing. <u>Journal of Perinatal Medicine, 10</u>, 203-208.

5.	Ohno, Y., Tsuji, M., Fujibayashi, H., Tomioka, M., Yanamoto, T., & Okada, H. (June 1986). Assessment of fetal heart rate variability with abdominal fetal electrocardiogram: Changes during fetal breathing movement. <u>Asia-Oceania Journal of Obstetrics and Gynaecology, 12</u>(2), 301-304.

6.	Guyton, A. C. (1986). <u>Textbook of medical physiology</u> (7th ed.). Philadelphia, PA: W. B. Saunders Company.

7.	Brown, J. S., Gee, H., Olah, K. S., Docker, M. F., & Taylor, E. W. (May 1992). A new technique for the identification of respiratory sinus arrhythmia in utero. <u>Journal of Biomedical Engineering, 14</u>(3), 263-267.

8.	Groome, L. J., Mooney, D. M., Bentz, L. S., & Wilson, J. D. (January 1994). Vagal tone in normal term fetuses during quiet sleep. <u>American Journal of Obstetrics and Gynecology, 170</u>(1, Pt. 2), 303. SPO abstracts #88.

9.	Donchin, Y., Caton, D., & Porges, S. W. (April 15, 1984). Spectral analysis of fetal heart rate in sheep: The occurrence of respiratory sinus arrhythmia. <u>American Journal of Obstetrics and Gynecology, 148</u>(8), 1130-1135.

10.	Viniker, D. A. (November 1979). The fetal EEG (detector of oxygen deprivation). <u>British Journal of Hospital Medicine, 22</u>(5), 504-507, 509-510.

11.	Dalton, K. J., Dawes, G. S., & Patrick, J. E. (June 15, 1983). The autonomic nervous system and fetal heart rate variability. <u>American Journal of Obstetrics and Gynecology, 146</u>(4), 456-462.

12.	Cabaniss, M. L. (1993). <u>Fetal monitoring interpretation.</u> Philadelphia, PA: J. B. Lippincott Company.

13.	Sherer, D. M., D'Amico, M. L., Arnold, C., Ron, M., & Abramowicz, J. S. (July 1993). Physiology of isolated long-term variability of the fetal heart rate. <u>American Journal of Obstetrics and Gynecology, 169</u>(1), 113-115.

14.	Ito, T., Maeda, K., Takahashi, H., Nagata, N., Nakajima, K., & Terakawa, N. (1994). Differentiation between physiologic and pathologic sinusoidal FHR pattern by fetal actocardiogram. <u>Journal of Perinatal Medicine, 22</u>, 39-43.

15.	Timor-Tritsch, I. E., Dierker, L. J., Zador, I., Hertz, R. H., & Rosen, M. G. (June 1, 1978). Fetal movements associated with fetal heart rate accelerations and decelerations. <u>American Journal of Obstetrics and Gynecology, 131</u>(3), 276-280.

16.	Sorokin, Y., Bottoms, S. F., Dierker, Jr., L. J., & Rosen, M. G. (August 15, 1982). The clustering of fetal heart rate changes and fetal movements in pregnancies between 20 and 30 weeks of gestation. <u>American Journal of Obstetrics and Gynecology, 143</u>(8), 952-957.

17.	Sorokin, Y., Dierker, L. J., Pillay, S. K., Zador, I. E., Schreinder, M. L., & Rosen, M. G. (June 1, 1982). The association between fetal heart patterns and fetal movements in pregnancies between 20 and 30 weeks' gestation. <u>American Journal of Obstetrics and Gynecology, 143</u>(3), 243-249.

18.	Mendoza, G. J., Almeida, O., & Steinfeld, L. (May 1989). Intermittent fetal bradycardia induced by midpregnancy fetal ultrasonographic study. <u>American Journal of Obstetrics and Gynecology, 160</u>(5, Pt. 1), 1038-1040.

19.	Matsuda, Y., Patrick, J., Carmichael, L., Fraher, L., & Richardson, B. (May 1994). Recovery of the ovine fetus from sustained hypoxia: Effects on endocrine, cardiovascular, and biophysical activity. <u>American Journal of Obstetrics and Gynecology, 170</u>(5, Pt. 1), 1433-1441.

20.	Nijhuis, J. G., Prechtl, H. F. R., Martin, Jr., C. B., & Bots, R. S. G. M. (1982). Are there behavioral states in the human fetus? <u>Early Human Development, 6</u>, 177-195.

21.	Brace, R. A., Wlodek, M. E., Cock, M. L., & Harding, R. (September 1994). Swallowing of lung liquid and amniotic fluid by the ovine fetus under normoxic and hypoxic conditions. <u>American Journal of Obstetrics and Gynecology, 171</u>(3), 764-770.

22.	Pillai, M., & James, D. (November 1990). The development of fetal heart rate patterns during normal pregnancy. <u>Obstetrics & Gynecology, 76</u>(5, Pt. 1), 812-816.

23.	Shaw, K. J., & Paul, R. H. (March 1990). Fetal body movement monitoring. <u>Obstetrics and Gynecology Clinics of North America, 17</u>(1), 95-110.

24.	Arduini, D., & Rizzo, G. (1990). Quantitative analysis of fetal rate: Its application in antepartum clinical monitoring and behavioral pattern recognition. <u>International Journal of Bio-Medical Computing, 25</u>(4), 247-252.

25. Sokol, R. J., Rosen, M. G., Borgstedt, A. D., Lawrence, R. A., & Steinbrecher, M. (April 1974). Abnormal electrical activity of the fetal brain and seizures of the infant. American Journal of Diseases of Children, 127(4), 477-483.

26. Ninomiya, Y., Murata, Y., Wakatsuki, A., Masaoka, N., Porto, M., & Tyner, J. G. (May 1994). Experimentally induced intermittent sinusoidal heart rate pattern and sleep cycle in fetal lambs. American Journal of Obstetrics and Gynecology, 170(5, Pt. 1), 1421-1424.

27. Richardson, B. S., Carmichael, L., Homan, J., & Patrick, J. E. (August 1992). Electrocortical activity, electroocular activity, and breathing movements in fetal sheep with prolonged and graded hypoxemia. American Journal of Obstetrics and Gynecology, 167(2), 553-558.

28. Cock, M. L., Wlodek, M. E., Hooper, S. B., McCrabb, G. J., & Harding, R. (May 1994). The effects of twenty-four hours of reduced uterine blood flow on fetal balance in sheep. American Journal of Obstetrics and Gynecology, 170(5, Pt. 1), 1442-1451.

29. Drummond, W. H., Rudolph, A. M., Keil, L. C., Gluckman, P. D., MacDonald, A. A., & Heymann, M. A. (1980). Arginine vasopressin and prolactin after hemorrhage in the fetal lamb. The American Physiological Society, E214-E219.

30. Dawes, G. S., & Redman, C. W. G. (December 1992). Automated analysis of the FHR: Evaluation? American Journal of Obstetrics and Gynecology, 167(6), 1912-1914.

31. Chaffin, D. G., Goldberg, C. C., & Reed, K. L. (November 1991). The dimension of chaos in the fetal heart rate. American Journal of Obstetrics and Gynecology, 165(5, Pt. 1), 1425-1429.

32. Breborowicz, G., Moczko, J., & Gadzinowski, J. (1988). Quantification of the fetal heart rate variability by spectral analysis in growth-retarded fetuses. Gynecologic & Obstetric Investigation, 25(3), 186-191.

33. Arnold-Aldea, S. A., & Parer, J. (1990). Fetal cardiovascular physiology. In R. D. Eden & F. H. Boehm (Eds.), Assessment and care of the fetus: Physiological, clinical and medicolegal principles (pp. 29-41). Norwalk, CT: Appleton & Lange.

34. Pincus, S. M., & Viscarello, R. R. (February 1992). Approximate entropy: A regularity measure for fetal heart rate analysis. Obstetrics & Gynecology, 79(2), 249-255.

35. Pappano, A. J. (March 1977). Ontogenetic development of autonomic neuroeffector transmission and transmitter reactivity in embryonic and fetal hearts. Pharmacological Reviews, 29(1), 3-33.

36. May, D. A., & Sturtevant, N. V. (October 1991). Embryonal heart rate as a predictor of pregnancy outcome: A prospective analysis. Journal of Ultrasound in Medicine, 10(10), 591-593.

37. Wakatsuki, A., Murata, Y., Minomiya, Y., Masaoka, M., Tyner, J. G., & Kutty, K. K. (August 1992). Autonomic nervous system regulation of baseline heart rate in the fetal lamb. American Journal of Obstetrics and Gynecology, 167(2), 519-523.

38. Ibarra-Polo, A. A., Guiloff, F. E., & Gomez-Rogers, C. (July 15, 1972). Fetal heart rate throughout pregnancy. American Journal of Obstetrics and Gynecology, 113(6), 814-818.

39. Newnham, J. P., Marshall, C. L., Padbury, J. F., Lam, R. W., Hobel, C. J., & Fisher, D. A. (August 15, 1984). Fetal catecholamine release with preterm delivery. American Journal of Obstetrics and Gynecology, 149(8), 888-893.

40. Weingold, A. B., Yonekura, M. L., & O'Kieff, J. (September 15, 1980). Nonstress testing. American Journal of Obstetrics and Gynecology, 138(2), 195-202.

41. Lavery, J. P. (December 1982). Nonstress fetal heart rate testing. Clinical Obstetrics and Gynecology, 25(4), 689-704.

42. Ware, D. J., & Devoe, L. D. (December 1994). The nonstress test. Reassessment of the "gold standard." Clinics in Perinatology, 21(4), 779-796.

43. Gagnon, R., Campbell, K., Hunse, C., & Patrick, J. (September 1987). Patterns of human fetal heart rate accelerations from 26 weeks to term. American Journal of Obstetrics and Gynecology, 157(3), 743-748.

44. Persianinov, L. S. (1973). The effect of normal and abnormal labour on the foetus. A survey. Acta Obstetricia et Gynecologica Scandinavica, 52(1), 29-36.

45. Ball, R. H., & Parer, J. T. (June 1992). The physiologic mechanisms of variable decelerations. American Journal of Obstetrics and Gynecology, 166(6, Pt. 1), 1683-1689.

46. O'Brien, W. F., Davis, S. E., Grissom, M. P., Eng, R. R., & Golden, S. M. (April 1984). Effect of cephalic pressure on fetal cerebral blood flow. American Journal of Perinatology, 1(3), 223-236.

47. Chung, F., & Hon, E. H. (June 1959). The electronic evaluation of fetal heart rate: I. With pressure on the fetal skull. Obstetrics & Gynecology, 13(6), 633-640.

48. Mann, L. I., Carmichael, A., & Duchin, C. (May 1972). The effect of head compression on FHR, brain metabolism and function. Obstetrics & Gynecology, 39(5), 721-726.

49. Kelly, J. V. (March 1, 1963). Compression of the fetal brain. American Journal of Obstetrics and Gynecology, 85(5), 687-694.

50. Harned, Jr., H. S., Wolkoff, A. S., Pickrell, J., & MacKinney, L. G. (August 1961). Hemodynamic observations during birth of the lamb. Studies of the unanesthetized full-term animal. American Journal of Diseases of Children, 102, 58-67.

51. Walker, D., Grimwade, J., & Wood, C. (March 1973). The effects of pressure on fetal heart rate. Obstetrics & Gynecology, 41(3), 351-354.

52. Maresh, M. (November 1987). Management of the second stage of labour. Midwife, Health Visitor & Community Nurse, 23(11), 498, 502-506.

53. Parer, J. T. (September/October 1976). Physiological regulation of fetal heart rate. JOGNN, 5(Suppl. 5), 25s-29s.

54. Abboud, S., & Sadeh, D. (March 1990). Power spectrum analysis of fetal heart rate variability using the abdominal maternal electro-cardiogram. Journal of Biomedical Engineering, 12(2), 161-164.

55. Pagani, M., Lombardi, F., Guzzetti, S., Sandrone, G., Rimoldi, O., & Malfatto, G. (1984). Power spectral density of heart rate variability as an index of sympatho-vagal interaction in normal and hypertensive subjects. Journal of Hypertension, 2(Suppl. 3), 383-385.

56. Akselrod, S., Gordon, D., Ubel, F. A., Shannon, D. C., Barger, A. C., & Cohen, R. J. (July 10, 1981). Power spectrum analysis of heart rate fluctuation: A quantitive probe of beat-to-beat cardiovascular control. Science, 213, 220-222.

57. Yeh, S-Y., Forsythe, A., & Hon, E. H. (March 1973). Quantification of fetal heart beat-to-beat interval differences. Obstetrics & Gynecology, 41(3), 355-363.

58. Ninomiya, Y., McMahan, P. C., Murata, Y., Wakatsuki, A., Masaoka, N., & Porto, M. (February 1993). Intermittent sinusoidal heart rate pattern in vagotomized fetal lambs. American Journal of Obstetrics and Gynecology, 168(2), 731-735.

59. Caldeyro-Barcia, R., Mendez-Bauer, C., Poseiro, J. J., Escarcena, L. A., Pose, S. V., & Bieniarz, J. (1966). Control of human fetal heart rate during labor. In D. E. Cassels (Ed.), The heart and circulation in the newborn and infants (pp. 7-38). New York, NY: Grune and Stratton.

60. Ayromlooi, I., Tobias, M., & Berg, P. (December 1980). The effects of scopolamine and ancillary analgesics upon the fetal heart rate recording. Journal of Reproductive Medicine, 25(6), 323-326.

61. Copper, R. L., & Goldenberg, R. L. (May/June 1990). Catecholamine secretion in fetal adaptation to stress [Principles and Practices]. JOGNN, 19(3), 223-226.

62. Cunningham, F. G., MacDonald, P. C., & Gant, N. F. (1989). Williams obstetrics (18th ed.). Norwalk, CT: Appleton & Lange.

63. Lagercrantz, H., & Bistoletti, P. (August 1977). Catecholamine release in the newborn infant at birth. Pediatric Resuscitation, 11(8), 889-893.

64. Gagnon, R., Challis, J., Johnston, L., & Fraher, L. (March 1994). Fetal endocrine responses to chronic placental embolization in the late-gestation ovine fetus. American Journal of Obstetrics and Gynecology, 170(3), 929-938.

65. Bistoletti, P., Nylund, L., Lagercrantz, H., Hjemdahl, P., & Strom, H. (December 1, 1983). Fetal scalp catecholamines during labor. American Journal of Obstetrics and Gynecology, 147(7), 785-788.

66. Milner, R. D. G., & De Gasparo, M. (1981). The autonomic nervous system and perinatal metabolism. Pitman Medical, London (CIBA Foundation Symposium), 83, 291-309.

67. Cohn, H. E., Piasecki, G. J., & Jackson, B. T. (December 1, 1982). The effect of β-adrenergic stimulation on fetal cardiovascular function during hypoxemia. American Journal of Obstetrics and Gynecology, 144(7), 810-816.

68. Garite, T. J., & Briggs, G. G. (1987). Effects on the fetus of drugs used in critical care. In S. L. Clark, J. P. Phelan, & D. B. Cotton (Eds.), Critical care obstetrics. Oradell, NJ: Medical Economics Books.

69. Verklan, M. T., Medoff-Cooper, B., & Shaman, P. (June 4-7, 1995). Cardiovascular indices (variability) predicting central nervous system maturation. In AWHONN 1995 Convention Session Resources. In tune with the country: no. 18. Nashville, TN.

70. Murata, Y., Miyake, Y., Yamamoto, T., Higuchi, M., Hesser, J., & Ibara, S. (November 15, 1985). Experimentally produced sinusoidal fetal heart rate pattern in the chronically instrumented fetal lamb. American Journal of Obstetrics and Gynecology, 153(6), 693-702.

71. Elliott, J. P., Castro, R. J., & O'Keeffe, D. F. (July 1988). Sinusoidal fetal heart rate associated with gastroschisis. American Journal of Perinatology, 5(3), 295-296.

72. Hanson, M., & Kumar, P. (1994). Chemoreceptor function in the fetus and neonate. In R. O'Regan, P. Nolan, D. S. McQueen, & D. J. Paterson (Eds.), Arterial chemoreceptors: Cell to system (pp. 99-108). New York, NY: Plenum Press.

73. Jackson, B. T., Piasecki, G. J., & Novy, M. J. (January 1987). Fetal responses to altered maternal oxygenation in rhesus monkey. American Journal of Physiology, 252(1, Pt. 2), R94-R101.

74. Scheid, P., & Shams, H. (1994). Chemosensitivity from the lungs of vertebrates. In R. O'Regan, P. Nolan, D. S. McQueen, & D. J. Paterson (Eds.), Arterial chemoreceptors: Cell to system (pp. 99-108). New York, NY: Plenum Press.

75. Edelstone, D. I. (July 1984). Fetal compensatory responses to reduced oxygen delivery. Seminars in Perinatology, 8(3), 184-191.

76. Itskovitz, J., La Gamma, E. F., & Rudolph, A. M. (October 1983). Heart rate and blood pressure responses to umbilical cord compression in fetal lambs with special reference to the mechanism of variable decelerations. American Journal of Obstetrics and Gynecology, 147(4), 451-457.

77. Itskovitz, J., La Gamma, E. F., & Rudolph, A. M. (April 1, 1983). The effect of reducing umbilical blood flow on fetal oxygenation. American Journal of Obstetrics and Gynecology, 145(7), 813-818.

78. Eggert, J. V., Weidner, W., Eggert, L. D., Woods, R. E., & Mattern, D. (October 1986). A simplified method of obtaining umbilical cord blood for pH using a heparinized vacutainer versus heparinized syringe. American Journal of Perinatology, 3(4), 311-314.

79. Parer, J. T. (February 1980). The effect of acute maternal hypoxia on fetal oxygenation and the umbilical circulation in the sheep. European Journal of Obstetrics, Gynaecology, and Reproductive Biology, 10(2), 125-136.

80.   Brubaker, K., & Garite, T. J. (December 1988). The lambda fetal heart rate pattern: An assessment of its significance in the intrapartum period. Obstetrics & Gynecology, 72(6), 881-885.

81.   Aladjem, S., Feria, A., Rest, J., & Stojanovic, J. (July 1977). Fetal heart rate responses to fetal movements. British Journal of Obstetrics and Gynaecology, 84(7), 487-491.

82.   Glanze, W. D., Anderson, K. N., & Anderson, L. E. (Eds.). (1990). Mosby's medical, nursing, & allied health dictionary (3rd ed.). St. Louis, MO: The C. V. Mosby Company.

83.   Yunek, M. J., & Lojek, R. M. (December 1978). Fetal and maternal monitoring: Intrapartal fetal monitoring. American Journal of Nursing, 78(12), 2102-2109.

84.   Giorlandino, C., Sibai, B., Bilancioni, E., Gambuzza, G., D'Alessio, P., & Nova, A. (January 1993). The importance of ductus venosus during prenatal life. American Journal of Obstetrics and Gynecology, 168(1, Pt. 2), 356. SPO abstracts #207.

85.   Economides, D. L., Nicolaides, K. H., & Campbell, S. (1991). Metabolic and endocrine findings in appropriate and small for gestational age fetuses. Journal of Perinatal Medicine, 19(1-2), 97-105.

86.   Kitanaka, T., Alonso, J. G., Gilbert, R. D., Siu, B. L., Clemons, G. K., & Long, L. D. (June 1989). Fetal responses to long-term hypoxemia in sheep. American Journal of Physiology, 256(6, Pt. 2), R1348-R1354.

87.   Kerr, D. R., Castro, M. I., Valego, N. K., Rawashdeh, N. M., & Rose, J. C. (December 1992). Corticotropin and cortisol responses to corticotropin-releasing factor in the chronically hypoxemic ovine fetus. American Journal of Obstetrics and Gynecology, 167(6), 1686-1690.

88.   Fujimori, K., Endo, C., Kin, S., Funata, Y., Araki, T., & Sato, A. (August 1994). Endocrinologic and biophysical responses to prolonged (24-hour) hypoxemia in fetal goats. American Journal of Obstetrics and Gynecology, 171(2), 470-477.

89.   Weiner, C. P. (August 1989). Nonhematologic effects of intravascular transfusion on the human fetus. Seminars in Perinatology, 13(4), 338-341.

90.   Cheung, C. Y. (November 1992). Autonomic and arginine vasopressin modulation of the hypoxia-induced atrial natriuretic factor release in immature and mature ovine fetuses. American Journal of Obstetrics and Gynecology, 167(5), 1443-1453.

91.   Ogundipe, O. A., Kullama, L. K., Stein, H., Nijland, M. J., Ervin M. G, & Padbury, J. (December 1993). Fetal endocrine and renal responses to in utero ventilation and umbilical cord occlusion. American Journal of Obstetrics and Gynecology, 169(6), 1479-1486.

92.   Kullama, L. K., Ross, M. G., Lam, R., Leake, R. D., Gore Ervin, M. G., & Fisher, D. A. (December 1992). Ovine maternal and fetal renal vasopressin receptor response to maternal dehydration. American Journal of Obstetrics and Gynecology, 167(6), 1717-1722.

93.   Shelley, H. J., Bassett, J. M., & Milner, R. D. G. (January 1975). Control of carbohydrate metabolism in the fetus and newborn. British Medical Bulletin, 31(1), 37-43.

94.   Parker, Jr., C. R., Favor, J. K., Carden, L. G., & Brown, C. H. (December 1993). Effects of intrapartum stress on fetal adrenal function. American Journal of Obstetrics and Gynecology, 169(6), 1407-1411.

95.   Socol, M. L., Garcia, P. M., & Riter, S. (April 1994). Depressed Apgar scores, acid-base status, and neurologic outcome. American Journal of Obstetrics and Gynecology, 170(4), 991-999.

96.   Romero, R., Munoz, H., Gomez, R., Ramirez, M., Araneda, H., & Cutright, J. (January 1994). Antibiotic therapy reduces the rate of infection-induced preterm delivery and perinatal mortality. American Journal of Obstetrics and Gynecology, 170(1, Pt. 2), 390.

97.   Sumioki, H., Shimokawa, H., Miyamoto, S., Uezono, K., Utsunomiya, T. & Nakano, H. (1989). Circadian variations of plasma atrial natriuretic peptide in four types of hypertensive disorder during pregnancy. British Journal of Obstetrics and Gynaecology, 96(8), 922-927.

98.   Meizner, I., Levy, A., & Katz, M. (February/March 1993). Assessment of uterine and umbilical artery velocimetry during latent and active phases of normal labor. Israel Journal of Medical Sciences, 29(2-3), 82-85.

99.   Bader, A. M., Datta, S., Arthur, G. R., Benvenuti, E., Courtney, M., & Hauch, M. (April 1990). Maternal and fetal catecholamines and uterine incision-to-delivery interval during elective cesarean. Obstetrics & Gynecology, 75(4), 600-606.

100.   Cooper, R. L., & Goldenberg, R. L. (May/June 1990). Catecholamine secretion in fetal adaptation to stress [Principles and Practice]. JOGNN, 19(3), 223-226.

101.   Richardson, B. S. (September 1989). Fetal adaptive responses to asphyxia. Clinics in Perinatology, 16(3), 595-611.

102.   Smith, J. H., Anand, K. J. S., Cotes, P. M., Dawes, G. S., Harkness, R. A., & Howlett, T. A. (October 1988). Antenatal fetal heart rate variation in relation to the respiratory and metabolic status of the compromised human fetus. British Journal of Obstetrics and Gynaecology, 95, 980-989.

103.   Cherrington, A. D., Frizzell, R. T., Biggers, D. W., & Connolly, C. C. (1991). Hypoglycemia, gluconeogenesis and the brain. In M. Vranic, S. Efendie, & C. H. Hollenberg (Eds.), Fuel homeostasis and the nervous system (pp. 197-211). New York, NY: Plenum Press.

104.   Schiff, E., Sivan, E., Terry, S., Dulitzky, M., Friedman, S. A., & Mashiach, S. (October 1993). Currently recommended oral regimens for ritodrine tocolysis result in extremely low plasma levels. American Journal of Obstetrics and Gynecology, 169(4), 1059-1064.

105.   Miodovnik, M., Peros, N., Holroyde, J. C., & Siddigi, T. A. (May 1985). Treatment of premature labor in insulin-dependent diabetic women. Obstetrics & Gynecology, 65(5), 621-627.

106. Carlan, S., Jones, M., Schorr, S., McNeill, T., Rawji, H., & Clark, K. (January 1994). Oral sulindac to prevent recurrence of preterm labor. American Journal of Obstetrics and Gynecology, 170(1, Pt. 2). SPO abstracts #337.

107. Meschia, G. (December 1, 1978). Evolution of thinking in fetal respiratory physiology. American Journal of Obstetrics and Gynecology, 132(7), 806-813.

108. Piquard, F., Schaefer, A., Dellenbach, P., & Haberey, P. (1990). Lactate movements in the term human placenta in situ. Biology of the Neonate, 58(2), 61-68.

109. Rosen, K. G., & Isaksson, O. (1976). Alterations in fetal heart rate and ECG correlated to glycogen, creatine phosphate and ATP levels during graded hypoxia. Biology of the Neonate, 30, 17-24.

110. Bissonnette, J. M. (May 31-June 4, 1981). Pathophysiology of altered placental transport. Placental transport - Mead Johnson symposium on perinatal and developmental medicine no. 18, 33-34. Vail, CO.

111. Hill, E. P., Hill, J. R., Power, G. G., & Longo, L. D. (March 1977). Carbon monoxide exchanges between the human fetus and mother: A mathematical model. American Journal of Physiology, 232(3), H311-H323.

112. Dancis, J. (May 31- June 4, 1981). Placental transport of amino acids, fats and minerals. Placental transport - Mead Johnson symposium on perinatal and developmental medicine no. 18, 25-31. Vail, CO.

113. Arulkumaran, S., Lilja, H., Lindecrantz, K., Ratnam, S. S., Thavarasah, A. S., & Rosen, K. G. (1990). Fetal ECG waveform analysis should improve fetal surveillance in labour. Journal of Perinatal Medicine, 18(1), 13-22.

114. Reece, E. A., Antoine, C., & Montgomery, J. (March 1986). The fetus as the final arbiter of intrauterine stress/distress. Clinical Obstetrics and Gynecology, 29(1), 23-32.

115. Lagercrantz, H., & Slotkin, T. A. (1986). The "stress" of being born. Scientific American, 254(4), 100-107.

116. Heerschap, A., & van den Berg, P. P. (1994). Proton magnetic resonance spectroscopy of human fetal brain. American Journal of Obstetrics and Gynecology, 170(4), 1150-1151.

117. Gimovsky, M. L., & Caritis, S. N. (June 1982). Diagnosis and management of hypoxic fetal heart rate. Clinics in Perinatology, 9(2), 313-324.

118. Cohen, W. R., & Schifrin, B. S. (1983). Clinical management of fetal hypoxemia. In W. R. Cohen & E. A. Friedman, (Eds.), Management of labor (pp. 163-188). Baltimore, MD: University Park Press.

119. Nicolaides, K. H. (1989). Studies on fetal physiology and pathophysiology in rhesus disease. Seminars in Perinatology, 13(4), 328-337.

120. Eguiluz, A., Lopez Bernal, A., McPherson, K., Parrilla, J. J., & Abad, L. (December 15, 1983). The use of intrapartum fetal blood lactate measurements for the early diagnosis of fetal distress. American Journal of Obstetrics and Gynecology, 147(8), 949-954.

121. Moll, W., & Kastendieck, E. (1985). Kinetics of lactic acid accumulation and removal in the fetus. In W. Kunzel (Ed.), Fetal heart rate monitoring. Clinical practice and pathophysiology (pp. 161-169). Berlin: Springer-Verlag.

122. Kamitomo, M., Alonso, J. G., Okai, T., Longo, L. D., & Gilbert, R. D. (September 1993). Effects of long-term, high-altitude hypoxemia on ovine fetal cardiac output and blood flow distribution. American Journal of Obstetrics and Gynecology, 169(3), 701-707.

123. Thomsen, S. G., & Weber, T. (November 1984). Fetal transcutaneous carbon dioxide tension during second stage of labour. British Journal of Obstetrics and Gynaecology, 91, 1103-1106.

124. Meschia, G. (April 1985). Safety margin of fetal oxygenation. Journal of Reproductive Medicine, 30(4), 308-311.

125. Mori, A., Trudinger, B., Mori, R., Reed, V., & Takeda, Y. (January 1995). The fetal central venous pressure waveform in normal pregnancy and in umbilical placental insufficiency. American Journal of Obstetrics and Gynecology, 172(1, Pt. 1), 51-57.

126. Eskes, T. K. A. B. (February 1993). Uterine contractions and their possible influence on fetal oxygenation. Gynakologe, 26(1), 39-45.

127. Schifrin, B. S. (September/October 1994). The ABCs of electronic fetal monitoring. Journal of Perinatology, 14(5), 396-402.

128. Creasy, R. K., & Resnik, R. (1984). Maternal-fetal medicine. Principles and practice. Philadelphia, PA: W. B. Saunders Company.

129. Parer, J. T. (1983). Handbook of fetal heart rate monitoring. Philadelphia, PA: W. B. Saunders Company.

130. Edelstone, D. I., Caine, M. E., & Fumia, F. D. (April 1, 1985). Relationship of fetal oxygen consumption and acid-base balance to fetal hematocrit. American Journal of Obstetrics and Gynecology, 151(7), 844-851.

131. Mallard, E. C., Gunn, A. J., Williams, C. E., Johnston, B. M., & Gluckman, P. D. (November 1992). Transient umbilical cord occlusion causes hippocampal damage in the fetal sheep. American Journal of Obstetrics and Gynecology, 167(5), 1423-1430.

132. Cohn, H. E., Sacks, E. J., Heymann, M. A., & Rudolph, A. M. (November 15, 1974). Cardiovascular responses to hypoxemia and acidemia in fetal lambs. American Journal of Obstetrics and Gynecology, 120(6), 817-824.

133. Rudolph, A. M., Itskovitz, J., Iwamoto, H., Reuss, M. L., & Heymann, M. A. (April 1981). Fetal cardiovascular responses to stress. Seminars in Perinatology, 5(2), 109-121.

134. Oeseburg, B., Ringalda, B. E., Crevels, J., Jonsma, H.W., Mannheimer, P., & Menssen, J. (1992). Fetal oxygenation in chronic maternal hypoxia: What's critical. Advances in Experimental Medicine & Biology, 317, 499-502.

135. Korones, S. B. (1981). <u>High-risk newborn infants. The basis for intensive nursing care</u> (3rd ed.). St. Louis, MO: The C. V. Mosby Company.

136. Henderson-Smart, D. J., & Read, D. J. C. (1979). Fetal cardio-respiratory physiology. In R. P. Shearman (Ed.). <u>Human reproductive physiology</u> (2nd ed.) (pp. 228-267). Blackwell Scientific Publications, Great Britain: The Alden Press, Oxford.

137. Young, B. K. (1990). Placental regulation of fetal oxygenation and acid-base balance. In R. D. Eden, F. H. Boehm, & M. Haire (Eds.), <u>Assessment and care of the fetus. Physiological, clinical, and medicolegal principles.</u> Norwalk, CT: Appleton & Lange.

138. Koga, S., Koga, Y., & Nagai, H. (February 26, 1988). Physiological significance of fetal blood gas changes elicited by different delivery postures. <u>Tohoku Journal of Experimental Medicine, 154</u>(4), 357-363.

139. Goodlin, R. C., Dobry, C. A., Anderson, J. C., Woods, R. E., & Quaife, M. (April 15, 1983). Clinical signs of normal plasma volume expansion during pregnancy. <u>American Journal of Obstetrics and Gynecology, 145</u>(8), 1001-1009.

140. Madsen, H. (April 1986). Fetal oxygenation in diabetic pregnancy. <u>Danish Medical Bulletin, 33</u>(2), 64-74.

141. Sibai, B. M. (1995). Hypertension in pregnancy: Life-threatening emergencies. [symposium handout].

142. Belfort, M. A., & Saade, G. R. (July 1994). Oxygen delivery and consumption in critically ill pregnant patients: Association with ophthalmic artery diastolic velocity. <u>American Journal of Obstetrics and Gynecology, 171</u>(1), 211-217.

143. Meschia, G. (October 1979). Supply of oxygen to the fetus. <u>Journal of Reproductive Medicine, 23</u>(4), 160-165.

144. Farquharson, R. G. (1983). Fetal oxygen affinity and its parameters in a random obstetric population. <u>Journal of Perinatal Medicine, 11</u>(1), 43-50.

145. Shailer, T. L., Harvey, C. J., & Guyer, F. (July/September 1992). Principles of oxygen transport in the critically ill obstetric patient. <u>NAACOG's Clinical Issues in Perinatal and Women's Health Nursing, 3</u>(3), 392-398.

146. Jepson, J. H. (December 1974). Factors influencing oxygenation in mother and fetus [Review]. <u>Obstetrics & Gynecology, 44</u>(6), 906-914.

147. Ship-Horowitz, T. (November/December 1983). Nursing care of the sickle cell anemic patient in labor [Principles and Practice]. <u>JOGNN,</u> 381-386.

148. Perry, Jr., K. G., & Morrison, J. C. (April 1990). The diagnosis and management of hemoglobinopathies during pregnancy. <u>Seminars in Perinatology, 14</u>(2), 90-102.

149. Ferguson, II, J. E., & O'Reilly, R. (July 1985). Hemoglobin E and pregnancy. <u>Obstetrics & Gynecology, 66</u>(1), 136-140.

150. Bardicef, M., Resnick, L. M., Bardicef, O., Sorokin, Y., & Cotton, D. B. (January 1994). P-NMR spectroscopy measurement of intracellular free magnesium and pH in erythrocytes of nonpregnant, pregnant, and gestational diabetic women. <u>American Journal of Obstetrics and Gynecology, 170</u>(1, Pt. 2), 309. SPO abstracts #114.

151. Tilkian, S. M., & Conover, M. H. (1975). <u>Clinical implications of laboratory tests.</u> Saint Louis, MO: The C. V. Mosby Company.

152. Battaglia, F. (May 31- June 4, 1981). Metabolism of the placenta: Its physiologic implications. <u>Placenta transport - Mead Johnson symposium on perinatal and developmental medicine no. 18,</u> 9-13. Vail, CO.

153. Mendoza, G. J. B., Calem-Grunat, J., Karmel, B. Z., LeBlanc, M. H., Brown, E. G., & Chervenak, F. (1989). Intrauterine growth retardation related to maternal erythrocyte oxygen transport. <u>Advances in Experimental Medicine & Biology, 248,</u> 377-386.

154. Jackson, B. T., & Piasecki, G. J. (1983). Fetal oxygenation. In W. R. Cohen, & E. A. Friedman (Eds.). <u>Management of labor</u> (pp. 117-142). Baltimore: University Park Press.

155. Saling, E. (1968). <u>Foetal and neonatal hypoxia in relation to clincial practice.</u> London: William Clowes & Sons, Ltd.

156. Brown, E. G., Mendoza, G. J. B., Chervenak, F. A., Karmel, B. Z., Krouskop, R. W., & LeBlanc, M. H. (January 1990). The relationship of maternal erythrocyte oxygen transport parameters to intrauterine growth retardation. <u>American Journal of Obstetrics and Gynecology, 162</u>(1), 223-229.

157. Gilbert, R. D., Lis, L., & Longo, L. D. (October 1985). Temperature effects on oxygen affinity of human fetal blood. <u>Journal of Developmental Physiology, 7</u>(5), 299-304.

158. Macaulay, J. H., Randall, N. R., Bond, K., & Steer, P. J. (March 1992). Continuous monitoring of fetal temperature by noninvasive probe and its relationship to maternal temperature, fetal heart rate, and cord arterial oxygen and pH. <u>Obstetrics & Gynecology, 79</u>(3), 469-474.

159. Cohn, H. E., Jackson, B. T., Piasecki, G. J., Cohen, W. R., & Novy, M. J. (October 1985). Fetal cardiovascular responses to asphyxia induced by decreased uterine perfusion. <u>Journal of Developmental Physiology, 7</u>(5), 289-297.

160. Pedron, S. L. (February 1994). Changes in total uterine blood flow do not always reflect changes in maternal placental blood flow [Letters]. <u>American Journal of Obstetrics and Gynecology,170</u>(2), 701-702.

161. Vorherr, H. (September 1, 1975). Placental insufficiency in relation to postterm pregnancy and fetal postmaturity. Evaluation of fetoplacental function, management of the postterm gravida [Current Developments]. <u>American Journal of Obstetrics and Gynecology, 123</u>(1), 67-102.

162. Longo, L. D., Dale, P. S., & Gilbert, R. D. (1986). Uteroplacental O_2 uptake: Continuous measurements during uterine quiescence and contractions. <u>American Journal of Physiology, 250</u>(Regulatory Integrative Comp. Physiol. 19), R1099-R1107.

163. Wilkening, R. B., & Meschia, G. (January/February 1992). Current topic: Comparative physiology of placental oxygen transport. <u>Placenta, 13</u>(1), 1-15.

164. Dennison, R. D. (July 1990). Understanding the four determinants of cardiac output. <u>Nursing90,</u> 35-41.

165. Clark, S. L., Cotton, D. B., Lee, W., Bishop, C., Hill, T., & Southwick, J. (December 1989). Central hemodynamic assessment of normal term pregnancy. American Journal of Obstetrics and Gynecology, 161(6, Pt. 1), 1439-1442.

166. Shortridge, L. A. (January/February 1983). Using ritodrine hydrochloride to inhibit preterm labor. MCN, 8, 58-61.

167. Aumann, G. M. E., & Blake, G. D. (March/April 1982). Ritodrine hydrochloride in the control of premature labor. JOGNN, 11(2), 75-79.

168. Fitzgerald, G. L. (1983). NAACOG update series: Preterm labor part 2: Management. Lesson 3, Volume 1. Continuing Professional Education Center, Inc., 1101 State Road, Building Q, Princeton, MJ 08540.

169. Haller, D. L. (November 1980). The use of terbutaline for premature labor. Drug Intelligence & Clinical Pharmacy, 14, 757-764.

170. Young, R. (January 1993). T-type and L-type calcium channels in freshly dispersed human uterine smooth muscle. American Journal of Obstetrics and Gynecology, 168(1, Pt. 2), 302. SPO abstracts.

171. Keeley, M. M., Wade, R. V., Laurent, S. L., & Hamann, V. D. (February 1993). Alterations in maternal-fetal doppler flow velocity waveforms in preterm labor patients undergoing magnesium sulfate tocolysis. Obstetrics & Gynecology, 81(2), 191-194.

172. Rayburn, W. F., & Zuspan, F. P. (1986). Drug therapy in obstetrics and gynecology (2nd ed.). Norwalk, CT: Appleton-Century-Crofts.

173. Binder, N. D., & Laird, M. R. (February 1994). Changes in total uterine blood flow do not always reflect changes in maternal placental blood flow [Letters]. American Journal of Obstetrics and Gynecology, 170(2), 701-702.

174. Burrow, G. N., & Ferris, T. F. (1995). Medical complications during pregnancy (4th ed.). Philadelphia, PA: The W. B. Saunders Company.

175. Dickinson, J. E., Andres, R. L., & Parisi, V. M. (May 1994). The ovine fetal sympathoadrenal response to the maternal administration of methamphetamine. American Journal of Obstetrics and Gynecology, 170(5, Pt. 1), 1452-1457.

176. Belfort, M. A., Anthony, J., Saade, G. R., Wasserstrum, N., Johanson, R., & Clark, S. (December 1993). The oxygen consumption/oxygen delivery curve in severe preeclampsia: Evidence for a fixed oxygen extraction state. American Journal of Obstetrics and Gynecology, 169(6), 1448-1455.

177. Larsen, L. G., Clausen, H. V., Andersen, B., & Graem, N. (February 1995). A stereologic study of postmature placentas fixed by dual perfusion. American Journal of Obstetrics and Gynecology, 172(2, Pt. 1), 500-507.

178. Williams, M. C., O'Brien, W. F. O., Porter, K. B., Lynch, C., & Casanova, C. (January 1994). Asymmetry correlates significantly with acidosis at birth. American Journal of Obstetrics and Gynecology, 372. SPO abstracts #344.

179. Nesse, R. E. (June 1983). Normal labor and the induction and augmentation of labor. Primary Care, 10(2), 253-267.

180. Girdina, B., Scatena, R., Clementi, M. E., Cerroni, L., Nuutinen, M., & Brix, O. (January 20, 1993). Physiology relevance of the overall delta H of oxygen binding to fetal human hemoglobin. Journal of Molecular Biology, 229(2), 512-516.

181. Castracane, V. D., Ramin, K., Pridjian, G., Chandler, P., Ramin, S., & Riffe, B. (January 1994). Endocrinology of twin pregnancy: Increases in maternal serum androgen. American Journal of Obstetrics and Gynecology, 170(1, Pt. 2). SPO Abstracts #95.

182. Panigel, M. (December 1, 1962). Placental perfusion experiments. American Journal of Obstetrics and Gynecology, 84(11, Pt. 2), 1664-1683.

183. Newman, W., Braid, D., & Wood, C. (January 1, 1967). Fetal acid-base status. I. Relationship between maternal and fetal PCO_2. American Journal of Obstetrics and Gynecology, 97(1), 43-51.

184. Martin, C. B., & Gingerich, B. (September/October 1976). Factors affecting the fetal heart rate: Genesis of FHR patterns. JOGNN (Suppl.), 30s-40s.

185. Altshuler, G. (May 31-June 4, 1981). Diseases of the placenta and their effect on transport. Placental transport - Mead Johnson symposium on perinatal and developmental medicine no. 18, 35-43. Vail, CO.

186. Benirschke, K. (1990). Placental implantation and development. In R. D. Eden, F. H. Boehm, & M. Haire (Eds). Assessment and care of the fetus. Physiological, clinical, and medicolegal principles. Norwalk, CT: Appleton & Lange.

187. Longo, L. D. (May 31 - June 4, 1981). Nutrient transfer in the placenta. Placenta transport - Mead Johnson symposium on perinatal and developmental medicine no. 18, 15-19. Vail, CO.

188. Jang, P. R., & Brace, R. A. (December 1992). Amniotic fluid composition changes during urine drainage and tracheoesophageal occlusion in fetal sheep. American Journal of Obstetrics and Gynecology, 167(6), 1732-1741.

189. Tropper, P. J., & Petrie, R. H. (1987). Placental exchange. In J. P. Lavery (Ed.), The human placenta: Clinical perspectives (pp. 199-206). Rockville, MD: Aspen.

190. Bawdon, R. E., Gravell, M., Roberts, S., Hamilton, R., Dax, J., & Sever, J. (February 1995). Ex vivo human placental transfer of human immunodefiency virus-1P24 antigen. American Journal of Obstetrics and Gynecology, 172(2, Pt. 1), 530-532.

191. Seeds, A. E. (November 1, 1981). Current concepts in amniotic fluid dynamics [Current Developments]. American Journal of Obstetrics and Gynecology, 138(5), 575-586.

192. Krishna, R. B., Levitz, M., & Dancis, J. (December 1993). Transfer of cocaine by the perfused human placenta: The effect of binding to serum proteins. American Journal of Obstetrics and Gynecology, 169(6), 1418-1423.

193. Dicke, J. M., Verges, D. K., & Polakoski, K. L. (September 1993). Cocaine inhibits alanine uptake by human placental microvillous membrane vesicles. American Journal of Obstetrics and Gynecology, 169(3), 515-521.

194. Guiet-Bara, A. (February 1980). Human placental oxygen transfer and consumption. Dissociation by cooling or use of respiratory enzyme inhibitors. European Journal of Obstetrics, Gynecology, and Reproductive Biology, 10(2), 83-98.

195. Oxorn-Foote, H. (1986). Human labor & birth (5th ed.). Norwalk, CT: Appleton-Century-Crofts.

196. Maguire, D. J., Cannell, G. R., & Addison, R. S. (1994). Oxygen supply and placental oxygen metabolism. In P. Vaupel, R. Zander, & D. F. Bruly (Eds.), Oxygen transport to tissue XV (pp. 709-715). New York, NY: Plenum Press.

197. Groome, L. J. (1991). A theoretical analysis of the effect of placental metabolism on fetal oxygenation under conditions of limited oxygen availability. BioSystems, 26(1), 45-56.

198. Crino, J. P., Harris, A. P., Parisi, V.M., & Johnson, T. R. B. (May 1993). Effect of rapid intravenous crystalloid infusion on uteroplacental blood flow and placental implantation-site oxygen delivery in the pregnant ewe. American Journal of Obstetrics and Gynecology, 168(5), 1603-1609.

199. Kay, H. H., Hawkins, S. R., Wang, Y., Mika, D. E., Ribeiro, A. A., & Spicer, L. D. (January 1993). Phosphorus 31 magnetic resonance spectroscopy of perfused human placental villi under varying oxygen concentrations. American Journal of Obstetrics and Gynecology, 168(1, Pt. 1), 246-252.

200. Ferguson, II, J. E., Seaner, R., Bruns, D. E., Redick, J. A., Mills, S. E., & Juppner, H. (April 1994). Expression of parathyroid hormone-related protein and its receptor in human umbilical cord: Evidence for a paracrine system involving umbilical vessels. American Journal of Obstetrics and Gynecology, 170(4), 1018-1026.

201. Schiff, E., Sibai, B. M., Weiner, E., Zalel, Y., & Shalev, E. (January 1993). Endothelin-1,2 levels in umbilical vein serum of second-trimester fetuses and growth-retarded third-trimester fetuses at time of cordocentesis. American Journal of Obstetrics and Gynecology, 168(1, Pt. 2), 329. SPO abstracts #104.

202. McCarthy, A. L., Woolfson, R. G., Evans, B. J., Davies, D. R., Raju, S. K., & Poston, L. (March 1994). Functional characteristics of small placental arteries. American Journal of Obstetrics and Gynecology, 170(3), 945-951.

203. Aladjem, S., Kahn, K., Dingfelder, J., Holzheimer, R., Cummings, S. R., & Michailov, D. (November 1971). Placental aspects of fetal heart rate patterns. Obstetrics & Gynecology, 38(5), 671-676.

204. Paulone, M. E., Edelstone, D. I., & Shedd, A. (January 1987). Effects of maternal anemia on uteroplacental and fetal oxidative metabolism in sheep. American Journal of Obstetrics and Gynecology, 156(1), 230-236.

205. Harvey, C. J., Hankins, G. D. V., & Synder, R. (January 1993). Maternal oxygen transport variables and fetal base excess in the sheep model: Determining predictors of fetal compromise. American Journal of Obstetrics and Gynecology, 168(1, Pt. 2), 329. SPO abstracts #105.

206. Hsieh, F., Chang, F., Ko, T., Kuo, P., Chang, D., & Chen, H. (December 1989). The antenatal blood gas acid-base status of normal fetuses and hydropic fetuses with Bart hemoglobinopathy. Obstetrics & Gynecology, 74(3), 722-725.

207. Yancy, M. K., Moore, J., Brady, K., Milligan, D., & Strampel, W. (April 1992). The effect of altitude on umbilical cord blood gases. Obstetrics & Gynecology, 79(4), 571-574.

208. Breathnach, C. S. (July 1991). The stability of the fetal oxygen environment. Irish Journal of Medical Science, 160(7), 189-191.

209. Elliott, B. D., & Langer, O. (January 1994). Fetal placental blood flow in a population at risk for growth abnormalitites and placental insufficiency. American Journal of Obstetrics and Gynecology, 170(1, Pt. 2), 314.

210. Mathews, D. D. (August 1967). The oxygen supply of the postmature foetus before the onset of labour. Journal of Obstetrics and Gynaecology of the British Commonwealth, 74(4), 523-527.

211. Alexander, L. L. (May/June 1987). The pregnant smoker: Nursing implications. JOGNN, 16(3), 167-173.

212. Fox, H. (December 1969). Pathology of the placenta in maternal diabetes mellitus. Obstetrics & Gynecology, 34(6), 792-798.

213. Dekker, G. A., & Sibai, B. M. (January 1993). Low-dose aspirin in the prevention of preeclampsia and fetal growth retardation: Rationale, mechanisms, and clinical trials. American Journal of Obstetrics and Gynecology, 168(1, Pt. 1), 214-227.

214. Hsu, C., Chan, D. W., Lriye, B., Johnson, T. R. B., Witter, F. R., & Hong, S. (1993). Elevated circulating thrombomodulin in severe preeclampsia. American Journal of Obstetrics and Gynecology, 169(1), 148-149.

215. Kilpatrick, D. C., Liston, W. A., Gibson, F., & Livingstone, J. (November 4, 1989). Association between susceptibility to pre-eclampsia within families and HLA DR4. The Lancet, 1063-1064.

216. O'Brien, W. F. (March 1990). Predicting preeclampsia. Obstetrics & Gynecology, 75(3, Pt. 1), 445-452.

217. Walsh, S. W. (April 1990). Physiology of low-dose aspirin therapy for the prevention of preeclampsia. Seminars in Perinatology, 14(2), 152-170.

218. Labarrere, C. A., & Faulk, W. P. (July 1994). Antigenic identification of cells in spiral artery trophoblastic invasion: Validation of histologic studies by triple-antibody immunocytochemistry. American Journal of Obstetrics and Gynecology, 171(1), 165-171.

219. Shimonovitz, S., Hurwitz, A., Dushnik, M., Anteby, E., Geva-Eldar, J., & Yagel, S. (September 1994). Developmental regulation of the expression of 72 and 92 Kd type IV collagenases in human trophoblasts: A possible mechanism for control of trophoblast invasion. American Journal of Obstetrics and Gynecology, 171(3), 832-843.

220. Kirschbaum, T. (April 1993). Antibiotics in the treatment of preterm labor. American Journal of Obstetrics and Gynecology, 168(4), 1239-1246.

221. Lockwood, C. J., Wein, R., Lapinski, R., Casal, D., Berkowitz, G., & Alverez, M. (October 1993). The presence of cervical and vaginal fetal fibronectin predicts preterm delivery in an inner-city obstetric population. <u>American Journal of Obstetrics and Gynecology, 169</u>(4), 798-804.

222. Mitchell, B. F., & Wong, S. (May 1993). Changes in 17, 20 -hydroxysteroid dehydrogenase activity supporting an increase in the estrogen/progesterone ratio of human fetal membranes at parturition. <u>American Journal of Obstetrics and Gynecology, 168</u>(5), 1377-1385.

223. Nageotte, M. P., Casal, D., & Senyei, A. E. (January 1994). Fetal fibronectin in patients at increased risk for premature birth. <u>American Journal of Obstetrics and Gynecology, 170</u>(1, Pt. 1), 20-25.

224. Blackburn, S. T., & Loper, D. L. (1992). <u>Maternal, fetal, and neonatal physiology. A clinical perspective.</u> Philadelphia, PA: W. B. Saunders Company.

225. Sorensen, T. K., Williams, M. A., Zingheim, R. W., Clement, S. J., & Hickok, D. E. (October 1993). Elevated second trimester human chorionic gonadotropin and subsequent pregnancy induced hypertension. <u>American Journal of Obstetrics and Gynecology, 169</u>(4), 834-838.

226. Roberts, W. E., Perry, Jr., K. G., Woods, J. B., Files, J. C., Blake, P. G., & Martin, Jr., J. N. (September 1994). The intrapartum platelet count in patients with HELLP (hemolysis, elevated liver enzymes, and low platelets) syndrome: Is it predictive of later hemorrhagic complications? <u>American Journal of Obstetrics and Gynecology, 171</u>(3), 799-804.

227. Salvesen, D. R., Higueras, M. T., Brudenell, J. M., Drury, P. L., & Nicolaides, K. H. (November 1992). Doppler velocimetry and fetal heart rate studies in nephropathic diabetics. <u>American Journal of Obstetrics and Gynecology, 167</u>(5), 1297-1303.

228. Seligman, S. P., Abramson, S. B., Young, B. K., & Buyon, J. P. (January 1994). The role of nitric oxide (NO) in the pathogenesis of preeclampsia. <u>American Journal of Obstetrics and Gynecology, 170</u>(1, Pt. 2). SPO abstracts #290.

229. Kraayenbrink, A. A., Dekker, G. A., Van Kamp, G. J., & Van Geijn, H. P. (July 1993). Endothelial vasoactive mediators in preeclampsia. <u>American Journal of Obstetrics and Gynecology, 169</u>(1), 160-165.

230. Mallozzi, A., Levesque, D., Vintzileos, A. M., Egan, J. F. X., Tsapanos, V., & Salafia, C. M. (January 1993). Placental pathology in discordant twins. <u>American Journal of Obstetrics and Gynecology, 168</u>(1, Pt. 2), 360. SPO abstracts #225.

231. Devedeux, D., Marque, C., Mansour, S., Germain, G., & Duchene, J. (December 1993). Uterine electromyography: A critical review. <u>American Journal of Obstetrics and Gynecology, 169</u>(6), 1636-1653.

232. Arlen, J. (December 1986). Cervical ripening and preterm labor. <u>Obstetrics & Gynecology, 68</u>(6), 875-876.

233. Rajabi, M., Dean, D. D., & Woessner, Jr., J. F. (February 1987). High levels of serum collagenase in premature labor-a potential biochemical marker. <u>Obstetrics & Gynecology, 69</u>(2), 179-186.

234. Romero, R., Baumann, P., Fidel, P., Ramirez, M., Araneda, H., & Cotton, D. B. (January 1993). Systemic and local cytokine profile in endotoxin induced preterm birth. <u>American Journal of Obstetrics and Gynecology, 168</u>(1, Pt. 2), 377. SPO abstracts #284.

235. Molnar, M., Romero, R., & Hertelendy, F. (October 1993). Interleukin-1 and tumor necrosis factor stimulate arachidonic acid release and phospholipid metabolism in human myometrial cells. <u>American Journal of Obstetrics and Gynecology, 169</u>(4), 825-829.

236. Barclay, C. G., Brennand, J. E., Kelly, R. W., & Calder, A. A. (September 1993). Interleukin-8 production by the human cervix. <u>American Journal of Obstetrics and Gynecology, 169</u>(3), 625-632.

237. Booker, S. S., Jayanetti, C., Karalak, S., Hsiu, J-G., & Archer, D. F. (July 1994). The effect of progesterone on the accumulation of leukocytes in the human endometrium. <u>American Journal of Obstetrics and Gynecology, 171</u>(1), 139-142.

238. Cherouny, P. H., Pankuch, G. A., Romero, R., Botti, J. J., Kuhn, D. C., & Demers, L. M. (November 1993). Neutrophil attractant/activating peptide-1/interleukin-8: Association with histologic chorioamnionitis, preterm delivery, and bioactive amniotic fluid leukoattractants. <u>American Journal of Obstetrics and Gynecology, 169</u>(5), 1299-1303.

239. Zuspan, F. P., Cibils, L. A., & Pose, S. V. (October 1, 1962). Myometrial and cardiovascular responses to alterations in plasma epinephine and norepinephine. <u>American Journal of Obstetrics and Gynecology, 84</u>(7), 841-851.

240. Morgan, M. A., Honnebier, M. B. O. M., Myers, T., Winter, J., Mecenas, C., & Nathaniels, P. W. (January 1994). Cocaine's effect on oxytocin in the baboon during late pregnancy. <u>American Journal of Obstetrics and Gynecology, 170</u>(1, Pt. 2). SPO abstracts #170.

241. Morgan, M. A., Wentworth, R. A., Silavin, S. L., Jenkins, S. L., Fishburne, Jr., J. I., & Nathaniels, P. W. (May 1994). Intravenous administration of cocaine stimulates gravid baboon myometrium in the last third of gestation. <u>American Journal of Obstetrics and Gynecology, 170</u>(5, Pt.1), 1416-1420.

242. Kofinas, A. D., Simon, N. V., Clay, D., & King, K. (January 1993). Functional asymmetry of the human myometrium documented by color and pulse-wave doppler ultrasonographic evaluation of uterine arcuate arteries during Braxton Hicks contractions. <u>American Journal of Obstetrics and Gynecology, 168</u>(1, Pt. 1), 184-188.

243. Oosterhof, H., Dijkstra, K., & Aarnoudse, J. G. (1992). Fetal doppler velocimetry in the internal carotid and umbilical artery during Braxton Hicks contractions. <u>Early Human Development, 30,</u> 33-40.

244. Shields, L. E., & Brace, R. A. (July 1994). Fetal vascular pressure responses to nonlabor uterine contractions: Dependence on amniotic fluid volume in the ovine fetus. <u>American Journal of Obstetrics and Gynecology, 171</u>(1), 84-89.

245. Initiation of labor workshop: Attempting to understand a perplexing process. (April 1988). <u>Research Reports for NICHD.</u>

246. Mazor, M., Romero, R., Chaim, W., Hershkowitz, R., Levy, J., & Sepulveda, W. (January 1993). Evidence for a local change in the progesterone/estrogen ratio in preterm parturition. American Journal of Obstetrics and Gynecology, 168(1, Pt. 2), 327. SPO abstracts #97.

247. Chow, L., & Lye, S. J. (March 1994). Expression of the gap junction protein connexin-43 is increased in the human myometrium toward term and with the onset of labor. American Journal of Obstetrics and Gynecology, 170(3), 788-795.

248. Lieppman, R. E., Williams, M. A., Cheng, E. Y., Resta, R., Zingheim, R., & Hickok, D. E. (June 1993). An association between elevated levels of human chorionic gonadotropin in the midtrimester and adverse pregnancy outcome. American Journal of Obstetrics and Gynecology, 168(6, Pt. 1), 1852-1857.

249. Jackson, G. M., Sharp, H. T., & Varner, M. W. (October 1994). Cervical ripening before induction of labor: A randomized trial of prostaglandin E_2 gel versus low-dose oxytocin. American Journal of Obstetrics and Gynecology, 171(4), 1092-1096.

250. Erny, R., Pigne, A., Prouvost, C., Gamerre, M., Malet, C., & Serment, H. (March 1986). The effects of oral administration of progesterone for premature labor. American Journal of Obstetrics and Gynecolgy, 154(3), 525-529.

251. Arnaudeau, S., Lepretre, N., & Mironneau, J. (August 1994). Chloride and monovalent ion-selective cation currents activated by oxytocin in pregnant rat myometrial cells. American Journal of Obstetrics and Gynecology, 171(2), 491-501.

252. Kulb, N. W. (1993). Preterm labor. In K. Buckley & N. W. Kulb (Eds.). High risk maternity nursing manual (2nd ed) (pp. 350-366). Baltimore, MD: Williams and Wilkins.

253. Higby, K., Xenakis, E. M. J., & Pauerstein, C. J. (April 1993). Do tocolytic agents stop preterm labor? A critical and comprehensive review of efficacy and safety. American Journal of Obstetrics and Gynecology, 168(4), 1247-1259.

254. Balducci, J., Risek, B., Gilula, N. B., Hand, A., Egan, J. F., & Vintzileos, A. M. (May 1993). Gap junction formation in human myometrium: A key to preterm labor? American Journal of Obstetrics and Gynecology, 168(5), 1609-1615.

255. Whitley, N. (September/October 1975). Uterine contractile physiology: Application in nursing care and patient teaching. JOGNN, 4(5), 54-58.

256. Freeman, R. K., & Garite, T. J., (1981). Fetal heart rate monitoring. Baltimore, MD: Williams & Wilkins.

257. Meizner, I., Levy, A., & Katz, M. (February/March 1993). Assessment of uterine and umbilical artery velocimetry during latent and active phases of normal labor. Israel Journal of Medical Sciences, 29(2-3), 82-85.

258. Bleker, O. P., Kloosterman, G. J., Mieras, D. J., Oosting, J., & Salle, H. J. A. (December 1, 1975). Intervillous space during uterine contractions in human subjects: An ultrasonic study. American Journal of Obstetrics and Gynecology, 123(7), 697-699.

259. Borell, U., Fernstrom, I., Ohlson, L., & Wiqvist, N. (September 1, 1965). Influence of uterine contractions on the uteroplacental blood flow at term. American Journal of Obstetrics and Gynecology, 93(1), 44-57.

260. Burke, M. E. (October 1989). Hypertensive crisis and the perinatal period. Journal of Perinatal and Neonatal Nursing, 3(2), 33-47.

261. Friedman, E.A. (1983). Physiology of labor. In W. R. Cohen & E. A. Friedman (Eds.). Managernent of labor (pp. 1-9). Baltimore, MD: University Park Press.

262. Brotanek, V., Hendricks, C. H., & Yoshida, T. (April 15, 1969). Changes in uterine blood flow during uterine contractions. American Journal of Obstetrics and Gynecology, 103(8), 1108-1116.

263. Peebles, D. M., Edwards, A. D., Wyatt, J. S., Bishop, A. P., Cope, M., & Delpy, D. T. (May 1992). Changes in human fetal cerebral hemoglobin concentration and oxygenation during labor measured by near-infrared spectroscopy. American Journal of Obstetrics and Gynecology, 166(5), 1369-1373.

264. Wallerstedt, C., Higgins, P., Kasnic, T., & Curet, L. B. (September 1994). Amnioinfusion: An update [Principles and Practice]. JOGNN, 23, 573-378.

265. Miller, Jr., J. M., Boudreaux, M. C., & Regan, F. A. (January 1995). A case-control study of cocaine use in pregnancy. American Journal of Obstetrics and Gynecology, 172(1, Pt. 1),180-185.

266. Dicke, J. M., Verges, D. K., & Polakoski, K. L. (April 1994). The effects of cocaine on neutral amnio acid uptake by human placental basal membrane vesicles. American Journal of Obstetrics and Gynecology, 171(2), 485-491.

267. Hurd, W. W., Gauvin, J. M., Dombrowski, M. P., & Hayashi, R. H. (September 1993). Cocaine selectively inhibits β-adrenergic receptor binding in pregnant human myometrium. American Journal of Obstetrics and Gynecology, 169(3), 644-649.

268. Monga, M., Weisbrodt, N. W., Andres, R. L., & Sanborn, B. M. (October 1993). The acute effect of cocaine exposure on pregnant human myometrial contractile activity. American Journal of Obstetrics and Gynecology, 169(4), 782-785.

269. Monga, M., Weisbrodt, N. W., Andres, R. L., & Sanborn, B. M. (December 1993). Cocaine acutely increases rat myometrial contractile activity by mechanisms other than potentiation of adrenergic pathways. American Journal of Obstetrics and Gynecology, 169(6), 1502-1506.

270. Morgan, B. (1994). Maternal anesthesia and analgesia in labor. In D. K. James, P. J. Steer, C. P. Weiner, & B. Gonik (Eds.), High risk obstetrics: Management options (pp. 1101-1108). Philadelphia, PA: W. B. Saunders Company.

271. Christmas, J. T., McGhee, P. H., Dinsmoor, M. J., Irons, S. J., Dawson, K. S., & Kish, C. W. (January 1993). Preterm labor: The effect of recent substance use on the occurrence of preterm delivery. American Journal of Obstetrics and Gynecology, 168(1, Pt. 2), 371. SPO abstracts #262.

272. Cowan, D. B. (August 30, 1980). Intrapartum fetal resuscitation. South African Medical Journal, 58(9), 376-379.

273. Goldsmith, J. (Fall 1995). Newborn research depends on partnerships. Reflections, 21(3), 6-8.

274. Siddiqi, T. A., Meyer, R.A., Lynch-Salamon, D., Rosenn, B., Jaekle, R. K., & Khoury, J. (January 1994). A prospective longitudinal study of human umbilical arterial blood flow. American Journal of Obstetrics and Gynecology, 170(1, Pt. 2).

275. Yeh, M-N., Morishima, H. O., Niemann, W. H., & James, L. S. (April 1, 1975). Myocardial conduction defects in association with compression of the umbilical cord [Fetus, Placenta, and Newborn]. American Journal of Obstetrics and Gynecology, 121(7), 951-957.

276. Vaughan, J. I., Warwick, R., Letsky, E., Nicolini, U., Rodeck, C. H., & Fisk, N. M. (July 1994). Erythropoietic suppression in fetal anemia because of kell alloimmunization. American Journal of Obstetrics and Gynecology, 171(1), 247-252.

277. Davis, L. E., Hohimer, A. R., & Brace, R. A. (January 1994). Lymph flow during chronic fetal anemia. American Journal of Obstetrics and Gynecology, 170(1, Pt. 2), 311. SPO abstracts #122.

278. Christmas, J. T., Vanner, L. V., Daniels, R. M., Bodurtha, J. N., Hays, P. M., & Redwine, F. O. (August 1994). The effect of fetomaternal bleeding on the risk of adverse pregnancy outcome in patients with elevated second-trimester maternal serum α-fetoprotein levels. American Journal of Obstetrics and Gynecology, 171(2), 315-320.

279. Hoag, R. W. (June 1986). Fetomaternal hemorrhage associated with umbilical vein thrombosis. American Journal of Obstetrics and Gynecology, 154(6), 1271-1274.

280. Ballas, S., Gitstein, S., & Kharasch, J. (1985). Fetal heart rate variation with umbilical haematoma. The Fellowship Postgraduate Medical Journal, 61, 753-755.

281. Bianchi, D. W., DeMaria, M. A., Shuber, A. P., Fougner, A. C., & Klinger, K. W. (January 1994). Fetal cells in maternal blood: Determination of purity and yield by quantitative PCR. American Journal of Obstetrics and Gynecology, 170(1, Pt. 2). SPO abstracts #38.

282. Willis, C., & Foreman, Jr., C. S. (March 1988). Chronic massive fetomaternal hemorrhage: A case report. Obstetrics & Gynecology, 71(3, Pt. 2), 459-461.

283. Welch, R., Rampling, M. W., Anwar, A., Talbert, D. G., & Rodeck, C. H. (March 1994). Changes in hemorheology with fetal intravascular transfusion. American Journal of Obstetrics and Gynecology, 170(3), 726-732.

284. Itskovitz, J., Goetzman, B. W., Roman, C., & Rudolph, A. M. (October 1984). Effects of fetal-maternal exchange transfusion on fetal oxygenation and blood flow distribution. American Journal of Physiology, 247(4, Pt. 2), H655-H660.

285. Thorp, J. A., Plapp, F. V., Cohen, G. R., Yeast, J. D., O'Kell, R. T., & Stephenson, S. (August 1990). Hyperkalemia after irradiation of packed red blood cells: Possible effects with intravascular fetal transfusion. American Journal of Obstetrics and Gynecology, 163(2), 607-609.

286. Weiner, C. P. (May 1990). The relationship between the umbilical artery systolic/diastolic ratio and umbilical blood gas measurements in specimens obtained by cordocentesis. American Journal of Obstetrics and Gynecology, 162(5), 1198-1202.

287. Gardner, K. (January/February 1993). Twin transfusion syndrome. JOGNN, 22(1), 64-71.

288. Wilcox, G. R., & Trudinger, B. J. (August 1993). Erythrocytes in fetuses with abnormal umbilical artery flow velocity waveforms. American Journal of Obstetrics and Gynecology,169(2, Pt. 1), 379-383.

289. Stevenson, D. K., Bucalo, R., Cohen, R. S., Vreman, H. J., Ferguson, II, J. E., & Schwartz, H. C. (January 1986). Increased immunoreactive erythropoietin in cord plasma and neonatal bilirubin production in normal term infants after labor. Obstetrics & Gynecology, 67(1), 69-73.

290. Widness, J. A., Clemons, G. K., Garcia, J. F., Oh, W., & Schwartz, R. (January 15, 1984). Increased immunoreactive erythropoietin in cord serum after labor. American Journal of Obstetrics and Gynecology, 148(2), 194-197.

291. Richey, S. D., Ramin, S. M., Bawdon, R. E., Roberts, S. W., Dax, J., & Roberts, J. (April 1995). Markers of acute and chronic asphyxia in infants with meconium-stained amniotic fluid. American Journal of Obstetrics and Gynecology, 172(4, Pt. 1), 1212-1215.

292. Duckworth, M. W. (1961). Tissue changes accompanying acclimatization to low atmospheric oxygen in the rat. Journal of Physiology, 156, 603-610.

293. Lemery, D., Santolaya, J., Serre, A., Denoix, S., Besse, G., & Jacquetin, B. (January 1993). Comparison between serum erythropoietin of AGA and SGA fetuses. American Journal of Obstetrics and Gynecology, 168(1, Pt. 2), 329. SPO abstracts #103.

294. Papile, L. A. (September 29-30, 1995). General session: The timing of perinatal brain injury. In Current concepts and controversies in perinatal care. Symposium conducted at the Sheraton Inn. Albuquerque, NM.

295. Phelan, J. P., Ahn, M. O., Korst, L., & Martin, G. I. (January 1994). Nucleated red blood cells: A marker for fetal asphyxia. American Journal of Obstetrics and Gynecology, 170(1, Pt. 2), 286. SPO abstracts #49.

296. Pleet, H. (June 1981). Central nervous system and facial defects associated with maternal hyperthermia at four to fourteen weeks of gestation. Pediatrics, 67(6), 785-789.

297. Yoneyama, Y., Shin, S. Iwasaki, T., Power, G. G., & Araki, T. (September 1994). Relationship between plasma adenosine concentration and breathing movements in growth-retarded fetuses. American Journal of Obstetrics and Gynecology, 171(3), 701-706.

298. Ball, R. H., Espinoza, M. I., Parer, J. T., Alon, E., Vertommen, J., & Johnson, J. (January 1994). Regional blood flow in asphyxiated fetuses with seizures. American Journal of Obstetrics and Gynecology, 170(1, Pt. 1), 156-161.

299. Harvey, C. J., & Hankins, G. D. V. (January 1994). The effect of pulmonary shunting (Qs/Qt) on fetal arterial hemoglobin saturation in the sheep model. American Journal of Obstetrics and Gynecology, 170(1, Pt. 2).

300. Gleason, C. A., Hamm, C., & Jones, Jr., M. D. (April 1990). Effect of acute hypoxemia on brain blood flow and oxygen metabolism in immature fetal sheep. American Journal of Physiology, 258(4, Pt. 2), H1064-H1069.

301. Egerman, R. S., & Bissonnette, J. M. (January 1993). The effects of centrally administered adenosine on fetal sheep heart rate accelerations. American Journal of Obstetrics and Gynecology, 168(1, Pt. 2), 327. SPO abstracts #98.

302. Egerman, R. S., Bissonnette, J. M., & Hohimer, A. R. (October 1993). The effects of centrally administered adenosine on fetal sheep heart rate accelerations. American Journal of Obstetrics and Gynecology, 169(4), 866-869.

303. Mason, B. A., Ogunyemi, D., Punla, O., & Koos, B. J. (May 1993). Maternal and fetal cardiorespiratory responses to adenosine in sheep. American Journal of Obstetrics and Gynecology, 168(5), 1558-1561.

304. Weiner, C. P., Power, G., & Yoneyama, Y. (January 1993). Adenosine in the human fetus. American Journal of Obstetrics and Gynecology, 168(1, Pt. 2), 328. SPO abstracts #99.

305. Yoneyama, Y., Wakatsuki, M., Sawa, R., Kamoi, S., Takahashi, H., & Shin, S. (February 1994). Plasma adenosine concentration in appropriate- and small-for-gestational-age fetuses. American Journal of Obstetrics and Gynecology, 170(2), 684-688.

306. Ortner, A., Zech, H., Humpeler, E., & Mairbaeurl, H. (1983). May high oxygen affinity of maternal hemoglobin cause fetal growth retardation? Archives of Gynecology, 234(2), 79-85.

307. Nicolaides, K. H., Bradley, R. J., Soothill, P. W., Campbell, S., Bilardo, C. M., & Gibb, D. (April 25, 1987). Maternal oxygen therapy for intrauterine growth retardation. The Lancet,1, 942-945.

308. Adamson, S. L., Morrow, R. J., & Ritchie, J. W. K. (December 1992). Vascular resistance and the umbilical arterial velocity waveforms [Letters]. American Journal of Obstetrics and Gynecology, 167(6), 1910-1912.

309. Forouzan, I. (January 1995). Hemodynamic changes in fetuses with absent end-diastolic velocity in umbilical artery [Letters]. American Journal of Obstetrics and Gynecology, 172(1, Pt. 1), 244.

310. Fleischer, A., Schulman, H., Farmakides, G., Bracero, L., Blattner, P., & Randolph, G. (February 15, 1985). Umbilical artery velocity waveforms and intrauterine growth retardation. American Journal of Obstetrics and Gynecology, 151(4), 502-505.

311. Collins, M. H., & James, L. S. (1990). Fetal respiratory physiology. In R. D. Eden, F. H. Bachm, & M. Haire (Eds.), Assessment and care of the fetus: Physiological, clinical and medicolegal principles (pp. 17-27). Norwalk, CT: Appleton & Lange.

312. Beksac, M. S., Onderoglu, L. S., Ozdemir, K., & Karakas, U. (November 3, 1991). The validation of a computerized system for the interpretation of the antepartum fetal heart rate tracings (version 89/2.34). European Journal of Obstetrics, Gynecology and Reproductive Biology, 42(1), 9-14.

313. Ferrazzi, E., Bellotti, M., Flisi, M. L., Barbera, A., & Pardi, G. (January 1993). Cardiac doppler velocimetry and acid base balance in IUGR fetuses. American Journal of Obstetrics and Gynecology, 168(1, Pt. 2), 328.

314. Ferrazzi, E., Bellotti, M., Barbera, A., Flisi, P., Bozzetti, P., & Pardi, G. (January 1994). Peak velocity of the outflow tract of the aorta and heart rate characteristics in growth retarded fetuses. American Journal of Obstetrics and Gynecology, 170(1, Pt. 2). SPO abstracts #94.

315. Snijders, R. J. M., Ribbert, L. S. M., Visser, G. H. A., & Mulder, E. J. H. (January 1992). Numeric analysis of heart rate variation in intrauterine growth-retarded fetuses: A longitudinal study. American Journal of Obstetrics and Gynecology, 166(1, Pt. 1), 22-27.

316. Emory, E. K., & Noonan, J. R. (August 1984). Fetal cardiac responding: A correlate of birth weight and neonatal behavior. Child Development, 55(4), 1651-1657.

317. Penning, D. H., Grafe, M. R., Hammond, R., Matsuda, Y., Patrick, J., & Richardson, B. (May 1994). Neuropathology of the near-term and midgestation ovine fetal brain after sustained in utero hypoxemia. American Journal of Obstetrics and Gynecology, 170(5, Pt. 1), 1425-1432.

318. Ang, C. K., Tan, T. H., Walters, W. A. W., & Wood, C. (October 25, 1969). Postural influence on maternal capillary oxygen and carbon dioxide tension. British Medical Journal, 4, 201-203.

319. Ogunyemi, D., Castro, L., Allen, L., Hobel, C., & Roll, K. (January 1994). Effects of tobacco use and tobacco + cocaine use on fetal growth and uterine flow velocity waveforms. American Journal of Obstetrics and Gynecology, 170(1, Pt. 2). SPO abstracts #467.

4

Extrinsic Factors that Affect Oxygen Delivery and the FHR

INTRODUCTION

The fetal heart rate (FHR) reflects *conduction* of an impulse from the brainstem to autonomic nerves to the heart and the state of fetal oxygenation. An appreciation of maternal and fetal anatomy and physiology is required to interpret the images on the fetal monitor paper. Skilled clinicians *identify maternal, placental, umbilical cord, and fetal factors that might limit fetal oxygen (O_2) delivery. They react to the probable physiology causing the tracing, not the images on the paper.* This chapter presents extrinsic factors that influence the FHR, such as maternal, placental, and umbilical cord factors related to acute and chronic fetal O_2 deprivation. The fetal compensatory response to hypoxia is also discussed.

EXTRINSIC FACTORS THAT AFFECT OXYGEN DELIVERY AND THE FHR

Obstacles to adequate O_2 delivery can cause acute or chronic fetal hypoxia. With chronic hypoxia, the supply of O_2 slowly decreases over time. The fetus decreases tissue metabolism and slows its growth (1). During acute hypoxia, neurohumoral compensatory mechanisms may be overwhelmed very quickly.

The clinician is challenged to determine which barriers to O_2 delivery exist so that the barrier can be removed or diminished. Analysis of the maternal history, physical manifestations of disease, and the FHR and uterine activity patterns often provide clues to the type of barriers that may be impeding O_2 delivery. Another challenge is to determine if the fetus will be better oxygenated by remaining in the uterus or if the fetus should become a newborn by expeditious delivery. The goal, of course, is to keep the fetus in the uterus as long as possible and to avoid operative delivery if at all possible.

Oxygen and Carbon Dioxide Diffusion

Oxygen diffuses from the atmosphere across maternal alveoli into maternal pulmonary capillary blood where it attaches to Hb. *The amount of O_2 women inhale during inspiration is called the inspiratory oxygen fraction (FIO_2)* (134). Room air is approximately 79 percent nitrogen and 21 percent oxygen, therefore the FIO_2 of room air is 21 percent (135).

Diffusion of gases, such as O_2 and CO_2, depends on five factors:
- partial pressure of the gas on either side of the exchange membrane
- surface area over which gases are exchanged
- permeability of the membrane through which gases must travel
- diffusion distance and
- blood flow rates on either side of the membrane (1, 136).

Partial pressure of the gas on either side of the membrane. Pressure is exerted by gas molecules bouncing against the membrane and/or the vessel wall. The pressure exerted by O_2 that is freely floating in plasma is denoted as PO_2. In the lungs, *O_2 diffusion* into maternal circulation is dependent upon the gradient between inspired oxygen (FIO_2) and pulmonary capillary PO_2, alveolar area and permeability, and pulmonary capillary permeability and blood flow.

The difference in pressure exerted by the gases on either side of the alveoli creates a gradient. *Gases travel from an area*

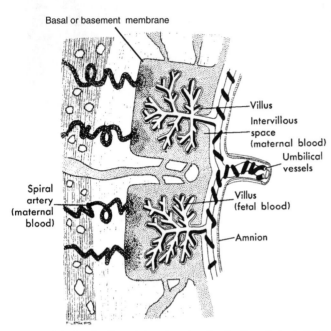

Figure 4.1: Section through the placenta, showing the spiral arteries that supply maternal blood to the intervillous spaces, the branching villi immersed in the intervillous space, and the umbilical vessels that branch repeatedly to terminate as villous capillaries. Spiral arteries run perpendicular to the basal exchange membrane, uterine veins run parallel to the basal membrane (modified from Netter: In E. Oppenheim (Ed.). (1965). Ciba collection of medical illustrations, vol. 2, Reproductive system. Reprinted with permission from The C. V. Mosby Company from Korones, S. B. (1981). *High-risk newborn infants. The basis for intensive nursing care. 3rd ed.*).

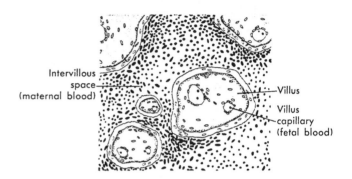

Figure 4.2: Microscopic transverse section of villi and the intervillous space. Fetal capillaries permeate the villi, which are immersed in maternal blood within the intervillous spaces (reproduced with permission of The C. V. Mosby Company from Korones, S. B. (1981). *High-risk newborn infants. The basis of intensive nursing care. 3rd ed.*).

of high pressure to an area of low pressure. At sea level, the PO_2 in room air is approximately 160 mm Hg. In the alveoli it is 104 mm Hg. Since the pressure of O_2 in the air is greater than that in the alveoli, O_2 will push its way through the alveolar membrane into maternal capillaries.

At higher altitudes, PO_2 in the air decreases (air is "thinner"). As a result, alveolar PO_2 decreases. In fact, at 30,000 feet, pilots need supplemental O_2 because without it their alveolar PO_2 would only be 21 mm Hg (6).

In the uterus, O_2 transfer from maternal to fetal blood is primarily by passive diffusion across the placental basal or basement membrane and villi (see Figure 4.1). Passive diffusion continues until gases reach equilibrium on either side of the villus exchange membrane. Oxygen *diffuses* from maternal blood in the intervillous space across the villous membrane into fetal capillaries inside the villi (see Figure 4.2). In the placenta, O_2 and CO_2 transfer will be affected by

- maternal/fetal PO_2 and PCO_2 gradients
- placental surface area
- maternal spiral artery O_2 delivery to intervillous spaces
- placental villi permeability
- placental lesions or villous edema
- fetal capillary quantity and permeability and
- maternal venous and fetal capillary blood flow.

CO_2, produced as a byproduct of aerobic glucose metabolism, combines with water in plasma to form carbonic acid ($H_2O + CO_2 = H_2CO_3$). The formation of carbonic acid is catalyzed by the enzyme carbonic anhydrase. Carbonic acid splits to form hydrogen (H^+) plus bicarbonate (HCO_3^-). Free H^+ ions attach to Hb which lowers blood pH. Thus, Hb is a powerful acid-base buffer.

$$CO_2 + H_2O \Rightarrow H_2CO_3 \text{ (carbonic acid)}$$

$$H_2CO_3 \Rightarrow H^+ + HCO_3^- \text{ (bicarbonate)}$$

$$H^+ + Hb \Rightarrow HbH$$

CO_2 is transported in the fetal bloodstream in three forms: 7 to 8 percent is dissolved in plasma (PCO_2), 23 to 30 percent is bound to Hb as carbaminohemoglobin ($HbCO_2$), and 62 to 70 percent is in the form of bicarbonate (HCO_3^-). When carbon monoxide (CO) binds with Hb, carboxyhemoglobin (HCO) is produced (6, 137).

CO_2 leaves the fetal body in umbilical arteries in the form of freely floating carbon dioxide ($P_{ua}CO_2$), carbon dioxide bound to hemoglobin ($HbCO_2$), and bicarbonate (HCO_3^-). In the placenta, free CO_2 leaves fetal capillaries and diffuses across the villous membrane to maternal blood in the intervillous spaces then across the basement membrane to maternal venous blood.

In maternal veins, CO_2 binds with Hb ($HbCO_2$), combines with water in plasma to form carbonic acid (H_2CO_3), and is carried by plasma proteins. Plasma proteins carry 1.5 ml of CO_2 per 100 ml of blood. CO_2 eventually reaches the maternal heart then lungs and is exhaled. The ratio of inhaled O_2 to exhaled CO_2 is 1:0.8, i.e., 20 percent more oxygen is inhaled than CO_2 is exhaled (6).

Oxygen Delivery to the Placenta and Fetus

Normal physiologic changes of pregnancy increase O_2 delivery to the placenta and fetus. These changes include:

- elevation of the maternal diaphragm 4 to 7 cm
- flaring of the lower ribs which increases the anterior-posterior and transverse diameters of the thorax
- minute ventilation increases 50% over nonpregnant norms (138)
- tidal volume increases from 500 to 700 ml
- PaO_2 increases by 10 mm Hg (138)
- O_2 consumption increases 20%
- $PaCO_2$ decreases from 40 mm Hg to 30 mm Hg (138)
- serum estrogen and estriol increase RBC 2,3-DPG production (139-140)
- the number of RBCs increases 20% (139)
- plasma volume increases 40 to 50% (139)
- blood volume increases 1600 ml in a singleton pregnancy and 2000 ml in multiple gestation
- colloid osmotic pressure (COP) decreases
- maternal heart rate (MHR) increases 20% (15 to 20 bpm by 38 to 42 weeks' gestation)
- stroke volume increases (25% at 24 to 26 weeks' gestation and 50% by term)
- cardiac output increases 30 to 50% (beginning at 10 weeks' gestation, peaking at 30 weeks' gestation), and
- systemic vascular resistance decreases 25% which is mediated by estrogen and progesterone.

Minute ventilation is the amount of gas exchanged between the lungs and the atmosphere per minute. There are four types of pulmonary volumes: tidal, inspiratory reserve, expiratory reserves, and residual volume. When two or more "volumes" are added together, their sum is called pulmonary capacity (6).

Table 1: Pulmonary Volumes and Capacities

TERM	DEFINITION
Tidal volume	amount of inspired or expired air during each normal breath.
Inspiratory reserve volume	amount of air that can be inspired above the normal tidal volume, which is less than 3000 ml in women.
Expiratory reserve volume	extra amount of air that can be exhaled by forceful expiration after the end of a normal tidal volume. This is less than 1100 ml in women.
Residual volume	the amount of air remaining in the lungs after the most forceful expiration. It is less than 1200 ml in women.
Functional residual capacity	sum of the expiratory reserve volume plus the residual volume.
Vital capacity	tidal volume plus the inspiratory reserve volume plus the expiratory reserve volume.
Total lung capacity	maximum volume to which the lungs can be expanded with the greatest possible inspiratory effort = the vital capacity plus residual volume (6).

Colloid Osmotic Pressure (COP)

Blood volume begins to increase about 4 to 6 weeks' gestation and plateaus about 33 weeks' gestation. Blood volume is related to estrogen, progesterone, and aldosterone. Colloids are proteins. Colloid osmotic pressure (COP) is the pressure measured between two solutions which are separated by a semipermeable membrane such as a capillary wall. Intravenous albumin and hetastarch (Hespan®) solutions are administered to increase COP.

The quantity of intravascular proteins, such as albumin, globulin, and fibrinogen, increases during pregnancy which increases COP. Albumin is a water-soluble, heat-coagulable protein that contains carbon, hydrogen, oxygen, nitrogen, and sulfur. Albumin is found in almost all tissues, blood, and urine. A loss of albumin in urine occurs when women are preeclamptic. The loss of albumin decreases intravascular COP. Globulin is a simple protein. Fibrinogen is a plasma protein that is essential for blood clot formation. Thrombin, produced by the liver, acts on fibrinogen to produce fibrin. Fibrin is a stringy, insoluble protein that is responsible for the semisolid character of a blood clot (82). The increase in plasma volume during pregnancy dilutes blood and diminishes the increase in RBC and protein volume which decreases blood viscosity and lowers COP.

Capillary Hydrostatic (Wedge) Pressure

The pressure exerted by fluid in capillaries is called capillary hydrostatic pressure or wedge pressure. *Capillary wedge pressure and COP are usually inversely related.* Capillary wedge pressure increases when COP decreases. Capillary wedge pressure decreases when COP increases. However, if a woman is given Hespan, the wedge pressure will increase as will the COP. *When blood becomes less viscous, capillary wedge pressure increases and blood flow increases.* Intravenous administration of crystalloid solutions, such as normal saline (NS), lactated Ringer's solution (LR), and 5% dextrose in water (D_5W), increase capillary wedge pressure and decrease COP and blood viscosity.

Increased wedge pressure. There is a fine line, however, between improving blood flow and iatrogenic fluid overload. If COP decreases below 15 mm Hg, the risk of pulmonary edema increases as increased wedge pressure forces fluid out of blood vessels. Wedge pressure can also increase if there is left ventricular dysfunction with impaired cardiac contractility during systole or impaired ventricular relaxation during diastole or a combination of the two. Maternal wedge pres-

200

sure increases after birth when extravascular fluid shifts back into blood vessels (141). Therefore, all post partum women are at increased risk for pulmonary edema.

Whole Blood Oxygen Content

Oxygen content in whole blood is measured as total O_2 in 100 ml of blood. Normal whole blood O_2 content is 20.6 ml%. The majority of O_2 is bound to Hb (20 ml%) and the rest (0.6 ml%) is floating freely in the plasma (6).

The erythrocyte or RBC carries O_2 and CO_2 (135). Oxygen binds with Hb to form oxyhemoglobin (HbO_2). When oxygen binds with Hb, Hb is saturated. Hb saturation is determined as the amount of Hb bound to oxygen (HbO_2) divided by the total amount of Hb that could bind with O_2 (HbO_2 + Hb).

$$SaO_2 = HbO_2 / HbO_2 + Hb$$

Whole blood Hb saturation can be directly measured by blood gases (SaO_2) or indirectly measured by a pulse oximeter (SpO_2). SvO_2 represents the percent of total venous hemoglobin saturated with O_2 (142). Unbound plasma O_2 is denoted as the partial pressure of oxygen or PO_2 (143).

SaO_2 depends on such factors as PO_2, carbon monoxide (CO), PCO_2, pH, temperature, and the affinity of Hb for O_2. An increase in PaO_2 usually increases SaO_2 and a decrease in PaO_2 decreases SaO_2. Carbon monoxide (CO) binds faster with Hb than O_2. When CO binds with Hb, carboxyhemoglobin is created (**HbCO**). HbCO decreases the quantity of Hb available for O_2 transport and decreases hemoglobin's oxygen-carrying capacity. *In addition, an increase in HbCO increases Hb oxygen affinity and decreases O_2 unloading which decreases tissue O_2 delivery* (140, 144).

Carbon dioxide (CO_2) also combines with Hb faster than O_2 to form carbaminohemoglobin (**HbCO_2**). CO_2 binds with plasma water to form carbonic acid (H_2CO_3), and carbonic acid splits into free H^+ and HCO_3^- (bicarbonate). The increase in hydrogen increases HbH which *decreases blood pH which decreases Hb oxygen affinity and increases unloading of O_2 which increases tissue O_2 delivery*. To summarize, maternal arterial O_2 content is related to:

FIO_2 = inspiratory oxygen fraction
PaO_2 = partial pressure of oxygen in arterial plasma
$PaCO_2$ = partial pressure of carbon dioxide in arterial plasma
HbO_2 = hemoglobin bound to oxygen, oxyhemoglobin
SaO_2 = ratio of oxyhemoglobin (HbO_2) to total Hb in the arteries
$HbCO$ = hemoglobin bound to carbon monoxide, carboxyhemoglobin
$HbCO_2$ = hemoglobin bound to carbon dioxide, carbaminohemoglobin
$HbCO$ decreases O_2 delivery
$HbCO_2$ increases O_2 delivery.

An increase in FIO_2 should increase maternal PaO_2. A decrease in FIO_2 should decrease maternal PaO_2. An increase

in HbCO increases Hb oxygen affinity and decreases O_2 available to tissues for oxidative metabolism. An increase in $HbCO_2$ decreases pH and Hb oxygen affinity and increases O_2 available for oxidative metabolism.

Hemoglobin Affinity and Oxygen-Carrying Capacity

Hemoglobin only carries a specific quantity of O_2. A gram of Hb can bind with 1.34 ml of O_2. In 100 ml of whole blood with a Hb of 11 gm, oxygen carrying capacity will be 11 x 1.34 or 14.74 ml% (135). This is well below the norm of 20.6 ml%.

Hemoglobin O_2 affinity is hemoglobin's ability to bond with O_2 (145). Hb oxygen affinity determines its oxygen-carrying capacity. Oxygen affinity is related to:

- hemoglobin type
- intraerythrocytic glycolytic metabolism (RBC glucose metabolism) and
- RBC 2,3 diphosphoglycerate (2,3-DPG) (146).

Hemoglobin (Hb) type. Adult hemoglobin A (HbA) is composed of four polypeptide chains. There are two alpha (globin) chains and two beta (globin) chains. Each chain is composed of amino acids. The chains attach to form a tetramer (see Figure 4.3).

The ability of Hb to carry and release O_2 depends on the type of globin chains. For example, Hb Bart is created by four gamma chains. HbH is created by four beta chains. Both types of Hb have a greater O_2 affinity than HbA. *An increase in Hb oxygen affinity decreases O_2 delivery to tissues*. Women with thalassemia are at high risk to deliver a child with Bart's Hb which is incompatible with life (146). Fetuses with Hb Bart's often develop hydrops and die before birth or soon thereafter (148). A Vietnamese woman with thalassemia major had immature RBCs (nucleated RBCs) and RBCs with

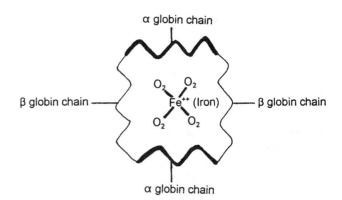

Figure 4.3: Illustration of adult Hb (HbA) which is created by four polypeptide chains composed of amino acids (globin). Each chain surrounds an iron (Fe^{++}) porphyrin atom (heme) to which oxygen, carbon monoxide, or carbon dioxide bind. Hb A can hold as many as four oxygen molecules or four carbon monoxide or carbon dioxide molecules. The combination of heme and globin creates hemoglobin (147).

anisocytosis (varying in size), poikilocytosis (abnormal variation in RBC shape), and hypochromia (less than normal color). Hemoglobin electrophoresis revealed Hb F (30 to 35 percent), a nonmigrating Hb (15 percent), an unknown Hb (50 percent) that migrated like HbA_2, no HbA, and HbE (40 percent) (149).

Oxygen Affinity (P_{50})

Pregnancy is associated with decreased plasma $PaCO_2$ which increases Hb oxygen affinity and decreases tissue O_2 delivery. However, pregnancy is also associated with a decrease in RBC pH, which decreases Hb oxygen affinity and increases O_2 delivery (150). These two factors offset one another so that there is no change in P_{50} between pregnant and nonpregnant women.

Oxygen affinity is expressed as P_{50}, the PaO_2 where half of all available Hb is saturated with O_2 at a pH of 7.40, a $PaCO_2$ of 40 mm Hg, and a temperature of 37° C (see Figure 4.4) (140). Hb oxygen affinity differs in maternal and fetal blood due to differences in:

- Hb type
- RBC glycolytic metabolism
- RBC 2,3-DPG
- pH
- PCO_2 and
- temperature.

Hemoglobin and Hematocrit

Normally during pregnancy, the maternal Hb and hematocrit (HCT) are adequate to deliver sufficient O_2 to the placenta and fetus (140). HCT is calculated by dividing the number of RBCs in 100 ml of blood by 100 ml (RBCs/RBCs + plasma) (151). The optimal Hb and HCT during pregnancy are:

Hb   11 - 12 gm/dl
HCT   33 - 35%.

If anemia is severe, or there is hemoconcentration, tissue oxygenation is impaired. Uterine, placental, and fetal hypoxia and nutritional deficits occur because of a lack of RBCs to carry O_2 (anemia) or due to sluggish blood flow due to the increase in blood viscosity (hemoconcentration). When Hb levels were less than 9 gm/dl or greater than 13 gm/dl, and HCT levels were less than 29 percent or greater than 39 percent, there was an increased incidence of low birth weight (LBW), preterm labor and birth, and stillbirth (139).

Intraerythrocytic glycolytic metabolism. Glucose metabolism in the RBC is called "the glycolytic pathway" or intraerythrocytic glycolytic metabolism. The glycolytic pathway affects the quantity of RBC 2,3 diphosphoglycerate and ATP. Oxidative glucose metabolism in the RBC increases 2,3-DPG levels and generates ATP. ATP stabilizes the RBC membrane. Glucose metabolism is affected by RBC pH and plasma pH (140, 146, 152).

Red blood cell 2,3 diphosphoglycerate (2,3-DPG). 2,3-DPG, with the help of ATP, binds to Hb on the β-chain in the central cavity of deoxygenated Hb. Glucose binds to the same site as 2,3-DPG. When glucose binds to the 2,3-DPG site, HbA becomes HbA_{1C} or glycosylated hemoglobin (140). When O_2 binds with Hb, 2,3-DPG is expelled, but O_2 cannot bind to glycosylated Hb. Thus, a decrease in 2,3-DPG is associated with an increase in oxygen-Hb affinity or oxyhemoglobin (HbO_2) (144). *An increase in HbA_{1C} decreases Hb oxygen-carrying capacity and limits tissue O_2 delivery.*

During pregnancy, the level of 2,3-DPG steadily increases 7 to 30 percent over nonpregnancy norms (153). The concentration of RBC 2,3-DPG is related to the level of thyroid stimulating hormone (TSH), thyroxine, serum phosphorus, and estrogen (146). 2,3-DPG is a highly charged anion. An anion is a negatively charged ion, a cation is a positively charged ion. It is also a metabolic intermediate in the anaerobic glycolytic pathway of the RBC.

Increase in 2,3-DPG. In women, estrogen and androgen levels increase during pregnancy. The increase in estrogen and/or androgens stimulates 2,3-DPG production. *When 2,3-DPG increases, there is a decrease in Hb oxygen affinity which increases O_2 unloading and tissue O_2 delivery* (140).

Normally, fetal Hb has a higher O_2 affinity than adult Hb. But O_2 affinity will decrease and O_2 unloading will increase when fetal plasma pH levels decrease. Carbon dioxide retention, e.g., when the umbilical cord is compressed, will lower plasma pH. Plasma pH also decreases with metabolic acidosis and asphyxia. The fetus compensates for hypoxemia by releasing androgens, cortisol and aldosterone, from the adrenal medullae. This should increase 2,3-DPG production and increase Hb oxygen unloading.

To summarize, factors that increase 2,3-DPG synthesis and increase P_{50} (a decrease in hemoglobin oxygen affinity) and *increase O_2 delivery to tissues include* an increase in:

- estrogen
- cortisol
- aldosterone
- carbon dioxide and
- a decrease in plasma pH.

Factors that increase metabolic rate such as *hyperthyrodism* or *hyperthermia* also increase P_{50} (140). The increase in 2,3-DPG causes *a right shift* in the oxygen-hemoglobin dissociation curve.

Decrease in 2,3-DPG. High pH levels inhibit 2,3-DPG synthesis. Maternal hyperventilation decreases $PaCO_2$ and increases pH. *Lower levels of 2,3-DPG can increase Hb oxygen affinity (P_{50} decreases) and decrease O_2 delivery to tissues* (140). This creates *a left shift* in the oxygen-hemoglobin dissociation curve. When the oxyhemoglobin dissociation curve shifts to the right or left due to changes in CO_2 and pH, the shift is called the *Bohr effect* (82, 140, 154-155).

To summarize, these factors decrease 2,3-DPG levels or P_{50} which *decreases O_2 delivery:*

- a rise in plasma pH
- a fall in plasma PCO_2

Factors that decrease metabolic rate such as *hypothyroidism* or *hypothermia* decrease P_{50} which increases O_2 affinity and decreases tissue O_2 delivery (140).

Fetal weight depends on the 2,3-DPG/Hb ratio (156). *A low 2,3-DPG increases Hb oxygen affinity, reduces tissue O_2 delivery, which may decrease tissue growth.* Diabetic pregnancy has been associated with anemia and an increase in 2,3-DPG synthesis. However, diabetics also had a high pH and low $PaCO_2$. Since the rise in 2,3-DPG should decrease Hb oxygen affinity and the high pH and low $PaCO_2$ should increase Hb oxygen affinity, there was no significant change in oxygen affinity (140).

Fetal Temperature. An increase in fetal temperature decreases oxygen-hemoglobin bonds. A decrease in fetal temperature increases O_2 binding to Hb. For each degree centigrade, the human fetal P_{50} value changes 0.0255 mm Hg (157). Warm fetuses release more O_2 to their tissues than cold fetuses. Therefore, if an amnioinfusion procedure includes the intrauterine instillation of *room temperature* normal saline or Lactated Ringer's solution, umbilical cord compression may be relieved but O_2 delivery to fetal tissues may be hindered. Therefore, it would be best if a blood warmer or infusion warmer device is used for a continuous drip amnioinfusion. The procedure is discussed in greater detail in Chapter 5.

Fetal skin temperature is 0.53 to 2.13° F (0.2 to 0.8° C) warmer than maternal temperature. The fetus cannot sweat and must lose 85 percent of its excess heat through the placenta. The rest is dissipated into the amniotic fluid. Contractions generate heat. As labor progresses, maternal temperature rises an average of 0.13° C and the fetal skin temperature increases an average of 0.21° C. Thus, labor is conductive to increased Hb oxygen unloading and tissue O_2 delivery. Maternal temperature also increases after epidural anesthesia by 0.37° C versus a 0.12° C decrease in women who did not have an epidural. Maternal temperature elevations after an epidural are probably due to sympathetic nerve blockade which diminishes sweating. The average rise in the FHR in women who had an epidural was 7.5 bpm. The FHR dropped an average of 5 bpm in women who did not have an epidural (158).

Fetal hyperthermia may be detrimental. If the fetus is excessively warm, the FHR often rises above 160 bpm, a tachycardic rate. Tachycardia has been associated with hypoxemia and acidosis (158). Hypoxemia stimulates the autonomic nervous system and the heart, muscles, glands, and organs respond to compensate for the decrease in blood O_2 levels. Therefore, when the fetus is tachycardic, clinicians should rule out the possibility of fetal hypoxemia versus hyperthermia. In the case of chorioamnionitis, both may be present.

Uterine Blood Flow

Blood flow may limit diffusion of gases (159). Uterine blood flow is abbreviated Q_{ut}. When researchers measure uterine artery blood flow, they are actually measuring myoendometrial and placental vessel blood flow. They assume placental vessels are maximally dilated (160). In humans, *normal uteroplacental blood flow is near 600 ml/minute. During contractions, Q_{ut} may decrease to 200 ml/minute* (161). In sheep, Q_{ut} is 1200 to 1500 ml/minute (124, 162). This represents about 15 to 16 percent of the left ventricular output when the pregnant ewe is at rest (124, 163).

Q_{ut} depends upon blood viscosity, blood vessel diameter, and maternal cardiac output. Each of these factors depends on the following:
Blood Viscosity
- hematocrit
- plasma proteins
Blood Vessel Diameter
- uterine artery diameter
- uterine intramural vessel and spiral artery diameter
Cardiac Output
Heart rate
Stroke volume
- preload
- afterload
- cardiac contractility (164).
Blood viscosity, the HCT, and plasma proteins have been discussed. Blood vessel diameter is self-explanatory.

Cardiac Output

Cardiac output (C.O.) is the product of heart rate (HR) and stroke volume (SV). Stroke volume is determined by preload, afterload, and cardiac contractility.

$$C.O. = HR \times SV$$

The four factors that determine C.O. may also be conceptualized as:
- *Heart rate* is a *chronotropic* response
- *Preload* is ventricular *volume*
- *Afterload* is vascular *resistance* and
- *Contractility* is an *inotropic* response (6).

C.O. is measured in liters per minute (L/min). In nonpregnant women, C.O. is 4 to 7 L/min (164). During pregnancy, C.O. increases to 5.2 to 7.3 L/min (161, 165). The increase in C.O. is primarily due to an increase in stroke volume not heart rate. Approximately 10 percent of C.O. (600 ml/min) reaches the uterus (161).

Heart Rate
Chronotropic applies to the number of times an event occurs over a specified period of time. Heart rate is chronotropic because it is measured as the number of times the heart beats per minute. During pregnancy, the maternal heart rate (MHR) should be 70 to 90 bpm (165). When the MHR increases, C.O. increases. When the MHR decreases, C.O. decreases

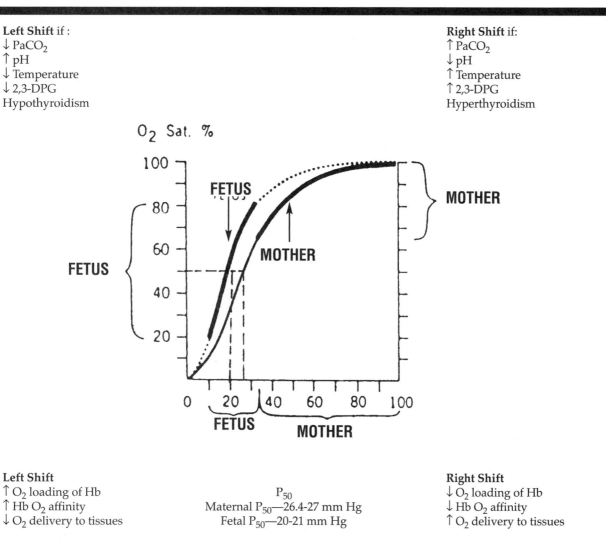

Left Shift if :
↓ $PaCO_2$
↑ pH
↓ Temperature
↓ 2,3-DPG
Hypothyroidism

Right Shift if:
↑ $PaCO_2$
↓ pH
↑ Temperature
↑ 2,3-DPG
Hyperthyroidism

Left Shift
↑ O_2 loading of Hb
↑ Hb O_2 affinity
↓ O_2 delivery to tissues

P_{50}
Maternal P_{50}—26.4-27 mm Hg
Fetal P_{50}—20-21 mm Hg

Right Shift
↓ O_2 loading of Hb
↓ Hb O_2 affinity
↑ O_2 delivery to tissues

Figure 4.4: Whole blood oxygen-hemoglobin dissociation curve. P_{50} denotes hemoglobin oxygen affinity. Maternal P_{50} is 26.4 to 27 mm Hg; fetal P_{50} is 20 to 21 mm Hg (111, 144). The P_{50} value shifts to the right or left depending on $PaCO_2$, pH, temperature, and red blood cell 2,3 diphosphoglycerate (2,3-DPG). A left shift decreases oxygen delivery to tissues as more is held by hemoglobin. A right shift decreases hemoglobin oxygen binding and more is available for tissue use (modified from Goodwin, Godwin, & Chance (Eds.). (1976). *Perinatal Medicine*. Reproduced with permission of Williams and Wilkins, Waverly, Inc., Baltimore, MD.).

(164). If the MHR increases to an abnormally high level, the duration of diastole decreases, which limits the amount of blood that enters the cardiac ventricles. For example, maternal supraventricular tachycardia, with a MHR greater than 150 bpm, may diminish C.O. due to inadequate time to completely fill the ventricles before systole.

Any drug that influences the sympathetic nervous system and increases the MHR has the potential for interfering with C.O. and uteroplacental blood flow (136). Tocolytics such as terbutaline (Brethine®) are ritodrine (Yutopar®) are β-sympathomimetics. If the MHR exceeds 120 bpm, there will be incomplete ventricular filling time which may decrease C.O. (6, 104, 166). Therefore, these drugs are discontinued when the MHR reaches 130 bpm (166).

MHR and the FHR may increase during inspiration or inspiratory movements, maternal exercise, maternal or fetal hyperthermia, hypoxia, or maternal hypotension. MHR and FHR may decrease during expiration or expiratory movements, maternal hypertension, or increased intracranial pressure. MHR also decreases because of athletic conditioning (164).

Stroke Volume: Preload, Afterload, and Cardiac Contractility
Preload (volume and force)
Preload is the force that stretches cardiac muscle fibers or myofibrils during diastole and is determined by venous return to the heart (164). *Preload is the major determinant of C.O.* (6).

The Frank Starling Law of the Heart. Cardiac myofibrils are like rubber bands: the more preload stretches them, the harder they spring back and increase contraction force and C.O. (164). The Frank Starling Law states that the heart will pump out all the blood that flows into it without significant buildup of back pressure within the right atrium (6, 45). To pump all the blood out, C.O. can increase by increasing the heart rate or myocardial contractility. Sometimes the heart cannot pump out all the blood that enters it because it is diseased, e.g., there is congestive heart failure, or it is overfilled, e.g., preload was excessive due to hypervolemia. Cardiac strength and contractility may be limited by a drug which blocks the contraction of cardiac muscle fibers.

For example, preeclamptic women are given magnesium sulfate ($MgSO_4$) to prevent seizures and women in preterm labor are given $MgSO_4$ as a tocolytic. $MgSO_4$ is also a T and L calcium channel blocker which prevents calcium from entering cells. Intracellular calcium is needed for myofibril contraction. $MgSO_4$ binds with calcium receptors and activates adenylate cyclase which converts ATP to cyclic adenosine monophosphate (cAMP). The increase in cAMP reduces intracellular calcium and decreases muscle contractions (167-171). If there is an overdose of $MgSO_4$ and maternal blood levels reach 15 mEq/L, cardiac impulse conduction decreases. Cardiac arrest may occur at concentrations in excess of 25 mEq/L because calcium is totally blocked from entering heart cells and is depleted within heart cells (172).

The measurement of preload. To measure *right ventricular preload*, a central venous catheter is inserted. The central venous pressure (*CVP*) reflects right preload. CVP ranges from 1 to 7 mm Hg during pregnancy (173). *Left ventricular preload, affected by venous return from the lungs to the left atrium,* is determined when a pulmonary artery catheter or Swan Ganz® catheter is in place to measure pulmonary capillary wedge pressure (*PCWP*). PCWP ranges from 6 to 10 mm Hg during pregnancy (165).

Low preload. To maintain cardiac output, preload must be normal. A low preload may be due to dehydration. Maternal preload may also be reduced with mechanical compression of the inferior vena cava (from maternal supine positioning and the weight of uterine contents on the vena cava), hypovolemia due to blood loss, a tachyarrhythmia, third spacing of fluids which creates maternal edema, restrictive cardiomyopathy, cardiac tamponade, and constrictive pericarditis (164). *A reduction in preload reduces C.O. and blood flow to the uterus which reduces O_2 delivery to the uterus, placenta, and fetus.* The reduction of blood flow to the uterus could cause uterine hypoxia, which may stimulate prostaglandin production and uterine activity.

CVP (right preload) = 1-7 mm Hg

PCWP (left preload) = 6-10 mm Hg

High preload. A high preload may be caused by hypervolemia which overstretches the cardiac muscle and may weaken it, reducing C.O. Preload may also be elevated as a result of iatrogenic fluid overload, bradyarrhythmias, or congestive cardiomyopathy or congestive heart failure. The latter condition is associated with a weak myocardium, decreased cardiac contractility and decreased C.O. (164). *The elevation in preload reduces C.O. and blood flow to the uterus which reduces O_2 delivery to the uterus, placenta, and fetus.*

Afterload (resistance and pressure)

Afterload is the pressure the ventricles must overcome to open up the pulmonic valve (between the right ventricle and the pulmonary artery) and the aortic valve (between the left ventricle and the aorta) to pump blood out of the heart. The heart ventricles exert pressure against resistance posed by the valves, the pulmonary artery, and the aorta. Opening the pulmonic and aortic valves is like opening a door (pressure) against a strong wind (resistance). Afterload is calculated as:

Afterload = Pressure / Resistance

Afterload affects C.O. and blood circulation. Afterload increases when the pressure the heart exerts to pump blood increases. If arterial resistance decreases, the pressure needed to eject blood decreases and afterload decreases.

Right afterload. Right afterload is the pressure the right ventricle must exert to pump blood out against resistance from the pulmonic valve and pulmonary artery. Right afterload is affected by pulmonary vascular resistance (**PVR**) and is measured with a pulmonary arterial line in place. The pulmonary arterial line can also be used to measure pulmonary artery blood pressure (**PAP**), PCWP, CVP, and C.O. (164). Systolic PAP should be 18 to 30 mm Hg, the diastolic PAP should be 6 to 10 mm Hg, and the mean PAP should be 11 to 15 mm Hg. Mean PAP is calculated as the systolic PAP + 2 times the diastolic PAP divided by 3. PVR during pregnancy is 56 to 100 dyne x sec x cm^{-5} (165).

Systolic	PAP	=	18-30 mm Hg
Diastolic	PAP	=	6-10 mm Hg
Mean	PAP	=	11-15 mm Hg
			(Systolic + (2 x Diastolic)/3
	PVR	=	56-100 dyne x sec x cm^{-5}

Increased right afterload. Pulmonary hypertension increases PVR and right afterload (164). Pulmonary hypertension may be due to a vascular abnormality or result from a congenital left-to-right intracardiac shunt (Eisenmenger's syndrome). Women with pulmonary hypertension have pathologic changes in the walls of small pulmonary arteries and arterioles with narrowing and even obliteration of the lumen of these vessels. Their right ventricle hypertrophies and they have an increased PVR and PAP. When pregnant women have pulmonary hypertension, approximately 50 percent of the women and 50 percent of the fetuses die (174). Right afterload also increases when women experience hypoxia, a pulmonary embolism, or there is pulmonic valve disease or polycythemia.

Left afterload. Left afterload is the pressure the left ventricle must exert to pump blood out against resistance from the aortic valve and aorta. Left afterload is affected by arterial diameter and systemic vascular resistance (SVR). *SVR is indirectly assessed by measuring diastolic blood pressure* (164). When cardiac output (C.O.) and mean arterial blood pressure (MAP) are known, SVR may be calculated. Maternal SVR is 944 to 1476 dyne x sec x cm^{-5} (165).

BP depends on the amount of blood pumped out of the heart (C.O.) and arterial resistance to blood flow (SVR) (6). BP is calculated as:

$$C.O. = SV \times HR$$

$$SVR = \left(\frac{MAP\text{-}CVP}{C.O.}\right) \times 80$$

Decreased left afterload. Left afterload and arterial blood pressure decrease when SVR decreases. An abnormal drop in SVR creates hypotension which reduces uteroplacental blood flow and O_2 delivery to the uterus, placenta, and fetus (75, 173). Antihypertensive drugs, such as nifedipine (Procardia®), have been used to stop premature labor. Hypotension is an adverse reaction. Left afterload may decrease when blood vessels abnormally dilate during anaphylaxis, septic shock, or neurogenic shock (164).

Increased left afterload. Vasoconstriction increases SVR, BP, and left afterload (164). The increase in left afterload is associated with a reduction in uteroplacental blood flow and O_2 delivery to the uterus, placenta, and fetus. Left afterload is increased in hypertensive women, and women who are polycythemic, hypothermic, or who have aortic valve disease.

Afterload is related to preload. A *low diastolic BP* may be caused by vasodilation which lowers resistance and *decreases SVR.* A reduction in SVR requires less pressure to eject blood from the heart (decreased pressure/decreased resistance). The decreased pressure and decreased resistance *decreases left afterload.*

A *high diastolic BP*, e.g., 90 mm Hg or higher, is often caused by vasoconstriction which *increases SVR. If the heart cannot increase ejection pressure, left afterload decreases (same pressure/increased resistance).* The decrease in left afterload decreases C.O., uteroplacental blood flow, and O_2 delivery. The reduction in blood leaving the heart decreases venous return to the heart which reduces preload. The reduction in preload perpetuates the reduction in C.O. and the reduction of O_2 delivered to the uterus, placenta, and fetus.

Cardiac Contractility

Cardiac contractility reflects the electrical-mechanical relationship between excitation of the heart's conductive nodes and fibers and contraction of cardiac myofibrils. The heart is two separate pumps: the right ventricle pumps blood to the lungs, the left ventricle pumps blood to the aorta (6).

If any atrial muscle fiber is stimulated by an electrical impulse, the entire atrium contracts. The contraction of myofibrils depends on intracellular calcium. Norepinephrine increases myofibril cell *permeability* to calcium. If extracellular calcium increases, cardiac contractility should increase (6).

Norepinephrine, from sympathetic nerve terminals or the adrenal medullae, binds with β_1-adrenergic receptors on the outer surface of the cardiac cell which activates the intracellular enzyme adenylate cyclase. Adenylate cyclase converts ATP to cAMP which "pushes" calcium out of the cell. The increased permeability of the cell allows calcium to reenter which increases myocardial contraction strength (6, 164).

Increase in cardiac contractility. Cardiac contractility increases in women who are hyperthyroid or who experience a sympathoadrenal stimulus. For example, amphetamines administered to pregnant ewes stimulated catecholamine release, an increase in glucose production, and a decrease in glucose utilization. Since *amphetamines* cross the placenta, the fetal lamb also had a sympathoadrenal response. Maternal and fetal plasma glucose and lactic acid levels increased. If the lamb was hypoxemic, hyperglycemia developed. Insulin levels initially dropped then increased. Amphetamine use was associated with an increase in LBW and preterm birth (175).

Decrease in cardiac contractility. Contractility decreases if β-blockers or antiarrhythmic drugs with β-blocking properties are used, or there is an electrolyte imbalance, congestive heart failure, a myocardial infarction, or abnormal acid-base balance, such as hypoxia, hypercarbia, or acidosis (164).

Cardiac Output and Uteroplacental Oxygen Delivery

Maternal cardiac output (C.O.) is the most important determinant of O_2 delivery to the uterus, placenta, and fetus (1, 176). Oxygen availability (O_2av) or delivery (DO_2) depends on C.O. and the total quantity of O_2 in maternal arteries ($SaO_2 + PaO_2 = CaO_2$).

O_2av or DO_2 (ml/min) = CaO_2 x C.O. x 10
(Oxygen availability or oxygen delivery)

Arterial O_2 reaches the uterus and placenta floating freely in the plasma (PaO_2) or bound to Hb (SaO_2). Oxygen delivery increases or decreases when maternal F^iO_2, PaO_2, or the Hb concentration change. For example, hyperoxygenation by application of a tight fitting face mask at an O_2 flow rate of 8 to 10 L/minute increases F^iO_2 which increases maternal PaO_2. Blood loss, as a result of hemorrhage, decreases Hb levels and limits the quantity of O_2 that can be delivered to the uterus, placenta, and fetus.

Maternal Tissue Oxygen Consumption

Cardiac output and total arterial oxygen content is related to O_2 consumption. Oxygen consumption is measured as the ml of O_2 consumed by tissues each minute. To determine maternal tissue oxygen consumption (VO_2), the following must be known:

- total artery O_2 content (CaO_2)
- total vein O_2 content (CvO_2)
- the arteriovenous O_2 difference ($avDO_2 = CaO_2 - CvO_2$) and
- cardiac output (C.O.)

Total artery or vein O_2 content is calculated by determining the quantity of Hb, the percent of Hb saturated with oxygen (SO_2), and the partial pressure of oxygen in the plasma (PO_2). A gram of Hb holds 1.34 ml of O_2, and there is 0.0031 ml of O_2 for every mm Hg of O_2 pressure.

$$CaO_2 \text{ (ml/dl)} = (1.34 \times Hb \times SaO_2) + (0.0031 \times PaO_2)$$
Total arterial oxygen content
$$CvO_2 \text{ (ml/dl)} = (1.34 \times Hb \times SvO_2) + (0.0031 \times PvO_2)$$
Total venous oxygen content
$$avDO_2 \text{ (ml/min)} = CaO_2 - CvO_2$$
Arteriovenous oxygen difference
$$VO_2 \text{ (ml/min/kg)} = avDO_2 \times C.O. \times 10/kg$$
Tissue oxygen consumption

In the adult, O_2 consumption is approximately 3.5 to 5 ml/min/kg (130). A significant reduction in C.O. and/or arterial O_2 content (CaO_2) decreases O_2 delivery and may reduce O_2 consumption if CaO_2 is below a "critical level" to meet tissue oxidative metabolic needs.

Maternal Oxygen Extraction

If O_2 consumption increases, but delivery remains the same, the O_2 extraction ratio ($O_2ER\%$) increases. Oxygen extraction is measured in ml/dl.

Oxygen Extraction = $O_2ER\%$(ml/dl) = Oxygen Consumption/Oxygen Delivery
$$O_2ER\% = VO_2/DO_2$$
$$O_2ER\% = avDO_2 \times C.O. \times 10/CaO_2 \times C.O. \times 10$$
$$O_2ER\% = avDO_2/CaO_2$$
$$O_2ER\% = CaO_2 - CvO_2/CaO_2$$

Based on these calculations, O_2 delivery can be measured by measuring the total arterial O_2 content and O_2 consumption can be measured as the arteriovenous O_2 difference. Total arterial O_2 content can be increased by supplemental inhalation of oxygen (hyperoxygenation).

Maternal brain oxygen delivery and consumption. Cardiac output delivers more than 4 liters of O_2 per minute per meter^2 (L/min/m^2) to the maternal body. Normally, the brain receives more than 600 ml/min/m^2 of O_2 and only consumes about 140 ml/min/m^2. Thus, the brain uses about 23 percent of the O_2 delivered to it (142). The rest could be considered "O_2 reserve."

A decrease in cerebral oxygenation activates the sympathoadrenal medullary system and β_2-receptors in cerebral blood vessels which causes vasodilation and increases cerebral blood flow up to 600 percent. The increase in blood flow increases O_2 delivery to maintain cerebral O_2 consumption (142).

Cerebral O_2 delivery in critically ill patients was measured by determining ophthalmic artery blood flow using Doppler ultrasound technology. Cerebral O_2 delivery (DO_2) was "critically low" at a level less than 600 ml/min/m^2 (142).

Uteroplacental oxygen delivery and consumption. The amount of O_2 consumed by the uterus and placenta affects fetal O_2 availability or delivery. Uteroplacental O_2 consumption is measured in ml/minute. The amount of O_2 consumed by the uterus and placenta (VO_{2ut}) depends on maternal C.O. which determines uterine blood flow (Q_{ut}). O_2 consumption also depends on the uterine arteriovenous difference (75). To determine uteroplacental O_2 consumption, the following must be known:

- total uterine artery O_2 content ($CaO_2 = SaO_2 + PaO_2$)
- total uterine vein O_2 content ($CvO_2 = SvO_2 + PvO_2$)
- the arteriovenous O_2 difference ($avDO_2 = CaO_2 - CvO_2$)
- uterine blood flow (Q_{ut})

Uteroplacental O_2 consumption is assumed to be constant and is determined based on the Fick Principle. The Fick Principle is an equation that includes blood flow and total arterial and venous O_2 content. O_2 consumption by uterine and placental tissues is calculated as:

$$VO_{2ut} \text{ (ml/dl)} = Q_{ut} \times (CaO_2 - CvO_2)$$
Uteroplacental Oxygen Consumption

Animal experiments provide an estimate of uteroplacental O_2 consumption because human CaO_2 and CvO_2 values have not been determined. For example, in pregnant sheep near term, the ewe's uteroplacental O_2 consumption was 6.5 to 10.3 ml/min/kilogram. Acute maternal hypoxia decreased fetal O_2 consumption to less than 50 percent of control values. The reduction in fetal O_2 consumption was proportional to maternal PaO_2 (79). Therefore, *an increase in maternal PaO_2 should increase fetal O_2 consumption.*

Uteroplacental oxygen availability or delivery

Cardiac output affects uteroplacental blood flow and O_2 delivery to the uterus, placenta, and fetus. If C.O. increases, O_2 delivery increases; if cardiac output decreases, O_2 delivery decreases (162, 176). *Uteroplacental sufficiency implies O_2 delivery was adequate to meet uterine, placental, and fetal oxidative metabolic needs.*

Uteroplacental Insufficiency (UPI). The uterus, placenta, and fetus require O_2 and nutrients to grow. If there is *uteroplacental insufficiency (UPI), blood flow to the uterus and placenta is inadequate to meet uterine, placental, and fetal O_2 and* *nutritive requirements* (177).

Uteroplacental insufficiency may be attributable to:
- low maternal FIO_2, SaO_2, and/or PaO_2
- elevated $PaCO_2$
- anemia or hemoconcentration
- high Hb oxygen affinity
- decreased preload, afterload, or cardiac contractility resulting in
- reduced cardiac output.

UPI may be related to a cessation of maternal and/or fetal blood flow. If blood flow on either side of the placenta ceases, the concentrations of CO_2 and O_2 on the two sides of placental villi rapidly achieve a state of equilibrium and transfer of gases and nutrients ceases (41).

UPI may be chronic or acute. Chronic UPI results in a small uterus, placenta and baby (159). The fetus may be IUGR. The newborn will be small for gestational age (SGA). IUGR fetuses have a LBW. They are often asymmetrical, with a large head, heart, and adrenal glands but a small body (178).

Acute UPI may be due to uterine contractions, supine hypotension, regional anesthesia such as a spinal or epidural, or maternal hemorrhage. To indirectly determine uteroplacental blood flow and maternal oxygenation, clinicians may assess the respiratory rate, pulse, BP, mean arterial pressure (MAP), pain level, and SpO_2. They may also observe for signs of maternal hypotension such as light-headedness. Signs of hemorrhage may include abnormal vaginal bleeding, a decrease in BP, and an increase in pulse. The changes in BP and pulse may reflect hypovolemic shock. In addition, the clinician may listen to lung and heart sounds and determine capillary refill and uterine activity.

Labor is associated with a decrease in maternal pH (due to a lack of food intake and metabolism of fats for energy) and pain (137, 146). Labor pain steadily intensifies as labor progresses and is a response to ischemia of the uterus, pressure on nerves, and traction of uterine ligaments (179). Sometimes women in labor hyperventilate which decreases $PaCO_2$ and increases plasma pH. Since the effect of hyperventilation may offset the drop in pH due to a lack of food, SaO_2 may not change. However, pain alone has been associated with decreased Hb oxygen saturation. If concerns exist about maternal SaO_2, it can be indirectly measured as SpO_2 with a pulse oximeter.

Direct measurements of the maternal Hb and HCT and blood gases may shed light on the possible causes of uteroplacental insufficiency. Hemodynamic monitoring of the critically ill pregnant woman can identify problems with preload, afterload, and cardiac contractility.

PLACENTAL ANATOMY AND PHYSIOLOGY

The placenta is a fetal hemochorial, chorioallantoic organ. It usually attaches to the maternal decidua on the inside of the uterus. The placenta is a heat exchanger, a protective barrier against infection, and an endocrine and respiratory organ (161). Heat is released when O_2 binds with fetal Hb. The placenta absorbs heat when maternal O_2 dissociates from Hb (180).

The placenta produces human chorionic gonadotropin (hCG), human placental lactogen, estrogen, estriol, estradiol, and progesterone (161). Estriol (E_3) is an estrogen and steroid which is synthesized by the placenta from fetal precursors. It is considered a marker of fetal and placental well-being and has been found in maternal and fetal serum (110, 181). Estradiol (E_2) is also an estrogen created by the placenta from maternal and fetal sources (181).

The placenta achieves its definitive form 8 to 10 weeks after conception and is fully formed by the end of the fourth month or early in the fifth month of gestation (161, 182). On one side of the placenta is the maternal decidua and spiral arteries. The spiral arteries perfuse the fetal basal or basement membrane and chorionic villi. Since maternal blood bathes fetal villi, the placenta is called a hemochorial organ.

On the fetal side of the placenta are fetal arterioles, venules, and capillaries (1, 182). Some fetal vessels are located in the allantois, a vascular fetal membrane located between the chorion and the amnion. Therefore, the hemochorial placenta is also called a chorioallantoic organ (112, 182).

Given enough time, virtually all circulating materials should be transported from maternal circulation through the placenta to fetal circulation (112). The placenta removes fetal metabolic byproducts, such as lactate and CO_2, and produces lactate and glucose for fetal consumption (85). Since the fetal lungs are inactive in utero, the placenta serves as the fetal respiratory organ. Some feel the placenta is an ineffective gas exchanger (124, 183).

Placental transport of gases and nutrients depends on placental surface area, the rate of blood flow on the maternal and fetal sides of the placenta, the diffusion distance gases must travel, vascular volume in maternal and fetal capillary beds, and the affinity of Hb for O_2 (1, 184).

Placental Villi

The chorion is the outer membrane of the trophoblast. About two weeks after conception it develops tiny projections called villi or microvilli. Fluid, gases, and nutrients pass through villi (82). Villi extend from the chorionic plate and are suspended in maternal blood. Placental villi have three layers: a basement membrane, a syncytiotrophoblast, and the cytotrophoblast. Placental villi also contain several other types of cells, including
- fibroblasts
- macrophages
- endothelial cells and
- trapped RBCs.

Fibroblasts are connective tissue cells. Macrophages are white blood cells. Endothelial cells are blood vessel wall cells, and RBCs are red blood cells.

A thin basal or basement membrane separates maternal veins and spiral arteries from the villous syncytiotrophoblast and cytotrophoblast. The basal membrane is a noncellular tissue layer (185).

The syncytiotrophoblast forms the outer surface of the

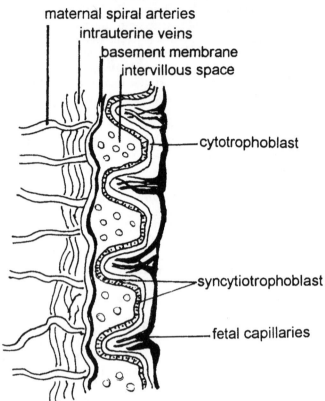

maternal spiral arteries
intrauterine veins
basement membrane
intervillous space

cytotrophoblast

syncytiotrophoblast

fetal capillaries

Figure 4.5: Illustration of maternal spiral arteries and intrauterine veins, the basal or basement membrane, and the syncytiotrophoblast and cytotrophoblast of placental villi. Maternal blood enters the basement membrane driven by spiral artery head pressure. Spiral arteries run perpendicular to the membrane. Maternal veins run parallel to the basement membrane.

villus which is in contact with maternal blood in intervillous spaces. The cytotrophoblast lies under the syncytiotrophoblast near the fibrous core of the villus. Syncytiotrophoblasts are metabolically active cells with a high O_2 consumption rate. These cells are nonreproductive and send out syncytial knots that eventually decrease in number as gestation advances. The presence of syncytial knots suggests placental immaturity (152, 186).

Together, the syncytiotrophoblast and cytotrophoblast are called the epithelial plate, the exchange membrane, the vasculosyncytial membrane, the villous chorionic membrane, the placental villous membrane, or the chorionic exchange membrane (177, 186). *Villous exchange surface area decreases when there is a placental infarction or placental separation from the uterine wall (abruption) or placenta previa* (where part of the placenta lies over the cervical os) (186).

Villi permeability and thickness and the number of capillaries in the villi affect O_2 transfer to the fetus (143). Villi that contain fetal capillaries are called tertiary villi. Capillaries proliferate during hypoxia. If villi and their capillaries break, fibrin clots form (186).

Placental Transport Mechanisms

The placenta has five transport mechanisms:
- *passive diffusion* of O_2, CO_2, fatty acids, steroids, nucleosides, electrolytes, fat soluble vitamins, water, and some medications,
- *facilitated diffusion* of D-glucose and other sugars,
- *active transport* of amino acids, water soluble vitamins, calcium, iron, and iodine,
- *pinocytosis* of maternal plasma microdroplets, serum proteins, and antibodies, and
- *bulk flow* across the chorionic and amniotic membranes of water, O_2, glucose, urea, sodium, chloride, potassium, and magnesium (101, 137, 184, 187-189).

Placental transfer depends on:
- molecular weight of the substance being transferred
- lipid solubility
- ionization
- protein binding
- placental surface area
- uteroplacental blood flow
- placental receptor sites and
- molecule consumption and degradation (189).

Passive Diffusion

During passive diffusion molecules, which weigh less than a molecular weight of 5000, pass through the chorionic exchange membrane alone or attached to proteins, such as albumin, amino acids, or fats (110, 190). O_2 and CO_2 passively diffuse in inverse proportion to the distance separating maternal blood in the intervillous spaces from fetal blood in the villous capillaries (110). O_2, CO_2, and nitrous oxide *peak in the fetus two to three minutes after maternal gas inhalation* (191).

Potassium, sodium, iron, and magnesium are transferred against a "chemical" gradient. Sodium attaches to proteins, amino acids, or fats. Proteins have a higher molecular weight than amino acids, therefore, anything bound to protein will take longer to transfer to fetal circulation than molecules bound to amino acids (110). Narcotics and free fatty acids (FFA) bind with protein in the blood.

FFA bound to albumin travels through placental vessels as lipoproteins, triglyceride, and cholesterol. In laboratory experiments with human placentas, an increase in "maternal" plasma albumin decreased the transfer of fats to the fetal side of the placenta (112). Therefore, an abnormally high maternal albumin level may impede FFA transfer.

The chorionic exchange membrane is lipophilic. FFA are lipids. They combine with protein molecules and form lipoproteins or phospholipids. The fetus synthesizes phospholipids from FFA. The placenta consumes a portion of maternal lipids and cholesterol and degrades phospholipids (112). Lipid-soluble compounds, such as narcotics or antibiotics, diffuse rapidly across the lipophilic exchange membrane, but not as fast as gases. For example, ampicillin peaks in the fetus 30 to 60 minutes after administration (191).

Cocaine transfer. During pregnancy, serum protein binding to cocaine decreases, increasing placental transfer of cocaine to the fetus. Cocaine is partially hydrolyzed by placenta cells where cholinesterase converts cocaine to benzoylecgonine. Cocaine also passively diffuses to the fetus and binds with fetal serum α_1-acid glycoprotein and albumin (192).

Facilitated Diffusion
Glucose is transported by facilitated diffusion, which is a strong carrier system that transports *faster* than passive diffusion (184). Actions to improve O_2 delivery to the fetus may include a maternal IV bolus and hyperoxygenation. Theoretically, if a glucose solution is infused during labor, rather than the recommended nonglucose-containing solution, some RBCs might bind with glucose instead of O_2 which would reduce tissue O_2 delivery.

Active Transport
Active transport of amino acids is sodium dependent and requires energy derived from ATP. Molecules are transferred based on an electrochemical concentration gradient (189, 193-194). Through a process of oxidative phosphorylation, villi produce ATP (194). In addition to ATP, O_2 is needed for active transport. Uteroplacental insufficiency is not only related to a decrease in O_2 delivery, it is also related to a decrease in amino acid transport and diminished fetal growth (112).

Pinocytosis
Microvilli on the syncytial surface of the villi engulf maternal plasma droplets and antibodies and bring them over to the fetal side of the placenta. Pinocytosis may be diminished in preeclamptics who have focal syncytial necrosis (185).

Bulk Flow
Bulk flow of water, ions, and low molecular weight solutes, such as urea, rapidly move across the chorion and amnion and allantoic fetal vessels based on a "chemical potential gradient." About 10 ml of water passes through this intramembranous pathway each day.

Amniotic fluid is mainly composed of a little water from maternal circulation, fetal lung fluid, and fetal urine. At term, it has been estimated that there is an average of 4 liters of water in the uterus: 2800 ml in the fetus, 400 ml in the placenta, and 800 in amniotic fluid (188, 191). Since 1 ml of water weighs 0.95 gm, water contributes the majority of weight to the fetus and placenta.

Human Immunodeficiency Virus: Maternal/Fetal Transmission
The human immunodeficiency virus-1 P24 (HIV-1 P24) antigen appears to enter the fetal circulation based on the quantity of the antigen in maternal circulation. Placentas differ in their permeability to the HIV-1 P24 antigen. Fortunately, the presence of the HIV-1 P24 antigen in neonatal blood is not synonymous with HIV infection (190).

Deficient Placental Transfer
The cause of deficient placental O_2 and nutrient transfer to the fetus is usually multifactorial and may be due to genetics, infection, ischemia, or anomalies. Anomalies may include a short cord or a long cord, velamentous insertion of the umbilical cord, a two vessel cord, chorioangiosis or a chorioangioma (185).

The normal umbilical cord measures between 32 to 100 cm (12.8 to 40 inches). If there is a velamentous insertion of the umbilical cord, the cord is inserted into the chorion and amnion rather than the placental disc. A velamentous insertion of cord vessels means vessels branch in the membranes before they reach the placenta (195). If a vessel is present in the membranes over the cervical os, vasa previa exists. If membranes are ruptured, a fetal vein or artery could rupture and the fetus would exsanguinate and die.

A two vessel cord occurs in about 1 percent of single births and 7 to 14 percent of multiple births (195). The absence of one umbilical artery has been associated with congenital anomalies such as Potter's syndrome or Pierre Rubin syndrome. These syndromes are associated with renal anomalies such as renal agenesis (Potter's syndrome) and micrognathia, which is underdevelopment of the jaw evidenced by a small chin.

Chorioangiosis is a condition where the basement membrane thickens (185). Chorioangioma is a vascular tumor with anastomoses between maternal and fetal vessels. When a chorioangioma is present, a fetomaternal transfusion of blood can occur which results in fetal anemia.

Placental Oxygen Consumption and Transfer
Placental cells need glucose and O_2 for oxidative (aerobic) metabolism. Oxidative metabolism generates ATP. ATP is needed for:
- placental transport of carbohydrates, glucose, lactate, and amino acids which supply carbon and nitrogen for fetal growth
- synthesis reactions to create proteins, peptides, and steroid hormones and
- skeletal muscle work (152).

When carbohydrates, glucose, lactate, and amino acids, such as lysine, are broken down, their byproducts include CO_2 and urea that pass through the placenta to maternal circulation as "waste." Maternal O_2 delivered to the placenta is partially consumed by the placenta and partially transferred to the fetal umbilical vein. In fetal lambs, *the placenta retains 30 to 75 percent of glucose it receives and consumes 50 percent of O_2 it receives in order to meet its own oxidative metabolic needs* (137, 152, 189, 196-197). Unlike glucose, maternal insulin crosses the placenta in trace amounts (189). In sheep, *the placenta consumes 400 percent more O_2 then the fetus per unit weight* (198). Term placenta *villi* consume O_2 at a rate of 1 ml/min/kg (199). The placenta delivers 50 percent of the O_2 it receives to the fetus.

Placenta life depends upon uteroplacental blood flow. Maternal O_2, not fetal O_2, is the primary O_2 source for living placenta trophoblastic cells (194). Maternal C.O. is related to placental

O_2 uptake. An increase in maternal blood flow to the placenta increases placental O_2 consumption. A decrease in fetal umbilical arterial flow to the placenta decreases placental O_2 consumption. The decrease in O_2 consumption is probably depressed as there is less need to remove fetal metabolic end products (196). *If placental O_2 delivery decreases, villi will become ischemic and increase anaerobic glucose consumption and lactic acid production.*

O_2 and CO_2 diffusion. Placental villi are the primary gas exchange site for O_2 and CO_2 diffusion (197). When there is a decrease in uteroplacental flow there will be a decrease in O_2 available for transfer which will be reflected in a decrease in umbilical vein $S_{uv}O_2$ and $P_{uv}O_2$ and an increase in $P_{uv}CO_2$ (124).

The placental villous membrane diffusing capacity is directly proportional to

* placental area
* the uneven placental perfusion pattern
* PO_2 differences between the umbilical vein and maternal venous blood
* PCO_2 differences between the umbilical artery and maternal venous blood (163).

Placental area. The size of the placenta and the number of blood vessels in the placenta and in the villi affect O_2 transfer to fetal circulation (143). Infarction, abruption, and placenta previa decrease the area for gas transfer.

At term, the placenta weighs 400 to 600 grams. It is round or oval and approximately 16 to 20 centimeters in diameter and 1.5 to 3 centimeter thick. Placental cotyledons are composed of blood vessels and millions of villi.

Fetal capillaries branch and penetrate each placental cotyledon forming a well-developed capillary bed (182). Each cotyledon has its own independent circulation. Therefore, if the placenta partially or marginally abrupts, there may still be enough intact fetal capillaries to transport adequate O_2 to the fetus. It is believed the placenta of a well-oxygenated fetus can lose 50 percent of its surface area, e.g., a 50 percent abruption, before the "critical level" is reached where fetal O_2 consumption decreases and the fetus decompensates (129).

O_2, CO_2 and Placental Vasoconstriction

Fetal placental vessels are normally dilated and have very low vascular resistance. Their diameter is at least 10 times greater than the diameter of maternal spiral arteries (126). Fetal placental blood vessel diameter may be affected by the level of O_2, CO_2, lactate, or parathyroid hormone. Fetal placental blood vessel diameter also appears to be affected by cooling, serotonin, histamine, endothelin, endoperoxides (prostaglandins G_2 and H_2), EDRF (nitric oxide), and prostaglandins I_2 and E_2. Endothelin (Et-1) is a potent vasoconstrictor (200). All fetuses produce Et-1 and Et-2, but the level of Et-1 and Et-2 was higher in the sera of IUGR fetuses (201). Fetal placental vasoconstriction due to increased endothelin levels partially explains the lack of fetal nutrient and O_2 delivery and LBW. Cooling, serotonin,

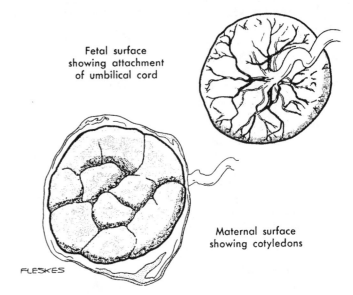

Figure 4.6: Maternal and fetal surfaces of the placenta. The cotyledons are visible on the maternal surface, which is implanted into the decidua and the uterine wall. After the birth of the neonate, if the placenta cotyledons (the maternal side) appear it is called the Duncan maneuver ("dirty Duncan"). The fetal surface glistens because it is covered by chorion and amnion. If this side of the placenta delivers, it is called the Shultz ("shiny Shultz") maneuver. Branches of the umbilical vessels can be seen under the amnion on the fetal surface of the placenta (modified from Netter: In E. Oppenheim (Ed.). (1965). Ciba collection of medical illustrations, vol. 2, Reproductive system. Reprinted with permission from The C. V. Mosby Company from Korones, S. B. (1981). *High-risk newborn infants. The basis for intensive nursing care.* 3rd ed.).

histamine, Et-1, Et-2, and prostaglandins G_2 and H_2 may cause vessels to spasm or constrict. EDRF and PGI_2 and E_2 cause vessels to dilate.

In laboratory experiments, human cotyledon vessels became constricted but never totally occluded when they were perfused with a solution containing a high concentration of O_2 or low level of CO_2 (182). At a PO_2 of 100 mm Hg, the umbilical artery, mainstem villous arteries, and small placental arteries contracted. Researchers thought high O_2 levels may decrease vascular sensitivity to natural vasodilators such as EDRF or prostacyclin (PGI_2), and increased sensitivity to vasoconstrictors such as PGG_2 and PGH_2 (endoperoxides), or thromboxane (TXA_2), which is a product of platelet cell wall arachidonic acid (202). These *in vitro* research findings created concern about the administration of supplemental O_2 to pregnant women. However, *none of these findings has ever been confirmed in vivo.* Chapter 5 addresses issues related to maternal hyperoxygenation.

An intravenous bolus of crystalloid increases maternal intravascular volume, preload, cardiac output and blood pressure and decreases placental vascular resistance at the site of placental implantation in sheep. When pregnant ewe's were given an intravenous bolus of 2000 to 2500 ml of normal saline (a quantity much greater than would be appropriate for women), uteroplacental blood flow increased 23 percent and placental O_2 delivery also increased. Placental implantation site blood flow increased 40 percent. Researchers speculated that placental vessel vasodilation was related to ANP and 17-estradiol. Estradiol may increase 2,3-DPG production and increase Hb unloading of O_2, increasing tissue O_2 delivery. Theoretically, the increase in cell O_2 would prevent a sympathomedullary response to hypoxia which would prevent vasoconstriction. As a result of the bolus, they also noted a decrease in the ewe's blood pH and Hb concentration (in 75 percent of the sheep), no change in PaO_2 or $PaCO_2$, an increase in mean arterial pressure, a 23 percent increase in renal blood flow (probably related to ANP), a 43 percent increase in skeletal blood flow, and a 60 percent increase in blood flow to the skin (198). *Perhaps any vasoconstrictive effect O_2 may exert on blood vessels is negated by an intravenous bolus of crystalloid.*

Lactate. Lactate causes fetal placental vasodilation (108). The placenta maintains fetal homeostasis by removing CO_2 and lactate from fetal blood and diffusing them into maternal blood. Lactate is transferred to maternal circulation by facilitated transport. A proton attaches to the lactate molecule and the gradient between maternal lactate and placental lactate determines the quantity of lactate that is transferred. Approximately 2/3rds of the lactate is transported to the maternal side of the placenta and 1/3rd is consumed by the placenta. Lactate consumption was inhibited in the placentas of preeclamptics (108).

The placenta also consumes maternal and fetal catecholamines and produces alanine. Alanine, an amino acid, is a precursor of gluconeogenesis (61, 107-108, 203). Researchers believe alanine is related to lactate metabolism but more studies are needed to clarify the relationship between alanine and lactate.

Prostaglandin I_2. PGI_2 is prostacyclin, a potent vasodilator created from the arachidonic acid of endothelial cell membranes. PGI_2 also decreases platelet adhesiveness. PGI_2 levels are lower than normal in the placentas of smokers, preeclamptic women, and women who have IUGR fetuses (200). Because of the decrease in PGI_2, uterine and placental vessels are vasoconstricted, which reduces nutrient and O_2 delivery to the fetus which explains the increased risk of LBW in the fetuses of preeclamptic women.

EDRF. Bradykinin, a small polypeptide from α_2-globulins in the plasma or tissue fluids, induces production of *endothelium-derived relaxing factor* (EDRF) or nitric oxide, a potent vasodilator. Bradykinin also increases capillary permeability. EDRF is produced by the amnion and chorion and has been found in umbilical cord vessels. EDRF levels were lower than normal in umbilical arteries of fetuses born to preeclamptic women (6, 200). Preeclamptics are vasoconstricted.

Parathyroid hormone-related protein receptors have been found in placental chorionic vessels and umbilical cord

vessels at the same site as **endothelin** (Et-1). Et-1 is a potent vasoconstrictor. Parathyroid hormone-related protein receptors have also been found in amnion epithelial cells. The level of this protein may affect placental and cord vessel diameter, however the relationship between these receptors and Et-1 has yet to be elucidated (200).

The Uneven Placental Perfusion Pattern:
The Concurrent Flow/Venous Equilibrium Exchange Model

The placenta is complex. It has a poorly defined vascular arrangement and vascular diffusion and perfusion shunts (137, 197). The placenta functions as an O_2 donor and CO_2 recipient. *The delivery of O_2 via the placenta, rather than the condition that might adversely affect the rate of delivery, is a primary predictor of fetal oxygenation (75).*

Placental transport of O_2 and nutrients is dependent upon both the maternal and fetal circulation of blood or perfusion, maternal and fetal Hb types, maternal and fetal shunting away from the placenta, and placental O_2 consumption (75, 204). Due to perfusion shunts, as much as 15 percent of uterine blood and 5 percent of fetal blood bypasses the placental gas exchange region (197). Perfusion shunts in placental blood vessels prevent exact equilibration of maternal and fetal O_2 and CO_2. Uneven placental perfusion contributes to the low O_2 diffusing capacity of the villous membrane which can be partially compensated for by increasing uteroplacental blood flow (163).

Maternal and fetal blood supply to the placenta is unevenly distributed. In late gestation, *uteroplacental blood flow* is divided as follows:

 3% to the uterus
 10% to the endometrium
 87% to placental cotyledons.

A greater portion of fetal blood perfuses the placenta than maternal blood. For example, in sheep, 16 percent of maternal cardiac output was delivered to the uterus and placenta but 40 percent of fetal cardiac output reached the placenta (107, 163). *Fetal blood* that perfuses the placenta is distributed as follows:

 93% to placental cotyledons
 7% to the intercotyledonary chorion (163).

Maternal cardiac output is the most important determinant of O_2 delivery to the placenta. But, O_2 delivery to the fetus by the placenta is primarily determined by O_2 content in umbilical arteries and the PO_2 diffusion gradient (1). If fetal $P_{ua}O_2$ drops, O_2 transfer increases (gases move from an area of high pressure to an area of low pressure). It was found that fetal blood flow to the placenta could decrease to 1 ml/minute and O_2 transfer from the placenta continued, but placental O_2 consumption decreased at least 50 percent (196). Thus, the placenta sacrifices its own oxidative metabolic needs, fails to remove fetal and placental metabolic end products, but continues to supply O_2 to the fetus.

Concurrent flow system. In spite of uneven perfusion, researchers believe the human placenta functions as a *concurrent flow system.* A concurrent flow model assumes two blood streams flow parallel to one another (154, 197). In this model, maternal and fetal arterial blood and maternal and fetal venous blood travel in the same direction (see Figure 4.7). In a *countercurrent* model, maternal arterial blood and fetal venous blood flow in the same direction.

The fetus, like the placenta, is entirely dependent upon maternal circulation and oxygenation for its O_2 and nutritive needs (144). One would think maternal PaO_2, which is 90 to 95 mm Hg, would predict fetal umbilical vein $P_{uv}O_2$. However, this is not the case. Homeostasis assumes that gases are in equilibrium on either side of the villous chorionic exchange membrane. But maternal PaO_2, near 90 mm Hg (torr), is not even close to fetal umbilical vein $P_{uv}O_2$ of 22 to 38 torr or fetal capillary PaO_2 of 30 to 35 torr (101, 111, 154). *Maternal uterine PvO_2 is near 40 torr. Therefore, maternal PaO_2 does not predict fetal $P_{uv}O_2$ nor PaO_2.*

The differences in PO_2 levels are explained by placental O_2 consumption and the concurrent model of O_2 and CO_2 exchange. *In humans, a concurrent, venous equilibrium exchange model exists. Maternal PvO_2 determines O_2 diffusion into the fetal umbilical vein. In this model, fetal $P_{uv}O_2$ cannot rise above maternal PvO_2* (143, 163). A concurrent equilibrium model also exists in sheep. The ewe's SvO_2 predicted the fetal lamb's SvO_2 (205).

In the concurrent model, $P_{ua}CO_2$ in fetal umbilical arteries determines maternal $PaCO_2$. $P_{ua}CO_2$ is about 48 torr, and $PaCO_2$ is about 32 torr, a difference of 16 mm Hg (111). This fetal-maternal difference increases to about 25 mm Hg at the beginning of the second stage of labor (10 cm dilatation), most likely due to the retention of CO_2 due to umbilical cord compression (117). When CO_2 accumulates in fetal umbilical arteries, the pressure difference between fetal and maternal blood should increase placental transfer of CO_2 to maternal circulation.

MATERNAL BLOOD FLOW

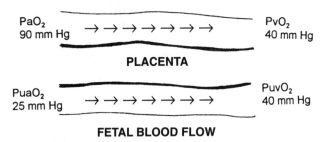

FETAL BLOOD FLOW

Figure 4.7: Illustration of concurrent model of maternal and fetal blood flow within the human placenta.

Fetal $P_{uv}O_2$ values are related to $S_{uv}O_2$ values. When $P_{uv}O_2$ is 30 to 35 torr, $S_{uv}O_2$ will be 80 to 90 percent. When $P_{uv}O_2$ drops to 20 to 25 torr, $S_{uv}O_2$ drops to 45 to 65 percent (124). Therefore, for maximum saturation of Hb in the umbilical vein, maternal PvO_2 should be near 35 mm Hg or higher.

Maternal venous PvO_2 and fetal capillary PO_2 and umbilical vein $P_{uv}O_2$ should reach equilibrium across the placental chorionic membrane exchange (see Figure 4.8) (162).

Fetal-Placental Blood Flow

Human fetal-placental blood flow has been estimated at 350 ml/min (111). Blood flow through the fetal lamb's umbilical cord was approximately 600 ml/min (124). Fetal-placental blood flow has been indirectly measured by umbilical vein Doppler velocimetry. Fetal-placental blood flow increases as gestational age and fetal weight increase. However, increments in blood flow become smaller as the fetus grows and matures. Fetal-placental flow decreases in women who are hypertensive, who have diabetes, who abuse drugs, who have twins, and/or who have abnormal placental development (209).

Fetal-placental blood flow can decrease 50 percent without a change in fetal O_2 consumption, umbilical cord vein O_2 content or fetal O_2 delivery. Fetal-placental blood flow and fetal O_2 decreases if maternal blood O_2 content or uteroplacental blood flow decrease or there is a lesion in the placenta, a decrease in fetal Hb concentration, or an increase in Hb oxygen affinity (1).

Placental Lesions

Placental growth normally continues throughout pregnancy (184). A postmature placenta, greater than 42 weeks old, has an increased risk of lesions which might impair placental function and fetal O_2 delivery. *Postmature placentas* have more villous edema and fibrosis, fibrin deposits, avascular villi, and syncytial hyperplasia. All these lesions increase the risk of fetal death (177). In 1975, as many as 40 percent of all fetal deaths were attributed to placental pathology (161).

As a result of placental lesions, postterm fetuses may be hypoxic, hypoglycemic, acidotic, dehydrated, and hypovolemic. It has been recommended that a pediatrician or neonatologist be present at the birth of a postterm fetus (161). On the other hand, some postmature placentas (42 to 43 weeks' gestation) still function well and deliver as much O_2 to fetal circulation as less mature placentas (210). Because the placenta and fetus continue to grow, a well-oxygenated post-term fetus may weigh over 4000 gms.

Women who are hypertensive, diabetic, or have chronic renal disease, have a high risk for placental pathology and degenerative changes in the walls of spiral arteries (184). Smokers have smaller placentas than nonsmokers, more fibrin deposits, and fewer fetal capillaries (211).

Hypertension and placental lesions. Hypertensive disorders are associated with uteroplacental insufficiency and placental:

- infarcts
- obliterative endarteritis, a non-inflammatory lesion which occludes placental vessels and may be caused by a viral infection, immunologic abnormalities, or hypoxia
- fibrinoid decidual ateriopathy
- villous cytotrophoblastic hyperplasia

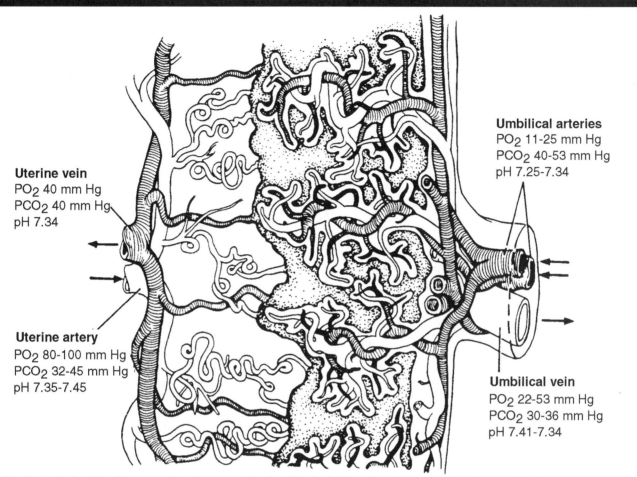

Uterine vein
PO_2 40 mm Hg
PCO_2 40 mm Hg
pH 7.34

Uterine artery
PO_2 80-100 mm Hg
PCO_2 32-45 mm Hg
pH 7.35-7.45

Umbilical arteries
PO_2 11-25 mm Hg
PCO_2 40-53 mm Hg
pH 7.25-7.34

Umbilical vein
PO_2 22-53 mm Hg
PCO_2 30-36 mm Hg
pH 7.41-7.34

Figure 4.8: Placental circulation. Compare maternal venous and fetal umbilical vein PO_2 values. In a concurrent exchange model, these values are similar (modified based on research from references 101, 111, 154, 206-208 and reproduced with permission of The C. V. Mosby Company from Tucker, S. M. (1978). *Fetal Monitoring and Fetal Assessment in High-Risk Pregnancy*).

- placental stem artery obliterative vasculopathy and
- thrombosis of placental vessels (185).

Diabetes and placental lesions. Lesions and placental vascular changes that impede transport of gases and nutrients have been identified in the placentas of diabetic women. They include:
- villous edema
- a large number of Hofbauer (stomal) cells
- villous fibrinoid necrosis and fibrosis
- marked villous congestion
- excess syncytial knot formation
- thickening of the basement membrane and
- thrombosis of fetal stem arteries (212).

Hofbauer cell physiology is poorly understood but they are found in the connective tissue of villi (186). Connective tissue lies between the syncytiotrophoblast and cytotrophoblast. Hofbauer cells, villous congestion with capillary proliferation, and large villi have been found with deficient syncytiotrophoblast growth (placental dysmaturity), chronic intrauterine infection, and fetal hemolytic anemia (185).

Villous edema. Even if uteroplacental blood flow is adequate, changes in villi can decrease O_2 delivery to the fetus. For example, *villous swelling or edema has been found in the placentas of women who have diabetes mellitus or fetuses with erythroblastosis fetalis or transplacental infections such as syphilis or chorioamnionitis* (184, 203). Chorioamnionitis is also associated with umbilical cord inflammation which impairs fetal O_2 delivery (161).

The increased diameter of edematous villi increases the distance O_2 has to travel between the intervillous space and fetal capillaries. This delays O_2 delivery. Plus, villous edema decreases the size of the intervillous space so that less blood and O_2 is available near the chorionic exchange membrane (184).

In addition to villous edema, diabetic women have retinal edema. Sorbitol produced by diabetics may be related to edema. Diabetics create sorbitol (a 5-chain sugar) when their blood glucose levels are elevated (personal communication, 1995, S. Fessler, M.D.). Sorbitol may elevate COP which would draw extravascular fluid into blood vessels. This excess fluid probably leaves maternal capillaries and enters retinal vessels and the villous membrane which swells the villi.

Avascular villi. The *placentas of preeclamptic women* may have avascular villi. Avascular villi have no vessels inside of them which results in a marked reduction in fetal capillaries (203). The lack of fetal capillaries in villi is related to fetal-placental vessel vasospasm and diminished uteroplacental blood flow which causes placental ischemia and fetal capillary necrosis. The lack of fetal capillaries diminishes fetal O_2 delivery.

Preeclampsia and spiral artery diameter. Preeclampsia manifests itself in the second or third trimester of pregnancy, yet the pathology of preeclampsia begins with conception. Preeclampsia is a trophoblast-dependent disease (213-214). In some women, preeclampsia appears to be related to HLA genes. Human lymphocyte antigens are tissue compatibility antigens important in tissue recognition (215). The human lymphocyte antigen DR4 (HLA DR4) and human lymphocyte antigen DR6 (HLA DR6) have been found in preeclamptic women, the fetus, and the placenta (215-217). Clearly, the spouse of a preeclamptic woman must also carry this recessive gene if the fetus has it. In preeclampsia, the trophoblast does not appear to be "compatible" with the uterus.

The trophoblast forms 6 to 8 days after fertilization and contains three types of cells: intermediate cells which are invasive, syncytiotrophoblast cells which are invasive, and cytotrophoblast cells which replace smooth muscle cells in spiral arteries (218). Because of invasive syncytiotrophoblast cells, the trophoblast normally changes uterine vessels from rigid structures to fully dilated vessels (186). Intermediate and syncytiotrophoblast cells secrete collagenases which invade the endometrium and decidua until the 20th week of gestation (219). Collagenases help strip the lamina from maternal spiral arteries.

Fibrin and fibronectin are deposited in the endometrium (128, 220). Fibronectin, a glycoprotein, attaches the trophoblast to the decidua and acts like glue that holds the placenta to the uterus (216, 221-223). Fibronectin is also a nonspecific attractor of leukocytes and macrophages which increases phagocytosis and attachment of these cells to microbes, antigens, and foreign bodies (216, 224). Plasma fibronectin levels are increased when there is vascular damage or inflammation (224-225). Fibronectin levels are higher in preeclamptic women than nonpreeclamptic women (226).

Fibronectin is also found in spiral arteries. Intermediate and syncytiotrophoblastic cells erode away the spiral artery lining and cytotrophoblastic cells replace the lining and lay down fibronectin (218, 226). In normal pregnancy, maternal spiral artery diameter increases during the first trophoblastic wave or invasion into the endometrium (126). Normally, spiral arteries are fully striped of their elastic lining and they fully dilate to perfuse the intervillous spaces (128). In the second trophoblastic wave, radial arteries, just below the myoendometrial junction in the uterus are stripped of their elastic lining (126).

In preeclamptic woman, the trophoblast does not completely strip maternal vessels of their elastic lamina. *In fact, the trophoblast fails to erode away the entire spiral artery lining and spiral artery diameter is 40 percent less than spiral artery diameter in normal* pregnancies (128, 217). Some spiral arteries show no changes at all and still retain their smooth muscle lamina and adrenergic nerves that secrete norepinephrine (218, 227). Norepinephrine in the placental bed was 500 percent higher in preeclamptics than nonpreeclamptics (217). Norepinephrine inhibits prostacyclin (PGI_2) production, a potent vasodilator, and stimulates β-adrenergic receptors to constrict blood vessels. Norepinephrine increases progesterone production by 36 to 49 percent (217). Progesterone further suppresses PGI_2 production.

EDRF synthesis is also decreased in the placentas of preeclamptic women (228-229). Decreased EDRF, a potent vasodilator and inhibitor of platelet adhesion and aggregation, increases placental vessel vasoconstriction and increases the risk of capillary stasis and clot formation (202). The production of EDRF or nitric oxide is mediated by tissue necrotic factor alpha (TNFα).

TNFα is a cytokine which is higher in the serum of preeclamptics than nonpreeclamptics. *High TNFα is associated with decreased EDRF.* The source of TNFα is unknown, but it is believed to be decidual or amniotic trophoblastic cells or macrophages. High levels of TNFα were found in IUGR fetuses (95). In addition, the vasoconstrictors endothelin-1 and endothelin-2 levels are significantly higher in IUGR fetuses than normally-grown fetuses (201). The lack of EDRF and the high levels of Et-1 and Et-2 are related to reduced placental blood flow, decreased nutritient and O_2 delivery, and IUGR (95).

Discordant Twins. There was a linear relationship between the percent of discordance in twin birth weights and the number of placental lesions in the smaller twin's placenta. The placentas of the smaller twin had infarctions, villous fibrosis, hypovascularity, and chronic villitis. Their weight difference was not related to placental size (230).

UTERINE ANATOMY AND PHYSIOLOGY
The Uterus
The uterus is a tubular organ lined with endometrium. The myometrium is the uterine muscle and the external serosa covers the outside of the uterus (179). The uterus is divided into three sections: the top is the uterine body, the bottom is the cervix, and in between the uterine body and the cervix lies the isthmus. At term, the uterine body contains about 65 percent of the smooth muscle fibers and the cervix contains 35 percent (231).

The Cervix
The cervix is also called the cervix uteri. During pregnancy, it is about 2.5 cm long and is closed (195). The cervix is mostly comprised of collagen (70 percent collagen) and smooth muscle (10 percent) (232). The rest (20 percent) has not been identified in the literature, but it is probably water. More

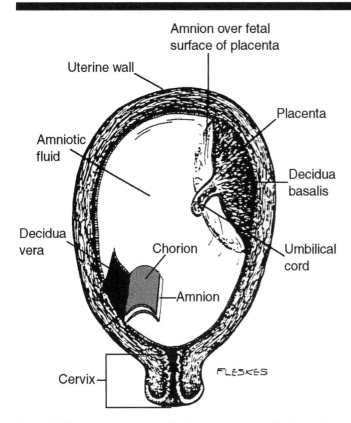

Figure 4.9: Uterine cavity at term. The chorion and amnion line the uterine wall and continue over the placenta and envelop the umbilical cord. Amniotic fluid surrounds the fetus (modified from Hillman, L. M., & Pritchard, J. A. (1971). Williams obstetrics, 14th ed., New York: Appleton-Century-Crofts, reproduced with permission of The C. V. Mosby Company from Korones, S. B. (1981). *High-risk newborn infants. The basis for intensive nursing care. 3rd ed.*).

uterine smooth muscle fibers are found at the top of the cervix (about 29 percent) than at the bottom of the cervix (about 6 percent) (231).

A ripe, soft cervix shortens to about 1.3 cm in length, opens to about 1 to 1½ cm, and is dilatable. Therefore, a ripe cervix that is 1 to 1½ cm dilated is about 50 percent effaced or thinned. A ripe cervix indicates the uterus is ready for labor. During labor, the cervix continues to shorten and dilate. At 10 cm, the term fetus can pass through the cervix to be delivered (195).

The cervix ripens when collagen bundles rearrange themselves in a more flexible pattern which allows smooth muscle fibers to slide over one another more freely (195). Collagenase breaks down collagen in the cervix. During labor, women had 66 percent more collagenase in their blood stream than when they were not in labor. The primary sources of collagenase appear to be the placenta and cervix (233). However, bacteria also produce collagenase, and women in preterm labor are often infected and have an 800 percent increase in collagenase over normal values (232-233).

Cervical ripening is cytokine/neutrophil-mediated (232, 234). Cytokines are found in cells. Cytokines in the amniotic membranes and cervix stimulate arachidonic acid metabolism. Arachidonic acid is in the cell wall. Cervical cell arachidonic acid is acted on by the enzyme cyclooxygenase to become prostaglandin E_2 (234-236).

The cytokine responsible for cervical ripening is interleukin-8 (IL-8). IL-8 is also called neutrophil-activating factor (236). IL-8 has been found in monocytes and endothelial cells and is a potent chemotaxic agent for leukocytes and macrophages (237). It was discovered (in vitro) that the cervix produced IL-8 and prostaglandin E_2 (PGE_2) (236). *IL-8 induces neutrophil migration into the chorion, decidua, and cervix and causes degranulation of collagenase-containing granules.* Neutrophils have been found in amniotic fluid, the chorion, and the placenta (221, 238). Prostaglandins work synergistically with IL-8 which speeds the cervical ripening process. Progesterone inhibits IL-8 production (220, 234).

Uterine Contractions

The myometrium is composed of diagonally interlaced smooth muscle fibers. Within these smooth muscle cells are calcium stores. When intracellular calcium increases, muscle cells contract (179). There are α-receptors and β_2-receptors on uterine smooth muscle cells. Simulation of α-receptors increases uterine activity. Stimulation of β_2-receptors activates uterine smooth muscle cell adenylate cyclase which increases cell cAMP and decreases intracellular calcium and uterine activity.

α- and β_2-receptors. Catecholamines bind with uterine α- and β_2-receptors. In a study with 30 women, who were 39 to 41 weeks pregnant, intravenous *epinephrine decreased uterine activity* and norepinephrine increased uterine contraction frequency, intensity, and resting tone (239). *Norepinephrine appears to selectively bind with α-adrenergic receptors (increasing uterine resting tone and contraction frequency, duration, and strength), and epinephrine binds with β_2-adrenergic receptors (decreasing contraction frequency, duration, and strength)* (240, 241).

Anxious women in labor secrete catecholamines which are primarily epinephrine (75 percent). Therefore, excessive *maternal anxiety and catecholamine release would mostly stimulate β_2-receptors and may decrease effective uterine activity which would slow labor.* Cocaine, on the other hand, augments α-adrenergic activity, inhibits β_2-adrenergic activity, and increases uterine activity (240-241).

Braxton Hicks Contractions. Beginning about 20 weeks' gestation, *high amplitude/low frequency* Braxton Hicks contractions occur about once every 2 to 4 hours and may increase in frequency as gestation advances (231). At 24 to 26 weeks' gestation, uterine artery resistance is at its lowest level (242). Braxton Hicks contractions can increase uterine artery resistance and diminish uteroplacental blood flow (126). Braxton Hicks contractions are not labor contractions. They are mild and only slightly diminish blood flow in the uterus. They are associated with an increase in maternal mean arterial pressure (126, 243).

During Braxton Hicks contractions, uterine vessels over the placenta were compressed less than other uterine vessels. Researchers speculated that placenta progesterone inhibited subplacental uterine activity (242).

Fetal effect of Braxton Hicks contractions. These contractions have little to no effect on fetal carotid artery, cerebral, or umbilical artery blood flow. They often coincide with an increase in fetal electrocortical activity, FM, and FHR baseline variability (243-244). In fetal lambs, "nonlabor" contractions were associated with mild, transient hypoxemia, decreased FBM, increased BP, and an increase in plasma angiotensin, AVP, and catecholamines. The increase in BP was related to the amount of amniotic fluid which affected the amount of pressure exerted by the uterus on the fetal body (244).

First stage of labor. In the United States, approximately 9,000 women are in labor each day. The biochemical trigger that initiates labor is still unknown, however, the change in the ratio of estrogen to progesterone is a primary labor stimulant (245). In addition to α-receptors and β₂-receptors, researchers have identified the following factors related to the initiation of labor:
- estrogen/progesterone ratio
- oxytocin receptors
- cytokines
- prostaglandin E_2
- prostaglandin $F_{2\alpha}$ and
- gap junctions.

Estrogen/progesterone. Estrogen and progesterone are secreted by the placenta, decidua, and membranes (6, 246). Uterine cells have estrogen and progesterone receptors (247). The ratio of estrogen to progesterone increases during the second trimester of pregnancy (248-249). Women in labor have significantly more estrogen than progesterone (249). *Estrogen stimulates cervical ripening and increases the concentration of oxytocin receptors* in the decidua and on uterine cells (250). Progesterone inhibits IL-8 production and cervical ripening (249).

Oxytocin receptors. Oxytocin receptors have been found in the decidua and on uterine smooth muscle cells prior to the onset of labor. During late pregnancy and in labor, they increase 500 percent even though there is no increase in the level of endogenous circulating oxytocin (128). When oxytocin binds with these receptors, calcium channels are opened, intracellular calcium increases, and prostaglandin production in the decidua increases (128, 251-253).

Prostaglandins E_2 and $F_{2\alpha}$. Prostaglandins produced in the decidua enter uterine cells (128). PGE_2 and $PGF_{2\alpha}$ have been found in uterine cells, amniotic fluid, maternal blood, and urine (220). *Estrogen and prostaglandins are needed for gap junction formation* (234). *Prostaglandins stimulate the release of sequestered intracellular calcium* (235).

Gap junctions. Estrogen stimulates the formation of gap junctions in uterine smooth muscle cells (252, 254). Gap junctions are present in late pregnancy, before labor, and they increase in number during labor (247). Gap junctions are raised areas on uterine smooth muscle cells that act like pores. They are composed of ribonucleic acid and protein (247, 254). These "pores" are low resistance pathways for charged ions which leave one cell and enter another cell. This spreads energy or an action potential from cell to cell. When gap junctions are forming, low amplitude, high frequency uterine activity waves are often seen. The uterine activity pattern is called uterine irritability. Within 24 to 72 hours following uterine irritability, uterine cells communicate through their gap junctions in a synchronous manner and uterine contractions occur.

Estrogen → Oxytocin receptors → Prostaglandin production → Gap junctions → Contractions ← ↑ intracellular calcium / Cervical ripening

First stage of labor. The first stage of labor is divided into three phases: the latent phase, active labor, and transition. The first stage ends at 10 cm. When descent of the fetus and dilatation of the cervix is plotted on a graph, active labor begins with the acceleratory phase of the dilatation labor curve. For some women that may be 3, 4 or 5 cm dilatation.

Contractions peak at 25 to 30 mm Hg during the latent phase, 25 to 70 mm Hg during the active phase, and 40 to 80 mm Hg during transition (182, 255). Intrauterine peak pressures with twins may never exceed 25 or 30 mm Hg, even in active labor with good progress (256).

Women in labor increase their heart rate and cardiac output (179). Blood flow to the uterus is constant before, during, and after contractions (257). Since maternal arteries and veins to and from the intervillous space pass through the uterine muscle, they are subject to compression during contractions. At the beginning of the contraction, maternal venous outflow from the uterus stops. Uterine intramural veins are squeezed, and arterial inflow continues to increase the volume of the intervillous space until intrauterine pressure exceeds arterial BP. As the uterus contracts, the length, thickness, and surface area of the placenta increases from distention of intervillous spaces with maternal blood. Contractions also apply pressure to the fetus and the umbilical cord (257). Wharton's jelly protects umbilical blood vessels from compression, but it is deficient in IUGR fetuses, who become more vulnerable to hypoxia (186). Fetal BP increases as intrauterine pressure increases (258).

The contracting uterus applies pressure to the maternal aorta and compresses uterine muscle intramural vessels and spiral arteries that supply the intervillous space with blood and O_2 (44, 243, 257, 259-260). During uterine contractions, intramyometrial and intrauterine pressure, maternal central venous pressure, BP, and cerebrospinal fluid pressure increase (261). *Blood flow to the placenta decreases at an intrauterine pressure (IUP) of 30 mm Hg. Placental blood flow totally ceases near 50 mm Hg,* limiting O_2 transfer (39, 259, 262).

In 5 term women in spontaneous labor, there was a slight decrease in uterine blood flow before the contraction began. Blood flow decreased again when IUP reached 30 mm Hg. Uterine blood flow was at its lowest level during the contraction peak and resumed a normal flow rate within 20 seconds after the contraction ended in the absence of excessive uterine activity (262). At an IUP of 57 mm Hg, uterine veins were almost totally occluded (259).

Because O_2 delivery to the placenta is curtailed during contractions, the fetus must rely on O_2 reserves contained on the fetal RBCs, in fetal tissues, or the O_2 that is already present in the intervillous spaces. *Fetal O_2 reserves normally last only one to two minutes.* Oxygen reserves are higher in well-grown fetuses and lower in IUGR fetuses (126). During "normal" contractions, fetal cerebral SaO_2 dropped in 6 of 8 human fetuses, but increased in 2 of 8. SaO_2 is related to cerebral blood volume. If contractions were seen in conjunction with FHR decelerations, *the deceleration reflected a transient drop in cerebral SaO_2 and a rise in deoxygenated Hb* (263).

Second stage of labor. At 10 cm dilatation, women begin the second stage of labor. During the second stage, maternal heart rate increases 20 percent and cardiac output increases 50 percent (179). Abdominal muscles and uterine contractions can create an intrauterine pressure as high as 110 mm Hg or more during pushing (255). "Normal" bearing down efforts and maternal hyperventilation do not seem to impair placental functioning, nor have an effect on newborn status (123). But prolonged contractions at pressures above 50 mm Hg could force the fetus to consume its O_2 reserves. Therefore, to prevent hypoxia and acidosis, adequate rest is needed between contractions and maternal ventilation is needed between each "push."

Resting tone. The lowest pressure between contractions is called uterine resting tone. Resting tone increases when the uterus is overstimulated by oxytocin or is overdistended by excessive intrauterine normal saline or Lactated Ringer's solution instilled during an amnioinfusion procedure (261, 264). Resting tone may be reduced if the uterus is malformed, overdistended by multiple fetuses, has fibroids, or when the woman has a debilitating disease, or has received narcotics, inhalation anesthesia, alcohol, magnesium, and tocolytic agents such as terbutaline (261). An abnormally high resting tone and contraction frequency (hypertonus with hyperstimulation) may be caused by oxytocin, placental abruption, or prostaglandins which are administered to ripen the cervix.

Cocaine. Cocaine addicts have an increased risk of preterm labor, premature rupture of membranes, abruption, meconium stained amniotic fluid, a LBW fetus (which is partly due to cigarette smoking), and sexually transmitted diseases such as syphilis, gonorrhea, and hepatitis B antigenemia (265). Fetuses of cocaine addicts are small because cocaine inhibits active placental transport of amino acids such as alanine. The placental affinity for cocaine is 10 to 20 times higher than the central nervous system's affinity for cocaine (193, 266).

Cocaine selectively inhibits β_2-receptor binding and cAMP production. It increases intracellular inositol phosphate, but has little effect on α-receptors, which alters the contractile equilibrium to increase uterine activity (267-269). Cocaine may also increase oxytocin receptor sensitivity or stimulate prostaglandin E_2 and prostaglandin F_2 production, the "prostaglandins of labor" (270).

β-mimetic tocolytics, such as terbutaline, bind with uterine cell β_2-receptors and inhibit contractions. Since cocaine inhibits β-receptor binding, tocolytics will be ineffective, resulting in "down regulation" and an increased risk of preterm labor (268-269, 271). In one study of *women in preterm labor, researchers found 45 percent of the women abused drugs. Seventy percent used cocaine and 30 percent used other drugs* (271). The effect of cocaine on the uterus is dose-dependent (270). If a woman is already in labor, cocaine will augment her uterine activity and increase the duration and force of contractions (268). When rats, cats, and rabbits are given cocaine, they have tetanic contractions that were strong and lasted more than 90 seconds (269).

FETAL OXYGEN DELIVERY

Maternal, placental, and umbilical cord factors determine fetal oxygenation. These factors include:
- uteroplacental blood flow (140)
- maternal venous SvO_2 and PvO_2 (140, 205)
- intervillous blood flow (140)
- placental O_2 consumption and transfer (140) and
- fetal umbilical vein $S_{uv}O_2$ and $P_{uv}O_2$ (140).

Umbilical Cord Blood Flow

Fetal factors that affect umbilical cord blood flow and fetal O_2 delivery include:
- fetal cardiac contractility
- systemic vascular resistance
- blood volume
- blood viscosity and
- umbilical vessel diameter.

Fetal blood pressure is proportional to umbilical vessel blood volume. If cord blood volume decreases, fetal BP decreases. If volume increases, BP increases (125). Therefore, fetal BP changes when the cord is compressed.

Blood viscosity and umbilical vessel diameter affect blood flow. Blood viscosity increases when RBC volume increases or protein content of blood increases. Blood flow in umbilical cord vessels can be measured with an ultrasound device that measures blood flow velocity.

Cord Compression

Umbilical cord compression reduces umbilical vein diameter and diminishes O_2 delivery to the fetus and CO_2 transfer across the placenta to maternal circulation. The fetus can become hypoxic and acidotic. Umbilical cord prolapse causes an acute fetal O_2 deficiency. Anoxia, with the accumulation of lactic acid and adenosine, will eventually cause fetal decompensation. The loss of compensatory mechanisms precedes fetal death (117, 272). Toxins, such as glutamate, destroy tissue and cause fetal death (273).

Umbilical vein O_2 delivery indirectly reflects uteroplacental blood flow, uteroplacental O_2 delivery, and placental function. Fetal tissue O_2 delivery depends on blood flow through the umbilical vein (Q_{umb}) and umbilical $S_{uv}O_2$ and $P_{uv}O_2$ (130). Umbilical artery blood flow increases as gestation advances (85, 274). As fetal weight increases, O_2 delivery increases to meet tissue metabolic needs.

$$DO_2 = Q_{umb} \times (S_{uv}O_2 + P_{uv}O_2)$$

$$DO_2 = Q_{umb} \times (C_{uv}O_2)$$

Umbilical Vein Oxygen Delivery

The umbilical cord should contain one vein and two arteries which are covered by Wharton's jelly. The average cord length in one study was 54 cm. The cord should be centrally inserted in the placenta. Cord length is related to fetal movement, i.e., cords are longer in fetuses who move a lot than in fetuses who move very little. Acardiac fetuses or fetuses with an amniotic band that limited their movement had very short cords (186).

Oxygen delivery to the fetus depends on umbilical vein blood flow, SvO_2 and PvO_2. If cord blood flow decreases, O_2 delivery decreases. If cord blood flow increases, O_2 delivery increases. Most cases of fetal hypoxia are due to umbilical cord compression or uteroplacental insufficiency (256). *If the fetal lamb's umbilical cord is compressed, the lamb will maintain O_2 consumption until flow is 50 percent or more below normal values.* If umbilical cord vessels are totally occluded, CO_2 accumulates, pH falls, tissue hypoxia may worsen, and metabolic acidosis and asphyxia can develop if O_2 delivery is not quickly reestablished (275).

Fortunately, umbilical cord compression is usually a transient event and O_2 delivery can be rapidly reestablished when cord compression ceases. Research with baboons found total umbilical cord vessel occlusion for 30 seconds to 12 minutes decreased O_2, increased CO_2, decreased pH, and decreased base excess. With cord release, there was a prompt rise in O_2 and a decrease in CO_2 levels (275).

Aside from mechanical compression of the cord, constriction of umbilical cord blood vessels or alterations of blood flow through the vessels may be associated with:
- severe maternal hypoxemia (182)
- acute or chronic uteroplacental insufficiency (182)
- maternal catecholamines (184, 256)
- thrombosis (161)
- prostaglandins (184)
- high O_2 or low CO_2 levels (182, 184)
- endothelium-derived relaxing factor (EDRF) or nitric oxide (200)
- parathyroid hormone-related protein receptors (200)
- possibly endothelin (200) and

- fetal hyperglycemia (209).

Fetal umbilical vein flow is a distal measure of total fetal placental blood flow. In diabetics, there was an inverse relationship between maternal serum glucose and umbilical vein blood flow. The cause and effect mechanism between glucose and umbilical vein flow was not explained. However, researchers believe maternal hyperglycemia may be related to uteroplacental insufficiency (209).

Fetal Hemoglobin (HbF)
Fetal hemoglobin, HbF, is composed of two alpha (α) and two gamma (λ) chains. The λ–chains have two fewer electrons than the β chains of adult HbA. This creates a weaker binding site for the negatively charged 2,3-DPG anion. *Thus, 2,3-DPG has a lower binding affinity for HbF than adult Hb.* HbF has less 2,3-DPG than HbA, which results in about 20 percent more O_2 being bound to HbF than is bound to adult HbA. *The greater O_2 affinity of HbF increases the oxygen-carrying capacity of fetal RBCs than adult RBCs* (146, 161, 157, 180). Because of its higher O_2 affinity, HbF in fetal capillaries in villi readily extracts O_2 (146). Beginning in the first trimester of pregnancy, the quantity of HbF begins to decrease and the quantity of HbA increases. At term, the fetus is born with approximately 75 percent HbF and 25 percent HbA (157).

As gestation advances, Hb and RBC volume decrease as does umbilical vein $P_{uv}O_2$. At term, 95 percent of the RBCs are produced in the bone marrow and fetal Hb averages 15.5 gm/dl (119). The placenta contains approximately 75 to 125 ml of fetal blood (111,135). The normal HCT is between 40 to 45% which is higher than the adult HCT (130). The high level of RBCs compensates for the low PaO_2. Fetal RBCs deliver 25 percent more O_2 per unit volume of blood than adult RBCs. For example, maternal blood O_2 capacity is 0.168 ml O_2/ml blood and fetal capacity is 0.208 ml O_2/ml blood (111). In addition, fetal cardiac output and blood flow are higher than adult cardiac output and blood flow per kg of body weight (184).

Fetal Anemia and Polycythemia
Fetal tissue O_2 delivery will be reduced when the fetus is anemic or polycythemic. For example, if the fetal lamb HCT was reduced 40 percent or increased 40 percent above control values, tissue O_2 delivery decreased (130). Anemia, with a decreased Hb concentration, decreases the quantity of O_2 that can be carried to tissues. Polycythemia, with an increased Hb and HCT, increases blood viscosity which decreases blood flow.

Anemia. Fetuses may be anemic and hypovolemic due to hemolysis or an acute blood loss. When the fetal lamb's HCT was reduced, there was no change in Q_{umb} until the HCT decreased by more than 40 percent. Then, oxygen delivery (DO_2) decreased (130). When the fetal HCT was near 19 percent, the number of new RBCs, nucleated RBCs (NRBCs), increased (276). The decrease in HCT was also related to a decrease in plasma protein, including lymph protein.

Thoracic duct lymph flow increased and doubled the amount of protein returning to the circulation, which increased COP as a compensatory response to blood loss (277).

As a result of anemia, the fetal response could include:

* intramedullary hemopoiesis within the bone marrow (with mild to moderate anemia)
* extramedullary hemopoiesis in the liver and spleen (with severe anemia)
* an increased number of NRBCs
* increased blood flow through the umbilical vein, inferior vena cava, descending thoracic aorta, and common carotid artery
* a decrease in FHR baseline variability
* *a sinusoidal pattern may appear if Hb is 3 to 12.3 gm/dl and blood O_2 content is 5 standard deviations below the mean* (i.e., a sinusoidal pattern is related to anemia, hypoxia, and asphyxia)
* fewer accelerations and
* decelerations (119, 276, 89).

Rh incompatibility and erythroblastosis fetalis. An Rh positive fetus has Rh D (Rho) antigens on its RBCs. An Rh negative mother, who is exposed to Rh positive RBCs, produces anti-D antibodies. Within 72 hours of the birth of a Rh positive baby, or following a miscarriage or abortion, the Rh negative mother should receive anti-D immunoglobulin (RhoGam®) which will coat any fetal Rh positive cells that entered her body at the time of placental separation and hemolyze and destroy them. If she does not receive anti-D immunoglobulin, and she becomes pregnant again and the fetus is Rh positive, her antibodies will enter the fetus via the placenta and cause fetal hemolysis or erythroblastosis fetalis. Amniotic fluid bilirubin levels will be elevated as a result of RBC destruction. Serial amniocentesis may be performed to assess bilirubin levels to estimate RBC destruction. To compensate for the destruction of RBCs, fetal kidneys, the liver, and the spleen will produce erythropoietin when Hb is less than 14 gm/dl. New RBCs (reticulocytes or nucleated RBCs) will appear when Hb is less than 9 gm/dl (276).

Hepatic blood flow sources include the umbilical vein flow (50 to 80 percent), portal venous blood flow (20 percent), and hepatic arterial flow (5 percent) (130, 189). The anemic fetus' liver will become enlarged due to the increase in hemopoietic tissue. *The enlarged liver can be visualized by ultrasound and is an early sign of fetal anemia.* Because of the severe fetal anemia and liver hyperplasia, the umbilical vein will be compressed where it enters the liver. The liver will be underperfused and may be damaged. Hypoalbuminemia, due to reduced production of albumin and other proteins by the liver, will lower COP, increase intravascular hydrostatic pressure, and increase the risk of fetal edema or hydrops (89,119). Liver hyperplasia and umbilical vein compression will also decrease umbilical vein drainage into the liver, resulting in distention and dilatation of the umbilical vein and an increase in placental thickness. Umbilical artery pressure will increase, as will right and left ventricular afterload. The fetus is at risk to develop pericardial effusion,

ascites, and hydrops. Rh-isoimmunized women's fetuses who had hydrops were hypoxic and some had myocardial dysfunction (89, 119). *Fetuses with hydrops are always anemic.*

Nonimmune hydrops has occurred in fetuses who did not have a Rh compatibility problem yet were edematous with pericardial and pleural effusions. They had inadequate cardiac output that failed to maintain adequate circulation. Plus, they had hypoxia-induced endothelial leakage (119). Their inadequate cardiac output was due to an arrhythmia such as supraventricular tachycardia (a FHR over 180 bpm) or congenital heart block (when the FHR was below 50 bpm).

Non-Rh alloimmunization. Sometimes during a transfusion, women receive blood with antigens that are foreign to their body. They then produce antibodies against these antigens. Other than anti-D antibodies (Rh positive antibodies), the two most common antibodies that can cause fetal anemia are anti-Kell and anti-c antibodies. The Kell protein may be a factor in RBC growth and differentiation and anti-Kell antibodies may interfere with RBC production. Unlike erythroblastosis, fetuses who are anemic from anti-Kell had lower levels of bilirubin in their amniotic fluid, and there was no relation in the number of NRBCs and their HCT. Researchers believe that fetal anemia from Kell alloimmunization is due to suppression of RBC synthesis rather than hemolysis. Through blood screening, anti-Kell antibodies can be identified in maternal serum. If she is anti-Kell positive, the father of the baby should also be tested. If he is Kell positive, the fetus' blood will need to be collected at 20 to 24 weeks for Hb, HCT, and the presence of the Kell antigen. Blood is collected by a percutaneous umbilical cord sample (PUBS). A needle is inserted through the maternal abdomen and uterus and into the umbilical cord and a blood sample is drawn. Serial ultrasounds will be used and possibly other PUBS will be done to determine fetal status during the pregnancy (276).

Fetomaternal transfusion. Sometimes anemia is a result of a fetomaternal transfusion where fetal blood enters maternal circulation due to breaks or anastamoses in the placenta. If the fetal blood type is incompatible with maternal blood, the woman may even develop a transfusion reaction (62). For example, the woman may become flushed, develop a rash or hives and itching. In extreme cases, she may develop asthmatic wheezing or laryngeal edema.

When fetal cells enter maternal circulation, maternal serum α-fetoprotein (AFP) increases (278). A fetal loss of 150 ml is considered a massive fetomaternal hemorrhage (279). In a case report, Hoag (279) described a rare example of fetal anemia caused by a thrombosis of the umbilical vein with a clot that totally occluded the vessel. As a clot forms in the umbilical vein, blood flow decreases. Venous blood stasis increases clot formation until the clot totally occludes the vein. On admission, the FHR pattern included variable and late decelerations, bradycardia to 90 bpm, and absent STV. Decreased fetal movement was reported. The FHR pattern also was sinusoidal and thick meconium was noted in the amniotic fluid. The fetus was stillborn and had cord blood gases consistent with a diagnosis of asphyxia. The fetus lost approximately 185 ml of blood and had a HCT of 16%. The autopsy revealed a small chambered heart, consistent with hypovolemia. The umbilical cord was dissected in 2 cm segments to reveal the thrombosis. The cause of the clot was not identified (279).

The umbilical cord can rapidly fill with blood when an umbilical vein or artery ruptures. In 1985, Ballas, Gitstein, and Kharasch (280) discovered only 50 case reports on umbilical cord hematoma, a rare condition. They reported a case of a baby that lived who had a 9 cm by 3 cm hematoma. They suggested umbilical cord hematoma may be caused by:
- torsion or traction on a short cord or
- looping of the cord around fetal body parts, especially if the hematoma is near the skin
- cord compression
- a congenitally weak vessel wall or
- syphilis.

Kleihauer-Betke test. It is rare to find fetal RBCs in maternal blood (281). To detect the ratio of fetal RBCs to maternal RBCs, a Kleihauer-Betke test is performed. The Kleihauer-Betke test is an acid elution test which was developed in 1957. Fetal RBCs are differentiated from adult RBCs to estimate the extent of the fetomaternal transfusion (279). The test gives a percentage of fetal RBCs in maternal blood. This percentage can be used to estimate fetal blood loss. A Kleihauer-Betke of 3 percent is considered a serious bleed. Some fetuses have serious bleeds and survive. For example, Willis and Foreman (282) reported a case of massive *chronic* fetomaternal hemorrhage with "remarkable" fetal compensation. The Kleihauer-Betke stain indicated 14.5% of RBCs were fetal in origin. The maternal HCT was 37.6%.

Based on this information, the total ml of whole blood (which would include maternal and fetal RBCs) can be calculated and the ml of fetal blood in maternal circulation can be estimated. A maternal HCT of 3% is approximately 500 ml of whole blood or 250 ml of packed RBCs. The maternal HCT can be used to estimate fetal blood loss.

HCT	ml of whole blood
3%	= 500 ml
37.6%	= ? ml

A proportion can be set up to calculate the total amont of whole blood represented by an HCT of 37.6%:

$$? \text{ ml}/37.6\% = 500 \text{ ml}/3\%$$

Then:

$$? \text{ ml} = 500 \text{ ml} \times 37.6\%/3\%$$
$$? \text{ ml} = 18,800/3 = 6266.67 \text{ ml}$$

The 6,267 ml represents 100% of maternal blood volume. If 14.5% of the RBCs found were fetal in origin, an estimate of fetal blood loss can be obtained by multiplying 14.5% x 6,267 ml.

$$14.5\% = 14.5/100$$
$$14.5/100 \times 6267 = 90871.5/100 = 908.71 \text{ ml}$$

Therefore, an estimated 909 ml of fetal blood was transfused into maternal circulation. However, Willis et al. (282) reported blood loss was approximately 700 ml. The FHR pattern had decreased STV and LTV and later developed persistant late decelerations. The male infant was delivered alive by cesarean section and had normal scalp and cord pH values. Chronic fetomaternal hemorrhage may be from a placenta previa with rupture of villi and fetal capillaries, abruption, trauma, amniocentesis, external and spontaneous version with placental disruption, and, as previously mentioned, umbilical vein thrombosis (282).

Sinusoidal pattern. Anemic fetuses may have a sinusoidal pattern or sinusoidal baseline. Features of a sinusoidal pattern include absent STV, absent accelerations, cyclic waves of LTV, and decelerations may be present. Pathologic sinusoidal patterns were created in lambs who had a vagotomy and their blood volume decreased. They became acidotic and intravenous arginine vasopressin (AVP) was administered. The level of AVP was related to the amplitude of the sinusoidal baseline (the baseline range). Fetal blood pressure increased and decreased as baseline cycles rose and fell above and below the average rate. The baseline cycled two to four times each minute. Researchers could not produce a sinusoidal pattern when atropine was administered to nonvagotomized lambs because atropine did not totally obliterate vagal activity. Thus, researchers concluded *a pathologic sinusoidal pattern exists only when there is absent efferent vagal control of the fetal heart* (70).

Loss of vagal tone ⇐ Anemia + Acidosis
▼ ▼ ▼
Absent short-term variability   AVP release and adenosine
▼ ▼
Pathologic sinusoidal pattern   Loss of sympathetic tone
2-4 cycles/minute ▼
+   Absent accelerations
BP fluctuates up and down as
FHR fluctuates up and down

Intrauterine transfusion. An intrauterine transfusion of blood is the most frequent treatment for Rh immune hemolytic anemia (89). The goal is to increase the fetal HCT to 40 to 50 percent (89, 130). There are three types of transfusions: direct, exchange, and intraperitoneal. A direct transfusion with adult blood takes 15 to 30 minutes to complete and has risks of volume overload and cardiac decompensation. An exchange transfusion takes more time, uses smaller amounts of blood, and removes sensitized RBCs. An intrauterine fetal transfusion of RBCs may:
- increase fetal Hb and HCT
- increase blood O_2 content
- increase tissue oxygenation
- increase blood viscosity
- decrease venous return to the heart and preload
- increase cardiac contractility but
- decrease cardiac output, especially if there is overloading

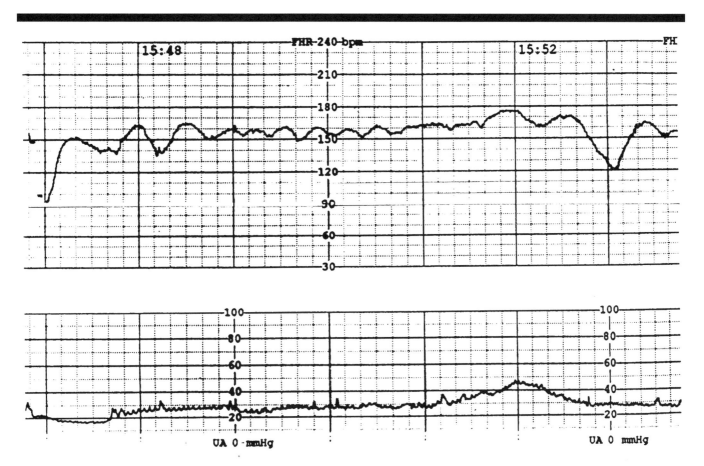

Figure 4.10: Pathologic sinusoidal pattern of Rh D (Rho) fetus whose G_4, P_2 Rh negative mother did not receive Rh D immunoglobulin (RhoGam®) following a previous pregnancy. She had five amniocenteses during this pregnancy and was seen in labor and delivery following a bloody amniocentesis. The variable decelerations on either side of the sinusoidal baseline may be due to retention of some vagal tone but are most likely a reflection of direct myocardial depression due to hypoxia and acidosis. An immediate cesarean section was performed with Apgar scores of 1, 1, and 1 at 1, 5, and 10 minutes. The severely anemic, hydropic neonate died 30 minutes after delivery.

or baroreceptor activity due to increased blood volume (119).

Adult blood is transfused through a 20 or 22 gauge needle that has been inserted into the umbilical vein at the placental-cord insertion site, or intrahepatically into the umbilical vein, or directly into the heart (283). Prior to transfusion, the fetus is given a drug such as pancuronium bromide for neuromuscular blockade. The fetus will be unable to move during the procedure. The fetus may also be given furosemide (Lasix®) which triggers AVP release.

Blood transfused into the fetus is typically O negative packed RBCs which are buffy coat poor, irradiated, washed twice in normal saline, and resuspended in saline for a HCT of 70%. Adult blood contains RBCs, proteins such as albumin and fibrinogen, and platelets. Platelets produce thromboxane A_2 (TXA_2), a potent vasoconstrictor, when they are activated or damaged (283, 284).

The transfusion of adult blood increases fetal RBC volume, systemic vascular resistance, left heart afterload, the HCT, blood viscosity, and capillary stasis. The *increase in blood viscosity and TXA_2* may increase umbilical venous pressure, decreasing umbilical blood flow and blood flow to all tissues except the brain and heart (283, 284).

Another goal of intrauterine transfusion is to improve tissue oxygenation without jeopardizing brain oxygenation. Transfused fetuses slightly increased blood flow to their brains; but, unlike hypoxic conditions where blood flow and O_2 delivery to the brain are maintained, the increase in blood viscosity *decreases O_2 delivery to the brain as much as 55 percent.* The reduction in O_2 delivery increases the O_2 extraction and the $O_2ER\%$ which increases the risk of fetal metabolic acidosis. As a result of decreased brain O_2 delivery, the fetus may have fewer GBM and FBM, which cannot be assessed until the effect of pancuronium bromide has faded (101, 284).

Within the first hour after the transfusion, cardiac output decreases due to the increase in afterload, HCT, and blood viscosity. But, within 24 hours, it returns to normal (283, 284). Most fetuses undergo electronic fetal monitoring for 2 to 4 hours post procedure. The transfusion may be repeated as indicated until 34 to 35 weeks' gestation. The risk of the procedure is umbilical cord trauma, cord hematoma, cord vasospasm, rapid expansion of intravascular volume, premature rupture of membranes, preterm labor, and fetal death (89, 283, 284). Many fetuses who had intrauterine transfusions grow normally and deliver without complications (1, 130).

Hyperkalemia and arrhythmias. A rare occurrence during intrauterine transfusion is a fetal arrhythmia from hyperkalemia. Potassium levels in packed RBCs ranged from 13.9 to 66.5 mEq/L. The high potassium level is caused by leakage of potassium from irradiated RBCs. The longer blood is stored prior to transfusion, the higher the potassium level. Fetal arrhythmias are also related to the temperature of the blood, the volume of blood transfused, and calcium and citrate levels in the blood (285).

Decreased umbilical artery resistence. Because the fetus is transfused with adult RBCs, which more freely unload O_2 than HbF, umbilical vein $S_{uv}O_2$ *decreases* after transfusions but $P_{uv}O_2$ *increases* (284). As a result of improved $P_{uv}O_2$, blood vessels dilate and the systolic/diastolic umbilical artery ratio decreases. The decline in the systolic/diastolic ratio was greater in fetuses who had the best PaO_2 and SaO_2 prior to transfusion (89, 286).

Increased umbilical venous pressure. The increase in blood volume and viscosity and the presence of TXA_2 may increase umbilical venous pressure. If pressure in the umbilical vein increases more than 10 mm Hg, there is an increased risk of fetal death due to volume overload and heart failure (283-284).

Polycythemia. Neonatal polycythemia is reflected in a Hb greater than 23 gm/dl and/or a HCT greater than 60 percent (135). Polycythemia may result from an intrauterine transfusion or be present in IUGR fetuses who have increased their NRBC volume in response to chronic hypoxia. Polycythemia may also be found in one of two identical twins who have a monochorionic, diamniotic membrane. Due to anastomoses in the placenta, e.g., vein to vein or artery to artery, the recipient twin becomes hypervolemic and polycythemic and the donor twin becomes anemic (135, 130, 287). The anemic twin becomes hypovolemic, IUGR, and develops oligohydramnios. The recipient twin diureses, probably due to increased ANP secretion in response to hemoconcentration. Diuresis increases amniotic fluid volume and the polycythemic twin usually has polyhydramnios, in addition to organomegaly, hydrops, pericardial and pleural effusion, and cardiomegaly. Treatment may include intraamniotic decompression by amniocentesis. The risk of decompression includes abruption, preterm labor, premature rupture of membranes, and amnionitis (287).

Polycythemia, with increased blood viscosity, is associated with decreased umbilical and hepatic blood flow. Oxygenated blood will be shunted past the liver through the ductus venosus (130). Singleton IUGR fetuses had polycythemia and abnormal Doppler umbilical artery blood flow with an increased systolic/diastolic ratio, greater than the 95th percentile (288). Elevated systolic/diastolic umbilical artery ratios were associated with neonatal intensive care admission after birth and stillbirth.

Absent or reversed umbilical artery blood flow. The absence or reversal of diastolic flow in the umbilical artery predicts fetal hypoxia. A reversal of flow means blood leaves the fetal body then backs up into the baby then leaves again as the heart pumps. Flow reversal suggests a problem with cardiac contractility, but is usually due to very high placental resistence (286). Direct myocardial failure or hypoxic myocardial failure can occur and late decelerations with absent baseline STV and LTV will be observed on the FHR pattern (129).

Erythropoietin and Nucleated Red Blood Cells (NRBCs)

Erythropoietin. Erythropoietin-glycoprotein hormone is created mainly by the kidneys but can be created by the liver and spleen. *Erythropoietin is the primary hormonal regulator of RBC production. Fetal hypoxemia and acidemia stimulate erythropoietin production.* There is an inverse relationship between fetal pH and erythropoietin level. As fetal umbilical artery pH drops in response to hypoxemia, the level of fetal erythropoietin increases (288).

Labor creates fetal hypoxemia (289). Fetuses who were 37 to 41 weeks' gestation and delivered vaginally had significantly higher levels of erythropoietin in mixed umbilical cord serum and umbilical cord plasma than fetuses who delivered by elective cesarean section (289, 290). The level of erythropoietin in fetuses born to women who had elective cesarean sections and no labor was 16 to 36 mU/ml. Fetuses, who delivered vaginally, had an erythropoietin level between 12 to 80 mU/ml (290).

Erythropoietin stimulates and regulates RBC production. Animal research suggests 3 to 4 hours of hypoxemia is needed before erythropoietin levels increase. Erythropoietin levels peak approximately 12 hours after the onset of hypoxia and return to normal 24 to 48 hours after O_2 levels are normalized (291). If hypoxemia is chronic, there will be an increase in erythropoietin and the number of fetal RBCs (292). Serum erythropoietin levels were significantly elevated in IUGR fetuses (293).

An increase in erythropoietin was related to the presence of meconium in amniotic fluid. Two theories exist as to why fetuses defecate and release meconium in utero. One theory concerns motilin, a peptide hormone that increases in quantity as the fetus ages. The belief is that the increase in motilin stimulates defecation. Another theory suggests hypoxia stimulates a vagal response, anal sphincter relaxation, and meconium release (291).

Term fetuses with normal FHR patterns and meconium in their amniotic fluid had significantly higher erythropoietin levels than term fetuses with normal FHR patterns and clear amniotic fluid. There was a significant elevation in erythropoietin with all consistencies of meconium, including thin and free-flowing or thick and particulate meconium. The researchers concluded that meconium-stained fluid is associated with a previous hypoxic insult, antedating labor, even when there are no FHR patterns that suggest fetal compromise (291).

Nucleated red blood cells (NRBCs). Erythropoietin production increases reticulocyte formation which increases the oxygen-carrying capacity of blood (102). Reticulocytes have a meshlike pattern of threads and particles at the former site of the cell nucleus. NRBCs have nuclei. *NRBCs become evident in fetal circulation two to three days after the onset of hypoxia.* A high neonatal NRBC count may be helpful in dating asphyxial brain injury because NRBCs are rarely present in newborns (294, 295).

NRBCs from umbilical artery blood are counted on a slide under the microscope (a blood smear). The ratio of NRBCs to 100 white blood cells determines the percent of NRBCs. NRBCs normally account for less than 1 percent of the circulating RBCs, therefore, a higher percentage of NRBCs reflects an increased rate of erythropoiesis (82). In normal neonates, the NRBC count was 0.6 to 3 percent. In neurologically impaired neonates, whose FHR pattern was persistently nonreactive (no accelerations), the NRBC count was 7.7 to 86.3 percent. NRBCs were cleared within 61.8 to 427.8 hours (295) .

Fetal Tissue Oxygen Consumption

Fetal tissues consume O_2 based on oxidative requirements determined by fetal size, activity, and metabolic processes. Severe anemia or polycythemia can decrease O_2 delivery and consumption. If the fetal HCT was 16 to 48 percent, there was no change in fetal lamb O_2 consumption. But, if the HCT dropped below 16 percent or increased to more than 48 percent, O_2 consumption decreased (130).

Oxygen requirements increase with fetal tissue hypoxia and an increase in the metabolic rate. Warm fetuses increase their metabolic rate and consume more O_2 as a result of maternal hyperthermia due to prolonged hot tub exposure, a heated whirlpool spa, sauna bathing, or maternal fever (143, 296). Maternal hyperthermia between 4 to 7 weeks' gestation may cause deficient tissue O_2 delivery and abnormal embryonic development. If maternal temperature was sustained at 102° F (38.9° C) for 1 or more days between 4 to 7 weeks' gestation, newborns had facial and CNS anomalies such as an abnormally small head, eyes, and or jaw, mental deficiency, seizures, hypotonia, cleft lip and/or cleft palate, midface hypoplasia, and ear anomalies (296).

Under normoxic conditions, the uterus, placenta and fetus consume O_2 at a constant rate to meet requirements for tissue oxidative metabolism (75). Fetal O_2 consumption increases with activity, such as FBM. For example, fetal lambs consume up to 20 percent of their total body oxygen during fetal breathing movements (297). Oxygen consumption is a product of umbilical vein blood flow (Q_{uv}) and the difference between umbilical vein and umbilical arterial O_2 content.

$$\text{Fetal } O_2 \text{ consumption in ml/dl } (VO_2) = Q_{uv} \times (C_{uv}O_2 - C_{ua}O_2)$$

Fetal Oxygen Reserves

Cells continue to consume O_2 even when O_2 delivery is curtailed. The difference between the amount of O_2 delivered and the "critical" amount consumed for oxidative metabolism is the O_2 reserve (75, 107).

$$\begin{array}{c} O_2 \text{ delivery/minute/kg} \\ - \ \underline{O_2 \text{ consumption/minute/kg}} \\ O_2 \text{ reserve} \end{array}$$

Oxygen reserves are a buffer for times of decreased O_2 delivery. Oxygen reserves are found in the placenta, umbilical cord, and fetus. Fetal lambs extract 34 percent of O_2 from their blood, leaving 66 percent in reserve (77). Human fetuses extract more O_2 than lambs (129). Normally, fetal O_2 delivery is 24 ml/min/kg. The fetus consumes 12 to 14 ml/min/kg for oxidative metabolism. The difference, 10 to 12 ml/min/kg is the O_2 reserve. *Oxygen delivery can be decreased at least 40 to 50 percent without an effect on O_2 consumption.* However, when O_2 delivery falls below 50 percent of normal, reserves become depleted, O_2 consumption must decrease, and anaerobic metabolism ensues (75).

Nicolaides (119) believes the O_2 critical level needed to meet oxidative metabolic needs is 2 mmol/L. At 1 mmol/L, even with an increase in cerebral blood flow, cerebral oxidative metabolism in the fetal lamb decreased (298). In sheep, uterine blood flow was decreased 30 to 90 percent for 60 minutes at which time fetal O_2 consumption decreased (1).

Fetal Oxygen Extraction Ratio

Oxygen extraction is related to the quantity of consumed O_2 and the quantity of delivered O_2. The ratio, consumption/delivery, is called the fractional oxygen extraction ratio and is abbreviated $O_2ER\%$ (75, 130).

[consumption] VO_2 (ml/dl) $= Q_{umb} \times (C_{uv}O_2 - CuaO_2)$
[delivery] $DO_2 = DO_2 = Q_{umb} \times (S_{uv}O_2 + P_{uv}O_2)$
$$DO_2 = Q_{umb} \times (C_{uv}O_2)$$

Consumption/delivery $= Q_{umb} \times (C_{uv}O_2 - C_{ua}O_2)/Q_{umb} \times C_{uv}O_2$
$$O_2ER\% = C_{uv}O_2 - C_{ua}O_2/ \ C_{uv}O_2$$

VO_2 is the amount of O_2 consumed by fetal tissues. Q_{umb} is blood flow through the umbilical vein. $C_{uv}O_2$ is the total O_2 content in the umbilical vein or $S_{uv}O_2 + P_{uv}O_2$. $C_{ua}O_2$ is the total O_2 content in the umbilical artery or $S_{ua}O_2 + P_{ua}O_2$. DO_2 is the amount of O_2 delivered to the fetus through the umbilical vein.

Fetal lambs extract 34 percent of O_2 delivered by the placenta (76). Initially fetal O_2 extraction is *independent* of O_2 supply and extraction depends on changes in the oxygen-hemoglobin dissociation curve (299). A decrease in O_2 delivery increases $O_2ER\%$. The increase in extraction and decrease in O_2 delivery may be related to such factors as a decrease in maternal FIO_2, placental O_2 diffusion, the O_2 exchange surface area, or umbilical vein blood flow (300, 130). In order to increase $O_2ER\%$, placental capillaries may proliferate. Placental O_2 must increase to increase the placental-fetal O_2 diffusion gradient. This should increase the fetal capillary to cell O_2 gradient to increase fetal tissue O_2 delivery (130).

Placental O_2 diffusion can be reduced by 50 percent without increasing $O_2ER\%$ (204). If maternal FIO_2 acutely decreases (in the ewe), the lamb's cerebral blood flow increases but not O_2 delivery. As a result, the lamb's fractional O_2 extraction ratio increases (300). The increase in the fractional O_2 extraction ratio is *a compensatory response* to the decrease in O_2 delivery (130).

The margin of safety. The O_2 "margin of safety" is the degree to which O_2 consumption can increase and O_2 delivery can decrease before cells become hypoxic and metabolic acidosis ensues (101). In fetal lambs, the "margin of safety" was depleted when umbilical cord blood flow was reduced 75 percent. At that point, their $O_2ER\%$ increased 80 percent above normal, their FHR decreased, PaO_2 and pH decreased, $PaCO_2$ increased, and the difference between umbilical cord SaO_2 and SvO_2 increased, indicating an increase in fetal O_2 consumption (76). With even greater reductions in umbilical cord blood flow, $O_2ER\%$ increased to a maximum of 86 percent (1). Therefore, tissues consumed 86 percent of available O_2.

Oxygen extraction and the "critical level." The increase in fractional O_2 extraction ($O_2ER\%$) depletes O_2 reserves. Eventually, O_2 supply will fall below the "critical level" needed to maintain oxidative metabolism. Below the "critical level," O_2 reserves are totally depleted, O_2 consumption decreases, anerobic metabolism occurs, and O_2 extraction and cell survival becomes entirely dependent on O_2 delivery.

The *"critical level" at which O_2 reserves are totally depleted and the human fetus decreases O_2 consumption* is not known. Some believe the critical level is reached in nonpregnant adults when $O_2ER\%$ is 70 percent. Perhaps the critical O_2 extraction level is higher than 70 percent in human fetuses because the O_2 extraction ratio of fetal lambs was greater than 80 percent when they developed significant changes in their blood gases (1, 76).

THE FHR AND HYPOXIA

Electronic fetal monitoring can be used to identify hypoxemic, acidotic, and asphyxiated fetuses. Hypoxia may cause a change in the fetal electrocardiogram and decrease the FHR. The FHR response partially depends on brain and heart O_2 and glucose and the accumulation of adenosine (109, 301, 302).

Adenosine

Normal substances found in fetal blood increase when there is a decrease in blood O_2 or hypoxemia. For example, AVP, lactate, and adenosine all increase in response to hypoxemia. Maternal adenosine does not cross the placenta (303).

Adenosine is produced from perivascular astrocytes and organ cells. Perivascular astrocytes are star-shaped cells that are found in nerve tissue (176, 82). Parenchymal cell mitochondria store ATP. Parenchymal cells are the functional cells of an organ, such as an adipocyte or hepatocyte (82). The degradation product of ATP is adenosine, a purine nucleoside (302, 303). Purines are nitrogenous compounds (82). Other sources of adenosine include S-adenosylhomocysteine and adenosine monophosphate (303).

Adenosine is a potent *vasodilator and metabolic regulator* that is found in normally grown human fetuses. It counteracts catecholamine stimulating effects to prevent overstimulation of the heart (176, 304, 305, 303). Adenosine binds with two types of cell receptors that contain guanine nucleotide-binding proteins, type A_1 and A_2. A_2 receptors mediate vasodilation (301).

Adenosine increases when fetal cells lack O_2 and H^+ ions accumulate. Both fetal and placental cells produce adenosine. Fetal lamb umbilical cord compression was associated with a 200 to 300 percent increase in adenosine. Adenosine is called a "retaliatory metabolite" because it retaliates for hypoxia by causing vasodilation in the heart and brain (305). In sheep, adenosine injection decreased diastolic blood pressure but did not change systolic blood pressure. Heart rate increased an average of 23 percent (303).

Adenosine may increase flow through the ductus arteriosus. It inhibits the central nervous system and decreases fetal eye and breathing movements. The decrease in movement decreases O_2 consumption. Adenosine inhibits thermoregulation. Adenosine also decreases adipose tissue metabolism and platelet aggregation (305).

RBCs pick up and release adenosine. When adenosine reaches the brainstem, it suppresses brainstem sympathetic outflow. Adenosine also modulates synaptic function at the level of the cell membrane by increasing potassium and calcium conductance which *inhibits neurotransmitter release* (302, 303). Thus, adenosine inhibits norepinephrine release from sympathetic nerve endings (302).

Adenosine can inhibit or activate adenylate cyclase which affects cAMP (303, 302). *The cardiac effects of adenosine decrease SA node activity, AV node conduction, atrial contractility, and ventricular automaticity* (303). The decrease in SA node activity decreases baseline variability. Adenosine in the brainstem decreases efferent sympathetic nerve impulses which decreases the number and size of accelerations.

Chronic Hypoxia, Malnutrition, and Intrauterine Growth Restriction (IUGR)

Maternal nutrition affects placental and fetal size, prompting the saying, "Big placenta, big baby." Perhaps the saying should be "Big mom, big placenta, big baby." A large placenta with a small baby suggests O_2 and nutrient delivery was impeded by the umbilical cord. A small placenta and small baby may be genetic or caused by uteroplacental insufficiency.

Oxygen affects growth. Oxygen receives electrons removed from food which provides energy for survival and growth (107). A chronically deficient O_2 supply will perpetuate fetal humoral effects and continual redistribution of cardiac output resulting in asymmetrical fetal growth (88). Due to chronic shunting of O_2 and nutrients to the brain, heart and adrenal glands, hyperplasia of these organs creates a fetus with a large head, heart, and adrenal glands but a small body. Adrenal glands may double in weight in the presence of chronic hypoxia (64).

IUGR has been defined as an estimated fetal weight less than 10 percent of the expected weight for that gestational age. Fetuses with severe IUGR have an abdominal circumference less than the 5th percentile. IUGR may be caused by maternal, placental, fetal, or unknown factors. Fetal causes may be genetic or infection related. Unknown causes are thought to be related to inadequate cell O_2 delivery (153).

Preterm and IUGR fetuses are more vulnerable to asphyxial injury as their reserve supply of O_2 is smaller than that of normally grown term fetuses. An IUGR fetus will be a small for gestational age (SGA) neonate. One third of all SGA neonates had mothers with vascular disease (185). SGA newborns are "starved for glucose and amino acids" and have abnormally high levels of triglycerides, abnormally low O_2, high CO_2, high lactic acid, and low pH levels. Due to chronic shunting, blood will be directed away from skeletal muscle, the liver, and adipose tissue which reduces glycogen and fat stores. Triglycerides may be abnormally elevated due to lipolysis, increased synthesis, or decreased utilization. IUGR fetuses also have high cortisol and low ACTH levels (85).

Normally, the ratio of insulin to glucose increases with gestational age. SGA neonates had deranged carbohydrates, lipid, and amino acid metabolism (227). IUGR fetuses may be hypoglycemic and hypoinsulinemic. Hypoinsulinemia is associated with hypoglycemia and possible pancreatic dysfunction (85). IUGR fetuses have a high risk of hypoglycemia because hypoxia increases glucagon which depletes liver glucose due to glycogenolysis (102). Hypoglycemia often causes hypoinsulinemia which stimulates protein breakdown, amino acid oxidation, and an increase in plasma alanine (102). Alanine is an amino acid which indirectly reflects hypoglycemia (102, 152). Hypoxia also precedes anaerobic metabolism and lactic acid production. Lactic acid interrupts the glucose-protein-alanine cycle by inhibiting liver uptake of alanine (102).

Beta-blockers, such as labetalol, prevent a rise in plasma glucose and have been associated with hypoglycemia of the newborn and IUGR. Beta-mimetic drugs, such as terbutaline, increase peripheral blood flow and improve placental perfusion, often resulting in fetal growth (66).

Maternal Causes of IUGR. Progressive maternal conditions such as hypertension, diabetes mellitus, and Rh incompatibility increase the risk the fetus will be chronically O_2 deprived and IUGR. *Women with IUGR fetuses had significantly higher Hb and HCT levels, lower P_{50} levels, and lower placental weights than women whose babies were normally grown* (306). It was suspected that women with IUGR fetuses had lower than normal 2,3-DPG levels due to decreased serum unconjugated estriol. The researchers suggested more research was needed to determine the association between maternal estriol, 2,3-DPG, oxygen affinity, and fetal IUGR (156). Five women with known IUGR at 23 or more weeks' gestation were given humidified O_2 via a tight fitting face mask at 8 liters per minute for 15 to 24 hours a day. After the first 10 minutes of hyperoxygenation, cordocentesis revealed a near normal fetal $P_{uv}O_2$ in the five normally grown and 5 IUGR fetuses. The normally grown fetal $P_{uv}O_2$ increased to above the 95th percentile, and the IUGR fetuses' $P_{uv}O_2$ increased to normal or near normal. In two of the IUGR fetuses who were acidotic, their $PuvO_2$ and pH increased and their $P_{uv}CO_2$ decreased after 10 minutes of O_2. Maternal arterial oxygen tension (PaO_2) increased to 280 to 360 mm Hg. In addition, blood flow increased in the fetal aorta and was sustained several weeks. Fetuses gained weight and were no longer IUGR (307).

Umbilical artery and placental causes of IUGR. Increased placental vascular resistance may cause IUGR due to impaired blood flow. Umbilical artery blood flow reflects placental vascular resistance and vasoconstriction in the umbilical arteries (308). Normally, the umbilical artery has low vascular resistance (67). The cause of increased umbilical vascular resistance may not be identified, but stimulation of β-adrenergic receptors dilates vessels to maintain blood flow (67). Possibly, these receptors are desensitized due to hypoxia or α-adrenergic receptors exert a stronger response and cause vasoconstriction in a low-oxygen environment. Umbilical artery blood flow may be impaired due to deficient cardiac output, decreased blood vessel diameter, and increased blood viscosity (33).

End diastolic blood flow. Using ultrasound technology to measure red blood cell flow velocity in the umbilical artery, *absent end diastolic flow was seen in arteries with high vascular resistance.* Extremely low end diastolic umbilical artery flow is considered abnormal, and is associated with extremely high umbilical artery and/or placental vascular resistance, and a high fetal morbidity and mortality rate (309).

If umbilical artery velocity ratios were normal, the test was 95 percent predictive of a well fetus. If ratios were abnormal, the test was 49 to 66 percent predictive of an IUGR fetus. The highest predictive values were found in hypertensive women (310).

Spontaneous decelerations and absent end-diastolic velocity. *Absent end-diastolic velocity may occur prior to the development of spontaneous decelerations in the FHR. Therefore, if the fetus is a known IUGR fetus, it may not be appropriate to wait to see decelerations if there is no end-diastolic blood flow in the umbilical artery* (309).

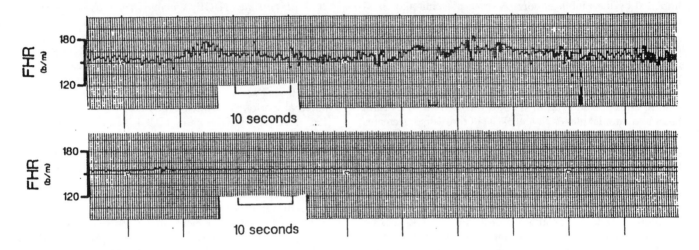

Figure 4.11: Baseline FHR pattern (top) and 20 minutes after administration of 0.5 µg of L-2-N^6-phenylisopropyl adenosine (bottom) (reproduced with permission from Egerman, R. S., Bissonnette, J. M., & Hohimer, A. R. (October 1993). The effects of centrally administered adenosine on fetal sheep heart rate accelerations. *American Journal of Obstetrics and Gynecology, 169*(4), 866-869.).

Fetal blood flow. Severe IUGR fetuses may have decreased aortic blood flow, renal blood flow, and oligohydramnios. Oligohydramnios has been defined as the lack of a pocket of amniotic fluid, observed by ultrasound, equal to or greater than 1 centimeter in depth (307).

Fetal behavior. Chronic fetal hypoxia is related to a lack of rapid eye movement (REM), limb movement, a reduction of lung fluid, and a decrease in FBM. In normoxic fetuses, FBM decreases with maternal hyperventilation with a reduction in maternal PaCO$_2$ and with hypothermia. FBM normally increases between 1 and 7 am, with increased maternal PaCO$_2$, and hyperthermia (311).

Adenosine Levels Are Elevated in IUGR Fetuses

Pregnancy is a progressive process and hypoxia can be too (312). *IUGR fetuses suffer from chronic hypoxia.* As a result of limited O$_2$ delivery, they have
- abnormal aortic and pulmonary artery blood flow
- abnormal umbilical cord vessel blood flow
- decreased FBM, REM, and limb movement
- fewer accelerations that are reduced in height and duration
- decreased baseline bandwidth and variability and
- more decelerations (42, 307, 313, 314).

Abnormal aortic blood flow and IUGR was related to an increase in the FHR baseline level, decreased STV and LTV, and fewer accelerations of shorter height and decreased duration compared with fetuses who had normal aortic blood flow (32, 314). The rise in the FHR baseline may be related to a chemoreceptor-brainstem-sympathetic nerve-cardiac response to hypoxia or a reduction in vagal tone. *The reduction in the FHR baseline, variability, and accelerations is related to adenosine.* Adenosine levels were higher in 30 to 38 week IUGR fetuses than appropriate for gestational age

(AGA) fetuses. IUGR adenosine levels were more than 100 percent higher than AGA levels. IUGR fetuses had significantly lower umbilical vein P$_{uv}$O$_2$, pH, and significantly higher P$_{uv}$CO$_2$ levels. The change in blood gases was proportional to their adenosine level (297, 305). The effects of adenosine are summarized in Table 2.

Table 2: Fetal Adenosine Effects
- **brainstem suppression**
- **inhibition of thermoregulation**
- **vasodilation**
- **decreased**
  cardiac contractility
  eye movements
  breathing movements
  sympathetic nerve norepinephrine release
  number, height, and duration of accelerations
  FHR baseline variability (STV and LTV)

Smaller or fewer accelerations. Adenosine suppresses central nervous system and sympathetic nervous system activity which decreases the number and size of accelerations (301, 302). The FHR pattern of IUGR hypoxemic and acidemic fetuses progresses from decreased height and duration of accelerations and decreased baseline variability to the presence of decelerations and eventually a rise in the FHR baseline level (315).

Increase in the baseline level. Dalton, Dawes, and Patrick (11) found the baseline of fetal lambs rose and STV decreased by 50 percent following epinephrine administration. LBW fetuses and preterm fetuses had fewer accelerations, more decelerations, and higher baselines than well grown fetuses (316). IUGR fetuses have more problems with thermoregulation and BP control (32). Perhaps, epinephrine released in response to hypoxia contributes to the rising baseline and problems with thermoregulation and BP.

Loss of variability. Fetal hypoxemia between 28 and 36 weeks' gestation was related to decreased STV and LTV (102). Variability decreases as a result of adenosine suppression of the medulla oblongata and sympathetic nerves (see Figure 4.11) (301, 302). Vagal tone and vagal activity decreases as a result of tissue hypoxia and acidosis, with lactic acid and adenosine accumulation (53, 129, 302, 317). The loss of baseline variability may precede terminal bradycardia (154).

Decelerations. When the fetus experiences an acute lack of O_2, the FHR may decelerate or increase baseline variability due to a chemoreceptor and baroreceptor response (33). The IUGR fetus may have variable, late, prolonged, and/or spontaneous decelerations. Examples of each type of deceleration appear in Chapter 5.

Bradycardia/Tachycardia. If O_2 levels become critically low, ATP is depleted, the fetus decompensates, and the FHR becomes bradycardic (33, 109). In the fetal goat subjected to prolonged, chronic hypoxemia, norepinephrine remained elevated while epinephrine normalized by 24 hours. The initial response to hypoxia was a *drop in the FHR for 2 to 15 minutes*, but by 20 minutes the FHR returned to the baseline or became tachycardic for as long as 5 hours. This is considered "rebound tachycardia." Fetal BP increased for 5 to 30 minutes after the bradycardic episode, and FBMs decreased. Within 40 minutes BP normalized. FBMs returned to 70 to 80 percent of normal after 4 hours (88).

CONCLUSION

Maternal and placental health determine fetal nutrient and oxygen delivery and removal of excess lactate and carbon dioxide. Any factor that decreases maternal partial pressure of oxygen (PaO_2) should be avoided if possible (318). Acute events, such as hyperventilation, uterine contractions, cord compression, or supine hypotension may diminish fetal oxygenation (1). *When uteroplacental blood flow, the maternal hematocrit, the placental exchange area, O_2 diffusion to maternal vessels or fetal capillaries, or umbilical cord blood flow decrease to less than 50 percent of normal, fetal O_2 cardiac output decreases and oxygen consumption decreases as oxygen extraction is insufficient to compensate for the lack of O_2 delivered to tissues* (1, 77, 205, 129, 124). Edelstone (75) pointed out it is not the condition that matters, but rather the amount of oxygen that reaches the fetus.

Chronic oxygen deficiencies can be related to maternal disease or addiction, such as hypertension, anemia, cigarette smoking, and cocaine use. Tobacco use begins to inhibit fetal growth about 31 weeks' gestation and is related to a decrease in uteroplacental blood flow and an increase in uterine artery resistance (319). Intrauterine growth restriction and oligohydramnios are chronic hypoxia markers. In these fetuses, catecholamine, lactate, and alanine levels remain elevated, red blood cell volume may increase 100 percent, and whole blood volume may increase 50 percent which will increase blood viscoscity and decrease tissue oxygen delivery (86).

Oxygen reserves are consumed to cope with insufficient oxygen delivery. The oxygen "margin of safety" is reduced in growth restricted fetuses. When oxygen reserves are depleted, oxygen consumption becomes dependent on oxygen supply. The decrease in supply decreases consumption. If oxygen delivery is not reestablished, the fetus may suffer irreversible tissue damage or even die (184).

The fetal heart rate pattern and fetal movement indirectly reflect the state of fetal oxygenation, compensation or decompensation. A sinusoidal pattern may be benign and associated with fetal breathing movements. Or, it may be pathological and associated with severe fetal anemia, acidosis, asphyxia, the lack of vagal tone and arginine vasopressin. When the fetus is hypoxemic, adenosine increases due to the breakdown of adenosine triphosphate. The rise in adenosine decreases the FHR bandwidth, variability, and the frequency and size of accelerations. Fetal heart rate decelerations may suggest the nature of the acute hypoxic insult. For example, late decelerations are related to uteroplacental insufficiency and variable decelerations occur when the umbilical cord is compressed. An appreciation of the physiology underlying the fetal heart rate and uterine activity patterns provides the clinician with a clear idea of the insult that must be removed to improve fetal oxygenation.

References

1.   Carter, A. M. (1989). Factors affecting gas transfer across the placenta and the oxygen supply to the fetus. Journal of Developmental Physiology, 12(6), 305-322.

2.   Hadi, H. A., Finley, J., Mallette, J. Q., & Strickland, D. (May 1994). Prenatal diagnosis of cerebellar hemorrhage: Medicolegal implications. American Journal of Obstetrics and Gynecology, 170(5, Pt. 1), 1392-1395.

3.   Dalton, K. J., Dawes, G. S., & Patrick, J. E. (February 15, 1977). Diurnal, respiratory, and other rhythms of fetal heart rate in lambs. American Journal of Obstetrics and Gynecology, 127(4), 414-424.

4.   Campogrande, M., Alemanno, M. G., Viora, E., & Bussolino, S. (1982). FHR short and long-term variability associated with fetal breathing. Journal of Perinatal Medicine, 10, 203-208.

5.   Ohno, Y., Tsuji, M., Fujibayashi, H., Tomioka, M., Yanamoto, T., & Okada, H. (June 1986). Assessment of fetal heart rate variability with abdominal fetal electrocardiogram: Changes during fetal breathing movement. Asia-Oceania Journal of Obstetrics and Gynaecology, 12(2), 301-304.

6.   Guyton, A. C. (1986). Textbook of medical physiology (7th ed.). Philadelphia, PA: W. B. Saunders Company.

7.   Brown, J. S., Gee, H., Olah, K. S., Docker, M. F., & Taylor, E. W. (May 1992). A new technique for the identification of respiratory sinus arrhythmia in utero. Journal of Biomedical Engineering, 14(3), 263-267.

8.   Groome, L. J., Mooney, D. M., Bentz, L. S., & Wilson, J. D. (January 1994). Vagal tone in normal term fetuses during quiet sleep. American Journal of Obstetrics and Gynecology, 170(1, Pt. 2), 303. SPO abstracts #88.

9.   Donchin, Y., Caton, D., & Porges, S. W. (April 15, 1984). Spectral analysis of fetal heart rate in sheep: The occurrence of respiratory sinus arrhythmia. American Journal of Obstetrics and Gynecology, 148(8), 1130-1135.

10.   Viniker, D. A. (November 1979). The fetal EEG (detector of oxygen deprivation). British Journal of Hospital Medicine, 22(5), 504-507, 509-510.

11.   Dalton, K. J., Dawes, G. S., & Patrick, J. E. (June 15, 1983). The autonomic nervous system and fetal heart rate variability. American Journal of Obstetrics and Gynecology, 146(4), 456-462.

12.   Cabaniss, M. L. (1993). Fetal monitoring interpretation. Philadelphia, PA: J. B. Lippincott Company.

13.   Sherer, D. M., D'Amico, M. L., Arnold, C., Ron, M., & Abramowicz, J. S. (July 1993). Physiology of isolated long-term variability of the fetal heart rate. American Journal of Obstetrics and Gynecology, 169(1), 113-115.

14.   Ito, T., Maeda, K., Takahashi, H., Nagata, N., Nakajima, K., & Terakawa, N. (1994). Differentiation between physiologic and pathologic sinusoidal FHR pattern by fetal actocardiogram. Journal of Perinatal Medicine, 22, 39-43.

15.   Timor-Tritsch, I. E., Dierker, L. J., Zador, I., Hertz, R. H., & Rosen, M. G. (June 1, 1978). Fetal movements associated with fetal heart rate accelerations and decelerations. American Journal of Obstetrics and Gynecology, 131(3), 276-280.

16.   Sorokin, Y., Bottoms, S. F., Dierker, Jr., L. J., & Rosen, M. G. (August 15, 1982). The clustering of fetal heart rate changes and fetal movements in pregnancies between 20 and 30 weeks of gestation. American Journal of Obstetrics and Gynecology, 143(8), 952-957.

17.   Sorokin, Y., Dierker, L. J., Pillay, S. K., Zador, I. E., Schreinder, M. L., & Rosen, M. G. (June 1, 1982). The association between fetal heart patterns and fetal movements in pregnancies between 20 and 30 weeks' gestation. American Journal of Obstetrics and Gynecology, 143(3), 243-249.

18.   Mendoza, G. J., Almeida, O., & Steinfeld, L. (May 1989). Intermittent fetal bradycardia induced by midpregnancy fetal ultrasonographic study. American Journal of Obstetrics and Gynecology, 160(5, Pt. 1), 1038-1040.

19.   Matsuda, Y., Patrick, J., Carmichael, L., Fraher, L., & Richardson, B. (May 1994). Recovery of the ovine fetus from sustained hypoxia: Effects on endocrine, cardiovascular, and biophysical activity. American Journal of Obstetrics and Gynecology, 170(5, Pt. 1), 1433-1441.

20.   Nijhuis, J. G., Prechtl, H. F. R., Martin, Jr., C. B., & Bots, R. S. G. M. (1982). Are there behavioral states in the human fetus? Early Human Development, 6, 177-195.

21.   Brace, R. A., Wlodek, M. E., Cock, M. L., & Harding, R. (September 1994). Swallowing of lung liquid and amniotic fluid by the ovine fetus under normoxic and hypoxic conditions. American Journal of Obstetrics and Gynecology, 171(3), 764-770.

22.   Pillai, M., & James, D. (November 1990). The development of fetal heart rate patterns during normal pregnancy. Obstetrics & Gynecology, 76(5, Pt. 1), 812-816.

23.   Shaw, K. J., & Paul, R. H. (March 1990). Fetal body movement monitoring. Obstetrics and Gynecology Clinics of North America, 17(1), 95-110.

24.   Arduini, D., & Rizzo, G. (1990). Quantitative analysis of fetal rate: Its application in antepartum clinical monitoring and behavioral pattern recognition. International Journal of Bio-Medical Computing, 25(4), 247-252.

25. Sokol, R. J., Rosen, M. G., Borgstedt, A. D., Lawrence, R. A., & Steinbrecher, M. (April 1974). Abnormal electrical activity of the fetal brain and seizures of the infant. <u>American Journal of Diseases of Children, 127</u>(4), 477-483.

26. Ninomiya, Y., Murata, Y., Wakatsuki, A., Masaoka, N., Porto, M., & Tyner, J. G. (May 1994). Experimentally induced intermittent sinusoidal heart rate pattern and sleep cycle in fetal lambs. <u>American Journal of Obstetrics and Gynecology, 170</u>(5, Pt. 1), 1421-1424.

27. Richardson, B. S., Carmichael, L., Homan, J., & Patrick, J. E. (August 1992). Electrocortical activity, electroocular activity, and breathing movements in fetal sheep with prolonged and graded hypoxemia. <u>American Journal of Obstetrics and Gynecology, 167</u>(2), 553-558.

28. Cock, M. L., Wlodek, M. E., Hooper, S. B., McCrabb, G. J., & Harding, R. (May 1994). The effects of twenty-four hours of reduced uterine blood flow on fetal balance in sheep. <u>American Journal of Obstetrics and Gynecology, 170</u>(5, Pt. 1), 1442-1451.

29. Drummond, W. H., Rudolph, A. M., Keil, L. C., Gluckman, P. D., MacDonald, A. A., & Heymann, M. A. (1980). Arginine vasopressin and prolactin after hemorrhage in the fetal lamb. <u>The American Physiological Society,</u> E214-E219.

30. Dawes, G. S., & Redman, C. W. G. (December 1992). Automated analysis of the FHR: Evaluation? <u>American Journal of Obstetrics and Gynecology, 167</u>(6), 1912-1914.

31. Chaffin, D. G., Goldberg, C. C., & Reed, K. L. (November 1991). The dimension of chaos in the fetal heart rate. <u>American Journal of Obstetrics and Gynecology, 165</u>(5, Pt. 1), 1425-1429.

32. Breborowicz, G., Moczko, J., & Gadzinowski, J. (1988). Quantification of the fetal heart rate variability by spectral analysis in growth-retarded fetuses. <u>Gynecologic & Obstetric Investigation, 25</u>(3), 186-191.

33. Arnold-Aldea, S. A., & Parer, J. (1990). Fetal cardiovascular physiology. In R. D. Eden & F. H. Boehm (Eds.), <u>Assessment and care of the fetus: Physiological, clinical and medicolegal principles</u> (pp. 29-41). Norwalk, CT: Appleton & Lange.

34. Pincus, S. M., & Viscarello, R. R. (February 1992). Approximate entropy: A regularity measure for fetal heart rate analysis. <u>Obstetrics & Gynecology, 79</u>(2), 249-255.

35. Pappano, A. J. (March 1977). Ontogenetic development of autonomic neuroeffector transmission and transmitter reactivity in embryonic and fetal hearts. <u>Pharmacological Reviews, 29</u>(1), 3-33.

36. May, D. A., & Sturtevant, N. V. (October 1991). Embryonal heart rate as a predictor of pregnancy outcome: A prospective analysis. <u>Journal of Ultrasound in Medicine, 10</u>(10), 591-593.

37. Wakatsuki, A., Murata, Y., Minomiya, Y., Masaoka, M., Tyner, J. G., & Kutty, K. K. (August 1992). Autonomic nervous system regulation of baseline heart rate in the fetal lamb. <u>American Journal of Obstetrics and Gynecology, 167</u>(2), 519-523.

38. Ibarra-Polo, A. A., Guiloff, F. E., & Gomez-Rogers, C. (July 15, 1972). Fetal heart rate throughout pregnancy. <u>American Journal of Obstetrics and Gynecology, 113</u>(6), 814-818.

39. Newnham, J. P., Marshall, C. L., Padbury, J. F., Lam, R. W., Hobel, C. J., & Fisher, D. A. (August 15, 1984). Fetal catecholamine release with preterm delivery. <u>American Journal of Obstetrics and Gynecology, 149</u>(8), 888-893.

40. Weingold, A. B., Yonekura, M. L., & O'Kieff, J. (September 15, 1980). Nonstress testing. <u>American Journal of Obstetrics and Gynecology, 138</u>(2), 195-202.

41. Lavery, J. P. (December 1982). Nonstress fetal heart rate testing. <u>Clinical Obstetrics and Gynecology, 25</u>(4), 689-704.

42. Ware, D. J., & Devoe, L. D. (December 1994). The nonstress test. Reassessment of the "gold standard." <u>Clinics in Perinatology, 21</u>(4), 779-796.

43. Gagnon, R., Campbell, K., Hunse, C., & Patrick, J. (September 1987). Patterns of human fetal heart rate accelerations from 26 weeks to term. <u>American Journal of Obstetrics and Gynecology, 157</u>(3), 743-748.

44. Persianinov, L. S. (1973). The effect of normal and abnormal labour on the foetus. A survey. <u>Acta Obstetricia et Gynecologica Scandinavica, 52</u>(1), 29-36.

45. Ball, R. H., & Parer, J. T. (June 1992). The physiologic mechanisms of variable decelerations. <u>American Journal of Obstetrics and Gynecology, 166</u>(6, Pt. 1), 1683-1689.

46. O'Brien, W. F., Davis, S. E., Grissom, M. P., Eng, R. R., & Golden, S. M. (April 1984). Effect of cephalic pressure on fetal cerebral blood flow. <u>American Journal of Perinatology, 1</u>(3), 223-236.

47. Chung, F., & Hon, E. H. (June 1959). The electronic evaluation of fetal heart rate: I. With pressure on the fetal skull. <u>Obstetrics & Gynecology, 13</u>(6), 633-640.

48. Mann, L. I., Carmichael, A., & Duchin, C. (May 1972). The effect of head compression on FHR, brain metabolism and function. <u>Obstetrics & Gynecology, 39</u>(5), 721-726.

49. Kelly, J. V. (March 1, 1963). Compression of the fetal brain. <u>American Journal of Obstetrics and Gynecology, 85</u>(5), 687-694.

50. Harned, Jr., H. S., Wolkoff, A. S., Pickrell, J., & MacKinney, L. G. (August 1961). Hemodynamic observations during birth of the lamb. Studies of the unanesthetized full-term animal. <u>American Journal of Diseases of Children, 102,</u> 58-67.

51. Walker, D., Grimwade, J., & Wood, C. (March 1973). The effects of pressure on fetal heart rate. <u>Obstetrics & Gynecology, 41</u>(3), 351-354.

52. Maresh, M. (November 1987). Management of the second stage of labour. <u>Midwife, Health Visitor & Community Nurse, 23</u>(11), 498, 502-506.

53. Parer, J. T. (September/October 1976). Physiological regulation of fetal heart rate. JOGNN, 5(Suppl. 5), 25s-29s.

54. Abboud, S., & Sadeh, D. (March 1990). Power spectrum analysis of fetal heart rate variability using the abdominal maternal electrocardiogram. Journal of Biomedical Engineering, 12(2), 161-164.

55. Pagani, M., Lombardi, F., Guzzetti, S., Sandrone, G., Rimoldi, O., & Malfatto, G. (1984). Power spectral density of heart rate variability as an index of sympatho-vagal interaction in normal and hypertensive subjects. Journal of Hypertension, 2(Suppl. 3), 383-385.

56. Akselrod, S., Gordon, D., Ubel, F. A., Shannon, D. C., Barger, A. C., & Cohen, R. J. (July 10, 1981). Power spectrum analysis of heart rate fluctuation: A quantitive probe of beat-to-beat cardiovascular control. Science, 213, 220-222.

57. Yeh, S-Y., Forsythe, A., & Hon, E. H. (March 1973). Quantification of fetal heart beat-to-beat interval differences. Obstetrics & Gynecology, 41(3), 355-363.

58. Ninomiya, Y., McMahan, P. C., Murata, Y., Wakatsuki, A., Masaoka, N., & Porto, M. (February 1993). Intermittent sinusoidal heart rate pattern in vagotomized fetal lambs. American Journal of Obstetrics and Gynecology, 168(2), 731-735.

59. Caldeyro-Barcia, R., Mendez-Bauer, C., Poseiro, J. J., Escarcena, L. A., Pose, S. V., & Bieniarz, J. (1966). Control of human fetal heart rate during labor. In D. E. Cassels (Ed.), The heart and circulation in the newborn and infants (pp. 7-38). New York, NY: Grune and Stratton.

60. Ayromlooi, I., Tobias, M., & Berg, P. (December 1980). The effects of scopolamine and ancillary analgesics upon the fetal heart rate recording. Journal of Reproductive Medicine, 25(6), 323-326.

61. Copper, R. L., & Goldenberg, R. L. (May/June 1990). Catecholamine secretion in fetal adaptation to stress [Principles and Practices]. JOGNN, 19(3), 223-226.

62. Cunningham, F. G., MacDonald, P. C., & Gant, N. F. (1989). Williams obstetrics (18th ed.). Norwalk, CT: Appleton & Lange.

63. Lagercrantz, H., & Bistoletti, P. (August 1977). Catecholamine release in the newborn infant at birth. Pediatric Resuscitation, 11(8), 889-893.

64. Gagnon, R., Challis, J., Johnston, L., & Fraher, L. (March 1994). Fetal endocrine responses to chronic placental embolization in the late-gestation ovine fetus. American Journal of Obstetrics and Gynecology, 170(3), 929-938.

65. Bistoletti, P., Nylund, L., Lagercrantz, H., Hjemdahl, P., & Strom, H. (December 1, 1983). Fetal scalp catecholamines during labor. American Journal of Obstetrics and Gynecology, 147(7), 785-788.

66. Milner, R. D. G., & De Gasparo, M. (1981). The autonomic nervous system and perinatal metabolism. Pitman Medical, London (CIBA Foundation Symposium), 83, 291-309.

67. Cohn, H. E., Piasecki, G. J., & Jackson, B. T. (December 1, 1982). The effect of β-adrenergic stimulation on fetal cardiovascular function during hypoxemia. American Journal of Obstetrics and Gynecology, 144(7), 810-816.

68. Garite, T. J., & Briggs, G. G. (1987). Effects on the fetus of drugs used in critical care. In S. L. Clark, J. P. Phelan, & D. B. Cotton (Eds.), Critical care obstetrics. Oradell, NJ: Medical Economics Books.

69. Verklan, M. T., Medoff-Cooper, B., & Shaman, P. (June 4-7, 1995). Cardiovascular indices (variability) predicting central nervous system maturation. In AWHONN 1995 Convention Session Resources. In tune with the country: no. 18. Nashville, TN.

70. Murata, Y., Miyake, Y., Yamamoto, T., Higuchi, M., Hesser, J., & Ibara, S. (November 15, 1985). Experimentally produced sinusoidal fetal heart rate pattern in the chronically instrumented fetal lamb. American Journal of Obstetrics and Gynecology, 153(6), 693-702.

71. Elliott, J. P., Castro, R. J., & O'Keeffe, D. F. (July 1988). Sinusoidal fetal heart rate associated with gastroschisis. American Journal of Perinatology, 5(3), 295-296.

72. Hanson, M., & Kumar, P. (1994). Chemoreceptor function in the fetus and neonate. In R. O'Regan, P. Nolan, D. S. McQueen, & D. J. Paterson (Eds.), Arterial chemoreceptors: Cell to system (pp. 99-108). New York, NY: Plenum Press.

73. Jackson, B. T., Piasecki, G. J., & Novy, M. J. (January 1987). Fetal responses to altered maternal oxygenation in rhesus monkey. American Journal of Physiology, 252(1, Pt. 2), R94-R101.

74. Scheid, P., & Shams, H. (1994). Chemosensitivity from the lungs of vertebrates. In R. O'Regan, P. Nolan, D. S. McQueen, & D. J. Paterson (Eds.), Arterial chemoreceptors: Cell to system (pp. 99-108). New York, NY: Plenum Press.

75. Edelstone, D. I. (July 1984). Fetal compensatory responses to reduced oxygen delivery. Seminars in Perinatology, 8(3), 184-191.

76. Itskovitz, J., La Gamma, E. F., & Rudolph, A. M. (October 1983). Heart rate and blood pressure responses to umbilical cord compression in fetal lambs with special reference to the mechanism of variable decelerations. American Journal of Obstetrics and Gynecology, 147(4), 451-457.

77. Itskovitz, J., La Gamma, E. F., & Rudolph, A. M. (April 1, 1983). The effect of reducing umbilical blood flow on fetal oxygenation. American Journal of Obstetrics and Gynecology, 145(7), 813-818.

78. Eggert, J. V., Weidner, W., Eggert, L. D., Woods, R. E., & Mattern, D. (October 1986). A simplified method of obtaining umbilical cord blood for pH using a heparinized vacutainer versus heparinized syringe. American Journal of Perinatology, 3(4), 311-314.

79. Parer, J. T. (February 1980). The effect of acute maternal hypoxia on fetal oxygenation and the umbilical circulation in the sheep. European Journal of Obstetrics, Gynaecology, and Reproductive Biology, 10(2), 125-136.

80. Brubaker, K., & Garite, T. J. (December 1988). The lambda fetal heart rate pattern: An assessment of its significance in the intrapartum period. Obstetrics & Gynecology, 72(6), 881-885.

81. Aladjem, S., Feria, A., Rest, J., & Stojanovic, J. (July 1977). Fetal heart rate responses to fetal movements. British Journal of Obstetrics and Gynaecology, 84(7), 487-491.

82. Glanze, W. D., Anderson, K. N., & Anderson, L. E. (Eds.). (1990). Mosby's medical, nursing, & allied health dictionary (3rd ed.). St. Louis, MO: The C. V. Mosby Company.

83. Yunek, M. J., & Lojek, R. M. (December 1978). Fetal and maternal monitoring: Intrapartal fetal monitoring. American Journal of Nursing, 78(12), 2102-2109.

84. Giorlandino, C., Sibai, B., Bilancioni, E., Gambuzza, G., D'Alessio, P., & Nova, A. (January 1993). The importance of ductus venosus during prenatal life. American Journal of Obstetrics and Gynecology, 168(1, Pt. 2), 356. SPO abstracts #207.

85. Economides, D. L., Nicolaides, K. H., & Campbell, S. (1991). Metabolic and endocrine findings in appropriate and small for gestational age fetuses. Journal of Perinatal Medicine, 19(1-2), 97-105.

86. Kitanaka, T., Alonso, J. G., Gilbert, R. D., Siu, B. L., Clemons, G. K., & Long, L. D. (June 1989). Fetal responses to long-term hypoxemia in sheep. American Journal of Physiology, 256(6, Pt. 2), R1348-R1354.

87. Kerr, D. R., Castro, M. I., Valego, N. K., Rawashdeh, N. M., & Rose, J. C. (December 1992). Corticotropin and cortisol responses to corticotropin-releasing factor in the chronically hypoxemic ovine fetus. American Journal of Obstetrics and Gynecology, 167(6), 1686-1690.

88. Fujimori, K., Endo, C., Kin, S., Funata, Y., Araki, T., & Sato, A. (August 1994). Endocrinologic and biophysical responses to prolonged (24-hour) hypoxemia in fetal goats. American Journal of Obstetrics and Gynecology, 171(2), 470-477.

89. Weiner, C. P. (August 1989). Nonhematologic effects of intravascular transfusion on the human fetus. Seminars in Perinatology, 13(4), 338-341.

90. Cheung, C. Y. (November 1992). Autonomic and arginine vasopressin modulation of the hypoxia-induced atrial natriuretic factor release in immature and mature ovine fetuses. American Journal of Obstetrics and Gynecology, 167(5), 1443-1453.

91. Ogundipe, O. A., Kullama, L. K., Stein, H., Nijland, M. J., Ervin M. G, & Padbury, J. (December 1993). Fetal endocrine and renal responses to in utero ventilation and umbilical cord occlusion. American Journal of Obstetrics and Gynecology, 169(6), 1479-1486.

92. Kullama, L. K., Ross, M. G., Lam, R., Leake, R. D., Gore Ervin, M. G., & Fisher, D. A. (December 1992). Ovine maternal and fetal renal vasopressin receptor response to maternal dehydration. American Journal of Obstetrics and Gynecology, 167(6), 1717-1722.

93. Shelley, H. J., Bassett, J. M., & Milner, R. D. G. (January 1975). Control of carbohydrate metabolism in the fetus and newborn. British Medical Bulletin, 31(1), 37-43.

94. Parker, Jr., C. R., Favor, J. K., Carden, L. G., & Brown, C. H. (December 1993). Effects of intrapartum stress on fetal adrenal function. American Journal of Obstetrics and Gynecology, 169(6), 1407-1411.

95. Socol, M. L., Garcia, P. M., & Riter, S. (April 1994). Depressed Apgar scores, acid-base status, and neurologic outcome. American Journal of Obstetrics and Gynecology, 170(4), 991-999.

96. Romero, R., Munoz, H., Gomez, R., Ramirez, M., Araneda, H., & Cutright, J. (January 1994). Antibiotic therapy reduces the rate of infection-induced preterm delivery and perinatal mortality. American Journal of Obstetrics and Gynecology, 170(1, Pt. 2), 390.

97. Sumioki, H., Shimokawa, H., Miyamoto, S., Uezono, K., Utsunomiya, T. & Nakano, H. (1989). Circadian variations of plasma atrial natriuretic peptide in four types of hypertensive disorder during pregnancy. British Journal of Obstetrics and Gynaecology, 96(8), 922-927.

98. Meizner, I., Levy, A., & Katz, M. (February/March 1993). Assessment of uterine and umbilical artery velocimetry during latent and active phases of normal labor. Israel Journal of Medical Sciences, 29(2-3), 82-85.

99. Bader, A. M., Datta, S., Arthur, G. R., Benvenuti, E., Courtney, M., & Hauch, M. (April 1990). Maternal and fetal catecholamines and uterine incision-to-delivery interval during elective cesarean. Obstetrics & Gynecology, 75(4), 600-606.

100. Cooper, R. L., & Goldenberg, R. L. (May/June 1990). Catecholamine secretion in fetal adaptation to stress [Principles and Practice]. JOGNN, 19(3), 223-226.

101. Richardson, B. S. (September 1989). Fetal adaptive responses to asphyxia. Clinics in Perinatology, 16(3), 595-611.

102. Smith, J. H., Anand, K. J. S., Cotes, P. M., Dawes, G. S., Harkness, R. A., & Howlett, T. A. (October 1988). Antenatal fetal heart rate variation in relation to the respiratory and metabolic status of the compromised human fetus. British Journal of Obstetrics and Gynaecology, 95, 980-989.

103. Cherrington, A. D., Frizzell, R. T., Biggers, D. W., & Connolly, C. C. (1991). Hypoglycemia, gluconeogenesis and the brain. In M. Vranic, S. Efendie, & C. H. Hollenberg (Eds.), Fuel homeostasis and the nervous system (pp. 197-211). New York, NY: Plenum Press.

104. Schiff, E., Sivan, E., Terry, S., Dulitzky, M., Friedman, S. A., & Mashiach, S. (October 1993). Currently recommended oral regimens for ritodrine tocolysis result in extremely low plasma levels. American Journal of Obstetrics and Gynecology, 169(4), 1059-1064.

105. Miodovnik, M., Peros, N., Holroyde, J. C., & Siddigi, T. A. (May 1985). Treatment of premature labor in insulin-dependent diabetic women. Obstetrics & Gynecology, 65(5), 621-627.

106. Carlan, S., Jones, M., Schorr, S., McNeill, T., Rawji, H., & Clark, K. (January 1994). Oral sulindac to prevent recurrence of preterm labor. American Journal of Obstetrics and Gynecology, 170(1, Pt. 2). SPO abstracts #337.

107. Meschia, G. (December 1, 1978). Evolution of thinking in fetal respiratory physiology. American Journal of Obstetrics and Gynecology, 132(7), 806-813.

108. Piquard, F., Schaefer, A., Dellenbach, P., & Haberey, P. (1990). Lactate movements in the term human placenta in situ. Biology of the Neonate, 58(2), 61-68.

109. Rosen, K. G., & Isaksson, O. (1976). Alterations in fetal heart rate and ECG correlated to glycogen, creatine phosphate and ATP levels during graded hypoxia. Biology of the Neonate, 30, 17-24.

110. Bissonnette, J. M. (May 31-June 4, 1981). Pathophysiology of altered placental transport. Placental transport - Mead Johnson symposium on perinatal and developmental medicine no. 18, 33-34. Vail, CO.

111. Hill, E. P., Hill, J. R., Power, G. G., & Longo, L. D. (March 1977). Carbon monoxide exchanges between the human fetus and mother: A mathematical model. American Journal of Physiology, 232(3), H311-H323.

112. Dancis, J. (May 31- June 4, 1981). Placental transport of amino acids, fats and minerals. Placental transport - Mead Johnson symposium on perinatal and developmental medicine no. 18, 25-31. Vail, CO.

113. Arulkumaran, S., Lilja, H., Lindecrantz, K., Ratnam, S. S., Thavarasah, A. S., & Rosen, K. G. (1990). Fetal ECG waveform analysis should improve fetal surveillance in labour. Journal of Perinatal Medicine, 18(1), 13-22.

114. Reece, E. A., Antoine, C., & Montgomery, J. (March 1986). The fetus as the final arbiter of intrauterine stress/distress. Clinical Obstetrics and Gynecology, 29(1), 23-32.

115. Lagercrantz, H., & Slotkin, T. A. (1986). The "stress" of being born. Scientific American, 254(4), 100-107.

116. Heerschap, A., & van den Berg, P. P. (1994). Proton magnetic resonance spectroscopy of human fetal brain. American Journal of Obstetrics and Gynecology, 170(4), 1150-1151.

117. Gimovsky, M. L., & Caritis, S. N. (June 1982). Diagnosis and management of hypoxic fetal heart rate. Clinics in Perinatology, 9(2), 313-324.

118. Cohen, W. R., & Schifrin, B. S. (1983). Clinical management of fetal hypoxemia. In W. R. Cohen & E. A. Friedman, (Eds.), Management of labor (pp. 163-188). Baltimore, MD: University Park Press.

119. Nicolaides, K. H. (1989). Studies on fetal physiology and pathophysiology in rhesus disease. Seminars in Perinatology, 13(4), 328-337.

120. Eguiluz, A., Lopez Bernal, A., McPherson, K., Parrilla, J. J., & Abad, L. (December 15, 1983). The use of intrapartum fetal blood lactate measurements for the early diagnosis of fetal distress. American Journal of Obstetrics and Gynecology, 147(8), 949-954.

121. Moll, W., & Kastendieck, E. (1985). Kinetics of lactic acid accumulation and removal in the fetus. In W. Kunzel (Ed.), Fetal heart rate monitoring. Clinical practice and pathophysiology (pp. 161-169). Berlin: Springer-Verlag.

122. Kamitomo, M., Alonso, J. G., Okai, T., Longo, L. D., & Gilbert, R. D. (September 1993). Effects of long-term, high-altitude hypoxemia on ovine fetal cardiac output and blood flow distribution. American Journal of Obstetrics and Gynecology, 169(3), 701-707.

123. Thomsen, S. G., & Weber, T. (November 1984). Fetal transcutaneous carbon dioxide tension during second stage of labour. British Journal of Obstetrics and Gynaecology, 91, 1103-1106.

124. Meschia, G. (April 1985). Safety margin of fetal oxygenation. Journal of Reproductive Medicine, 30(4), 308-311.

125. Mori, A., Trudinger, B., Mori, R., Reed, V., & Takeda, Y. (January 1995). The fetal central venous pressure waveform in normal pregnancy and in umbilical placental insufficiency. American Journal of Obstetrics and Gynecology, 172(1, Pt. 1), 51-57.

126. Eskes, T. K. A. B. (February 1993). Uterine contractions and their possible influence on fetal oxygenation. Gynakologe, 26(1), 39-45.

127. Schifrin, B. S. (September/October 1994). The ABCs of electronic fetal monitoring. Journal of Perinatology, 14(5), 396-402.

128. Creasy, R. K., & Resnik, R. (1984). Maternal-fetal medicine. Principles and practice. Philadelphia, PA: W. B. Saunders Company.

129. Parer, J. T. (1983). Handbook of fetal heart rate monitoring. Philadelphia, PA: W. B. Saunders Company.

130. Edelstone, D. I., Caine, M. E., & Fumia, F. D. (April 1, 1985). Relationship of fetal oxygen consumption and acid-base balance to fetal hematocrit. American Journal of Obstetrics and Gynecology, 151(7), 844-851.

131. Mallard, E. C., Gunn, A. J., Williams, C. E., Johnston, B. M., & Gluckman, P. D. (November 1992). Transient umbilical cord occlusion causes hippocampal damage in the fetal sheep. American Journal of Obstetrics and Gynecology, 167(5), 1423-1430.

132. Cohn, H. E., Sacks, E. J., Heymann, M. A., & Rudolph, A. M. (November 15, 1974). Cardiovascular responses to hypoxemia and acidemia in fetal lambs. American Journal of Obstetrics and Gynecology, 120(6), 817-824.

133. Rudolph, A. M., Itskovitz, J., Iwamoto, H., Reuss, M. L., & Heymann, M. A. (April 1981). Fetal cardiovascular responses to stress. Seminars in Perinatology, 5(2), 109-121.

134. Oeseburg, B., Ringalda, B. E., Crevels, J., Jonsma, H.W., Mannheimer, P., & Menssen, J. (1992). Fetal oxygenation in chronic maternal hypoxia: What's critical. Advances in Experimental Medicine & Biology, 317, 499-502.

135. Korones, S. B. (1981). High-risk newborn infants. The basis for intensive nursing care (3rd ed.). St. Louis, MO: The C. V. Mosby Company.

136. Henderson-Smart, D. J., & Read, D. J. C. (1979). Fetal cardio-respiratory physiology. In R. P. Shearman (Ed.). Human reproductive physiology (2nd ed.) (pp. 228-267). Blackwell Scientific Publications, Great Britain: The Alden Press, Oxford.

137. Young, B. K. (1990). Placental regulation of fetal oxygenation and acid-base balance. In R. D. Eden, F. H. Boehm, & M. Haire (Eds.), Assessment and care of the fetus. Physiological, clinical, and medicolegal principles. Norwalk, CT: Appleton & Lange.

138. Koga, S., Koga, Y., & Nagai, H. (February 26, 1988). Physiological significance of fetal blood gas changes elicited by different delivery postures. Tohoku Journal of Experimental Medicine, 154(4), 357-363.

139. Goodlin, R. C., Dobry, C. A., Anderson, J. C., Woods, R. E., & Quaife, M. (April 15, 1983). Clinical signs of normal plasma volume expansion during pregnancy. American Journal of Obstetrics and Gynecology, 145(8), 1001-1009.

140. Madsen, H. (April 1986). Fetal oxygenation in diabetic pregnancy. Danish Medical Bulletin, 33(2), 64-74.

141. Sibai, B. M. (1995). Hypertension in pregnancy: Life-threatening emergencies. [symposium handout].

142. Belfort, M. A., & Saade, G. R. (July 1994). Oxygen delivery and consumption in critically ill pregnant patients: Association with ophthalmic artery diastolic velocity. American Journal of Obstetrics and Gynecology, 171(1), 211-217.

143. Meschia, G. (October 1979). Supply of oxygen to the fetus. Journal of Reproductive Medicine, 23(4), 160-165.

144. Farquharson, R. G. (1983). Fetal oxygen affinity and its parameters in a random obstetric population. Journal of Perinatal Medicine, 11(1), 43-50.

145. Shailer, T. L., Harvey, C. J., & Guyer, F. (July/September 1992). Principles of oxygen transport in the critically ill obstetric patient. NAACOG's Clinical Issues in Perinatal and Women's Health Nursing, 3(3), 392-398.

146. Jepson, J. H. (December 1974). Factors influencing oxygenation in mother and fetus [Review]. Obstetrics & Gynecology, 44(6), 906-914.

147. Ship-Horowitz, T. (November/December 1983). Nursing care of the sickle cell anemic patient in labor [Principles and Practice]. JOGNN, 381-386.

148. Perry, Jr., K. G., & Morrison, J. C. (April 1990). The diagnosis and management of hemoglobinopathies during pregnancy. Seminars in Perinatology, 14(2), 90-102.

149. Ferguson, II, J. E., & O'Reilly, R. (July 1985). Hemoglobin E and pregnancy. Obstetrics & Gynecology, 66(1), 136-140.

150. Bardicef, M., Resnick, L. M., Bardicef, O., Sorokin, Y., & Cotton, D. B. (January 1994). P-NMR spectroscopy measurement of intracellular free magnesium and pH in erythrocytes of nonpregnant, pregnant, and gestational diabetic women. American Journal of Obstetrics and Gynecology, 170(1, Pt. 2), 309. SPO abstracts #114.

151. Tilkian, S. M., & Conover, M. H. (1975). Clinical implications of laboratory tests. Saint Louis, MO: The C. V. Mosby Company.

152. Battaglia, F. (May 31- June 4, 1981). Metabolism of the placenta: Its physiologic implications. Placenta transport - Mead Johnson symposium on perinatal and developmental medicine no. 18, 9-13. Vail, CO.

153. Mendoza, G. J. B., Calem-Grunat, J., Karmel, B. Z., LeBlanc, M. H., Brown, E. G., & Chervenak, F. (1989). Intrauterine growth retardation related to maternal erythrocyte oxygen transport. Advances in Experimental Medicine & Biology, 248, 377-386.

154. Jackson, B. T., & Piasecki, G. J. (1983). Fetal oxygenation. In W. R. Cohen, & E. A. Friedman (Eds.). Management of labor (pp. 117-142). Baltimore: University Park Press.

155. Saling, E. (1968). Foetal and neonatal hypoxia in relation to clincial practice. London: William Clowes & Sons, Ltd.

156. Brown, E. G., Mendoza, G. J. B., Chervenak, F. A., Karmel, B. Z., Krouskop, R. W., & LeBlanc, M. H. (January 1990). The relationship of maternal erythrocyte oxygen transport parameters to intrauterine growth retardation. American Journal of Obstetrics and Gynecology, 162(1), 223-229.

157. Gilbert, R. D., Lis, L., & Longo, L. D. (October 1985). Temperature effects on oxygen affinity of human fetal blood. Journal of Developmental Physiology, 7(5), 299-304.

158. Macaulay, J. H., Randall, N. R., Bond, K., & Steer, P. J. (March 1992). Continuous monitoring of fetal temperature by noninvasive probe and its relationship to maternal temperature, fetal heart rate, and cord arterial oxygen and pH. Obstetrics & Gynecology, 79(3), 469-474.

159. Cohn, H. E., Jackson, B. T., Piasecki, G. J., Cohen, W. R., & Novy, M. J. (October 1985). Fetal cardiovascular responses to asphyxia induced by decreased uterine perfusion. Journal of Developmental Physiology, 7(5), 289-297.

160. Pedron, S. L. (February 1994). Changes in total uterine blood flow do not always reflect changes in maternal placental blood flow [Letters]. American Journal of Obstetrics and Gynecology,170(2), 701-702.

161. Vorherr, H. (September 1, 1975). Placental insufficiency in relation to postterm pregnancy and fetal postmaturity. Evaluation of fetoplacental function, management of the postterm gravida [Current Developments]. American Journal of Obstetrics and Gynecology, 123(1), 67-102.

162. Longo, L. D., Dale, P. S., & Gilbert, R. D. (1986). Uteroplacental O_2 uptake: Continuous measurements during uterine quiescence and contractions. American Journal of Physiology, 250(Regulatory Integrative Comp. Physiol. 19), R1099-R1107.

163. Wilkening, R. B., & Meschia, G. (January/February 1992). Current topic: Comparative physiology of placental oxygen transport. Placenta, 13(1), 1-15.

164. Dennison, R. D. (July 1990). Understanding the four determinants of cardiac output. Nursing90, 35-41.

165. Clark, S. L., Cotton, D. B., Lee, W., Bishop, C., Hill, T., & Southwick, J. (December 1989). Central hemodynamic assessment of normal term pregnancy. American Journal of Obstetrics and Gynecology, 161(6, Pt. 1), 1439-1442.

166. Shortridge, L. A. (January/February 1983). Using ritodrine hydrochloride to inhibit preterm labor. MCN, 8, 58-61.

167. Aumann, G. M. E., & Blake, G. D. (March/April 1982). Ritodrine hydrochloride in the control of premature labor. JOGNN, 11(2), 75-79.

168. Fitzgerald, G. L. (1983). NAACOG update series: Preterm labor part 2: Management. Lesson 3, Volume 1. Continuing Professional Education Center, Inc., 1101 State Road, Building Q, Princeton, MJ 08540.

169. Haller, D. L. (November 1980). The use of terbutaline for premature labor. Drug Intelligence & Clinical Pharmacy, 14, 757-764.

170. Young, R. (January 1993). T-type and L-type calcium channels in freshly dispersed human uterine smooth muscle. American Journal of Obstetrics and Gynecology, 168(1, Pt. 2), 302. SPO abstracts.

171. Keeley, M. M., Wade, R. V., Laurent, S. L., & Hamann, V. D. (February 1993). Alterations in maternal-fetal doppler flow velocity waveforms in preterm labor patients undergoing magnesium sulfate tocolysis. Obstetrics & Gynecology, 81(2), 191-194.

172. Rayburn, W. F., & Zuspan, F. P. (1986). Drug therapy in obstetrics and gynecology (2nd ed.). Norwalk, CT: Appleton-Century-Crofts.

173. Binder, N. D., & Laird, M. R. (February 1994). Changes in total uterine blood flow do not always reflect changes in maternal placental blood flow [Letters]. American Journal of Obstetrics and Gynecology, 170(2), 701-702.

174. Burrow, G. N., & Ferris, T. F. (1995). Medical complications during pregnancy (4th ed.). Philadelphia, PA: The W. B. Saunders Company.

175. Dickinson, J. E., Andres, R. L., & Parisi, V. M. (May 1994). The ovine fetal sympathoadrenal response to the maternal administration of methamphetamine. American Journal of Obstetrics and Gynecology, 170(5, Pt. 1), 1452-1457.

176. Belfort, M. A., Anthony, J., Saade, G. R., Wasserstrum, N., Johanson, R., & Clark, S. (December 1993). The oxygen consumption/oxygen delivery curve in severe preeclampsia: Evidence for a fixed oxygen extraction state. American Journal of Obstetrics and Gynecology, 169(6), 1448-1455.

177. Larsen, L. G., Clausen, H. V., Andersen, B., & Graem, N. (February 1995). A stereologic study of postmature placentas fixed by dual perfusion. American Journal of Obstetrics and Gynecology, 172(2, Pt. 1), 500-507.

178. Williams, M. C., O'Brien, W. F. O., Porter, K. B., Lynch, C., & Casanova, C. (January 1994). Asymmetry correlates significantly with acidosis at birth. American Journal of Obstetrics and Gynecology, 372. SPO abstracts #344.

179. Nesse, R. E. (June 1983). Normal labor and the induction and augmentation of labor. Primary Care, 10(2), 253-267.

180. Girdina, B., Scatena, R., Clementi, M. E., Cerroni, L., Nuutinen, M., & Brix, O. (January 20, 1993). Physiology relevance of the overall delta H of oxygen binding to fetal human hemoglobin. Journal of Molecular Biology, 229(2), 512-516.

181. Castracane, V. D., Ramin, K., Pridjian, G., Chandler, P., Ramin, S., & Riffe, B. (January 1994). Endocrinology of twin pregnancy: Increases in maternal serum androgen. American Journal of Obstetrics and Gynecology, 170(1, Pt. 2). SPO Abstracts #95.

182. Panigel, M. (December 1, 1962). Placental perfusion experiments. American Journal of Obstetrics and Gynecology, 84(11, Pt. 2), 1664-1683.

183. Newman, W., Braid, D., & Wood, C. (January 1, 1967). Fetal acid-base status. I. Relationship between maternal and fetal PCO_2. American Journal of Obstetrics and Gynecology, 97(1), 43-51.

184. Martin, C. B., & Gingerich, B. (September/October 1976). Factors affecting the fetal heart rate: Genesis of FHR patterns. JOGNN (Suppl.), 30s-40s.

185. Altshuler, G. (May 31-June 4, 1981). Diseases of the placenta and their effect on transport. Placental transport - Mead Johnson symposium on perinatal and developmental medicine no. 18, 35-43. Vail, CO.

186. Benirschke, K. (1990). Placental implantation and development. In R. D. Eden, F. H. Boehm, & M. Haire (Eds). Assessment and care of the fetus. Physiological, clinical, and medicolegal principles. Norwalk, CT: Appleton & Lange.

187. Longo, L. D. (May 31 - June 4, 1981). Nutrient transfer in the placenta. Placenta transport - Mead Johnson symposium on perinatal and developmental medicine no. 18, 15-19. Vail, CO.

188. Jang, P. R., & Brace, R. A. (December 1992). Amniotic fluid composition changes during urine drainage and tracheoesophageal occlusion in fetal sheep. American Journal of Obstetrics and Gynecology, 167(6), 1732-1741.

189. Tropper, P. J., & Petrie, R. H. (1987). Placental exchange. In J. P. Lavery (Ed.), The human placenta: Clinical perspectives (pp. 199-206). Rockville, MD: Aspen.

190. Bawdon, R. E., Gravell, M., Roberts, S., Hamilton, R., Dax, J., & Sever, J. (February 1995). Ex vivo human placental transfer of human immunodefiency virus-1P24 antigen. American Journal of Obstetrics and Gynecology, 172(2, Pt. 1), 530-532.

191. Seeds, A. E. (November 1, 1981). Current concepts in amniotic fluid dynamics [Current Developments]. American Journal of Obstetrics and Gynecology, 138(5), 575-586.

192. Krishna, R. B., Levitz, M., & Dancis, J. (December 1993). Transfer of cocaine by the perfused human placenta: The effect of binding to serum proteins. American Journal of Obstetrics and Gynecology, 169(6), 1418-1423.

193. Dicke, J. M., Verges, D. K., & Polakoski, K. L. (September 1993). Cocaine inhibits alanine uptake by human placental microvillous membrane vesicles. American Journal of Obstetrics and Gynecology, 169(3), 515-521.

194. Guiet-Bara, A. (February 1980). Human placental oxygen transfer and consumption. Dissociation by cooling or use of respiratory enzyme inhibitors. European Journal of Obstetrics, Gynecology, and Reproductive Biology, 10(2), 83-98.

195. Oxorn-Foote, H. (1986). Human labor & birth (5th ed.). Norwalk, CT: Appleton-Century-Crofts.

196. Maguire, D. J., Cannell,G. R., & Addison, R. S. (1994). Oxygen supply and placental oxygen metabolism. In P. Vaupel, R. Zander, & D. F. Bruly (Eds.), Oxygen transport to tissue XV (pp. 709-715). New York, NY: Plenum Press.

197. Groome, L. J. (1991). A theoretical analysis of the effect of placental metabolism on fetal oxygenation under conditions of limited oxygen availability. BioSystems, 26(1), 45-56.

198. Crino, J. P., Harris, A. P., Parisi, V.M., & Johnson, T. R. B. (May 1993). Effect of rapid intravenous crystalloid infusion on uteroplacental blood flow and placental implantation-site oxygen delivery in the pregnant ewe. American Journal of Obstetrics and Gynecology, 168(5), 1603-1609.

199. Kay, H. H., Hawkins, S. R., Wang, Y., Mika, D. E., Ribeiro, A. A., & Spicer, L. D. (January 1993). Phosphorus 31 magnetic resonance spectroscopy of perfused human placental villi under varying oxygen concentrations. American Journal of Obstetrics and Gynecology, 168(1, Pt. 1), 246-252.

200. Ferguson, II, J. E., Seaner, R., Bruns, D. E., Redick, J. A., Mills, S. E., & Juppner, H. (April 1994). Expression of parathyroid hormone-related protein and its receptor in human umbilical cord: Evidence for a paracrine system involving umbilical vessels. American Journal of Obstetrics and Gynecology, 170(4), 1018-1026.

201. Schiff, E., Sibai, B. M., Weiner, E., Zalel, Y., & Shalev, E. (January 1993). Endothelin-1,2 levels in umbilical vein serum of second-trimester fetuses and growth-retarded third-trimester fetuses at time of cordocentesis. American Journal of Obstetrics and Gynecology, 168(1, Pt. 2), 329. SPO abstracts #104.

202. McCarthy, A. L., Woolfson, R. G., Evans, B. J., Davies, D. R., Raju, S. K., & Poston, L. (March 1994). Functional characteristics of small placental arteries. American Journal of Obstetrics and Gynecology, 170(3), 945-951.

203. Aladjem, S., Kahn, K., Dingfelder, J., Holzheimer, R., Cummings, S. R., & Michailov, D. (November 1971). Placental aspects of fetal heart rate patterns. Obstetrics & Gynecology, 38(5), 671-676.

204. Paulone, M. E., Edelstone, D. I., & Shedd, A. (January 1987). Effects of maternal anemia on uteroplacental and fetal oxidative metabolism in sheep. American Journal of Obstetrics and Gynecology, 156(1), 230-236.

205. Harvey, C. J., Hankins, G. D. V., & Synder, R. (January 1993). Maternal oxygen transport variables and fetal base excess in the sheep model: Determining predictors of fetal compromise. American Journal of Obstetrics and Gynecology, 168(1, Pt. 2), 329. SPO abstracts #105.

206. Hsieh, F., Chang, F., Ko, T., Kuo, P., Chang, D., & Chen, H. (December 1989). The antenatal blood gas acid-base status of normal fetuses and hydropic fetuses with Bart hemoglobinopathy. Obstetrics & Gynecology, 74(3), 722-725.

207. Yancy, M. K., Moore, J., Brady, K., Milligan, D., & Strampel, W. (April 1992). The effect of altitude on umbilical cord blood gases. Obstetrics & Gynecology, 79(4), 571-574.

208. Breathnach, C. S. (July 1991). The stability of the fetal oxygen environment. Irish Journal of Medical Science, 160(7), 189-191.

209. Elliott, B. D., & Langer, O. (January 1994). Fetal placental blood flow in a population at risk for growth abnormalitites and placental insufficiency. American Journal of Obstetrics and Gynecology, 170(1, Pt. 2), 314.

210. Mathews, D. D. (August 1967). The oxygen supply of the postmature foetus before the onset of labour. Journal of Obstetrics and Gynaecology of the British Commonwealth, 74(4), 523-527.

211. Alexander, L. L. (May/June 1987). The pregnant smoker: Nursing implications. JOGNN, 16(3), 167-173.

212. Fox, H. (December 1969). Pathology of the placenta in maternal diabetes mellitus. Obstetrics & Gynecology, 34(6), 792-798.

213. Dekker, G. A., & Sibai, B. M. (January 1993). Low-dose aspirin in the prevention of preeclampsia and fetal growth retardation: Rationale, mechanisms, and clinical trials. American Journal of Obstetrics and Gynecology, 168(1, Pt. 1), 214-227.

214. Hsu, C., Chan, D. W., Lriye, B., Johnson, T. R. B., Witter, F. R., & Hong, S. (1993). Elevated circulating thrombomodulin in severe preeclampsia. American Journal of Obstetrics and Gynecology, 169(1), 148-149.

215. Kilpatrick, D. C., Liston, W. A., Gibson, F., & Livingstone, J. (November 4, 1989). Association between susceptibility to pre-eclampsia within families and HLA DR4. The Lancet, 1063-1064.

216. O'Brien, W. F. (March 1990). Predicting preeclampsia. Obstetrics & Gynecology, 75(3, Pt. 1), 445-452.

217. Walsh, S. W. (April 1990). Physiology of low-dose aspirin therapy for the prevention of preeclampsia. Seminars in Perinatology, 14(2), 152-170.

218. Labarrere, C. A., & Faulk, W. P. (July 1994). Antigenic identification of cells in spiral artery trophoblastic invasion: Validation of histologic studies by triple-antibody immunocytochemistry. American Journal of Obstetrics and Gynecology, 171(1), 165-171.

219. Shimonovitz, S., Hurwitz, A., Dushnik, M., Anteby, E., Geva-Eldar, J., & Yagel, S. (September 1994). Developmental regulation of the expression of 72 and 92 Kd type IV collagenases in human trophoblasts: A possible mechanism for control of trophoblast invasion. American Journal of Obstetrics and Gynecology, 171(3), 832-843.

220. Kirschbaum, T. (April 1993). Antibiotics in the treatment of preterm labor. American Journal of Obstetrics and Gynecology, 168(4), 1239-1246.

221. Lockwood, C. J., Wein, R., Lapinski, R., Casal, D., Berkowitz, G., & Alverez, M. (October 1993). The presence of cervical and vaginal fetal fibronectin predicts preterm delivery in an inner-city obstetric population. American Journal of Obstetrics and Gynecology, 169(4), 798-804.

222. Mitchell, B. F., & Wong, S. (May 1993). Changes in 17, 20 -hydroxysteroid dehydrogenase activity supporting an increase in the estrogen/progesterone ratio of human fetal membranes at parturition. American Journal of Obstetrics and Gynecology, 168(5), 1377-1385.

223. Nageotte, M. P., Casal, D., & Senyei, A. E. (January 1994). Fetal fibronectin in patients at increased risk for premature birth. American Journal of Obstetrics and Gynecology, 170(1, Pt. 1), 20-25.

224. Blackburn, S. T., & Loper, D. L. (1992). Maternal, fetal, and neonatal physiology. A clinical perspective. Philadelphia, PA: W. B. Saunders Company.

225. Sorensen, T. K., Williams, M. A., Zingheim, R. W., Clement, S. J., & Hickok, D. E. (October 1993). Elevated second trimester human chorionic gonadotropin and subsequent pregnancy induced hypertension. American Journal of Obstetrics and Gynecology, 169(4), 834-838.

226. Roberts, W. E., Perry, Jr., K. G., Woods, J. B., Files, J. C., Blake, P. G., & Martin, Jr., J. N. (September 1994). The intrapartum platelet count in patients with HELLP (hemolysis, elevated liver enzymes, and low platelets) syndrome: Is it predictive of later hemorrhagic complications? American Journal of Obstetrics and Gynecology, 171(3), 799-804.

227. Salvesen, D. R., Higueras, M. T., Brudenell, J. M., Drury, P. L., & Nicolaides, K. H. (November 1992). Doppler velocimetry and fetal heart rate studies in nephropathic diabetics. American Journal of Obstetrics and Gynecology, 167(5), 1297-1303.

228. Seligman, S. P., Abramson, S. B., Young, B. K., & Buyon, J. P. (January 1994). The role of nitric oxide (NO) in the pathogenesis of preeclampsia. American Journal of Obstetrics and Gynecology, 170(1, Pt. 2). SPO abstracts #290.

229. Kraayenbrink, A. A., Dekker, G. A., Van Kamp, G. J., & Van Geijn, H. P. (July 1993). Endothelial vasoactive mediators in preeclampsia. American Journal of Obstetrics and Gynecology, 169(1), 160-165.

230. Mallozzi, A., Levesque, D., Vintzileos, A. M., Egan, J. F. X., Tsapanos, V., & Salafia, C. M. (January 1993). Placental pathology in discordant twins. American Journal of Obstetrics and Gynecology, 168(1, Pt. 2), 360. SPO abstracts #225.

231. Devedeux, D., Marque, C., Mansour, S., Germain, G., & Duchene, J. (December 1993). Uterine electromyography: A critical review. American Journal of Obstetrics and Gynecology, 169(6), 1636-1653.

232. Arlen, J. (December 1986). Cervical ripening and preterm labor. Obstetrics & Gynecology, 68(6), 875-876.

233. Rajabi, M., Dean, D. D., & Woessner, Jr., J. F. (February 1987). High levels of serum collagenase in premature labor-a potential biochemical marker. Obstetrics & Gynecology, 69(2), 179-186.

234. Romero, R., Baumann, P., Fidel, P., Ramirez, M., Araneda, H., & Cotton, D. B. (January 1993). Systemic and local cytokine profile in endotoxin induced preterm birth. American Journal of Obstetrics and Gynecology, 168(1, Pt. 2), 377. SPO abstracts #284.

235. Molnar, M., Romero, R., & Hertelendy, F. (October 1993). Interleukin-1 and tumor necrosis factor stimulate arachidonic acid release and phospholipid metabolism in human myometrial cells. American Journal of Obstetrics and Gynecology, 169(4), 825-829.

236. Barclay, C. G., Brennand, J. E., Kelly, R. W., & Calder, A. A. (September 1993). Interleukin-8 production by the human cervix. American Journal of Obstetrics and Gynecology, 169(3), 625-632.

237. Booker, S. S., Jayanetti, C., Karalak, S., Hsiu, J-G., & Archer, D. F. (July 1994). The effect of progesterone on the accumulation of leukocytes in the human endometrium. American Journal of Obstetrics and Gynecology, 171(1), 139-142.

238. Cherouny, P. H., Pankuch, G. A., Romero, R., Botti, J. J., Kuhn, D. C., & Demers, L. M. (November 1993). Neutrophil attractant/activating peptide-1/interleukin-8: Association with histologic chorioamnionitis, preterm delivery, and bioactive amniotic fluid leukoattractants. American Journal of Obstetrics and Gynecology, 169(5), 1299-1303.

239. Zuspan, F. P., Cibils, L. A., & Pose, S. V. (October 1, 1962). Myometrial and cardiovascular responses to alterations in plasma epinephine and norepinephine. American Journal of Obstetrics and Gynecology, 84(7), 841-851.

240. Morgan, M. A., Honnebier, M. B. O. M., Myers, T., Winter, J., Mecenas, C., & Nathaniels, P. W. (January 1994). Cocaine's effect on oxytocin in the baboon during late pregnancy. American Journal of Obstetrics and Gynecology, 170(1, Pt. 2). SPO abstracts #170.

241. Morgan, M. A., Wentworth, R. A., Silavin, S. L., Jenkins, S. L., Fishburne, Jr., J. I., & Nathaniels, P. W. (May 1994). Intravenous administration of cocaine stimulates gravid baboon myometrium in the last third of gestation. American Journal of Obstetrics and Gynecology, 170(5, Pt.1), 1416-1420.

242. Kofinas, A. D., Simon, N. V., Clay, D., & King, K. (January 1993). Functional asymmetry of the human myometrium documented by color and pulse-wave doppler ultrasonographic evaluation of uterine arcuate arteries during Braxton Hicks contractions. American Journal of Obstetrics and Gynecology, 168(1, Pt. 1), 184-188.

243. Oosterhof, H., Dijkstra, K., & Aarnoudse, J. G. (1992). Fetal doppler velocimetry in the internal carotid and umbilical artery during Braxton Hicks contractions. Early Human Development, 30, 33-40.

244. Shields, L. E., & Brace, R. A. (July 1994). Fetal vascular pressure responses to nonlabor uterine contractions: Dependence on amniotic fluid volume in the ovine fetus. American Journal of Obstetrics and Gynecology, 171(1), 84-89.

245. Initiation of labor workshop: Attempting to understand a perplexing process. (April 1988). Research Reports for NICHD.

246. Mazor, M., Romero, R., Chaim, W., Hershkowitz, R., Levy, J., & Sepulveda, W. (January 1993). Evidence for a local change in the progesterone/estrogen ratio in preterm parturition. American Journal of Obstetrics and Gynecology, 168(1, Pt. 2), 327. SPO abstracts #97.

247. Chow, L., & Lye, S. J. (March 1994). Expression of the gap junction protein connexin-43 is increased in the human myometrium toward term and with the onset of labor. American Journal of Obstetrics and Gynecology, 170(3), 788-795.

248. Lieppman, R. E., Williams, M. A., Cheng, E. Y., Resta, R., Zingheim, R., & Hickok, D. E. (June 1993). An association between elevated levels of human chorionic gonadotropin in the midtrimester and adverse pregnancy outcome. American Journal of Obstetrics and Gynecology, 168(6, Pt. 1), 1852-1857.

249. Jackson, G. M., Sharp, H. T., & Varner, M. W. (October 1994). Cervical ripening before induction of labor: A randomized trial of prostaglandin E$_2$ gel versus low-dose oxytocin. American Journal of Obstetrics and Gynecology, 171(4), 1092-1096.

250. Erny, R., Pigne, A., Prouvost, C., Gamerre, M., Malet, C., & Serment, H. (March 1986). The effects of oral administration of progesterone for premature labor. American Journal of Obstetrics and Gynecolgy, 154(3), 525-529.

251. Arnaudeau, S., Lepretre, N., & Mironneau, J. (August 1994). Chloride and monovalent ion-selective cation currents activated by oxytocin in pregnant rat myometrial cells. American Journal of Obstetrics and Gynecology, 171(2), 491-501.

252. Kulb, N. W. (1993). Preterm labor. In K. Buckley & N. W. Kulb (Eds.). High risk maternity nursing manual (2nd ed) (pp. 350-366). Baltimore, MD: Williams and Wilkins.

253. Higby, K., Xenakis, E. M. J., & Pauerstein, C. J. (April 1993). Do tocolytic agents stop preterm labor? A critical and comprehensive review of efficacy and safety. American Journal of Obstetrics and Gynecology, 168(4), 1247-1259.

254. Balducci, J., Risek, B., Gilula, N. B., Hand, A., Egan, J. F., & Vintzileos, A. M. (May 1993). Gap junction formation in human myometrium: A key to preterm labor? American Journal of Obstetrics and Gynecology, 168(5), 1609-1615.

255. Whitley, N. (September/October 1975). Uterine contractile physiology: Application in nursing care and patient teaching. JOGNN, 4(5), 54-58.

256. Freeman, R. K., & Garite, T. J., (1981). Fetal heart rate monitoring. Baltimore, MD: Williams & Wilkins.

257. Meizner, I., Levy, A., & Katz, M. (February/March 1993). Assessment of uterine and umbilical artery velocimetry during latent and active phases of normal labor. Israel Journal of Medical Sciences, 29(2-3), 82-85.

258. Bleker, O. P., Kloosterman, G. J., Mieras, D. J., Oosting, J., & Salle, H. J. A. (December 1, 1975). Intervillous space during uterine contractions in human subjects: An ultrasonic study. American Journal of Obstetrics and Gynecology, 123(7), 697-699.

259. Borell, U., Fernstrom, I., Ohlson, L., & Wiqvist, N. (September 1, 1965). Influence of uterine contractions on the uteroplacental blood flow at term American Journal of Obstetrics and Gynecology, 93(1), 44-57.

260. Burke, M. E. (October 1989). Hypertensive crisis and the perinatal period. Journal of Perinatal and Neonatal Nursing, 3(2), 33-47.

261. Friedman, E.A. (1983). Physiology of labor. In W. R. Cohen & E. A. Friedman (Eds.). Managernent of labor (pp. 1-9). Baltimore, MD: University Park Press.

262. Brotanek, V., Hendricks, C. H., & Yoshida, T. (April 15, 1969). Changes in uterine blood flow during uterine contractions. American Journal of Obstetrics and Gynecology, 103(8), 1108-1116.

263. Peebles, D. M., Edwards, A. D., Wyatt, J. S., Bishop, A. P., Cope, M., & Delpy, D. T. (May 1992). Changes in human fetal cerebral hemoglobin concentration and oxygenation during labor measured by near-infrared spectroscopy. American Journal of Obstetrics and Gynecology, 166(5), 1369-1373.

264. Wallerstedt, C., Higgins, P., Kasnic, T., & Curet, L. B. (September 1994). Amnioinfusion: An update [Principles and Practice]. JOGNN, 23, 573-378.

265. Miller, Jr., J. M., Boudreaux, M. C., & Regan, F. A. (January 1995). A case-control study of cocaine use in pregnancy. American Journal of Obstetrics and Gynecology, 172(1, Pt. 1),180-185.

266. Dicke, J. M., Verges, D. K., & Polakoski, K. L. (April 1994). The effects of cocaine on neutral amnio acid uptake by human placental basal membrane vesicles. American Journal of Obstetrics and Gynecology, 171(2), 485-491.

267. Hurd, W. W., Gauvin, J. M., Dombrowski, M. P., & Hayashi, R. H. (September 1993). Cocaine selectively inhibits β-adrenergic receptor binding in pregnant human myometrium. American Journal of Obstetrics and Gynecology, 169(3), 644-649.

268. Monga, M., Weisbrodt, N. W., Andres, R. L., & Sanborn, B. M. (October 1993). The acute effect of cocaine exposure on pregnant human myometrial contractile activity. American Journal of Obstetrics and Gynecology, 169(4), 782-785.

269. Monga, M., Weisbrodt, N. W., Andres, R. L., & Sanborn, B. M. (December 1993). Cocaine acutely increases rat myometrial contractile activity by mechanisms other than potentiation of adrenergic pathways. American Journal of Obstetrics and Gynecology, 169(6), 1502-1506.

270. Morgan, B. (1994). Maternal anesthesia and analgesia in labor. In D. K. James, P. J. Steer, C. P. Weiner, & B. Gonik (Eds.), High risk obstetrics: Management options (pp. 1101-1108). Philadelphia, PA: W. B. Saunders Company.

271. Christmas, J. T., McGhee, P. H., Dinsmoor, M. J., Irons, S. J., Dawson, K. S., & Kish, C. W. (January 1993). Preterm labor: The effect of recent substance use on the occurrence of preterm delivery. American Journal of Obstetrics and Gynecology, 168(1, Pt. 2), 371. SPO abstracts #262.

272. Cowan, D. B. (August 30, 1980). Intrapartum fetal resuscitation. South African Medical Journal, 58(9), 376-379.

273. Goldsmith, J. (Fall 1995). Newborn research depends on partnerships. Reflections, 21(3), 6-8.

274. Siddiqi, T. A., Meyer, R.A., Lynch-Salamon, D., Rosenn, B., Jaekle, R. K., & Khoury, J. (January 1994). A prospective longitudinal study of human umbilical arterial blood flow. American Journal of Obstetrics and Gynecology, 170(1, Pt. 2).

275. Yeh, M-N., Morishima, H. O., Niemann, W. H., & James, L. S. (April 1, 1975). Myocardial conduction defects in association with compression of the umbilical cord [Fetus, Placenta, and Newborn]. American Journal of Obstetrics and Gynecology, 121(7), 951-957.

276. Vaughan, J. I., Warwick, R., Letsky, E., Nicolini, U., Rodeck, C. H., & Fisk, N. M. (July 1994). Erythropoietic suppression in fetal anemia because of kell alloimmunization. American Journal of Obstetrics and Gynecology, 171(1), 247-252.

277. Davis, L. E., Hohimer, A. R., & Brace, R. A. (January 1994). Lymph flow during chronic fetal anemia. American Journal of Obstetrics and Gynecology, 170(1, Pt. 2), 311. SPO abstracts #122.

278. Christmas, J. T., Vanner, L. V., Daniels, R. M., Bodurtha, J. N., Hays, P. M., & Redwine, F. O. (August 1994). The effect of fetomaternal bleeding on the risk of adverse pregnancy outcome in patients with elevated second-trimester maternal serum α-fetoprotein levels. American Journal of Obstetrics and Gynecology, 171(2), 315-320.

279. Hoag, R. W. (June 1986). Fetomaternal hemorrhage associated with umbilical vein thrombosis. American Journal of Obstetrics and Gynecology, 154(6), 1271-1274.

280. Ballas, S., Gitstein, S., & Kharasch, J. (1985). Fetal heart rate variation with umbilical haematoma. The Fellowship Postgraduate Medical Journal, 61, 753-755.

281. Bianchi, D. W., DeMaria, M. A., Shuber, A. P., Fougner, A. C., & Klinger, K. W. (January 1994). Fetal cells in maternal blood: Determination of purity and yield by quantitative PCR. American Journal of Obstetrics and Gynecology, 170(1, Pt. 2). SPO abstracts #38.

282. Willis, C., & Foreman, Jr., C. S. (March 1988). Chronic massive fetomaternal hemorrhage: A case report. Obstetrics & Gynecology, 71(3, Pt. 2), 459-461.

283. Welch, R., Rampling, M. W., Anwar, A., Talbert, D. G., & Rodeck, C. H. (March 1994). Changes in hemorheology with fetal intravascular transfusion. American Journal of Obstetrics and Gynecology, 170(3), 726-732.

284. Itskovitz, J., Goetzman, B. W., Roman, C., & Rudolph, A. M. (October 1984). Effects of fetal-maternal exchange transfusion on fetal oxygenation and blood flow distribution. American Journal of Physiology, 247(4, Pt. 2), H655-H660.

285. Thorp, J. A., Plapp, F. V., Cohen, G. R., Yeast, J. D., O'Kell, R. T., & Stephenson, S. (August 1990). Hyperkalemia after irradiation of packed red blood cells: Possible effects with intravascular fetal transfusion. American Journal of Obstetrics and Gynecology, 163(2), 607-609.

286. Weiner, C. P. (May 1990). The relationship between the umbilical artery systolic/diastolic ratio and umbilical blood gas measurements in specimens obtained by cordocentesis. American Journal of Obstetrics and Gynecology, 162(5), 1198-1202.

287. Gardner, K. (January/February 1993). Twin transfusion syndrome. JOGNN, 22(1), 64-71.

288. Wilcox, G. R., & Trudinger, B. J. (August 1993). Erythrocytes in fetuses with abnormal umbilical artery flow velocity waveforms. American Journal of Obstetrics and Gynecology,169(2, Pt. 1), 379-383.

289. Stevenson, D. K., Bucalo, R., Cohen, R. S., Vreman, H. J., Ferguson, II, J. E., & Schwartz, H. C. (January 1986). Increased immunoreactive erythropoietin in cord plasma and neonatal bilirubin production in normal term infants after labor. Obstetrics & Gynecology, 67(1), 69-73.

290. Widness, J. A., Clemons, G. K., Garcia, J. F., Oh, W., & Schwartz, R. (January 15, 1984). Increased immunoreactive erythropoietin in cord serum after labor. American Journal of Obstetrics and Gynecology, 148(2), 194-197.

291. Richey, S. D., Ramin, S. M., Bawdon, R. E., Roberts, S. W., Dax, J., & Roberts, J. (April 1995). Markers of acute and chronic asphyxia in infants with meconium-stained amniotic fluid. American Journal of Obstetrics and Gynecology, 172(4, Pt. 1), 1212-1215.

292. Duckworth, M. W. (1961). Tissue changes accompanying acclimatization to low atmospheric oxygen in the rat. Journal of Physiology, 156, 603-610.

293. Lemery, D., Santolaya, J., Serre, A., Denoix, S., Besse, G., & Jacquetin, B. (January 1993). Comparison between serum erythropoietin of AGA and SGA fetuses. American Journal of Obstetrics and Gynecology, 168(1, Pt. 2), 329. SPO abstracts #103.

294. Papile, L. A. (September 29-30, 1995). General session: The timing of perinatal brain injury. In Current concepts and controversies in perinatal care. Symposium conducted at the Sheraton Inn. Albuquerque, NM.

295. Phelan, J. P., Ahn, M. O., Korst, L., & Martin, G. I. (January 1994). Nucleated red blood cells: A marker for fetal asphyxia. American Journal of Obstetrics and Gynecology, 170(1, Pt. 2), 286. SPO abstracts #49.

296. Pleet, H. (June 1981). Central nervous system and facial defects associated with maternal hyperthermia at four to fourteen weeks of gestation. Pediatrics, 67(6), 785-789.

297. Yoneyama, Y., Shin, S. Iwasaki, T., Power, G. G., & Araki, T. (September 1994). Relationship between plasma adenosine concentration and breathing movements in growth-retarded fetuses. American Journal of Obstetrics and Gynecology, 171(3), 701-706.

298. Ball, R. H., Espinoza, M. I., Parer, J. T., Alon, E., Vertommen, J., & Johnson, J. (January 1994). Regional blood flow in asphyxiated fetuses with seizures. American Journal of Obstetrics and Gynecology, 170(1, Pt. 1), 156-161.

299. Harvey, C. J., & Hankins, G. D. V. (January 1994). The effect of pulmonary shunting (Qs/Qt) on fetal arterial hemoglobin saturation in the sheep model. American Journal of Obstetrics and Gynecology, 170(1, Pt. 2).

300. Gleason, C. A., Hamm, C., & Jones, Jr., M. D. (April 1990). Effect of acute hypoxemia on brain blood flow and oxygen metabolism in immature fetal sheep. American Journal of Physiology, 258(4, Pt. 2), H1064-H1069.

301. Egerman, R. S., & Bissonnette, J. M. (January 1993). The effects of centrally administered adenosine on fetal sheep heart rate accelerations. American Journal of Obstetrics and Gynecology, 168(1, Pt. 2), 327. SPO abstracts #98.

302. Egerman, R. S., Bissonnette, J. M., & Hohimer, A. R. (October 1993). The effects of centrally administered adenosine on fetal sheep heart rate accelerations. American Journal of Obstetrics and Gynecology, 169(4), 866-869.

303. Mason, B. A., Ogunyemi, D., Punla, O., & Koos, B. J. (May 1993). Maternal and fetal cardiorespiratory responses to adenosine in sheep. American Journal of Obstetrics and Gynecology, 168(5), 1558-1561.

304. Weiner, C. P., Power, G., & Yoneyama, Y. (January 1993). Adenosine in the human fetus. American Journal of Obstetrics and Gynecology, 168(1, Pt. 2), 328. SPO abstracts #99.

305. Yoneyama, Y., Wakatsuki, M., Sawa, R., Kamoi, S., Takahashi, H., & Shin, S. (February 1994). Plasma adenosine concentration in appropriate- and small-for-gestational-age fetuses. American Journal of Obstetrics and Gynecology, 170(2), 684-688.

306. Ortner, A., Zech, H., Humpeler, E., & Mairbaeurl, H. (1983). May high oxygen affinity of maternal hemoglobin cause fetal growth retardation? Archives of Gynecology, 234(2), 79-85.

307. Nicolaides, K. H., Bradley, R. J., Soothill, P. W., Campbell, S., Bilardo, C. M., & Gibb, D. (April 25, 1987). Maternal oxygen therapy for intrauterine growth retardation. The Lancet, 1, 942-945.

308. Adamson, S. L., Morrow, R. J., & Ritchie, J. W. K. (December 1992). Vascular resistance and the umbilical arterial velocity waveforms [Letters]. American Journal of Obstetrics and Gynecology, 167(6), 1910-1912.

309. Forouzan, I. (January 1995). Hemodynamic changes in fetuses with absent end-diastolic velocity in umbilical artery [Letters]. American Journal of Obstetrics and Gynecology, 172(1, Pt. 1), 244.

310. Fleischer, A., Schulman, H., Farmakides, G., Bracero, L., Blattner, P., & Randolph, G. (February 15, 1985). Umbilical artery velocity waveforms and intrauterine growth retardation. American Journal of Obstetrics and Gynecology, 151(4), 502-505.

311. Collins, M. H., & James, L. S. (1990). Fetal respiratory physiology. In R. D. Eden, F. H. Bachm, & M. Haire (Eds.), Assessment and care of the fetus: Physiological, clinical and medicolegal principles (pp. 17-27). Norwalk, CT: Appleton & Lange.

312. Beksac, M. S., Onderoglu, L. S., Ozdemir, K., & Karakas, U. (November 3, 1991). The validation of a computerized system for the interpretation of the antepartum fetal heart rate tracings (version 89/2.34). European Journal of Obstetrics, Gynecology and Reproductive Biology, 42(1), 9-14.

313. Ferrazzi, E., Bellotti, M., Flisi, M. L., Barbera, A., & Pardi, G. (January 1993). Cardiac doppler velocimetry and acid base balance in IUGR fetuses. American Journal of Obstetrics and Gynecology, 168(1, Pt. 2), 328.

314. Ferrazzi, E., Bellotti, M., Barbera, A., Flisi, P., Bozzetti, P., & Pardi, G. (January 1994). Peak velocity of the outflow tract of the aorta and heart rate characteristics in growth retarded fetuses. American Journal of Obstetrics and Gynecology, 170(1, Pt. 2). SPO abstracts #94.

315. Snijders, R. J. M., Ribbert, L. S. M., Visser, G. H. A., & Mulder, E. J. H. (January 1992). Numeric analysis of heart rate variation in intrauterine growth-retarded fetuses: A longitudinal study. American Journal of Obstetrics and Gynecology, 166(1, Pt. 1), 22-27.

316. Emory, E. K., & Noonan, J. R. (August 1984). Fetal cardiac responding: A correlate of birth weight and neonatal behavior. Child Development, 55(4), 1651-1657.

317. Penning, D. H., Grafe, M. R., Hammond, R., Matsuda, Y., Patrick, J., & Richardson, B. (May 1994). Neuropathology of the near-term and midgestation ovine fetal brain after sustained in utero hypoxemia. American Journal of Obstetrics and Gynecology, 170(5, Pt. 1), 1425-1432.

318. Ang, C. K., Tan, T. H., Walters, W. A. W., & Wood, C. (October 25, 1969). Postural influence on maternal capillary oxygen and carbon dioxide tension. British Medical Journal, 4, 201-203.

319. Ogunyemi, D., Castro, L., Allen, L., Hobel, C., & Roll, K. (January 1994). Effects of tobacco use and tobacco + cocaine use on fetal growth and uterine flow velocity waveforms. American Journal of Obstetrics and Gynecology, 170(1, Pt. 2). SPO abstracts #467.

Notes

5

Acid-Base Balance

INTRODUCTION

Fetal acid-base equilibrium is reflected by fetal movement, fetal heart rate (FHR) accelerations, and baseline short-term variability (1-2). This chapter defines terms related to acid-base balance and describes animal and human fetal responses to biochemical changes. Fetal heart rate patterns that reflect acid-base changes are presented. Maternal factors and/or conditions that may limit fetal oxygen delivery are discussed.

ACIDS, BASES, AND BUFFERS

An *acid* is a hydrogen (H^+) ion donor. For example, carbonic acid (H_2CO_3) in the plasma splits into H^+, an acid, and bicarbonate (HCO_3^-), a base and buffer. *Bases* are H^+ ion acceptors (3). HCO_3^- can recombine with H^+ forming carbonic acid. This maintains a normal pH (4). pH reflects acidity of body fluids and is calculated as the negative logarithm of the grams of H^+ ions. A pH of 5 is a concentration of .00001 or 10^{-5} grams of H^+ in a liter of solution (5). As the H^+ level increases, pH decreases, and acidity increases.

The formula for pH is pH = pK + log HCO_3^-/CO_2. pK reflects the potassium (K^+) concentration in body fluids. pH increases or decreases as HCO_3^- and carbon dioxide (CO_2) increase or decrease. HCO_3^- is the metabolic component of pH; CO_2 is the respiratory component. With metabolic acidosis, HCO_3^- molecules are consumed and pH decreases. With respiratory acidosis, CO_2 increases, creating carbonic acid, free H^+ ions, and pH decreases (6). Blood H^+, HCO_3^-, oxygen (SO_2 and PO_2), carbon dioxide (PCO_2), lactate, buffer base, and base excess (BE) may be analyzed to determine fetal acid-base status. BE, a measurement of metabolic acidosis or alkalosis, expresses the amount of acid or alkali needed to titrate 1 liter of fully oxygenated blood to a pH of 7.40 at a temperature of 37° C and a PCO_2 of 40 mm Hg (7). A negative BE is a positive base deficit (BD). For example a BE of -15 mEq/L is the same as a BD of 15 mEq/L. The only difference in BD or BE is the sign (8). BE, rather than BD, will be consistently used in this chapter.

Buffers are weak acids and bases which bind with excess H^+ to maintain fetal tissue and blood acid-base balance. The principle buffer systems that regulate pH are the bicarbonate-carbonic acid system which is present in all body fluids, the phosphate system in the kidneys, the hemoglobin-oxyhemoglobin system, and the protein buffer system in cells and plasma. Examples of buffers include HCO_3^- and proteins in the plasma, and hemoglobin (Hb) in the red blood cells (RBCs) (9). The placenta and kidneys remove excess H^+ from fetal blood (10-11). For example, intracellular phosphate or ammonia binds with H^+ and is excreted in the urine as a weak acid (12-13).

DEFINITION OF TERMS

Oxygen deprivation may precede the development of any one of the following acid-base disorders:
1. hypoxemia
2. hypoxia
3. acidemia
4. hypercapnia (hypercarbia)
5. respiratory acidosis
6. metabolic acidosis
7. mixed acidosis
8. anoxia or
9. asphyxia.

Figure 5.1 illustrates the continuum from aerobic metabolism to asphyxia.

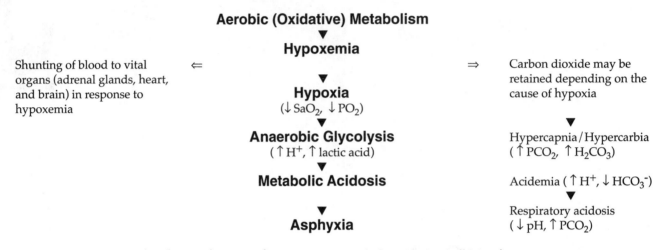

(Asphyxia = hypoxia + hypercapnia + metabolic acidosis + cell injury)

Figure 5.1: The continuum from hypoxemia to asphyxia. Aerobic metabolism ceases without oxygen. Tissue hypoxia precedes anaerobic glycolysis and ATP depletion and the development of metabolic acidosis and asphyxia.

Asphyxiated fetuses develop flat electroencephalograms (EEGs) (14). Prior to changes in their EEG, they change their FHR (15). If the FHR pattern is frequently evaluated, for example, every 15 minutes in a high-risk pregnancy, it is possible to discover a fetus suffering from hypoxia prior to the onset of metabolic acidosis and asphyxia.

Hypoxemia

Hypoxemia is an *arterial blood* O_2 deficiency (16-17). Fetal hypoxemia differs from hypoxia (18). *Hypoxemia precedes hypoxia*, acidemia, metabolic acidosis, and asphyxia (19).

Hypoxia

Hypoxia is a *tissue* O_2 deficiency, indirectly measured as an abnormally low SaO_2 and PaO_2 (16-17, 20-22). During hypoxia, tissue O_2 is inadequate to meet oxidative metabolic demands (21). **Isocapnic hypoxia** is hypoxia with normal PCO_2. **Hypercapnic hypoxia** is hypoxia with an accumulation of CO_2 (23).

Total blood O_2 content may be measured to diagnose hypoxia. The mass weight of ions is measured as millimoles per liter (mmol/L). The valence of ions is measured as milliequivalents per liter (mEq/L). Hypoxia exists when fetal blood O_2 content is less than 4.2 mmol/L or 4.2 mEq/L (24). Progressive, untreated intrapartum hypoxia precedes acidemia, metabolic acidosis, and asphyxia (25).

Acidemia: Whose Hydrogen Is It?

Acidemia is an abnormally high *blood* H^+ ion concentration (16, 20). A change in pH may change tissue O_2 availability if there is a right or left shift of the oxyhemoglobin dissociation curve (26). **Lacticemia** is the accumulation of lactic acid, accompanied by a pH drop (23). The decrease in pH causes a right shift in the oxyhemoglobin dissociation curve, decreasing hemoglobin O_2 affinity, freeing O_2 for tissue use.

Infusion Acidosis. Sometimes fetal scalp blood pH is very low, the baby is delivered by cesarean section, and is born undamaged with high Apgar scores. In this case, the low pH was probably a mix of maternal and fetal H^+ ions. Infusion acidosis is a process where maternal H^+ enters fetal circulation and lowers fetal pH (1). Since fetal pH is lower than maternal pH (7.25 to 7.35 versus 7.35 to 7.52), a chemical gradient exists. Maternal H^+ enters the fetal circulation in the placenta (moving from a high concentration to a low concentration) to establish an equilibrium, especially when women are hypoxic or metabolically acidotic (27). If a woman is acidemic, it takes approximately four hours for her pH and fetal pH to equilibrate (28).

While different samples of pregnant women may have slightly different blood gases, they are similar. The following maternal (non-laboring) norms were created from the work of several physicians (3, 9, 13, 29-32):

Table 1: Maternal Arterial Norms

pH	7.35 - 7.52
Lactate	0.1 - 0.5 mEq/L
Pa0$_2$	76 - 105.4 mm Hg
SaO$_2$	95 - 97%
PaCO$_2$	23.9 - 49 mm Hg
Bicarbonate	15.7 - 26 mEq/L
Base excess	-4.7 - -0.7 mEq/L

Maternal position does not alter *maternal* arterial blood gases. Ten normotensive women spent 30 minutes on their left side prior to turning to a left lateral, right lateral, supine, sitting, standing, or knee-chest position for 10 minutes, at which time a sample of arterial blood was drawn. In all these positions, there was no significant difference in maternal arterial blood gases (31).

Maternal alkalosis. *Women in labor may become alkalotic.* *Metabolic* alkalosis may be a result of excessive vomiting which causes a relative increase in HCO_3^- due to the loss of H^+ in stomach acid. Maternal hyperventilation, due to progesterone stimulation of respiratory centers, may cause *respiratory* alkalosis which is diagnosed by an abnormally low extracellular $PaCO_2$, and a high pH. Intracellular pH values decrease during pregnancy (33-34). Maternal and fetal $PaCO_2$ decrease when women hyperventilate due to the change in the CO_2 fetal-maternal gradient (35). A drop in fetal $PaCO_2$ has no negative consequences (36).

If women become uncomfortable or light headed as a result of hyperventilation, it may be helpful to instruct them to put their hands together and cover their mouth and nose while slowing down their respiratory rate. Ask them to breathe deeply and slowly. Short-term application of an operating room mask over the woman's nose and mouth or the classic "brown paper bag" may increase CO_2 inhalation.

Maternal ketoacidosis. The prolonged lack of food during labor or dehydration results in an increase in blood lactate lowering maternal pH. For example, during early labor 1.4% of women were acidemic, during transition (7 to 10 centimeters (cm) dilatation) 2.4% were acidemic, and, during the second stage 9.6% were acidemic (37). In addition to the rise in lactate and fall in pH, the deprivation of food results in metabolism of fat stores with ketone production and metabolism of glucose stores which increases CO_2.

Ketoacidosis, secondary to the burning of fat for energy, is seen in its most severe form during starvation and uncontrolled diabetes mellitus. A diabetic woman, with ketoacidosis as a result of anaerobic lipolysis, has a lower than normal pH (38). Severe ketoacidosis can cause maternal coma or death. Ketoacidosis may be treated by administering intravenous (IV) dextrose, such as a solution of 5% or 10% dextrose in lactated Ringers and large doses of insulin. IV dextrose may correct maternal ketonemia but at the same time decrease pH as it increases maternal and fetal lactate (39-40). In addition, aerobic glucose metabolism produces CO_2, increasing maternal CO_2 levels. The high maternal $PaCO_2$ changes the transplacental maternal-fetal gradient and the fetus accumulates CO_2. The additional fetal CO_2 combines with water (H_2O) in the plasma to form carbonic acid (H_2CO_3) which releases H^+ and decreases fetal pH (41). Thus, maternal ketoacidosis, even when treated, may create a false low pH.

If the woman is diabetic or has an intrauterine growth restricted (IUGR) fetus, there is an increased risk of fetal asphyxia in the presence of ketoacidosis. Fetuses of diabetic women also have an increased risk of hyperinsulinemia, hypoglycemia, and asphyxial damage (41). IUGR fetuses may also be hypoglycemic and hypoinsulinemic with oligohydramnios, increasing their risk of asphyxial damage (42-44). A low pH in these fetuses should be perceived as a true low pH until complete blood gases are obtained.

Acidosis

Acidosis is a pathologic condition defined as increased H^+ ions *in the tissues* and a pH less than 7.20 (16, 20). There are two types of acidosis, respiratory and metabolic. A pH value without other blood gases can only describe the presence or absence of acidemia. When the blood pH is less then 7.20, the fetus is acidemic and may have acidosis. If the other acid-base parameters are known, the diagnosis of respiratory, metabolic, or mixed acidosis can be made.

Table 2: Umbilical Artery pH and Description from the Literature

pH	Description
7.10 to 7.20	Lower limit of normal
7.15	Moderate acidemia
7.10	Significant acidemia
7.05-7.10	Less acidotic than a pH of 7.04
7.05	Severe acidosis, severe acidemia
7.04	Very acidotic
< 7.00	Extreme acidemia, severe acidemia, severe intrapartum asphyxia, clinically significant acidosis (16, 31, 44-49).

Severe Acidosis: pH 7.05 or less, BE -10 mEq/L or less. Severely acidemic preterm fetuses are more likely to have developmental delays than severely acidemic term fetuses. For example, 8.2% of term neonates with these pH and BE values had a neurologic deficit at the time of hospital discharge. But, 46.9% of preterm neonates with these values had a neurologic deficit at the time of hospital discharge. Follow up evaluation of impaired neonates at 1 year of age revealed 4.5% of the infants born at term had a minor developmental delay of tone but no major motor or cognitive abnormality. However, 18.75% of the impaired preterm neonates had a minor developmental delay at 1 year of age. 8.2% of term neonates and 43.8% of preterm neonates had mild developmental delays or tone abnormalities during their first year of life. Fortunately, the majority of infants who had a pH of 7.05 or less at birth (91.8% of the term newborns and 53.1% of the preterm newborns) had no neurologic deficits at the time of discharge from the hospital (48). Of course, any impairment, even those classified as "minor," is major to the parents.

pH less than 7.00. An umbilical artery pH less than 7.00 has been considered severe acidemia or asphyxia and may be related to neurologic impairment (46, 50). At a pH of 7.00,

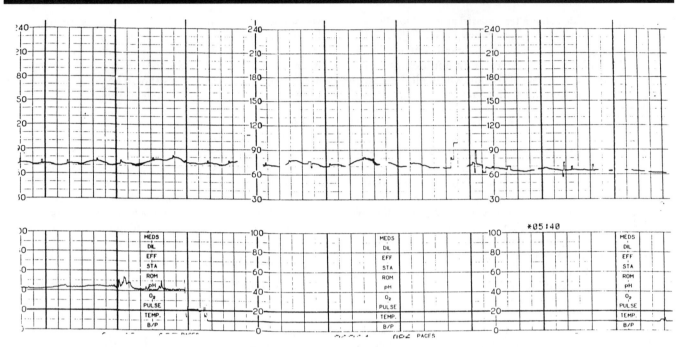

Figure 5.2: Fetal pH less than 7.00. At 39 weeks' gestation, following 2 days of an induction attempt with no cervical change, the woman checked out of the hospital against medical advice (AMA). She returned 11 days later, after a trip out of the country, with this fetal heart rate pattern. Fetal scalp pH was 6.9, terbutaline 0.25 milligrams (mg) was administered subcutaneously. An emergency cesarean section was performed. A complete abruption was noted and the fetus was stillborn.

preterm fetal lambs had a terminal fall in O_2 consumption, a rise in lactic acid, and metabolic acidemia (51). Most term human neonates with an umbilical artery pH less than 7.00 are neurologically normal. Of 129 term neonates with an umbilical artery pH less than 7.00, 4% died, 30% had an abnormal neurologic outcome including early seizures, *but 66% were neurologically normal at the time of discharge from the hospital* (45). In another study, 30 newborns with an umbilical artery pH less than 7.00 were admitted to the neonatal intensive care unit (NICU) but discharged without major problems. They had a "good outcome" at their 19 month follow-up examination. Four of the infants (14%) had mild hypertonia or a mild motor delay (52).

A pH less than 7.00, a BE less than -20 mEq/L, and a 10 minute Apgar score less than 3 can be expected when a normal FHR pattern precedes a sudden catastrophic event such as a complete placental abruption, uterine rupture, umbilical cord prolapse, or maternal cardiopulmonary arrest. Often birth is preceded by a prolonged deceleration near 60 beats per minute (bpm) (53-54).

If the pH is 7.00 or less and the 1 minute Apgar score is 3 or less, the risk of neonatal complications and seizures is high. A pH less than 7.00 was associated with a 5 minute Apgar score of 7 or less, intubation, respiratory and neurologic complications, NICU admission, meconium aspiration syndrome, and hypotonia (23, 55). If the pH was *7.00 or higher* and the 1 minute Apgar score was 3 or less, 14% of neonates were hypotonic and 4% seized. If the pH was *7.00 or less* and the 1

minute Apgar was 3 or less, 100% of the neonates needed resuscitation and 50% had neurologic dysfunction with hypotonia and seizures (23). In the very small neonate, who weighs 1000 or fewer grams, the pH and BE were inversely related to the number of days with intubation and mechanical ventilation (56). Of 28 preterm fetuses who were *34 or more weeks' gestation* with an umbilical artery pH less than 7.00, there were:

3 neonatal deaths (10.7%)
24 with a 1 minute Apgar score less than 7 (85.7%)
15 with a 5 minute Apgar score less than 7 (53.6%)
11 with a 1 minute Apgar score of 3 or less (39.3%)
6 with a 5 minute Apgar score of 3 or less (21.4%)
9 with *no significant morbidity* who were admitted
    to the normal nursery (32.2%)
19 were admitted to the NICU (42.8%) (57).

These findings suggest that 1 out of 10 neonates who are more than 34 weeks' gestation with a pH less than 7.00 may die but almost 1/3rd will have no significant problems. Newborns admitted to the NICU have an increased incidence of organ dysfunction. In this sample, 12 of the 19 babies admitted to the NICU had organ dysfunction (42.8%). *Seizures occurred in all babies who had an Apgar score of 3 or less at 1 minute.* About a third (32.1%) had pulmonary dysfunction and 2 babies (17.8%) developed hypoxic-ischemic encephalopathy (57).

Hypercapnia

Hypercapnia, also called hypercarbia, is increased blood CO_2 (20). Fetal hypercapnia may have a maternal or fetal cause. For example, CO_2 and H^+ are retained during maternal hypoventilation, e.g., following a drug overdose. Excess maternal CO_2 will be transferred to the fetus. If the umbilical cord is compressed repeatedly or the placenta abrupts, fetal CO_2 accumulates. When CO_2 increases, pH decreases and there will be *fewer accelerations* in the FHR (58). After birth, hypercapnia and hypoxemia rapidly resolve during positive pressure ventilation (59).

Respiratory Acidosis

Hypercapnia precedes respiratory acidosis. The retention of CO_2 and H^+ causes *respiratory* acidosis. Respiratory acidosis has occurred in as many as 91% of fetuses that had a nuchal cord (49). Respiratory acidosis is evident by an umbilical artery PCO_2 greater than 65 mm Hg, a pH less than 7.20, a BE greater than -9 mEq/L, and a HCO_3^- level greater than or equal to 22 mEq/L (16). When CO_2 accumulates in the plasma and combines with plasma water, carbonic acid (H_2CO_3) increases. Accumulated H_2CO_3 is rapidly excreted across the placenta if blood flow is restored in a reasonable period of time (60).

Respiratory acidosis is NOT associated with damage to the neonate's central nervous system (CNS), cardiovascular, respiratory, or renal systems (45, 61). On the other hand,

severe *metabolic* acidosis and asphyxia can damage these systems (62). *Recurrent variable decelerations or a prolonged deceleration* of the FHR due to umbilical cord compression may precede respiratory acidosis. As is true with hypercapnia, a neonate born with respiratory acidosis is usually responsive to positive pressure ventilation (59).

Metabolic Acidosis

Hypoxia precedes anaerobic metabolism which causes the accumulation of L-lactic acid and the development of metabolic acidosis. Anaerobic glycolysis produces L-lactic acid, which lowers pH (20, 63). Fetal metabolic acidosis is diagnosed when there is an umbilical artery PCO_2 less than 65 mm Hg, a BE of -13 mEq/L or less, and a HCO_3^- level of 17 mEq/L or less (16, 44, 48). Others have defined metabolic acidosis by a BE less than -9 mm Hg and a pH less than 7.15 (64).

Mixed Acidosis

Mixed acidosis is respiratory and metabolic acidosis. The umbilical artery pH will be less than 7.20. PCO_2 will be 65 or more mm Hg with a BE less than -13 mEq/L and HCO_3^- of 17 mEq/L or less. Mixed respiratory and metabolic acidosis *without* hypoxia may occur when a fetus has a combination of simultaneously occurring metabolic and respiratory acidosis but O_2 delivery has been reestablished by interventions such as hyperoxygenation and an IV bolus. The nonhypoxic fetus will have a PO_2 of 18 mm Hg or more (16).

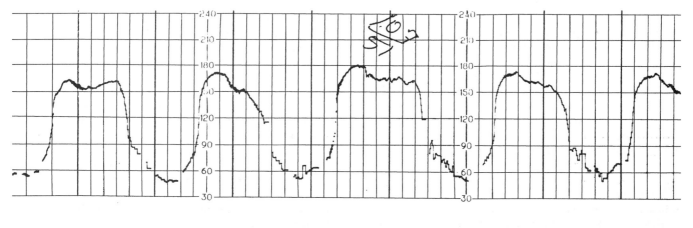

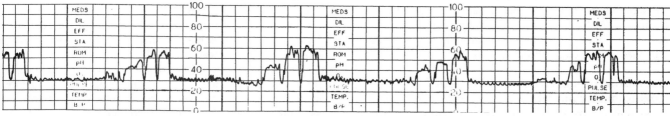

Figure 5.3: Acidemia and hypercapnia. This was the second pregnancy of a woman who had a previous cesarean section after pushing two hours and a failed vacuum extraction. This tracing was observed when she was completely dilated with the fetus at a zero station in a right occiput anterior position. She had an epidural, membranes were ruptured, and she pushed approximately one hour with this pattern. Following a successful vaginal birth after cesarean (VBAC), the Apgar scores were 7, 8, and 9 at 1, 5, and 10 minutes. The newborn required blow-by oxygen and weighed 7 lbs 12 ounces. Umbilical artery blood gases revealed acidemia with hypercapnia: pH 7.19, PO_2 23 mm Hg, PCO_2 62 mm Hg, bicarbonate 22 mEq/L, and base excess of -7.5 mEq/L.

Anoxia

Anoxia is the *total lack of tissue O_2*. Postmature fetuses have an increased risk of anoxia due to placental insufficiency (65). Hypoglycemic IUGR fetuses are more prone to tissue damage during periods of anoxia than euglycemic fetuses because they lack glucose for anaerobic metabolism (66).

Cerebral anoxia can precede circulatory collapse with decreased cerebral blood flow. Anoxia precedes metabolic acidosis, lactate accumulation, a drop in pH, glucose and adenosine triphosphate (ATP) depletion, and brain damage (66). *Nerve damage occurs after 10 to 12 minutes of anoxia (in rhesus monkeys). Hypoxia and metabolic acidosis that last two or more hours also cause nerve damage* (67). Umbilical cord prolapse, uterine rupture, and amniotic fluid embolism are examples of acute anoxic insults. All require immediate delivery after maternal stabilization. Delivery is usually by cesarean section.

ASPHYXIA AND TISSUE DAMAGE
Asphyxia

Asphyxia results from cessation of placental gas exchange with subsequent damaging acidemia, hypoxia, hypercapnia, metabolic acidosis, and tissue ischemia. Ischemia is decreased blood flow with reduced tissue perfusion and oxygenation (16, 20, 23, 50, 54, 68-70, 72). Tissue ischemia precedes an increase in intracellular calcium (Ca^{++}) and the release of toxins, such as glutamate, which cause cell death. Brain cell death precedes seizures (73-74).

In July, 1995, the American College of Obstetricians and Gynecologists (ACOG) defined asphyxia as hypoxia with metabolic acidosis (20). While hypoxia and metabolic acidosis contribute to asphyxia, they are not asphyxia. The diagnosis of asphyxia is based on evidence of ischemia, i.e., organ dysfunction such as cardiovascular, renal, hematologic, gastrointestinal, and/or pulmonary system disturbances (75). Asphyxia may precede fetal death due to irreversible cell damage (69). The process preceding cell damage and death includes the accumulation of glutamate, the loss of adenosine triphosphate (ATP), and the production of oxygen free radicals.

Glutamate

Glutamate is an excitatory amino acid and brain nerve impulse transmitter. As the fetus becomes progressively more metabolically acidotic, glutamate levels increase and become neurotoxic. At the same time, ATP production decreases and ATP is degraded for anaerobic metabolism (74). Glutamate damaged animal brain cells (76).

Adenosine Triphosphate (ATP) Depletion and Adenosine Accumulation

Persistent hypoxia and anaerobic metabolism precedes depletion of phosphates and ATP. ATP byproducts include adenosine diphosphate, adenosine monophosphate (AMP), and adenosine. An *AMP* byproduct is hypoxanthine, a marker of hypoxia found in cord blood. *Hypoxanthine is* catabolized by xanthine oxidase in blood vessel endothelial cells to produce oxygen free radicals. *Oxygen free radicals* damage tissue and can injure the brain (77).

Plasma adenosine and endorphins are present in asphyxiated neonates (67, 78). Adenosine is released by placental and vascular endothelium parenchymal cells and taken up by RBCs and body cells. Umbilical vein adenosine increases when there is placental ischemia, fetal hypoxia and acidemia (79). *Adenosine limits glutamate release*, therefore its accumulation may be seen as a compensatory response to hypoxia (77). A high umbilical vein adenosine level *with normal blood gases* suggests there was severe, nonlethal hypoxia more than 24 hours prior to blood gas analysis followed by normalization of pH and HCO_3^- (80). High adenosine levels impair regulation of brain blood flow. Adenosine decreases neuron signal firing and slows brain cell metabolism (81). In the heart, adenosine depresses sinoatrial node activity, atrioventricular node conduction, atrial contractility, and ventricular automaticity (82). *Adenosine accumulation will be related to a decrease in fetal brain activity, fetal movement, accelerations, and FHR variability* (12).

The half-life of adenosine is 0.6 to 1.5 seconds. In normoxic fetuses adenosine levels were 0.58 ± 0.14 μmol/L. In hypoxic neonates, umbilical vein adenosine was 1.78 ± 0.18 μmol/L. The elevation of umbilical vein adenosine suggests a significant hypoxic insult occurred and more adenosine was released than could be consumed. If umbilical artery Doppler velocimetry was abnormal, suggesting there was increased placental vascular resistance, adenosine levels were significantly higher, even in normoxic fetuses of preeclamptic women (79).

Preeclamptic women have an increased risk of fetal asphyxia due to chronic placental ischemia, placental lesions, and vasospasm (83). Chronic inflammatory lesions in the decidual vessels and basal plate of placentas of preterm fetuses born to preeclamptic women included decidual vasculitis, chronic villitis, avascular villi, and focal hemorrhagic endovasculitis (84). In spite of the increased risk of asphyxia, if preeclamptic women were managed well during their pregnancy they had a healthy neonate (85).

Potassium Leakage and Intracellular Calcium Accumulation

As a result of continuing tissue hypoxia and anaerobic metabolism, K^+ ions leak out of cells into the brain's extracellular spaces. Fetuses may become flaccid and bradycardic due to the high extracellular K^+ (12).

Sodium enters cells and depolarizes the cell membrane opening Ca^{++} channels. Ca^{++} entry into cells increases. At the same time, Ca^{++} leaves cell stores in mitochondria and the sarcoplasmic reticulum which increases intracellular Ca^{++}. *Intracellular Ca^{++} is toxic in high concentrations* and its accumulation affects enzyme function, such as the function of phospholipases (77).

Release of Free Fatty Acids and Oxygen Free Radicals

Ca^{++} activates phospholipases A and C. Phospholipases break down cell membranes causing the release of free fatty acids. Free fatty acids are converted by the enzyme cyclooxygenase to *lipid peroxides or oxygen free radicals*. Oxygen free radicals attack phospholipids in the cell wall and damage cells. The placenta does not clear lipid peroxides so umbilical artery levels will be higher than normal in acidemic fetuses (77).

Thromboxane

Cell wall destruction also causes the conversion of cell wall arachidonic acid to the prostaglandin thromboxane, a potent vasoconstrictor. The rise in thromboxane worsens ischemia (73). The following diagram summarizes these destructive events:

Hypoxia
▼
Redistribution of blood
▼
Tissue Ischemia
▼
ATP consumption
AMP accumulation ➤ hypoxanthine ➤ oxygen free radicals
➤ tissue injury
Adenosine accumulation ➤ ↓ fetal movement, ↓ variability
↓ accelerations,
▼
↑ Glutamate ➤ damages brain cells
▼
Acidemia (↑ H⁺, ↓ pH)
▼
Na⁺ and K⁺ leave cells ➤ CNS depression, flaccidity,
bradycardia
▼
↑ Cell membrane permeability
K⁺ continues to leave cells
Na⁺ enters cells
▼
Cell wall depolarization
▼
Ca^{++} channels open
▼
↑ intracellular Ca^{++}
▼
↑ Phospholipase A and C activity ➤ cell wall breakdown ➤
release of free fatty acids
▼
↑ Cyclooxygenase activity
Cyclooxygenase + free fatty acids ➤ oxygen free radicals ➤
tissue injury
Cyclooxygenase + arachidonic acid ➤ ↑ thromboxane ➤
ischemia worsens
▼
Cell wall breakdown continues ➤ intracellular edema ➤
cell damage and death
▼

Organ dysfunction
▼
Death

Figure 5.4: Glutamate, intracellular calcium, and oxygen free radicals cause cell damage. If asphyxia continues, organs become damaged and the fetus may die.

THE DIAGNOSIS OF ASPHYXIA
Partial Fetal Asphyxia

Maternal hypotension, uterine hyperstimulation, carbon monoxide inhalation, and anxiety may create partial fetal asphyxia due to diminished gas exchange within the placenta (86). Asphyxia from partial umbilical cord occlusion will be less severe than asphyxia due to uteroplacental insufficiency (87). Within five minutes of initial fetal lamb umbilical cord compression, there was an increase in blood flow to the skin, bones, and muscles (88). Eventually, blood flow diminishes and the animal becomes bradycardic and hypotensive. In partially asphyxiated monkeys, bradycardia lasting 30 or more minutes was related to fetal brain injury such as cerebral necrosis and white matter hemorrhage (86).

Acute Total Fetal Asphyxia

Anoxia precedes total fetal asphyxia. There will be a sudden increase in peripheral vascular resistance and BP followed by bradycardia and a fall in BP for a minute, a rise in BP for two minutes, then a permanent fall in BP. Within four minutes of anoxia, gasping occurs. By the *12th to 14th minute* there is a lack of brain blood flow which causes brainstem damage. The heart rate fell to 60 to 70 bpm for as long as 35 minutes, but most of the monkeys in this study died by the 20th minute after total asphyxia began. *The severity of asphyxia required to produce brain damage was of slightly less duration than asphyxia that preceded death* (86).

Biochemical and Clinical Asphyxia

By themselves, blood gases and Apgar scores do not confirm the diagnosis of neonatal asphyxia. The diagnosis of neonatal asphyxia requires blood gases reflective of hypoxia and metabolic acidosis, low Apgar scores, and organ dysfunction (16, 47). If there is no evidence of umbilical artery metabolic acidosis, *intrapartum* asphyxia did not occur (89). In 1994, in an ACOG committee opinion on fetal distress, it was stated that a neonate who had hypoxia proximate to delivery severe enough to cause hypoxic encephalopathy would have *all* of the following:
- profound metabolic or mixed acidemia (pH less than 7.00) on an umbilical cord arterial blood sample, if obtained
- a persistent Apgar score of 0 to 3 for longer than 5 minutes and
- evidence of neonatal neurologic sequelae (e.g., seizures, coma, hypotonia, and one or more of the following: cardiovascular, gastrointestinal, hematologic, pulmonary, or renal system dysfunction) (72).

Profound metabolic or mixed acidemia. *Blood gases are the biochemical component of asphyxia. Apgar scores and the condition of the neonate are the clinical component of asphyxia.* Asphyxial blood gases usually include an umbilical artery pH less than 7.20, PO_2 less than 11 mm Hg, a BE less than -10 mEq/L, and a PCO_2 greater than 65 mm Hg (90-91). Other researchers diagnose asphyxia when the pH is less than 7.15 and the HCO_3^- is less than 15 mEq/L (61).

When the fetus is hypoxic, lactate increases as a result of anaerobic glucose metabolism. The rise in lactate causes a fall in pH, BE, and the buffer base (92). A buffer base less than 30 mEq/L is equivalent to a blood BE of -16 mEq/L and an extracellular BE of -12 mEq/L. This has been classified as moderate asphyxia (59). When the buffer base is less than 34 mEq/L, there is "significant" or severe fetal asphyxia (67, 93).

Persistent Apgar score of 0 to 3 for longer than 5 minutes. *The best use of Apgar scores is to direct attention to immediate neonatal needs (70).* Apgar scores reflect the neonate's condition and may reflect intrauterine acid-base status just prior to birth (94). To predict the neonate's condition at birth, clinicians review the FHR pattern. To their surprise, a nonreassuring pattern may precede the birth of a neonate with normal blood gases which often occurs when there is a fetal anomaly (95). If the fetus is well-oxygenated, it is reasonable to expect high Apgar scores (96). A hypoxemic fetus, with a low SpO_2 during the last hour of labor, often has low Apgar scores (97). But, the best predictors of Apgar scores were birth weight and gestational age (48, 98) (see Table 3).

Table 3: Relationship Between Low Apgar Scores (< 7) at 1 and 5 minutes and Birth Weight

Weight (Grams)	Apgar < 7 at 1 minute	Apgar < 7 at 5 minutes
500-999	87%	57%
1000-1500	77%	41%
> 1500	68%	19%

In general, *Apgar scores poorly correlate with fetal acid-base status.* Fetal pH did not predict Apgar scores, Apgar scores did not predict neonatal complications, and pH did not predict neonatal complications (45-46, 71). Preterm fetuses have the lowest Apgar scores (71). Preterm fetuses who were 32 weeks' gestation or less and who weighed less than 2000 grams, and fetuses with abnormal FHR patterns, meconium, oligohydramnios, polyhydramnios, or mothers with hypertension, have low Apgar scores (73). Neonates with normal acid-base status may be born impaired (47). Acidotic fetuses may have high or low Apgar scores (71, 98-99).

When the 5 minute Apgar score is 0 to 3, it is more likely that umbilical artery blood gases will reflect biochemical asphyxia. Yet, 60.7% of neonates with a 5 minute Apgar score of 0 to 3 had a pH of 7.00 or higher and 53.6% had a pH greater than 7.10 (100). Therefore, *without confirmation of blood gases, the Apgar score cannot be used to confirm asphyxia* (16).

A 5 minute Apgar score of 0 to 3 was associated with a 1600% increased risk of fetal death and a 17 fold increased risk of cerebral palsy (70). In spite of the risks, survival following a 0 to 3 Apgar score at 10 minutes of age usually results in a good outcome, with 80% of children being free of a *major* handicap by early school age (48, 70).

Evidence of neurologic sequelae: clinical asphyxia. *Clinical asphyxia may occur in the absence of biochemical asphyxia.* In a study by Chowdhary, Narang, and Bhakoo, 60% of preterm fetuses with clinical asphyxia evidenced by low Apgar scores, did *not* have biochemical asphyxia. Some vigorously crying infants had severe acidosis (42%); others had low Apgar scores with normal pH values (93). Fetal pH poorly predicted immediate neonatal complications. However, *pH and BE were related to developmental delays* found during a follow-up examination at six months of age.

Table 4: Developmental Delay and Severity of Asphyxia (93)

Asphyxia	pH	BE (mEq/L)	6 month follow-up
Mild	7.101-7.25	-8 to -15	no evidence of delay
Moderate	7.001-7.10	-16 to -23	developmental delay
Severe	7.00	< -23	developmental delay

Some neonates, whose umbilical artery pH was greater than 7.00, were impaired with persistent hypotonia, renal or cardiac dysfunction or persistently low Apgar scores (100). Therefore, to diagnose neonatal asphyxia, ACOG suggested that all three requirements be met: the umbilical artery pH is less than 7.00, there is evidence of metabolic acidosis, and the neonatal course is abnormal (72). The abnormal neonatal course usually includes cardiopulmonary, renal, and cerebral injury evident shortly after birth (45). Cerebral injury may be diagnosed as hypoxic-ischemic encephalopathy (HIE) which includes abnormalities of consciousness, tone, and primitive reflexes, such as sucking and rooting. In severe cases of HIE, the brain is edematous, necrotic, with intracranial bleeding, and a decrease in density (101-102). Even though the neonate meets criteria and is diagnosed with asphyxia, asphyxial damage may not result in cerebral palsy. Instead, the infant may have abnormal tone or persistence of neonatal reflexes (93).

Substantiating the Diagnosis of Neonatal Asphyxia

According to the American Academy of Pediatrics, an abnormal neonatal course due to asphyxia includes early neonatal seizures, prolonged hypotonia, and an Apgar score of 0 to 3 at 10 minutes (89).

Early neonatal seizures. Seizures are not predictable based on Apgar scores. Many term neonates who seized had a 5 minute Apgar score of 7 to 10 (103). The onset of seizures does not help time the neurologic injury (104). Early seizures, during the first 24 hours of life, portend a poor outcome and are related to developmental deficits at 1 year of age in 20 to 49% of infants (105).

Blood gases do not always account for the *significance* of the asphyxial episode preceding neonatal seizures (67). In fact, the degree of acidemia required to cause fetal neurologic damage was unknown in 1991 (50). FHR, BP, biophysical behaviors, such as electroocular and nuchal muscle activities, pH, and lactate were not reflective of *the extent* of fetal lamb brain injury, because after brain injury cardiovascular parameters normalized (19, 67). Seizures have many causes besides asphyxia, such as intracranial hemorrhage, trauma, drug withdrawal, cerebral infarcts, cerebral malformations, infection such as meningitis or congenital syphilis, sepsis, and metabolic disorders such as hypoglycemia, hypocalcemia, hyponatremia, or hypomagnesemia (23, 49, 70, 103, 105).

Hypoxic-ischemic encephalopathy. Cerebral dysfunction occurs as a result of hypoxic-ischemic injury or encephalopathy. HIE is a syndrome of altered consciousness, tone, and primitive reflexes. Babies with HIE may seize (50). HIE may be diagnosed by ultrasound, computerized tomography (CT scan), magnetic resonance imaging (MRI), or a radionucleotide brain scan, but not blood gases or Apgar scores (23, 106-107). The ultrasound of the neonate's brain might reveal edema, increased echogenicity, loss of anatomical landmarks, decreased pulsations in blood vessels, compressed ventricles, and hemorrhage. The CT scan might demonstrate hypodensity, infarcts, periventricular leukomalacia (PVL), cysts (porencephaly), and ventricular dilation. The MRI might confirm infarcts, PVL, porencephaly, and even indicate a congenital anomaly (106).

Although fetal compensatory mechanisms for hypoxia act to spare the brain from permanent damage, a significant asphyxial insult can damage the brain and other organs (48). Evidence of multisystem organ dysfunction might be decreased urine output, cardiac dysfunction, impaired liver function, gastrointestinal dysfunction, coagulopathy such as disseminated intravascular coagulopathy (DIC), and lung abnormalities such as respiratory distress syndrome. Neonates with HIE usually have 1 or more of the following: persistent fetal circulation, renal dysfunction with a blood urea nitrogen of 20 or more mg/dl and a serum creatinine of 1.5 mg/dl or more, a grade III or IV intraventricular hemorrhage, and/or respiratory distress syndrome (48). HIE has three stages: mild, moderate, and severe (59). *Fetuses can pass through these stages in utero.*

Table 5: Stages of Hypoxic-Ischemic Encephalopathy

MILD	*hyperalertness,* hyperexcitable, staring, decreased blinking, normal to decreased spontaneous motor activity, decreased tolerance of stimuli, easy to elicit startle (Moro) reflex, jittery. This state reflects sympathetic/adrenergic responses and is usually self limiting and not associated with permanent disability or death.
MODERATE	*lethargic,* abnormal tone, hypotonia, suppressed primitive reflexes such as sucking, decreased spontaneous movement. Seizures will depend on extent of brain injury. There will be selective neuronal necrosis of the cerebral cortex and parts of the brain supplied by the anterior and middle cerebral arteries, e.g., the basal ganglia. This stage reflects vagal responses. In the fetus, bradycardia will be evident.
SEVERE	*seizures, stupor,* flaccidity, no primitive reflexes, subcortical and cortical infarcts, brain necrosis due to ischemia/hypoperfusion (107).

Babies with HIE will be hypotonic or floppy for 24 to 48 hours (23). Neonates with severe asphyxia and moderate or severe HIE have an increased risk for long-term neurologic disorders and death (50). *Neonatal seizures with other signs of severe neonatal encephalopathy are the strongest predictors of long-term adverse neurologic outcome* (101). In one study, a neonate with severe HIE had a 12.5% risk of dying, a 15.4% risk of neurologic impairment, and a 25% risk of neurologic handicap followed by death at an early age (107).

Table 6: Hypoxic-Ischemic Encephalopathy (HIE) and Risk of a Neurologic Deficit

MILD HIE	**MODERATE HIE**	**SEVERE HIE**
No deficits at discharge	20% adverse outcome 5% die 15% disabled	82% died, 18% disabled. Possible long term disability: spastic quadraparesis, CP, mental retardation cortical blindness, seizure disorder, neurosensory deafness (107)

ANTEPARTAL CAUSES OF CEREBRAL PALSY (CP)

Cerebral palsy is a *nonprogressive* disorder of movement, posture, and position which appears early in life. CP is also a complex set of symptoms not a disease which may manifest as spastic quadriparesis with mental retardation. However, mental retardation and seizures may not be related to birth events or CP (101). More than 300,000 children in the United States have CP (108). There are no clinical findings, such as meconium or a FHR pattern, that can be consistently linked to CP (101). Asphyxia, severe enough to cause CP, may *not* include a pH less than 7.00, Apgar scores less than 3, HIE, and multiple organ dysfunction (101, 108). To link CP to intrapartal events and birth asphyxia, Nelson (101) felt the following questions had to answered in the affirmative:

1. Was there intrapartal evidence of severe and prolonged distress?
2. Was the newborn severely ill?
3. Does the child have CP?
4. Have all other causes of CP been excluded?

Approximately 2.2 per 1000 neonates develop CP as a result of *intrapartal* asphyxia (109). Blair, Stanley & Hockey (110) found 7.65% of children with CP had asphyxia in and around the time of delivery. Combining these two statistics, it appears that approximately 5.45% of children with CP were asphyxiated prior to labor and delivery. Other causes of CP include, but are not limited to, congenital malformations, infections, metabolic abnormalities, familial disease, microcephaly, substance abuse, and thyroid disease. There may be a maternal risk factor for having a child with CP such as a seizure disorder or mental retardation.

CP is more common in low birth weight (LBW) preterm neonates who also had PVL. Twins who weighed less than 2500 grams and had a LBW for their gestational age had a high risk of developing CP (21.4/1000 pregnancies) (19, 111). Fetuses at high risk for asphyxia and CP include the IUGR fetus, the fetus in a breech presentation, and fetuses born to women who have third trimester bleeding or preeclampsia (101). CP was significantly less frequent if women received magnesium sulfate ($MgSO_4$) to treat preeclampsia or preterm labor prior to the birth of their 24 to 25 week 500 to 1000 gram neonate (6% versus 33%). CP was half as frequent if $MgSO_4$ was administered when gestation was greater than 26 weeks (112). Researchers did not speculate why this happened but, perhaps the vasodilatory effects of $MgSO_4$ and its Ca^{++} channel blocking properties improved cerebral blood flow and limited Ca^{++} entry into brain cells which prevented cell damage and CP.

Periventricular Leukomalacia (PVL)

Periventricular leukomalacia (also spelled leucomalacia) is necrosis of the brain's white matter lateral to the ventricles. PVL is a common lesion in preterm neonates and a major risk factor for CP (108, 113-115). Fetuses with middle cerebral artery or internal carotid artery perfusion failure from "serious" hypoxemia are at risk for PVL (108). In monkeys, Myers (86) found PVL was associated with hypoxia and white matter hemorrhage.

Infection, such as chorioamnionitis, increases the risk of PVL. PVL may be the result of cytokine mediated brain injury. WBCs, such as macrophages, produce cytokines as part of the inflammatory response to infection (116). IL-6 is a cytokine that is present when there is an infection. In 94% of autopsied neonatal brains that had evidence of PVL, astrocytes produced cytokines, primarily IL-6 and IL-1. IL-6, more so than IL-1, appears to be the mediator of neuronal injury (113). IL-6 has also been found in cord blood and was significantly higher in those babies with PVL. A cord blood IL-6 level of more than 0.54 ng/ml had a 78% specificity, i.e., it identified PVL in 107 of 138 neonates (117). In addition to cord blood IL-6, amniotic fluid may contain a significantly elevated IL-6 level. Researchers confirmed that IL-6 was significantly elevated in amniotic fluid of preterm neonates who developed PVL and intraventricular hemorrhage (IVH). Neonates without PVL and IVH had a higher gestational age, birth weight, and a lower incidence of infection or chorioamnionitis (118). Chorioamnionitis and an IL-6 level greater than 5000 pg/ml in pregnancies less than 37 weeks' gestation was associated with significantly more neonates who had PVL or IVH or IVH with PVL. If IL-6 was less than or equal to 5000 pg/ml babies did not have PVL (119, 120).

Steroids administered to women to mature the preterm fetal lungs prior to preterm delivery prevent PVL and IVH, *except when chorioamnionitis is present* (121). In fetuses who weighed 1750 grams or less, betamethasone decreased the incidence of IVH and PVL in women who had preterm premature rupture of membranes (PPROM) with preterm labor (122). The incidence of major handicaps decreased as preterm fetuses aged and was lower in neonates whose mothers received steroids to mature fetal lungs prior to preterm birth (123).

IUGR fetuses have less risk of developing PVL. In the absence of chorioamnionitis, IUGR preterm babies, born at 34 or fewer weeks' gestation weighing 1750 grams or less, had a decreased risk of IVH and PVL than babies who were not IUGR but were a similar weight and gestational age (124-125).

Intraventricular Hemorrhage (IVH)

An intracranial hemorrhage may be subdural, parenchymal, or intraventricular. PVL and IVH may be diagnosed by ultrasound imaging (126). *Risk factors for IVH, seizures, and an abnormal neurologic examination include deficient vitamin-K-dependent clotting factors, LBW, prematurity, and hypercapnia* (28, 127-128). A deficiency of clotting factors may be due to maternal diphenylhydantoin and phenobarbital which was prescribed for epilepsy (128). Compression of the cord increases the risk of hypercapnia and IVH. Preterm fetuses, less than 29 weeks' gestation, were more likely to develop PVL or IVH when the umbilical cord was compressed for periods of one or more minutes at a time, e.g., repetitive severe variable decelerations prior to birth (129). *Therefore, if the fetus is preterm, umbilical cord compression and other causes of hypercapnia should be promptly treated to prevent IVH.*

Chorioamnionitis increases the risk of IVH in preterm fetuses who weigh 1000 or fewer grams (22% if chorioamnionitis was present versus 11% if noninfected). If chorioamnionitis is confirmed, e.g., by amniotic fluid analysis, delivery may prevent IVH or PVL. Severe preeclampsia, IUGR, and the physician's willingness to perform a cesarean section for distress were protective against IVH (127). *The risk of IVH decreases in the IUGR fetus and as gestation increases* (130-131). Thirty to 40% of preterm fetuses weighing less than 1500 grams had IVH. If the preterm fetus was also IUGR, the incidence of IVH was less (131). The cause of this difference is unknown, but may be related to vasodilation due to adenosine and the brain-sparing effect of chronic hypoxia in IUGR fetuses.

Preterm fetuses have an increased risk for PVL and IVH. However, it is not clear if they have less risk, more risk, or the same risk for asphyxial brain damage than term fetuses. Preterm lambs were *more vulnerable* to hypoxic-ischemic injury because they could not adequately dilate their cerebral blood vessels to increase brain O_2 delivery. Instead, they relied on increasing the fractional O_2 extraction ratio (132). In a more recent study, preterm lambs seemed to have an *increased resistance* to brain damage and recovered faster than term lambs after occlusion of their umbilical cord (115). In experiments where the ewe was deprived of O_2, the extent of injury to the fetal lamb was not related to the degree of hypoxemia or metabolic acidosis. Lambs developed white matter necrosis and focal cortical infarcts following maternal ewe hypoxemia (19).

Asymmetry decreases the risk of IVH. Asymmetrical fetuses may or may not be IUGR. An asymmetrical baby has a big head and a lean body, usually as a result of chronic redistribution of blood flow to the head, heart, and adrenal glands. After reviewing data from 47,922 births, researchers found *IUGR fetuses and asymmetrical fetuses without IUGR had an increased morbidity rate but less risk of IVH.* Morbidity included the presence of meconium, an Apgar score of 0 to 3 at 1 minute and 0 to 4 at 5 minutes, and death prior to one year of age (133). Although they had less risk of IVH, *asymmetrical fetuses had an increased risk for CP* (134). Symmetrical but small for gestational age neonates, born prior to 34 weeks' gestation, had an increased risk of mental retardation and a lower intelligent quotient (IQ) but not CP (135).

Survival after IVH increases as gestational age increases. Forty four percent of 23 week old neonates with IVH survived. Beyond 27 weeks' gestation, 85% of neonates with IVH survived. Eighty eight to 100% of survivors had no major neurologic injury at the time of hospital discharge (136). These survival rates reflect the significant advances in neonatal care over the last decade, which have pushed the age of viability down to at least 24 weeks' gestation. Some would suggest the age of viability is 23 weeks' gestation.

Prevention of Cerebral Palsy

Sometimes it is better to deliver a hypoxic or hypercapnic preterm fetus than to continue the pregnancy and risk the development of PVL or IVH. When babies were delivered preterm because of biochemical or biophysical indications, there was a decreased incidence of IVH, retinopathy of prematurity, and seizures (137). Severe preeclampsia is associated with impaired fetal oxygenation, increased O_2 extraction, and increased risk of metabolic acidosis (138). Severe preeclampsia, IUGR, and the physician's willingness to perform a cesarean section for "fetal distress" were protective against neonatal neurological morbidity (127).

The words "fetal distress" poorly define the fetal condition. Some have used these words to suggest fetal physiology is so altered as to make *death or permanent injury* a probability within a relatively short period of time. In that case, fetal distress would be associated with asphyxia. However, the authors described FHR patterns associated with hypoxemia, hypoxia, and acidemia and not metabolic acidosis or aphyxia. For example, they suggested patterns of the distressed fetus included:

- a baseline rate greater than 160 bpm or less than 120 bpm
- no accelerations for 40 or more minutes
- decreased or absent variability and/or
- decelerations (77).

These FHR characteristics do *not* portend death and perman-ent injury. Instead, they suggest fetal hypoxia, acidemia, and a risk of metabolic acidosis. Therefore, it may be best to think of fetal distress as impending fetal ill health which requires action to avert damage (32).

In 1996, it was reported that labor, delivery, and birth records of 155,636 children born in California were reviewed. The rate of CP was 1.1/1000 births. Cerebral palsy was related to late decelerations and/or decreased STV in only 0.19% of children who had CP at three years of age. No other specific FHR pattern appeared to be related to CP. A flaw of this study was only physician notes were reviewed regarding the FHR pattern and no fetal monitor tracings were analyzed. Based only on review of the medical record, the researchers found the FHR baseline was not related to CP. They recommended that a randomized trial is needed to explore the relationship of specific FHR patterns and CP. Researchers also need to identify which interventions, if any, prevent CP or decrease the incidence of CP (139).

IUGR babies whose birth weight was less than the 10th percentile most frequently had FHR "abnormalities." FHR abnormalities after more than 40 weeks' gestation and a weight of 2500 gms or more created a five-fold increase in the risk of CP. CP was also related to the presence of vaginal bleeding during pregnancy, breech presentation, delivery before 37 weeks', meconium in the amniotic fluid, or a maternal infection (139).

THE FETAL CONTINUUM FROM OXYGENATED TO ASPHYXIATED

Fetal acid-base status is assumed based on knowledge about the condition of the fetus prior to the onset of labor, the probable hypoxic source, the duration of hypoxia, the placenta's ability to transfer gases, and maternal health. A well oxygenated, *nonhypoxic* fetus should have *a reassuring FHR pattern*. Depletion of O_2 moves the fetus through three stages of deterioration: transient hypoxemia without metabolic acidosis, tissue hypoxia with a risk of metabolic acidosis, and hypoxia with metabolic acidosis or asphyxia (140). Fetuses with transient hypoxemia have *compensatory FHR patterns*. Fetuses with hypoxia and a risk of metabolic acidosis have *nonreassuring FHR patterns*. Fetuses with metabolic acidosis or asphyxia have *ominous FHR patterns*. By reviewing the FHR pattern, clinicians mentally place the fetus on this continuum then act according to their classification of the tracing as reassuring, compensatory, nonreassuring, or ominous.

Transient Hypoxemia Without Metabolic Acidosis

During *transient hypoxemia without metabolic acidosis*, fetal homeostasis is maintained by compensatory mechanisms. Cardiac output is redistributed and cerebral blood flow increases to avert permanent brain damage (19, 71, 141). Peripheral vessels constrict, a baroreceptor and chemoreceptor/vagal response, and fetal bradycardia may occur (141). Women perceive more weak fetal movements. Fetal blood flow to peripheral tissues, such as the skeleton, skin, intestines, and kidneys decreases. Fetal growth may slow if hypoxemia is chronic (18, 140).

Tissue Hypoxia

In the second stage of physiologic deterioration, O_2 levels drop more than 30% below normal and homeostatic mechanisms become inadequate to meet cell oxidative metabolic needs. To avert brain damage, the hypoxic fetus compensates by redistributing left ventricular cardiac output and increasing coronary and cerebral blood flow, a brain-sparing compensatory mechanism (67, 142). If hypoxia is unrelieved, eventually fetal autoregulation of brain blood flow becomes impaired, increasing the risk of brain damage (29, 67). In monkeys, hypoxia without acidosis damaged white matter which was accompanied by hemorrhage and focal areas of PVL. Hypoxia with acidosis damaged the cerebral cortex. Anoxia damaged basal ganglia in the caudate nucleus located under the ventricles (86). Basal ganglia affect muscle coordination (143).

When the fetus is hypoxic, movements such as swallowing and limb flexion and extension decrease, acceleration frequency decreases, tachycardia may occur, and low voltage electrocortical activity decreases (144). Hypoxia is believed to *decrease* chorionic villi syncytiotrophoblast production of prostacyclin (PGI_2), a vasodilator (145). This increases the risk of placental vessel vasoconstriction which may hasten the onset of metabolic acidosis. Therefore, any sign of fetal hypoxia should be promptly treated.

As the pH falls, the FHR changes. Average long-term variability may become marked or saltatory with a baseline bandwidth greater than 25 bpm. Short-term variability (STV) will be present but eventually there will be a loss of variability as acidemia worsens (60, 146). The risk of acidosis increases as the pH decreases. Although a low pH in and of itself is not an indication for immediate delivery, the belief that acidemia is worsening and the risk of acidosis is increasing would support a decision to deliver the fetus as soon as possible (147). The loss of STV is nonreassuring.

Hypoxia with Frank Metabolic Acidosis

O_2 consumption continues until O_2 delivery is 50% below normal. At that point, O_2 extraction increases. When fetal lamb blood O_2 content was less than 2 mmol/L, SaO_2 was 20 to 30% and hemoglobin was 6 to 10 mmol/L (46, 148). Brain oxygenation decreased and the probability of neurologic damage increased. Lambs, with a blood O_2 content less than 1 mmol/L (the critical level) decompensated (149). Below the critical level, O_2 consumption depends entirely on supply. O_2 reserves are totally depleted and *hypoxia with frank metabolic acidosis* occurs (19, 149-152). Cardiac output significantly decreases (152). Brain O_2 consumption decreases and the brain becomes vulnerable to asphyxial insult. Organs are damaged and some lambs seized in utero (149).

In response to hypoxia and acidemia, nucleated RBCs (NRBCs) proliferate as fetal pH decreases (154-155). The time required to produce new NRBCs is unknown. *Usually there are less than 10 NRBCs per 100 white blood cells (WBCs) in a sample of mixed venous and arterial umbilical cord blood.* In neurologically impaired neonates there were 34 to 103 NRBCs per 100 WBCs. If the asphyxial event was close to the time of birth there were fewer NRBCs than if the event occurred long before the birth (156).

An acute event, such as uterine rupture, is associated with fewer than 30 NRBCs per 100 WBCs. If the FHR pattern was reactive, but later developed tachycardia, there were also fewer than 30 NRBCs per 100 WBCs in the cord blood sample (156). Since IUGR is a result of chronic hypoxia, NRBCs will be increased (157-158). *Neurologically impaired neonates have significantly more NRBCs in their cord blood than well neonates and may have a persistently nonreactive FHR pattern or a reactive admission pattern but later develop tachycardia or an acute prolonged deceleration.* The highest number of NRBCs were found in fetuses who had a *persistently nonreactive* FHR pattern (67.3 ± 128 per 100 WBCs). The next highest number of NRBCs were found in fetuses who had reactive admission strips but developed *tachycardia* (13.4 ± 10.2 per 100 WBCs) or an *acute prolonged deceleration* (12.4 ± 9.1 per 100 WBCs) (156).

THE FETAL RESPONSE TO ACID-BASE CHANGES

The Condition of the Fetus Prior to Labor

The acid-base status of the fetus at the onset of labor influences the fetal response to O_2 deprivation during labor. Awareness of maternal and fetal risk factors determines the intensity and frequency of FHR monitoring. For example, women at high risk for fetal demise who require intensive fetal monitoring are single, black, undereducated teenagers who live in a rural area (159). These women would be best monitored electronically with FHR assessments every 15 minutes during active labor and every 5 minutes during the second stage of labor (16). Table 7 is a list of some risk factors associated with intrapartal fetal hypoxemia and asphyxia (20, 46, 160-161). If risk factors are present, electronic fetal monitoring (EFM) is a better choice for fetal assessment than auscultation.

Table 7: Fetal and Maternal Risk Factors Associated with Intrapartal Fetal Hypoxemia and Asphyxia

Antepartal Factors
- prior stillbirth or neonatal death
- fetal anomalies
- IUGR
- prematurity
- oligohydramnios
- polyhydramnios
- maternal medical complications, e.g., diabetes
- maternal obstetric complications, e.g., hemorrhage
- regular painful contractions that spontaneously ceased 24 hours prior to the onset of active labor (associated with an increase in arrest of labor disorders and cesarean section)

Intrapartal Factors
- maternal hypoxia
- uterine artery occlusion
- umbilical vessel occlusion
- fetal anemia
- preterm or postterm labor
- meconium
- abnormal labor (prolonged, unfavorable progress) and
- a "major" malpresentation.

IUGR and Preterm Fetuses: The Most Vulnerable to Hypoxia

IUGR and preterm fetuses have a decreased O_2 reserve compared to term, well grown fetuses (47). There is a greater O_2 diffusion distance in preterm placentas than term placentas (162). This delays O_2 delivery and limits preterm O_2 reserves. IUGR fetuses lack O_2 reserves due to chronic O_2 deprivation.

IUGR fetuses are more likely to be born preterm, become hypoxic, and have neonatal complications such as meconium aspiration syndrome, myocardial infarction, and heart failure (73, 163-164). Fetuses with abnormal umbilical artery Doppler velocimetry, a low estimated weight, and prematurity are at risk for asphyxia. Preterm IUGR fetuses who weighed 1000 grams or less had a higher incidence of umbilical artery acidemia, hypoxia, and hypercapnia than normally grown fetuses at a similar gestational age (165). IUGR and preterm fetuses have a higher incidence of abnormal FHR patterns and acidosis than term, normally grown fetuses (94).

Acidosis developed when their transcutaneous PO_2 decreased with 72% or more uterine contractions (166). Although all babies are important, heroic measures to salvage pregnancies with IUGR and preterm fetuses with an estimated weight of less than 550 grams has been discouraged due to the rare chance of survival (167).

The Admission Test
One fourth of fetuses who had biochemical intrapartal asphyxia, with a buffer base less than 34 mmol/L and a BE less than -12 mEq/L, had mothers with no known risk factors (160). Therefore, low-risk women should be electronically monitored at the time of admission to confirm fetal well-being. An abnormal FHR pattern may indicate fetal disease, and the midwife and/or physician should be notified of any abnormality in a timely manner (94). A well oxygenated, nonacidemic fetus has at least one acceleration and moves twice within a 20 minute observation period, whereas compromised fetuses do not accelerate 15 bpm above the baseline FHR. If the admission FHR pattern indicates fetal well-being, the monitor may be removed and the fetus may be auscultated the rest of the labor, until a FHR is heard that warrants application of the electronic fetal monitor. For example, if the auscultated rate is irregular or decreased during or following contractions, EFM may be reapplied to assess the FHR pattern. If, on the other hand, the admission strip is *nonreactive* (accelerations are less than 15 seconds in duration from baseline to baseline and 15 bpm above the baseline at their acme) *or if the fetus has a history of absent end diastolic pressure in the umbilical artery*, fetal surveillance should be heightened and EFM should be continuous (168).

HYPOXEMIA
Fetal hypoxemia may be the result of maternal, placental, or fetal causes (20, 49, 169). Umbilical cord compression is a common cause of hypoxemia. When a fetus is hypoxemic, spontaneous accelerations are usually present. STV is present. Long-term variability (LTV) is present but may be decreased at times. Signs of a chemoreceptor response to hypoxemia include tachycardia, uniform or periodic accelerations (in response to umbilical vein compression), and variable decelerations. Hypoxemic preterm fetuses, 20 to 26 weeks' gestation, had a tachycardic rate, decreased baseline variability, with variable decelerations that lasted 60 or more seconds (170). Late decelerations may occur, but accelerations and STV will be present. If hypoxemia is acute and reversible, actions to improve fetal O_2 delivery should change the FHR pattern from a compensatory pattern to a reassuring pattern. To summarize, the hypoxemic fetus will demonstrate:
- spontaneous accelerations with
- short-term variability and
- long-term variability, although it may be decreased
There may be
- uniform accelerations
- variable decelerations
- tachycardia
- late decelerations with short-term variability and accelerations.

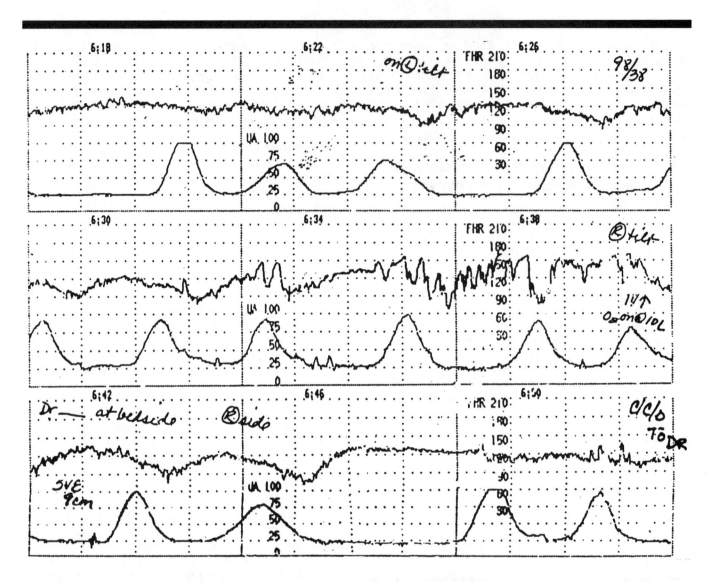

Figure 5.5: Fetal hypoxemia. Maternal hypotension was related to the presence of late decelerations. Accelerations are clearly evident as well as short-term variability. An occasional variable deceleration occurred. After turning the woman, increasing intravenous fluids, and administering oxygen, the fetus recovered from the hypoxemia caused by uteroplacental insufficiency and cord compression and was delivered vaginally with Apgar scores of 8 and 9 at 1 and 5 minutes.

HYPOXIA WITH A RISK OF METABOLIC ACIDOSIS

The hypoxic fetus decreases movements. Accelerations may become smaller and fewer in number (171). *The presence of accelerations and STV suggests the fetus is not yet acidotic (20).* Activation of chemoreceptors may be noted as uniform accelerations, or variable, late, or prolonged decelerations. In the past, some physicians believed that the fetus should be delivered at once when late decelerations were observed (168). However, immediate delivery would be an overreaction if late decelerations were due to maternal hypotension. A hypoxic fetus may not have late decelerations but may have *tachycardia, flattening of the baseline, and variable decelerations.* Decelerations usually precede the loss of variability (20). To

summarize, the hypoxic fetus will have:
- smaller and fewer spontaneous accelerations
- short-term variability
- absent to minimal long-term variability

The hypoxic fetus may have:
- tachycardia
- uniform accelerations
- variable decelerations
- late decelerations.

The main differences between FHR patterns that reflect hypoxemia and those that reflect hypoxia is the decrease in acceleration height and frequency and the decrease in long-term variability.

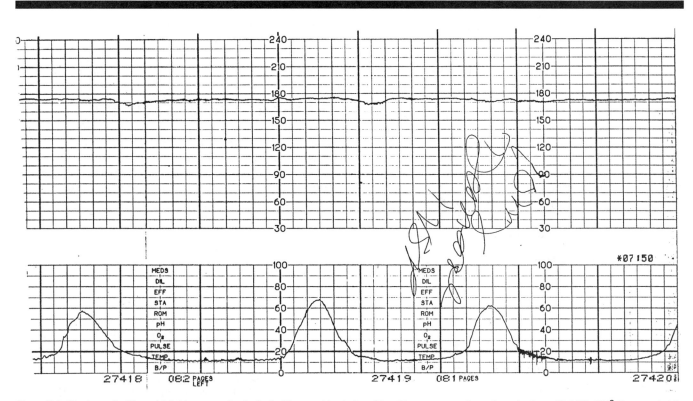

Figure 5.6: Chorioamnionitis and fetal hypercapnia. A single 22 year old primigravida with severe preeclampsia and a fever (172/90, 101° F) presented to labor and delivery at 40 weeks' gestation with a fetus who had tachycardia, absent variability, and late decelerations. She was delivered by cesarean section. Apgar scores were 8 and 9 at 1 and 5 minutes. Umbilical artery gases revealed hypercapnia: pH 7.25, PO_2 21 mm Hg, PCO_2 71 mm Hg. Carbon dioxide retention was most likely due to placental inflammation and chorioamnionitis. The lack of accelerations can be attributed to hypercapnia (58).

ACIDEMIA
Acidemia and Chorioamnionitis

Chorioamnionitis is inflammation of the placenta evidenced by villous edema. Villous edema can cause *fetal hypoxia* due to the delay in O_2 transfer created by an increased transfer distance (172). Chorioamnionitis increases the risk of acid-base disorders because of bacterial endotoxins, hypoxemia, acidemia, or prolonged labor (173). The cause of chorioamnionitis is usually a maternal infection rather than a fetal infection (173). Bacterial endotoxins *lower fetal pH*. Because the cause of chorioamnionitis is usually maternal, it does not predict fetal or neonatal sepsis (174). Chorioamnionitis is related to a significant *prolongation of labor* in women who have a temperature greater than 38° C (100° F), abdominal tenderness, fetal or maternal tachycardia, and leukocytosis (abnormally elevated WBCs). Women with chorioamnionitis had a first stage that lasted 1 to 19 hours versus 2 to 10 hours in noninfected women. The second stage was 12 to 98 minutes in infected women and 8 to 82 minutes in noninfected women (175). Leukocytosis is defined as a WBC count greater than 20,000/mm³. Evidence of chorioamnionitis may include a purulent vaginal discharge or foul smelling amniotic fluid (174). Although researchers did not speculate on how chorioamnionitis slows labor, the infection probably interferes with normal uterine cell function.

Chorioamnionitis may be predicted by measurement of cytokines such as interleukin 6 (IL-6). IL-6 is a cytokine found in cervical secretions of infected women who were in preterm labor. There is an inverse relationship between umbilical artery pH and BE and the IL-6 level. *As IL-6 increased, pH and BE decreased.* However, there was no relationship between the IL-6 level and neonatal sepsis (176). Women with chorioamnionitis had 10 times more granulocyte colony stimulating factor (GCSF) in their amniotic fluid than noninfected women (177). Perhaps, in the future, clinicians will have a quick way to test for IL-6 or GCSF during labor to confirm chorioamnionitis.

Acidemia and a Straight Umbilical Cord or a Nuchal Cord

A straight umbilical cord may be seen with real-time ultrasound. Color Doppler assessment allows differentiation of single and multiple loops of nuchal cord (178). A straight cord lacks coils and Wharton's Jelly, is prone to compression with fetal descent, and is related to an umbilical artery pH less than 7.16. Straight umbilical cords are more common in women who have preeclampsia, gestational diabetes, chronic hypertension, or syphilis. Women, whose fetus had a short umbilical cord, were more likely to have meconium in their amniotic fluid, a preterm delivery prior to 34 weeks' gestation, a LBW neonate with a 5 minute Apgar score less than 5, admission to the NICU, or a fetal demise (179). *LBW was related to the location of the placenta.* A low-lying placenta and placenta previa at 14 to 24 weeks' gestation was associated with preterm delivery and LBW (180). Fetal weight was greater when the placenta was centrally located in the uterus or on the left lateral side. Lower weights were found when the placenta was on the maternal right side (181).

The nuchal notch is a small protrusion at the posterior base of the skull above the neck. A nuchal cord is an umbilical cord that is looped around the fetal neck, below the nuchal notch. Significant acidemia, with a pH between 7.00 and 7.10, was more likely if there were two or more loops of nuchal cord.

Table 8: Incidence of Nuchal Cord Loops (182)

Loops of Nuchal Cord	Incidence (%)
1	22.9
2	3.0
3	0.5
4	0.07

In another study, 51.8% of babies had a single loop (178). As many as seven loops of nuchal cord have been observed with good outcomes. These statistics suggest that almost one in four women will have a fetus with at least one loop of nuchal cord. When a nuchal cord is present, variable decelerations and "abnormal" FHR patterns will be evident as labor progresses, increasing the risk of a low or midforceps delivery and "mild umbilical artery acidosis" at birth (182). When there are multiple loops of nuchal cord, there is a significantly higher incidence of meconium-stained amniotic fluid, cesarean section, one minute Apgar scores less than seven, umbilical artery pH less than 7.16, umbilical vein pH less than 7.20, neonatal resuscitation, and NICU admission (178).

THE FHR RESPONSE TO ACIDEMIA

FHR patterns suggest fetal well-being or acidemia. Electronic fetal monitoring predicted normal fetal pH in 97% of well fetuses, whereas auscultation only predicted normal pH in 34% of well fetuses (183). FHR patterns present 20 minutes prior to scalp blood pH determination resulted in distinct pH values (see Table 9) (184).

Based on these findings, it appears that the depth and duration of the variable or late decelerations were associated with fetal scalp pH, i.e., *the bigger the deceleration, the lower the pH.*

Tachycardia

Fetal tachycardia, with a baseline rate greater than 160 bpm, may be a response to hypoxemia (185). In that case, pH would be lower than the tachycardia that represents sympathetic nerve stimulation, e.g., following acoustic stimulation. Forty-three percent of acidemic preterm fetuses were tachycardic, 39% had decreased variability, 55 to 70% had variable decelerations. Decreased variability was defined as a baseline 5 to 10 bpm wide. In preterm fetuses, late decelerations were associated with acidemia in five of six babies, especially if the late decelerations were severe. *A combination of tachycardia, decreased variability, and variable or late decelerations was always associated with acidemia* (186).

Tachycardia usually reflects a compensatory, chemoreceptor and catecholamine response to chorioamnionitis, hypoxemia, and acidemia. As the fetus becomes acidemic,

Table 9: Scalp Capillary Blood pH in Relation to Different FHR Patterns

pH	Pattern
7.26-7.34	No Decelerations Early Decelerations
> and < 7.25	Tachycardia
7.24-7.34	mild and moderate Variable Decelerations mild = less than 30 seconds duration or nadir above 80 bpm or nadir 70 to 80 bpm but deceleration less than 60 seconds moderate = 30 to 60 seconds duration, nadir above 70 bpm or nadir 70 to 80 bpm but deceleration more than 60 seconds
7.16-7.28	mild and moderate Late Decelerations mild = less than 15 bpm drop in FHR moderate = 15 to 45 bpm drop in FHR
7.05-7.22	severe Variable Decelerations (more than 60 seconds duration, nadir below 70 bpm) severe Late Decelerations (more than 45 bpm drop in FHR)

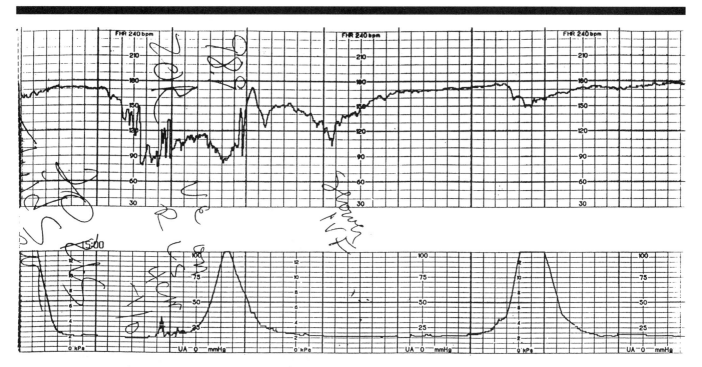

Figure 5.7: FHR pattern suggestive of acidemia and chorioamnionitis. A primigravida diet-controlled gestational diabetic at 40 weeks' gestation presented to labor and delivery with a complaint of leaking fluid for 2 days. Her pulse was 108 bpm, her temperature was 99.9° F. She was dilated 2 cm with a ballottable vertex presentation. Now at 4 cm/-1 station, the FHR pattern reveals tachycardia and variable decelerations. A cesarean section was performed with Apgar scores of 8 and 9 at 1 and 5 minutes. A very small placenta and cord were found. Tachycardia is most likely the result of infection, hypoxemia, and acidemia. Variable decelerations suggest umbilical cord compression due to insufficient amniotic fluid.

there may be changes in the electrocardiogram (ECG). Metabolically acidemic fetal lambs had a shorter PR interval, decreased P wave duration, and a rise in P wave height. T wave changes were related to the level of catecholamines (187). If, in the 10 minutes prior to birth, the fetus had a tachycardic rate or a rate less than 120 bpm, there was an increased chance of an umbilical artery pH less than 7.20 (49). A pH less than 7.20 preceded the birth of a depressed neonate 50 to 70% of the time (37). Neonatal resuscitation should be anticipated and prepared for prior to the birth of a tachycardic fetus.

Whenever the fetus is tachycardic, chorioamnionitis should be suspected until it is excluded. Maternal temperature and maternal heart rate should be obtained. Women may be afebrile yet infected. Chorioamnionitis may be associated with a maternal heart rate greater than 100 bpm. Amniotic fluid should be assessed for a foul odor. Abdominal tenderness should be assessed. Findings should be reported to the midwife and/or physician. Delivery decisions must be based on the maternal risks related to chorioamnionitis and the fetal risks such as myocardial fatigue, heart failure, and sepsis. If the fetus is infected, neonatal resuscitation is usually required (37).

Decelerations

In another study, 75% of preterm LBW fetuses, who weighed less than 1500 grams and had late decelerations, were hypox-

emic but not acidemic. The depth of the late decelerations in relation to pH was not described. Their average pH was 7.24 when there was "absent short-term variability" with a baseline greater of 150 or more bpm. The equipment used to assess STV was not described, nor was the criteria for absent and present STV. The average pH was 7.17 when there was absent STV with a baseline less than 150 bpm. When LTV was present, the average pH was 7.31. pH dropped to an average of 7.28 when LTV was absent. Combination deceleration patterns, such as early and variable decelerations, were not related to pH. However, early plus late decelerations were associated with a pH less than 7.20 in these LBW preterm fetuses (146).

Term, acidemic fetuses who were appropriate for gestational age (AGA) or large for gestational age (LGA) with "healthy, low-risk" mothers had:
• late decelerations and/or
• variable decelerations and/or
• a flat tracing.
The time required *for a well fetus to become acidemic* (scalp pH less than 7.25) varied in relation to the observed FHR pattern. The median time to become acidemic was:
• 1.92 hours of *late decelerations*
• 2.42 hours of *variable decelerations*
• 3.08 hours of a *flat tracing*.
Some well fetuses became acidemic in as little as 30 minutes when late decelerations were observed (94).

Decreased Variability

Acidemic lambs have increased STV and LTV (188). However, acidemic IUGR human fetuses have *decreased variability* (188-189). A flat FHR baseline *in a normal range* has been found in fetuses whose umbilical vein and artery pH values were less than 7.20 (190). As long as the umbilical artery pH is greater than 7.12, all acidemic neonates should be neurologically normal (191). A breech presentation has no effect on umbilical artery gases (192). However, a breech, IUGR fetus with a lack of variability will have a lower pH than a normoxic breech fetus. Postterm fetuses should move 15 to 20 times in a 10 minute observation period (193). Acidemic postterm fetuses moved less and had severe variable decelerations (184, 194). Acidemic postterm fetuses may be *tachycardic with no decelerations* (194).

Bradycardia

Hypoxia, acidemia, and hypercapnia have preceded fetal bradycardia (195). When the fetus is acidemic, excess H^+ enters cells, K^+ leaves cells, and intravascular K^+ increases. The high K^+ level prolongs the cardiac PR interval, widens the QRS waveform, impairs neural excitability, and causes CNS depression and bradycardia. An extremely high K^+ level also causes *flaccidity* (12). Fetal movement decreases (151). Many *severely acidemic babies* are born limp and blue and require resuscitation. If the fetal pH is less than 7.20, and maternal pH is normal, the acidemic fetus may have:

- accelerations, until metabolic acidosis develops
- short-term variability, until metabolic acidosis develops
- absent long-term variability, i.e., a flat tracing

- late decelerations
- variable decelerations
- tachycardia
- bradycardia.

METABOLIC ACIDOSIS

Metabolically acidotic fetuses eventually:

- stop moving
- stop accelerating
- may have long-term variability, e.g., a sinusoidal pattern
- *have absent short-term variability.*

There may have:

- late decelerations or
- variable decelerations or
- tachycardia
- bradycardia.

L-lactic acid removal from fetal circulation may require 15 minutes or more after normal O_2 levels have been restored (196). Consequently, it is rare for a fetus to tolerate the effects of metabolic acidosis for the time required to correct it. Therefore, when fetal metabolic acidosis is suspected, or interventions to relieve fetal hypoxia are not improving the FHR pattern, expeditious delivery should be considered.

Absent Short-term Variability

Short-term variation greater than 2.5 milliseconds (msec), calculated by computer over 1/16th of a minute, suggests fetal well-being. *However, short-term variation 2.5 or less msec predicts metabolic acidemia and impending fetal death, even if the*

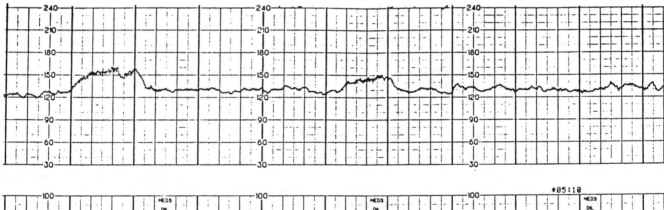
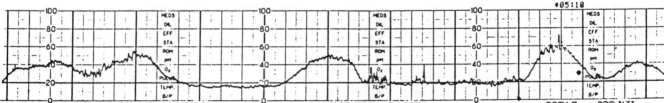

Figure 5.8: Fetal compensatory pattern. A low risk, gravida 1 woman at 39 weeks' gestation was admitted at 3 cm dilatation, 85% effacement, and a -2 station with normal vital signs. Over the course of labor, she received epidural anesthesia and developed a temperature of 101.5° F. Her admission strip revealed uniform accelerations, suggestive of umbilical vein compression. One hour and 40 minutes later, she had a higher fetal heart rate baseline (a sign of hypoxia) probably due to chorioamnionitis.

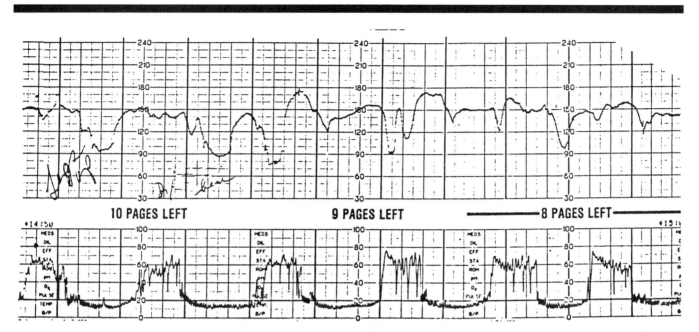

Figure 5.9: Nonreassuring fetal heart rate pattern associated with metabolic acidosis. Four hours and forty minutes after admission, variable decelerations were noted with thick meconium. Seven hours and forty minutes after admission, during maternal pushing there was absent short-term variability, variable decelerations with overshoots, and absent to minimal long-term variability. Apgars were 2 at 1 minute and 6 at 5 minutes. The fetus had mixed respiratory and metabolic acidosis but was not hypoxic. Acute chorioamnionitis, a Battledore placenta and subchorionic fibrosis were noted by the pathologist. The neonate was treated for a beta hemolytic streptococcus infection and did well following antibiotic therapy.

baseline is in a normal range with NO decelerations (197). When the fetus is becoming metabolically acidotic, accelerations disappear and STV and LTV decrease. Eventually, STV will be absent (198). LTV may be present, e.g., the baseline could be sinusoidal. *The loss of variability is a sign of depleted cardiac glycogen* (199). Fetal breathing movements and swallowing movements decrease and eventually cease (198, 200-201).

Decelerations

Metabolic acidosis has been predicted by a biophysical profile score of six or less, an abnormal umbilical artery systolic/diastolic (S/D) ratio, and a nonreactive FHR pattern with late decelerations or severe variable decelerations or "reduced" variability (64).

Variable decelerations. Both variable and late decelerations can precede fetal acidemia, acidosis, and asphyxia. Since umbilical cord compression does not decrease uteroplacental blood flow, acidemia from umbilical cord compression may be less severe and asphyxial injury may be "more benign" than when there is uteroplacental insufficiency (87).

Late decelerations. Isolated late decelerations, i.e., there may be just one, were associated with a decrease in transcutaneous ($tcPO_2$) of five to eight mm Hg. Repetitive late decelerations were associated with a "mild to marked decline" in $tcPO_2$, however *the size of the deceleration was not associated with the size of the $tcPO_2$ decline* (166).

Bradycardia

Hypoxia eventually depletes ATP, creatine-phosphate, and glycogen stores in the brain, heart, and liver which precedes ECG changes and bradycardia (199). The fetal T/QRS ratio increases to greater than 0.25 and is inversely related to the fall in HCO_3^- (61). Bradycardia, especially at a rate near 60 bpm, is a late finding and may be associated with fetal asphyxia.

ASPHYXIA

Fetal asphyxia may be *acute or chronic*. An acute asphyxial insult would be uterine rupture or maternal hemorrhage. Other acute causes of asphyxia include umbilical cord compression with interruption of umbilical blood flow, abruption or placental insufficiency with impaired placental gas exchange, and maternal hypotension or abnormal uterine contractions with insufficient placental perfusion (54).

Use of continuous electronic fetal monitoring (EFM) versus auscultation may suggest an increased risk of metabolic acidosis or asphyxia and prompt interventions to lower the risk of neonatal seizures (202). Therefore, any fetus at increased risk for asphyxia, i.e., a high-risk fetus, should be closely monitored throughout labor. For example, if the fetus is known to be IUGR with oligohydramnios, the FHR should be assessed every 15 minutes in active labor and every 5 minutes during the second stage of labor (16). Other chronic causes of fetal asphyxia include maternal cardiopulmonary disease or severe anemia. Impaired transition from fetal to

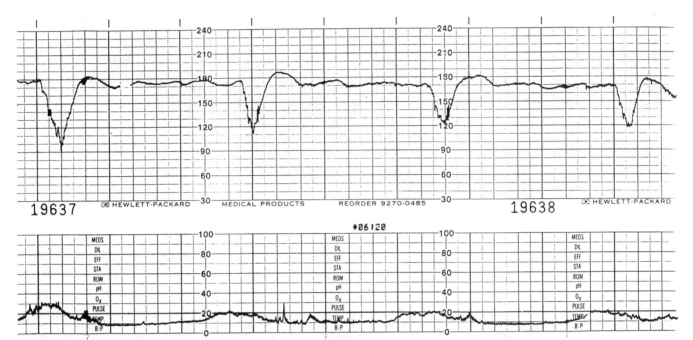

Figure 5.10: Ominous fetal heart rate pattern and a good outcome. A primigravida woman with a history of kidney stones during this pregnancy presented to labor and delivery at 38 weeks' gestation, dilated 3 cm and 80% effaced with a vertex presentation. This tracing was obtained five hours after admission when she was completely dilated. Note the tachycardia with absent short-term variability, absent to minimal long-term variability, and "small variable decelerations" with overshoots. A 5 pound 15 ounce baby was vaginally delivered. Apgar scores were 8 and 9 at 1 and 5 minutes. Blood gases were not obtained.

neonatal cardiopulmonary circulation can cause neonatal asphyxia (54).

The Fetal Response to Asphyxia

Signs and symptoms of asphyxia during labor and after birth include:
- an abnormal FHR pattern
- meconium staining
- low Apgar scores
- early onset seizures
- gross abnormalities of tone, movement, and reflexes and
- signs of cerebral irritation (109).

If asphyxia is suspected, it may be helpful to assess umbilical artery NRBCs. Acute changes in the FHR, such as a prolonged deceleration, were associated with fewer NRBCs than chronic changes, such as a flat tracing (203). In preterm neonates who weighed 500 to 1750 grams, there was no significant difference in the number of NRBCs between neonates who had PVL or IVH and babies without PVL and IVH. But, if the preterm neonate was LBW, there were significantly more NRBCs than normally grown babies (158).

Fetuses who were asphyxiated and neurologically impaired had four distinct FHR patterns:
- a reactive admission FHR followed by *bradycardia lasting at least 15 minutes* or

- a persistent nonreactive tracing from admission to delivery or
- bradycardia on admission to the hospital or
- a reactive admission FHR followed by tachycardia with decelerations and a *loss of variability* (157).

If the FHR drops below 80 bpm and is not rising or if any of these patterns are observed, the physician should be immediately summoned to the bedside to make management decisions. Intrauterine resuscitative measures should be instituted and nurses should be prepared to assist with an expeditious delivery. Newborn resuscitation personnel should be present at delivery.

Reactive FHR Followed by a Prolonged Deceleration and Bradycardia For 15 or More Minutes

By the *12th to 14th minute* of asphyxia, monkeys had brainstem damage. Most of the monkeys died by the 20th minute after total asphyxia began (86). If after a reactive admission strip there was *sudden prolonged bradycardia for 15 to 81 minutes, neonates were brain damaged* (157).

Persistent Nonreactive FHR

Asphyxiated fetuses *lack baseline variability* (108). *The lack of variability is due to direct myocardial depression* (204). When *absent variability and meconium* are present, the fetus is at high risk for seizures. Forty-two percent of fetuses with meconium and absent variability that seized during the first 24 hours after birth were diagnosed with spastic diplegia or quadriplegia at 6 months of age (205).

Reactive FHR Followed by Tachycardia with Decelerations and a Loss of Variability

Asphyxiated fetuses *may have* absent baseline variability, small variable decelerations with an overshoot, and a normal baseline rate (73). Overshoots immediately follow a variable deceleration. Rather than a shoulder or secondary acceleratory phase that is within a 20 second by 20 bpm box, an overshoot is greater that 20 bpm high *or* longer than 20 seconds in duration. Some physicians believe brain injury following this FHR pattern is potentially preventable (157).

MECONIUM

Fetal stool is called meconium, a word derived from the Greek word meconium-arion meaning opium-like. Aristotle believed meconium induced fetal sleep (206). Meconium is formed in the fetal bowel between the 10th and 16th week of gestation (206-208). It is viscous, dark green, and consists of gastrointestinal secretions, bile, bile acids, mucus, pancreatic juice, cellular debris, amniotic fluid, swallowed vernix caseosa, lanugo, and blood (208-209). As gestation advances, the amount of meconium increases (207).

The Incidence of Meconium Passage

The passage of meconium follows fetal peristalsis and anal sphincter relaxation. Sphincter relaxation may occur following compression of the fetal head and/or umbilical cord due to a vagal response (210-212). Sporadic or repetitive cord compression can cause hypoxia, hypercapnia, and a chemoreceptor-vagal response with meconium passage (213). Meconium passage is associated with a higher incidence of abnormal labor, fetal hypoxia, delivery by cesarean section, and low Apgar scores (207).

Preterm fetuses rarely pass meconium due to their immature gut musculature (214-215). However, they are more likely to pass meconium following maternal betamethasone and thyroxine which was administered to increase fetal lung maturity prior to preterm birth. Theoretically, the gut matured as well as the lungs and meconium was more readily released (215). *Betamethasone administration has also been associated with a decrease in FHR variability for 48 hours and a decrease in the number and episodes of fetal breathing movements and limb and gross body movements* (216). After betamethasone administration, real-time ultrasound biophysical evaluation may *erroneously* suggest fetal asphyxia.

Meconium-stained amniotic fluid most often occurs in fetuses at 34 or more weeks' gestation, and is more prevalent at 37 or more weeks' gestation. If the fetus was postterm, 35% released meconium (213). Meconium-stained amniotic fluid occurs in 1 to 22% of low-risk and high-risk pregnancies (207, 217-221). Meconium passage is more common if women have cholestasis or interruption of bile flow through their biliary system. Cholestasis may be due to hepatitis, drug and alcohol

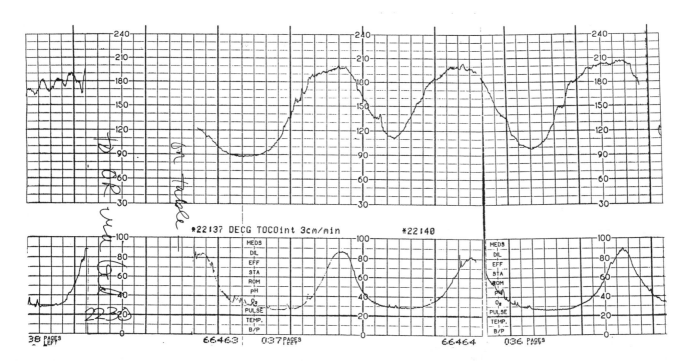

Figure 5.11: Ominous fetal heart rate pattern and biochemical asphyxia. Tachycardia, absent short-term variability, and late decelerations prior to the birth of a 6 lb 14 ounce female with Apgar scores of 1, 6, and 8 at 1, 5, and 10 minutes. Asphyxial blood gases were obtained from the umbilical artery: pH 7.07, PO_2 5 mm Hg, PCO_2 75.8 mm Hg, BE -12.1 mEq/L, bicarbonate 20.8 mEq/L. After 5 days in neonatal intensive care, the baby went home without disability.

abuse, gallstones, a tumor in the common bile duct, or metastatic cancer. Signs of cholestasis include jaundice, intense itching, dark urine, and pale, fatty stools (222). The cause and effect relationship, if any, between cholestasis and meconium is unclear.

The Color and Consistency of Meconium

In addition to evaluation of labor progress, uterine activity, and the FHR pattern, nurses assess the *color, amount, and odor* of amniotic fluid (223). When the fetus defecates in utero, the amniotic fluid may look yellow, light green (split pea soup color), dark green, or almost black. The color depends on the dilution of the meconium in the amniotic fluid and the time it was passed in relation to the time of delivery.

When the fetus spontaneously passes meconium before the onset of labor, it may be swallowed and reabsorbed with no subsequent complications (224-225). However, thick meconium poses a greater risk to the fetus. "Fresh,"thick meconium can be wiped off the umbilical cord after delivery and is usually passed less than 20 hours prior to delivery (226). Meconium-stained fluid has been described as *early light, early heavy, and late meconium* (207, 220). Passage of early light meconium is more common than passage of late meconium (47.5 versus 27.5%) (220). Early heavy (particulate) meconium is associated with an increased risk of fetal and neonatal morbidity, low Apgar scores, meconium aspiration syndrome, and perinatal death (227). Late meconium is often passed in the second stage of labor and is associated with oxytocin augmentation, prolonged labor, a prolonged second stage, and forceps deliveries (207).

Meconium may also be classified as *thin and watery, moderate, thick, particulate, and "pea-soup" like. Thick meconium plus an abnormal FHR pattern* was associated with a poor perinatal outcome, lower Apgar scores, lower pH values, increased risk of metabolic acidosis at all weights and gestational ages, and an increased cesarean section rate when compared with fetuses who had clear amniotic fluid (94, 224, 228-230).

Others have classified meconium as

1+ thin or light
2+ thin with particulate matter
3+ moderate to thick green and
4+ greenish yellow, pea-soup thick with cord and placental staining or late meconium or heavy meconium with particles (210, 220, 231).

Unless the chart form contains a legend that clearly defines 1+ to 4+ meconium, numbers should not be used to describe meconium as each health care provider may have a different idea of what the number means. Based on a review of the literature, 4+ had three different meanings.

Meconium Aspiration Syndrome

Hypoxia and hypercapnia may precede fetal gasping and in utero aspiration of meconium or the neonate may aspirate meconium from the pharynx during the initial breaths of life (213, 217). Figure 5.12 illustrates this process.

Hypoxia
▼
Sympathoadrenal response
▼
Vasoconstriction of blood vessels supplying the fetal bowel
▼
↓ Oxygen supply to the gut
▼
Chemoreceptor-vagal stimulation
▼
Sphincter relaxation
▼
Meconium passage
▼
Continued hypoxia and hypercapnia
▼
Gasping
▼
Meconium aspiration

Figure 5.12: Meconium passage and aspiration may occur in utero, especially after continued hypoxia and hypercapnia.

The amount and thickness of meconium appear to be directly related to the severity of neonatal respiratory symptoms. As many as 62% of meconium-stained neonates may manifest respiratory illness (232). The degree of symptoms is related to the viscosity of meconium-stained fluid, while bile salts contribute to a *"chemical" pneumonitis* (233). It appears that the chemical pneumonitis caused by meconium can occur and create meconium aspiration syndrome (MAS) even when meconium is dilute and thin. From 5 to 41% of neonates with MAS were born through thin meconium (234-236).

Meconium in the lungs diminishes aeration. As many as 28% of neonates with MAS die (236). Meconium correlates poorly with the neonate's initial acid-base status. Even the nonacidemic fetus is prone to MAS. More nonacidemic neonates (2%) than acidemic neonates (1%) developed MAS (49).

Amnioinfusion for Thick Meconium

If the fetus is not acidemic, and delivery is not imminent, thick meconium may be diluted and flushed out of the fetal lungs, and umbilical cord compression from thick meconium may be relieved, by the administration of intrauterine normal saline or lactated Ringer's solution. These solutions are normally used for IV administration (238-239). The solution should be warmed to no greater than 104° F (40° C) if a continuous infusion is used for a preterm woman (personal communication Abbott Laboratories, November 14, 1994 and Baxter Healthcare Corporation, November 11, 1994). A blood warmer or infusion warmer, such as the Flo Tem IIe® from DataChem, Inc. in Indianapolis, Indiana, is the proper device for fluid warming. Both Abbott and Baxter *recommend the microwave not be used to warm IV solutions*. IV fluids should *not* be placed in a blanket warmer because it exceeds the manufacturer's recommended storage temperature.

Prophylactic amnioinfusion dilutes thick meconium and decreases the incidence of meconium below the cords, *but may not decrease the incidence of meconium aspiration syndrome* (217, 240). In fact, it may increase the incidence of MAS (240).

Benefits of amnioinfusion include reduction of umbilical cord compression and repetitive variable decelerations, fewer cesarean sections for "fetal distress," and higher Apgar scores compared to women who had no amnioinfusion for thick meconium or women who had an amnioinfusion for variable decelerations (240). Complications of amnioinfusion include uterine hypertonus, FHR decelerations, and umbilical cord prolapse (241-242).

Meconium Increases the Risk of Chorioamnionitis

Acid-base disorders may precede the release of meconium and meconium increases the risk of acid-base disorders. Meconium enhances bacterial growth and increases the risk of chorioamnionitis because meconium inhibits neutrophil phagocytosis (207, 243). There were significantly more intraamniotic infections associated with all consistencies of meconium-stained amniotic fluid (244).

Early light meconium, following initially clear amniotic fluid, and early heavy meconium have been associated with *fetal tachycardia*, decreased FHR variability, amnionitis, prolonged labor, and a decreased likelihood of prolonged rupture of membranes (207). Prolonged labor and tachycardia are associated with chorioamnionitis (175). If the FHR was tachycardic or bradycardic, there was a 1 in 4 chance the fetus would be delivered by cesarean section or forceps (207). Meconium

▼

Chorioamnionitis

▼

Prolonged labor, tachycardia, decreased variability

▼

Increased risk of fetal acid-base disorders and bradycardia

▼

Increased risk of meconium aspiration

▼

Increased risk of cesarean section or forceps delivery

Figure 5.13: Meconium increases the risk of chorioamnionitis, fetal acid-base disorders, nonreassuring FHR patterns, and meconium aspiration syndrome.

Airway Cleansing During and After Birth

In 1992, the American Heart Association's (AHA) Committee on Neonatal Ventilation and Meconium recommended all neonates who are born through meconium should have pharyngeal suctioning. This is done after delivery of the fetal head, prior to the delivery of the body. They also recommended intratracheal suctioning should be performed immediately after birth prior to the first breath if:

1. there was evidence of fetal distress
2. the infant is depressed or requires positive pressure ventilation
3. meconium is thick or particulate
4. and/or obstetrical pharyngeal suctioning was not performed (245).

Since aspiration of early light meconium is rare, intratracheal suction is not required (220). However, some researchers have reported thin meconium caused a number of cases of MAS and they recommend all meconium-stained babies undergo both nasopharyngeal suctioning with delivery of the baby's head then intratracheal suctioning after birth (246). Even with airway cleansing, MAS may still occur (221).

Meconium and Nonreassuring FHR Patterns

Postterm fetuses have an increased risk of placental infarctions, calcifications, villous stomal edema, fibrosis, fibrin deposition, avascular villi, and syncytial hyperplasia (247). These lesions increase the risk of asphyxia and meconium release (248). Late decelerations may be more prevalent when there is meconium-stained amniotic fluid (6% versus 2% when there was clear fluid). Meconium-stained neonates had a lower umbilical artery pH, PO_2, HCO_3^-, and BE than babies born through clear amniotic fluid (226). Apgar scores were lower in neonates who passed meconium in utero than those who did not pass meconium (249).

In response to late decelerations and meconium, women were placed in a left lateral position, given supplemental O_2 by mask at 5 liters per minute (LPM), and an IV bolus of 10% dextrose in water ($D_{10}W$). They were then taken to the operating room for a cesarean section (226). At 5 LPM, maternal PaO_2 increased 100% without a significant change in maternal pH, PCO_2, or BE. Intervillous blood flow *decreased* from 190 ± 66 ml/minute to 125 ± 58 ml/minute, which was still within the normal range. A pathologic intervillous blood flow level is less than 100 ml/minute. *There was a slight increase in umbilical vein blood flow following these interventions* (87 ± 25 ml/min/kg prior to O_2 therapy, 90 ± 29 ml/min/kg after hyperoxygenation) (250). To summarize, in response to late decelerations and meconium, a left lateral position, IV bolus, and hyperoxygenation with 5 LPM by face mask:

- increases maternal PaO_2
- does not change maternal pH, PCO_2, or BE
- decreases intervillous blood flow to a normal level
- increases umbilical vein blood flow.

If the nurse observes meconium in the amniotic fluid, it should be reported as soon as possible to the midwife or physician along with other observations such as decelerations and maternal vital signs. Maternal temperature should be taken and reevaluated at least every two hours due to the increased risk of chorioamnionitis when meconium is present. A spiral electrode, although not required, may be applied and rarely fetal pH is determined. A vaginal examination should be done to rule out a breech presentation. If the fetus is vertex, thick meconium should be considered a warning sign of fetal compromise (219). Some physicians have recommended that additional hypoxic stressors, such as oxytocin administration, should be avoided when thick meconium is observed, to avoid the risk of fetal hypoxia due to uterine hyperstimulation and/or hypertonus and to reduce the risk of MAS (227, 229). However, amnioinfusion may dilute thick meconium and some physicians will choose to administer oxytocin to decrease labor duration, decrease the risk of chorioamnionitis, and to increase the likelihood of a vaginal birth.

Metabolic Acidosis and Meconium

Fetal metabolic acidosis increases the incidence of meconium-stained fluid (33% versus 18% in the meconium-stained, nonacidotic fetus), operative delivery by forceps or cesarean section (40% versus 20% in nonacidotic fetuses), an Apgar score less than 7 at 1 minute (64% versus 13%), an Apgar score less than 8 at 5 minutes (41% versus 4%), and neonatal complications (78% versus 27%). Neonatal complications included CNS, respiratory, cardiovascular, and renal abnormalities (62). While the passage of meconium does not always correlate with neonatal outcome nor portend neurologic problems, "normal" fetuses who passed meconium and who had an Apgar score of five or less at one minute had subclinical renal injury (230). To summarize, metabolic acidosis was related to an increased incidence of:

- meconium
- forceps deliveries
- cesarean sections
- Apgar score less than seven at one minute
- Apgar score less than eight at five minutes
- neonatal complications.

Based on the association between metabolic acidosis and meconium, some physicians have advocated an urgent delivery when meconium is fresh or increasing (251). Others suggest that meconium plus late decelerations and a low scalp pH warrant active intervention (248-249). Thus,

delivery decisions are based on a number of data points and physician preference. When meconium is present in the amniotic fluid, delivery personnel should provide suction equipment to the physician or midwife for suctioning of the baby's mouth and nose prior to birth of the baby's body. Equipment to intubate the newborn and suction meconium from below the vocal cords, e.g., endotracheal tubes, should be readily available. In spite of all efforts to prevent MAS, in utero aspiration of meconium may not be preventable, especially if the woman presents with thick meconium and an abnormal FHR pattern or a rising FHR baseline rate and decreased variability (219, 252).

MATERNAL FACTORS THAT IMPACT FETAL ACID-BASE BALANCE

Medical and obstetric conditions can disrupt maternal and fetal acid-base equilibrium. The fetus depends on its mother and the placenta to meet its nutritive and O_2 needs. The journey of O_2 from the atmosphere through maternal alveoli to the maternal blood stream to uterine and placental vessels to the umbilical vein to the fetal blood stream may be smooth or it may be perilous. If it is smooth, fetal well-being will be evident in a reassuring FHR pattern. All too often, there are numerous obstacles which impair O_2 delivery. Table 10 lists maternal factors that may limit O_2 and nutrient delivery to the placenta and fetus, i.e., high-risk factors related to an increased fetal risk for hypoxia and/or asphyxia. For example, noncardiogenic pulmonary edema, a respiratory infection, or aspiration of gastric contents may cause maternal hypoxemia, hypotension, decreased cardiac output, and decreased uterine perfusion (253). *A risk factor is any condition that decreases F^IO_2, uteroplacental blood flow, or blood O_2 content.* Risk factors may diminish placental and fetal growth, decrease placental perfusion, and reduce fetal O_2 delivery. High-risk conditions often result in preterm delivery, IUGR, and oligohydramnios. Oligohydramnios is a sign of insufficient placental function (254).

Table 10: Maternal Risk Factors that Limit Fetal Oxygen Delivery

Decreased Oxygen Content in Inspired Air
    Altitude
    Hypoventilation
    Breath-holding During the Second Stage
    Pulmonary Disease
    Noncardiogenic Pulmonary Edema
    Adult Respiratory Distress Syndrome (ARDS)
    Seizures
    Respiratory Arrest/High Spinal Anesthesia
    Air Embolism
Increased Blood Carbon Monoxide
    Air Pollution, Suicide Attempts, Fires
    Smoking
Decreased Blood Carbon Dioxide
    Hyperventilation
Cardiac Contractility/Cardiac Output
    Cyanotic Heart Disease
    Amphetamines
    Maternal Exercise
Blood Flow and Blood Volume
    Hypovolemia
Venous Return to the Heart
    Hypotension
    Supine Position
    Position for Cesarean Section: Supine Versus Left Tilt
    Hypertension
    Preeclampsia and Spiral Artery Diameter
    Cocaine
Hemoglobin and Blood Viscosity
    Glycosylated Hemoglobin
    Blood Viscosity
    Hemoglobinopathies and Anemia
    Anemia and HbE
    Anemia and HbS
    Hemoconcentration
The Uterus
    Braxton Hicks Contractions
    Contractions
    Resting Tone
    Labor
    Uterine Rupture

Other factors, not on this list, that can increase the risk of maternal pulmonary compromise include a drug overdose, hemorrhage, DIC, congestive heart failure, cardiomyopathy, a myocardial infarction, aspiration, pulmonary embolism, and amniotic fluid embolism (255-256).

DECREASED OXYGEN CONTENT IN INSPIRED AIR
Altitude

At sea level, the PO_2 in pulmonary venules equilibrates with alveolar PO_2 (257). The mean SaO_2 level of pregnant women between 8 and 42 weeks' gestation at sea level is 98% (258). SaO_2 is stable during pregnancy. At sea level, maternal and fetal PO_2 values were as follows:

Table 11: Maternal and Fetal PO$_2$ at Sea Level

MATERNAL		FETAL	
PaO_2 90 to 100 mm Hg		P_aO_2 10-35 mm Hg	
		$P_{ua}O_2$ 10-20 mm Hg (umbilical arteries)	
PvO_2 40 mm Hg		$P_{uv}O_2$ 22-38 mm Hg (umbilical vein) (259-262).	

Notice that the maternal venous PO_2 and the umbilical vein PO_2 are very close due to the concurrent model of placental gas exchange.

Airline travel and high altitude (in animal studies) has been associated with slightly higher, but within normal, umbilical vein and artery pH, lower PCO_2, a 10 to 20% drop in fetal PaO_2, and lower birth weight compared to values obtained at sea level (259-260, 263-264). The decrease in pH and PCO_2 in umbilical cord vessels was thought to be due to maternal hyperventilation as a compensatory response to decreased O_2 levels in the air (264). Residence at high altitude creates a long-term fetal hypoxemia which may cause an increase in RBCs and blood volume, venous return to the heart, arginine vasopressin (AVP), and catecholamines. At high altitude, fetal O_2 consumption may decrease (260).

When ama fisher women of Japan and South Korea dive to harvest awabi fish, they hyperventilate before the dive. Prior to the dive, their alveolar PO_2 may reach 149 mm. However, after a 15 to 30 second dive, their PO_2 drops to 41 mm Hg (259).

Scuba divers breath in a mixture of nitrogen and O_2. Henry's Law states the amount of gas dissolved in a liquid (such as the maternal blood stream) is proportional to the pressure of the gas. The partial pressure of nitrogen is approximately 600 mm Hg. The partial pressure of O_2 is approximately 160 mm Hg. Therefore, more nitrogen than O_2 enters the diver's lungs and blood stream. At deeper levels, a higher air flow from the scuba tanks is needed to wash CO_2 out of the lungs (265). To diminish the risk of respiratory acidosis when pregnant women dive with scuba gear, it has been recommended that they limit their dives to a depth of 60 feet for half the duration recommended in the United States Navy Decompression Table (263).

266

Scuba divers also have a risk of decompression sickness from nitrogen retention. If nitrogen is not exhaled, partial pressure remains high in maternal blood and nitrogen bubbles form in tissue and body fluids. Decompression sickness occurs when nitrogen is not eliminated and bubbles form in the venous system. While the placenta is relatively impermeable to HCO_3^-, it is not impermeable to nitrogen gas. Some nitrogen bubbles enter the fetus and can damage tissue, increasing the risk of anomalies (263).

Hypoventilation

Hypoventilation results from a decreased respiratory rate and/or a decrease in the amount of inhaled O_2. Animal and human research demonstrated a *reduction in maternal F^IO_2 was associated with fetal hypoxia and acidemia and an increase in fetal AVP, renin, lactic acid and decrease in BE.* Fetal lambs significantly decreased their breathing movement time. Swallowing movements, the amount of amniotic fluid swallowed, and urine production also significantly decreased as arterial PO_2 dropped (169, 201, 266).

When women hypoventilate, CO_2 is retained and maternal and fetal PCO_2 increase. There is an increased risk of hypoventilation and orthostatic hypotension after narcotic administration. General anesthetics and CNS depressant drugs increase the risk of hypoventilation and Hb desaturation (255). Morphine sulfate, a narcotic and respiratory depressant, dilates blood vessels which lowers maternal BP. Five milligrams of IM morphine decreased the maternal respiratory rate and minute ventilation, decreased maternal PaO_2 an average of 8 mm Hg, and increased maternal $PaCO_2$ (267). When women decreased their F^IO_2 from the normal 21% to 10% for 10 minutes their fetuses had 1 of 3 possible fetal responses: *no change in the FHR, a rise in the baseline FHR of 5 to 10 bpm, or a fall in the baseline FHR of more than 20 bpm.* The smallest fetuses had a rise or fall in their FHR. Their small size suggests they were deprived of nutrients and O_2 during the pregnancy and lacked O_2 reserves to cope with maternal hypoventilation (268).

Breath-holding During The Second Stage

When six healthy people held their breath for 10 to 25 seconds their SaO_2 levels dropped (269). When a woman is pushing in a lithotomy position, on her back with her legs up in stirrups, the uterus and its contents compress the inferior vena cava, aorta, and iliac vessels. This traditional birthing position decreases maternal PaO_2. The drop in PaO_2 was not found when women pushed in an upright position (270).

If women are in lithotomy position and also hold their breath when they push, the risk of maternal and fetal PaO_2 reduction heightens. Women who were asked to hold their breath for a count of 10 had a lower PaO_2 then women who pushed based on their own physiologic need. If they held their breath during their pushing efforts they had a greater fall in their PaO_2 and rise in their $PaCO_2$ than when they breathed between pushing efforts. When women were not instructed in how to push, their *average pushing effort lasted 5

seconds with an average of 4.29 pushing efforts during each contraction. They began spontaneous pushing at an intrauterine pressure of 32 mm Hg (270).

The "count to 10" pushing method requires women to perform a Valsalva maneuver while someone counts to 10. Williams and Wilson (271) used a noninvasive hemodynamic monitoring technique to measure maternal cardiac output during four contractions and during pushing with the *Valsalva Maneuver.* They could not find a significant change in maternal cardiac output during the contractions or pushing, however, they did find maternal heart rate and mean arterial pressure increased and there was *a decrease in stroke volume* (271). The decrease in stroke volume could limit O_2 delivery to the uterus, placenta, and fetus.

Since the count to 10 method of pushing may create fetal hypoxemia, it has been recommended that any factor that decreases maternal PO_2 should, if possible, be avoided (272). Pushing techniques, other than the count to 10 method, should be encouraged. An alternate technique to breath holding during pushing is to moan, creating the sound of "Oh" or a deep humming sound. Using this alternative technique significantly shortened the second stage of labor (A. Threlfall-Mase, personal communication, September 1995).

Rest prior to pushing and open glottal pushing, where the woman makes noise, may diminish interventions, improve fetal status, diminish maternal fatigue, and improve neonatal status. Open glottal pushing may result in a shorter second stage and fewer forceps deliveries and episiotomies (273-275). Allowing primigravida women at 10 cm dilatation to rest 2 hours and multigravida women to rest 1 hour prolongs the second stage up to 4.9 hours but results in significantly fewer variable decelerations, less maternal fatigue, a significant decrease in pushing time, and a trend towards higher Apgar scores (276).

Pulmonary Disease

Interstitial and restrictive lung disease includes acute and chronic disorders of inflammation and fibrosis of the pulmonary parenchyma. Antenatal fetal surveillance may include fetal movement counting beginning at 28 weeks' gestation, and, in severe cases, ultrasound evaluation of fetal growth may occur on a regular basis (277).

Asthma. Asthma is a restrictive lung disease and acute airway obstruction that occurs in 0.4 to 1.3% of all pregnancies (278). Women with asthma hyperventilate and become hypocapnic, alkalotic, hypoxic, and anxious. Catecholamines are released and blood is shunted away from their "nonvital" uterus to their brain, heart, and adrenal glands, the "vital" organs. Uterine artery constriction and hypoxia diminish O_2 delivery to the uterus, placental, and fetus and increase the risk of fetal demise. Pregnant asthmatics may receive corticosteroids to inhale, intravenous β_2-agonists, and theophylline (279). Corticosteroids were associated with a higher than normal spontaneous abortion rate, placental insufficiency, and cleft palate. Theophylline toxicity may manifest as neonatal malformations. Malformations were more common if women received epinephrine during the first four lunar months of pregnancy. In asthmatics, histamine can provoke bronchospasm and trigger an asthma attack, increasing the risk of fetal hypoxia. Narcotics depress the respiratory rate, inhibit the cough reflex, dry secretions, and cause histamine release (30). Therefore, during labor, women with a history of asthma who receive narcotics should be closely monitored after drug administration for symptoms of asthma.

Pneumonia. Pneumonia limits maternal and fetal oxygenation. Risk factors for pneumonia include: cigarette smoking, cocaine use, asthma, human immunodeficiency virus (HIV) infection, epilepsy, and sickle cell anemia (280). In a sample of 2135 women from a Fetal Alcohol Center, 93 (4.38%) had pneumonia, 23 were HIV positive, 550 (25.88%) had endometritis during their pregnancy, and 225 (10.59%) had pyelonephritis during their pregnancy. Pneumonia was more common in women who drank alcohol and smoked cigarettes during their pregnancy, and was most common in binge drinkers and cigarette smokers (281). Alcohol consumption increases the risk of having an IUGR baby. As the number of alcoholic drinks per day increases, the risk of IUGR and oligohydramnios increases (282). The cause and effect relationship between alcohol and IUGR is unclear. However, placental insufficiency was not a major determinant of IUGR in infants who had fetal alcohol syndrome.

Noncardiogenic Pulmonary Edema

Women who have preeclampsia or iatrogenic pulmonary overload may have decreased intravascular colloid osmotic pressure (COP). The decrease in COP encourages fluid to leak out of the vasculature into the lungs (253). O_2 and CO_2 diffusion will be impaired. Impaired diffusion, ventilation-perfusion inequalities, and alveolar collapse can cause pulmonary shunting and deficient O_2 delivery to the uterus, placenta, and fetus.

Pulmonary shunting. In a critical care setting, pulmonary function may be determined by measurement of pulmonary shunting. Normally during breathing, there is a physiologic shunting of blood within pulmonary vessels so that some blood (Qs) is not returned to the left side of the heart for distribution throughout the maternal body. Qt is the abbreviation for total cardiac output. P_B is barometric pressure. PH_2O is pressure of water vapor in the lungs. <u>a</u> is a standard value (0.0031) of O_2 solubility in plasma. CaO_2 is the total amount of O_2 in the arteries and CvO_2 is the total amount of O_2 in the veins (283). The formula to calculate the right to left pulmonary shunt or Qs/Qt is:

$$Qs/Qt = \frac{100 + [1 + CaO_2 - CvO_2)/\underline{a}(P_B - PH_2O - PaCO_2 - PaO_2)}{100}$$

Qs/Qt is an indirect measure of oxygenation efficacy. *A low intrapulmonary shunt suggests more O_2 was made available to tissues such as the uterus, placenta, and fetus. A high intrapulmonary shunt suggests an inability to increase PaO_2 and O_2 delivery to the tissues.* Pulmonary or cardiac problems may create a high Qs/Qt ratio and cause an inadequate PO_2 increase (283). In *nonpregnant* healthy adults, Qs/Qt is usually 3 to 5% or 0.03 to 0.05 (284).

When Qs/Qt is abnormally high, blood and O_2 are being diverted away from the uterus, placenta, and fetus (284-285). In pregnant ewes, a Qs/Qt of 0.36 was related to decreased fetal SaO_2 and metabolic acidosis (284). In critically ill pregnant women, the average Qs/Qt ratio was as high as 180/100 or 1.80 (286). A decrease in maternal SaO_2 of 3 to 20% was related to a 21% increase in intrapulmonary shunting (255).

Intrapulmonary shunt (Qs/Qt) and position. An increase in cardiac output (Qt) reflects a decrease in the right to left pulmonary shunt. Maternal position may increase or decrease cardiac output and impact tissue O_2 delivery. To determine the normal Qs/Qt in pregnancy, 10 healthy normotensive women between 36 and 38 weeks' gestation participated in a study. *Cardiac output was significantly higher and the intrapulmonary shunt was significantly lower following 30 minutes in a left lateral position then 10 minutes in a knee-chest (on elbows and knees) position than following 30 minutes in a left*

Table 12: Intrapulmonary Shunt and Maternal Position

POSITION	AVERAGE Qs/Qt	STANDARD DEVIATION (SD)	SD ERROR
Knee-chest	0.101	0.054	0.022
Left lateral	0.152	0.033	0.01
Right lateral	0.154	0.024	0.008
Standing	0.135	0.069	0.024
Supine	0.138	0.016	0.005
Sitting	0.141	0.019	0.006

lateral position then 10 minutes in a left or right lateral position. The average intrapulmonary shunt value was nearly identical in the left and right lateral positions, therefore *either side* provides the same maternal cardiac output and O_2 delivery efficacy. There was no significant difference in the intrapulmonary shunt between a lateral, sitting, supine, or standing position. *These preliminary findings suggest a change to a knee-chest position would more likely increase uteroplacental blood flow and O_2 delivery than a sustained lateral position or a sitting, supine, or standing position* (286) (see Table 12).

Although this research suggests the best position to enhance O_2 delivery to the uterus, placenta, and fetus is knee-chest, knee-chest is awkward and is usually reserved for use when the umbilical cord prolapses. Additional research is needed to measure Qs/Qt when pregnant women have spent at least 10 minutes on their hands and knees ("on all fours"), or in a kneeling, squatting, or Trendelenburg position.

A lateral or sitting position during labor and delivery are better for fetal O_2 delivery than a supine position. Maternal cardiac output increased when women turned from a supine position to their right side. A sitting up position for 10 minutes increased maternal PO_2 an average of 13 mm Hg and *decreased* PCO_2 an average of 2.4 mm Hg. After 20 minutes in a supine position, maternal PO_2 decreased and maternal PCO_2 *increased* (272). Therefore, the risk of maternal respiratory acidosis increases after 20 minutes in a supine position.

When women were turned from a lateral position to a supine position, fetal cerebral oxygenation decreased within 10 minutes but only 5 of 14 fetuses changed their FHR in response to decreased brain oxygenation (288). When supine hypotension occurs and there is a significant fall in fetal cerebral O_2 delivery, the FHR becomes bradycardic (289-290).

A supine position during delivery decreases fetal and maternal blood O_2 content. When women sat at a 55 to 60 degree angle during delivery, fetal umbilical vein and artery O_2 content were higher than if they were supine. In spite of the differences in cord blood gases, they were still within normal limits in the sitting and supine groups. Women who sat upright had a shorter second stage than women who were supine, which might have contributed to higher O_2 levels. Women who delivered sitting up had a reduced incidence of postpartum hemorrhage (291). A maternal standing position decreased fetal lamb PaO_2 and SaO_2 (292).

Adult Respiratory Distress Syndrome (ARDS)

Adult respiratory distress occurs in 7 of 10,000 births and almost 25% of women who have ARDS die (293). Women who have ARDS are critically ill (294). ARDS may be preceded by gram negative sepsis, preeclampsia with HELLP syndrome, preterm labor and tocolysis with pulmonary edema, aspiration, or obstetric hemorrhage. Women die from multisystem organ failure, sepsis, or DIC (293).

During pregnancy, O_2 consumption increases to 245 to 340 ml/minute at term. CO_2 consumption is less than O_2 consumption at 194 to 284 ml/minute at term. Usually the O_2 delivered to maternal tissues is 400 to 500% greater than is needed to meet oxidative metabolic needs, which creates a large O_2 reserve (295). In women with ARDS, the O_2 reserve is rapidly depleted, increasing the risk of metabolic acidosis.

Women with ARDS have deficient FiO_2 and O_2 levels (294). They are hypoxemic and they hyperventilate. They become hypotensive with decreased systemic vascular resistance. Their cardiac output decreases and their risk of cardiopulmonary arrest increases. Decreased cardiac output diminishes uteroplacental perfusion and reduces O_2 delivery to the fetus (253).

Respiratory support is often necessary with endotracheal intubation and mechanical ventilation at a respiratory rate of 10 to 16 respirations per minute. Table 13 provides mechanical ventilation parameters for pregnant women who were mechanically ventilated.

Seizures

Cerebral anoxia, as a result of an air embolism or amniotic fluid embolism, may cause seizures. During the seizure, women become hypotensive. Catecholamines are released and blood is diverted away from the uterus, placenta, and fetus. The fetus will suffer an acute asphyxial insult evidenced by fetal bradycardia. Women who seize as a complication of preeclampsia become eclamptic. The seizure usually lasts about one minute but may recur (297). Eclampsia is associated with an increased risk of placental abruption, hemolysis, elevated liver enzymes, low platelets (HELLP syndrome), and DIC (298).

When women seize, they stop breathing. To prevent aspiration, women should be positioned on their side. A bite

Table 13: Mechanical Ventilation Parameters During Pregnancy (296)

FACTOR	PARAMETERS
Minute ventilation	$10,500 \pm 2496.5$ ml/minute
Tidal volume goal	9.4 ± 1 ml/kg for a $PaCO_2$ of approximately 30 mm Hg
Dynamic compliance	26.6 ± 10 ml/cm H_2O, at extubation 37.6 ± 15.8 ml/cm H_2O
Peak inspiratory pressure	34.2 ± 10.1 cm H_2O
Negative inspiratory force	39.7 ± 13.9 cm H_2O

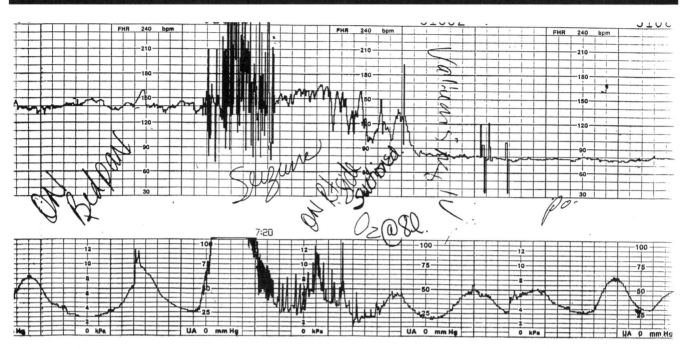

Figure 5.14: Fetal response to maternal eclampsia. The fetus had a normal heart rate until the eclamptic seizure (see artifact) occurred in this primigravida woman whose admission blood pressure was 140/105. She had a trace of proteinuria, 3+ bilateral reflexes, and no clonus. Her seizure occurred when she was receiving 2 grams/hour of magnesium sulfate. Oxytocin was immediately discontinued and a cesarean section was performed. The drop in the FHR is due to the acute asphyxial insult created by the seizure. There was one loop of nuchal cord. The baby had a lusty cry at the time of birth. Apgar scores were 9 and 9 at 1 and 5 minutes.

stick may be placed between the teeth and tongue if the jaw has not already tightened. Since the priority is to stop the seizure, a fetal monitor need not be applied at this time. If the monitor was on and is not recording, it should be ignored until the seizure has stopped and medication has been administered to prevent a recurrent seizure. Following a seizure, a tight fitting face mask should be applied and 100% O_2 at 8 to 10 LPM should be administered.

$MgSO_4$ is the best drug to stop eclamptic seizures and prevent future seizures. *$MgSO_4$, 6 grams given slowly in a vein over 15 minutes, rather than phenytoin (Dilantin), 1000 to 1500 mg via an IV drip, more often decreased the risk of recurrent seizures* (299). Instead of a 6 gram loading dose, 4 grams of a 20% solution of $MgSO_4$ in 20 ml may be administered over 3 or more minutes to stop seizures. The $MgSO_4$ loading dose should then be followed by a continuous IV infusion of one to three grams of $MgSO_4$ per hour (300).

Depending on the severity of preeclampsia, cardiac output may be half of normal, normal, or elevated (301-303). When Ca^{++} enters endothelial smooth muscle cells, blood vessels constrict. $MgSO_4$ is a Ca^{++} channel blocker. When Ca^{++} entry into cells is blocked by $MgSO_4$, blood vessels dilate. When systemic blood vessels dilate, as a result of $MgSO_4$ administration, intravascular volume and preload increase. Cardiac output and perfusion to maternal tissues should increase. In the uterus, $MgSO_4$ acts as a tocolytic by inhibiting Ca^{++} from entering uterine cells (301, 304-307). The

combination of vasodilation, increased intravascular volume, increased cardiac output, and decreased uterine activity should increase O_2 delivery to the uterus, placenta, and fetus.

During the seizure, the FHR abruptly decreases in response to the anoxic insult. Uterine hyperactivity, with increased contraction frequency and elevated resting tone, occurs because anoxic uterine cells release cytokines which stimulate prostaglandin F_2 production by the placenta and uterus (308). The surge of prostaglandins causes uterine hyperstimulation and hypertonus. Uterine hyperactivity gradually subsides over 10 to 12 minutes after the eclamptic seizure ends (297). After the seizure, the FHR usually rebounds to a tachycardic level. Fetuses that have rebound tachycardia are often delivered in good condition. Unfortunately in some cases, even with prompt intervention, eclampsia may precede fetal death. For example, in one case report, eclampsia preceded severe fetal asphyxia and the following umbilical artery blood gases: pH 6.62, PO_2 2 mm Hg, PCO_2 169 mm Hg, and HCO_3^- 15 mEq/L. The fetus died from ischemia and irreversible cardiac damage (50).

There are many other causes of maternal seizures besides eclampsia. For example, women may have epilepsy or Sturge-Weber syndrome, a rare disorder involving a port-wine facial nevus associated with intracranial venous malformation (309). Women may seize during an epidural anesthesia procedure when they accidentally receive an IV injection of an anesthetic agent such as bupivacaine (Marcaine®) and develop cardiovascular toxicity. They will initially become tachycardic, hypertensive, nauseated, they may vomit, feel tingling lips and hands, become agitated and twitch prior to the seizure. During the seizure, they may develop hypotension and arrhythmias. They need an IV bolus of crystalloid and an IV dose of ephedrine to increase their BP. They may need to be intubated and given 100% O_2. Following the seizure they may be light-headed, have slurred speech, and convulse again. They could suffer cardiorespiratory collapse and require cardiopulmonary resuscitation.

Respiratory Arrest/High Spinal Anesthesia

According to ACOG's Standards for Obstetric-Gynecologic Services, p. 38:

> "Persons administering or supervising obstetric anesthesia should be qualified to manage infrequent but occasional life-threatening complications of major regional anesthesia, such as respiratory and cardiovascular failure, toxic local anesthetic, convulsions, or vomiting and aspiration. It is preferable, however, for an anesthesiologist or anesthetist to provide obstetric anesthesia so that the obstetrician may devote undivided attention to the delivery."

A life-threatening emergency occurs when anesthesia enters the brainstem by way of the spinal canal. There will be an immediate subarachnoid block and CNS toxicity which causes a massive motor block, hypotension, and a respiratory arrest. This is obviously a medical emergency. The woman should be immediately intubated while someone holds pressure on the cricoid cartilage in the neck to compress the esophagus and prevent aspiration. She must have an IV line. A pulse oximeter should be applied to assess capillary S_pO_2. The woman will need to be manually and/or mechanically ventilated until the anesthetic dissipates. She may need medication to increase her BP and heart rate as well as chest compressions. She may seize if she develops cerebral hypoxia. The fetal response to a high spinal is nearly immediate (see Figure 5.15).

Air Embolism and the Vaginal Insufflation Syndrome

Air embolism is a rare, life-threatening emergency. An air embolism is *always* caused by air entering a vein. As little as 100 ml of air can create an air embolism. Symptoms of air embolism include:
- millwheel heart murmur with a loud, transient, churning sound over the heart
- wheezing due to acute bronchospasm
- hypotension
- confusion, obtundation, loss of consciousness and
- cyanosis.

Treatment for an air embolism includes:
- left lateral positioning or Trendelenburg so that air can rise to the top of the right ventricle and
- 100% O_2 by tight fitting face mask or intubation and 100% O_2 (310)
- placement of a right-sided heart line to aspirate air.

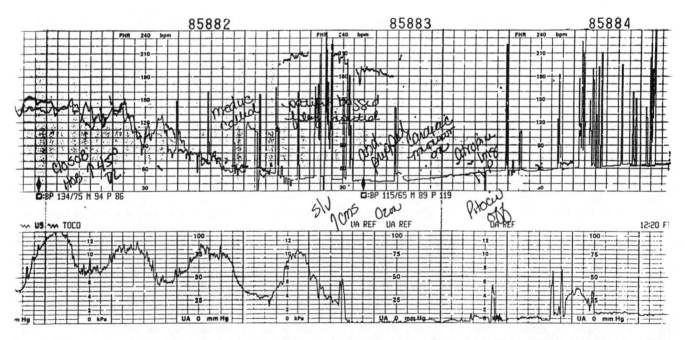

Figure 5.15: After requesting her epidural be redosed, 3 ml of 0.25% Marcaine was injected into the epidural catheter. Within four minutes she suffered a complete respiratory arrest and hypotension. Note uterine hyperstimulation and probable hypertonus following respiratory arrest. The twins were delivered by cesarean section within minutes of this tracing. Both survived without permanent injury. Their mother also survived after spending several days in intensive care. She seized after delivery and required mechanical ventilation. She suffered no residual effects from the high spinal or her seizure.

Between 1935 and 1985 there were 15 case reports of vaginal insufflation syndrome in pregnant women. They suffered a massive venous air embolism during the second or third trimester. In 93% of cases the fetus died and in 87% of cases the woman died. Vaginal insufflation syndrome occurs as a result of orogenital sex, i.e., someone blew air into the vagina. According to Geist (311), a woman's vagina can accommodate one to two liters of air under pressure. No reference to the source of this measurement was provided. Theoretically, if air passes through the cervix between the membranes and the uterine wall, it can dissect the chorion off the uterine wall and pass into veins under the placenta. Once entering maternal veins, air can travel to the right atrium, the right ventricle, the pulmonary circulation, and the left ventricle. Air in the ventricles displaces blood and decreases cardiac output. Air may enter blood vessels and cause cerebral vessel occlusion, bronchospasm, and DIC. Air embolism in pregnant women who suffered from vaginal insufflation syndrome included the previously mentioned symptoms plus chest pain, seizures, vaginal bleeding, tachypnea, focal neurologic deficits, collapse, and death. To avoid vaginal insufflation syndrome, pregnant women and their partners should be counseled to avoid the sexual practice of blowing air into the vagina. However, "routine cunnilingus is safe."

INCREASED CARBON MONOXIDE
Air Pollution, Suicide Attempts

Air pollution and smoking increase carbon monoxide levels in maternal and fetal blood. A suicide attempt with inhalation of automobile exhaust in a closed garage increases carbon monoxide levels and plasma carboxyhemoglobin (HbCO) content. The rise in HbCO increases Hb oxygen affinity and decreases tissue O_2 delivery (312). HbCO levels will be even higher in the fetus than the mother (262). Fetal and/or maternal death from hypoxia and eventual asphyxia may occur.

Smoking
Cigarette smoking, nicotine and carbon monoxide:
- reduce uteroplacental blood flow
- increase plasma carbon monoxide
- reduce placental O_2 diffusion
- create tissue hypoxia
- decrease uterine, placental, and fetal growth
- decrease fetal movement and
- lower birth weight (313-314).

In 1989, it was estimated that 20 to 30% of women of childbearing age smoked and 20 to 30% of LBW babies were born to smokers. Smokers have an increased risk of preterm birth. If women smoked 20 cigarettes per day, i.e., 1 pack per day, their babies weighed an average of 290 grams less than the babies of nonsmokers. Smokers have a reduced plasma volume but a high hematocrit which increases blood viscosity and reduces uteroplacental blood flow. Maternal spiral artery

diameter decreases and there a reduction in placental blood flow (314).

Nicotine. Nicotine and carbon monoxide diffuse across the placenta into fetal circulation. Uteroplacental blood flow is also reduced due to *nicotine*-induced vasospasm (315). Nicotine stimulates the release of epinephrine and norepinephrine from the adrenal medullae resulting in blood vessel α-receptor stimulation and vasoconstriction (316). In the placenta, nicotine increases the level of thromboxane B_2, a potent vasoconstrictor (317). Placental vasoconstriction decreases fetal O_2 delivery and birth weight. Nicotine also stimulates the release of maternal and fetal acetylcholine which inhibits SA node activity. In the fetus, nicotine is related to *decreased STV* (318). In fetal lambs, an increase in nicotine preceded an increase in BP, a decrease in umbilical blood flow, fetal hypoxia, and *a decrease in the FHR* (319).

Carbon monoxide. A decrease in O_2 affinity increases O_2 release to tissues (320). However, in smokers, there is an increase in HbCO, a decrease in P_{50}, an increase in Hb oxygen affinity, and *a decrease in O_2 delivery* to tissues (312). Cigarette smoke contains carbon monoxide. Carbon monoxide increases the level of HbCO. HbCO has been found in fetal cord blood after birth when woman smoked one cigarette within one hour before delivery (292).

Maternal hyperoxygenation expedites removal of carbon monoxide from fetal circulation. At room air, it takes approximately 7 to 9 hours to halve fetal HbCO levels, and 20 to 24 hours to remove it all. In one woman, hyperoxygenation decreased the time required to halve fetal HbCO from 3 to 4 hours at room air to 45 minutes (262).

The placenta. Smokers had more placental cystic lesions, IUGR fetuses, and oligohydramnios than nonsmokers (321). Similar lesions have been found in the placentas of diabetic women (322). Other placental lesions found in smokers include marginal *decidual necrosis which heightens the risk of abruption*, shortened microvilli, a thickened basement membrane, a decreased number of villous capillaries, and endothelial injury (314, 323). Placental O_2 transfer decreases due to trophoblastic basement membrane thickening. The placentas of smokers have decreased metabolic activity, decreased human placental lactogen production, and enlargement of the intervillous spaces. Basement membrane thickening and the enlarged intervillous space increase the distance O_2 has to travel to reach fetal capillaries, which predisposes the fetus to hypoxia (292, 315).

Biochemical synthesis of vasodilators is reduced in the umbilical arteries of babies born to women who smoke cigarettes. Umbilical arteries have a reduced capacity to generate prostacyclin (PGI_2), a vasodilator, from endothelial cells, and nitric oxide (also called endothelium-derived relaxing factor), a potent vasodilator. Nitric oxide production is reduced due to the reduction in its precursor, L-arginine (324). Therefore, the umbilical circulation is exposed to nicotine and its vasoconstrictive effect, but also there is a deficiency of vasodilators.

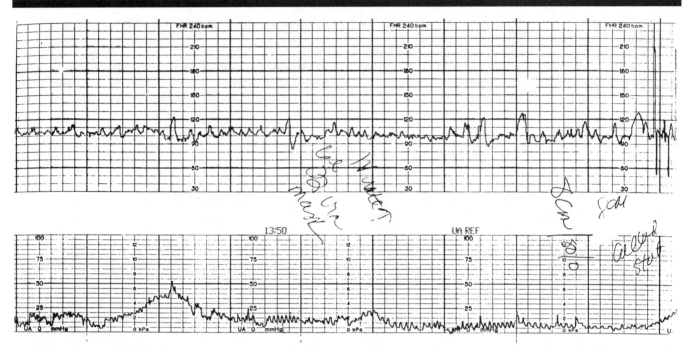

Figure 5.16: Smoking decreases the fetal heart rate. A woman who was gravida 7, para 3 with a history of 3 low birth weight babies presented at 39 weeks' gestation. She is a diet-controlled gestational diabetic who smokes 1 to 2 packs per day. Her total weight gain was 15 lbs. She presented with spontaneous rupture of membranes and clear fluid. Her cervical examination revealed a dilatation of 4 cm, 70% effacement and a vertex presentation at -1 station. Smoking decreases the fetal heart rate and increases the risk of placenta previa. Note fetal bradycardia. Apgar scores were 8, 9, and 9 at 1, 5, and 10 minutes.

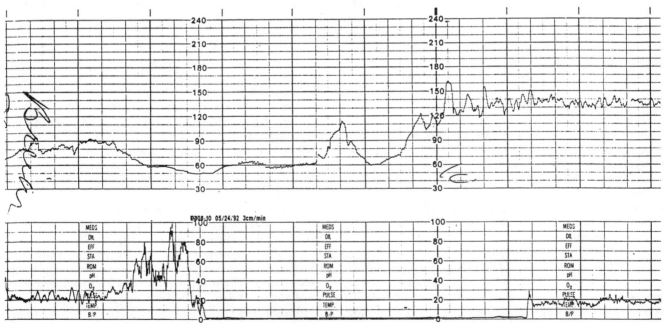

Figure 5.17: Smoking increases the risk of asphyxia. A gravida 3 para 0 single woman who smokes 2 packs per day was admitted at 41 weeks' gestation. Her cervical examination revealed 3 cm, 0 station, and vertex. Her temperature was 99° F, blood pressure was 130/88, and pulse was 90 bpm. At the time of admission, "moderate stained" meconium fluid and variable decelerations were noted. Following this prolonged deceleration, a cesarean section was performed. The baby had a nuchal cord and Apgar scores of 7, 8, and 9 at 1, 5, and 10 minutes.

Smoking increases the risk of placenta previa. When the placenta is over the internal os of the cervix, placenta previa exists. Placenta previa occurs in approximately 6 of 1000 women. In response to hypoxia, placental capillaries and villi proliferate. This increases placental diameter and thickness and increases the risk of placenta previa. As women age and their number of pregnancies increases, their risk of placenta previa also increases. The risk of placenta previa increases in woman with a history of a spontaneous or induced abortion, cesarean section, or in women who use alcohol, cigarettes, and/or illicit drugs (325).

Smoking cessation is difficult. Even though women say they quit smoking, urine cotinine tests supported the lack of smoking cessation in 5,572 women who participated in a smoking cessation program in public clinics (326). Use of the nicotine patch may not be helpful since it was associated with higher maternal blood pressures (327). Some believe smoking cessation is more likely if women are informed of the fetal risks of their smoking and the physician reinforces instructions at each prenatal visit. It seemed helpful for women to met regularly with a smoking cessation counselor. As a result of the combined physician/counselor interventions, 27% of women decreased the number of cigarettes they smoked, 36% stopped smoking, and there was an increase in birth weight compared with babies of women who did not limit their smoking (328). Even without a smoking cessation counselor, physicians who followed a scripted intervention were apparently able to decrease the number of women who smoke during their pregnancy. Biochemical confirmation of smoking cessation was verified by breath carbon monoxide levels (329). Some women will relapse and smoke again, often to assuage their strong feelings of deprivation (330).

DECREASED CARBON DIOXIDE
Hyperventilation
During pregnancy, women increase their respiratory rate over prepregnant norms (331). When the respiratory rate increases, maternal PCO_2 levels decrease which creates a state of respiratory alkalosis (312). Respiratory alkalosis is secondary to the effect of progesterone. Increased renal HCO_3^- excretion partially compensates for the drop in PCO_2 and the rise in H^+ (332). Hyperventilation and maternal alkalosis may cause *vasoconstriction of uterine and umbilical blood vessels* (33, 254, 333).

Decrease in PO_2 and PCO_2, increase in lactate. When women were asked to hyperventilate for 18 minutes or less, there was *a drop in fetal scalp capillary PCO_2* (331). During the first stage of labor as many as 32% of women were alkalotic, but only 19.2% were alkalotic during the second stage (37). During the first stage of labor, the average fetal PCO_2 was 33.8 mm Hg, and the average maternal PCO_2 was 29.9 mm Hg, a difference of 3.9 torr. Maternal and fetal PCO_2 increased during the second stage of labor and this gradient slightly decreased from an average fetal PCO_2 of 45.2 mm Hg

and maternal PCO_2 of 41.9 mm Hg, a difference of 3.3 mm Hg (35).

General anesthesia and a fall in pH. If the induction-to-delivery time was more than 8 minutes and the *uterine incision-to-delivery time was more than 3 minutes, there was a significant decrease in the umbilical artery pH* (from an average of 7.31 to 7.22) and more 1-minute Apgar scores that were less than 7 (73 versus 4%). If women had a spinal, a uterine incision-to-delivery time greater than 3 minutes was associated with lower umbilical artery pH (7.18 versus 7.30) and Apgar scores less than 7 (62% versus 0%). All women received 1000 ml of 5% dextrose in lactated Ringer's solution prior to either type of anesthesia. The researchers recommended prolongation of the uterine incision-to-delivery interval should be avoided to minimize the risk of fetal acidemia (334).

General anesthesia and a rise in pH. During general anesthesia, women were purposefully hyperventilated. Their PCO_2 decreased and their pH increased with no ill effect on the fetus. Fetal scalp PO_2 decreased from 24.8 mm Hg to 19.3 mm Hg. A bolus of IV fluid prior to anesthesia diminished the drop in fetal PO_2 (30, 331). The bolus of IV fluid given prior to anesthesia increases uteroplacental blood flow. Concomitant inhalation of O_2 maintains high fetal PO_2 levels (30).

Animal studies with fetal lambs, guinea pigs, and pigs found maternal *hyperventilation resulted in a fall in fetal PCO_2, PO_2, and BE and a rise in lactate, pyruvate, and pH* (36). In humans, lactate increases in the fetal umbilical vein when maternal PCO_2 is less than 23 mm Hg. In addition, there may be *a small but significant drop in umbilical vein PO_2, an increase in pH*, but no change in the buffer base or HCO_3^-. The small drop in umbilical vein PO_2 is innocuous (333).

CARDIAC CONTRACTILITY/CARDIAC OUTPUT
Pregnant women with a mitral valve prosthesis, mechanical aortic prosthesis, atrial fibrillation, or a combination of these are at high risk for systemic arterial embolization, often from valve thrombosis (335). Ventricular fibrillation may precede cardiac arrest, maternal and fetal anoxia, and bradycardia (see Figure 5.18).

Cyanotic Heart Disease
Women with cyanotic heart disease are hypoxemic (259). They shunt blood away from their uterus which decreases uteroplacental blood flow. The placenta continues to consume O_2, increasing the risk of fetal hypoxemia. In lab experiments, placental blood flow could be significantly reduced to a level of 25 ml/minute before O_2 transfer to fetal circulation became inadequate to meet fetal oxidative metabolic needs (336).

Amphetamines
S(+) methamphetamine hydrochloride, known as "ice," can be smoked in a pipe. Amphetamines interact with

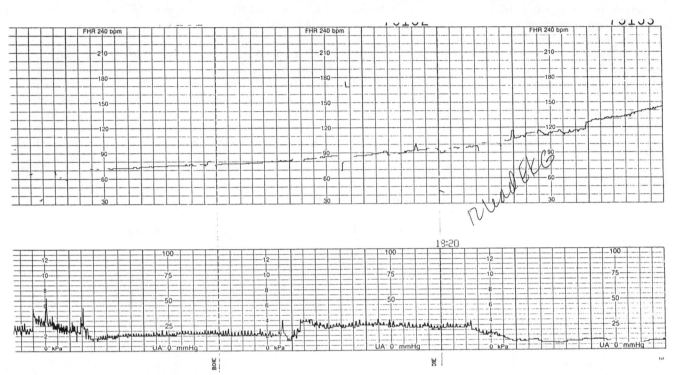

Figure 5.18: Maternal ventricular fibrillation then defibrillation preceded this fetal heart rate pattern. The fetus rebounded to a flat baseline rate of 170 bpm and later developed late decelerations with a baseline near 150 bpm. The woman was intubated and hyperoxygenated. Maternal pH was 7.35. Fetal pH was 7.25 three hours after this fetal heart rate pattern. After the vaginal birth, umbilical artery gases revealed hypoxia and respiratory acidosis with the following blood gases: pH 7.129 PO_2 14.9 PCO_2 66.4 Base excess -8.8 Bicarbonate 22 mEq/L.

neuronal monoamine transporters in the CNS. They block the neuronal reuptake of catecholamines which causes cardiac stimulation and vasoconstriction. Serotonin and norepinephrine levels increase in the intervillous space. Both of these are monoamines and potent vasoconstrictors (337). Amphetamines administered to pregnant ewes decreased uteroplacental blood flow and fetal lamb PaO_2 (338). Methamphetamine administration increased systemic vascular resistance (SVR), the mean arterial pressure (MAP), but did not change the heart rate. The increase in SVR decreased uteroplacental perfusion (339). Amphetamines cause maternal hypertension, fetal IUGR, preterm labor, and placental abruption (337). The fetal lamb response to maternal methamphetamine administration is an increase in plasma glucose, insulin, and lactate and a decrease in umbilical artery pH (340).

Maternal Exercise

Strenuous exercise may reduce uteroplacental blood flow, create fetal hypoxemia, and reduce birth weight. Women who were 25 to 36 weeks pregnant performed isometric extensor exercises of their legs. Their heart rate, SVR, and MAP increased. However, their cardiac output did not change (341). Experiments with pregnant ewes who walked on a treadmill found fetal oxygenation was compromised by reduced uterine blood flow during moderate exercise and maternal and fetal glucose concentrations increased due to glycogenolysis. Glycogenolysis was most likely a consequence of exercise-induced hypoxemia (342).

If fetal O_2 delivery is decreased, birth weight will be adversely affected. In human fetuses, *birth weight was lower in women who had the highest exertion and lowest relaxation at work, at home, and during fitness exercise* (343). Concern existed that maternal respiratory alkalosis might be induced by exercise and that would decrease placental O_2 transfer due to a left shift in the oxyhemoglobin dissociation curve. Concern also existed that fetal hypocapnia (as a result of maternal hypocapnia during exercise) might decrease umbilical blood flow, a finding in fetal lambs when the ewe exercised to exhaustion (342). However, strenuous bicycling by 15 "in shape" women had no effect on umbilical artery blood flow or fetal cardiac diastolic ventricular filling (344).

BLOOD FLOW AND BLOOD VOLUME

Blood flow and Hb concentration affect tissue O_2 delivery. *Blood flow is more important than intravascular volume, because uncirculated RBCs cannot reach their destination to deliver O_2* (345). Blood flow is dependent on hemodynamic factors including blood volume and blood viscosity.

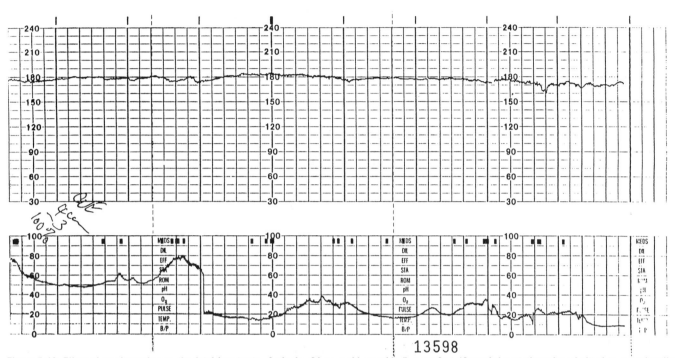

Figure 5.19: Effect of amphetamine on the fetal heart rate. A single, 21 year old, gravida 5, para 3 at 40 weeks' gestation who admitted to occasionally smoking but denied alcohol consumption during the pregnancy had a positive urine toxicology screen for amphetamines (> 8,000). She was admitted with spontaneous rupture of membranes at home, 4 cm, vertex, -3 station. She delivered within 1 hour of admission. Her heart rate was 120 to 130 bpm. Temperature was 97.8° F. Note fetal tachycardia. Even after her positive urine screen for amphetamines, she denied drug use. The baby also tested positive for amphetamines. The Apgar scores were 6, 7, and 7 at 1, 5, and 10 minutes.

Hypovolemia

Hypovolemia is deficient blood volume. Hypervolemia is rare and is excessive blood volume. Hypervolemia is usually iatrogenic and due to IV fluid overload and the inability of the kidneys to excrete excess water. Hypervolemia may occur during prolonged administration of oxytocin given in conjunction with 5% dextrose in water (D_5W). The resulting water intoxication can cause maternal death (346).

The amount of fluid in blood vessels depends on the balance between colloid osmotic pressure (COP), capillary hydrostatic pressure, interstitial fluid osmotic pressure, interstitial hydrostatic pressure, and capillary permeability (345). Preeclamptic women have decreased COP due to proteinuria and a reduction in plasma colloids. Capillary permeability is also increased in preeclamptic women and fluid leaks into interstitial spaces causing edema. The loss of plasma into interstitial spaces causes hemoconcentration and hypovolemia. Hypovolemia worsens if preeclamptic women develop HELLP syndrome with hemolysis (H), liver ischemia and elevated liver enzymes (EL), and abnormal platelet consumption with a low platelet count (LP).

Hypovolemia was found in 64.5% of women who had either preterm labor, preeclampsia, an IUGR fetus, oligohydramnios, or polyhydramnios (345). Hypovolemia limits nutrient and O_2 delivery to tissues resulting in *IUGR and a LBW neonate*. Women with preeclampsia have an increased preterm birth rate and more IUGR fetuses than non-preeclamptic women (347).

Indirect evidence of hypovolemia includes a failure of the hematocrit to decrease between 24 and 36 weeks' gestation, no dependent ankle edema, *diminished uterine growth*, no cardiac systolic ejection murmur, no increase in heart size, and a serum blood urea nitrogen (BUN)/creatinine ratio greater than 15. Supine and upright positions limit renal excretion of BUN and creatinine (348). Therefore, if treatment for hypovolemia includes bed rest, women should be instructed to lay in a lateral position. IV crystalloids may be administered to increase intravascular volume and albumin or Hespan® may be administered to increase COP.

VENOUS RETURN TO THE HEART
Hypotension

Hypotension occurs in 5 to 25% of women undergoing regional anesthesia, such as an epidural or spinal (20). The risk of hypotension is highest after spinal anesthesia which occurred in 25 to 95% of women. Maternal hypotension can decrease the delivery of O_2 to the uterus, placenta, and fetus. Following administration of regional anesthetics, fetal cerebral hemoglobin O_2 saturation fell as much as 8% without a significant change in cerebral blood flow (288). Hypotension may be detected best in the legs versus the arms (288, 349).

The risk of hypotension increases if a woman is supine following regional anesthetic administration. Normally, sympathetic nerves compensate for hypotension by causing peripheral vasoconstriction. However, after epidural or spinal anesthesia, sympathetic blockade prevents vasoconstriction. Instead, blood vessels dilate and BP falls. Vasodilation causes blood to pool in the lower extremities, decreasing preload, cardiac output, and uteroplacental blood flow (288, 350-351). Hypotension may be prevented by fluid preloading with 1000 to 1500 of a nondextrose crystalloid solution. When the woman is supine, the uterus should be shifted to the left by insertion of a wedge or pillow under the right side or hip (290, 350, 352).

Epidural anesthesia may precede a significant drop in fetal cerebral O_2 delivery. Therefore, some physicians advocate continuous fetal monitoring during and following regional anesthesia (73). It is reasonable to monitor the fetus after regional anesthetic drugs have been administered. It may not be reasonable to monitor the fetus during the insertion of the needle into the spinal column or epidural space. Depending on the preference of the anesthesiologist or certified nurse anesthetist (CRNA), the fetal monitor may be removed during the insertion of the needle into the spine. Even if a fetal monitor were on the woman during needle insertion and there was a change in the FHR pattern that caused concern, the woman cannot be moved until the needle is out of her back. Because of the risk of hypotension, the fetal monitor should be applied as soon as possible after needle removal, and preferably prior to injection of anesthetic drugs used for spinal anesthesia.

Supine Position

It has been recommended that the supine or back-lying position be avoided in labor and in pregnant women who have an acute blood loss, preeclampsia, or hypovolemic shock (272). If a woman has an acute blood loss, in may be helpful to raise her legs while measures are being taken to increase RBC and/or intravascular volume. A supine position may decrease lung expiratory reserve volume and ventilation in lower lung zones. When women were given morphine sulfate and placed in a supine position, their capillary PO_2 decreased (353).

Pregnant women have an exaggerated lumbar lordotic curvature in their spine which facilitates compression of their vena cava and aortoiliac vessels when they lie on their back (20). *Iliac artery compression* in the pregnant ewe decreased uterine perfusion, decreased fetal PaO_2, pH and BE, increased serum lactate, and there was no significant rise in $PaCO_2$ (354). *Compression of the ewe's aorta* decreased uterine perfusion and caused hypoxia, CO_2 retention, and a decrease in the pH. The fetal lamb's *heart rate decreased 30%*, umbilical blood flow decreased 22%, PO_2 decreased, PCO_2 increased, and pH decreased (195). *Mechanical compression* on the aorta, inferior vena cava, and iliac vessels can potentially increase venous pressure in the lower body and decrease venous return to the heart, decreasing preload, cardiac output, BP,

and uterine blood flow (20, 288, 354-355). *Aortocaval compression is associated with fetal respiratory acidosis, metabolic acidosis, and bradycardia* (288-290).

Position for Cesarean Section: Supine Versus Left Tilt

In 1971, Waldron and Wood (349) discovered that a supine position for cesarean section decreased uteroplacental blood flow and umbilical vein PO_2 (29.7 to 15.7 mm Hg). When women were tilted 10 degrees to the left, umbilical vein PO_2 values were higher (23.9 to 36.1 mm Hg). If the time from *uterine* incision to delivery took longer than three minutes, neonatal catecholamine levels were higher, arterial pH was lower, and Apgar scores were lower than in neonates who were delivered in less than three minutes from uterine incision to delivery (356).

Hypertension

Blood flow is chronically reduced in hypertensive women such as preeclamptics, severe diabetics, and women with chronic renal disease, underlying vascular disease, or autoimmune diseases (357-358). Preeclampsia is a disease of vasospasm, hypertension, and spiral artery vasoconstriction (359). Organ and placental perfusion are decreased. To compensate, preeclamptic women have a high O_2 extraction ratio (consumption/delivery). In spite of increased O_2 extraction, they are often unable to meet tissue needs and tissues become ischemic (294). Autoimmune diseases that affect pregnancy outcome include systemic lupus erythematosus, Sjögren's syndrome, and antiphospholipid antibody syndromes such as anticardiolipin antibody (ACA) syndrome. ACA is also associated with hypertension and clot formation which can limit O_2 delivery to the fetus.

Antihypertensive drugs, such as hydralazine (Apresoline®), had a greater effect on maternal blood vessel diameter than placental vascular resistance (360). When blood vessel smooth muscles relax, diastolic pressure falls. As long as the diastolic BP is maintained near 90 mm Hg, there will be no significant change in uteroplacental blood flow. A drop below 90 mm Hg is a *relative hypotension* for a hypertensive pregnant women, and blood will be shunted away from the uterus to meet her tissue O_2 needs.

Cocaine

Cocaine is the most commonly abused illicit drug during pregnancy (361). The statistics of cocaine addiction in the United States are shocking: 2.2 million people or 1 out of every 100 Americans is a cocaine addict. There were over 400,000 cocaine addicts in the state of New York (362). *Fifty-six million American women between 15 and 44 years of age are substance abusers (361). Every day more than 1000 babies are born addicted to an illicit drug (363). Approximately 1 out of every 10 live-born babies in the United States is exposed in utero to cocaine* (364). Cocaine use may be as low as 3.9% during pregnancy in rural areas and 11% or more in urban areas (365). Cocaine use may be as high as 45% of women surveyed (366-367). If cocaine-addicted women remained in a chemical dependency program for three or more months during their pregnancy, they had better pregnancy outcomes and were drug-free at delivery compared to women who did not receive these services prior to 28 weeks' gestation (368).

Women with a history of substance abuse during their pregnancy were more likely to be single (81%), smoke cigarettes (60%), drink alcohol (50%), have a drug exposed neonate (45%), have preterm labor (19%), and have syphilis (15%) (369). In a survey of pregnant inner-city women, 65% smoked and 50% used illicit drugs. They also had a limited understanding of neonatal risks of maternal HIV infection (370). Sex for drugs was prevalent among pregnant women who binged on crack or cocaine every 5 to 7 days. Prostitution was common among women who binged every 3 to 5 days (366).

The predominant route of cocaine administration is inhalation by smoking. Crack cocaine, the solid, rock-like, alkaloidal form of cocaine, may be rolled in a tobacco or marijuana cigarette or freebased. Intranasal snorting of cocaine was the next most common. Polydrug use occurred in 94.2% of women who used cocaine (366). Marijuana and heroin use are increasing (371).

Cocaine abuse is associated with poor nutrition, indiscriminate sexual activity, and decreased use of health services (366). Women who are addicted may never seek prenatal care or they may begin care in the late second or third trimester. They may become agitated, anxious, excited, or defensive when asked about illicit drug use (372). Women may smuggle hashish, heroin, or cocaine in their vagina. One woman who did so died. Another woman needed the physician to use a small Elliot forceps to remove a vaginal package of cocaine. This is known as body packing. If the package ruptures, the vagina should be immediately flushed with a large amount of saline irrigation solution to prevent absorption of the drug (373).

Cocaine use within 48 hours of testing may be confirmed by urine or serum toxicology screening for benzoylecgonine, a cocaine metabolite (365, 374). The level of urine benzoylecgonine was strongly related to the level of serum benzoylecgonine (r = 0.92) (374). Cocaine is metabolized primarily by esterases and by cytochromic P_{450} enzymes, which may be reduced during pregnancy. Cocaine levels were considerably higher in pregnant than nonpregnant ewes (375). Cocaine metabolites include ecgonine methyl ester and norcocaine which may be detected in amniotic fluid (376). Placental transfer of cocaine is by simple diffusion (361). Cocaine travels to the fetus via the umbilical vein (376). Drug concentration in the fetus is usually 50 to 100% of maternal levels (361).

Some hospitals have universal drug screening of all women in labor. Others screen when women verbalize recent drug use or have no prenatal care, a positive blood test for HIV, or a sexually transmitted disease (364). Cocaine addicts have mood swings and are often reluctant to provide a sample of urine (372). When drug addiction is suspected, it is best to observe the woman urinate or obtain a specimen by sterile catheterization. Some women have been caught placing toilet bowl water in their specimen cup prior to urination. Others have had a sample of someone else's urine with them in anticipation of a drug screen.

Cocaine blocks the reuptake of epinephrine and norepinephrine in presynaptic nerve terminals and extraneuronal sites. This causes vasoconstriction increasing maternal and fetal BP (366, 377-378). Between 24 and 36 weeks' gestation, *fetal cerebral blood flow decreased* following maternal cocaine use (379). Chronic cocaine use is associated with IUGR and LBW (29 versus 12% in noncocaine users) (380). Babies born to cocaine addicts had an increased risk of limb defects, abdominal wall defects, cleft lip, and poor neurodevelopment (366, 381).

Cocaine stimulates the medulla oblongata which increases the respiratory rate. Breathing will be rapid and shallow (361). Cardiovascular complications of cocaine use include anemia, hypertension, myocardial ischemia and infarction, arrhythmias, and death from cardiotoxicity and cardiovascular collapse (366-367). The acute, life-threatening cardiac events often appear in the first minute after cocaine use. In the pregnant ewe, IV cocaine produced tachycardia, increased myocardial O_2 demand and O_2 consumption, decreased cardiac output, and after the first minute, increased systemic vascular resistance (375). Systemic infections, such as pneumonia, hepatitis B, and urinary tract infections increase as the frequency of cocaine binging increases. Cocaine users are more likely to have syphilis or HIV than nondrug users (366). Cerebrovascular hemorrhage may occur (366-367). If "crack" cocaine is smoked, the risk of asthma, chronic cough, and pneumothorax increase. Cocaine addicts are at risk for platelet deficiency (thrombocytopenia) and hemorrhage. The reason for the platelet deficiency is unknown. *A platelet count is needed when cocaine use has been confirmed and/or the following are noted: petechiae, a bloody nose, blood in the urine or stool, and bleeding gums* (367).

Cocaine use is associated with spontaneous abortions, abruption, *preterm labor, preterm birth, and prelabor rupture of membranes* (366-367, 380, 382-383). Cocaine use increases the risk of *preterm labor* by 20 to 50% and increases uterine activity because it

- stimulates oxytocin secretion in a dose-dependent manner
- inhibits cAMP or β-adrenergic uterine receptor activity and
- stimulates α -adrenergic uterine receptors
- increases myometrial prostaglandin production (351, 366, 378, 382, 384-385).

In women with a history of cesarean section, "crack" abuse has been associated with uterine rupture (378). Cocaine addicts have a risk of precipitous delivery. The time from rupture of membranes to labor and rupture of membranes to delivery is significantly shorter in cocaine users versus nonusers. For example, rupture of membranes to delivery was 17.8 to 60.4 hours in the cocaine users and 18 to 137.2 hours in the nonusers (383). During pregnancy, labor, delivery, and post partum, a supportive and caring nursing approach will provide comfort to the cocaine-addicted woman (386).

HEMOGLOBIN AND BLOOD VISCOSITY
Glycosylated Hemoglobin (HbA$_{1C}$)

Glucose binds to the same site on Hb that 2,3-DPG binds to. When Hb is bound to glucose, it is called glycosylated hemoglobin. When O$_2$ is bound to Hb, Hb takes longer to become glycosylated. Deoxygenated Hb (Hb) binds with glucose twice as fast as oxygenated Hb (HbO$_2$). A high level of HbA$_{1C}$ in the first seven weeks of pregnancy depletes cell phospholipids and causes malformations (387-388). There were fewer malformations in rat fetuses when their mothers were given myoinositol and arachidonic acid by mouth. This experimental regimen restored membrane phospholipid integrity and prevented embryopathy and might be available some day for human fetuses (387). The level of HbA$_{1C}$ is associated with the preceding one to two month period. Pregnant diabetic women should have their HbA$_{1C}$ levels examined every two to four weeks during pregnancy and a minimum of one nonstress test a week (312). Even with "good" metabolic control and HbA$_{1C}$ levels of 6.2 to 7.6%, newborns were hypoglycemic and hyperbilirubinemic (389). The cytokine interleukin 1 (IL-1) mediates vascular endothelial injury in diabetics. The concentration of IL-1 was weakly associated with the concentration of HbA$_{1C}$ (r = 0.597). *As HbA$_{1C}$ increases, the risk of vascular injury increases.* Women who had an elevated HbA$_{1C}$ level between 16 and 20 weeks' gestation had significantly more preeclampsia than women with lower HbA$_{1C}$ levels (390). Glucose control should decrease the risk of vascular injury and may decrease the incidence of preeclampsia (391-392). Use of an insulin pump resulted in lower HbA$_{1C}$ levels in class B to R diabetics than in diabetics who did not use the pump (393).

Diabetes

Elevated glucose levels after ingestion of 100 grams of glucola are:

- Fasting glucose >105 mg/dl
- 1 hour post prandial glucose > 190 mg/dl
- 2 hour post prandial glucose > 165 mg/dl
- 3 hour post prandial glucose > 145 mg/dl (394).

A one hour 50 gram glucola test is often used to screen for gestational diabetes. If it is greater than 190 mg/dl, the diagnosis is usually made (395). Women with elevated glucose screening tests were at higher risk for macrosomia and shoulder dystocia (394). Babies of insulin-dependent diabetic women have an increased risk of myocardial hypertrophy (396). If the 1 hour post prandial level was 220 mg/dl and the 3 hour post prandial glucose was greater than 200 mg/dl, as many as 90% of gestational diabetes were identified (395, 397).

Diabetics have excessive HbA$_{1C}$ and thromboxane, a potent vasoconstrictor (398). Glycosylation lowers RBC 2,3-DPG, lowers the P$_{50}$ level, increases Hb oxygen affinity and decreases O$_2$ delivery to maternal and fetal tissues (312). *Excessive HbA$_{1C}$ has been associated with chronic tissue hypoxia,* *fetal acidosis, asphyxia, and stillbirth.* Acidosis was more common in fetuses who weighed more than 4000 grams versus less than 4000 grams, possibly due to poor glucose control and a lower pH (399). Neonates of insulin-dependent diabetics (Type I) also had a higher rate of hypoglycemia and respiratory distress syndrome than neonates of adult onset diabetics (Type II) (400). Evidence of chronic hypoxia includes extramedullary hematopoietic tissue, significant increases in umbilical cord erythropoietin, and an abnormally high number of NRBCs. Hypoxia of growing embryonic or fetal tissues increases the risk of birth defects (312, 389). Therefore, it is important for diabetic women to decrease their HbA$_{1C}$ levels prior to conception.

Villous changes related to diabetes hinder O$_2$ diffusion. Diabetics also have a significant risk of ketoacidosis. As many as 75% of all stillbirths prior to 36 weeks' gestation have been associated with ketoacidosis (312). Sodium bicarbonate may be administered to treat maternal ketoacidosis. Sodium bicarbonate does not cross the placenta, but it does increase maternal PCO$_2$ and fetal PCO$_2$. In one woman, fetal PCO$_2$ increased from 21 to 76 mm Hg after maternal sodium bicarbonate administration (35).

Pregnancy and labor management of the diabetic. The three goals of management of diabetes during pregnancy and/or labor include avoidance of ketoacidosis, optimal weight gain, and maintenance of a fasting glucose and 2 hour post prandial glucose between 61 and 150 mg/dl (388). Diet therapy improves insulin secretion in gestational diabetics (401). Amylase, secreted by the fetal pancreas, can be measured in amniotic fluid. A high amylase level was associated with an elevation of maternal HbA$_{1C}$ (402).

When goals are met during pregnancy, diabetic women should be able to reach full term. Even class F diabetics with significant loss of renal function are delivering after 34 weeks' gestation when they are well managed during pregnancy. As many as 53.1% of these women had preeclampsia and 12% had a small for gestational age (SGA) neonate (403). Catopril improved renal function and resulted in favorable fetal outcomes (404). However, angiotensin-converting enzyme inhibitors should be avoided in pregnancy due to their association with oligohydramnios and neonatal anuria.

With close glucose control, diabetic women may be counseled to expect favorable outcomes in spite of the increased risk of neonatal malformations, maternal hypertension, and pre-eclampsia (405). Between 1978 and 1993, the number of vaginal births in diabetic women increased from 14% to 32% in one medical center. The cesarean section rate fell from 80% between 1978 and 1983 to 61% between 1988 and 1993 (406).

The risk of neonatal respiratory distress is higher in diabetic women due to the delay in the appearance of phosphatidylglycerol (PG) until after the 37th week of gestation. After the 37th week, there was no significant increase in neonatal pulmonary disease (407).

Blood Viscosity

Blood viscosity is related to O_2 delivery in all vascular beds (408). The hematocrit is independent of blood flow yet it affects blood flow (285). A change in the hematocrit affects tissue O_2 delivery. The hematocrit is the ratio of RBCs to plasma volume and is the primary determinant of blood viscosity. An abnormally high or low hematocrit will increase or decrease blood viscosity. In either case, *O_2 delivery to tissues decreases due to diminished perfusion.* For example, IUGR fetuses may be polycythemic due to increased NRBC production in response to chronic hypoxia (292). The increase in their blood viscosity due to their elevated hematocrit perpetuates their hypoxia. Maternal anemia decreases O_2 delivery to the uterus, placenta, and fetus and increases the risk of fetal hypoxia and death.

Hemoglobinopathies and Anemia

There are over 325 hemoglobinopathies and 6 types of Hb alpha (α), beta (β), gamma (γ), delta (δ), epsilon (ϵ), and zeta (ζ)). Adult Hb, HbA, is composed of two alpha chains and two beta chains. Adult HbA_2 is composed of two alpha chains and two delta chains (409).

Two hemoglobinopathies can cause maternal anemia: thalassemia and sickle cell disease (409). Maternal anemia may be chronic or acute. Thalassemia major and sickle cell disease are associated with *chronic anemia.*

Acute anemia may be caused by maternal hemorrhage. As long as the hematocrit was not less than 50% below the normal level, *acute blood loss in the ewe* caused cardiac output to increase, coronary blood vessels dilated, and tissue O_2 delivery remained constant or slightly dropped. Blood flow to the brain and adrenal glands increased slightly less than coronary blood flow and there was a slight drop in O_2 delivery to the heart. Blood flow to the kidneys, internal organs, uterus, placenta, and fetus all decreased due to vasoconstriction (406). When the ewe's hematocrit dropped below 50% of normal, fetal O_2 reserves became depleted, O_2 consumption decreased, and the fetal lamb became hypoxic and acidemic (292, 408).

Anemia and HbE

Thalassemia is a disorder of autosomal dominant inheritance which may be heterozygous (on one chromosome) or homozygous (on two chromosomes). Women with thalassemia have decreased production of alpha or beta globin chains (409). HbE, an abnormal Hb, is found in Southeast Asians from Cambodia, Thailand, and Laos, and in people from northeast India. Women with homozygous HbE/HbE blood do not suffer from anemia. However, women with heterozygous HbE/Hb β-thalassemia will be diagnosed with thalassemia major and will suffer from severe anemia.

Women with thalassemia have decreased hemoglobin-O_2 binding due to high levels of 2,3 DPG. There may be a marked increase in the number of NRBCs. They often have extra spinal tissue (extramedullary hematopoiesis) that produce RBCs. Extramedullary tissue may also be found in

their spleen, liver, and lymph nodes. Their fetuses may be anomalous or be IUGR due to chronic hypoxia. They often deliver preterm (163).

Anemia and HbS

When the two beta globin chains are abnormal, HbS exists with sickle cell disease. When only one beta chain is abnormal, women have HbAS and sickle cell trait. Sickle cell trait is present in approximately 8% of Americans of African and Mediterranean descent (410-411).

Sickle cell life span. The life span of a sickle cell is 20 days versus a normal RBC life span of 120 days (411). Women with sickle cell disease and sickle cell trait often have high levels of HbF. The level of HbF was inversely associated with birth weight (412).

Complications of sickle cell disease. In addition to anemia, women with sickle cell disease may be hypertensive, edematous, and have proteinuria, yet they are not preeclamptic. During their pregnancy, they may receive biweekly ultrasounds to measure amniotic fluid volume and monitor fetal behavior and growth. If they go into preterm labor, they may be given betamethasone to mature fetal lungs and diminish the risk of respiratory distress syndrome and IVH (413).

Women with sickle cell disease are prone to infections (414). They may have multiple urinary tract infections and pyelonephritis (410). To prevent infection and treat anemia, they are often given prophylactic antibiotics (414). Most women are not iron deficient due to their history of multiple transfusions. All women, however, need additional folate supplementation.

Anemia and the fetus. Often, women with sickle cell disease have an Hb of only 7 gm/dl. *The goal of care is to maintain their Hb at or above 10 gm/dl* in order to provide sufficient O_2 carrying capacity to meet maternal, placental, and fetal needs (413). A Hb level less than 10 mg/dl significantly decreases O_2 delivery resulting in fetal hypoxemia and decreased FHR baseline variability (see Figure 5.20).

Labor management. During labor, the Hb and hematocrit of anemic women should be measured every four to six hours (415). Women with sickle cell disease should be well hydrated. Their room should be comfortable and well ventilated with limited stimuli. To prevent infectious morbidity, vaginal examinations should be limited. If membranes are ruptured, a spiral electrode should be applied to improve patient comfort (one less belt) and to continuously monitor the fetus. She may need a transfusion of washed packed RBCs which are warmed to no greater than 42°C. The goal is to maintain the Hb above 7 gm/dl and the hematocrit above 20% (413-414). Blood must not be warmed above 42° C (personal communication, American Association of Blood Banks, Bethesda, MD

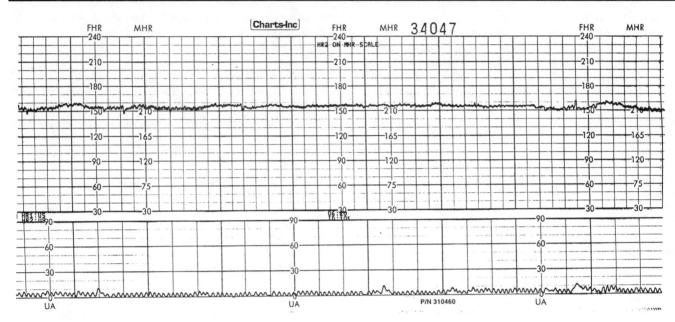

Figure 5.20: Severe anemia limits oxygen delivery to the fetus. A single economically disadvantaged gravida 3, para 2 woman with a history of gestational diabetes and 2 previous cesarean sections was admitted at 36 weeks' gestation with a hemoglobin of 6.5 gm/dl and a hematocrit of 21.7%. Small spontaneous accelerations were present as well as small uniform accelerations (see the first and last minute of this example). She was given a tocolytic and supplemental vitamins and iron.

December 1994). She will need analgesia for pain. Warm compresses should be applied to painful bones or joints. She may require O_2 by mask at 8 to 10 liters per minute and heparin therapy. A pediatrician or neonatologist should be present at the birth. Some women may receive sodium bicarbonate. In the past, women with sickle cell disease were given urea or cyanate in invert sugar to decrease the risk of sickling and a crisis (411, 414).

Sickle cell crisis. Sickle cells are distorted RBCs that become elongated and crescent-shaped. They are slow moving and cause blood stasis which causes more sickling (411). When the Hb is 7 gm/dl or less, the risk of a sickle cell crisis heightens. Sickle cell crisis is a painful vasoocclusive condition. During sickle cell crisis, sickle cells aggregate and blood flow diminishes through capillaries. There is localized tissue hypoxia and acidosis and woman in crisis feel pain in the ischemic areas (414).

Dehydration, hypotension, exertion, sudden cooling, overheating, anesthesia, air pollution, high altitude, and infection can trigger a crisis in a woman with sickle cell disease (411, 414). Under conditions of extreme stress, e.g., dehydration, hypoxia, and metabolic acidosis, even RBCs with HgAS will sickle. Thus, even women with sickle cell trait can have a sickle cell crisis (411).

When women have sickle cell disease, a sickle cell crises may occur as many as six times during the pregnancy (416). During a sickle cell crisis, women are apprehensive. They may be uncooperative, unmanageable, and extremely sensitive to pain (417). As a result, it can be expected that their cat-

echolamine levels rise and there will be uterine artery vasoconstriction and a fall in uteroplacental perfusion. The placenta may become infarcted and may abrupt, increasing the fetal risk of asphyxia (411).

Pain management during a sickle cell crisis may include IM meperidine (Demerol) every three hours, or a continuous Demerol or morphine sulfate drip via a patient-controlled analgesia (PCA) pump. Oral methadone or codeine may be ordered (417). Women in sickle cell crisis may die if sickle cells block their arteries, veins and cause pulmonary edema and/or cerebral edema (410-411).

Hemoconcentration

Hemoconcentration may be due to an abnormally high level of RBCs or an abnormally low plasma level. Hemoconcentration increases blood viscosity (359). Pregnant women are hemoconcentrated when their *Hb is 13 gm/dl or higher or their hematocrit is 39% or higher* (345).

Women with mild preeclampsia have an increased risk of hemoconcentration due to the shift of fluid from within blood vessels to tissue outside of blood vessels. Their hematocrits rise, and they often have an increase in their thrombin-antithrombin complex level as well as their fibrinopeptide A levels. These changes in clotting factor levels predisposes them to clots and thromboemboli (335). Clots and increased blood viscosity limit O_2 and nutrient delivery to the uterus, placenta, and fetus. This increases the risk of LBW, preterm labor and birth, and stillbirth (345). Uterine hypoxia precedes contractions (preterm labor), and deficient O_2 and nutrient delivery to the fetus causes LBW and/or stillbirth.

THE UTERUS

Braxton Hicks Contractions

Beginning about 20 weeks' gestation, high amplitude/low frequency contractions occur about once every 2 to 4 hours (418). These are different from the low amplitude/high frequency (LAHF) waves known as uterine irritability. Braxton Hicks contractions last 30 or more seconds.

As gestation advances, Braxton Hicks contractions increase in frequency and amplitude. They are associated with an increase in MAP, an increase in uterine vascular resistance and a decrease in uteroplacental perfusion (419-420). However, they have little to no effect on fetal carotid artery, cerebral, or umbilical artery blood flow. Braxton Hicks contractions often coincide with fetal movement and an increase in baseline variability (420).

Contractions

During uterine contractions, there is an increase in intramyometrial and intrauterine pressure, maternal central venous pressure, BP, and cerebrospinal fluid pressure (421). At the beginning of the contraction maternal venous outflow from the uterus stops. Uterine intramural veins are squeezed, and arterial inflow continues to increase the volume of the intervillous space until intrauterine pressure (IUP) exceeds arteri-

al blood pressure (422). *Maternal blood flow to the intervillous spaces ceased at an IUP of 50 to 60 mm Hg (423).*

When the uterus contracts, the length, thickness, and surface area of the placenta increase due to distention of intervillous spaces with maternal blood. Fetal BP increases when IUP increases (422). The fetus will use O_2 reserves contained on RBCs, in tissues, or in the intervillous spaces. *Fetal O_2 reserves normally last one to two minutes (419).*

O_2 reserves are higher in well-grown fetuses and lower in fetuses who are small for their gestational age (419). During "normal" contractions, fetal cerebral SaO_2 dropped in 6 out of 8 human fetuses, but increased in 2 out of 8 fetuses. SaO_2 was dependent on cerebral blood volume. If contractions were seen in conjunction with FHR *decelerations*, the deceleration reflected a *transient drop in cerebral SaO_2* and a rise in deoxygenated Hb (424).

Resting tone

The lowest uterine pressure between contractions is called uterine resting tone. Resting tone may be reduced in the presence of a uterine anomaly, overdistention, e.g., with multiple gestation, fibroids, debilitating disease, narcotics, inhalation anesthesia, alcohol, magnesium, and tocolytic agents such as terbutaline (421).

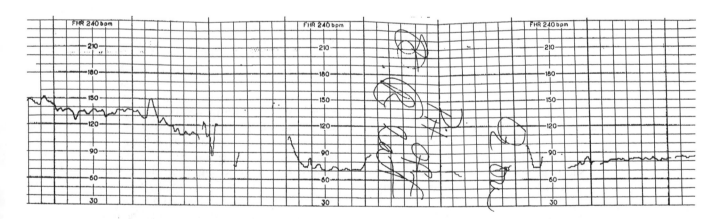

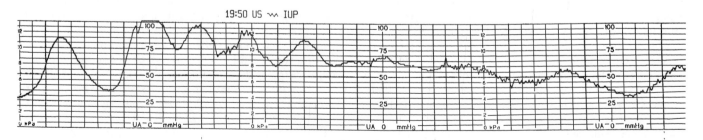

Figure 5.21: The fetal response to hyperstimulation and hypertonus is immediate. The woman was gravida 4, para 2 at 40 2/7 weeks' gestation with oligohydramnios and a oxytocin augmentation. The fetus was delivered vaginally with a vacuum extraction assist. Apgar scores were 2, 4, and 5 at 1, 5, and 10 minutes.

Resting tone may be increased due to IV oxytocin (Pitocin®) administration or overdistention during an amnioinfusion (421, 425). An abnormally high resting tone and frequency of contractions may be caused by oxytocin, placental abruption, or prostaglandins. The fetal response to hyperstimulation with hypertonus is immediate (see Figure 5.21).

LABOR
Anxiety
The fetus is more vulnerable to hypoxia during times of maternal anxiety (66, 426). As a response to anxiety and fear, adrenal glands secrete catecholamines. Maternal epinephrine binds with uterine β-receptors, diminishing effective uterine contractions and increasing the risk of a dysfunctional labor, increasing the duration of the first stage of labor, and decreasing Montevideo units (427-428). The increase in maternal catecholamines increases her:
- heart rate
- BP
- blood glucose
- blood flow to the brain, heart, and adrenal glands and decreases
- blood flow to the uterus and
- perfusion of intervillous spaces.

Oxygen delivery to the fetus decreases and fetal PaO_2, SaO_2, and pH may decrease and PCO_2 will increase. Fetal BP may decrease and there will be decelerations or bradycardia (66, 96, 426, 429-430). Fetal movement decreases in anxious women (431). About 10 to 12% of maternal catecholamines are transferred to fetal circulation, which may contribute to fetal vasoconstriction and the development of fetal hypoxemia, hypoxia, and acidemia (358, 432-433).

Pain
A similar catecholamine response can occur with pain during contractions. Laboring women increase their O_2 consumption an average of 281 ml/minute. They expend approximately 1200 kcal during an 8 to 10 hour labor (30). Pain and anxiety increase hyperventilation and the risk of maternal respiratory alkalosis. PaO_2 may slightly increase.

Analgesics counterbalance maternal catecholamine release during labor by decreasing sympathetic nervous system activity and uterine blood vessel tone. Uterine vasodilation increases uterine blood flow and fetal O_2 delivery. Analgesics also decrease the forces of labor, which increases placental O_2 transfer and the release of moderate to large amounts of maternal and fetal serum glucose (434).

In response to pain, nulliparous women *increase* their respiratory rate, minute ventilation, and *PaO_2*, and decrease their $PaCO_2$ and pulmonary residual capacity (429). The increase in minute ventilation increases tidal volume (30).

Analgesia administration may decrease maternal SaO_2. Fifty to 100 mg of IM meperidine (Demerol), given to nulliparous women in conjunction with inhalation of a mixture of O_2/nitrous oxide, lowered their SaO_2 5 to 9%. SaO_2 decreased less (0.3 to 3.1%) following epidural anesthesia. Multiparous women did not demonstrate similar SaO_2 changes. Umbilical artery pH was higher after epidural anesthesia (7.23 to 7.35) than after Demerol and O_2/nitrous oxide (7.11 to 7.31). Apgar scores were similar between the groups (429).

The fetal response to maternal pain and analgesics. Fetal pain, O_2 deprivation, and catecholamine release during contractions appear to affect the fetal T/QRS ratio. The T/QRS ratio increases during the ascending limb of the contraction and decreases during the descending limb of the contraction (44).

Variability may increase or decrease as fetal PO_2 changes in response to maternal anesthesia and analgesia. Transcutaneous scalp PO_2 (tcPO$_2$) decreased and variability increased approximately 7.5 minutes after a paracervical block. Variability decreased following Demerol administration due to a short-lived 60 to 80% decline in fetal tcPO$_2$. The decline in tcPO$_2$ began 3.2 minutes after the slow IV push injection. tcPO$_2$ reached its lowest level 5.3 minutes after drug administration.

If the fetus is hypoxemic at the time of narcotic administration, the risk of hypoxia and acidemia increases. Timing of drug administration affects the quantity that reaches the fetus. If the IV drug is administered *between* contractions, fetal drug levels will be higher than maternal drug levels. *Placental drug transfer is reduced when IV doses are injected at the beginning of a contraction because contractions limit intervillous space perfusion.* During a contraction, maternal distribution of the drug plus protein binding in the plasma rapidly lower maternal plasma concentration before placental circulation is reestablished between contractions (435-436). Theoretically, only 10 to 20% of the drug should be transferred to the fetus (the percentage of maternal cardiac output) (436). About 64% of Demerol binds with plasma proteins in maternal plasma, and 36% is available for transport to the fetus (435). Maximal neonatal depression would be expected if delivery occurs 2 hours after IM morphine and 1 to 3 hours after 100 mg of IM Demerol. Milligram per mg, Butorphanol (Stadol) is 5 times more potent than morphine and 40 times more potent than Demerol. One to two mg of Stadol provides effective analgesia for labor pain. Maximum neonatal depression following Stadol administration is similar to Demerol. Fentanyl (Sublimaze) is an ultrashort duration, fast-acting opiate with analgesic activity 100 times that of morphine. Analgesia peaks 20 to 40 minutes after IM administration and dissipates during the second hour. The risk of neonatal depression depends on the dose administered (436).

Narcotics accumulate in the fetal bloodstream in the presence of acidemia (435). *If there are any signs of fetal hypoxemia, e.g., tachycardia or variable decelerations, prior to narcotic administration, it would be reasonable for the nurse to observe the FHR pattern at least 6 minutes after medication administration.* tcPO$_2$ should return to normal within 15 minutes after narcotic injection (437-438). If there is a reassuring or compensatory FHR pattern after 15 minutes, there most likely will not be an adverse fetal response to maternal narcotic administration. Narcotics should be withheld by the nurse, and the physician should be notified, if concern exists that the fetus is acidemic and will be further compromised by drug administration.

UTERINE RUPTURE

Uterine rupture is a separation in the uterine wall which requires operative intervention (439-440). Uterine rupture may appear as a small tear, dehiscence of the old scar from a previous cesarean section, or, as one nurse put it, "she blew a hole out the backside of her uterus." In one study, 59% of uterine ruptures included extension of the previous uterine scar. Uterine rupture was related to longer durations of oxytocin, at greater doses, prolonged labor, and a high station on admission (441). The risk of uterine rupture also increases with abdominal trauma, a congenital anomaly of the uterus, placenta percreta (where placental tissue grows into the uterine muscle), forceps use, internal podalic version, shoulder dystocia, and prostaglandin gel use (442). Trauma may result from a motor vehicle accident, domestic violence, falls, burns, or bites. *A minimum of four hours of electronic fetal monitoring and observation should follow maternal trauma.* Following trauma, less than 2% of women suffered an abruption, 3% of fetuses had an abnormal FHR pattern, and 5.3% of the fetuses died (443).

The Incidence of Uterine Rupture

It has been estimated that 1 in 2,000 women who undergo a trial of labor after cesarean (TOLAC) will have a uterine rupture (444). Uterine scar dehiscence during labor occurs in 0.84% to 3% of women (445-446). There is a higher rate of uterine dehiscence in women who have two or more previous cesarean sections. Uterine scar dehiscence may be associated with severe variable and late decelerations and prolapse of the umbilical cord through the site of uterine rupture (445). The risk of rupture increases when oxytocin is used, even if it is at a low dose (439). The risk of uterine rupture increases as the number of cesarean sections women have had increases. The risk of rupture was three times greater after two cesarean sections than after one cesarean section (447). The risk of rupture was lower if Vicryl® sutures were used for uterine closure during the previous cesarean birth (448-449).

Women who have had no prior cesarean section may rupture their uterus, e.g., during a pregnancy years after uterine perforation during a hysteroscopic examination or following the use of prostaglandin gel for cervical ripening (450-453). One in 8,000 to 15,000 women spontaneously rupture their unscarred uterus. Risk factors for rupture of an unscarred uterus include:
- 5 or more births (grand multiparity)
- advanced maternal age (which usually means 35 or more years of age)
- undiagnosed fetopelvic disproportion with obstructed labor, e.g., failure to progress

- oxytocin augmentation with hypertonicity
- macrosomia with hydrocephalus
- a prior instrumental abortion or invasive hydatidiform mole
- placenta percreta
- a midtrimester version, where a breech baby is turned in utero to a head down position and
- uterine anomalies such as a rudimentary horn (454).

Judicious use of oxytocin and careful monitoring of labor progress are essential in women at risk for spontaneous uterine rupture.

Trial of Labor After Cesarean (TOLAC)

With the push to lower the cesarean section rate in the United States, more and more women are encouraged to have a TOLAC. Women who had a vaginal delivery after cesarean (VBAC) appreciated active participation in their "natural" childbirth, the shorter recovery time, and the presence of their partner during the entire birth experience. The most negative memories about the VBAC experience were the pain of labor, perineal discomfort, and technology, such as the IV line (455). Women who were unable to VBAC were more likely to be a gestational diabetic, have a 12 hour or longer labor, or have had a cesarean section for dystocia (456). Women with a history of a failed TOLAC, who were delivered by cesarean section, had almost three times more risk of uterine dehiscence and rupture than women who had an elective cesarean section (445).

Women should be counseled about the risk of uterine rupture by their midwife and/or physician. Because women with a history of cesarean section have an increased risk of uterine rupture, any woman undergoing a TOLAC needs ready access to surgical facilities and a surgeon (440).

An epidural does not mask signs or symptoms of uterine scar separation (457). Signs and symptoms of uterine rupture may include:
- abdominal pain, sudden pain, sharp pain
- palpation through the abdomen of fetal body parts
- no fetal descent or an elevation in the presenting part, e.g. from a -1 cm station to a higher station (a *higher* station than previously noted on vaginal examination is associated with extrusion of the fetus into the abdomen)
- maternal tachycardia and/or hypotension and a rapid pulse (hypovolemic shock)
- decreased intensity of uterine contractions, very few women stop contracting
- the sound of crepitus (due to blood collecting between the uterus and subcutaneous tissue)
- referred pain in the shoulder (with epidural anesthesia)
- vaginal bleeding may occur
- an "erratic" FHR pattern
- decelerations or bradycardia
- sudden anxiety and restlessness
- thrashing in the bed
- incoherent conversation

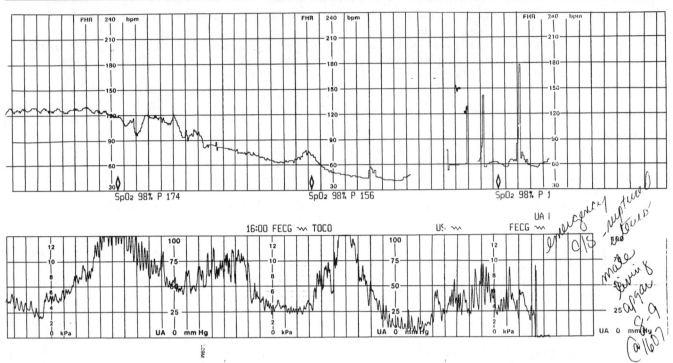

Figure 5.22: Uterine rupture of an unscarred uterus. A gravida 4, para 1 gestational diabetic at 38 to 39 weeks' gestation was induced with oxytocin. Her first baby was vaginally delivered. When she reached 5 to 6 cm, and 8 mU/minute of oxytocin, her pulse was 174 bpm, blood pressure was 90/50, respiratory rate was 32/minute and the fetus was out of the pelvis. An emergency cesarean section was initiated. The uterus was ruptured and Apgar scores were 8, 9, and 9 at 1, 5, and 10 minutes. Note the uterine hyperactivity prior to terminal bradycardia.

- a change in dilatation, e.g. from 8 cm to 3 cm
- a change in the presenting part, e.g. from vertex to elbows or footling breech
- hematuria with blood in the foley catheter (personal communication, R. Chaney, RN, November, 1995, 442, 454).

If no decelerations of the FHR are present prior to rupture of the uterus, and delivery occurs *within 17 minutes of the onset of the prolonged deceleration, no significant perinatal morbidity will occur.* If the prolonged deceleration is preceded by severe, repetitive late decelerations, asphyxia occurred as early as 10 minutes between the onset of the prolonged deceleration and delivery (458). *Thus, to prevent asphyxial brain damage, the fetus should be delivered within 10 to 17 minutes of the onset of the prolonged deceleration.* If no decelerations were present prior to uterine rupture, there is a little more time between rupture and delivery before significant neonatal morbidity occurs.

With uterine rupture, women may also rupture their bladder and develop hypovolemic shock. They may need blood transfusions and a hysterectomy if the uterus is unrepairable. Bladder rupture occurs in 0.05 to 11.7% of women who rupture their uterus. Hysterectomies occur in 0.1% of women who rupture their uterus (458-459). Complications of uterine rupture also include abruption of the placenta and total extrusion of the fetus into the abdomen.

Uterine rupture may prompt legal action against the hospital and health care providers. In March of 1993, a child died as a result of brain damage sustained following birth after a uterine rupture. The baby was in a breech position. The woman was a finger tip dilated (less than 1 cm), not in labor, and contracting. About four hours later she had an urge to have a bowel movement, a sharp pain, and within moments after the pain, vaginal bleeding and a FHR in the 60s to 70s. She told her nurse she felt like "her stomach had ripped open and the baby had moved up towards the ceiling." The physician called for an emergency cesarean section. The infant died during the first month of life. The family sued the hospital and physician. Sixteen breaches of the standard of care were cited by the plaintiff's medical expert. Two important breaches were:
- "the woman should have been typed and cross matched for blood upon admission"
- "the nurse should have started oxygen to get increased oxygen to the baby."

The physician expert also said, "The nurse should have notified a physician of anything deviant from the regular course of labor...particularly, at around 4:40 (a.m.), when Mrs.... complained of the rectal pain or pressure. In my opinion, at that point she was showing evidence of a uterine rupture and should have been related to Dr...." The nurse described the cervix as being completely dilated when she called the physician. In actuality, her cervix was not dilated. The plaintiff

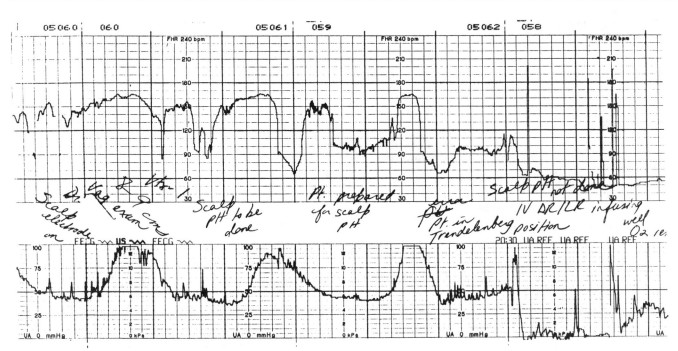

Figure 5.23: Uterine rupture of a scarred uterus. A gravida 2, para 1 woman who delivered her first child by cesarean section had a normal labor until she was 8 to 9 cm and -1 station. Variable decelerations were repetitive and nonperiodic in their timing. The FHR became severely bradycardic and a cesarean section was performed under general anesthesia. Apgar scores were 1, 3, 9, and 9 at 1, 5, 10, and 15 minutes. The umbilical vein pH was 7.19. The umbilical artery pH was 6.90. The baby went home with his mother with no abnormal sequelae. The uterine scar had separated and there was a tear down through the cervix and up to the left with a laceration of the left uterine artery. There was also a 10% abruption and a 1500 ml estimated blood loss. The baby was in the peritoneal cavity (extruded) with its head in the "birth canal."

expert also said, "Based on the improperly performed vaginal examination, Dr.... proceeded to manage Mrs.... in the way he did... It is the standard of care that when the fetal heart rate drop(s) down from the normal range, as it did in this case, oxygen is started automatically by the nurse without a doctor's order." The jury awarded the plaintiff $600,000 and the case was appealed. The Supreme Court affirmed the judgment against the hospital (460).

Based on this case, women who are attempting to deliver vaginally after a previous cesarean section should be type and cross matched for a minimum of two units of blood. *Prevention of uterine rupture requires early recognition of labor disorders and fetal compromise.* Oxytocin should be judiciously managed because oxytocin use increases the risk of uterine rupture (461). If oxytocin is infusing and signs or symptoms of uterine rupture occur, it should be immediately discontinued and the physician should be notified. *Any woman who is having a TOLAC should have close monitoring of labor progress. It may be helpful to plot her labor curve.* Arrest of dilatation or descent should be reported to the midwife or physician. Decelerations of the FHR or bradycardia should be promptly reported and aggressively treated. If fetal bradycardia occurs, O_2 should be applied without a doctor's order at 8 to 10 liters

per minute by tight face mask (20). A simple mask may be used. Complaints of rectal pain and/or vaginal bleeding should be immediately reported to the physician. Failure to deliver the fetus in a timely manner when the uterus has ruptured may cause fetal asphyxia and even death.

CONCLUSION

The healthy fetus is well prepared for the normal stresses of labor and birth. Compensatory mechanisms allow the fetus to readily respond to temporary epidsodes of oxygen deprivation. Changes in acid-base status are often reflected in the fetal heart rate pattern and fetal behavior. The continuum from a reassuring pattern to an ominous pattern may occur prior to hospital admission. In that case, periventricular leukomalacia, intraventricular hemorrhage, and cerebral palsy may not be preventable. Maternal factors prior to or during labor may limit fetal oxygenation. Clinicians who understand how the maternal condition impacts fetal oxygen delivery will more vigilantly monitor the fetus. Their ability to recognize compensatory, nonreassuring, and ominous fetal heart rate patterns and intervene in a timely manner should prevent intrapartal fetal asphyxia and its sequelae.

References

1. Reece, E. A., Antoine, C., & Montgomery, J. (March 1986). The fetus as the final arbiter of intrauterine stress/distress. Clinical Obstetrics and Gynecology, 29(1), 23-32.

2. Gonser, M., & Marzusch, K. (May 1995). Correlation of doppler-detected fetal body movements with fetal heart rate parameters and perinatal outcome: A reevaluation. American Journal of Obstetrics and Gynecology, 172(5), 1635.

3. Goldberger, E. (1986). A primer of water, electrolyte and acid-base balance. Philadelphia, PA: Lea & Febiger.

4. Cohen, A. V., Schulman, H., & Romney, S. L. (1970). Maternal acid-base metabolism in normal human parturition. American Journal of Obstetrics and Gynecology, 107(6), 933-938.

5. Barnhart, C. L., & Stein, J. (Eds.). (1964). The American College Dictionary. New York: Random House.

6. West, J., Chez, B. F., & Miller, F. C. (1993). Fetal heart rate. In R. A. Knuppel, & J. E. Drukker (Eds.), High risk pregnancy a team approach (pp. 316-336). Philadelphia, PA: W. B. Saunders Company.

7. Glanze, W. D., Anderson, K. N., Anderson, L. E. (Eds.). (1990). Mosby's medical, nursing, and allied health dictionary (3rd. ed.). St. Louis, MO: The C. V. Mosby Company.

8. Martin, R. W., & McColgin, S. G. (March 1990). Evaluation of fetal and neonatal acid-base status. Obstetrics and Gynecology Clinics of North America, 17(1), 223-233.

9. Stringfield, Y. N. (November 1993). Back to basics. Acidosis, alkalosis, and ABGs. American Journal of Nursing, 93(1), 43-44.

10. Blechner, J. N. (March 1993). Maternal-fetal acid-base physiology. Clinical Obstetrics and Gynecology, 36(1), 3-12.

11. Creasy, R. K., & Resnik, R. (1984). Maternal-fetal medicine. Philadelphia, PA: W. B. Saunders Company.

12. Janusek, L. W. (July 1990). Metabolic acidosis: Pathophysiology, signs, and symptoms [Clinical Insights]. Nursing, 52-53.

13. Jauniaux, E., Jurkovic, D., Gulibis, B., Collins, W. P., Zaidi, J., & Campbell, S. (May 1994). Investigation of the acid-base balance of coelomic and amniotic fluids in early human pregnancy. American Journal of Obstetrics and Gynecology, 170(5, Pt. 1), 1365-1369.

14. Viniker, D. A. (November 1979). The fetal EEG (detection of oxygen deprivation). British Journal of Hospital Medicine, 22(5), 504-507, 509-510.

15. Sureau, C. (February 1987). Fetal monitoring present and future-discussion. European Journal of Obstetrics, Gynecology and Reproductive Biology, 24(2), 119-121.

16. Assessment of fetal and newborn acid-base status. (April 1989). Technical bulletin number 127, 1-4. Washington, DC: ACOG.

17. Urdang, L. (Ed. in Chief). (1983). Mosby's medical and nursing dictionary. St. Louis: The C. V. Mosby Company.

18. Richardson, B. S. (September 1989). Fetal adaptive responses to asphyxia. Clinics in Perinatology, 16(3), 595-611.

19. Penning, D. H., Grafe, M. R., Hammond, R., Matsuda, Y., Patrick, J., & Richardson, B. (May 1994). Neuropathology of the near-term and midgestation ovine fetal brain after sustained in utero hypoxemia. American Journal of Obstetrics and Gynecology, 170(5, Pt. 1), 1425-1432.

20. Fetal heart rate patterns: Monitoring interpretation, and management (July 1995). Technical bulletin number 207, 1-11. Washington, DC: ACOG.

21. Hankins, G. D. V., & Harvey, C. J. (January 1994). Decreased SaO_2 produces hind limb hypertension and reduced oxygen extraction in the fetal sheep. American Journal of Obstetrics and Gynecology, 170(1, Pt. 2), 312. SPO abstracts #126.

22. Thomas, C. L. (Ed.). (1976). Taber's cyclopedic medical dictionary. Philadelphia: F. A. Davis Company.

23. Gilstrap, L. C., Leveno, K. J., Burris, J., Williams, M. L., & Little, B. B. (September 1989). Diagnosis of birth asphyxia on the basis of fetal pH, Apgar score, and newborn cerebral dysfunction. American Journal of Obstetrics and Gynecology, 161(3), 825-830.

24. Pardi, G., Cetin, I., Marconi, A. M., Lan Franchi, A., Bozzetti, P., & Ferrazzi, E. (March 11, 1993). Diagnostic value of blood sampling in fetuses with growth retardation. The New England Journal of Medicine, 328(10), 692-696.

25. Cowan, D. B. (August 30, 1980). Intrapartum fetal resuscitation. South African Medical Journal, 58(9), 376-379.

26. Jepson, J. H. (December 1974). Factors influencing oxygenation in mother and fetus [Review]. Obstetrics & Gynecology, 44(6), 906-914.

27. Blechner, J. N., Stenger, V. G., Eitzman, D. V., & Prystowsky, H. (September 1, 1970). Oxygenation of the human fetus and newborn infant during maternal metabolic acidosis. American Journal of Obstetrics and Gynecology, 108(1), 47-55.

28. Sakes, G. S., Johnson, P., Ashworth, F., Molloy, P. M., Gu, W., & Stirrat, G. M. (February 27, 1982). Do Apgar scores indicate asphyxia? The Lancet, 494-495.

29. Rorke, M. J., Davey, D. A., & Du Toit, H. J. (October 1968). Foetal oxygenation during caesarean section. Anaesthesia, 23(4), 585-596.

30. Turner, E. S., Greenberger, P. A., & Patterson, R. (December 1980). Management of the pregnant asthmatic patient. Annals of Internal Medicine, 93(6), 905-918.

31. Hankins, G., Clark, S., Uckan, E., Harvey, C., & Cotton, D. (January 1996). Arterial blood gas analysis during normal third-trimester pregnancy and the effect of position changes. American Journal of Obstetrics and Gynecology, 174(1, Pt. 2), 376. SPO abstracts #233.

32. Crawford, J. S. (February 18, 1984). Fetal distress and the condition of newborn infants. British Medical Journal, 288, 567-568.

33. Rankin, J. H. G. (1973). Maternal alkalosis and fetal oxygenation. Advances in Experimental Medicine & Biology, 37, 1067-1073.

34. Bardicef, O., Bardicef, M., Sorokin, Y., Cotton, D. B., & Resnick, L. M. (September 1995). "Physiologic" intracellular acidosis in pregnancy. American Journal of Obstetrics and Gynecology, 173(3, Pt. 1), 879-880.

35. Newman, W., Braid, D., & Wood, C. (January 1, 1967). Fetal acid-base status. I. Relationship between maternal and fetal PCO_2. American Journal of Obstetrics and Gynecology, 97(1), 43-51.

36. Miller, F. C., Petrie, R. H., Arcs, J. J., Paul, R. H., & Hon, E. H. (October 15, 1974). Hyperventilation during labor. American Journal of Obstetrics and Gynecology, 120(4), 489-495.

37. Bowen, L. W., Kochenour, N. K., Ream, N. E., & Woollen, F. R. (April 1986). Maternal-fetal pH difference and fetal scalp pH as predictors of neonatal outcome. Obstetrics & Gynecology, 67(4), 487-495.

38. Young, B.K. (1990). Placental regulation of fetal oxygenation and acid-base balance. In R. D. Eden, F. H. Boehm, & M. Haire, (Eds.), Assessment and care of the fetus. Physiological, clinical, and medicolegal principles. Norwalk, CT: Appleton & Lange.

39. Lawrence, G. F., Brown, V. A., Parsons, R. J., & Cooke, I. D. (January 1982). Feto-maternal consequences of high-dose glucose infusion during labour. British Journal of Obstetrics and Gynaecology, 89(1), 27-32.

40. Rutter, N., Spencer, A., Mann, N., & Smith, M. (July 19, 1980). Glucose during labour. The Lancet, 2(8186), 155.

41. Langer, O., Berkus, M., Elliott, B., McFarland, M., & Xenakis, E. M-J. (January 1995). Diabetes in pregnancy: The relationship of amniotic fluid insulin, diabetic class and lung maturity profiles. American Journal of Obstetrics and Gynecology, 172(1, Pt. 2), 329. SPO abstracts #246.

42. Economides, D. L., Nicolaides, K. H., & Campbell, S. (1991). Metabolic and endocrine findings in appropriate and small for gestational age fetuses. Journal of Perinatal Medicine, 19(1-2), 97-105.

43. Brown, E. G., Mendoza, G. J. B., Chervenak, F. A., Karmel, B. Z., Krouskop, R. W., & LeBlanc, M. H. (January 1990). The relationship of maternal erythrocyte oxygen transport parameters to intrauterine growth retardation. American Journal of Obstetrics and Gynecology, 162(1), 223-229.

44. Deans, A. C., & Steer, P. J. (January 1994). The use of the fetal electrocardiogram in labour. British Journal of Obstetrics and Gynaecology, 101, 9-17.

45. Goodwin, T. M., Belai, I., Hernandez, P., Durand, M., & Paul, R. H. (December 1992). Asphyxial complications in the term newborn with severe umbilical acidemia. American Journal of Obstetrics and Gynecology, 167(6), 1506-1512.

46. Ball, R. H., Espinoza, M. I., Parer, J. T., Alon, E., Vertommen, J., & Johnson, J. (January 1994). Regional blood flow in asphyxiated fetuses with seizures. American Journal of Obstetrics and Gynecology, 170(1, Pt. 1), 156-161.

47. Dennis, J., Johnson, A., Mutch, L., Yudkin, P., & Johnson, P. (July 1989). Acid-base status at birth and neurodevelopmental outcome at four and one-half years. American Journal of Obstetrics and Gynecology, 161(1), 213-220.

48. Fee, S. C., Malee, K., Deddish, R., Minogue, J. P., & Socol, M. L. (March 1990). Severe acidosis and subsequent neurologic status. American Journal of Obstetrics and Gynecology, 162(3), 802-806.

49. Goldaber, K. G., & Gilstrap, III, L. C. (March 1993). Correlations between obstetric clinical events and umbilical cord blood acid-base and blood gas values. Clinical Obstetrics and Gynecology, 36(1), 47-59.

50. Winkler, C. L., Hauth, J. C., Tucker, J. M., Owen, J., & Brumfield, C. G. (February 1991). Neonatal complications at term as related to the degree of umbilical artery acidemia. American Journal of Obstetrics and Gynecology, 164(2), 637-641.

51. Asano, H., Homan, J., Carmichael, L., Korkola, S., & Richardson, B. (March 1994). Cerebral metabolism during sustained hypoxemia in preterm fetal sheep. American Journal of Obstetrics and Gynecology, 170(3), 939-944.

52. Nagel, H. T. C., Vandenbussche, F. P. H. A., Oepkes, D., Jennekens-Schinkel, A., Laan, L. A. E. M., & Gravenhorst, J. B. (December 1995). Follow-up of children born with an umbilical arterial blood pH < 7. American Journal of Obstetrics and Gynecology, 173(6), 1758-1764.

53. Phelan, J., Korst, L., Ahn, M. O., & Martin, G. (January 1995). Intrapartum fetal asphyxia: Could the brain be injured first? American Journal of Obstetrics and Gynecology, 172(1, Pt. 2), 364. SPO abstracts #379.

54. Carter, B. S. (February 1996). Asphyxia update. NRP News Intermountain West, 3(1),1-2.

55. van den Berg, P. P., Jongsma, H. W., Nijhuis, J. G., & Eskes, T. K. A. B. (January 1995). Neonatal complications in newborns with an umbilical artery. American Journal of Obstetrics and Gynecology, 172(1, Pt. 2), 363. SPO abstracts #378.

56. Kimberlin, D., Hauth, J. C., Goldenberg, R. L., MacPherson, C., Thom, E., & Bottoms, S. F. (January 1996). Relationship of acid-base status and neonatal morbidity in ≤1000 g infants. American Journal of Obstetrics and Gynecology, 174(1, Pt. 2), 382. SPO abstracts #260.

57. Drake, K., Randolph, G., Weiss, N., Fern, S., Mikhail, M., & Anyaegbunam, A. (January 1995). Neonatal complications associated with severe acidemia. American Journal of Obstetrics and Gynecology, 172(1, Pt. 2), 363. SPO abstracts #377.

58. Henson, G. L., Dawes, G. S., & Redman, C. W. G. (March 1983). Antenatal fetal heart-rate variability in relation to fetal acid-base status at caesarean section. British Journal of Obstetrics and Gynaecology, 90, 516-521.

59. Low, J. A., Panagiotopoulos, C., & Derrick, E. J. (March 1995). Newborn complications after intrapartum asphyxia with metabolic acidosis in the preterm fetus. American Journal of Obstetrics and Gynecology, 172(3), 805-810.

60. Parer, J. T. (1983). Handbook of fetal heart monitoring. Philadelphia, PA: W. B. Sanders Company.

61. Arulkumaran, S., Lilja, H., Lindecrantz, K., Ratnam, S. S., Thavarasah, A. S., & Rosen, K. G. (1990). Fetal ECG waveform analysis should improve fetal surveillance in labour. Journal of Perinatal Medicine, 18(1), 13-22.

62. Low, J. A., Panagiotopoulos, C., & Derrick, E. J. (April 1994). Newborn complications after intrapartum asphyxia with metabolic acidosis in the term fetus. American Journal of Obstetrics and Gynecology, 170(4), 1081-1087.

63. Martin, C. B., & Gingerich, B. (September/October 1976). Factors affecting the fetal heart rate: Genesis of FHR patterns. JOGNN, 5(5, Suppl.), 16s-25s, 30s-40s.

64. Weiner, Z., Divon, M. Y., Katz, N., Minior, V. K., Nasseri, A., & Girz, B. (January 1996). Multivariant analysis of antepartum fetal tests in predicting neonatal outcome of growth retarded fetuses. American Journal of Obstetrics and Gynecology, 174(1, Pt. 2), 339. SPO abstracts #94.

65. Mathews, D. D. (August 1967). The oxygen supply of the postmature foetus before the onset of labour. Journal of Obstetrics and Gynaecology of the British Commonwealth, 74(4), 523-527.

66. Myers, R. E. (September 1985). Basic principles of perinatal brain damage. Paper presented at the meeting of the Neonatal Asphyxia and the Brain Damaged Newborn, Issues in 1985, Albuquerque, New Mexico.

67. Low, J. A. (November 1988). The role of blood gas and acid-base assessment in the diagnosis of intrapartum fetal asphyxia [Current Development]. American Journal of Obstetrics and Gynecology, 159(5), 1235-1240.

68. Clark, S. L., & Paul, R. H. (December 1, 1985). Intrapartum fetal surveillance: The role of fetal scalp blood sampling. American Journal of Obstetrics and Gynecology, 153(7), 717-720.

69. Paneth, N., & Stark, R. (1983). Mental retardation, cerebral palsy, and intrapartum asphyxia. In W. R. Cohen & E. A. Friedman (Eds.). Management of labor (pp 143-162). Baltimore: University Park Press.

70. Freeman, J. M. (Ed.) (April 1985). Prenatal and perinatal factors associated with brain disorders. NIH Publication No. 85-1149, 240-250, 288-299.

71. Ruth, V. J., & Raivio, K. O. (July 2, 1988). Perinatal brain damage: Predictive value of metabolic acidosis and the Apgar score. British Medical Journal, 297, 24-27.

72. Fetal distress and birth asphyxia. (April 1994). ACOG committee opinion number 137. Washington, DC: ACOG.

73. van Geijn, H. P., Copray, F. J. A., Donkers, D. K., & Bos, M. H. (December 1991). Diagnosis and management of intrapartum fetal distress. European Journal of Obstetrics, Gynecology and Reproductive Biology, 42(Suppl.), s63-s72.

74. Espinoza, M. I., & Parer, J. T. (June 1991). Mechanisms of asphyxial brain damage, and possible pharmocologic interventions, in the fetus. American Journal of Obstetrics and Gynecology, 164(6, Pt. 1), 1582-1591.

75. Tucker, S. (1992). Pocket guide to fetal monitoring. St. Louis: Mosby Year Book.

76. Monosodium glutamate (January 1996). FDA Medical Bulletin, 3.

77. Wang, W., Pang, C. C. P., Rogers, M. S., & Chang, A. M. Z. (January 1996). Lipid peroxidation in cord blood at birth. American Journal of Obstetrics and Gynecology, 174(1, Pt. 1), 62-65.

78. Dawes, G. S., Moulden, M., & Redman, C. W. G. (May 1990). Criteria for the design of fetal heart rate analysis systems. International Journal of Bio-Medical Computing, 25(4), 287-294.

79. Yoneyama, Y., Sawa, R., Suzuki, S., Shin, S., Power, G. G., & Araki, T. (January 1996). The relationship between uterine artery doppler velocimetry and umbilical venous adenosine levels in pregnancies complicated by preeclampsia. American Journal of Obstetrics and Gynecology, 174(1, Pt. 1), 267-271.

80. Wilkening, R. B., Boyle, D. W., & Meschia, G. (1993). Fetal pH improvement after 24 h of severe, nonlethal hypoxia [Brief Communication]. Biology of the Neonate, 63(2), 129-132.

81. Goldsmith, J. (Fall 1995). Newborn research depends on partnerships. Reflections, 21(3), 6-8.

82. Mason, B. A., Ogunyemi, D., Punla, O., & Koos, B. J. (May 1993). Maternal and fetal cardiorespiratory responses to adenosine in sheep [Basic Science Section]. American Journal of Obstetrics and Gynecology, 168(5), 1558-1561.

83. Salafia, C. M., Sherer, D. M., Vintzileos, A. M., Pezzullo, J. C., Minior, V. K., & Romero, R. (January 1995). Relationship of placental histology to umbilical cord blood gases in preterm gestations. <u>American Journal of Obstetrics and Gynecology, 172</u>(1, Pt. 2), 419. SPO abstracts #582.

84. Salafia, C. M., Pezzullo, J. C., Vintzileos, A. M., Minior, V. K., & Romero, R. (January 1995). Preterm preeclampsia has major pathology distinct from uteroplacental insufficiency. <u>American Journal of Obstetrics and Gynecology, 172</u>(1, Pt. 2), 373. SPO abstracts #406.

85. Paidas, M. J., Turtulici, P., Winslow, J., Chelmow, D., Morin, L., & Frantz, I. (January 1995). Neonatal outcome of preeclamptic (PE) women delivered ≤34 weeks gestation. <u>American Journal of Obstetrics and Gynecology, 172</u>(1, Pt. 2), 375. SPO abstracts #416.

86. Myers, R. E. (1975). Four patterns of perinatal brain damage and their conditions of occurrence in primates. In B. S. Meldrum, & C. D. Marsden (Eds.), <u>Advances in neurology, 10</u> (pp. 223-234). New York, NY: Raven Press.

87. Ball, R. H., Parer, J. T., Caldwell, L. E., & Johnson, J. (January 1994). Cerebral oxidative metabolism during severe umbilical cord occlusion. <u>American Journal of Obstetrics and Gynecology, 170</u>(1, Pt. 2), 270. SPO abstracts #17.

88. Bobby, P., Divon, M. Y., Yun, E., & Santos, A. (January 1996). Skin blood flow response to stable asphyxia in the premature fetal lamb. <u>American Journal of Obstetrics and Gynecology, 174</u>(1, Pt. 2), 383. SPO abstracts #261.

89. Use and abuse of the Apgar score. American academy of pediatrics, committee on fetus and newborn. (1986). <u>Pediatrics 78,</u> 1148-1149.

90. Hankins, G. D. V. (February 15, 1991). Apgar scores: Are they enough? <u>Contemporary OB/GYN, 36,</u> 13-25.

91. Blackstone, J., & Young, B. K. (March 1993). Umbilical cord blood acid-base values and other descriptors of fetal condition. <u>Clinical Obstetrics and Gynecology, 36</u>(1), 33-46.

92. Westgren, M., Divon, M., Horal, M., Ingemarsson, I., Kublickas, M., & Markus, C. (January 1995). Routine measurements of umbilical artery lactate in the prediction of perinatal outcome. <u>American Journal of Obstetrics and Gynecology, 172</u>(1, Pt. 2), 364. SPO abstracts #380.

93. Chowdhary, J., Narang, A., & Bhakoo, O. N. (January 1987). Study of biochemical asphyxia at birth. <u>Indian Pediatrics, 24</u>(1), 63-68.

94. Fleischer, A., Schulman, H., Jagani, N., Mitchell, J., & Randolf, G. (September 1, 1982). The development of fetal acidosis in the presence of an abnormal fetal heart rate tracing. I. The average for gestational age fetus. <u>American Journal of Obstetrics and Gynecology, 144</u>(1), 55-60.

95. Johnson, J. W. C., Richards, D. S., & Wagaman, R. A. (March 1990). The case for routine umbilical acid-base studies at delivery. <u>American Journal of Obstetrics and Gynecology, 162</u>(3), 621-625.

96. Persianinov, L. S. (1973). The effect of normal and abnormal labour on the foetus. A survey. <u>Acta et Obstetricia Gynecologica Scandinavica, 52</u>(1), 29-36.

97. Schaffer, I., Knitza, R., Pahl, C., Schlamp, K., Rall, G., & Mainz, S. (January 1995). Fetal pulse oximetry: Correlation of O_2 saturation during labor and the fetal outcome. <u>American Journal of Obstetrics and Gynecology, 172</u>(1, Pt. 2), 365. SPO abstracts #385.

98. Perkins, R. P., & Papile, L. (April 1985). The very low birthweight infant: Incidence and significance of low Apgar scores, "asphyxia," and morbidity findings at delivery. <u>American Journal of Perinatology, 2</u>(2), 108-113.

99. Rothberg, A. D., Cooper, P. A., Fisher, H. M., & Shaw, J. J. (May 10, 1986). Apgar scores and asphyxia. Results of a study and proposal for a clinical grading system. <u>South African Medical Journal, 69,</u> 605-607.

100. Socol, M. L., Garcia, P. M., & Riter, S. (April 1994). Depressed Apgar scores, acid-base status, and neurologic outcome. <u>American Journal of Obstetrics and Gynecology, 170</u>(4), 991-999.

101. Nelson, K. B. (1989). Perspective on the role of perinatal asphyxia in neurologic outcome. <u>Canadian Medical Association Journal, 141</u>(Suppl.), 3-10.

102. Dickenson, J. E., Eriksen, N. L., Meyer, B. A., & Parisi, V. M. (April 1992). The effect of preterm birth on umbilical cord blood gases. <u>Obstetrics & Gynecology, 79</u>(4), 575-578.

103. Lien, J. M., Towers, C. V., Quilligan, E. J., de Veciano, M., Toohey, J. S., & Morgan, M. A. (January 1994). Term neonatal seizures: Evaluation of obstetrical factors. <u>American Journal of Obstetrics and Gynecology, 170</u>(1, Pt. 2), 373. SPO abstracts #350.

104. Ahn, M. O., Korst, L., Phelan, J., & Martin, G. (January 1995). Are early neonatal seizures a sign of acute intrapartum asphyxia? <u>American Journal of Obstetrics and Gynecology, 172</u>(1, Pt. 2), 269. SPO abstracts #44.

105. Low, J. A., Galbraith, R. S., Muir, D. W., Killen, H. L., Pater, E. A., & Karchmar, E. J. (June 1, 1985). The relationship between perinatal hypoxia and newborn encephalopathy. <u>American Journal of Obstetrics and Gynecology, 152</u>(3), 256-260.

106. Korst, L. M., Phelan, J. P., Martin, G. I. (October 1, 1996). Nucleated red blood cells: An update on the marker for fetal asphyxia. <u>American Journal of Obstetrics and Gynecology, 175</u> (4, Part 1), 843.

107. Robertson, C. M. T., & Finer, N. N. (June 1993). Long-term follow-up of term neonates with perinatal asphyxia. <u>Clinics in Perinatology, 20</u>(2), 483-499.

108. Goodlin, R. C. (June 1995). Do concepts of causes and prevention of cerebral palsy require revision? <u>American Journal of Obstetrics and Gynecology, 172</u>(6), 1830-1836.

109. Grant, A., Joy, M-T., O'Brien, N., Hennessy, E., & MacDonald, D. (November 25, 1989). Cerebral palsy among children born during the Dublin randomised trial of intrapartum monitoring. <u>The Lancet.</u>(8674), 1233-1236.

110. Blair, E., Stanley, F., & Hockey, A. (July 1992). Intrapartum asphyxia and cerebral palsy. <u>Journal of Pediatrics, 121</u>(1), 170-171.

111. Rydhstroem, H. (September 1995). The relationship of birth weight and birth weight discordance to cerebral palsy or mental retardation later in life for twins weighing less than 2500 grams [General Obstetrics & Gynecology/Fetus-Placenta-Newborn]. American Journal of Obstetrics and Gynecology, 173(3, Pt. 1), 680-686.

112. Hauth, J. C., Goldenberg, R. L., Nelson, K. G., DuBard, M. B., Peralta, M. A., & Gaudier, F. L. (January 1995). Reduction of cerebral palsy with maternal $MgSO_4$ treatment in newborns weighing 500-1000 g. American Journal of Obstetrics and Gynecology, 172(1, Pt. 2), 419. SPO abstracts #581.

113. Yoon, B. H., Romero, R., Kim, C. J., Park, K. H., Hong, S. A., & Jun, J. K. (January 1996). High expression of interleukin-6, interleukin-1, and tumor necrosis factor-α in periventricular leukomalacia. American Journal of Obstetrics and Gynecology, 174(1, Pt. 2), 399. SPO abstracts #319.

114. Yoon, B. H., Romero, R., Jun, J. K., Park, K. H., Yang, S. H., & Kim, I. O. (January 1996). Amniotic fluid concentrations of interleukin-6 identify fetuses at risk for the development of periventricular leukomalacia. American Journal of Obstetrics and Gynecology, 174(1, Pt. 2), 330. SPO abstracts #68.

115. Mallard, E. C., Williams, C. E., Johnston, B. M., & Gluckman, P. D. (January 1994). Increased vulnerability to neuronal damage after umbilical cord occlusion in fetal sheep with advancing gestation. American Journal of Obstetrics and Gynecology, 170(1, Pt. 1), 206-214.

116. Irive, B. K., Rumney, P. J., Adhoot, D., Asrat, T., Towers, C. V., & Carroll, S. F. (January 1996). Differences in the concentration of an endotoxin binding protein help explain sensitivity to septic complications in pregnancy. American Journal of Obstetrics and Gynecology, 174(1, Pt. 2), 390. SPO abstracts #291.

117. Yoon, B. H., Romero, R., Yang, S. H., Jun, J. K., Choi, J. H., & Kim, I. O. (January 1995). Interleukin-6 concentrations in umbilical cord plasma identify infants at risk for the development of white matter brain lesions associated with periventricular leukomalacia. American Journal of Obstetrics and Gynecology, 172(1, Pt. 2), 268. SPO abstracts #37.

118. Figueroa, R., Martinez, E., Sehgal, P., Garry, D., Patel, K., & Verma, U. (January 1996). Elevated amniotic fluid interleukin-6 predicts neonatal periventricular leukomalacia and intraventricular hemorrhage. American Journal of Obstetrics and Gynecology, 174(1, Pt. 2), 330. SPO abstracts #67.

119. Verma, U., Tejani, N., Klein, S., Reale, M., Beneck, D., & Jeanty, M. (January 1995). Maternal chorioamnionitis increases risk of major intraventricular hemorrhage (IVH) & periventricular leucomalacia (PVL). American Journal of Obstetrics and Gynecology, 172(1, Pt. 2), 370. SPO abstracts #403.

120. Martinez, E., Figueroa, R., Sehgal, P., Verma, U., Patel, K., & Hsu, E. (January 1995). Elevated amniotic fluid interleukin 6 (AFIL6) is a better predictor of neonatal periventricular leucomalacia (PVL) and grades 3 & 4 intraventricular hemorrhage (IVH) than positive amniotic fluid culture (AF) cultures. American Journal of Obstetrics and Gynecology, 172(1, Pt. 2), 369. SPO abstracts #402.

121. Canterino, J., Verma, U., Jejani, N., Klein, S., Reale, M., & Jeanty, M. (January 1996). Antepartum maternal steroids and the risk of intraventricular hemorrhage and periventricular leucomalacia. American Journal of Obstetrics and Gynecology, 174(1, Pt. 2), 399. SPO abstracts #318.

122. Canterino, J., Verma, U., Tejani, N., Klein, S., Reale, M., & Jeanty, M. (January 1996). Maternal steroids, chorioamnionitis and the risk of periventricular leucomalacia in the preterm neonate. American Journal of Obstetrics and Gynecology, 174(1, Pt. 2), 475. SPO abstracts #607.

123. Goldenberg, R., Gaudier, F., Nelson, K., Peralta, M., Dubard, M., & Cliver, S. (January 1994). The relationship of maternal and neonatal characteristics to major handicap at ≥ one year of age. American Journal of Obstetrics and Gynecology, 372. SPO abstracts #346.

124. Verma, U., Canterino, J., Tejani, N., Beneck, D., Klein, S., & Jeanty, M. (January 1996). Preeclampsia and the risk of intraventricular hemorrhage and periventricular leucomalacia in the preterm neonate. American Journal of Obstetrics and Gynecology, 174(1, Pt. 2), 452. SPO abstracts #524.

125. Verma, U., Tejani, N., Klein, S., & Reale, M. (January 1995). Intrauterine growth restriction (IUGR) decreases the risk of intraventricular hemorrhage (IVH) and periventricular leucomalacia. American Journal of Obstetrics and Gynecology, 172(1, Pt. 2), 369. SPO abstracts #399.

126. Nores, J., Roberts, A., & Carr, S. (January 1996). Prenatal diagnosis and management of fetuses with intracranial hemorrhage. American Journal of Obstetrics and Gynecology, 174(1, Pt. 2), 424. SPO abstracts #419.

127. Goepfert, A. R., Goldenberg, R. L., Hauth, J. C., Owen, J., MacPherson, C., & Thom, E. (January 1996). Obstetrical determinants of neonatal neurological morbidity. American Journal of Obstetrics and Gynecology, 174(1, Pt. 2), 470. SPO abstracts #586.

128. Gimovsky, M. L., & Petrie, R. (January 1986). Maternal anticonvulsants and fetal hemorrhage. A report of two cases. Journal of Reproductive Medicine, 31(1), 61-62.

129. Bryant, D., Batton, D., Sloan, C., & Lorenz, R. (January 1995). Variable decelerations and the risk of intraventricular hemorrhage/periventricular leukomalacia: A case control study. American Journal of Obstetrics and Gynecology, 172(1, Pt. 2), 418. SPO abstracts #578.

130. Mercer, B., Bottoms, S., Paul, R., Iams, J., MacPherson, C., & Jones, P. (January 1996). The utility of ultrasound in the prediction of neonatal outcome after delivery 1,000 grams. American Journal of Obstetrics and Gynecology, 174(1, Pt. 2), 421. SPO abstracts #405.

131. Mari, G., Abuhamad, A., Keller, M., Ment, L., Uerpairojkit, B., & VandeKerkhove, K. (January 1995). Is the fetal brain sparing effect a risk factor for the development of intraventricular hemorrhage in the preterm infant? American Journal of Obstetrics and Gynecology, 172(1, Pt. 2), 268. SPO abstracts #40.

132. Gleason, C. A., Hamm, C., & Jones, Jr., M. D. (April 1990). Effect of acute hypoxemia on brain blood flow and oxygen metabolism in immature fetal sheep. American Journal of Physiology, 258(4, Pt. 2), H1064-H1069.

133. Williams, M. C., & O'Brien, W. F. (January 1995). Asymmetric growth restriction is associated with neonatal morbidity in non-growth retarded neonates. American Journal of Obstetrics and Gynecology, 172(1, Pt. 2), 268. SPO abstracts #39.

134. Williams, M. C., O'Brien, W. F., & Oechsli, F. W. (January 1995). Low ponderal index is associated with cerebral palsy independent of intrauterine growth retardation. <u>American Journal of Obstetrics and Gynecology, 172</u>(1, Pt. 2), 268. SPO abstracts #38.

135. Goldenberg, R., DuBard, M., Cliver, S., Nelson, K., Blankson, K., & Ramey, S. (January 1995). Pregnancy outcome and intelligence at age five. <u>American Journal of Obstetrics and Gynecology, 172</u>(1, Pt. 2), 270. SPO abstracts #45.

136. Batton, D., Roberts, C., & Swails, T. (January 1996). Survival of premature babies without major neurologic injury. <u>American Journal of Obstetrics and Gynecology, 172</u>(1, Pt. 2), 472. SPO abstracts #595.

137. Kimberlin, D., Hauth, J., Guinn, D., Owen, J., Thom, E., & Bottoms, S. F. (January 1996). Indication versus spontaneous preterm delivery: An evaluation of neonatal morbidity in ≤1000 g infants. <u>American Journal of Obstetrics and Gynecology, 174</u>(1, Pt. 2), 470. SPO abstracts #585.

138. Wheeler, T., Graves, C., Troiano, N., & Reed, G. (January 1995). Severe preeclampsia: Base deficit predicts oxygen transport status. <u>American Journal of Obstetrics and Gynecology, 172</u>(1, Pt. 2), 381. SPO abstracts #439.

139. Nelson, K. B., Dambrosia, J. M., Ting, T. Y., & Grether, J. K. (March 7, 1996). Uncertain value of electronic fetal monitoring in predicting cerebral palsy. <u>The New York Journal of Medicine, 334</u>(10), 613-618.

140. Fetal oxygen physiology. (1993). Hayward, CA: Nellcor, Inc.

141. Fujimori, K., Endo, C., Kin, S., Funata, Y., Araki, T., & Sato, A. (August 1994). Endocrinologic and biophysical responses to prolonged (24-hour) hypoxemia in fetal goats. <u>American Journal of Obstetrics and Gynecology, 171</u>(2), 470-474.

142. Jackson, B. T., Piasecki, G. J., & Novy, M. J. (January 1987). Fetal responses to altered maternal oxygenation in rhesus monkey. <u>American Journal of Physiology, 252</u>(1, Pt. 2), R94-R101.

143. Cunningham, F. G., MacDonald, P. C., & Gant, N. F. (1989). <u>Williams obstetrics</u> (18th ed.). Norwalk, CT: Appleton & Lange.

144. Kjellmer, I., Karlsson, K., Olsson, T., & Rosen, K. G. (1974). Cerebral reactions during intrauterine asphyxia in the sheep. I. Circulation and oxygen consumption in the fetal brain. <u>Pediatric Research, 8</u>(1), 50-57.

145. Lim, K. H., Mishell, J. M., DiFederico, E. M., Gallery, E. D. M., & Fisher, S. J. (January 1995). Oxygen regulates trophoblast and decidual endothelial cell prostanoid production. <u>American Journal of Obstetrics and Gynecology, 172</u>(1, Pt. 2), 272. SPO abstracts #49.

146. Zanini, B., Paul, R. H., & Huey, J. R. (January 1, 1980). Intrapartum fetal heart rate: Correlation with scalp pH in the preterm fetus [Fetus, Placenta, and Newborn]. <u>American Journal of Obstetrics and Gynecology, 136</u>(1), 43-47.

147. Berry, S. M., Field, S. J., Dombrowski, M. P., Lanouette, J. M., Brown, C. L., & Cotton, D. B. (January 1996). Expectant management in pregnancies complicated by growth retardation and acidemia? <u>American Journal of Obstetrics and Gynecology, 174</u>(1, Pt. 2), 382. SPO abstracts #257.

148. Nijland, R., Jongsma, H. W., Nijhuis, J. G., van den Berg, P. P., & Oeseburg, B. (March 1995). Arterial oxygen saturation in relation to metabolic acidosis in fetal lambs. <u>American Journal of Obstetrics and Gynecology, 172</u>(3), 810-819.

149. Low, J. A., Cox, M. J., Karchmar, M. J., McGrath, M. J., Pancham, S. R., & Piercy, W. N. (February 1, 1981). The prediction of intrapartum fetal metabolic acidosis by fetal heart rate monitoring. <u>American Journal of Obstetrics and Gynecology, 139</u>(3), 299-305.

150. Itskovitz, J., La Gamma, E. F., & Rudolph, A. M. (April 1, 1983). The effect of reducing umbilical blood flow on fetal oxygenation. <u>American Journal of Obstetrics and Gynecology, 145</u>(7), 813-818.

151. Richardson, B. S., Carmichael, L., Homan, J., & Patrick, J. E. (August 1992). Electrocortical activity, electroocular activity, and breathing movements in fetal sheep with prolonged and graded hypoxemia. <u>American Journal of Obstetrics and Gynecology, 167</u>(2), 553-558.

152. Gagnon, R., & Johnston, L. (January 1995). Fetal heart rate patterns during umbilical placental hypoperfusion. <u>American Journal of Obstetrics and Gynecology, 172</u>(1, Pt. 2), 337. SPO abstracts #278.

153. Cohn, H. E., Sacks, E. J., Heymann, M. A., & Rudolph, A. M. (November 15, 1974). Cardiovascular responses to hypoxemia and acidemia in fetal lambs [Fetus, Placenta, and Newborn]. <u>American Journal of Obstetrics and Gynecology, 120</u>(6), 817-824.

154. Tucker, C., Cook, V., & Weeks, J. (January 1995). Arterial umbilical cord pH, gestational age, and nucleated red blood cell count. <u>American Journal of Obstetrics and Gynecology, 172</u>(1, Pt. 2), 320. SPO abstracts #212.

155. Bonebrake, R., Fleming, A., & Dutton, K. (January 1995). Nucleated red blood cells as an indicator of fetal asphyxia. <u>American Journal of Obstetrics and Gynecology, 172</u>(1, Pt. 2), 321. SPO abstracts #214.

156. Phelan, J. P., Ahn, M. O., Korst, L. M., & Martin, G. I. (November 1995). Nucleated red blood cells: A marker for fetal asphyxia? <u>American Journal of Obstetrics and Gynecology, 173</u>(5), 1380-1384.

157. Phelan, J. P., Ahn, M. O., Korst, L., & Martin, G. I. (January 1996). Is intrapartum fetal brain injury in the term fetus preventable? <u>American Journal of Obstetrics and Gynecology, 174</u>(1, Pt. 2), 318. SPO abstracts #38.

158. Leikin, E., Verma, U., Klein, S., & Tejani, N. (January 1996). Relationship between nucleated red blood cell (NRBC) counts and intraventricular hemorrhage (IVH) and periventricular leucomalacia (PVL). <u>American Journal of Obstetrics and Gynecology, 174</u>(1, Pt. 2), 399. SPO abstracts #317.

159. Menard, M., Hulsey, T. C., Ebeling, M., & Newman, R. (January 1995). Urban/rural and ethnic disparities in fetal mortality. <u>American Journal of Obstetrics and Gynecology, 172</u>(1, Pt. 2), 400. SPO abstracts #516.

160. Low, J. A., Simpson, L. L., Tonni, G., & Chamberlain, S. (March 1995). Limitations in the clinical prediction of intrapartum fetal asphyxia. <u>American Journal of Obstetrics and Gynecology, 172</u>(3), 801-804.

292

161. Henderson, C. E., Cardonick, E., & Divon, M. Y. (January 1995). Obstetrical outcome following spurious labor. <u>American Journal of Obstetrics and Gynecology, 172</u>(1, Pt. 2), 292. SPO abstracts #108.

162. Salafia, C. M., Minior, V. K., Lopez-Zeno, J. A., Whittington, S. S., Pezzullo, J. C., & Vintzileos, A. M. (October 1995). Relationship between placental histologic features and umbilical cord blood gases in preterm gestations. <u>American Journal of Obstetrics and Gynecology, 173</u>(4), 1058-1064.

163. Ferguson, II, J. E., & O'Reilly, R. (July 1985). Hemoglobin E and pregnancy. <u>Obstetrics & Gynecology, 66</u>(1), 136-140.

164. Pardi, G., Marconi, A. M., Cetin, I., Baggiani, A. M., Lan Franchi, A., & Bozzetti, P. (1991). Fetal oxygenation and acid base balance during pregnancy. <u>Journal of Perinatal Medicine, 19</u>(Suppl. 1), 139-144.

165. Gaudier, F. L., Goldenberg, R. L., Du Bard, M., Nelson, K. G., & Hauth, J. C. (January 1994). Acid-base status at birth in small for gestational age vs appropriate for gestational age ≤ 1,000 grams infants. <u>American Journal of Obstetrics and Gynecology, 170</u>(1, Pt. 2), 309. SPO abstracts #112.

166. Baxi, L. V. (June 1982). Symposium on fetal monitoring. Current status of fetal oxygen monitoring. <u>Clinics in Perinatology, 9</u>(2), 423-431.

167. Lee, M. J., Charafeddine, L., Woods, Jr., J. R., & Del Priore, G. (January 1995). Birthweight determines survival in premature severely growth retarded newborns. <u>American Journal of Obstetrics and Gynecology, 172</u>(1, Pt. 2), 367. SPO abstracts #394.

168. Nyholm, H. C., Hansen, T., & Neldam, S. (1983). Fetal activity acceleration during early labor. <u>Acta Obstetricia et Gynecologica Scandinavica, 62,</u> 131-133.

169. Cock, M. L., Wlodek, M. E., Hooper, S. B., McCrabb, G. J., & Harding, R. (May 1994). The effects of twenty-four hours of reduced uterine blood flow on fetal fluid balance in sheep. <u>American Journal of Obstetrics and Gynecology, 170</u>(5, Pt. 1), 1442-1451.

170. Nicolaides, K. H., Sadovsky, G., & Visser, G. H. (May 1989). Heart rate patterns in normoxemic, hypoxemic, and anemic second-trimester fetuses. <u>American Journal of Obstetrics and Gynecology, 160</u>(5, Pt. 1), 1034-1037.

171. Scherjon, S. A., Smolders-DeHaas, H., Kok, J. H., & Zondervan, H. A. (July 1993). The "brain-sparing" effect: Antenatal cerebral doppler findings in relation to neurologic outcome in very preterm infants. <u>American Journal of Obstetrics and Gynecology, 169</u>(1), 169-175.

172. Klima, H., Jones, D., & Morotti, R. (January 1995). The rise and fall of villous edema as a function of time from initiation of intrauterine infection. <u>American Journal of Obstetrics and Gynecology, 172</u>(1, Pt. 2), 312. SPO abstracts #186.

173. McNamara, M., Wallis, T., Qureshi, F., Jacques, S., & Gonik, B. (January 1996). Determining maternal vs fetal immunologic contribution to chorioamnionitis (CHORIO). <u>American Journal of Obstetrics and Gynecology, 174</u>(1, Pt. 2), 404. SPO abstracts #337.

174. Salafia, C., Minior, V. K., Pezzullo, J. C., Spong, C. Y., Sherer, D. M., & Ghidini, A. (January 1996). Histologic acute intrauterine inflammation versus clinical chorioamnionitis: Which best predicts neonatal sepsis. <u>American Journal of Obstetrics and Gynecology, 174</u>(1, Pt. 2), 490. SPO abstracts #665.

175. Miller, H. S., & Aqua, K. A. (January 1996). Intraamniotic infection: Its effect on duration of labor. <u>American Journal of Obstetrics and Gynecology, 174</u>(1, Pt. 2), 483. SPO abstracts #640.

176. Smulian, J. C., Campbell, W. A., Vintzileos, A. M., & Rodis, J. F. (January 1996). Correlation of umbilical artery levels of interleukin-6 (IL-6) and soluble intracellular adhesion molecule-1 (SICAM-1) with umbilical arterial blood gas measurements. <u>American Journal of Obstetrics and Gynecology, 174</u>(1, Pt. 2), 371. SPO abstracts #216.

177. Raynor, D., Clark, P., & Duff, P. (January 1995). Granulocyte colony stimulating factor (GCSF) in amniotic fluid. <u>American Journal of Obstetrics and Gynecology, 172</u>(1, Pt. 2), 280. SPO abstracts #70.

178. Jauniaux, E., Ramsay, B., Peellaerts, C., & Scholler, Y. (1996). Perinatal features of pregnancies complicated by nuchal cord. <u>American Journal of Perinatology, 12,</u> 255-258 in <u>Capsules & Comments in Perinatal and Women's Health Nursing, 2</u>(1), 61-62.

179. Del Valle, G. O., Santerini, K., Sanchez-Ramos, L., Gaudier, F. L., & Delke, I. (January 1995). The straight umbilical cord: Significance and perinatal implications. <u>American Journal of Obstetrics and Gynecology, 172</u>(1, Pt. 2), 286. SPO abstracts #83.

180. Davis, R. O., Goldenberg, R. L., Brumfield, C. G., Owen, J., Wenstrom, K. D., & DuBard, M. (January 1995). Placental location and pregnancy outcome. <u>American Journal of Obstetrics and Gynecology, 172</u>(1, Pt. 2), 346. SPO abstracts #310.

181. Castro, L. C., Hobel, C. J., Walla, C., Ortiz, L., & Platt, L. D. (January 1995). Placental migratory patterns and birthweight. <u>American Journal of Obstetrics and Gynecology, 172</u>(1, Pt. 2), 346. SPO abstracts #309.

182. Larson, J., Rayburn, W., Crosby, S., & Thurnau, G. (January 1995). Multiple nuchal cord entanglements and perinatal outcomes. <u>American Journal of Obstetrics and Gynecology, 172</u>(1, Pt. 2), 364. SPO abstracts #382.

183. Vintzileos, A., Nochimson, D., Guzman, E., & Knuppel, R. (January 1995). Comparison of intrapartum electronic fetal heart rate monitoring versus intermittent auscultation in detecting fetal acidemia at birth. <u>American Journal of Obstetrics and Gynecology, 172</u>(1, Pt. 2), 367. SPO abstracts #391.

184. Kubli, F. W., Hon, E. H., Khazin, A. F., & Takemura, H. (August 15, 1969). Observations on heart rate and pH in the human fetus during labor. <u>American Journal of Obstetrics and Gynecology, 104</u>(8), 1190-1206.

185. Heymann, M. A. (1989). Biophysical evaluation of fetal status. Fetal cardiovascular physiology. In R. K. Creasy, & R. Resnik (Eds.), <u>Maternal-fetal medicine: Principles and practice</u> (2nd ed., pp. 288-302). Philadelphia, PA: W. B. Saunders Company.

186. Westgren, M., Holmquist, P., Svenningsen, N. W., & Ingemarsson, I. (July 1982). Intrapartum fetal monitoring in preterm deliveries: Prosecutive study. Obstetrics & Gynecology, 60(1), 99-106.

187. Murray, H. G. (January 1996). The fetal ECG: PR waveform changes associated with metabolic acidemia. American Journal of Obstetrics and Gynecology, 174(1, Pt. 2), 323. SPO abstracts #52.

188. Chaffin, D., Barnard, J., Phemetton, T., Newman, A., & Reed, K. (January 1996). The effect of acidemia on fetal heart rate variability. American Journal of Obstetrics and Gynecology, 174(1, Pt. 2), 382. SPO abstracts #259.

189. Guzman, E., Vintzileos, A., Egan, J., Benito, C., Lake, M., & Lai, Y. (January 1996). Antenatal prediction of fetal pH in intrauterine growth restricted fetuses using computer analysis of the fetal heart rate. American Journal of Obstetrics and Gynecology, 174(1, Pt. 2), 335. SPO abstracts #80.

190. Pincus, S. M., & Viscarello, R. R. (February 1992). Approximate entropy: A regularity measure for fetal heart rate analysis. Obstetrics & Gynecology, 79(2), 249-255.

191. Dildy, G. A., van den Berg, P. P., Katz, M., Clark, S. L., Jongsma, H. W., & Nijhuis, J. G. (January 1994). Intrapartum fetal pulse oximetry: Fetal oxygen saturation trends during labor with normal neonatal outcome. American Journal of Obstetrics and Gynecology, 170(1, Pt. 2), 391. SPO abstracts #420.

192. Zinger, K., Guzman, E., & Scorza, W. (January 1996). The effect of breech presentation on umbilical artery acid-base status at birth. American Journal of Obstetrics and Gynecology, 174(1, Pt. 2), 348. SPO abstracts #130.

193. Monteiro, H. A., Miller, D. A., & Paul, R. H. (January 1995). Fetal movement profile: A useful predictive tool? American Journal of Obstetrics and Gynecology, 172(1, Pt. 2), 337. SPO abstracts #279.

194. Shaw, K., & Clark, S. L. (December 1988). Reliability of intrapartum fetal heart rate monitoring in the postterm fetus with meconium passage. Obstetrics & Gynecology, 72(6), 886-889.

195. Cohn, H. E., Jackson, B. T., Piasecki, G. J., Cohen, W. R., & Novy, M. J. (October 1985). Fetal cardiovascular responses to asphyxia induced by decreased uterine perfusion. Journal of Developmental Physiology, 7(5), 289-297.

196. Moll, W., & Kastendieck, E. (1985). Kinetics of lactic acid accumulation and removal in the fetus. In W. Kunzel (Ed.), Fetal heart rate monitoring. Clinical practice and pathophysiology (pp. 161-169). Berlin, Heidelberg: Germany. Springer-Verlag.

197. Dawes, G. S. (December 1991). Computerised analysis of the fetal heart rate. European Journal of Obstetrics, Gynecology and Reproductive Biology, 42(Suppl.), s5-s8.

198. Meschia, G. (December 1, 1978). Evolution of thinking in fetal respiratory physiology. American Journal of Obstetrics and Gynecology, 132(7), 806-813.

199. Rosen, K. G., & Isaksson, O. (1976). Alterations in fetal heart rate and ECG correlated to glycogen, creatine phosphate and ATP levels during graded hypoxia. Biology of the Neonate, 30, 17-24.

200. Wittmann, B. K., Davison, B. M., Lyons, E., Frohlich, J., & Towell, M. E. (April 1979). Real-time ultrasound observation of fetal activity in labour. British Journal of Obstetrics and Gynaecology, 86, 278-281.

201. Sherman, D. J., Ross, M. G., Day, L., Humme, J., & Ervin, M. G. (November 1991). Fetal swallowing: response to graded maternal hypoxemia. Journal of Applied Physiology, 71(5), 1856-1861.

202. McGlashan, H. E. (August 1994). Electronic fetal heart rate monitoring with epidural analgesia [Letters to the editor]. Australian and New Zealand Journal of Obstetrics and Gynaecology, 34(4), 499-500.

203. Korst, L. M., Ahn, M. O., & Phelan, J. P. (January 1996). Nucleated red blood cells: An update on the marker for fetal asphyxia. American Journal of Obstetrics and Gynecology, 174(1, Pt. 2), 318. SPO abstracts #40.

204. Smith, J. H., Anand, K. J. S., Cotes, P. M., Dawes, G. S., Harkness, R. A., & Howlett, T. A. (October 1988). Antenatal fetal heart rate variation in relation to the respiratory and metabolic status of the compromised human fetus. British Journal of Obstetrics and Gynaecology, 95, 980-989.

205. Keegan, Jr., K. A., Waffarn, F., & Quilligan, E. J. (December 1, 1985). Obstetric characteristics and fetal heart rate patterns of infants who convulse during the newborn period. American Journal of Obstetrics and Gynecology, 153(7), 732-737.

206. Antonowicz, I., & Schwachman, H. (1979). Meconium in health and disease. Advanced Pediatrics, 26, 275.

207. Meis, P. J., Hall III, M., Marshall, J. R., & Hobel, C. J. (July 1, 1978). Meconium passage: A new classification for risk assessment during labor. American Journal of Obstetrics and Gynecology, 131(5), 509-513.

208. Holtzman, R. B., Banzhaf, W. C., Silver, R. K., Hageman, J. R. (December 1989). Perinatal management of meconium staining of the amniotic fluid. Clinics in Perinatology, 16(4), 825-838.

209. Hobbes, J. F., & Eidelman, A. L. (1979). The meconium aspiration syndrome. In G. F. Marx (Ed.), Clinical management of mother and newborn, (137). New York, NY: Springer-Verlag.

210. Carson, B. S., Losey, R.W., Bowes, Jr., W. A.,& Simmons, M. A. (November 15, 1976). Combined obstetric and pediatric approach to prevent meconium aspiration syndrome. American Journal of Obstetrics and Gynecology, 126(6), 712-715.

211. Miller, F. C., & Read, J. A. (November 1, 1981). Intrapartum assessment of the postdate fetus. <u>American Journal of Obstetrics and Gynecology, 141,</u> 516-520.

212. Miller, Jr., J. M., Bernard, M., Brown, H. L., St. Pierre, J. J., & Gabert, H. A. (April 1990). Umbilical cord blood gases for term healthy newborns. <u>American Journal of Perinatology, 7</u>(2), 157-159.

213. Wiswell, T. E., & Bent, R. C. (October 1993). Meconium staining and the meconium aspiration syndrome-unresolved issues. <u>Pediatric Clinics of North America, 40</u>(5), 955-981.

214. Kimble, F. W. (April 1986). The clinical significance of meconium stained liquor during the first stage of labour-A retrospective study of 114 patients admitted to Harare Maternity Hospital as compared to a control group. <u>The Central African Journal of Medicine, 32</u>(4), 91-94.

215. Ross, B., Bradley, K., Kullama, L., Nijland, M. J. M., & Ross, M. G. (January 1996). Increased fetal colonic muscle contractility following glucocorticoid and thyroxine (T_4) therapy: Implications for meconium passage. <u>American Journal of Obstetrics and Gynecology, 174</u>(1, Pt. 2), 385. SPO abstracts #270.

216. Rotmensch, S., Liberati, M., Sahavi, Z., Lev, S., Efrat, Z., & Kobo, M. (January 1996). Suppression of fetal biophysical activity and false diagnosis of asphyxia following antenatal steroid administration. <u>American Journal of Obstetrics and Gynecology, 174</u>(1, Pt. 2), 336. SPO abstracts #83.

217. Eriksen, N. L., Hostetter, M., Parisi, U. M. (October 1994). Prophylactic amnioinfusion in pregnancies complicated by thick meconium. <u>American Journal of Obstetrics and Gynecology, 171,</u> 1026-30.

218. Wong, W. S. F., Wong, K. S., & Chang, A. (May 1985). Epidemiology of meconium staining of amniotic fluid in Hong Kong. <u>Australian and New Zealand Journal of Obstetrics and Gynaecology, 25</u>(2), 90-93.

219. Davis, R. O., Philips, J. B., Harris, B. A., Wilson, E. R., & Huddleston, J. F. (March 15, 1985). Fatal meconium aspiration syndrome occurring despite airway management considered appropriate. <u>American Journal of Obstetrics and Gynecology, 151</u>(6), 731-736.

220. Gupta, S., Mathur, S. V., & Gupta, P. (February 1984). Foetal outcome in cases of meconium stained amniotic fluid during labour. <u>Journal of the Indian Medical Association, 82</u>(2), 47-49.

221. Bhutta, Z. A., Jalil, S. (1992). Meconium aspiration syndrome: The role of resuscitation and tracheal suction in prevention. <u>Asia-Oceania Journal of Obstetrics/Gynecology, 18</u>(1), 13-17.

222. Alsulyman, O., Ouzounian, J., Castro, M. A., Paul, R., & Goodwin, T. M. (January 1996). Cholestasis of pregnancy: Perinatal outcome associated with expectant management. <u>American Journal of Obstetrics and Gynecology, 174</u>(1, Pt. 2), 393. SPO abstracts #301.

223. <u>Standards for the nursing care of women and newborns</u> (4th ed.). (1991). Washington, DC: Nurses' Association of the American College of Obstetricians and Gynecologists.

224. Wong, F. W. S., Loong, E. P. L., & Chang, A. M. Z. (June 1, 1985). Ultrasound diagnosis of meconium-stained amniotic fluid. <u>American Journal of Obstetrics and Gynecology, 52</u>(3), 359.

225. Miller, P. W., Coen, R. W., & Penirschke, K. (October 1985). Dating the time interval from meconium passage to birth. <u>Obstetrics & Gynecology, 66</u>(4), 459-462.

226. Ramachandra, K., Bhargava, V. L., Pande, Y., & Goel, B. K. (1984). Significance of meconium during labour and its correlation with umbilical cord blood studies. <u>Indian Journal of Pediatrics, 51,</u> 149-153.

227. Arulkumaran, S., Yeoh, S. C., Gibb, D. M. F., Ingemarsson, I., & Ratnam, S. S. (December 1985). Obstetric outcome of meconium stained liquor in labour. <u>Singapore Medical Journal, 26</u>(7), 523-526.

228. Low, J. A., Karchmar, J., Broekhoven, L., Leonard, T., McGrath, M. J., & Pancham, S. R. (December 15, 1981). The probability of fetal metabolic acidosis during labor in a population at risk as determined by clinical factors. <u>American Journal of Obstetrics and Gynecology, 141</u>(8), 941-951.

229. Mitchell, J., Schulman, H., Fleisher, A., Farmakides, G., & Nadeau, D. (March 1985). Meconium aspiration and fetal acidosis. <u>Obstetrics & Gynecology, 65</u>(3), 352-355.

230. Cole, J. W., Portman, R. J., Lim, Y., Perlman, J. M., & Robson, A. M. (December 1985). Urinary β_2-microglobulin in full-term newborns: Evidence for proximal tubular dysfunction in infants with meconium-stained amniotic fluid. <u>Pediatrics, 76</u>(6), 958-964.

231. Goodlin, R. C. (August 1, 1984). Detrimental perinatal associations with increased fetal reactivity. <u>American Journal of Obstetrics and Gynecology, 149</u>(7), 801-802.

232. Burke-Strickland, M. (1973). Meconium aspiration of the newborn. <u>Minnesota Medicine, 56,</u> 1031.

233. Oelberg, D. G., Downey, S. A., & Flynn, M. M. (1990). Bile salt-induced intracellular Ca^{++} accumulation in type II pneumocytes. <u>Lung, 168</u>(6), 297-308.

234. Katz, V. L., & Bowes, W. A. (January 1992). Meconium aspiration syndrome: Reflections on a murky subject. <u>American Journal of Obstetrics and Gynecology, 166,</u> 171-183.

235. Gregory, G. A., Gooding, C. A., Phibbs, R. H., & Tooley, W. H. (December 1974). Meconium aspiration in infants: A prospectus study. <u>Journal of Pediatrics, 85</u>(6), 848-852.

236. Yeh, T.F., Harris, V., Srinivasan, G., Lilien, L., Payati, S., & Pildes, R. S. (July 6, 1979). Roentgenographic findings in infants with meconium aspiration syndrome. JAMA, 242(1), 60-63.

237. Vidyasagar, D., Harris, V., & Pildes, R. S. (August 1975). Assisted ventilation in infants with meconium aspiration syndrome. Pediatrics, 56(2), 208-213.

238. Bar-Tao, W., Li-Jun, S., & Lo-Yun, T. (1991). Intrapartum amnioinfusion for replacement of meconium-stained amniotic fluid to prevent MAS. Chinese Medical Journal, 104, 221.

239. Macri, C. J., Schrimmer, D. B., Leung, A., Greenspoon, J. S., & Paul, R. H. (1992). Prophylactic amnioinfusion improves outcomes of pregnancy complicated by thick meconium and oligohydramnios. American Journal of Obstetrics and Gynecology, 167(1), 117-121.

240. Spong, C. Y., Ogundipe, A., & Ross, M. G. (August 1995). Amnioinfusion and the intrauterine prevention of meconium aspiration. American Journal of Obstetrics and Gynecology, 173(2), 671-672.

241. Wenstrom, K. D., Parsons, M. T. (1989). The prevention of meconium aspiration in labor using amnioinfusion. Obstetrics & Gynecology, 73(4), 647-651.

242. Sadovsky, Y., Amon, E., Bade, M. E., & Petrie, R. H. (September 1989). Prophylactic amnioinfusion during labor complicated by meconium: A preliminary report. American Journal of Obstetrics and Gynecology, 161(3), 613-617.

243. Clark, P., & Duff, P. (January 1995). Inhibition of neutrophil oxidative burst and phagocytosis by meconium. American Journal of Obstetrics and Gynecology, 172(1, Pt. 2), 300. SPO abstracts #140.

244. Piper, J. M., Newton, E. R., Berkus, M. D., & Peairs, W. A. (January 1995). Is meconium a marker for peripartum infection? American Journal of Obstetrics and Gynecology, 172(1, Pt. 2), 305. SPO abstracts #158.

245. Wiswell, T. E. (December 1992). Meconium aspiration syndrome made murkier [Letters]. American Journal of Obstetrics and Gynecology, 167(6), 1914-1915.

246. Suresh, G. K., & Subrata, S. (October 1994). Delivery room management of infants born through thin meconium-stained liquor. Indian Pediatrics, 3(10), 1177-1181.

247. Larsen, L. G., Clausen, H. V., Andersen, B., & Graem, N. (February 1995). A stereologic study of postmature placentas fixed by dual perfusion. American Journal of Obstetrics and Gynecology, 172(2, Pt. 1), 500-507.

248. Yeh, S., Bruce, S. L., & Thorton, Y. S. (June 1982). Intrapartum monitoring and management of the postdate fetus. Clinics in Perinatology, 9(2), 381-386.

249. Miller, F. C., Sacks, D. A., Yeh, S., Paul, R. H., Schifrin, B. S., & Martin, C. B. (July 1, 1975). Significance of meconium during labor. American Journal of Obstetrics and Gynecology, 122(5), 573-580.

250. Jouppila, P., Kirkinen, P., Koivula, A., & Jouppila, A. (1983). The influence of maternal oxygen inhalation on human placental and umbilical venous blood flow. European Journal of Obstetrics, Gynaecology and Reproductive Biology, 16, 151-156.

251. Molcho, J., Leiberman, J. R., Hagay, Z., & Hagay, Y. (April 1986). Spectrophotometric determination of meconium concentration in amniotic fluid. Journal of Biomedical Engineering, 8(2), 162-165.

252. Dooley, S. L., Pesavento, D. J., Depp, R., Socol, M. L., Tamura, R. K., & Wiringa, K. S. (December 1, 1985). Meconium below the vocal cords at delivery: Correlation with intrapartum events. American Journal of Obstetrics and Gynecology, 153(7), 767-770.

253. Surratt, N., & Troiano, N. H. (November/December 1994). Adult respiratory distress in pregnancy: Critical care issues [Principles and Practice]. JOGNN, 23(9), 773-780.

254. Vorherr, H. (September 1, 1975). Placental insufficiency in relation to postterm pregnancy and fetal postmaturity. Evaluation of fetoplacental function, management of the postterm gravida [Current Developments]. American Journal of Obstetrics and Gynecology, 123(1), 67-102.

255. Shailer, T. L., Harvey, C. J., & Guyer, F. (July/September 1992). Principles of oxygen transport in the critically ill obstetric patient. NAACOG's Clinical Issues in Perinatal and Women's Health Nursing, 3(3), 392-398.

256. Powrie, R., Larson, L., & Montella, K. R. (January 1996). Alveolar-arterial oxygen gradient in acute pulmonary embolism in pregnancy. American Journal of Obstetrics and Gynecology, 174(1, Pt. 2), 390. SPO abstracts #289.

257. Meschia, G. (October 1979). Supply of oxygen to the fetus. Journal of Reproductive Medicine, 23(4), 160-165.

258. Hook, J. V., & Harvey, C. (January 1994). The effect of pregnancy on maternal SaO_2 values at biweekly intervals at sea level. American Journal of Obstetrics and Gynecology, 170(1, Pt. 2), 313.

259. Breathnach, C. S. (July 1991). The stability of the fetal oxygen environment. Irish Journal of Medical Science, 160(7), 189-191.

260. Kitanaka, T., Alonso, J. G., Gilbert, R. D., Siu, B. L., Clemons, G. K., & Long, L. D. (June 1989). Fetal responses to long-term hypoxemia in sheep. American Journal of Physiology, 256(6, Pt. 2), R1348-R1354.

261. Wilkening, R. B., & Meschia, G. (January/February 1992). Current topic: Comparative physiology of placental oxygen transport. Placenta, 13(1), 1-15.

262. Hill, E. P., Hill, J. R., Power, G. G., & Longo, L. D. (March 1977). Carbon monoxide exchanges between the human fetus and mother: A mathematical model. American Journal of Physiology, 232(3), H311-H323.

263. Newhall, Jr., J. F. (August 15, 1981). Scuba diving during pregnancy: A brief review. <u>American Journal of Obstetrics and Gynecology, 140,</u> 893-894.

264. Yancey, M. K., Moore, J., Brady, K., Milligan, D., & Strampel, W. (April 1992). The effect of altitude on umbilical cord blood gases. <u>Obstetrics & Gynecology, 79</u>(4), 571-574.

265. Guyton, A. C. (1986). <u>Textbook of medical physiology</u> (7th ed.). Philadelphia, PA: W. B. Saunders Company.

266. Oeseburg, B., Biny, E. M., Ringnalda, M., Crevels, J. H. W., Jongsma, P., & Mannheimer, J. (May 1992). Fetal oxygenation in chronic maternal hypoxia: What's critical? In W. Erdmann, & D. F. Bruley (Eds.), <u>Advances in experimental medicine & biology, vol. 317. Oxygen transport to tissue XIV</u> (pp. 499-502). New York, NY: Plenum Press.

267. Krins, A. J., Mitchells, W. R., & Wood, C. (April 1969). Effect of morphine upon maternal capillary blood oxygen and carbon dioxide tension. <u>Journal of Obstetrics and Gynaecology of the British Commonwealth, 76,</u> 359-361.

268. Dolezal, L., Zavodny, P., Krikal, Z., Gazarek, F., Pohanka, J., & Machovska, K. (1987). Examination of fetal oxygenation by controlled hypoxia. <u>Acta Universitatis Palackianae Olomucensis Facultatis Medicae 116,</u> 395-400.

269. Strohl, K. P., & Altose, M. D. (February 1984). Oxygen saturation during breath-holding and during apnea in sleep. <u>Chest, 85</u>(2), 181-186.

270. Caldeyro-Barcia, R., Giussi, G., Storch, E., Poseiro, J. J., Lafaurie, N., & Kettenhuber, K. (1981). The bearing-down efforts and their effects on fetal heart rate, oxygenation and acid base balance. <u>Journal of Perinatal Medicine, 9</u>(Suppl. 1), 63-67.

271. Williams, K., & Wilson, S. (January 1996). Effect of epidural anaesthesia on maternal cerebral hemodynamics during labour. <u>American Journal of Obstetrics and Gynecology, 174</u>(1, Pt. 2), 484. SPO abstracts #642.

272. Ang, C. K., Tan, T. H., Walters, W. A. W., & Wood, C. (October 25, 1969). Postural influence on maternal capillary oxygen and carbon dioxide tension. <u>British Medical Journal, 4,</u> 201-203.

273. Caldeyro-Barcia, R. (Spring 1979). The influence of maternal bearing-down efforts during second stage on fetal well-being. <u>Birth and the Family Journal, 6</u>(1), 17-21.

274. Yeates, D. A., & Roberts, J. E. (January/February 1984). A comparison of two bearing-down techniques during the second stage of labor. <u>Journal of Nurse-Midwifery, 29</u>(1), 3-10.

275. Roberts, J. E., Goldstein, S. A., Gruener, J. S., Maggio, M., & Mendez-Bauer, C. (January/February 1987). A descriptive analysis of involuntary bearing-down efforts during the expulsive phase of labor [Research and Studies]. <u>JOGNN, 17,</u> 48-54.

276. Hansen, S. L., & Clark, S. L. (January 1996). Rest & descend vs. pushing with epidural anesthesia in the 2nd stage of labor. <u>American Journal of Obstetrics and Gynecology, 174</u>(1, Pt. 2), 479. SPO abstracts #621.

277. Boggess, K. A., Easterling, T. R., & Raghu, G. (October 1995). Management and outcome of pregnant women with interstitial and restrictive lung disease. <u>American Journal of Obstetrics and Gynecology, 173</u>(4), 1007-1014.

278. Boggess, K., Gill, P., Raghu, G., & Easterling, T. (January 1995). Restrictive lung disease in pregnancy. <u>American Journal of Obstetrics and Gynecology, 172</u>(1, Pt. 2), 334. SPO abstracts #266.

279. Wendel, P. J., Ramin, S. M., Hamm, C. B., Rowe, T. F., & Cunningham, F. G. (January 1995). A randomized controlled study of the management of asthma complicating pregnancy. <u>American Journal of Obstetrics and Gynecology, 172</u>(1, Pt. 2), 253. SPO abstracts #2.

280. Briggs, R. G., Mabie, W. C., & Sibai, B. M. (January 1996). Community-acquired pneumonia in pregnancy. <u>American Journal of Obstetrics and Gynecology, 174</u>(1, Pt. 2), 389. SPO abstracts #287.

281. Whitty, J. E., Dombrowski, M. P., Martier, S. S., & Sokol, R. J. (January 1996). Alcohol and cigarette use increases risk of pneumonia during gestation. <u>American Journal of Obstetrics and Gynecology, 174</u>(1, Pt. 2), 400. SPO abstracts #321.

282. Martier, S., Wolfe, H. M., Ager, J., & Sokol, R. (January 1996). Decreased amniotic fluid volume: Suggestive but not predictive of FAS. <u>American Journal of Obstetrics and Gynecology, 174</u>(1, Pt. 2), 439. SPO abstracts #470.

283. Hodgson, R. J. R., Leadon, D. P., & Rossdale, P. D. (1983). Effect of intranasal oxygen administration on arterial blood gas and acid base parameters in spontaneous delivered, term induced and induced premature foals. <u>Research in Veterinary Science, 34,</u> 159-162.

284. Harvey, C. J., & Hankins, G. D. V. (January 1, 1994). Critical oxygen extraction in the pregnant ewe undergoing acute hypoxemia. <u>American Journal of Obstetrics and Gynecology, 170</u>(1, Pt. 2), 313. SPO abstracts #127.

285. Paulone, M. E., Edelstone, D. I., & Shedd, A. (January 1987). Effects of maternal anemia on uteroplacental and fetal oxidative metabolism in sheep. <u>American Journal of Obstetrics and Gynecology, 156</u>(1), 230-236.

286. Harvey, C., Van Hook, J., Shailer, T., & Anderson, G. (January 1995). The accuracy of a/A ratio in the assessment of intrapulmonary shunting compared to QS/QT in acutely ill pregnant patients. <u>American Journal of Obstetrics and Gynecology, 172</u>(1, Pt. 2), 281. SPO abstracts #73.

287. Hankins, G., Harvey, C., Clark, S., & Uckan, E. (January 1996). Intrapulmonary shunt (QS/Qt) and position in healthy third-trimester pregnancy. <u>American Journal of Obstetrics and Gynecology, 174</u>(1, Pt. 2), 322. SPO abstracts #49.

288. Aldrich, C. J., D'Antona, D., Spencer, J. A., Wyatt, J. S., Peebles, D. M., & Delpy, D. T. (January 1995). The effect of maternal posture on fetal cerebral oxygenation during labour. <u>British Journal of Obstetrics & Gynaecology, 102</u>(1), 14-19.

289. Goodlin, R. C. (February 1, 1979). History of fetal monitoring. <u>American Journal of Obstetrics and Gynecology, 133</u>(3), 323-352.

ANTEPARTAL AND INTRAPARTAL FETAL MONITORING

290. Caritis, S. N., Abouleish, E., Edelstone, D. I., & Mueller-Heubach, E. (November 1980). Fetal acid-base state following spinal or epidural anesthesia for cesarean section. Obstetrics & Gynecology, 56(5), 610-615.

291. Koga, S., Koga, Y., & Nagai, H. (1988). Physiological significance of fetal blood gas changes elicited by different delivery postures. Tohoku Journal of Experimental Medicine, 154(4), 357-363.

292. Carter, A. M. (1989). Factors affecting gas transfer across the placenta and the oxygen supply to the fetus. Journal of Developmental Physiology, 12(6), 305-322.

293. Perry, Jr., K. G., Martin, R. W., Blake, P. G., Roberts, W. E., & Martin, Jr., J. N. (January 1996). Maternal outcome associated with adult respiratory distress syndrome. American Journal of Obstetrics and Gynecology, 174(1, Pt. 2), 391. SPO abstracts #293.

294. Belfort, M. A., & Saade, G. R. (July 1994). Oxygen delivery and consumption in critically ill pregnant patients: Association with ophthalmic artery diastolic velocity. American Journal of Obstetrics and Gynecology, 171(1), 211-217.

295. Kramer, W., Saade, G., Leibman, B., Kirshon, B., Adam, K., & Baker, W. (January 1995). Maternal oxygen consumption and CO_2 production during the peripartum period in normal gestation. American Journal of Obstetrics and Gynecology, 172(1, Pt. 2), 319. SPO abstracts #205.

296. Van Hook, J., Harvey, C., & Uckan, E. (January 1995). Mechanical ventilation in pregnancy and postpartum minute ventilation and weaning. American Journal of Obstetrics and Gynecology, 172(1, Pt. 2), 326. SPO abstracts #234.

297. Paul, R. H., Koh, K. S., & Bernstein, S. G. (January 15, 1978). Changes in fetal heart rate-uterine contraction patterns associated with eclampsia. American Journal of Obstetrics and Gynecology, 130(2), 165-169.

298. Frangieh, A. Y., Friedman, S. A., Audibert, F., Usta, I., & Sibai, B. M. (January 1996). Maternal outcome in women with eclampsia. American Journal of Obstetrics and Gynecology, 174(1, Pt. 2), 453. SPO abstracts #528.

299. Friedman, S. A., Schiff, E., Kao, L., & Sibai, B. M. (January 1995). Phenytoin versus magnesium sulfate in patients with eclampsia: Preliminary results from a randomized trial. American Journal of Obstetrics and Gynecology, 172(1, Pt. 2), 384. SPO abstracts #452.

300. Management of preeclampsia. (February 1996). Technical bulletin number 91, 1-5. Washington, DC: ACOG.

301. Mabie, W. C., Ratts, T. E., & Sibai, B. M. (1989). The central hemodynamics of severe preeclampsia. American Journal of Obstetrics and Gynecology, 161, 1443-1448.

302. Easterling, T. R., Benedetti, T. J., Schmucker, B. C., & Millard, S. P. (December 1990). Maternal hemodynamics in normal and preeclamptic pregnancies: A longitudinal study. Obstetrics & Gynecology, 76(6), 1061-1069.

303. Hines, T., & Jones, M. B. (September/October 1994). Can aspirin prevent and treat pre-eclampsia. MCN, 258-263.

304. Haller, D. L. (November 1980). The use of terbutaline for premature labor. Drug Intelligence & Clinical Pharmacy, 14, 757-764.

305. Aumann, G. M. E., & Blake, G. D. (March/April 1982). Ritodrine hydrochloride in the control of premature labor. JOGNN, 11(2), 75-79.

306. Fitzgerald, G. L. (1983). NAACOG update series: Preterm labor part 2: Management. Lesson 3, Volume 1. Continuing Professional Education Center, Inc., 1101 State Road, Building Q, Princeton, ME 08540.

307. Young, R. (January 1993). T-type and L-type calcium channels in freshly dispersed human uterine smooth muscle. American Journal of Obstetrics and Gynecology, 168(1, Pt. 2), 302. SPO abstracts.

308. Valenzuela, G. J., Norburg, M., & Ducsay, C. A. (November 1992). Acute intrauterine hypoxia increases amniotic fluid prostaglandin F metabolites in the pregnant sheep. American Journal of Obstetrics and Gynecology, 167(5), 1459-1464.

309. Dolkart, L. A., & Bhat, M. (September 1995). Sturge-Weber syndrome in pregnancy. American Journal of Obstetrics and Gynecology, 173(3, Pt. 1), 969-971.

310. Volk, M. D., & Morgan, M. D. (September 1, 1990). Medical malpractice series. Medical malpractice handling obstetric and neonatal cases. The Logical First Choice, (1990 cumulative Suppl.).

311. Gist, R. F. (August 1988). Sexually related trauma. Emergency Medicine Clinics of North America, 6(3), 439-443.

312. Madsen, H. (April 1986). Fetal oxygenation in diabetic pregnancy. Danish Medical Bulletin, 33(2), 64-74.

313. Rayburn, W. F. (December 15, 1982). Clinical implications from monitoring fetal activity [Current Developments]. American Journal of Obstetrics and Gynecology, 144(8), 967-980.

314. Aaronson, L. S. & MacNee, C. (July/August 1989). Tobacco, alcohol, and caffeine use during pregnancy. JOGNN, 18(4), 279-287.

315. Yancey, M. K., & Harlass, F. E. (March 1993). Extraneous factors and their influences on fetal acid-base status. Clinical Obstetrics and Gynecology, 36(1), 60-72.

316. Henderson-Smart, D. J., & Read, D. J. C. (1979). Fetal cardio-respiratory physiology. In R. P. Shearman (Ed.). Human reproductive physiology (2nd ed.) (pp. 228-267). Great Britain: Blackwell Scientific Publications, The Alden Press, Oxford.

317. Boley, T., Markenson, G., Maslow, A., Kopelman, J., & Read, J. (January 1995). Does nicotine affect levels of thromboxane and prostacyclin in the dually perfused human placental cotyledon model? American Journal of Obstetrics and Gynecology, 172(1, Pt. 2), 274. SPO abstracts #55.

318. Pappano, A. J. (March 1977). Ontogenetic development of autonomic neuroeffector transmission and transmitter reactivity in embryonic and fetal hearts. Pharmacological Reviews, 29(1), 3-33.

319. Clark, K. E., & Irion, G. L. (December 1992). Fetal hemodynamic response to maternal intravenous nicotine administration. American Journal of Obstetrics and Gynecology, 167(6), 1624-1631.

320. Farquharson, R. G. (1983). Fetal oxygen affinity and its parameters in a random obstetric population. Journal of Perinatal Medicine, 11(1), 43-50.

321. Pinette, M. G., Pan, Y., Pinette, S. G., Blackstone, J., & Chard, R. (January 1996). Associations of non-doppler-flow placental cystic lesion with smoking, elevated maternal serum alphafetoprotein and pregnancy outcomes. American Journal of Obstetrics and Gynecology, 174(1, Pt. 2), 414. SPO abstracts #379.

322. Fox, H. (December 1969). Pathology of the placenta in maternal diabetes mellitus. Obstetrics & Gynecology, 34(6), 792-798.

323. Altshuler, G. (May 31-June 4, 1981). Diseases of the placenta and their effect on transport. Placental transport - Mead Johnson symposium on perinatal and developmental medicine no. 18, 35-43. Vail, CO.

324. Ulm, M. R., Plockinger, B., Pirich, C., Gryglewski, R. J., & Sinzinger, H. F. (May 1995). Umbilical arteries of babies born to cigarette smokers generate less prostacyclin and contain less arginine and citrulline compared with those of babies born to control subjects. American Journal of Obstetrics and Gynecology, 172(5), 1485-1487.

325. Handler, A. S., Mason, E. D., Rosenberg, D. L., & Davis, F. G. (March 1994). The relationship between exposure during pregnancy to cigarette smoking and cocaine use and placenta previa. American Journal of Obstetrics and Gynecology, 170(3), 884-889.

326. Kendrick, J. S., Zahniser, S. C., Miller, N., Salas, N., Stine, J., & Gargiullo, P. M. (1995). Integrating smoking cessation into routine public prenatal care: The smoking cessation in pregnancy project. American Journal of Public Health, 85, 217-222 in Capsules & Comments in Perinatal and Women's Health Nursing, 1(4), 248.

327. Hardardottir, H., Oncken, C., Lupo, V. R., Daragjati, C., Chang, R. & Smeltzer, J. S. (January 1996). Maternal and fetal cardiovascular effects of a nicotine-patch versus maternal smoking. American Journal of Obstetrics and Gynecology, 174(1, Pt. 2), 367. SPO abstracts #198.

328. Cook, C., Ward, S., Myers, S., & Spinnato, J. (January 1995). A prospective randomized evaluation of intensified therapy for smoking reduction in pregnancy. American Journal of Obstetrics and Gynecology, 172(1, Pt. 2), 290. SPO abstracts #98.

329. Hartmann, K., Thorp, J., Pahel-Short, L., & Koch, M. (January 1995). A randomized controlled trial of smoking cessation intervention in pregnancy. American Journal of Obstetrics and Gynecology, 172(1, Pt. 2), 287. SPO abstracts #86.

330. O'Connell, K. A., Gerkovich, M. M., & Cook, M. R. (Winter 1995). Reversal theory's mastery and sympathy states in smoking cessation. IMAGE: Journal of Nursing Scholarship, 27(4), 311-316.

331. Lumley, J., Renou, P., Newman, W., & Wood, C. (March 15, 1969). Hyperventilation in obstetrics. American Journal of Obstetrics and Gynecology, 103(6), 847-855.

332. Mendoza, G. J. B., Calem-Grunat, J., Karmel, B. Z., LeBlanc, M. H., Brown, E. G., & Chervenak, F. (1989). Intrauterine growth retardation related to maternal erythrocyte oxygen transport. Advances in Experimental Medicine & Biology, 248, 377-386.

333. Low, J. A., Boston, R. W., & Cervenko, F. W. (April 1, 1970). Effect of low maternal carbon dioxide tension on placental gas exchange. American Journal of Obstetrics and Gynecology, 106(7), 1032-1043.

334. Datta, S., Ostheimer, G. W., Weiss, J. B., Brown, Jr., W. U., & Alper, M. H. (September 1981). Neonatal effect of prolonged anesthetic induction for cesarean section. Obstetrics & Gynecology, 58(3), 331-335.

335. Sipes, S. Z., & Weiner, C. P. (April 1990). Venous thromboembolic disease in pregnancy. Seminars in Perinatology, 14(2), 103-118.

336. Maguire, D. J., Cannell, G. R., & Addison, R. S. (1994). Oxygen supply and placental oxygen metabolism. In P. Vaupel, R. Zander, & D. F. Brul (Eds.), Oxygen transport to tissue XV (pp. 709-715). New York, NY: Plenum Press.

337. Ramamoorthy, J. D., Ramamoorthy, S., Leibach, F. H., & Ganapathy, V. (December 1995). Human placental monoamine transporters as targets for amphetamines. American Journal of Obstetrics and Gynecology, 173(6), 1782-1787.

338. Stek, A. M., Baker, S., Fisher, B. K., Lang, U., & Clark, K. E. (November 1995). Fetal responses to maternal and fetal methamphetamine administration in sheep. American Journal of Obstetrics and Gynecology, 173(5), 1592-1598.

339. Shields, L. E., & Brace, R. A. (July 1994). Fetal vascular pressure responses to nonlabor uterine contractions: Dependence on amniotic fluid volume in the ovine fetus. American Journal of Obstetrics and Gynecology, 171(1), 84-89.

340. Ramirez, M. M., Andres, R. L., & Parisi, V. (January 1994). The sympathoadrenal response of the ovine fetus to the direct intravascular administration of methamphetamine. American Journal of Obstetrics and Gynecology, 170(1, Pt. 2), 270.

341. Van Hook, I., Easterling, T., Schmucker, B., Braeteng, D., Carlson, K., & DeLateur, B. (January 1993). The hemodynamic effects of isometric exercise during late pregnancy. American Journal of Obstetrics and Gynecology, 168(1, Pt. 2), 330. SPO abstracts #107.

342. Chandler, K. D., & Bell, A. W. (June 1981). Effects of maternal exercise on fetal and maternal respiration and nutrient metabolism in the pregnant ewe. Journal of Developmental Physiology, 3(3), 161-176.

343. Woo, G., Castro, L., Dunkel-Schetter, C., Walla, C., & Hobel, C. (January 1996). Exertion, employment, and relaxation during pregnancy: Associations with birth outcomes. American Journal of Obstetrics and Gynecology, 174(1, Pt. 2), 477. SPO abstracts #613.

344. Veille, J. C., Kitzman, D. R., Tatum, K., Stewart, K., & Milsaps, P. (January 1996). Effects of advancing pregnancy on the umbilical artery (UA) pulsitility index (PI) after strenuous non-weight bearing (bicycle) exercise (bex). American Journal of Obstetrics and Gynecology, 174(1, Pt. 2), 377. SPO abstracts #237.

345. Goodlin, R. C., Dobry, C. A., Anderson, J. C., Woods, R. E., & Quaife, M. (April 15, 1983). Clinical signs of normal plasma volume expansion during pregnancy. American Journal of Obstetrics and Gynecology, 145(8), 1001-1009.

346. Blackwell, S., Tomlinson, M. W., Gonik, B., Mason, B. A., Whitty, J. E., & Cotton, D. B. (January 1996). Maternal mortality at a tertiary center with critical care obstetrics. American Journal of Obstetrics and Gynecology, 174(1, Pt. 2), 388. SPO abstracts #281.

347. Sibai, B. M., & Ramadan, M. K. (June 1993). Acute renal failure in pregnancies complicated by hemolysis, elevated liver enzymes, and low platelets. American Journal of Obstetrics and Gynecology, 168(6, Pt. 1), 1682-1690.

348. Huddleston, J. E., Huggins, W. F., Williams, G. S., & Flowers, Jr., C. E. (September 1993). A prospective comparison of two endogenous creatine clearance testing methods in hospitalized hypertensive gravid women. American Journal of Obstetrics and Gynecology, 169(3), 576-581.

349. Waldron, K. W., & Wood, C. (May 1971). Cesarean section in the lateral position. Obstetrics & Gynecology, 37(5), 706-710.

350. Umstad, M. P., Ross, A., Rushford, D. D., & Permezel, M. (August 1993). Epidural analgesia and fetal heart rate abnormalities. Australian & New Zealand Journal of Obstetrics & Gynaecology, 33(3), 269-272.

351. Morgan, B. (1994). Maternal anesthesia and analgesia in labor. In D. K. James, P. J. Steer, C. P. Weiner, & B. Gonik (Eds.), High risk obstetrics: Management options (pp. 1101-1108). Philadelphia, PA: W. B. Saunders Company.

352. Roberts, S. W., Leveno, K. J., Sidawi, J. E., Lucas, M. J., & Kelly, M. A. (January 1995). Fetal acidemia associated with regional anesthesia for elective cesarean delivery. Obstetrics & Gynecology, 85(1), 79-83.

353. Lumley, J., & Wood, C. (1974). Effect of changes in maternal oxygen and carbon dioxide tensions on the fetus [Review]. Clinical Anesthesia, 10(2), 121-137.

354. de Haan, H. H., Ijzermans, A. C. M., de Haan, J., & Hasaart, T. H. M. (January 1995). The T/QRS ratio of the electrocardiogram does not reliably reflect well-being in fetal lambs. American Journal of Obstetrics and Gynecology, 172(1, Pt. 1), 35-43.

355. Lee, W., & Cotton, D. B. (1987). Cardiorespiratory changes during pregnancy. In S. L. Clark, J. P. Phelan, & D. B. Cotton (Eds.), Critical care obstetrics (pp. 39-53). Oradell, NJ: Medical Economics Books.

356. Bader, A. M., Datta, S., Arthur, G. R., Benvenuti, E., Courtney, M., & Hauch, M. (April 1990). Maternal and fetal catecholamines and uterine incision-to-delivery interval during elective cesarean. Obstetrics & Gynecology, 75(4), 600-606.

357. Ware Branch, D. (1994). Autoimmune disease. In D. K. James, P. J. Steer, C. P. Weiner, & B. Gonik, (Eds.), High risk pregnancy management options (pp. 433-447). Philadelphia, PA: W. B. Saunders Company.

358. Martin, C. B., & Gingerich, B. (September/October 1976). Factors affecting the fetal heart rate: Genesis of FHR patterns. JOGNN(Suppl.), 30s-40s.

359. Burke, M. E. (October 1989). Hypertensive crisis and the perinatal period. Journal of Perinatal and Neonatal Nursing, 3(2), 33-47.

360. Pedron, S. L. (February 1994). Changes in total uterine blood flow do not always reflect changes in maternal placental blood flow [Letters]. American Journal of Obstetrics and Gynecology, 170(2), 701-702.

361. Dattel, B. J. (April 1990). Substance abuse in pregnancy. Seminars in Perinatology, 14(2), 179-187.

362. One out of 100 americans called cocaine addict. (October 1990). Albuquerque Journal.

363. Gemma, Jr., P. B. (October 23, 1990). Threat of jail can cure junkie moms [An Opposing View]. Albuquerque Journal.

364. Birchfield, M., Scully, J., & Handler, A. (1995). Perinatal screening for illicit drugs: Policies in hospitals in a large metropolitan area. Journal of Perinatology, 15, 208-214 in Capsules & Comments in Perinatal and Women's Health Nursing, 1(4), 313-314.

365. Matti, L. K., & Caspersen, V. M. (November/December 1993). Prevalence of drug use among pregnant women in a rural area [JOGNN Clinical Studies]. JOGNN, 22(6), 510-514.

366. Burkett, G., Yasin, S. Y., Palow, D., LaVoie, L., & Martinez, M. (August 1994). Patterns of cocaine binging: Effect on pregnancy. American Journal of Obstetrics and Gynecology, 171(2), 372-379.

367. Kain, Z. N., Mayes, L. C., Pakes, J., Rosenbaum, S. H., & Schottenfeld, R. (September 1995). Thrombocytopenia in pregnant women who use cocaine. American Journal of Obstetrics and Gynecology, 173(3, Pt. 1), 885-890.

368. Watts, D. H., Krohn, M. A., Farrow, J., Martens, S., Frest, M., & Stark, K. (January 1993). Pregnancy outcomes and duration of chemical dependency treatment. American Journal of Obstetrics and Gynecology, 168(1, Pt. 2), 405. SPO abstracts #389.

369. Andres, R. L., & Wilson, P. D. (January 1995). Associated risk factors for poor obstetrical outcome in the drug using population. American Journal of Obstetrics and Gynecology, 172(1, Pt. 2), 300. SPO abstracts #137.

370. Silverman, N., Rohner, D., Markson, L., & Turner, B. (January 1996). Attitudes toward health care and human immunodeficiency virus infection among pregnant inner-city women. American Journal of Obstetrics and Gynecology, 174(1, Pt. 2), 411. SPO abstracts #365.

371. U. S.: Heroin, marijuana use is rising. Cocaine holds steady, spot checks indicate. (May 12, 1994). Chicago Tribune, 16(Section 1).

372. Williams, D. (1990). Management of cocaine patient. Perinatal Nurses Council Newsletter, Albuquerque, New Mexico.

373. Benjamin, F., Guillaume, A. J., Chao, L. P., & Jean, G. A. (November 1994). Vaginal smuggling of illicit drug: A case requiring obstetric forceps for removal of the drug container. American Journal of Obstetrics and Gynecology, 171(5), 1385-1387.

374. Monga, M., Wong, S., Larrabee, K. D., & Andres, R. L. (January 1996). Correlation of urine and serum benzoylecgonine levels in pregnant women. American Journal of Obstetrics and Gynecology, 174(1, Pt. 2), 432. SPO abstracts #441.

375. Woods, Jr., J. R., Scott, K. J., & Plessinger, M. A. (April 1994). Pregnancy enhances cocaine's actions on the heart and within the peripheral circulation. American Journal of Obstetrics and Gynecology, 170(4), 1027-1035.

376. Mahone, P. R., Scott, K., Sleggs, G., D'Antoni, T., & Woods, Jr., J. R. (August 1994). Cocaine and metabolites in amniotic fluid may prolong fetal drug exposure. American Journal of Obstetrics and Gynecology, 171(2), 465-469.

377. Chan, K., Dodd, P. A., Day, L., Kullama, L., Gore Ervin, M., & Padbury, J. (December 1992). Fetal catecholamine, cardiovascular, and neurobehavioral responses to cocaine. American Journal of Obstetrics and Gynecology, 167(6), 1616-1623.

378. Mishra, A., Landzberg, B. R., & Parente, J. T. (July 1995). Uterine rupture in association with alkaloidal ("crack") cocaine abuse. American Journal of Obstetrics and Gynecology, 173(1), 243-244.

379. Whiteman, V. E., Stanell, W., & Reece, E. A. (January 1996). Prospective evaluation of the effect of maternal cocaine use on fetal cerebral blood flow. American Journal of Obstetrics and Gynecology, 174(1, Pt. 2), 460. SPO abstracts #556.

380. Sprauve, M., Lindsay, M., Herbert, S., & Graves, W. (January 1995). Adverse perinatal outcome in crack-cocaine using parturients. American Journal of Obstetrics and Gynecology, 174(1, Pt. 2), 337. SPO abstracts #277.

381. Hume, R. F., Martin, L. S., Hassan, S. S., Collins, K. B., Tomlinson, M., & Bottoms, S. F. (January 1995). Vascular disruption birth defects and history of prenatal cocaine exposure: A case control study. American Journal of Obstetrics and Gynecology, 172(1, Pt. 2), 396. SPO abstracts #500.

382. Cardonick, E., Comfort, M., Kaltenbach, K., & Silverman, N. (January 1996). Pregnancy complication rates in an inner-city prenatal drug treatment program. American Journal of Obstetrics and Gynecology, 174(1, Pt. 2), 389. SPO abstracts #285.

383. Dinsmoor, M. J., Irons, S. J., & Christmas, J. T. (August 1994). Preterm rupture of the membranes associated with recent cocaine use. American Journal of Obstetrics and Gynecology, 171(2), 305-309.

384. Christmas, J. T., McGhee, P. H., Dinsmoor, M. J., Irons, S. J., Dawson, K. S., & Kish, C. W. (January 1993). Preterm labor: The effect of recent substance use on the occurrence of preterm delivery. American Journal of Obstetrics and Gynecology, 168(1, Pt. 2), 371. SPO abstracts #262.

385. Monga, M., Weisbrodt, N. W., Andres, R. L., & Sanborn, B. M. (December 1993). Cocaine acutely increases rat myometrial contractile activity by mechanisms other than potentiation of adrenergic pathways. American Journal of Obstetrics and Gynecology, 169(6), 1502-1506.

386. Collins, B. A., McCoy, S. A., Sale, S., & Weber, S. E. (May 1994). Descriptions of comfort by substance-using and nonusing postpartum women [JOGNN Clinical Studies]. JOGNN, 23(4), 293-300.

387. Khandelwal, M., Wu, Y. K., Bronstein, M., & Reece, E. A. (January 1995). Dietary phospholipid therapy, hyperglycemia-induced membrane changes and associated diabetic embryopathy. American Journal of Obstetrics and Gynecology, 172(1, Pt. 2), 265. SPO abstracts #32.

388. Kramer, R., Gilson, G., Izquierdo, L., & Curet, L. (January 1995). Not so intensive treatment of insulin-requiring diabetes in pregnancy. American Journal of Obstetrics and Gynecology, 172(1, Pt. 2), 330. SPO abstracts #250.

389. Teramo, K., Ammala, P., Ylinen, K., & Raivio, K. O. (May 1983). Pathologic fetal heart rate associated with poor metabolic control in diabetic pregnancies. Obstetrics & Gynecology, 61(5), 559-565.

390. Hsu, C. D., Tan, H. Y., Hong, S. F., & Copel, J. A. (January 1995). The role of glycosylated hemoglobin (HbA_1C) in the pathogenesis of insulin-dependent diabetes mellitus (IDDM) pregnancies complicated with preeclampsia. American Journal of Obstetrics and Gynecology, 172(1, Pt. 2), 380. SPO abstracts #434.

391. Magriples, U., Hsu, C. D., Copel, J. A., Nickless, N., & Chan, D. W. (January 1995). Circulating interleukin-1 as a clinical marker in pregnant diabetics. American Journal of Obstetrics and Gynecology, 172(1, Pt. 2), 331. SPO abstracts #253.

392. Mentakis, A., Kuboshige, J., Brinkman, III, C. R., & Cabalum, M. T. (January 1996). Glycemic control in pregestational diabetics influences the incidence of preeclampsia. American Journal of Obstetrics and Gynecology, 174(1, Pt. 2), 396. SPO abstracts #314.

393. Silverman, R., & Artal, R. (January 1996). 3-year experience with insulin pump therapy during pregnancy. American Journal of Obstetrics and Gynecology, 174(1, Pt. 2), 396. SPO abstracts #315.

394. Major, C. A., Cohen, B. F., & Reimbold, T. (January 1996). Patients with elevated glucose screening tests are at higher risk for cesarean section, macrosomia and birth trauma despite a normal 3 hour glucose tolerance test. American Journal of Obstetrics and Gynecology, 174(1, Pt. 2), 394. SPO abstracts #307.

395. Svendsen, T., Abuhamad, A., de Veciana, M., Morgan, J., & Evans, A. T. (January 1996). How predictive is the degree of abnormality of the glucola test for gestational diabetes? American Journal of Obstetrics and Gynecology, 174(1, Pt. 2), 395. SPO abstracts #310.

396. Gandhi, J., Zhang, X., & Maidman, J. (January 1996). Cardiac and somatic growth in infants of insulin controlled diabetics. American Journal of Obstetrics and Gynecology, 174(1, Pt. 2), 420. SPO abstracts #403.

397. Harris, J. L., Brown, P., Bazargan, M., & Kendricks, B. (January 1995). The prevalence of gestational diabetes in gravidas with screening glucose value >200 mg/dl. American Journal of Obstetrics and Gynecology, 172(1, Pt. 2), 330. SPO abstracts #249.

ANTEPARTAL AND INTRAPARTAL FETAL MONITORING

398. Star, J., Rosene, K., Carpenter, M. W., Ferland, J., Ray, V., & DiLeone, G. (January 1996). Platelet activation in diabetic pregnancy. <u>American Journal of Obstetrics and Gynecology, 174</u>(1, Pt. 2), 394. SPO abstracts #306.

399. Hod, M., Langer, O., McFarland, M., Xenakis, E. M-J., & Elliott, B. (January 1995). The effect of diabetes on cord blood gas at term. <u>American Journal of Obstetrics and Gynecology, 172</u>(1, Pt. 2), 330. SPO abstracts #252.

400. Rosenn, B., Miodovnik, M., Holan, J., Khoury, J., & Siddiqui, T. (January 1995). Delivery in mothers with type I diabetes: Changing trends over fifteen years. <u>American Journal of Obstetrics and Gynecology, 172</u>(1, Pt. 2), 333. SPO abstracts #264.

401. Berkus, M., McFarland, M., & Langer, O. (January 1995). Improved insulin secretion after diet therapy in GDM. <u>American Journal of Obstetrics and Gynecology, 172</u>(1, Pt. 2), 332. SPO abstracts #258.

402. Gollin, Y., Marks, C., Marks, W., & Copel, J. (January 1995). The effect of maternal diabetes on the fetal exocrine pancreas. <u>American Journal of Obstetrics and Gynecology, 172</u>(1, Pt. 2), 325. SPO abstracts #231.

403. Gordon, M., Landon, M. B., Samuels, P., Hissrich, S., Boyle, J., & Gabbe, S. G. (January 1995). Perinatal outcome and long-term follow-up associated with modern management of diabetic (DM) nephropathy (class F). <u>American Journal of Obstetrics and Gynecology, 172</u>(1, Pt. 2), 329. SPO abstracts #247.

404. Hod, M., van Dyk, D. J., Karp, M., Kalter, O., Bar, J., & Peled, Y. (January 1995). Ace-1 treatment of IDDM nephrotic patients prior to pregnancy: Maternal-fetal outcome. <u>American Journal of Obstetrics and Gynecology, 172</u>(1, Pt. 2), 330. SPO abstracts #251.

405. Sivan, E., Homko, C., & Reece, E. A. (January 1996). Outcomes in pregnancies complicated by diabetes (class B to FR) versus non-diabetic controls. <u>American Journal of Obstetrics and Gynecology, 174</u>(1, Pt. 2), 393. SPO abstracts # 302.

406. Rosenn, B. M., Miodovnik, M., Khoury, J. C., & Siddiqi, T. A. (January 1996). Pregnancy outcome in women with type II diabetes mellitus. <u>American Journal of Obstetrics and Gynecology, 174</u>(1, Pt. 2), 394. SPO abstracts #305.

407. Piper, J., & Langer, O. (January 1996). Delayed pulmonary maturation is associated with poor glucose control in diabetic pregnancies. <u>American Journal of Obstetrics and Gynecology, 174</u>(1, Pt. 2), 396. SPO abstracts #313.

408. Edelstone, D. I., Paulone, M. E., Maljovec, J. J., & Hagberg, M. (March 1987). Effects of maternal anemia on cardiac output, systemic oxygen consumption, and regional blood flow in pregnant sheep. <u>American Journal of Obstetrics and Gynecology, 156</u>(3), 740-748.

409. Perry, Jr., K. G., & Morrison, J. C. (April 1990). The diagnosis and management of hemoglobinopathies during pregnancy. <u>Seminars in Perinatology, 14</u>(2), 90-102.

410. Pastorek, II, J. G., & Seiler, B. (February 1, 1985). Maternal death associated with sickle cell trait. <u>American Journal of Obstetrics and Gynecology, 151</u>(3), 295-297.

411. Richardson, E. A.W., & Milne, L. S. (November/December 1983). Sickle-cell disease and the childbearing family: An update. <u>MCN, 8,</u> 417-422.

412. Fuentes, A., Kalter, C., & Chez, R. A. (January 1995). The relationship of maternal fetal hemoglobin level to perinatal outcome in pregnancies with sickle cell disease. <u>American Journal of Obstetrics and Gynecology, 172</u>(1, Pt. 2), 336. SPO abstracts #275.

413. Gimovsky, M. L. (1990). Perinatal/Neonatal casebooks: Fetal heart rate monitoring casebook. <u>Journal of Perinatology, 10</u>(2), 198-201.

414. Ship-Horowitz, T. (November/December 1983). Nursing care of the sickle cell anemic patient in labor [Principles and Practice]. <u>JOGNN,</u> 381-386.

415. Anyaegbunam, A., & Mikhail, M. S. (January 1994). Uterine artery velocity waveforms during postpartum in women with sickle cell disease. <u>American Journal of Obstetrics and Gynecology, 170</u>(1, Pt. 2). SPO abstracts #460.

416. Anyaegbunam, A., Mikhail, M. S., Jadali, D., & Billett, H. (January 1996). The lack of association between selected hematologic paramaters and frequency of painful sickle cell crisis during pregnancy. <u>American Journal of Obstetrics and Gynecology, 174</u>(1, Pt. 2), 390. SPO abstracts #292.

417. Kresevic, D., & Whitman, S. (July 1990). Sickle cell anemia. Managing the pain. <u>Nursing 90,</u> 71.

418. Devedeux, D., Marque, C., Mansour, S., Germain, G., & Duchene, J. (December 1993). Uterine electromyography: A critical review. <u>American Journal of Obstetrics and Gynecology, 169</u>(6), 1636-1653.

419. Eskes, T. K. A. B. (February 1993). Uterine contractions and their possible influence on fetal oxygenation. <u>Gynakologe, 26</u>(1), 39-45.

420. Oosterhof, H., Dijkstra, K., & Aarnoudse, J. G. (August 1992). Fetal doppler velocimetry in the internal carotid and umbilical artery during Braxton Hicks contractions. <u>Early Human Development, 30</u>(1), 33-40.

421. Friedman, E.A. (1983). Physiology of labor. In W. R. Cohen & E. A. Friedman (Eds.). <u>Mangernent of labor</u> (pp. 1-9). Baltimore, MD: University Park Press.

422. Bleker, O. P., Kloosterman, G. J., Mieras, D. J., Oosting, J., & Salle, H. J. A. (December 1, 1975). Intervillous space during uterine contractions in human subjects: An ultrasonic study. <u>American Journal of Obstetrics and Gynecology, 123</u>(7), 697-699.

423. Newnham, J. P., Marshall, C. L., Padbury, J. F., Lam, R. W., Hobel, C. J., & Fisher, D. A. (August 15, 1984). Fetal catecholamine release with preterm delivery. <u>American Journal of Obstetrics and Gynecology, 149</u>(8), 888-893.

424. Peebles, D. M., Edwards, A. D., Wyatt, J. S., Bishop, A. P., Cope, M., & Delpy, D. T. (May 1992). Changes in human fetal cerebral hemoglobin concentration and oxygenation during labor measured by near-infrared spectroscopy. <u>American Journal of Obstetrics and Gynecology, 166</u>(5), 1369-1373.

425. Wallerstedt, C., Higgins, P., Kasnic, T., & Curet, L. B. (September 1994). Amnioinfusion: An update [Principles and Practice]. JOGNN, 23, 573-378.

426. Myers, R. E. (May 1, 1975). Maternal psychological stress and fetal asphyxia: A study in the monkey. American Journal of Obstetrics and Gynecology, 122(1), 47-59.

427. Lederman, R. P., Lederman, E., Work, Jr., B. A., & McCann, D. S. (November 1, 1978). The relationship of maternal anxiety, plasma catecholamines, and plasma cortisol to progress in labor. American Journal of Obstetrics and Gynecology, 132(5), 495-500.

428. Simkin, P. (December 1986). Stress, pain, and catecholamines in labor: Part 1. A review. Birth, 13(4), 227-232.

429. Deckardt, R., Fembacher, P. M., Schneider, K. T. M., & Graeff, H. (July 1987). Maternal arterial oxygen saturation during labor and delivery: Pain-dependent alterations and effects on the newborn. Obstetrics & Gynecology, 70(1), 21-25.

430. Arnold-Aldea, S. A., & Parer, J. (1990). Fetal cardiovascular physiology. In R. D. Eden & F. H. Boehm (Eds.), Assessment and care of the fetus: Physiological, clinical and medicolegal principles (pp. 29-41). Norwalk, CT: Appleton & Lange.

431. Groome, L. J., Swiber, M. J., Bentz, L. S., Holland, S. B., & Atterbury, J. L. (January 1995). The relationship between maternal trait anxiety and fetal behavior. American Journal of Obstetrics and Gynecology, 172(1, Pt. 2), 318. SPO abstracts #201.

432. Freeman, R. K., & Garite, T. J. (1981). Fetal heart rate monitoring. Baltimore: Williams and Wilkins.

433. Lagercrantz, H., & Bistoletti, P. (August 1977). Catecholamine release in the newborn infant at birth. Pediatric Resuscitation, 11(8), 889-893.

434. Myers, R. E., & Myers, S. E. (January 1, 1979). Use of sedative, analgesic, and anesthetic drugs during labor and delivery: Bane or boon? American Journal of Obstetrics and Gynecology, 133(1), 83-104.

435. Fishburne, J. I. (February 1982). Systemic analgesia during labor. Clinics in Perinatology, 9(1), 29-49.

436. Albright, G. A., Joyce, T. H., & Stevenson, D. K. (1986). Systemic medication. In G. A. Albright, J. E. Ferguson, T. H. Joyce, & D. K. Stevenson (Eds.), Anesthesia in obstetrics (pp. 167-176). Boston, MA: Butterworths.

437. Willcourt, R. J., King, J. C., & Queenan, J. T. (July 15, 1983). Maternal oxygenation administration and the fetal transcutaneous PO_2. American Journal of Obstetrics and Gynecology, 146(6), 714-715.

438. Baxi, L. V. (June 1982). Effect of maternal administration of oxygen on fetal oxygenation. Clinics in Perinatology, 9(2), 426-231.

439. Esplin, M. S., Jackson, G. M., Clark, M. H., Varner, M. W., & Scott, J. R. (January 1995). Uterine rupture in modern obstetrics. American Journal of Obstetrics and Gynecology, 172(1, Pt. 2), 295. SPO abstracts #119.

440. Miller, D. A., McClain, C. J., & Paul, R. H. (January 1995). Trial of labor in a selected, low-risk population: A hospital-based birthing center staffed by certified nurse-midwives. American Journal of Obstetrics and Gynecology, 172(1, Pt. 2), 297. SPO abstracts #126.

441. Benito, C. W., Smullian, J. C., Gray, S. E., & Scorza, W. E. (January 1996). A case control study of uterine rupture during pregnancy. American Journal of Obstetrics and Gynecology, 174(1, Pt. 2), 485. SPO abstracts #647.

442. Moskovitz, H., O'Grady, J. P., & Gimovsky, M. (March/April 1994). Fetal heart rate monitoring casebook. Denouement and discussion. Uterine rupture and sinusoidal heart rate. Journal of Perinatology, 14(2), 154-158.

443. Connolly, A. M., & Katz, V. L. (January 1995). Trauma in pregnancy. American Journal of Obstetrics and Gynecology, 172(1, Pt. 2), 328. SPO abstracts #241.

444. Naef, III, R. W., Ray, M. A., Chauhan, S. P., Roach, H., Blake, P. G., & Martin, Jr., J. N. (June 1995). Trial of labor after cesarean delivery with a lower-segment, vertical uterine incision: Is it safe? American Journal of Obstetrics and Gynecology, 172(6), 1666-1674.

445. Stone, J., Lockwood, C. J., Berkowitz, G. S., Lynch, L., Alvarez, M., & Lapinski, R. H. (December 1992). Morbidity of failed labor in patients with prior cesarean section. American Journal of Obstetrics and Gynecology, 167(6), 1513-1517.

446. Phelan, J. P., Ahn, M. O., Diaz, F., Brar, H. S., & Rodriguez, M. H. (February 1989). Twice a cesarean, always a cesarean? Obstetrics & Gynecology, 73(2), 161-165.

447. Kornfeld, I., Amankwha, K., & Kung, R. (January 1996). Trial of labor after multiple cesarean birth-a meta-analysis. American Journal of Obstetrics and Gynecology, 174(1, Pt. 2), 357. SPO abstracts #166.

448. Zuidema, L., Elderkin, R., Cook, C., & Jelsema, R. (January 1996). Is vicryl suture closure of uterine wounds associated with more dehiscence? American Journal of Obstetrics and Gynecology, 174(1, Pt. 2), 357. SPO abstracts #167.

449. Pruett, K. M., Kirshon, B., & Cotton, D. B. (October 1988). Unknown uterine scar and trial of labor. American Journal of Obstetrics and Gynecology, 159(4), 807-810.

450. Yaron, Y., Shenhav, M., Jaffa, A. J., Lessing, J. B., & Peyser, M. R. (1994). Uterine rupture at 33 weeks' gestation subsequent to hysteroscopic uterine perforation. American Journal of Obstetrics and Gynecology, 170(3), 786-787.

451. Azem, F., Jaffa, A., Lessing, J. B., & Peyser, M. R. (May 1993). Uterine rupture with the use of a low-dose vaginal PGE_2 tablet. Acta Obstetricia et Gynecologica Scandinavica, 72(4), 316-317.

452. Maymon, R., Haimovich, L., Shulman, A., Pomeranz, M., Holtzinger, M., & Bahary, C. (May 1992). Third-trimester uterine rupture after prostaglandin E_2 use for labor induction. Journal of Reproductive Medicine, 37(5), 449-452.

453. Maymon, R., Shulman, A., Pomeranz, M., Holtzinger, M., Haimovich, L., & Bahary, C. (August 1991). Uterine rupture at term pregnancy with the use of intracervical prostaglandin E_2 gel for induction of labor. <u>American Journal of Obstetrics and Gynecology, 165</u>(2), 368-370.

454. Sweeten, K. M., Graves, W. K., & Athanassiou, A. (1996). Spontaneous rupture of the unscarred uterus. <u>American Journal of Obstetrics and Gynecology, 172,</u> 1851-1856 in <u>Capsules & Comments in Perinatal and Women's Health Nursing, 2</u>(1), 64-65.

455. Fawcett, J., Tulman, L., & Spedden, J. P. (March/April 1994). Responses to vaginal birth after cesarean section [Clinical Studies]. <u>JOGNN, 23</u>(3), 253-259.

456. Jackson, G. M., Clark, M. H., Esplin, M. S., Varner, M. W., & Scott, J. R. (January 1995). Attempted vaginal birth after cesarean section: Predictors of failure. <u>American Journal of Obstetrics and Gynecology, 172</u>(1, Pt. 2), 297. SPO abstracts #127.

457. Clark, S. L. (December 1988). Rupture of the scarred uterus. <u>Obstetrics and Gynecology of North America, 15</u>(4), 737-744.

458. Leung, A. S., Leung, E. K., & Paul, R. H. (October 1993). Uterine rupture after previous cesarean delivery: Maternal and fetal consequences. <u>American Journal of Obstetrics and Gynecology, 169</u>(4), 945-950.

459. Benito, C. W., Smullian, J. C., Gray, S. E., & Scorza, W. E. (January 1996). A case control study of uterine rupture during pregnancy. <u>American Journal of Obstetrics and Gynecology, 174</u>(1, Pt. 2), 485. SPO abstracts #647.

460. <u>Baptist Medical Center Montclair v. Myra Wilson, et al.</u> (S. C. AL. March 26, 1993).

461. Lao, T. T., & Leung, B. F. (July 1987). Rupture of the gravid uterus. <u>European Journal of Obstetrics, Gynecology, & Reproductive Biology, 25</u>(3), 175-180.

Notes

6

Prediction and Prevention of Intrapartal Fetal Asphyxia

INTRODUCTION

"The object of intrapartum fetal monitoring is to protect the fetus from the damaging effects of hypoxia." (1, p. 1118)

The fetus may be monitored by electronic or auscultatory devices (2). Electronic fetal monitoring (EFM) is cardiotocography. Cardio refers to a heart rate, toco is derived from the Greek word for birth and refers to uterine activity. EFM flourished in the United States of America and the United Kingdom in the late 1970s and 1980s (3-6). Today, EFM is performed in physician offices, clinics, hospitals, and homes. EFM, rather than intermittent auscultation, has been the primary fetal surveillance tool for labor lasting more than five hours, labor that was augmented or induced, when there was a multiple gestation or thick meconium in the amniotic fluid, intrauterine growth restriction (IUGR), preterm labor, or when decelerations were heard by auscultation (7-8). This chapter presents the purpose of EFM, benefits and limitations of EFM and auscultation, and fetal monitoring practice implications.

PURPOSE

The purpose of EFM is to evaluate the fetal heart rate (FHR) response with and without uterine activity (UA) (9-10). FHR and UA information is interpreted so that interventions to prevent fetal or maternal injury or death may be performed in a timely manner (11-14). EFM is a screening tool used to detect hypoxia or acidemia related to fetal brain injury of an already compromised fetus or a fetus who is dying (15-17). EFM has limitations (18). EFM use may not guarantee a perfect outcome nor prevent neonatal seizures or cerebral palsy (CP) not related to care (19). However, EFM use should reduce the number of stillbirths and the number of neonates who have seizures (20). EFM data can be used to predict fetal asphyxia or a risk of death in preterm fetuses (21). EFM can provide an accurate and continuous measurement of fetal well-being when frequent auscultation is not possible (22).

ELECTRONIC FETAL MONITOR-HUMAN INTERACTION

The electronic fetal monitor's paper printout is called a strip, tracing, or cardiotocogram. Interpretation differences occur, possibly because FHR patterns may be too complex to interpret visually in a consistent and accurate way. To limit interpretation error, computer analysis of the FHR pattern has been advocated (11). Despite the risk of misinterpretation, the most common practice is to have human beings interpret the data produced by the electronic fetal monitor.

In order to prevent bad outcomes, proper surveillance is required. Proper surveillance is dependent on adequate staffing and education (23). If the data produced by EFM is not seen or correctly interpreted in a timely manner, injury can occur. The potential for errors increases with inadequate staffing, increased patient loads, and overtime shifts (24). The lack of nursing staff or the lack of education in EFM may create obstacles to implement desirable care (25). The result may be suboptimal care and injury or death.

Suboptimal care preceded neonatal seizures, the development of CP, and even fetal and maternal death. Suboptimal care was an inappropriate response to social, medical or fetal risk factors such as the omission of an ultrasound or antepartal testing. The lack of continuous intrapartal EFM and an inappropriate or inadequate response to signs of distress with an additional test such as fetal scalp pH sampling was suboptimal care (26).

Neonates who had seizures within 48 hours after birth were more likely than not to have received suboptimal care. The care of 54 term neonates who were born in Cardiff, England between 1976 and 1979 and who had seizures was compared with 41,090 who did not have seizures. Researchers found that the seizures would have been avoidable had action been taken earlier in response to bradycardia, severe variable decelerations, and/or late decelerations (27).

FHR PATTERNS AND ACID-BASE BALANCE

Electronic fetal monitors detect FHR changes due to hypoxemia and hypoxia (14, 31-33). Fetal hypoxia results from lack of oxygen delivery to the uterus and/or placenta or through the umbilical cord. Asphyxia can develop if hypoxia persists and a normal acid-base balance cannot be reestablished. Late decelerations, variable decelerations, and prolonged decelerations with decreased or absent baseline variability have been associated with asphyxia or previous brain damage (34-35). Asphyxia is diagnosed when there is an abnormally low PO_2, high PCO_2 and low pH (33, 36). ACOG, the American College of Obstetricians and Gynecologists, equated asphyxia with hypoxia with metabolic acidosis (37). Asphyxia can cause cerebral palsy (38-39).

In most cases, the FHR reflects a nonhypoxic fetus but changes in the FHR pattern influence clinical management decisions (40). In order to evaluate the fetus during the antepartal period, antepartal testing has begun between 20 and 26 weeks of gestation (41-42). Analysis of the FHR pattern suggests the presence of hypoxia, acidosis, or asphyxia (43-46). Asphyxia should be absent when there is a "normal" FHR pattern, stable baseline FHR in a normal range, baseline long-term variability, and no late decelerations or "significant" decelerations (43). Fetal hypoxia will be suspected when the FHR baseline rises to 180 or more bpm, has decreased variability, few to no accelerations, and late decelerations (46).

For ethical reasons, no human fetal research has defined the degree and duration of hypoxia that precedes nerve cell injury (31, 47). EFM data has a very limited ability to predict permanent neurologic injury because neonatal information during the first days of life is needed to predict long-term outcome (48). Our understanding of the duration of oxygen deprivation needed to cause permanent injury comes from prospective animal research or retrospective human studies. In humans, it is believed that if hypoxemia is suspected, actions to improve fetal oxygenation should prevent metabolic acidosis, asphyxia, and/or brain damage (47, 49-50).

SPECIFICITY AND SENSITIVITY

Research has consistently shown that EFM detects the absence of fetal hypoxia better than it detects signs of hypoxemia, acidosis, and asphyxia (40, 51-52). In other words, the specificity of EFM to predict a good outcome or the absence of disease (number of normal outcomes divided by number with false abnormal outcomes plus normal outcomes) is higher than its sensitivity to predict a bad outcome or the presence of disease (number of abnormal outcomes divided by abnormal outcomes plus false normal outcomes) (53).

An example of specificity is the ability of a normal pattern to predict a normal outcome. For example, a "normal" FHR pattern in preterm fetuses who weighed less than 1750 grams was related to a normal neurologic status at one year of age (54). The problem with the sensitivity of EFM to predict a bad outcome is that a FHR pattern may have more than one meaning. For example, a FHR pattern of a stable tachycardic or bradycardic baseline with present short-term variability and no decelerations was associated with a normal fetal scalp pH 90 to 95% of the time (14, 52, 55).

In spite of the imperfect sensitivity of EFM, abnormal FHR patterns can reflect developing metabolic acidosis and precede neonatal neurologic depression, an abnormal neurologic examination or abnormal neurologic development at one year of age (37, 47). Therefore, any abnormal FHR pattern requires action to prevent potential injury.

Abnormal deceleration patterns preceded an abnormal neonatal neurological evaluation in as many as 41% of term appropriate for gestational age babies (TAGA) babies. If there is a pattern of late decelerations for 130 minutes, there will be an increased risk for hearing loss at one year of age (47). TAGA with an increased risk of metabolic acidosis had an abnormal FHR pattern of
- late decelerations or
- moderate variable decelerations (30 to 60 seconds, nadir below 80 bpm) and
- **severe variable decelerations (60 or more seconds, nadir below 70 bpm) and**
- a loss of variability and
- no reactive accelerations (peaking 15 bpm above the baseline and lasting 15 seconds at their base) or
- a flat tracing.

Metabolic acidosis develops sooner in fetuses that have late decelerations than in those with variable decelerations (56-57). Hypoxemia in fetuses 28 to 36 weeks of gestation was related to a computer determined FHR decrease in short- and long-term variation (58).

DURATION AND SEVERITY OF OXYGEN DEPRIVATION

Late decelerations which persisted for 15 minutes did not cause long-term neurologic injury based on examinations completed at six to nine years of age (12). When the abnormal FHR pattern lasted 2 or more hours, 78% of term neonates were acidotic (56). There was a 20% incidence of CP in preterm infants who weighed less than 1750 gms with an average abnormal FHR pattern lasting 104 minutes prior to delivery. In a similar preterm infant group who were auscultated, only 8% developed CP but the average duration from recognition of an abnormality to delivery was much shorter, only 60 minutes (19, 54).

FETAL DISTRESS

Fetal distress have been part of obstetric jargon for many years (59). The ACOG Committee on Obstetric Practice was concerned that "fetal distress" was imprecise, limited, non-specific, and implied an ill fetus (39). In spite of their concern and their desire to change the language to "nonreassuring fetal status" the words "fetal distress" remained on the list in 2003 as an International Classification of Diseases (ICD) code (656.3 fetal distress affecting management of mother).

What is fetal distress? Is it equivalent to a nonreassuring fetal status? In 1997, Goodlin and Haesslein (60) proposed that fetal distress reflected acid-base abnormalities or cardiovascular dysfunction. To others, fetal distress was synonymous with a FHR pattern suggestive of fetal compromise and/or developing metabolic acidosis (61). Drs. Parer and Livingston suggested fetal distress was "progressive fetal asphyxia that, if not corrected or circumvented, will result in decompensation of the physiologic responses (primarily redistribution of blood flow to preserve oxygenation of vital organs) and cause permanent central nervous system and other damage or death" (62, p. 1424). Drs. Rosen and Dickinson equated fetal distress with a fetal risk for significant fetal asphyxia (63).

Patterns have been equated with fetal distress, such as persistent late decelerations, severe variable decelerations, or prolonged bradycardia (38). Fetal distress reflects certain FHR patterns obtained by EFM since auscultatory criteria for fetal distress do not exist (64). Therefore, auscultation should not be used to diagnose fetal distress (65). Even though some believe audible FHR changes might suggest variable and late decelerations, auscultation cannot be used to diagnose fetal distress (66).

When a FHR pattern suggests fetal distress, additional information should be acquired to confirm fetal acid-base status and avoid unnecessary surgery (14, 61, 67-68). The number of cesarean sections for a nonreassuring pattern reported in 169 studies published between 1990 and 2000 was 3% but only 10% of the babies had an umbilical artery pH less than 7.00 (69). At nine medical centers in the United States, women at term in active labor with abnormal FHR patterns had significantly more than a 50% reduction in cesarean sections for nonreassuring fetal status when the fetal SpO$_2$ (FSpO$_2$) was continuously recorded (70).

Another technique to rule out metabolic acidosis by evoking FHR accelerations is fetal scalp stimulation which is done between contractions and decelerations (71). To perform scalp stimulation, the cervix must be sufficiently dilated to introduce the gloved fingers and touch the fetal scalp. Skupski, Rosenberg, and Eglinton (72) reviewed articles related to intrapartum stimulation tests published between 1966 to 2000 and performed a meta-analysis on 11 studies that met their criteria. They found that gentle digital scalp stimulation for 15 seconds was the easiest to use routinely because no device was required and the membranes could be intact. If the fetus failed to accelerate at least 10 bpm x 10 seconds which was related to a scalp pH greater than 7.20, a scalp pH was recommended to provide additional information.

THE DEVELOPMENT OF EFM

In 1958, Dr. Edward Hon wrote the first report on EFM. He described a continuous recording of the FHR calculated from a fetal electrocardiogram (ECG) which had been obtained from maternal abdominal leads. In 1967, the first clinically useful fetal monitor was created with a phonotransducer for sound detection of the fetal heartbeat (73). By 1968, the first commercially available fetal monitor was produced (74).

Before EFM was available for use, many physicians believed that preventable intrapartal asphyxia caused CP, a disorder of movement and posture caused by a lesion or injury of the brain (3, 75-77). At that time, intrapartal assessment of the fetal condition was limited to auscultation and a fetal scalp blood pH. In 1969, after EFM was available to hospitals, it was discovered that an abnormal fetal pH was related to late decelerations or severe variable decelerations that occurred during the 20 minutes preceding the pH sample (78).

Naturally, there was enthusiasm among obstetricians in the early 1970s, that EFM would significantly decrease the incidence of CP by its ability to detect signs of hypoxia early and prompt actions to prevent asphyxia. This early optimism prompted hospitals to purchase electronic fetal monitors even though research had not validated their safety nor benefit. However, their enthusiasm was short-lived when, by the end of the decade, the Department of Health, Education, and Welfare concluded, "The effectiveness of electronic fetal monitoring has not been proven scientifically (79)." In spite of this report, the belief persisted that intrapartal hypoxic events accounted for 20 to 40% of children with CP (14). Therefore, EFM continued to be a desired technique to prevent asphyxia.

By 1984, EFM was in widespread use as a screening technique in the United States, in spite of concerns that EFM was overused and was only intended for use with high risk or at-risk pregnant women (46, 80-81). Research findings published in 1977 and 1988 changed the perception regarding CP and intrapartal asphyxia (82-83). Between 1959 and 1966 the National Institute of Neurological and Communicative Disorders and Stroke Collaborative Perinatal Project (NCPP) collected auscultated FHR data and followed children born at 12 urban teaching hospitals in the United States. Of the 40,057 singletons born between 1959 and 1966, 90 children later developed CP. There were distinct differences in intrapartal findings compared with the children who did not develop CP. For example, Nelson and Broman reported that children with CP versus those who did not have CP had:

more meconium (41% vs. 19%)
a lower auscultated FHR during the second stage of labor (95 to 118 bpm vs. 110 to 146 bpm)
more arrested labor (78% vs. 6.6%)
more midforceps deliveries (23% vs. 8%)
more Apgar scores of 3 or less at 1 minute (33% vs. 5%)
more respiratory problems including apnea
more intracranial hemorrhage (6% vs. 0.0029%)
more seizures in the first month of life (30% vs. 0.3%) (82).

The estimates of the number of children who developed CP solely from intrapartal asphyxia has ranged from 3 to 22%

(76, 83-84). In 1991, the exact proportion of neonatal encephalopathy caused by intrapartal asphyxia was unknown (85). However, based on randomized clinical trials it was clear that intrapartal EFM of low risk and high risk women did not reduce the overall incidence of CP (7, 86-95). This is because CP has many causes including antepartal asphyxia (38, 44, 83, 85, 96-97). Therefore, in spite of the use of EFM the overall incidence of CP has not declined which may be partly related to the increased survival of very premature infants (98).

Abnormal FHR patterns preceded neonatal seizures (99). A clear benefit of EFM is the reduction of fetal deaths and neonatal seizures. As many as 55% more neonates had seizures when intermittent auscultation was used during labor rather than EFM with scalp pH sampling (7-8, 76, 87, 94, 100-101). However, there was no difference in the number of infants who developed CP in either the auscultated or EFM group at one year and four years of age (7, 76). In one study, there was no difference in the number of fetal or neonatal deaths when auscultation or EFM were used in low risk women (102).

EFM AND THE CESAREAN SECTION RATE

In 1979, the National Institute of Child Health and Human Development (NICHD) Task Force of the National Institutes of Health believed EFM had a potential to destroy the process of normal childbirth. At that time there was no standard of care requiring EFM use for low risk women. The standard of care for low risk women was to auscultate the FHR every 15 minutes during the first stage of labor and every 5 minutes duringthe second stage of labor for 30 seconds after a contraction (103).

During the 1970s the cesarean section rate was rising which alarmed researchers. For example, between 1970 and 1978, the cesarean section rate in the United States rose from 5.5% to 15.2% (104). At the end of the decade, in 1979, the NICHD Task Force recommended EFM use should not be routine to avoid the significant increase in the number of cesarean sections when the woman was electronically monitored (103, 105). In one report from 1979, the cesarean section rate for fetal distress was near 1% (106). EFM had no impact on the cesarean section rate at one medical center when they compared the three years before they instituted EFM with the two years following EFM use (107). In fact, the medical diagnosis of dystocia was responsible for 29.2% of the increase, repeat cesarean sections for 27% of the increase, and breech presentation for 15.7% of the increase. Overall, the diagnosis of fetal distress was only responsible for 10 to 15% of the increase in the cesarean section rate (104). Between 1976 and 1980, 46.5% of cesareans at one Detroit hospital were for dystocia and only 11.1% were for fetal distress (108). The cesarean rate did not change when the obstetrician was in the hospital versus at home (109).

In September, 1980, the NIH Consensus Development Conference Task Force on Cesarean Childbirth did little to dispel the myth that EFM was responsible for a significant increase in the cesarean section rate when they wrote, "The use of monitoring techniques is associated with an increase in cesarean delivery (110)." However, they did acknowledge the increase was related to dystocia, having had a previous cesarean birth, and breech presentation, more so than "fetal distress."

During the 1980s, the cesarean rate continued to rise from 16.9% in 1980 to 22.7% in 1985 (111). In 1982, it was believed that the incidence of fetal distress during labor was approximately 2% (112). Dystocia and a prior cesarean continued to be the major factors related to the increase in the overall cesarean section rate, even though some studies suggested EFM when used, versus auscultation, increased the number of cesareans because of the "diagnosis" of fetal distress (86, 89, 92). When an additional test of fetal status was used in conjunction with EFM, there was no difference in the number of cesarean sections for low risk or high risk term and preterm laboring women. For example, women who were monitored electronically when scalp pH sampling was available compared with women whose fetus was auscultated had a similar number of cesarean sections (86, 88, 90, 93). Results from research in Dublin, Ireland with over 10,000 women whose fetus was either auscultated or electronically monitored during labor revealed no difference in the cesarean section rate between the two groups (7). It was finally becoming obvious that the type of fetal surveillance tool was not related to the increasing cesarean section rate.

Between 1986 and 1992, the cesarean section rate dropped 5.5% in the United States and the cesarean section rate for fetal distress remained unchanged (near 2%) (113). Cesareans were more often a result of failure to progress than fetal distress (114). EFM and the diagnosis of fetal distress remained minor contributors to the overall cesarean rate (113). Poma suggested that the cesarean section rate was due to individual obstetrician characteristics (115). Lidegaard et al. found that inexperienced physicians would perform more cesarean sections than experienced physicians (116). The management of labor, not the use of EFM, had a significant impact on cesarean reduction. There was a 52% decrease in the cesarean section rate of primigravida women at 34 or more weeks of gestation who were augmented with oxytocin (starting at 2 mU/minute and increasing by 2 mU/minute ever 15 minutes unless there were 7 contractions in 15 minutes). If there was a nonreassuring pattern, a fetal scalp pH was obtained, oxygen was administered and there was a position change prior to surgery (117).

By 1998, the cesarean section rate in the United States had risen to 20.2% (118). The primary reason for a cesarean section was still failure to progress due to cephalopelvic disproportion (119). "Fetal distress" continued to be a minor contributor to the overall cesarean section rate. After reviewing 4,721 cesarean sections done between December 1, 1998 and July 1, 1999, researchers in Norway found 32% were due to a combination of failure to progress and fetal "stress," and 14% were due solely to failure to progress (120). Between July 1995 and June 1998 at one specialty hospital, the cesarean section rate for a persistent nonreassuring pattern was 3.6%. It might have been lower had additional tests been done to confirm fetal acid-base status. Unfortunately, only 15% had a fetal scalp pH, 37% had fetal scalp or acoustic stimulation, and 25% received a tocolytic prior to surgery (121).

The search for ways to lower the cesarean section rate continued into the next decade. Dr. Emily Hamilton and her colleagues at LMS Medical Systems Ltd. in Montreal, Canada found a 3% reduction in cesarean sections when their Computer-Assisted Labor Monitoring, CALM™, system was used to provide physicians with a consistent way to evaluate labor progress (122). Other factors that might contribute to loweringthe cesarean section rate include one-to-one supportive nursing care during active labor, effective multidisciplinary teams, and a strong commitment to evidence-based practice (123). A one-to-one nurse-patient ratio was related to a decrease in the number of cesarean sections of primigravida women who received oxytocin (124). After reviewing fourteen randomized controlled trials on the effects of labor support, Sauls found labor support was related to a reduction in the number of cesarean sections and operative vaginal deliveries (125). The inability of the nurse to provide enough labor support may indeed have increased the cesarean section rate.

Another change that probably contributed to the increase in the cesarean section rate was ACOG's change in their vaginal birth after cesarean (VBAC) practice bulletin. In July 1999, ACOG changed their position on VBAC and recommended that "because uterine rupture may be catastrophic, VBAC should be attempted in institutions equipped to respond to emergencies with physicians immediately available to provide emergency care" (126, p. 5). Since many physicians could not be immediately available in the hospital during the trial of labor after cesarean and would be unable to fulfill this recommendation, the number of repeat cesarean sections increased. By 2002, the total cesarean delivery rate was 26.1%, the highest level ever reported in the United States (127).

In addition to a drop in VBACs, fetal gender may play a role in the increase in cesarean sections as more males are delivered by cesarean section than females. In the United States nulliparous women at low risk from 109 obstetric and family practices in Illinois, Indiana, Iowa, Massachusetts, Missouri, and Wisconsin participated in a randomized clinical trial that found their cesarean section rate was higher if they had a male fetus (3.3% more cesareans) (128). In the Netherlands, more males than females were delivered by cesarean section for distress (129).

Maternal characteristics can increase the risk of cesarean section. For example, there were more cesarean sections when women were shorter than 5 feet 3 inches and/or gained 43 or more pounds during pregnancy. In California, the four leading risks for cesarean section were age (35 years or higher) and ethnicity (black women had the highest risk). In addition, preterm gestation, hypertension, diabetes, and malpresentation increased the risk of cesarean section (130).

In women with premature rupture of the membranes, independent risk factors for cesarean section were nulliparity, labor lasting more than 12 hours, a previous cesarean section, epidural anesthesia, clinical chorioamnionitis, spiral electrode use, an infant who weighed 4000 or more grams, oxytocin use, age of 35 years or higher, a latent phase of labor lasting 12 or more hours, and meconium stained amniotic fluid (131).

Although the number of cesarean sections done for non-reassuring fetal status is small, it may be possible to prevent unnecessary surgery if a test of fetal acid-base status is done prior to the decision to operate. For example, when scalp pH sampling was used in conjunction with EFM, the cesarean section rate decreased (14). After a review of 9 prospective randomized clinical trials, Neilson found that when scalp pH analysis was *not* available, there was a fourfold increase in the risk of an emergency cesarean section and a nearly threefold increase in the risk of a nonemergency cesarean section, but no increase in the use of forceps or vacuum extraction (8). The cesarean section rate also dropped when continuous EFM was used with pH determinations or ST analysis of the fetal ECG (106, 132).

No matter what the reason was for the cesarean section, it is still clear that the use of EFM has not significantly contributed to the rise in the rate. Sometimes the decision is influenced by other factors such as the presence of the attending physician or resident in the hospital, residency training, FHR pattern interpretation skill, continuing medical education attendance, defensive medical practice, and management style (133-134). Clearly, physicians and physician groups have different cesarean section rates (134). The cesarean section rate declined when physicians were given information about their total and repeat cesarean section rate and coded information about the cesarean sections of their peers. It appears that scrutiny of individual practice patterns and behaviors was the key determinant of cesarean birth reduction (135). Physician presence in the hospital may affect the cesarean section rate. For example, when the attending physician was in hospital, the cesarean section rate dropped in private service patients (136). When care is organized to include certified nurse midwives and nurse practitioners there may be a reduction in the cesarean section rate (137).

The physician may be influenced to perform a cesarean section by fear or patient demands. Ferri and Sofer have suggested the rising cesarean section rate in the United States may be due in part to a fear of lawsuits (138). In Tawain, physicians performed cesarean sections when women had a fear of labor pain or they desired to plan and control their birth experience or their fortune teller determined their destiny and fate, which is called ba-tzu (139).

The presence of a circulating nurse is needed to perform a cesarean section. Perhaps there was a shortage of circulating nurses when Canadian nurses went on strike, because the cesarean rate decreased 13.2% for breech presentation and 6.2% for distress (140). Nurses who collected psychosocial data and who had patients with significantly shorter labors saw fewer cesarean sections in their patients (141).

PREDICTIONS BASED ON THE FHR

EFM use escalated during the 1980s from 33.5 to 44.6% in 1980 to being the most widely used test of fetal surveillance in 1986 (81, 142-143). In 1987, 78.8% of pregnant women were electronically monitored, which decreased in 1988 to 62.2% (81). In 1990, Dr. Jick commented in *Ob. Gyn. News* that he was not aware of a single practicing obstetrician who was even considering giving up EFM (144). Estimates in both 1993 and 1994 were that 75% of pregnant women were electronically monitored (3, 81). By 2001, EFM was the standard of practice in 80% of labors (145).

EFM is still used to predict fetal status and prevent fetal morbidity and mortality. Critics of EFM will continue to discuss EFM's inability to prevent all perinatal morbidity and mortality (3, 15, 146). However, for EFM to be 100% valid, an abnormal FHR pattern would always be associated with a particular adverse outcome which is unrealistic. Users of EFM can increase the predictability of FHR patterns when they know the research associated with changes in the pattern from admission to delivery. For example, in a retrospective review of 21 deaths of singleton term fetuses, Drs. Golditch, Ahn, and Phelan found fetal death could be preceded by a reactive 30 minute admission strip followed by a catastrophic event such as uterine rupture; a reactive 30 minute admission strip followed by a rising baseline, loss of variability, decelerations, then a falling baseline or bradycardia; or, a nonreactive admission strip (147).

For EFM to be 100% reliable, there would be 100% agreement on pattern interpretation (143). This is an impossible goal due to the diversity of educational and work experiences of electronic fetal monitor users. Interobserver interpretation variations will always exist due to poor teaching, superficial teaching, or a lack of clinical experience (148-149). Just having the technology does not mean there will be an improvement in medical standards (150). To gain the most value from EFM, a knowledgeable user who properly interprets the FHR pattern and predicts fetal acid-base status is required. EFM data can be analyzed to predict fetal well-being or fetal compromise (146, 151).

Predicting Fetal or Neonatal Demise

EFM predicts the current status of the fetus, not long-term outcomes such as which babies might later develop CP (152). In 1963, Drs. Hon and Lee found certain FHR patterns predicted fetal death, e.g., prolonged bradycardia or a smooth and/or flat baseline with decelerations that had a slow recovery (153). Fetal demise was related to fetal bradycardia less than 100 bpm or a fixed tachycardic rate of 180 or more bpm for 30 or more minutes followed by a profound, unremitting bradycardia (154).

The type of device used to assess the FHR may increase the risk of fetal death. EFM use is better than auscultation in preventing fetal death. In a 1974 retrospective review of 28,621 births, Drs. Hon and Paul found a lower fetal death rate in the EFM group (6 per 10,000 babies weighing 1500 or more grams) versus the auscultated group (14 per 10,000 babies) (155). EFM use plus fetal scalp blood sampling (pH) also lowered the fetal mortality rate (52). Data from Greece suggested that there were fewer perinatal deaths due to hypoxia in the EFM group than in the auscultated group (2 deaths versus 9) (94).

Predicting Hypoxemia and Hypoxia

Dr. James Low and his colleagues have suggested that fetuses are on a "continuum of casualty" between being well or nonhypoxic to becoming hypoxemic, hypoxic, acidotic, and asphyxiated (156). Neurologic injury will be related to the degree and duration of hypoxia (157). Hypoxemia might be reflected by intermittent late decelerations due to excessive uterine activity or prolonged decelerations, loss of short-term variability, or a sinusoidal pattern (158). Hypoxia is often suspected when there is bradycardia, decreased or increased long-term variability or severe variable decelerations (45). However, to appreciate the meaning of the FHR baseline, the user must have a depth of knowledge since a tachyarrhythmia or bradyarrhythmia is usually not related to hypoxia. In addition, decreased variability may be related to the fetal quiescent (1F) behavioral state. Variability by itself did not predict good or bad outcomes (159).

Predicting Acidemia (Low pH)

Acidemia has been defined as an umbilical artery pH less than or equal to 7.15 and a base excess less than or equal to -8 mmol/L (160). The presence of spontaneous or evoked accelerations ruled out acidemia. Accelerations were related to an umbilical artery pH greater than 7.15 (nonacidemic) (159).

Although variability of the FHR baseline may not predict outcomes, preterm infants weighing 1500 or fewer grams with "good" baseline variability had a normal umbilical artery pH. When variability was "decreased," 71% had an acidemic cord artery pH (161). If for 2 or more hours prior to delivery there was decreased long-term variability (less than or equal to a 5 bpm baseline bandwidth), umbilical artery pH averaged 7.01. However, when there was "normal" long-term variability, the average pH was 7.18. If there was decreased long-term variability for 1 or more hours but less than 2 hours prior to delivery, the average umbilical artery pH was 7.15 (162).

If acidemia is severe, i.e., umbilical artery pH less than 7.0, there is an increased risk of neonatal death (163). A pH less than 7.0 is known as "pathologic acidemia" (164-165). In addition to increasing the risk of neonatal death, pathologic acidemia was related to a 5 minute Apgar score less than 7, neonatal seizures, intraventricular hemorrhage, respiratory distress, necrotizing enterocolitis, increased liver enzymes, and/or sepsis (165). Therefore, it is important to rule out acidemia by finding signs of fetal well-being such as accelerations with "normal" baseline long-term variability.

Predicting Metabolic Acidosis

Acidosis has been defined as a fetal scalp pH less than 7.20 (166). However, it also includes an abnormal base excess and bicarbonate level. An abnormally low base excess and bicarbonate value predicts the risk of hypoxic ischemic encephalopathy (HIE) better than an umbilical artery pH. Neonates who had seizures and who developed HIE had an average base excess of -20.6 mmol/L. They did not develop HIE if their base excess was between -12 and -18 mmol/L (164). A base excess of -12 mmol/L or lower was related to an increased risk of admission to the neonatal intensive care unit (167).

The risk of metabolic acidosis increases when there is tachycardia, decreased baseline short-term and long-term variability, variable decelerations and/or late decelerations. For example, in an intrapartum computerized analysis of the FHR, researchers found a weak correlation between metabolic acidosis and decelerations that dropped more than 20 bpm but a stronger correlation between metabolic acidosis and decreased short-term and long-term variability (168). Tachycardia during the two hours prior to delivery was associated with metabolic acidosis in 80% of fetuses (169). In fetuses who were 37 or more weeks of gestation, decreased baseline long-term variability and moderate and severe variable decelerations during the last 90 minutes prior to delivery had an increased risk of metabolic acidemia (170). Variable decelerations (dropping to 60 bpm or lower or lasting 60 seconds or longer) and late decelerations in fetuses who were postdates (more than 294 days of gestation) and who had meconium stained amniotic fluid increased the chance of an acidotic scalp pH (166). Variable decelerations that dropped below 70 bpm and late decelerations predicted metabolic acidosis in fetuses who were 37 to 42 weeks of gestation (171-172). Late decelerations during the four hours prior to delivery predicted metabolic acidosis in 48% of fetuses born to high risk women. In other women, as the number of variable decelerations increased, there was an increased association with hypoxia. If decelerations were present with 30% or more of the contractions, 25% of the fetuses were acidotic (46). To rule out metabolic acidosis, one must rule out acidemia. To rule out acidemia, digital scalp stimulation could be done for 15 seconds. If the fetus responds with an acceleration that is at least 10 bpm high that lasts at least 10 seconds at its base, there is no acidemia (173).

Fetal Acoustic Stimulation

Fetuses begin to hear at about 26 weeks of gestation. A fetus that responds to sound would be a viable fetus. When the FHR is at the baseline, a 3 to 5 second sound stimulus at 82 to 120 decibels may be used to elicit an acceleration. If the acceleration peaks at least 15 or more bpm above its base and lasts 15 or more seconds at its base (15 x 15), researchers have found the fetus was not acidemic and the fetal scalp pH was greater than 7.25 (174).

As many as 50% will not accelerate in response to sound, even though they are not acidemic (174-176). For example, maternal narcotic administration may diminish the fetal response or prevent a fetal acceleration (174). If there is no response to acoustic stimulation, another test should be performed to assess fetal status. Neonatal hearing will not be impaired by acoustic stimulation (175).

Fetal Scalp Stimulation

Fetal scalp stimulation with application of gentle digital pressure over one of the parietal bones for no more than 15 seconds or the tug of an Allis clamp on the fetal scalp, has been used between contractions and between decelerations to elicit a FHR acceleration to rule out acidemia. When an acceleration occurred within 10 minutes of stimulation, the fetal pH was greater than 7.19 (57, 177-179). Scalp stimulation predicted fetal well-being more often than it predicted fetal compromise. Like acoustic stimulation, 50% of fetuses did not respond with

an acceleration but only 34% of the nonresponders were acidemic (176).

Fetal Electrode Stimulation Test

Pulling gently on the spiral electrode five times over a period of five or fewer seconds is believed to cause fetal pain. This stimulus elicited fetal movement and at least one 15 x 15 acceleration in nearly 95% of full term fetuses in the minute following stimulation (180). A reactive acceleration rules out metabolic acidosis.

Fetal Scalp pH

Obtaining a fetal scalp blood sample is time-consuming and inconvenient for busy obstetricians (181). However, the technique is still practiced in some hospitals, especially when continuous EFM is used. If there is only one prolonged deceleration, it is not likely that the scalp pH will be less than 7.20 (182). However, a fetus who is metabolically acidotic will not accelerate following the painful stimulus of a scalp puncture. Seventy three percent of fetuses tested who did not have a 15 x 15 acceleration were acidemic (pH less than 7.20). The remaining 27% were not acidemic (183). Therefore, the failure to accelerate following scalp puncture may not be related to acidemia.

Fetal Pulse Oximetry

Although the Food and Drug Administration in the United States approved the Nellcor N-400® Fetal Oxygen Saturation Monitoring System, ACOG's Committee on Obstetric Practice in 2001 did not endorse the adoption of the device due to concerns related to increasing medical costs without a concomitant improvement in clinical outcomes, i.e., the overall cesarean section rate did not decrease (184). The device provided additional information to discern fetuses at risk for metabolic acidosis (185). When the $FSpO_2$ of a term fetus was less than 30%, the fetus was hypoxic with an increased risk of fetal scalp and umbilical vessel acidemia and neonatal compromise, especially when there were 10 episodes at less than 30% lasting 10 seconds (186-188).

The Nellcor® device was no longer sold in 2006. It was inserted after rupture of membranes and at least 3 centimeters of dilatation and placed on the fetal temple or cheek. Some women found sensor placement uncomfortable and they needed to stay in bed after placement (189). The $FSpO_2$ was less than 30% if late decelerations lasted more than 10 minutes, there were severe variable decelerations, or there was "decreased" long-term variability (190).

Fetal ECG ST Analysis

The T/QRS ratio and the PR interval may be influenced by oxygenation and acid-base balance (191). For example, hypoxia may precede a surge of catecholamines, beta-adrenoceptor activation, and myocardial glycogenolysis (192). Eventually, there will be a depletion of cardiac creatine-phosphate, an increase in lactic acid, and a decrease in pH which will liberate potassium ions and change the sodium pump resulting in a change in the action potentials across the myocardial cell membranes. The result will be a change in the ST segment and T wave (ventricular repolarization). The ST segment elevates and the T wave amplitude increases or becomes inverted with hypoxia and acidemia (193). For example, in fetal lamb experiments, the ST segment rose and the T/QRS ratio increased when there was hypotension and acidosis after umbilical cord occlusion. A negative or biphasic ST waveform was found when there was myocardial ischemia and during reoxygenation between cord occlusions (194).

To analyze human fetal ECG changes, a device known as a STAN® recorder was developed by Neoventa Medical in Gothenburg, Sweden. It is used to produce continuous information on the ECG response during labor with continuous FHR and uterine activity data. Use of the STAN® recorder resulted in better 1 minute Apgar scores and fewer neonates with metabolic acidosis than EFM alone (using a criteria for acidosis of umbilical artery pH less than 7.05 and base excess less than 12 mmol/L) (195). Another device known as the Nottingham fetal ECG analyzer has been used to process raw fetal ECG signals in the 30 minutes prior to delivery. Researchers found no association between the T/QRS ratio and birth asphyxia (196). In 10 European centers with a medical teaching program, the rate of metabolic acidosis based on umbilical artery sampling decreased from 1.44% to 0.57% when EFM was used with the STAN® recorder (197). Use of the STAN® recorder increased agreement between physicians regarding the significance of FHR patterns from 87% to 96% (198). In addition, ECG analysis plus EFM decreased the number of operative deliveries, cesarean sections, and babies with metabolic acidosis (199). It appears that both FSpO$_2$ and ST analysis can detect early stages of intermittent hypoxia (200).

The illustration in Figure 6.1 depicts the ECG with a schematic presentation of hypoxia related to changes in the ECG waveform. The T/QRS ratio measure is on the right. This ratio, together with the occurrence of biphasic ST changes, form the basis for the automatic detection of significant ST events. Using the STAN® recorder with EFM can alert nurses and physicians in cases of nonreassuring FHR patterns to reduce the risk of term neonates developing metabolic acidosis. ST analysis plus EFM increases specificity to detect the lack of hypoxia without decreasing sensitivity to detect hypoxia (192).

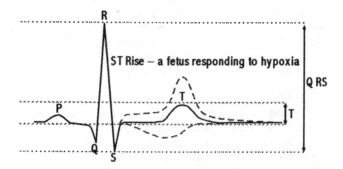

Figure 6.1: ST segment rise - a fetus responding to hypoxia. Negative ST segment - a fetus who is unable to respond or has not had time to react to hypoxia (Data from Rosén, K. G., with permission).

The Significance of Meconium

Acute asphyxia which causes brain damage may not be related to the release of meconium or multiorgan system dysfunction (201-202). However, the presence of meconium in the amniotic fluid may be related to hypoxia and/or metabolic acidosis. To determine the significance of meconium, actions should be taken to determine fetal acid-base status (31-102). Fetal SpO$_2$ was determined even in the presence of meconium (203). A high level of anxiety was also related to the presence of meconium (204). In a study of 59 metabolically acidotic term fetuses, 33% had meconium, 64% had a low (< 7) one minute Apgar score, and 78% had neonatal complications of their cardiovascular, respiratory, renal, and/or central nervous system(s) (67). The presence of meconium increases the risk of meconium aspiration syndrome (205). A long-standing intrauterine infection with chorion vasculitis, funisitis, and villitis may be related to meconium aspiration syndrome (206). Naturally, a vigorous newborn will have no excess morbidity from meconium (207). However, even in a study of 43,625 women who were classified as low risk at 37 to 42 weeks of gestation, the presence of meconium instead of clear fluid increased the risk for

- fetal and neonatal death (0.2 vs. 0.001%)
- fetal distress (6.5 vs. 2.1%)
- cesarean section (5.6 vs. 2.3%)
- instrumental delivery (3.2 vs. 1.8%)
- chorioamnionitis (0.2 vs. 0.1%)
- postpartum infection (0.5 vs. 0.2%) and
- 1 and 5 minute Apgar scores less than 3 (1.9 and 0.4% vs. 1 and 0.1%) (208).

Forty five percent of newborns who were asphyxiated during labor had meconium stained amniotic fluid and/or an abnormal FHR pattern (209).

Predicting Asphyxia

Drs. Low, Pancham, and Worthington believed that EFM was based on the premise that careful assessment of FHR patterns would indicate the presence of fetal asphyxia with metabolic acidosis, especially during the last two hours of labor (210). The diagnosis of asphyxia could be confirmed after delivery when blood gases were analyzed. For example, asphyxia was diagnosed based on an umbilical artery buffer base less than 34 mmol/L. Marked metabolic acidosis was defined as a buffer base of 25 to 32 mEq/L with a pH of 6.68 to 7.125 (209). A normal value was greater than 38 mmol/liter (211-212). As the number of decelerations increased, the umbilical artery buffer base decreased.

Asphyxia is a condition of impaired blood gas exchange leading to progressive hypoxemia and hypercapnia with a significant metabolic acidosis (213). Significant metabolic acidosis includes an umbilical artery base excess less than or equal to -10 mmol/L. This increases the risk of neurologic disorders in nonanomalous neonates (214). When the base excess was less than -16 mmol/L, 40% of term fetuses had moderate or severe brain, lung, or renal complications. When the base excess was between -12 and -16, only 10% of neonates had moderate or severe complications (213).

Although asphyxia may be severe enough to cause CP in 10% of term neonates, there is no way to tell when asphyxia will cause CP (215). Asphyxia can be ruled out by fetal movement accompanied by a "normal" FHR pattern (77). FHR patterns of late decelerations of any depth, variable decelerations with a duration of 40 or more seconds and/or a depth of 60 or fewer bpm, or a smooth baseline were associated with asphyxia in fetuses less than 33 weeks' gestation (216). When decelerations occur with 38% or more of the contractions in the 2 hours before delivery, there is an increased risk of asphyxia (217). Absent long-term variability with deep late decelerations with 30 or more seconds to their nadir or prolonged decelerations (2 minutes to 5 minutes) during 20 or more minutes in the hour prior to delivery was associated with moderate to severe asphyxia (218). Bradycardia occurred prior to the birth of 61% of neonates with Apgar scores of 0 at 1 and 5 minutes and increased the risk of neonatal death (67%) or seizures within the first 48 hours of life (219).

When fetal asphyxia is suspected a cesarean section may be performed. However, a cesarean section does not necessarily prevent the birth of an asphyxiated neonate (220). Anoxia for 10 to 12 minutes can cause brain damage. Therefore, there is a very small window of time to prevent injury when asphyxia is suspected. Preterm and intrauterine growth restricted (IUGR) fetuses have a higher rate of asphyxia than normally grown term neonates (18-21% vs. 6-10%) (217).

Predicting Neonatal Seizures

Cerebral dysfunction may be a result of asphyxia (221). However, organ injury may be transient or permanent (222). In one study of 100,000 fetuses who were "well" on admission, 27 or 0.027% were born with a central nervous system injury (68% intrapartal insult, 41% antepartal insult) (223). A review of 109,981 deliveries between 1985 to 2000 revealed an increased cesarean section rate from 5.1% to 14.2%, with no change in the number of neonates who seized, i.e., 2.7/1,000 seized and 1.7/1,000 died (224). Therefore, a cesarean section does not necessarily prevent neonatal seizures.

In a study of 10,089 women, labor duration, late decelerations, and meconium were related to neonatal seizures. Seizures were more common if labor lasted more than 5 hours or there was failure to progress. Seizures were also related to the number of fetal scalp blood samples and the use of oxytocin (7, 101, 114). Bradycardia lasting 20 or more minutes at a rate less than 100 bpm increased the risk of neonatal seizures (225). In a study with a small sample, i.e. 25 neonates who were diagnosed with seizures due to hypoxic ischemic encephalopathy, the presence of minimal long-term variability for an average of 72 minutes was more common (64%) than in a similar matched sample of neonates who did not have seizures (36%) and who had an average of 36 minutes of minimal long-term variability. However, this difference was not statistically significant (226).

Even if the newborn seizes, more than half should have no long-term brain damage. For example, 51 to 80% of neonates who had seizures were normal at one year of age. This is partly due to the fact that neonatal seizures have causes other than intrapartal asphyxia, such as intracranial hemorrhage, infection, and metabolic and developmental disorders (227).

Predicting Cerebral Palsy

CP is a chronic neuromuscular disorder with many possible causes. CP has been diagnosed in 1 to 2 children per 1,000 live births (7, 76, 228). However, CP was related to intrapartal asphyxia in only 2 children per 10,000 infants born in western Australia (229). Preterm babies have a higher incidence of CP (17/1,000 if birth weight was less than 2 kilograms) (230). CP in preterm fetuses who weighed less than 1750 grams was not related to the type of fetal surveillance (EFM versus auscultation) but was related to the time from recognition of an abnormal FHR pattern to delivery (19, 54). If the neonate weighed 2.5 or more kilograms, the CP rate decreased to less than 1 per 1,000 live births but was nearly tripled to quadrupled when there were multiple late decelerations and/or decreased "beat-to-beat" variability (231). Tight nuchal cord may be related to CP. For example, Nelson and Grether (232-233) found 6% of children with CP had a tight nuchal cord and spastic quadripegia (CP) but not with diplegia or hemiplegia. Williams and O'Brien found no association between a tight nuchal cord and CP (234). An increase in the cesarean section rate was not associated with a decrease in the number of children who had CP (235).

An international consensus statement supported by American, Australian, British, Canadian, Chinese, Irish, and New Zealand midwife, obstetrician, perinatologist, pediatrician, and pathologist groups was published in 1999 which defined the causal relationship between acute intrapartal events and CP (236). The type of CP attributable to an acute intrapartum event was believed to be associated with the following factors:

1. Evidence of metabolic acidosis of pH < 7.00 and base excess less than or equal to -12 mmol/L
2. Early onset severe or moderate neonatal encephalopathy (if 34 or more weeks of gestation)
3. Spastic quadriplegia or dyskinetic CP.

There were no specific FHR pattern characteristics that the group felt should be used to predict CP. However they did agree that a baseline between 110 to 160 bpm with baseline long-term variability between 6 to 25 bpm (bandwidth) and absent decelerations represented a fetus who had no risk of acidemia. They also recognized that the absence of variability in the presence of persistent late or variable decelerations or bradycardia was evidence of potentially damaging acidemia (236). They failed to recognize the importance of accelerations as a critical sign of the absence of acidemia.

HIGH RISK VS. LOW RISK: WHAT DOES IT MEAN?

Knowing a woman's risk level may help clinicians predict outcomes. Physicians have classified their patients as low risk, moderate risk, at risk, and high risk. High risk usually means the pregnancy has an increased risk of a poor outcome (237). The assumption is women who are at low to moderate risk have a somewhat less risk of a poor outcome than at risk or high risk women. The distinction between at risk or high risk versus low risk is important since fetuses of at risk or high risk women are more vulnerable to develop metabolic acidosis or asphyxia sooner than the fetuses of low risk women (209).

Knowing a woman's risk category may help predict the risk of neonatal metabolic acidosis and impact impact clinical decisions (238). Low, Simpson, Tonni, and Chamberlain studied 100 women and used a clinical risk scoring tool to determine their risk level (239). They looked at the relationship between the level of risk and neonatal metabolic acidosis. They found that antepartal risk factors had a 64% specificity to predict the absence of metabolic acidosis and antepartal plus intrapartal risk factors had a 42% specificity.

Risk factors for fetal asphyxia may be maternal, fetal, or placental (240-241). An example of a maternal risk factor is asthma. Women with asthma had more TAGA newborns with higher nucleated red blood cells and lymphocytes than babies of women who did not have asthma, i.e., babies of asthmatic women had a greater risk of hypoxia (242). Umbilical cord compression or chronic uteroplacental insufficiency are examples of fetal and placental factors than can increase the risk of fetal jeopardy (243).

Risk status may change from low risk to high risk during labor. Herbst and Ingemarsson found that 4,044 low risk women between 33 and 42 weeks of gestation who had a reactive admission test (20 minute tracing with at least 2 accelerations in 10 of the minutes) could be monitored continuously or intermittently with EFM for 10 to 30 minutes every 2 hours and with a stethoscope (auscultation) every 15 to 30 minutes between intermittent EFM assessments and still deliver babies with similar umbilical artery pHs, Apgar scores, and neonatal intensive care (NICU) admissions. They also found no difference in the number of cesarean sections between the groups. Even though the women were classified as low risk at the beginning of the study, 6.3 - 6.6% developed ominous FHR patterns during labor. Thus, some women change from low risk to high risk during labor (244).

To determine risk status of the mother and her fetus, a risk-screening tool may be helpful (245). However, the predictive validity of risk profiles has been challenged and many clinicians use no formal tool for antepartal or intrapartal risk assessment (246-247). The lack of a risk profile has created a dilemma as to how to best determine risk status. The lack of a formal risk assessment may lead clinicians to apply a fetal monitor continuously. Some physicians have advocated continuous fetal monitoring and routine umbilical artery blood gas and acid-base assessment in women with no clinical risk factors (239, 248).

Risk During Pregnancy

The lack of prenatal care significantly increased the risk of thick meconium stained amniotic fluid, low birth weight, and neonatal death. Just one prenatal visit lowered the perinatal death rate 20% (249-250).

Examples of low risk factors are a maternal age of 18 to 35, parity of 0 to 3, 37 to 42 weeks of gestation, a singleton pregnancy, cephalic presentation, prenatal care by the 5th month of pregnancy with at least 5 visits, no obstetric or medical problems, and no drug or alcohol abuse (81). During pregnancy, a low risk woman can become high risk for fetal asphyxia (251). For example, physical abuse, a fall, or a motor vehicle accident increases her risk for abruptio placentae and changes her low risk status to high risk until the abruption is ruled out. If there has been trauma and the fetus is viable, continuous EFM up to 48 hours after admission has been recommended (252). However, with normal FHR activity, no contractions, and no vaginal bleeding or significant uterine tenderness, four to six hours of monitoring have been considered adequate (253-255).

Risk During Labor

The initial decision of how frequently to assess the FHR during labor is based on the perception of risk prior to the onset of labor (6). In 1979, the NICHD Task Force on Predictors of Intrapartum Fetal Distress found no evidence that EFM decreased the fetal or neonatal morbidity or mortality rate in low risk women during labor (14). Newborns of low risk women had no different outcomes when intermittent rather than continuous EFM was used during labor (89). However, even low and "medium" risk women need to have appropriate interpretation of FHR data. Suboptimal interpretation or failure to use continuous EFM was related to moderate to severe neonatal encephalopathy and significant metabolic acidemia within five hours after birth in 8 out of 12 babies (256).

The fetal risk for asphyxia increased when there was a malpresentation, abnormal labor, cord prolapse, meconium, and a trial of forceps (248). When these things exist, the woman should be classified as a high risk patient. Of the 738 women who were classified as low risk their during pregnancy, 20% became high risk during labor. Another 46% were low risk during pregnancy and labor, and 18% were high risk during pregnancy but low risk for fetal asphyxia during labor. The remaining 16% were high risk during their pregnancy and labor. High risk women who were low risk during labor had babies with Apgar scores at 5 minutes that were 5 or higher, fewer resuscitations, fewer cases of hypoglycemia, and fewer neonates who seized than in women who were high risk during labor. Woman with a high risk pregnancy and labor had the greatest neonatal morbidity and mortality (247).

During labor of a low risk woman, the Society of Obstetricians and Gynecologists of Canada (SOGC) has endorsed auscultation with a hand-held ultrasound Doppler for 1 minute immediately following a contraction every 30 minutes during the latent phase, every 15 to 30 minutes during the active phase, and every 5 minutes during the second stage of labor. They also support continuous and close support from an appropriately trained professional for 80 to 90% of active labor (257).

The American Academy of Pediatrics and ACOG had recommended that there be a one-to-one nurse:high risk (ill with complications) laboring woman ratio, and a one-to-two nurse:low risk laboring women ratio (258). However, in their 2002 5th edition of *Guidelines for Perinatal Care*, they changed their recommendation to one nurse for any two women in labor even during induction or augmentation with oxytocin. They did not identify intrapartal risk factors but increased the recommended nurse:patient ratio. They obviously recognize risk can exist in labor and delivery. For example, on pages 25 to 26, they wrote "A registered nurse with advanced training and experience in routine and high risk obstetric care should be assigned to the labor and delivery area at all times" at a specialty (level II) facility. On page 125 they wrote "Because intrapartum complications can arise, sometimes quickly and without warning, ongoing risk assessment and surveillance of the mother and the fetus is essential." On pages 129 to 130 they acknowledged "At all times in the hospital labor and delivery area, the safety and well-being of the mother and the fetus are the primary concern and responsibility of the obstetric staff." Yet, they did not differentiate the frequency to assess and record the FHR between low risk and high risk women. Currently, they recommend the following if risk factors are present:

Active labor: determine and record the FHR every 15 minutes

Second stage of labor: determine and record the FHR every 5 minutes (259).

The SOGC recommendations are more in line with prior recommendations, i.e., for low risk woman in labor, assess and record the FHR
- periodically during the latent phase
- every 30 minutes during the active phase
- every 15 minutes during the second stage (260-262)

"Periodically" and the frequency of assessment of the high risk woman in the latent phase of labor should be defined by hospital protocol and the FHR should be recorded at specified intervals.

ADMISSION TEST STRIP: IS IT NECESSARY?

Intrapartal fetal distress was not reliably predicted by pregnancy risk assessment (263). At least 20% of low risk women became high risk during labor, and as many as 30% of "healthy" fetuses developed a nonreassuring FHR pattern during labor. To detect "fetal distress" on admission and avoid fetal death Ingemarrson and his colleagues recommended a 20 minute admission screening test before allocating a woman to continuous EFM or intermittent auscultation. They considered 2 accelerations in 10 minutes during the 20 minute screening period to be a reflection of fetal well-being (264).

Today, the admission fetal monitor strip is the standard of care and a 20 to 30 minute EFM strip should be obtained to assess fetal well-being and to document fetal admission status (32, 247, 265-266). In the past, some physicians were unsure if an admission FHR screening strip was useful (267). In the first randomized control trial of Doppler auscultation versus EFM as a means to assess the fetus on admission, more babies in the auscultated group had hypoxic ischemic encephalopathy (19.19%) than in the EFM group (9.8%). The researchers never addressed this clinically significant finding (268). Some physicians thought that if the admission strip or intermittent EFM had "decreased" baseline variability it might be "more dangerous" than continuous EFM (6). Conversely, others believed EFM should always be used to screen at risk women and may be helpful in screening low risk women because the lack of fetal well-being on admission could be due to fetal asphyxia or injury that occurred prior to admission (52, 269-270). Twins need an admission strip to evaluate well-being (270).

The admission strip has a higher specificity than sensitivity. If the woman was in the latent phase of labor, the admission strip predicted a well fetus during labor with 98% specificity. However, it predicted a fetus who would develop fetal distress with only 57% sensitivity. Researchers recommended admission of the woman whose fetus had an abnormal admission test (271). Dai and Fox examined the first and last 30 minutes of monitoring in 559 deliveries and reported the first 30 minutes do reflect the fetal status in labor and predict a vigorous fetus at 37 to 42 weeks of gestation. They used scalp pH sampling to predict a compromised fetus (272). Umstad found a 30 minute admission test when the woman was 4 or fewer centimeters was helpful in allocating women to a low or high risk group (272). An IUGR fetus will have a worse admission strip than a normally grown fetus and is more prone to perinatal asphyxia due to their history of chronic hypoxia (274).

A 20 minute admission strip was obtained from 130 women who were classified as low risk during their pregnancy. Almost 1% (0.9 %) of the fetuses were asphyxiated at the time of admission, and another 3.9% developed acidosis during labor. Auscultation failed to detect any of the fetuses that became acidotic, but auscultation was performed every 30 minutes for only 15 seconds (264). Kulkarni and Shrotri studied 100 high risk women who were 3 or fewer centimeters dilated in labor at 37 or more weeks of gestation. There research was conducted in India where they had limited access to continuous EFM, even for high risk women in labor. Of the 100 high risk women, 58 had fetuses who had 2 accelerations in 10 minutes and fetal well-being appeared to last for five hours. Based on this finding, they recommended repeat EFM every 4 to 5 hours. Of the 100 high risk women, 35 had an equivocal tracing of no accelerations in 20 minutes or long-term variability of 5 to 10 bpm (bandwidth) or variable decelerations. Fetuses with an equivocal admission test accounted for 31.42% of the perinatal morbidity. The 7 women with an ominous admission tracing, less than 5 bpm long-term variability or late decelerations or severe variable decelerations or bradycardia, accounted for 85.71% of the perinatal morbidity (275).

Based on the admission test research findings, if time and the maternal condition allow, verbal informed consent to use the electronic fetal monitor should be given and an admission FHR tracing should be obtained soon after a woman arrives on the labor unit (6). A nonreactive 40 minute admission strip (less than 2 accelerations that are 15 x 15 in 20 minutes) was associated with a five times higher risk of intrapartal fetal distress than a reactive admission strip (276). A nonreactive FHR pattern for a period of 60 minutes was associated with an increased risk of hypoxemia and acidemia, particularly in the lower birth weight or preterm fetus (267). Auscultation may not be an acceptable method of admission fetal surveillance because auscultation does not identify fetal distress as early as EFM. EFM also identified twice as many fetuses with abnormal FHRs (32, 277).

A minimum of a 10 minute strip can be used to screen the fetus on admission if there are two 15 x 15 accelerations during that 10 minutes (264, 278-279). However, only one reactive acceleration is needed to rule out metabolic acidosis. If the woman is low risk, waiting for a second reactive acceleration will needlessly prolong EFM. Since some protocols require an admission strip that lasts 20 or more minutes and has at least 2 accelerations, nurses should know and follow their institution's protocol (280).

HUMAN VS. ELECTRONIC SURVEILLANCE (AUSCULTATION VS. EFM)

In 1984, an attorney expressed concern about the adequacy of human surveillance of the fetus (80). Auscultation at the beginning of a contraction and for 30 seconds after the end of the contraction every 15 minutes during the first stage of labor and every 5 minutes during the second stage of labor was unable to detect sudden changes in the FHR, a fixed (flat) FHR of a compromised fetus, short-term variability, subtle late decelerations, or predict a metabolically acidotic fetus. In fact, 392 of the 423 women could not be monitored every 15 miutes during the first stage of labor and every 5 minutes during the second stage of labor. Researchers concluded that it was not possible to use auscultation as the primary means of fetal surveillance during labor in the majority of women (281). Hankins, Leicht, Anderson, & Rowe found that in 34 low risk women assessing the FHR every 30 minutes during active labor and every 15 minutes during the second stage with auscultation was only achieved 97% of the time and even less in high risk women who needed more frequent assessments (282).

The Association of Women's Health, Obstetrics, and Neonatal Nurses (AWHONN) published a clinical position statement suggesting there is no research literature consensus that EFM provides superior assessment of laboring women without risk factors (283). In 2001, Banta and Thacker published their findings after a review of 10 randomized controlled trials plus 600 books and articles on EFM and auscultation to evaluate the efficacy, safety, costs, and social implications of EFM. They concluded EFM had limited and marginal benefits over auscultation (284).

Clearly, EFM and auscultation are not equivalent in the data they collect or the predictions that can be made from that data (285). Fetuses who were monitored by EFM had fewer deaths than fetuses monitored by auscultation (286-287). Baseline variability cannot be heard with auscultation (288). EFM is superior to auscultation in predicting umbilical artery acidemia at birth (289). Most of the auscultated baselines were inaccurate and were 20 to 30 bpm faster than the actual baseline assessed by EFM (290).

In a study of 54,000 women from 12 university hospitals, the only auscultation finding related to CP was a rate less than 60 bpm (291). In 1995, Dr. Barry Schifrin summarized the problems with auscultation, i.e., auscultation cannot determine fetal status except where there is severe asphyxia, it is inaccurate, incapable of detecting large decelerations, not a useful admission screening tool, vulnerable to more subjective interpretation than visual analysis of the FHR pattern, difficult to verify, can only identify major FHR changes, and is hard to use due to staffing logistics (292). In addition, use of a Pinard stethoscope requires skill and it is difficult to hear the FHR with fetal descent behind the symphysis pubis (293). In fact, many hospitals in the United States do not have a fetoscope in their labor and delivery units and there are limited numbers of hand-held Dopplers.

Auscultation may miss late decelerations. Schifrin, Amsel, and Burdorf used a computer simulation of late decelerations that lasted one to two minutes and found that late decelerations were easiest to detect by auscultation if they lasted longer or occurred late in the contraction (294). Miller, Pearse, and Paul found nurses and physicians who used auscultation failed to identify late decelerations with and without long-term variability 18.4 to 33% of the time (295).

The failure to hear late decelerations when auscultation is used may be responsible for the birth of more babies who had seizures. In two of the eight randomized controlled trials that compared auscultation with EFM, the auscultated fetus had more seizures (7, 87, 296). When researchers examined data from 12,964 women who participated in the Dublin trial, late decelerations were the most powerful predictor of neonatal seizures, but they were often missed when auscultation was used (7, 297). This finding may explain why auscultation preceded the birth of more babies who had seizures. They also found that marked bradycardia could be heard with auscultation and preceded the birth of neurologically abnormal neonates.

Because auscultation provides limited information about the fetus, it cannot be used to detect fetal distress except when the fetus is dying. In the days prior to the use of EFM in hospitals, Benson and his colleagues evaluated auscultation data collected from 24,863 fetuses who were assessed every 15 minutes during the first stage of labor and every 5 minutes during the second stage of labor. They acknowledged there was no one auscultatory indicator of fetal distress and no agreement on the seriousness of FHR changes (298).

In spite of the limitations of auscultation, the fetus of a low risk or high risk woman may be monitored during labor by auscultation, preferably after the admission test strip has been evaluated. Following an admission strip, the fetuses of low risk women were auscultated with a hand-held Doppler or the EFM tracing was checked every 30 minutes during labor. There were no differences in the number of stillbirths, NICU admissions, or neonatal seizures between the low risk and high risk groups (92). On the other hand, Renou found that neonates of high risk women who were auscultated during labor had more twitching, apneic episodes, hypotonia or hypertonia, seizures, tachypnea, and high-pitched crying than fetuses monitored by EFM (87). Therefore, the choice to not use EFM as the primary assessment tool during the labor of high risk women may increase the risk of neonatal morbidity.

Several factors should be considered when choosing a method of intrapartal fetal surveillance:

- Do you have a fetoscope, stethoscope, Pinard, or hand-held Doppler?
- Do you have the education and training to use the device?
- Can you provide one-to-one care during active labor?
- Do you have a protocol for auscultation?
- What is the woman's preference for her desired birth experience: technical vs. nontechnical?
- How much does she weigh? It is difficult to auscultate with a fetoscope when a woman is obese.
- What are her risk factors?
- What was the FHR on the admission strip?
- What is the risk of fetal oxygen deprivation during labor?
- Do you have the time to assess and record the FHR?

In Denmark, 655 women in their 36th week of pregnancy were interviewed. One-third preferred EFM, one-third preferred auscultation, and one-third were undecided as to which intrapartal surveillance technique they desired. High risk women mostly preferred continuous, precise, electronic surveillance of their fetus, feeling it promoted their partner's involvement and contributed to the possibility of a quick intervention. Women who desired a natural childbirth and a nontechnological environment preferred auscultation over EFM. They thought they would be more comfortable, mobile, and less disturbed by the signal from the fetal monitor. Women desired auscultation as they had less fear about potential fetal trauma posed by EFM (299-300).

The fetal heart rate may be auscultated with a fetoscope, Pinard stethoscope, or hand-held Doppler device. If a hand-held Doppler is used, assess the maternal heart rate simultaneously to confirm the auscultated rate is fetal in origin. Auscultate for a minimum of 30 seconds following a contraction (54, 301). Auscultation may last for longer periods or occur more frequently, e.g. for 60 seconds after a contraction during the first stage of labor and between every contraction during the second stage of labor (7, 101).

In studies where there was no difference in the "fetal condition" whether or not EFM or auscultation was used during active labor and the second stage, there was a one-to-one nurse/woman ratio (302). This is the "adequate nursing care" needed for auscultation, and the hospital may be held liable if harm could have been prevented by having adequate numbers of trained personnel (80). Even if auscultation was used for intrapartal surveillance, the fetal monitor may be applied prior to delivery as a normal FHR pattern at that time may help refute claims that acidosis or asphyxia caused neurologic injury (281).

ACOG, in July 1995, suggested that intermittent auscultation of the FHR was equivalent to continuous electronic monitoring in assessing the fetal condition when auscultation was performed at specific intervals with a 1:1 nurse-to-patient ratio (37). ACOG based this opinion on six controlled randomized clinical trials in which both high risk and/or low risk women participated (7, 86-90). "Fetal condition" was not defined, but may refer to fetal blood gas values obtained from an umbilical artery (262). Results from the Dublin trial revealed auscultation prevented fetal or neonatal morbidity or mortality from asphyxia in labor *until labor lasted more than five hours*. Then, auscultation was not as effective as EFM in preventing hypoxic ischemic encephalopathy (7, 102).

The belief by ACOG that FHR monitoring is equally effective whether done electronically or by auscultation is not true for all women in all circumstances (37). "Equivalence" in assessing the fetal condition between intermittent auscultation and continuous EFM is more likely when the woman is low risk. Low risk status usually meant no pregnancy risk factors for fetal stress, no intrapartal signs of fetal stress, no meconium in the amniotic fluid, no oxytocin use, no prolonged labor, and no failure to progress (114).

IS EFM BETTER THAN AUSCULTATION?

In the 1980s, EFM was considered an essential diagnostic technique and the most reliable method for intrapartum fetal evaluation (90, 303). Sentiment has changed. Critics of continuous EFM feel it is an imperfect, unreliable technique with unproven clinical value (152, 304). They advocate auscultation instead. However, if auscultation is chosen for fetal surveillance, the user must be cognizant of its limitations.

A combination of intermittent auscultation and intermittent EFM will lessen the time a woman is electronically monitored. In a study of 4044 *low risk* women, auscultation by stethoscope between contractions was performed every 15 to 30 minutes. EFM was used every 10 to 30 minutes for 2 to 2 1/2 minutes during labor until the second stage of labor when continuous EFM was used. The time women were on the electronic monitor decreased almost 40%. Compared to other low risk women who received continuous fetal monitoring, there was no difference in Apgar scores, NICU admissions, fetal umbilical cord artery pH, or the cesarean section rate (244). Reflecting the current sentiment about continuous monitoring of low risk women, The Society of Obstetricians and Gynecologists of Canada advised physicians to stop routine continuous monitoring of low risk women and to auscultate instead (305).

EFM only has advantages over auscultation when its use is coupled with skilled interpretation and prompt intervention. EFM provided both auditory and visual information and detected more FHR abnormalities than auscultation (95, 261, 306-307). EFM, unlike auscultation, also provides a hard copy of records (261).

Nurse staffing levels may be insufficient to auscultate laboring women every 15 minutes, although sometimes auscultation standards have been met (4, 281, 308). Auscultation is best used to:

- confirm the FHR prior to placement of the external ultrasound transducer
- monitor the fetal condition of low risk women during labor (after obtaining an admission EFM tracing), and
- confirm the FHR when abnormal or questionable FHR tracings are obtained by EFM, e.g. if artifact or an arrhythmia are suspected (309).

During labor, the auscultated FHR should be assessed for at least 30 seconds immediately following a contraction (14). The rate can be counted 5 times, each for 6 seconds, then multiplied by 10 to give 5 rates during the 30 second period. This might help to conceptualize an increase or decrease in the rate (66). If a fetoscope or Pinard stethoscope is used during a contraction, it is often difficult to hear the FHR, especially if the woman is obese. Many nurses prefer a hand-held Doppler device with a digital readout in these cases (100).

Some believe sound transmission through a fetoscope is enhanced by bone conduction (310). However, that concept originated in 1917, and is unsupported by scientific research. When a fetoscope or stethoscope is used, the fetal heart sounds (fetal souffle), uterine (placental) souffle or bruit, and funic (umbilical cord) souffle may be heard. The fetal souffle represents sounds from the fetal heart and is due to flow through the foramen ovale. The uterine or placental souffle is a rushing sound of maternal blood in the placental bed and is synchronous with the maternal heart rate. The funic souffle is due to fetal blood flow in the umbilical arteries, occurred in about 15% of pregnancies, and may represent compression of the umbilical cord. The funic souffle is synchronous with the FHR (73).

Auscultation criteria for "fetal distress" originated in 1893 and included a FHR greater than 160 bpm or less than 100 bpm, an irregular FHR, gross alterations of fetal movements (which was not defined), and/or meconium with a vertex presentation. By 1968, following review of 25,000 deliveries, it was concluded that auscultation had no reliable indicator of "fetal distress" (73). Not so surprisingly, in the same year electronic fetal monitors were manufactured for clinical use.

Advocates of EFM recognized that the human ear may miss subtle changes in the FHR (8). One cannot hear fluctuation or variability in the FHR nor distinguish short-term from long-term variability (8, 45). Auscultation may fail to detect absent short-term variability of the metabolically

acidotic fetus or distinguish a sinusoidal pattern of an asphyxiated fetus. Auscultation may be painful to the woman. Thirty-two percent of more than 6000 women auscultated with a Pinard stethoscope felt its application was painful and they would have preferred EFM in a future labor. Only 8% who were electronically monitored would have preferred auscultation (102).

Although auscultation was used to recognize significant accelerations and decelerations during contractions, it missed some decelerations which would have been electronically recorded (100, 264). Thus, some believe it best to use the electronic fetal monitor to detect FHR abnormalities or to apply it when a deceleration is heard to clarify the FHR pattern (100).

EFM detects abnormal FHR patterns better than auscultation. Use of the electronic monitor detected more abnormal FHR patterns than auscultation with a stethoscope. Fetal blood gases were better in the EFM group than the auscultation group. There was no difference in the cesarean section rate or Apgar scores between the groups (91).

Many childbearing families desire a nontechnical birth experience. If the woman is low risk during her labor, auscultation is a reasonable choice for fetal surveillance (following a short admission strip). The careful determination of who should be monitored by electronic means rather than by auscultation is necessary prior to discussion of the use of this technology with the woman and her family.

APGAR SCORES AND ACID-BASE BALANCE

Apgar scores do not rule out the presence of acid-base disturbances, including asphyxia severe enough to cause CP. Low Apgar scores of 7 or less may be related to severe metabolic acidosis, asphyxia, or CP (36, 77, 311-313), but so might high Apgar scores (61, 313). Apgar scores are often lower at 1, 5, and 15 minutes in asphyxiated neonates (312). Yet, even Apgar scores between 0 and 3 at 1 and 5 minutes were only related to CP less than 26% of the time (36). In a prospective study of 1210 women, 19 to 21% of neonates with low 1 and 5 minute Apgar scores and 73% with high Apgar scores had "severe acidosis" (pH less than 7.20, base excess -13 mEq/L) (313). In a retrospective study of 347 women, an abnormal pattern predicted a low 1 minute Apgar 43% of the time and a low 5 minute Apgar 20% of the time (67). In a larger retrospective study of 31,578 neonates, 53.6% with an Apgar score of 3 or less at 5 minutes had a cord artery pH greater than 7.10 (33).

Most studies confirmed that a normal FHR pattern predicted a high 1 minute Apgar more than 90% of the time, but an abnormal FHR predicted a low 1 minute Apgar less than 50% of the time. In a prospective study of 6,825 women, 93.4% of the neonates who had a normal FHR had a high 1 minute Apgar score (314). However, in one study of healthy, term fetuses, the FHR pattern was not related to Apgar scores (315).

An abnormal FHR pattern related to low Apgar scores included a baseline that rose to a level greater than 180 bpm, severe variable decelerations, and/or late decelerations (113).

When the FHR pattern was abnormal for 2 hours or longer, the incidence of a low Apgar score less than 7 was 27% or greater (56). In a 1982 study of low risk and high risk women, an abnormal FHR pattern preceded a low 5 minute Apgar score 99% of the time (316). An abnormal FHR pattern has been a poor predictor of low Apgar scores because Apgar scores are affected by how well physicians and/or nurses resuscitate the newborn (56, 64). Neonatal sepsis, trauma, maternal drugs, or an anomaly, not acidosis or asphyxia, may also contribute to low Apgar scores (32, 36).

The finding that abnormal patterns preceded a low 5 minute Apgar most of the time has not been supported by research (316). For example, an abnormal FHR pattern preceded a low 1 minute Apgar score in only 27.4% of neonates with only 35.2% needing positive pressure ventilation (314). In another study, fetuses diagnosed as having fetal distress were delivered by cesarean section, but only 25% had low 1 and 5 minute scores (106). Other researchers found only 47% of fetuses delivered by cesarean due to an abnormal FHR pattern had a low 1 minute Apgar score (314).

The Apgar score in intubated neonates is a poor guide to the presence or absence of acidosis. Fifty-seven percent of neonates who were 32 or more weeks of gestation who were intubated during the first minute or two of extrauterine life had a normal FHR pattern and/or were not acidotic (317). Since the FHR pattern did not predict the need for intubation in 43% of cases, it is best to be ready to resuscitate all neonates. Neonates may need to be intubated due to the presence of thick meconium in the amniotic fluid or following a traumatic birth, a tight nuchal cord, or a cesarean section. Low birth weight, low scalp pH, acidosis, NICU admissions, seizures, an abnormal electroencephalogram, an abnormal intracranial ultrasound, and spastic diplegia or hemiplegia were related to an abnormal FHR pattern (317).

The relationship between FHR patterns and Apgar scores is similar between term and preterm fetuses. In the preterm fetus, normal FHR patterns near the time of delivery predicted a high five minute Apgar score well. Abnormal FHR patterns near the time of delivery predicted a low five minute Apgar scores poorly (318-319). If the last 30 minutes of the FHR pattern prior to delivery of a preterm neonate (26 to 30 weeks' gestation) was "normal," the 5 minute Apgar score was high and there was a normal umbilical vein pH (318). If, on the other hand, the pattern was abnormal, e.g. tachycardic, no accelerations, and variable or late decelerations, approximately 52% had low 5 minute scores.

Low birth weight was related to the Apgar score more so than gestational age (317). In addition, the method of monitoring was related to the Apgar score. Continuous EFM of the very low birth weight infant predicted the five minute Apgar score and arterial pH better than auscultation (319).

FETAL ASSESSMENT PRACTICE IMPLICATIONS
Accountability
Accountability is being responsible and answerable for actions or inactions of oneself and others (320). To know

which actions are necessary, proper interpretation of FHR and UA data is required. EFM requires the user to know the paper speed to avoid misinterpretation. Times of the EFM record should be correct. The FHR and UA patterns should be systematically evaluated and documented (321-322).

In 1997, AWHONN recommended that the application of the FHR monitor, auscultation of the FHR, and/or the initial and ongoing assessments of maternal-fetal status, including auscultaton and FHR pattern interpretation, should not be delegated to unlicensed assistive personnel (320). Should the nurse choose to delegate tasks, the nurse will be legally responsible for that delegation (323).

Anyone who monitors a pregnant women needs to know how to operate and maintain the equipment and interpret the FHR tracing (324-325). Physician and nurses who use fetal monitors are responsible for understanding the significance of FHR patterns, physiology of the patterns, and the mechanics of the fetal monitor. They need to be able to offer a reasonable interpretation of the pattern and their plan of action.

Nurses are as liable as residents and attending physicians in their evaluation and interpretation of FHR tracings (326). Nurses and physicians are responsible for assessment and interpretation of the fetal and/or maternal status. Nurses must be capable of taking appropriate actions, monitoring and using oxytocin properly, completing an initial history and physical including risk status, and communicating changes in the woman's or fetus' condition. Their documentation should be "adequate" as should the provision of informed consent (327-328). The physician should write the plan in the record. The nurse should record actions in the nurses' notes or on a flow sheet (32). If a nurse writes on the tracing it must be retained. Some nurses use the tracing for notations when situations are rapidly unfolding. They may use the mark button on the fetal monitor to denote the time of events which will later be transcribed into their nursing notes (322).

Risk reduction related to EFM includes
- common EFM language in communications and documentation
- joint nurse-physician EFM education
- competence, collaboration, and mutual respect
- a clear definition of fetal well-being
- admission and ongoing assessments of fetal status and the maternal heart rate
- use of intrauterine resuscitation measures
- appropriate FHR and UA monitoring with EFM
- accurate FHR and UA interpretation
- support for timely interventions when there are nonreassuring FHR patterns
- neonatal resuscitation team at the birth if fetal compromise is suspected and
- interdisciplinary case reviews for potential and actual adverse outcomes (329-330).

Education
Fetal monitors were sold to hospitals in 1968 when there were no universally accepted classification of FHR changes and few references to guide health care providers or educators in the

use of electronic fetal monitors or interpretation of the tracing (55). Naturally, problems arose regarding education and interpretation. By 1986, there still was no sanctioned nomenclature, minimal interpretation standards, standardized certification test, uniform education curriculum, or authority to define minimal standards of application, interpretation, or paper speed (142).

In 1988 in response to the need for EFM nursing education, the Nurse's Association of the American College of Obstetricians and Gynecologists (NAACOG) created and sold the first educational videotape series on EFM which was accompanied by the first edition of *Antepartal and Intrapartal Fetal Monitoring*. In 1992, NAACOG changed their name to the Association of Women's Health, Obstetric, and Neonatal Nurses (AWHONN). In that same year, Dr. Michelle Murray created the first Fetal Monitoring Certification (FMC) course with valid and reliable pretests and post tests (331). Dr. Murray presented the course to over 9000 nurses between 1992 and 2005. Certification attests to a one's ability to demonstrate a distinct knowledge base (326). Once certified, nurses often have increased confidence, competence, credibility, and control which are attributes of high-quality care givers (332).

The 1980s were a time of rapid EFM use, yet there was no requirement that physicians be proficient in EFM use or interpretation (142). Unlike AWHONN, ACOG never created a formal EFM course for physicians. In fact, nurses often attend a fetal monitoring course yearly or biannually but physicians who review EFM tracings as part of their daily clinical practice have never sought the same breath nor depth of education in EFM. The lack of education in EFM may foster conflict between physicians and nurses when there are differences in FHR or UA pattern interpretation. Nurses have reported instances where a physician told them they could not or should not name the deceleration in their documentation. However, it is clear that both nurses and physicians should name the FHR component they see. For example, *Guidelines for Perinatal Care*, a book published by the American Academy of Pediatrics and ACOG states:

> "Terms that describe the fetal heart rate pattern (eg, early, late, or variable decelerations; accelerations; and beat-to-beat variability) should be used in both medical record entries and verbal communication among obstetric personnel" (259, p. 134).

The ability to properly interpret FHR patterns is related to the qualify of EFM education. Only Kinnick and Murray have studied how well nursing students learned basic fetal monitoring concepts from lecture and/or computer-assisted instruction (333-334). How concepts are presented affects the amount of learning that takes place. Murray found that nursing students learned equally well from a computer disk as from a lecture with transparencies which contained identical content (334).

Physicians and nurses are responsible for their EFM competence. It has been recommended that continuing education

opportunities to gain competence must be provided by each institution (335). But, hospital education programs may not exist or may vary in their design and instructor qualifications. Few to no hospital-based educational programs arose from a cognitive psychology theoretical framework, which is imperative to maximize learning of visual images such as FHR patterns (333-334). In addition, the knowledge base and experience of the learner should be considered when preparing EFM courses. McCartney found expert and novice labor and delivery nurses differed in their EFM pattern analysis ability. Experts were better at analyzing the pattern and intervening than novices (336).

Institutions are expected to validate competency in EFM use, yet there is no standardized method to do so (262, 325, 335). "Skills validation" rather than "competency validation" has been the language of choice. Yet, in preparation for competency validation, curricula, prerequisite training, and nomenclature for fetal monitoring interpretation may vary from institution to institution or state to state. Skills that were validated in one institution may not be skills required for validation at another institution. Standardization will most likely never occur as there is no national or international authority that standardizes practice or education in EFM (337).

Education can be a risk management strategy. Many concerned and skilled individuals have worked to provide excellent learning experiences for users of fetal monitors. For example, simulators have been created to teach application of spiral electrodes (57). Programs have been developed that use computer-assisted instructional disks, skills checklists, in-house educational courses, written examinations, and tracing assessments. Nurses have also attended annual EFM recredentialing that included review of tracings and a multiple choice test. Monthly one-half hour inservice discussions of cases and strip review have been used for ongoing education (335, 338). Nurses and physicians have attended all day seminars. In Canada, nurses took a pretest, attended a one day workshop, then took a post test after the course and six months later (339). Organizations, such as the Association of Women's Health, Obstetric, and Neonatal Nurses (AWHONN), were concerned about the lack of standardization in EFM education and have developed guidelines for clinical competency, a book and courses for skills validation and fetal monitoring (340-341).

Interpretation

Interpretation is an important nursing and medical function (303, 342). Labor management is partly based on interpretation of the FHR pattern (343). Proper interpretation may be the most reliable determinant of neonatal outcome (45). Following a systematic review of the tracing, nurses might diagnose "potential for fetal compromise," and physicians might diagnose "fetal distress" or "nonreassuring fetal status" (37, 303).

A lack of skill in FHR pattern interpretation may be "legal suicide" (344). In a review of obstetric malpractice cases, 17% of claims were related to a failure or delay in the identification of "fetal distress" (345). Often, an added allegation was delay to deliver by cesarean section. Physicians and nurses have been accused of delaying delivery. Conversely, they have also been accused of unnecessary surgery due to incompetent interpretation (262).

In 1982, Dr. Edward Hon felt an obstetrician's competence to read and understand FHR patterns was of paramount importance but there was a remarkable degree of incompetence in reading FHR patterns. Physicians often disagree among themselves regarding FHR patterns. For example, in the Netherlands 21 experienced obstetricians reviewed 13 fetal monitor tracings. They had good agreement for the baseline, fair agreement for accelerations, and poor agreement for decelerations, baseline variability, and obstetric management (346).

Since the inception of EFM, concern has existed about interpretation ability and management decisions based on that interpretation. Interpretation is subjective and depends on one's ability to recognize FHR and UA patterns. Conflict may arise between physicians and/or nurses when there are differences in interpretation of EFM data (100, 344). For example, junior residents indicated a need for a cesarean section 30% more often than senior residents following their interpretation of 11 FHR patterns. Depending on the pattern, there was only 26 to 80% agreement on the classification of the tracing as nonstressed, slightly stressed, moderately stressed, or severely stressed (116).

Even if auscultation is used instead of EFM, physicians and nurses did not agree on the pattern that would exist based on audiotones. Late decelerations and the lack of baseline variability were missed by more than a third of the nurses and physicians. Marked long-term variability was correctly identified by only 31% of the nurses and physicians (143). In another study, auscultated baseline rates and accelerations with contractions were correctly identified 84 to 97% of the time. But, auscultation could not be used to evaluate variability or confirm whether or not an acceleration was "reactive" (307). In a lab simulation, registered nurses and second to fourth year residents listened to six tracings that lasted three minutes. They significantly underestimated the baseline, had considerable interobserver variation, and could not reliably assess variability (347).

Standards of Care

The standard of care reflects a consensus as to what the average, reasonable practicing physician or nurse would do in a similar circumstance (348-349). Physicians and nurses are held to their prevailing standards of care and they have a duty to be aware of hospital systems, protocols, and to use their best judgment (19, 80, 350). They must possess a reasonable degree of skill and learning commonly possessed and exercised by others who are of the same school and who practice in a similar situation (80).

To determine what is "reasonable" one needs to consider the recommended nurse:patient ratio, the needs of the patients, circumstances that may alter what is reasonable, and written sources or case law (258, 349). To meet the standard of care the practice should be safe and appropriate (351). It should be based on the best available research, i.e., evidence-based (352).

The standard of care may vary depending on the presence or absence of a certified nurse midwife or physician in the hospital or the labor setting. Rooks, Weatherby, and Ernst examined the care provided to 17,856 patients of certified nurse midwives between 1985 to 1987. 11,814 were admitted to birth centers where registered nurses, student nurse midwives (SNMs), and certified nurse midwives (CNMs) provided labor support. The majority of the women (78.6%) were supported during their labor by SNMs and CNMs. Obstetricians delivered only 13% of the women. In that setting less then 9% were monitored by EFM if their labor lasted less than 7 hours. Only 10.3% were monitored by EFM when their labor lasted more than 10 hours. A hand-held Doppler was the primary fetal surveillance tool. In a hospital setting where the physician is not "in house," nurses assume a major role in the management of labor (353).

The United States has been moving towards a nationally recognized standard of care versus a state or local standard of care (354). In some situations, the national standards of care will be applied to questions of malpractice (344, 349). Recommended practices have been suggested by organizations such as AWHONN, ACOG, and the Joint Commission on Accreditation of Healthcare Organizations (JCAHO). Regionally, state practice acts and rules and regulations suggest appropriate care. Locally, practice guidelines are defined by hospital documents such as job descriptions, employment manuals, contracts, and handbooks (355). Institutions also provide guidelines, policies, procedures, and/or protocols for health care providers. These should be updated and reviewed on a regular basis (356). When a deviation from the protocol is required, that deviation should be explained in the medical record (355).

Nurses and physicians have a duty to meet the standard of care. If they do not meet the standard of care, they may be found negligent in the performance of that duty (348). An example of duty is the need to monitor the woman and her fetus during labor (357). When EFM is used, nurses are responsible for recognizing and identifying FHR patterns and instituting nursing interventions in an attempt to correct any problems (358). Their assessments should be communicated to the primary care provider which is often the link in the chain of action that facilitates an optimal outcome (359). If the FHR tracing suggests a compromised fetus who requires medical attention, immediate nursing intervention is necessary and the physician must be notified (360). Failure to communicate may cause harm which may precede litigation. For example, when the nurse failed to request the presence of the attending physician at the bedside of a woman who was induced and who had an abnormal FHR pattern 90 minutes after admission, there was a delay to perform a cesarean section that resulted in a child who has CP and a $30 million jury verdict (361).

Registered nurses share responsibility with physicians in the care of patients (362). However, the nurse usually functions as the patient's advocate (358, 363). When the physician or certified nurse midwife do not agree with the nurse's actions, the nurse is responsible for implementation of the conflict resolution procedure and following the chain of command to protect the patient from harm. The charge nurse, supervisor, or team leader should be called to assist the nurse in promoting safe patient care (364).

Some believe liability is reduced when EFM is used instead of auscultation (365). However, EFM may not be the standard of care for all patients (366). For example, if the physician orders the nurse to auscultate the low risk woman's FHR after an admission strip demonstrating fetal well-being has been obtained, and staffing permits a one-to-one nurse/woman ratio, the nurse should follow the physician's order and auscultate the FHR until a need arises for EFM.

If EFM is chosen for fetal surveillance, the standard in the United States, confirmed by the Supreme Court of Alabama, is that the monitor paper printout speed should be set at 3 cm/minute (37, 102, 367). A setting at a slower rate, such as 1 cm or 2 cm/minute would be a violation of that standard in the United States.

AWHONN and ACOG have suggested practices regarding EFM (240, 258, 319, 368). For example, the intrapartum nurse may:

1. monitor the FHR and its characteristics at specified intervals by selected methods and document findings using appropriate terminology
2. monitor UA patterns using palpation and/or the electronic fetal monitor
3. apply the spiral electrode and/or intrauterine pressure catheter in accordance with nurse practice acts, institutional policy, and medical orders
4. recognize normal and abnormal FHRs or nonreassuring characteristics and promptly initiate appropriate nursing interventions, and
5. recognize normal and abnormal UA and intervene accordingly (240).

Appropriate terminology may vary depending on definitions adopted by the user or the institution. In 1997, the NICHD Research Planning Workshop published recommendations for definitions of FHR concepts for research purposes (369-370). When a registered nurse, certified nurse midwife, obstetrician, and maternal-fetal faculty member used their terminology to evaluate a one hour tracing, there was no improvement in agreement on most FHR features beyond those expected by chance or that noted in previous reports (371).

An additional standard of care is to assess the woman's comfort level and pain tolerance. To promote comfort, it may be helpful to move the transducer belts at least every two hours or wash the abdomen with warm water to remove any dry coupling (ultrasonic) gel. To increase comfort, the woman's position might be changed every half hour, she should try to urinate at least every two hours, and she may eat ice chips or take small sips of water or clear liquids during labor.

The current standard of care requires frequent monitoring of the FHR prior to delivery. As many as 50% of injuries occurred just prior to delivery (372-373). In a study of 277

women who had a cesarean section, researchers found that 92 were at risk from unexpected worsening of the fetal condition in the operating room (374). To be more aware of the fetal condition in that situation, fetal surveillance with the external ultrasound transducer should continue until the abdominal sterile preparation has begun. If a spiral electrode is on the fetus, it should be removed after the abdominal sterile preparation is completed (259).

Nurses have a duty to foresee harm and act to allay harm (375). There should be timely and proper fetal evaluations (376). By frequently using a systematic approach to tracing review, harm should be prevented. When the nurse or physician identify signs of fetal compromise, the standard of care requires nonsupine positioning, such as a lateral position. An intravenous bolus of a nonglucose containing solution, such as Lactated Ringers, might be infused to decrease uterine activity. Oxygen may be administered at 8 or more liters per minute by a tight-fitting face mask (37, 368). No specific written order is needed for these actions. In fact, the nurse usually initiates actions based on the identified FHR pattern then notifies the physician. The nurse should then evaluate the fetal response. Oxygen should reach the fetus between one to nine minutes after its initiation (54, 377-378). Depending on the pattern, oxytocin may be decreased or discontinued. Tocolytics, such as 0.25 mg of terbutaline given subcutaneously or intravenously, may be ordered to reduce uterine hypercontractility not caused by an abruption. When actions are taken for a nonreassuring pattern, EFM should be continued (379-380).

Prompt communication of changes in the maternal or fetal status is an imperative aspect of the nurse's role. When the nurse contacts the physician, the FHR pattern and all actions taken should be communicated (381). Should they not agree with the nurse's interpretation of the FHR pattern, not respond as expected, or not respond in a timely manner, a policy should exist to resolve this conflict (258, 325, 383). The nurse should document the provider's failure to respond and take actions for the best interest of the patient (376).

Informed Consent

External monitoring is not an invasive medical procedure that requires a formal, written informed consent. However, prior to use the woman should be aware of the purpose of EFM and consent to its use. Her well-informed decisions may be the best defense in future litigation (383). An informed consent discussion includes four factors:

- the proposed intervention
- risks and benefits of the proposed intervention
- treatment alternatives
- risks if there is no intervention (384).

Informed consent should also include a discussion of the woman's wishes and her concerns and questions. To avoid confusion regarding intrapartal EFM use, it is best to discuss fetal surveillance techniques during the course of prenatal care and again upon admission to the labor suite (80).

If the woman refuses EFM for an admission test, the physician should be immediately informed. Although legal precedents have been set in which the fetal rights superseded maternal rights, in the majority of cases the maternal right to informed consent and her rights related to her own body superseded fetal rights (161). If a waiver (an Against Medical Advice (AMA) form) was signed, the nurses and physicians could still be held liable for negligence if the infant is believed to be injured before or after birth. The AMA form does not protect physicians and nurses from being accused of negligence or malpractice. Therefore, it is best to document the informed consent discussion with the woman's quoted verbal response if she refused EFM.

An informed consent discussion prior to EFM of either low or high risk women might be: "I would like to place the electronic fetal monitor on your abdomen to obtain information about your baby's heart rate and your contractions. This will not cause harm to you or your baby. If I do not use this device, I will need to use a (hand-held ultrasound, stethoscope, fetoscope, or Pinard device) to listen to your baby's heartbeat and feel your uterus when it contracts. Since you just arrived, using this electronic fetal monitor will help me see if anything is affecting oxygen levels in your baby. I will also be able to see what your baby's heartbeat does when you have a contraction. Once I determine your baby is well, I will take the monitor off and use the (auscultation device) to monitor your baby. If I hear a drop in the baby's heart rate, I will need to put the monitor back on for a while to see exactly what is happening during your contractions. Do you have any questions? Is this acceptable to you?"

Some believe all high risk patients require EFM rather than auscultation. It has been recommended that if EFM is not used, the reasons should be documented after discussion with the woman (32). The option of auscultation and palpation should not be encouraged if one-to-one care cannot be provided (80). Silence may violate one's duty to the patient. Therefore, the nurse should disclose relevant facts which affect the woman's condition (372). In this case, the woman should be told why auscultation may not be possible throughout her entire labor.

Documentation

Documentation, whether on the tracing, in the computer, or in the medical record, reflects the standard of care provided. If the tracing will be saved on computer disk, anything written by hand on the paper printout will not be saved on the disk. If there are hand-written notations on the tracing, it is wise to store and eventually microfilm the tracing. Some hospitals shred the tracing if there are no hand-written entries and it is stored on disk (385). However, prior to shredding, it is essential to confirm the entire strip is stored on the disk. It has been recommended that "if electronic fetal monitoring is used, all fetal heart tracings should be identified with the patient's name, hospital number, and the date and time of admission. All fetal heart rate tracings should be easily retrievable from storage so that the events of labor can be studied in proper relationship to the tracings" (259, p. 134).

During monitoring, times should appear on the tracing, as well as events related to her care (368, 382). Ensure the time printed by the fetal monitor is accurate. It helps medical records' personnel who need to microfilm the tracing if the tracing parts are numbered as #1, #2, #3, etc., as tracings are collected.

Additional items that may be documented on the tracing include the woman's expected date of delivery (EDD), delivery time with infant gender and Apgar scores, physician's name(s), high risk condition(s), purpose of monitoring, e.g., NST, status of membranes, and time and type of rupture of membranes, i.e., spontaneous or artificial, with the color, amount, and odor of the fluid (240). The FHR should be assessed and recorded immediately following rupture of membranes. Maternal movement may be recorded on the tracing, e.g. left side, to bathroom. Scalp or acoustic stimulation and vaginal examinations may be recorded on the tracing. Other interventions that might affect the FHR or UA tracing may be recorded on the tracing. This assists the reader in relating the FHR and UA to events. A continuous tracing then becomes a self-contained story. Without the delivery data, e.g. time of delivery, infant gender, cord gases and Apgar scores, the story has no ending until the chart is read. There is no doubt that nurses will double chart at times. All entries on the tracing should appear in the nurse's notes and/or on the flow sheet.

Nurses are responsible for the quality of the tracing (342). If it is unclear, it is the responsibility of the nurse to institute measures to gain a clear tracing. For example, coupling gel may need to be reapplied to the ultrasound transducer or the ultrasound transducer may need repositioning. In some cases, a spiral electrode must be applied to the fetal presenting part, especially when the woman is obese. Some have suggested that a difficult to read tracing may be a greater legal hazard than no recording at all (386). If the tracing is inadequate, it may be helpful to perform a manual test of the fetal monitor to assess the printer quality or test the transducers. In the event equipment problems cannot be resolved, the FHR may need to be auscultated and/or the abdomen palpated for uterine activity until new equipment can be obtained.

In 1990, Pat McMullen, a practicing attorney and faculty member in a school of nursing, suggested that a nurse should press the fetal monitor's "mark" button and write their initials on the strip to serve as evidence that the nurse evaluated the client at regular intervals (328). Since initials could be added to a strip after delivery, they usually do not prove the nurse or physician actually analyzed the FHR or UA at that time (373). Better documentation than initials would be timely entries in the nursing or progress notes.

If the woman is preterm, the hospital fetal monitor tocotransducer may not detect UA accurately as it is rare to find a tocotransducer for preterm gestations in the hospital setting. Therefore, it is important to palpate uterine contractions and record the woman's subjective complaints such as groin aches, intermittent low backache, or cramps. The strength of palpated contractions is usually recorded as mild, moderate, or strong. Relaxation or resting tone between contractions might be documented as soft or firm between contractions (240).

The tracing should be saved as long as the law requires. Both the discovery period and the statute of limitations help define this time frame. For example, state statutes of limitations define periods during which specified types of legal actions must be filed with the court (387). The period of discovery is the time frame within which the injury must be discovered. Consult with the hospital risk manager or attorney to determine how long records should be saved. In some cases, physicians and nurses may be sued up to 21 years after the birth (388).

The strip does not "stand alone." Evidence the FHR was assessed and the type of monitoring used should be documented (37, 382, 389). The auscultated FHR when a fetoscope is used might be documented as, "FHR 150 bpm by fetoscope, regular rhythm, accelerated to 170 bpm between contractions, no decreases in the FHR heard." Documentation should also include signs of the lack of hypoxia and acidemia such as accelerations that have occurred since the last FHR assessment and reports of fetal movement or palpated fetal movement. If the electronic fetal monitor is used, document if the tracing is lost, the acceleration will confirm fetal well-being at that time. Since tracings may be lost, it may be best to document the baseline rate as a range, e.g. 132-136 bpm. If only one number is recorded, the reader might assume the baseline was flat. Documentation of baseline variability may include long-term variability and/or short-term variability. If decelerations are present, it is best to name the type of deceleration(s). There are 2 types of accelerations (uniform and spontaneous) and 5 types of decelerations (early, variable, late, prolonged, and spontaneous). When variable decelerations are observed, it is more descriptive to describe their duration and depth (nadir), e.g., variable decelerations x 40-60 seconds to 70 to 90 bpm. The size of the variable deceleration has more predictive value than the recovery time. However, some entries may describe the recovery as prompt or slow (389). Because their physiology is clear, usually the duration, depth, and recovery times of early, late, and spontaneous decelerations are not described. Because prolonged decelerations last 2 to 10 minutes, their duration and depth is usually documented. In addition to the FHR pattern, UA assessments such as the frequency, duration, and strength of contractions or uterine irritability (low amplitude, high frequency waves) should be recorded, especially when decelerations are observed. If the tracing is lost, comprehensive documentation reflecting the visualized patterns of the FHR and UA will help the reader better visualize the frequency of decelerations that occurred with contractions (periodic decelerations). Documenting of a systematic review of the tracing is critical if, in the future, the tracing is missing and the experts in the case have to recreate the tracing using blank fetal monitor paper.

Document procedures done to confirm fetal status such as scalp blood pH determinations, acoustic or scalp stimulation, and if the FHR accelerated following the procedure. If the heart rate accelerated, describe its size. If there was no response, note the lack of an acceleration. If the FHR pattern suggested hypoxia or acidosis, document actions to improve fetal oxygenation, and the content of communications with the CNM or physician. Document the FHR and uterine response following actions.

"The chart is a witness that never dies and never lies" (327). It is a "witness" of medical care and the nursing process. It is believed that the nurses' notes, not the tracing, provide the most reliable record of nursing care (390). Documentation is a written form of communication. It provides evidence of assessments, actions, communications, and patient responses. Nurses often document in narrative notes, flow sheets, and other medical records forms. Assessments, actions, maternal and fetal responses to actions, and diagnostic procedures are usually documented soon after they occur. Nurses are accountable for documenting FHR and contraction data and their actions when changes in the FHR occur (310). However, sometimes assessments and actions cannot be documented in a timely manner due to patient care needs. Some entries are delayed until patient care needs are met (37, 382). Ideally, these late entries should be written as close to the event as possible (376). If late entries are written, they should be designated as a "late entry," and the date and time of the late entry should be written prior to specifying the time of the events being documented. Never backdate, tamper with, or add to notes that were previously written (391).

A modified form of charting by exception accompanied by care pathways has been created to decrease nursing documentation in a LDRP (labor-delivery-recovery-post partum) setting (372, 392). Pure charting by exception is not a good idea since only abnormalities are recorded in narrative notes. If abnormalities are recorded in narrative notes, flow sheets or computer annotations or notes should be used to record FHR pattern assessments, actions, and responses to actions. If this is done, the reader should be able to visualize labor and delivery assessments, interventions, communications, actions, and evaluations from admission through delivery.

Communication is a critical aspect of patient care. Policies, procedures, and/or protocols should guide nurses as to when, how, and to whom to communicate, reducing the risk of failure to communicate or miscommunication (303). To enhance the clarity of the communication, computers may be used to compose, deliver, and process messages or store EFM data on disk (393). Since EFM uses a visual medium, the tracing, the best communication of the images seen requires transmittal of the picture versus a verbal description. Tracings have been transmitted via the telephone lines as facsimiles (FAX) or physicians have accessed the images using a modem (394-395). Hospitals should not expect to save money once computers are installed at the bedside (392).

In 1990 and even 2002, there was no final determination of the legal status of computer-archived FHR records existed as they were close facsimiles but not exact copies (396). In 1995, ACOG suggested that computer storage of FHR patterns on laser disks which do not permit overwriting or revision was a reasonable way to store fetal monitor records (21).

It is also reasonable and the standard of care to run the paper during patient care. Images on the fetal monitor paper may be held in one's hands to enhance interpretation or they may be brought to different healthcare providers for a second opinion. Sometimes it helps to turn the image upside down to differentiate uniform from spontaneous accelerations. It may be helpful to hold the tracing in one hand and pull it up towards the shoulder to visualize subtle late decelerations. To go "paperless" at the bedside and rely only on a computer monitor for tracing analysis has not been tested scientifically but it probably diminishes the quality of interpretation. Since there is no research that shows it is safe or reasonable to go "paperless" at the bedside, it would not be evidence-base practice to not run the paper during care and should be discouraged.

CONCLUSION

EFM is a surveillance tool that may be used to predict fetal well-being, fetal death, or suggest the presence of hypoxemia, hypoxia, acidosis, and/or asphyxia. However, neither EFM or auscultation are used to predict CP or reduce the indicence of CP. EFM is better than auscultation for the detection of FHR variability, late decelerations, and abnormalities that might be called fetal distress. EFM use also precedes fewer perinatal deaths and neonatal seizures than auscultation.

The majority of fetuses with an abnormal FHR pattern will have high Apgar scores, partly because of excellent resuscitation. Apgar scores do not rule out the presence or absence of acidosis, asphyxia, or the later development of CP related to intrapartal asphyxia. When an abnormal FHR pattern is observed, additional data is needed to rule out fetal acidemia, such as obtaining a scalp pH. Accelerations can be evoked by acoustic stimulation, scalp stimulation, or the spiral electrode. If acoustic or scalp stimulation is used to rule out acidosis, as many as 50% of fetuses will not respond to the stimuli but only 34% of the nonresponders will be acidemic.

As of 2001, there were 12 randomized controlled trials of EFM versus auscultation during labor (86-95, 244, 277, 268). In these studies, little attention was paid to the research design, patient population, EFM interpretation skills of those who analyzed and classified the tracings, the type of fetal monitor used, having a consistent assessment time or duration for auscultation, or the clinical management of patterns (45, 263). Eight studies had small samples, no power analysis, or changed their power analysis prior to publication which limits the applicability of their findings for generalization to other groups of women. In spite of these limitations, researchers suggested that EFM was related to more cesarean sections, forceps, and vacuum extractions, but acknowledged that fetal death was significantly less in the EFM group versus the auscultated group (263).

It is clear that EFM in and of itself does not increase the risk of cesarean section or operative delivery.

Dystocia remains the most common reason for a cesarean section. The decisions of physicians, the availability of nurses, and the demands of women may impact the cesarean section rate. Adjunct technology, such as CALM™ or ST analysis may enhance physician decision-making and decrease the cesarean section rate.

Research is lacking that supports the continuous use of EFM in women whose fetus is nonacidotic and "low risk" based on the admission strip. However, even a tracing of a fetus that demonstrates a nonhypoxic fetus on admission has limited predictive value. Somewhere between two and five hours after admission, the fetus should again be monitored electronically to demonstate a reactive tracing and confirm continued fetal well-being. Whether or not auscultation or EFM is the chosen monitoring method, standards of care should guide practice. Nurses and physicians should know their profession's standards and are accountable for protecting their patients from harm.

Interpretation of FHR and UA patterns is an acquired and learned skill. EFM is not a substitute for hands-on patient care or close surveillance of the mother and her unborn baby (356). Should injury occur, either by omission (the nurse or physician knew what to do and did not do it) or by commission (the performed action was not the appropriate action in that situation) and proximate cause can be demonstrated, the nurse, CNM, physician, and/or hospital may be held liable for negligence and malpractice.

Continuous emotional support during labor has been associated with better maternal and neonatal outcomes (5, 397-398). Nurses should encourage physical and emotional support by significant others. In some hospitals, birth attendants (doulas) stay with the woman throughout the labor. It is the nurse, CNM, and physician at the bedside, not the use of an electronic monitor that can prevent fetal death (103). EFM is not a substitute for certified nurse midwives or labor nurses (8, 356). It has been suggested that money should be spent on training good midwives as "personal monitors" rather than on electronic fetal monitors or other machines (6). Health care providers should continue to provide supportive and comprehensive care to the woman and her family, rather than appear to focus primarily on fetal surveillance and information gathering (146). Rather than looking first at the fetal monitor after entering the room, perhaps nurses and physicians should look at the woman and her family instead (399).

Lastly, EFM can be a useful tool when the user is able to properly interpret FHR and UA patterns, acts to clarify the meaning of nonreassuring patterns, and takes an active role in the prevention of fetal and neonatal injury related to metabolic acidosis and asphyxia. Since there is yet no research that interpretation using a computer monitor screen is equivalent to interpretation of the tracing printed on fetal monitor paper, paper should be run at the bedside until evidence exists to go "paperless."

References

1. Beard, R. W., & Rivers, R. P. A. (November 24, 1979). Fetal asphyxia in labour. *Lancet, 2*(8152), 1117-1119.

2. Freeman, R. K. (October 2002). Problems with intrapartum fetal heart rate monitoring interpretation and patient management. *Obstetrics and Gynecology, 100*(4), 813-826.

3. Paul, R. H. (1994). Electronic fetal monitoring and later outcome: A thirty-year overview. *Journal of Perinatology, 14*(5), 393-395.

4. Sandmire, H. F. (December 1990). Whither electronic fetal monitoring? *Obstetrics & Gynecology, 76*(6), 1130-1134.

5. Sosa, R., Kennell, J., Klaus, M., Robertson, S., & Urrutia, J. (September 11, 1980). The effect of a supportive companion on perinatal problems, length of labor, and mother-infant interaction. *The New England Journal of Medicine, 303*(11), 597-600.

6. Spencer, J. A. D. (June 1994). Electronic fetal monitoring in the United Kingdom. *Birth, 21*(2), 106-108.

7. MacDonald, D., Grant, A., Sheridan-Pereira, M., Boylan, P., & Chalmers, I. (July 1, 1985). The Dublin randomized controlled trial of intrapartum fetal heart rate monitoring. *American Journal of Obstetrics and Gynecology, 152*(5), 524-539.

8. Neilson, J. P. (June 1994). Round table discussion: Controversies in electronic fetal monitoring. Electronic fetal heart rate monitoring during labor: Information from randomized trials. *Birth, 21* (2), 101-104.

9. Cetrulo, C. L., & Schifrin, B. S. (November 1976). Fetal heart rate patterns preceding death. *Obstetrics and Gynecology, 48*(5), 521-527.

10. Gabbe, S. G. (September 1996). The electronic evaluation of the fetal heart rate. Preliminary report. 1958. *American Journal of Obstetrics and Gynecology, 175*(3, Pt. 1), 747-748.

11. Redman, C. W. G. (March 1993). Communicating the significance of the fetal heart rate record to the user. *British Journal of Obstetrics and Gynaecology, 100*(Suppl. 9), 24-27.

12. Painter, M. J., Scott, M., Hirsch, R. P., O'Donoghue, P., & Depp, R. (October 1988). Fetal heart rate patterns during labor: Neurologic and cognitive development at six to nine years of age. *American Journal of Obstetrics and Gynecology, 159*(4), 854-858.

13. Jongsma, H. W., & Nijhuis, J. G. (1991). Critical analysis of the validity of electronic fetal monitoring. *Journal of Perinatal Medicine, 19*(1-2), 33-37.

14. Zuspan, F. P., Quilligan, E. J., Iams, J. D., & van Geijn, H. P. (December 1979). NICHD consensus development task force report: Predictors of intrapartum fetal distress-the role of electronic fetal monitoring. *The Journal of Pediatrics, 95*(6), 1026-1030.

15. Depp, R. (March 1995). Perinatal asphyxia: Assessing its causal role and timing. *Seminars in Pediatric Neurology, 2*(1), 3-36.

16. Ellison, P. H., Foster, M., Sheridan-Pereira, M., & MacDonald, D. (May 1991). Electronic fetal heart monitoring, auscultation and neonatal outcome. *American Journal of Obstetrics and Gynecology, 14*(5, Pt. 1), 1281-1289.

17. Nelson, K. B., Dambrosia, J. M., Ting, T. Y., & Grether, J. K. (March 7, 1996). Uncertain value of electronic fetal monitoring in predicting cerebral palsy. *The New England Journal of Medicine, 334*(10), 613-618.

18. van Geign, H. P. (June 1996). Developments in CTG analysis. *Baillière's Clinical Obstetrics and Gynecology, 10*(2), 185-209.

19. American College of Obstetricians and Gynecologists. (September 1988). Risk management in the hospital setting. *The Assistant*, Washington, DC: author.

20. Parer, J. T., & King, T. (April 2000). Fetal heart rate monitoring. Is it salvageable? *American Journal of Obstetrics and Gynecology, 182*(4), 982-987.

21. Low, J. A., Killen, H., & Derrick, E. J. (February 2002). The prediction and prevention of intrapartum fetal asphyxia in preterm pregnancies. *American Journal of Obstetrics and Gynecology, 186*(2), 279-282.

22. Henderson-Smart, D. (May 6, 1991). Throwing the baby out with the fetal monitoring? Obstetric care, birth asphyxia and brain damage. *Medical Journal of Australia, 154*(9), 576-578.

23. Koh, K. S., Greves, D., Yung, S., & Peddle, L. J. (February 1975). Experience with fetal monitoring in a university teaching hospital. *Canadian Medical Association Journal, 112*(4), 455-456, 459-460.

24. Foley, M. (2000, January 26). *Written testimoney of the American Nurses Association before the senate committee on health, education, labor and pensions on medical errors*. Washington, DC: The Association. Retrieved from http://www.nursingworld.org/gova/federal/legis/testimon/2000/mf0126/htm.

25. Gennaro, S., Hodnett, E., & Kearney, M. (September/October 2001). Making evidence-based practice a reality in your institution. Evaluating the evidence and using the evidence to change clinical practice. *MCN, 26*(5), 236-245.

26. Niswander, K., Henson, G., Elbourne, D., Chalmers, I., Redman, C., MacFarlane, A., & Tizard, P. (October 13, 1984). Adverse outcome of pregnancy and the quality of obstetric care. *The Lancet, 8407,* 827-831.

27. Minchom, P., Niswander, K., Chalmers, I., Dauncey, M., Newcombe, R., Elbourne, D., et al. (May 1987). Antecedents and outcome of very early neonatal seizures in infants born at or after term. *British Journal of Obstetrics and Gynaecology, 94*(5), 431-439.

28. Gaffney, G., Sellers, S., Flavell, V., Squier, M., & Johnson, A. (March 19, 1994). Case-study of intrapartum care, cerebral palsy, and perinatal death. *British Medical Journal, 308*(6931), 743-750.

29. Kline, C., Watts, D. H., & Krieger, J. (January 1999). Modified obstetrics care factors associated with infant mortality. *American Journal of Obstetrics and Gynecology, 180*(1, Pt. 2), S66. Abstract No. 202.

30. de Swiet, M. (April 2000). Maternal mortality: Confidential enquiries into maternal deaths in the United Kingdom. *American Journal of Obstetrics and Gynecology, 182*(4), 760-766.

31. Low, J. A., Karchmar, J., Broekhoven, L., Leonard, T., McGrath, M. J., Pancham, S. R., & Piercy, W. N. (December 15, 1981). The probability of fetal metabolic acidosis during labor in a population at risk as determined by clinical factors. *American Journal of Obstetrics and Gynecology, 141*(8), 941-951.

32. Schifrin, B. S., Weissman, H., & Wiley, J. (June 1985). Electronic fetal monitoring and obstetrical malpractice. *Law, Medicine & Health Care,* 100-105.

33. Socol, M. L., Garcia, P. M., & Riter, S. (April 1994). Depressed Apgar scores, acid-base status, and neurologic outcome. *American Journal of Obstetrics and Gynecology, 170*(4), 991-999.

34. Low, J. A., Pancham, S. R., & Worthington, D. N. (April 1, 1977). Intrapartum fetal heart rate profiles with and without fetal asphyxia. *American Journal of Obstetrics and Gynecology, 127*(7), 729-737.

35. Schifrin, B. S. (April 1992). Details of electronic fetal monitoring randomized control trials [Letter to the editor]. *American Journal of Obstetrics and Gynecology, 166*(4), 1308-1309.

36. Hankins, G. D. V. (February 15, 1991). Apgar scores: Are they enough? *Contemporary OB/GYN, 36.* 13-25.

37. American College of Obstetricians and Gynecologists. (July 1995). Fetal heart rate patterns: Monitoring, interpretation, and management. *ACOG Technical bulletin number 207.* Washington DC: author.

38. American College of Obstetricians and Gynecologists. (January 1992). Fetal and neonatal neurologic injury. *ACOG Technical bulletin number 163.* Washington, DC: ACOG.

39. American College of Obstetricians and Gynecologists. (April 1994). Fetal distress and birth asphyxia. *ACOG Committee Opinion Number 137.* Washington, DC: ACOG.

40. American College of Obstetricians and Gynecologists. (June 1975). Fetal heart rate monitoring. *ACOG Technical bulletin number 32.* Washington, DC: ACOG.

41. Druzin, M. L., Fox, A., Kogut, E., & Carlson, C. (October 15, 1985). The relationship of the nonstress test to gestational age. *American Journal of Obstetrics and Gynecology, 153*(4), 386-389.

42. Eganhouse, D. J., & Burnside, S. M. (September/October 1992). Nursing assessment and responsibilities in monitoring the preterm pregnancy. *JOGNN, 21*(5), 355-363.

43. Shields, J. R., & Schifrin, B. S. (June 1988). Perinatal antecedents of cerebral palsy. *Obstetrics & Gynecology, 71*(6), 899-905.

44. Rosen, M. G., & Dickinson, J. C. (March 1993). The paradox of electronic fetal monitoring: More data may not enable us to predict or prevent infant neurologic morbidity [Review]. *American Journal of Obstetrics and Gynecology, 168*(3, Pt.1), 745-751.

45. Schifrin, B. S. (September/October 1994). The ABCs of electronic fetal monitoring. *Journal of Perinatology, 14*(5), 396-402.

46. Low, J. A., Cox, M. J., Karchmar, E. J., McGarth, M. J., Pancham, S. R., & Piercy, W. N. (February 1, 1981). The prediction of intrapartum fetal metabolic acidosis by fetal heart rate monitoring. *American Journal of Obstetrics and Gynecology, 139*(3), 299-305.

47. Painter, M. J., Depp, R., & O'Donoghue, P. D. (October 1, 1978). Fetal heart rate patterns and development in the first year of life. *American Journal of Obstetrics and Gynecology, 132*(3), 271-277.

48. Nelson, K. B. (1989). Relationships of intrapartum and delivery room events to long-term neurologic outcome. *Clinics in Perinatology, 16*(4), 995-1007.

49. Espinosa, M. I., & Parer, J. T. (June 1991). Mechanism of asphyxiated brain damage, and possible pharmacologic interventions, in the fetus. *American Journal of Obstetrics and Gynecology, 164*(6, Pt. 1), 1582-1591.

50. Parer, J. T. (June 1986). Roundtable: Part 1. The Dublin trial of fetal heart rate monitoring: The final word? *Birth, 13*(2), 119-121.

51. Evenhouse, R., & McConathy, D. (Winter 1989). Development and construction of a fetal monitoring simulator. *The Journal of Biocommunication, 16*(1), 2-9.

52. Tejani, N., Mann, L. I., Bhakthavathsalan, A., & Weiss, R. R. (October 1975). Correlation of fetal heart rate-uterine contraction patterns with fetal scalp blood pH. *Obstetrics & Gynecology, 46*(4), 392-396.

53. Lumley, J. (October 1988). Does continuous intrapartum fetal monitoring predict long-term neurologic disorders? *Paediatric and Perinatal Epidemiology, 2*(4), 299-307.

54. Shy, K. K., Luthy, D. A., Bennett, F. C., Whitfield, M., Larson, E. B., van Belle, G., Hughes, J. P., Wilson, J. A., & Stenchever, M. A. (March 1, 1990). Effects of electronic fetal heart-rate monitoring, as compared with periodic auscultation, on the neurologic development of premature infants. *The New England Journal of Medicine, 322*(9), 588-593.

55. Beard, R. W., Filshie, G. M., Knight, C. A., & Roberts, G. M. (October 1971). The significance of the changes in the continuous fetal heart rate in the first stage of labour. *Journal of the Obstetrics and Gynaecology of the British Commonwealth, 78*(10), 865-881.

56. Fleischer, A., Schulman, H., Jagani, N., Mitchell, J., & Randolph, G. (September 1, 1982). The development of fetal acidosis in the presence of an abnormal fetal heart rate tracing. I. The average for gestational age fetus. *American Journal of Obstetrics and Gynecology, 144*(1), 55-60.

57. Clark, S. L., Gimovsky, M. L., & Miller, F. C. (February 1, 1984). The scalp stimulation test: A clinical alternative to fetal scalp blood sampling. *American Journal of Obstetrics and Gynecology, 148*(3), 274-277.

58. Smith, J. H., Anand, K. J. S., Cotes, P. M., Dawes, G. S., Harkness, R. A., Howlett, T. A., Rees, L. H., & Redman, C. W. G. (October 1988). Antepartal fetal heart rate variation in relation to the respiratory and metabolic status of the compromised human fetus. *British Journal of Obstetrics and Gynaecology, 95*, 980-989.

59. Gilstrap III, L. C. (March 1996). A guest editorial: Distress over fetal distress. *Obstetrical and Gynecological Survey, 51*(3), 143-144.

60. Goodlin, R. C., & Haesslein, H. C. (June 15, 1977). When is it fetal distress? *American Journal of Obstetrics and Gynecology, 128*(4), 440-447.

61. Reece, E. A., Antoine, C., & Montgomery, J. (March 1986). The fetus as the final arbiter of intrauterine stress/distress. *Clinical Obstetrics and Gynecology, 29*(1), 23-32.

62. Parer, J. T., & Livingston, E. G. (June 1990). What is fetal distress? *American Journal of Obstetrics and Gynecology, 162*(6), 1421-1425.

63. Rosen, M. G., & Dickinson, J. C. (March 1993). The paradox of electronic fetal monitoring: More data may not enable us to predict or prevent infant neurologic morbidity. *American Journal of Obstetrics and Gynecology, 168*(3, Pt. 1), 745-751.

64. Schifrin, B. S., & Dame, L. (March 6, 1972). Fetal heart rate patterns. Prediction of Apgar score. *Journal of the American Medical Association (JAMA), 219*(10), 1322-1325.

65. Skyes, G. S., Molloy, P. M., Johnson, P., Stirrat, G. M., & Turnbull, A. C. (October 1, 1983). Fetal distress and the condition of newborn infants. *British Medical Journal, 287*(6397), 943-945.

66. Lawrence, L. (Winter 1992-1993). Fetal heart monitoring with a fetoscope. *Midwifery Today, 24*, 30-37.

67. Low, J. A., Panagiotopoulos, C., & Derrick, E. J. (April 1994). Newborn complications after intrapartum asphyxia with metabolic acidosis in the term fetus. *American Journal of Obstetrics and Gynecology, 170*(4), 1081-1087.

68. Lavin, Jr., J. P., & Miodovnik, M. (December 1981). Delayed abruption after maternal trauma as a result of an automobile accident. *Journal of Reproductive Medicine, 26*(12), 621-624.

69. Chauhan, S., Magann, E., Hendrix, N., Scott, J., Scardo, J., & Martin Jr., J. (December 2002). Cesarean delivery for fetal distress: Review of 392 articles. *American Journal of Obstetrics and Gynecology, 187*(6), S146. Abstract No. 313.

70. Garite, T. J., Dildy, G. A., McNamara, H., Nageotte, M. P., Boehm, F. H., Dellinger, E. H., et al. (November 2000). A multicenter controlled trial of fetal pulse oximetry in the intrapartum management of nonreassuring fetal heart rate patterns. *American Journal of Obstetrics and Gynecology, 183*(5), 1049-1058.

71. Clark, S. L., & Paul, R. H. (December 1, 1985). Intrapartum fetal surveillance: The role of fetal scalp blood sampling. *American Journal of Obstetrics and Gynecolog,. 153*(7), 717-720.

72. Skupski, D. W., Rosenberg, C. R., & Eglinton, G. S. (January 2002). Intrapartum fetal stimulation tests: A meta-analysis. *Obstetrics and Gynecology, 99*(1), 129-134.

73. Goodlin, R. C. (February 1, 1979). History of fetal monitoring. American Journal of Obstetrics and Gynecology, 133(3), 323-352.

74. Flamm, B. L. (June 1994). Electronic fetal monitoring in the United States. *Birth, 2*(2), 105-106.

75. Scheller, J. M. (November 1992). Preterm versus term asphyxia [Letter to the editor]. *American Journal of Obstetrics and Gynecology, 167*(5), 1481.

76. Grant, A., O'Brien, N., Joy, M-T., Hennessy, E., & MacDonald, D. (November 25, 1989). Cerebral palsy among children born during the Dublin randomised trial of intrapartum monitoring. *The Lancet, 8674*, 1233-1235.

77. Goodlin, R. C. (June 1995). Do concepts of causes and prevention of cerebral palsy require revision? *American Journal of Obstetrics and Gynecology, 172*(6), 1830-1836.

78. Kubli, F. W., Hon, E. H., Khazin, A. F., & Takemura, H. (August 15, 1969). Observations on heart rate and pH in the human fetus during labor. *American Journal of Obstetrics and Gynecology, 104*(8), 1190-1206.

79. Fetal monitoring labeled risky. (1979, Spring). *ICEA News, 18*(1), 1.

80. Gilfix, M. G. (Spring 1984). Electronic fetal monitoring: Physician liability and informed consent. *American Journal of Law & Medicine, 10*(1), 31-90.

81.   Albers, L. L., & Krulewitch, C. J. (July 1993). Electronic fetal monitoring in the United States in the 1980s. *Obstetrics & Gynecology, 82*(1), 8-10.

82.   Nelson, K. B., & Broman, S. H. (November 1977). Perinatal risk factors in children with serious motor and mental handicaps. *Annals of Neurology, 2*(5), 371-377.

83.   Blair, E., & Stanley, F. J. (April 1988). Intrapartum asphyxia: A rare cause of cerebral palsy. *Journal of Pediatrics, 112*(4), 515-519.

84.   Nelson, K. B. (April 1988). What proportion of cerebral palsy is related to birth asphyxia? *Journal of Pediatrics, 112*(4), 572-574.

85.   Nelson, K. B., & Leviton, A. (November 1991). How much of neonatal encephalopathy is due to birth asphyxia? *American Journal of Diseases of Children, 145*(11), 1325-1331.

86.   Haverkamp, A. D., Thompson, H. E., McFee, J. G., & Cetrulo, C. (June 1,1976). The evaluation of continuous fetal heart rate monitoring in high-risk pregnancy. *American Journal of Obstetrics and Gynecology, 125*(3), 310-320.

87.   Renou, P., Chang, A., Anderson, I., & Wood, C. (October 15, 1976). Controlled trial of fetal intensive care. *American Journal of Obstetrics and Gynecology, 126*(4), 470-475.

88.   Haverkamp, A. D., Orleans, M., Langendoerfer, S., McFee, J., Murphy, J., & Thompson, H. E. (June 15, 1979). A controlled trial of the differential effects of intrapartum fetal monitoring. *American Journal of Obstetrics and Gynecology, 134*(4), 399-412.

89.   Kelso, I. M., Parsons, R. J., Lawrence, G. F., Arora, S. S., Edmonds, D. K., & Cooke, I. D. (July 1, 1978). An assessment of continuous fetal heart rate monitoring in labor. A randomized trial. *American Journal of Obstetrics and Gynecology, 131*(5), 526-532.

90.   Wood, C., Renou, P., Oats, J., Farrell, E., Beischer, N., & Anderson, I. (November 1, 1981). A controlled trial of fetal heart rate monitoring in a low-risk obstetric population. *American Journal of Obstetrics and Gynecology, 141*(5), 527-534.

91.   Neldam, S., Osler, M., Hansen, P. K., Nim, J., Smith, S. F., & Hertel, J. (1986). Intrapartum fetal heart rate monitoring in a combined low- and high-risk population: *A controlled clinical trial. European Journal of Obstetrics, Gynecology, and Reproductive Biology, 23,* 1-11.

92.   Leveno, K. J., Cunningham, F. G., Nelson, S., Roark, M., Williams, M. L., Guzick, D., Dowling, S., Rosenfeld, C. R., & Buckley, A. (September 4, 1986). A prospective comparison of selective and universal electronic fetal monitoring in 34,995 pregnancies. *New England Journal of Medicine, 315*(10), 615-619.

93.   Luthy, D. A., Shy, K. K., van Belle, G., Larson, E. B., Hughes, J. P., Benedetti, T. J., Brown, Z. A., Effer, S., King, J. F., & Stenchever, M. A. (May 1987). A randomized trial of electronic fetal monitoring in preterm labor. *Obstetrics & Gynecology, 69*(5), 687-695.

94.   Vintzileos, A. M., Antsaklis, A., Varvarigos, I., Papas, C., Sofatzis, I., & Montgomery, J. T. (June 1993). A randomized trial of intrapartum electronic fetal heart rate monitoring versus intermittent auscultation. *Obstetrics & Gynecology, 81*(6), 899-907.

95.   Mahomed, K., Nyoni, R., Mulambo, T., Kasule, J., & Jacobus, E. (February 19, 1994). Randomised controlled trial of intrapartum fetal heart rate monitoring. *British Medical Journal, 308,* 497-500.

96.   Carter, B. S., Haverkamp, A. D., & Merenstein, G. B. (June 1993). The definition of acute perinatal asphyxia. *Clinics in Perinatology, 20*(2), 287-304.

97.   Niswander, K. R. (February 15, 1991). EFM and brain damage in term and post-term infants. *Contemporary OB/GYN, 36,* 39-50.

98.   Phelan, J. P. (1991). Confronting medical liability. *Contemporary OB/GYN,* 70-81.

99.   Keegan, Jr., K. A., Waffarn, F., & Quilligan, E. J. (December 1, 1985). Obstetric characteristics and fetal heart rate patterns of infants who convulse during the newborn period. *American Journal of Obstetrics and Gynecology, 153*(7), 732-737.

100. Anthony, M. Y., & Levene, M. I. (1990). An assessment of the benefits of intrapartum fetal monitoring for low-risk full-term fetus. *Developmental Medicine and Child Neurology, 32,* 547-553.

101. Shearer, M. H. (Ed.). (June 1986). Roundtable: Part 1. Summary of the Dublin trial. *Birth,13*(2), 117-118.

102. Boylan, P. (March 1987). Intrapartum fetal monitoring. *Bailliere's Clinical Obstetrics and Gynaecology, 1*(1), 73-95.

103. Shearer, M. H. (Spring 1979). Auscultation is "acceptable" in low-risk women according to National Institute of Child Health and Human Development Task Force [Editorial]. *Birth and the Family Journal, 6*(1), 3-6.

104. Task force recommendations could help stem rising cesarean rate. (October 20, 1980). *The Federal Monitor, 3*(6), 1, 5-7.

105. Koszalka, M. F., Haverkamp, A. D., Orleans, M., & Murray, J. (October 1982). The effect of internal electronic fetal heart rate monitoring on maternal and infant infections in high risk pregnancies. *The Journal of Reproductive Medicine, 27*(10), 661-665.

106. Zalar, Jr., R. W., & Quilligan, E. J. (September 15, 1979). The influence of scalp sampling on the cesarean section rate for fetal distress. *American Journal of Obstetrics and Gynecology, 135*(2), 239-246.

107. Boehm, F. H., Davidson, K. K., & Barrett, J. M. (June 1, 1981). The effect of electronic fetal monitoring on the incidence of cesarean section. *American Journal of Obstetrics and Gynecology, 140*(3), 295-298.

108. Chuong, C. J., Lee, C. Y., Chuong, M. C., & Drukker, B. H. (September 1986). Does 24-hour supervisory staff coverage in the labour and delivery area change the emergency caesarean section rate? *British Journal of Obstetrics and Gynaecology, 93*(9), 938-942.

109. Chuong, C. J., Lee, C. Y., Chuong, M. C., & Drukker, B. H. (June 1988). Does 24-hour supervisory staff coverage in the labour and delivery area change the fetal outcome? A preliminary observation. *British Journal of Clinical Practice, 42*(6), 238-240.

110. Consensus development conference on cesarean childbirth. (1980). *Draft report of the task force on cesarean childbirth.* Washington, DC: U. S. Department of Health and Human Services, Public Health Service, NIH.

111. Notzon, F. C., Cnattingius, S., Bergsjo, P., Cole, S., Taffel, S., Irgens, L., & Daltveit, A. K. (February 1994). Cesarean section delivery in the 1980s: International comparison by indication. *American Journal of Obstetrics and Gynecology, 170*(2), 495-504.

112. Hon, E. H. (Fall 1982). The impact of fetal heart rate monitoring. *Journal of the California Perinatal Association, 2*(2), 79-80.

113. Paul, R. H., & Miller, D. A. (June 1995). Cesarean birth: How to reduce the rate. *American Journal of Obstetrics and Gynecology, 172*(6), 1903-1911.

114. Ellison, P. H., Foster, M., Sheridan-Pereira, M., & MacDonald, D. (May 1991). Electronic fetal heart monitoring, auscultation, and neonatal outcome. *American Journal of Obstetrics and Gynecology, 164*(5, Pt. 1), 1281-1288.

115. Poma, P. A. (June 1999). Effects of obstetrician characteristics on cesarean delivery rates: A community hospital experience. *American Journal of Obstetrics and Gynecology, 180*(6, Pt. 1), 1364-1372.

116. Lidegaard, O., Bottcher, L. M., & Weber, T. (January 1992). Description, evaluation and clinical decision making according to various fetal heart rate patterns. Inter-observer and regional variability. *Acta Obstetricia et Gynecologica Scandinavica, 71*(1), 48-53.

117. Gerhardstein, L. P., Allswede, M. T., Sloan, C. T., & Lorenz, R. P. (January 1995). Reduction in the rate of cesarean birth with active management of labor and intermediate-dose oxytocin. *Journal of Reproductive Medicine, 40*(1), 4-8.

118. National Center for Health Statistics. (1998). *Fast stats a to z, births-method of delivery.* Retrieved from http://www.cdc.gov/nchs/faststats/delivery.htm.

119. Naiden, J., & Deshpande, P. (June 2001). Using active management of labor and vaginal birth after previous cesarean delivery to lower cesarean section rates: A 10-year experience. *American Journal of Obstetrics and Gynecology, 184*(7), 1535-1543.

120. Kolås, T., Hofoss, D., Daltveit, A. K., Nilsen, S. T., Henriksen, T., Häger, R., et al. (April 2003). Indications for cesarean deliveries in Norway. *American Journal of Obstetrics and Gynecology, 188*(4), 864-870.

121. Hendrix, N. W., Chauhan, S. P., Scardo, J. A., Ellings, J. M., & Devoe, L. D. (December 2000). Managing nonreassuring fetal heart rate patterns before cesarean delivery. Compliance with ACOG recommendations. *Journal of Reproductive Medicine, 45*(12), 995-999.

122. Office of Technology Transfer. (2002, October 30). *LMS Medical Systems.* McGill University, Montreal, Canada.

123. Lowe, N. K. (May/June 2002). The institutional factor in cesarean section rates [Editorial]. *JOGNN, 31*(3), 245.

124. Gagnon, A. J., & Waghorn, K. (July/August 1999). One-to-one nurse labor support of nulliparous women stimulated with oxytocin. *JOGNN, 28*(4), 371-376.

125. Sauls, D. J. (November/December 2002). Effects of labor support on mothers, babies, and birth outcomes. *JOGNN, 31*(6), 733-741.

126. American College of Obstetricians and Gynecologists. (July 1999). Vaginal birth after previous cesarean delivery. *ACOG Practice Bulletin. Clinical Management Guidelines for Obstetrician-Gynecologists,* 1-8. Washington, DC: author.

127. U. S. Department of Health and Human Services. (2003). *U.S. birth rate reaches record low. Birth to teens continue 12-year decline; cesarean deliveries reach all-time high.* Retrieved from http://www.cdc.gov/nchs/releases/03news/lowbirth.htm.

128. Harlow, B. L., Frigoletto, F. D., Cramer, D. W., Evans, J. K., Bain, R. P., Ewigman, B., McNellis, D., & The RADIUS Study Group. (January 1995). Epidemiologic predictors of cesarean section in nulliparous patients at low risk. *American Journal of Obstetrics and Gynecology, 172*(1, Pt. 1), 156-162.

129. Bekedam, D. J., Engelsbel, S., Mol, B. W. J., Buitendijk, S. E., & van der Pal-de Bruin, K. M. (December 2002). Male predominance in fetal distress during labor. *American Journal of Obstetrics and Gynecology, 187*(6), 1605-1607.

130. Gregory, K. D., & Korst, L. M. (June 2003). Age and racial/ethnic differences in maternal, fetal and placental conditions in laboring patients. *American Journal of Obstetrics and Gynecology, 188*(6), 1602-1608.

131. Peleg, D., Hannah, M. E., Hodnett, E. D., Foster, G. A., Willan, A. R., & Farine, D. (June 1999). Predictors of cesarean delivery after prelabor rupture of membranes at term. *Obstetrics and Gynecology, 93*(6), 1031-1035.

132. deHaan, H. H., Ijzermans, A. C. M., de Haan, J., & Hasaart, T. H. M. (January 1995). The T/QRS ratio of the electrocardiogram does not reliably reflect well-being in fetal lambs. *American Journal of Obstetrics and Gynecology, 172*(1, Pt. 1), 35-43.

133. Danforth, D. N. (February 8, 1985). Cesarean section. *Journal of the American Medical Association, 253*(6), 811-818.

134. Sandmire, H. F., & DeMott, R. K. (June 1994). The Green Bay cesarean section study. III. Falling cesarean birth rates without a formal curtailment program. *American Journal of Obstetrics and Gynecology, 170*(6), 1790-1802.

135. Main, E. (January 1999). Reducing cesarean birth rate with data-driven quality improvement activities. *Pediatrics, 103*(1), 374-383.

136. Klasko, S. K., Cummings, R. V., Balducci, J., DeFulvio, J. D., & Reed III, J. F. (February 1995). The impact of mandated in-hospital coverage on primary cesarean delivery rates in a large nonuniversity teaching hospital. *American Journal of Obstetrics and Gynecology, 172*(2, Pt. 1), 637-642.

137. Schimmel, L. M., Schimmel, L. D., & DeJoseph, J. (September 1997). Toward lower cesarean birth rates and effective care: Five years' outcomes of joint private obstetric practice. *Birth, 24*(3), 181-187.

138. Ferri, R. S., & Sofer, D. (April 2003). Do vaginal births need a good push? *American Journal of Nursing, 103*(4), 19.

139. Chen, C. H., & Wang, S. Y. (2002). Psychosocial outcomes of vaginal and cesarean births in Taiwanese primiparas. *Research in Nursing and Health, 25*, 452-458.

140. Mustard, C. A., Harman, C. R., Hall, P. F., & Derksen, S. (February 1995). Impact of a nurses' strike on the cesarean birth rate. *American Journal of Obstetrics and Gynecology, 172*(2, Pt. 1), 631-636.

141. Holland-Toftness, C., & Dowling-Quarles, S. (June 4-7, 1995). Nurses' care during labor: Its effect on the cesarean birth rate of healthy, nulliparous women: A replication. *In Tune With the Country. AWHONN 1995 Convention Session Resources.* Nashville: TN.

142. Moore, Jr., R. M., Jeng, L. L., Kaczmarek, R. G., & Placek, P. J. (September/October 1990). Use of diagnostic imaging procedures and fetal monitoring devices in the care of pregnant women. *Public Health Reports, 105*(5), 471-475.

143. Schifrin, B. S. (1986). Polemics in perinatology: The future of fetal monitoring. *Journal of Perinatology, 6*(4), 331-332.

144. Jick, B. S. (1990). EFM: Would you give it up? [Letter to the editor]. Ob. Gyn. News, 25(11).

145. Banta, D. H., & Thacker, S. B. (November 2001). Historical controversy in health technology assessment: The case of electronic fetal monitoring. *Obstetrical and Gynecological Survey, 56*(11), 707-719.

146. Paneth, N., Bommarito, M., & Stricker, J. (1993). Electronic fetal monitoring and later outcome. *Clinical and Investigative Medicine, 16*(2), 159-165.

147. Golditch, B. D., Ahn, M. O., & Phelan, J. P. (April 1998). The fetal admission test and intrapartum fetal death. *American Journal of Perinatology, 15*(4), 273-276.

148. Beckmann, C. A., Van Mullen, C., Beckmann, C. R., & Broekhuizen, F. F. (1997). Interpreting fetal heart rate tracings: Is there a difference between labor and delivery nurses and obstetricians? *Journal of Reproductive Medicine, 42*(10), 647-650.

149. Cibils, L. A. (November 1996). On intrapartum fetal monitoring. *American Journal of Obstetrics and Gynecology, 174*(4), 1382-1389.

150. Beller, F. K. (February 1995). The cerebral palsy story: A catastrophic misunderstanding in obstetrics [Editorial]. *Obstetrical and Gynecological Survey, 50*(2), 83.

151. Dawes, G. S., & Redman, C. W. G. (1985). Antenatal heart rate analysis at the bedside using a microprocessor. In W. Kunzel (Ed.), *Fetal heart rate monitoring* (pp. 63-65). Berlin: Springer-Verlag.

152. Albers, L. L. (June 1994). Clinical issues in electronic fetal monitoring. *Birth, 21*(2), 108-110.

153. Hon, E. H., & Lee, S. T. (November 15, 1963). Electronic evaluation of the fetal heart rate. VIII. Patterns preceding fetal death further observations. *American Journal of Obstetrics and Gynecology, 87*(6), 814-826.

154. Lilien, A. A. (June 15, 1970). Term intrapartum fetal death. *American Journal of Obstetrics and Gynecology, 107*(4), 595-603.

155. Paul, R. H., & Hon, E. H. (1974). Clinical fetal monitoring. V. Effect on perinatal outcome. *American Journal of Obstetrics and Gynecology, 118*(4), 529-533.

156. Low, J. A., Muir, D. W., Pater, E. A., & Karchmar, E. J. (October 1990). The association of intrapartum asphyxia in the mature fetus with newborn behavior. *American Journal of Obstetrics and Gynecology, 163*(4, Pt. 1), 1131-1135.

157. Low, J. A., Galbraith, R. S., Muir, D. W., Killen, H. L., Pater, E. A., & Karchmar, E. J. (January 15, 1983). Intrapartum fetal hypoxia: A study of long-term morbidity. *American Journal of Obstetrics and Gynecology, 145*(2), 129-134.

158. Gimovsky, M. L., & Caritis, S. N. (June 1982). Diagnosis and management of hypoxic heart rate patterns. *Clinics in Perinatology, 9*(2), 313-324.

159. Berkus, M. D., Langer, O., Samueloff, A., Xenakis, E. M. J., & Field, N. T. (January 1999). Electronic fetal monitoring: What's reassuring? *Acta Obstetricia et Gynecologica Scandinavica, 78*(1), 15-21.

160. Strachan, B. K., Sahota, D. S., van Wijngaarden, W. J., James, D. K., & Chang, A. M. Z. (August 2001). Computerised analysis of the fetal heart rate and relation to acidaemic at delivery. *British Journal of Obstetrics and Gynaecology, 108*(8), 848-852.

161. Bowes, Jr., W. A., Gabbe, S. G., Bowes, C. (August 1, 1980). Fetal heart rate monitoring in premature infants weighing 1,500 grams or less. *American Journal of Obstetrics and Gynecology, 137*(7), 791-796.

162. Williams, K., & Galerneau, F. (December 2001). The significance of the duration of intrapartum fetal heart rate variability in predicting the development of significant neonatal acidosis. *American Journal of Obstetrics and Gynecology, 185*(6), S130. Abstract No. 183.

163. Van de Riet, J. E., Vandenbussche, F. P. H. A., Le Cessie, S., & Keirse, M. J. N. C. (April 1999). Newborn assessment and long-term adverse outcome: A systematic review. *American Journal of Obstetrics and Gynecology, 180*(4), 1024-1029.

164. Andres, R. L., Saade, G., Gilstrap III, L. C., Wilkins, I., Witlin, A., Zlatnik, F., & Hankins, G. V. (October 1999). Association between umbilical blood gas parameters and neonatal morbidity and death in neonates with pathologic fetal acidemia. *American Journal of Obstetrics and Gynecology, 181*(4), 867-871.

165. Sehdev, H. M., Stamilio, D. M., Macones, G. A., Graham, E., & Morgan, M. A. (November 1997). Predictive factors for neonatal morbidity in neonates with an umbilical arterial cord pH less than 7.00. *American Journal of Obstetrics and Gynecology, 177*(5), 1030-1034.

166. Shaw, K., & Clark, S. L. (December 1988). Reliability of intrapartum fetal heart rate monitoring in the postterm fetus with meconium passage. *Obstetrics and Gynecology, 72*(6), 886-889.

167. Sheiner, E., Hadar, A., Hallak, M., Katz, M., Shoham-Vardi, I., Mazor, M., et al. (January 2001). The significance of fetal heart rate monitoring during the second stage of labor. *American Journal of Obstetrics and Gynecology, 184*(1), S98. Abstract No. 0306.

168. Agrawal, S., Doucette, F., Sachdeva, H., Gagnon, R., Gratton, R., & Richardson, B. (January 1999). Intrapartum computerized fetal heart rate (FHR) analysis: Effects of labor and the relationship to measures of acidosis. *American Journal of Obstetrics and Gynecology, 180*(1, Pt. 2), S91. Abstract No. 302.

169. Low, J. A., Boston, R. W., & Pancham, S. R. (March 15, 1971). The role of fetal heart patterns in the recognition of fetal asphyxia with metabolic acidosis. *American Journal of Obstetrics and Gynecology, 109*(6), 922-929.

170. Blackwell, S., Field, S., Refuerzo, J., Hassan, S., Redman, M., Naccasha, N., et al. (January 2001). Pathologic acidemia at birth: Correlation with intrapartum electronic fetal heart rate patterns. *American Journal of Obstetrics and Gynecology, 184*(1), S99. Abstract No. 0312.

171. Hadar, A., Sheiner, E., Hallak, M., Katz, M., Shoham-Vardi, I., & Mazor, M. (January 2001). Abnormal fetal heart rate tracing patterns during the first stage of labor: Effect on perinatal outcome. *American Journal of Obstetrics and Gynecology, 184*(1), S 98. Abstract No. 0308.

172. Hadar, A., Sheiner, E., Hallak, M., Katz, M., Mazor, M., & Shoham-Vardi, I. (October 2001). Abnormal fetal heart rate tracing patterns during the first stage of labor: Effect on perinatal outcome. *American Journal of Obstetrics and Gynecology, 185*(4), 863-868.

173. Elimian, A., Figueroa, R., & Tejani, N. (March 1997). Intrapartum assessment of fetal well-being: A comparison of scalp stimulation with scalp blood pH sampling. *Obstetrics and Gynecology, 89*(3), 373-376.

174. Smith, C. V., Nguyen, H. N., Phelan, J. P., & Paul, R. H. (1986). Intrapartum assessment of fetal well-being: A comparison of fetal acoustic stimulation with acid-base determinations. *American Journal of Obstetrics and Gynecology, 155*(4), 726-728.

175. Read, J. A., & Miller, F. C. (November 1, 1977). Fetal heart rate acceleration in response to acoustic stimulation as a measure of fetal well-being. *American Journal of Obstetrics and Gynecology, 129*(5), 512-517.

176. Richards, D. S., Cefalo, R. C., Thorpe, J. M., Salley, M., & Rose, D. (April 1988). Determinants of fetal heart rate response to vibroacoustic stimulation in labor. *Obstetrics & Gynecology, 71*(4), 535-540.

177. A simple check on fetal distress. (December 15, 1984). *Emergency Medicine,* 101,

178. Harvey, C. J. (July 1987). Fetal scalp stimulation: Enhancing the interpretation of fetal monitor tracings. *Journal of Perinatal and Neonatal Nursing, 1*(1), 13 -21.

179. Miller, F. C. (1990). Fetal scalp stimulation. In E. J. Quilligan & F. P. Zuspan (Eds.) *Current therapy in obstetrics and gynecology* (pp. 332-333). Philadelphia: W. B. Saunders Company.

180. Zimmer, E. Z., & Vadasz, A. (January 1989). Influence of the fetal scalp electrode stimulation test on fetal heart rate and body movements in quiet and active behavioral states during labor. *American Journal of Perinatology, 6*(1), 24-29.

181. Paul, R. H., & Hon, E. H. (January 1970). Endoscopic examination of fetal scalp and fetal electrocardiography value of lateral position. *Obstetrics and Gynecology, 35*(1), 111-113.

182. Tejani, N., Mann, L. I., Bhakthavathsalan, A., & Weiss, R. R. (August 15, 1975). Prolonged fetal bradycardia with recovery-its significance and outcome. *American Journal of Obstetrics and Gynecology, 122*(8), 975-978.

183. Clark, S. L., Gimovsky, M. L., & Miller, F. C. (November 15, 1982). Fetal heart response to scalp blood sampling. *American Journal of Obstetrics and Gynecology, 144*(6), 706-708.

184. American College of Obstetricians and Gynecologists. (September 2001). Fetal pulse oximetry. *ACOG Committee Opinion No. 258.* Washington, DC: author.

185. Dildy, G. A., Clark, S. L., & Loucks, C. A. (July 1996). Intrapartum fetal pulse oximetry: Past, present, and future. American *Journal of Obstetrics and Gynecology, 175*(1), 1-9.

186. Gorenberg, D., Patillo, C., Hendi, P., Rumney, P., & Garite, T. (December 2001). Fetal pulse oximetry: Correlation between oxygen desaturation, duration and frequency and neonatal outcomes. *American Journal of Obstetrics and Gynecology, 185*(6), S129. Abstract No. 180.

187. Kühnert, M., Seelbach-Göebel, B., & Butterwegge, M. (February 1998). Predictive agreement between the fetal arterial oxygen saturation and fetal scalp pH: Results of the German multicenter study. *American Journal of Obstetrics and Gynecology, 178*(2), 330-335.

188. Seelbach-Göbel, B., Heupel, M., Kühnert, M., & Butterwegge, M. (January 1999). The prediction of fetal acidosis by means of intrapartum fetal pulse oximetry. *American Journal of Obstetrics and Gynecology, 180*(1, Pt. 1), 73-81.

189. East, C. E., & Colditz, P. B. (1996). Women's evaluations of their experience with fetal intrapartum oxygen saturation monitoring and participation in a research project. *Midwifery, 12*, 93-97.

190. Lee, R., Moore, M., Brewster, W., Hendi, P., Pattillo, C., Ziogas, A., & Garite, T. (December 2001). Late decelerations and severe variables are predictive of fetal hypoxia. *American Journal of Obstetrics and Gynecology, 185*(6), S130. Abstract No. 184.

191. Lewinsky, R. M., Sharf, M., Dejani, S., & Eibschitz, I. (September-November 1992). Prediction of pregnancy outcome by combined analysis of the fetal electrocardiogram and systolic time intervals. *American Journal of Perinatology, 9*(5-6), 348-352.

192. Norén, H., Amer-Wåhlin, I., Hagberg, H., Herbst, A., Kjellmer, I., Mar_ál, K., et al. (January 2003). Fetal electrocardiography in labor and neonatal outcome: Data from the Swedish randomized controlled trial on intrapartum fetal monitoring. *American Journal of Obstetrics and Gynecology, 188*(1), 183-192.

193. Deans, A. C., & Steer, P. J. (January 1994). The use of the fetal electrocardiogram in labour. *British Journal of Obstetrics and Gynaecology, 101*(1), 9-17.

194. Westgate, J. A., Bennet, L., Brabyn, C., Williams, C. E., & Gunn, A. J. (March 2001). ST waveform changes during repeated umbilical cord occlusions in near-term fetal sheep. *American Journal of Obstetrics and Gynecology, 184*(4), 743-751.

195. Rosén, K., Kjellmer, I., & Marsál, K. (December 2001). Perinatal outcome and fetal surveillance – Data from Swedish RCT of CTG versus CTG plus analysis of the ST waveform of the fetal ECG. *American Journal of Obstetrics and Gynecology, 185*(6), S131. Abstract No. 188.

196. Strachan, B., Sahota, D., van Wijngaarden, W. J., James, D. K., & Chang, A. Z. M. (May 2000). The fetal electrocardiogram: Relationship with acidemia at delivery. *American Journal of Obstetrics and Gynecology, 182*(3), 603-606.

197. Luzietti, R., Rosén, K. G., & Direnzo, G. C. (December 2001). A knowledge based system for appropriate intervention during labor based on fetal electrocardiogram. *American Journal of Obstetrics and Gynecology, 185*(6), S129. Abstract No. 177.

198. Ross, M. G., Devoe, L., & Rosén, K. (December 2002). ST-segment analysis of the fetal ECG improves fetal heart rate tracing interpretation. *American Journal of Obstetrics and Gynecology, 187*(6), S149. Abstract No. 325.

199. Hagberg, H., Amer-Wåhlin, I., Hellsten, C., Norén, H., Hagberg, A., & Herbst, A. (January 2001). Intrapartum fetal monitoring. Cardiotocography versus cardiotocography plus fetal ECG ST waveform analysis. A Swedish randomized controlled trial. *American Journal of Obstetrics and Gynecology, 184*(1), S19. Abstract No. 0041.

200. Luttkus, A. K., Stupin, J. H., Foertsch, I., Porath, M., & Dudenhausen, J. W. (December 2001). Agreement between fetal pulse oximetry and fetal ECG in episodes of suspected hypoxia. *American Journal of Obstetrics and Gynecology, 186*(6), S129. Abstract No. 179.

201. Kirkendall, C., & Phelan, J. (December 2002). Is meconium a sign of fetal distress? *American Journal of Obstetrics and Gynecology, 187*(6), S148. Abstract No. 323.

202. Phelan, J., Korst, L., Ahn, M. O., Martin, G., & Kirkendall, C. (January 2000). Intrapartum uterine rupture and permanent brain injury: A retrospective analysis of current indicators. *American Journal of Obstetrics and Gynecology, 182*(1, Pt. 2), S185. Abstract No. 604.

203. Szabó, I., Halvax, L., & Kiss, T. (May 1998). Clinical value of intrapartum fetal pulse oximetry in cases complicated with meconium-stained amniotic fluid [Letter to the editor]. *American Journal of Obstetrics and Gynecology, 178*(5), 1100-1101.

204. Bhagwanani, S. G., Seagraves, K., & Kierker, L. (January 1997). Relationship between prenatal anxiety, social support and perinatal outcome. *American Journal of Obstetrics and Gynecology, 176*(1, Pt. 2), S126. Abstract No. 432.

205. Goodlin, R. C. (December 1997). How about meconium? [Letter to the editor]. *American Journal of Obstetrics and Gynecology, 177*(6), 1565-1566.

206. Scorza, W. E., Shen-Schwarz, S., Smulian, J. C., Oksov, K., Ananth, C. V., & Vintzileos, A. M. (January 1998). The mystery surrounding meconium aspiration syndrome: Does the clue lie in placental histopathology? *American Journal of Obstetrics and Gynecology, 178*(1, Pt. 2), S208. Abstract No. 750.

207. Peng, T. C. C., Gutcher, G. R., & Van Dorsten, J. P. (August 1996). A selective aggressive approach to the neonate exposed to meconium-stained amniotic fluid. *American Journal of Obstetrics and Gynecology, 175*(2), 296-303.

208. Maymon, E., Haim, W., urman, B., Shoham-Vardi, I., & Mazors, M. (January 1998). Meconium stained amniotic fluid in a low risk population at term is a predictor of peripartum complications and maternal morbidity. *American Journal of Obstetrics and Gynecology, 178*(1, Pt. 2), S99. Abstract No. 330.

209. Low, J. A., Pancham, S. R., Worthington, D., & Boston, R. W. (February 15, 1975). Clinical characteristics of pregnancies complicated by intrapartum fetal asphyxia. *American Journal of Obstetrics and Gynecology, 121*(4), 452-455.

210. Low, J. A., Pancham, S. R., & Worthington, D. (January 1976). Fetal heart deceleration patterns in relation to asphyxia and weight–gestational age percentile of the fetus. *Obstetrics and Gynecology, 47*(1), 14-20.

211. Low, J. A. (November 1988). The role of blood gas and acid-base assessment in the diagnosis of intrapartum fetal asphyxia. *American Journal of Obstetrics and Gynecology, 159*(5), 1235-1240.

212. Low, J. A., Wood, S. L., Killen, H. L., Pater, E. A., & Karchmar, E. J. (February 1990). Intrapartum asphyxia in the preterm fetus < 2000 gm. *American Journal of Obstetrics and Gynecology, 162*(2), 378-382.

213. Low, J. A., Lindsay, B. O., & Derrick, E. J. (December 1997). Threshold of metabolic acidosis associated with newborn complications. *American Journal of Obstetrics and Gynecology, 177*(6), 1391-1394.

214. van den Berg, P. P., Pasker-de Jong, P. G. M., Nelen, W. L. D. M., Wüstefeld, K., & Jongsma, H. W. (January 1997). What are the determinants of neonatal neurologic dysfunction. *American Journal of Obstetrics and Gynecology, 176*(1, Pt. 2), S116. Abstract No. 392.

215. American College of Obstetricians and Gynecologists. (January 1992). Fetal and neonatal neurologic injury. *ACOG Technical bulletin number 163*. Washington, DC: author.

216. Westgren, L. M., Malcus, P., & Sevenningsen, N. W. (April 1986). Intrauterine asphyxia and long-term outcome in preterm fetuses. *Obstetrics & Gynecology, 67*(4), 512-516.

217. Low, J. A., Pancham, S. R., Piercy, W. N., Worthington, D., & Karchmar, J. (December 15, 1977). Intrapartum fetal asphyxia: Clinical characteristics, diagnosis and significance in relation to pattern of development. *American Journal of Obstetrics and Gynecology, 129*(8), 857-872.

218. Low, J. A., Victory, R., & Derrick, E. J. (February 1999). Predictive value of electronic fetal monitoring for intrapartum fetal asphyxia with metabolic acidosis. *Obstetrics and Gynecology, 93*(2), 285-291.

219. Haddad, B., Mercer, B. M., Livingston, J. C., Talati, A., & Sibai, B. M. (May 2000). Outcome after successful resuscitation of babies born with Apgar scores of 0 at 1 and 5 minutes. *American Journal of Obstetrics and Gynecology, 182*(5), 1210-1214.

220. Bailit, J. L., Garrett, J. M., Miller, W. C., McMahon, M. J., & Cefalo, R. C. (September 2002). Hospital primary cesarean delivery rates and the risk of poor neonatal outcomes. *American Journal of Obstetrics and Gynecology, 187*(3), 721-727.

221. Gilstrap III, L. C., Leveno, K. J., Burris, J., Willaims, M. L., & Little, B. B. (September 1989). Diagnosis of birth asphyxia on the basis of fetal pH, Apgar score, and newborn cerebral dysfunction. *American Journal of Obstetrics and Gynecology, 161*(3), 825-830.

222. Koen, S., Gei, A., Lopez, S., Van Hook, J., Anderson, G., & Hankins, G. (January 2001). Prevalence of organ system injury in acute birth asphyxia. *American Journal of Obstetrics and Gynecology, 184*(1), S133. Abstract No. 0439.

223. Greenberg, J., Economy, K., Mark, A., & Ringer, S. (December 2001). In search of "true" birth asphyxia: Labor characteristics associated with the asphyxiated term infant. *American Journal of Obstetrics and Gynecology, 185*(6), S94. Abstract No. 54.

224. Foley, M., Alarab, M., & O'Herlihy, C. (December 2002). Neonatal seizures and peripartum deaths: Lack of correlation with cesarean rate. *American Journal of Obstetrics and Gynecology, 187*(6), S102. Abstract No. 151.

225. Murphy, K. W., Johnson, P., Moorcraft, J., Pattinson, R., Russell, V., & Turnbull, A. (June 1990). Birth asphyxia and the intrapartum cardiotocograph. *British Journal of Obstetrics and Gynaecology, 97*, 470-479.

226. Williams, K., & Galerneau, F. (December 2002). Comparison of intrapartum fetal heart rate tracings in patients with neonatal seizures vs. no seizures. What are the differences? *American Journal of Obstetrics and Gynecology, 187*(6), S149. Abstract No. 324.

227. Low, J. A., Galbraith, R. S., Muir, D. W., Killen, H. L., Pater, E. A., & Karchmar, E. J. (June 1, 1985). The relationship between perinatal hypoxia and newborn encephalopathy. *American Journal of Obstetrics and Gynecology, 152*(3), 256-260.

228. Ramin, S. M., & Gilstrap III, L. C. (June 2000). Other factors/conditions associated with cerebral palsy. *Seminars in Perinatology, 24*(3), 196-199.

229. Badawi, N., Kurinczuk, J. J., Keogh, J. M., Alessandri, L. M., O'Sullivan, F., Burton, P. R., et al. (December 1998). Intrapartum risk factors for newborn encephalopathy: The western Australian case-control study. *British Medical Journal, 317*(7172), 1554-1558.

230. Churchill, J. A., Masland, R. L., Naylor, A. A., & Ashworth, M. R. (April 1974). The etiology of cerebral palsy in pre-term infants. *Developmental Medicine and Child Neurology, 16*(2), 143-149.

231. Nelson, K. B., Dambrosia, J. M., Ting, T. Y., & Grether, J. K. (March 1996). Uncertain value of electronic fetal monitoring in predicting cerebral palsy. *The New England Journal of Medicine, 334*(10), 613-618.

232. Nelson, K. B., & Grether, J. K. (August 1998). Potentially asphyxiating conditions and spastic cerebral palsy in infants of normal birth weight. *American Journal of Obstetrics and Gynecology, 179*(2), 507-513.

233. Nelson, K. B., & Grether, J. K. (December 1999). Causes of cerebral palsy. *Current Opinions in Pediatrics, 11*(6), 487-491.

234. Williams, M., & O'Brien, W. (December 2002). Single tight cord entanglements are not associated with perinatal depression or long term morbidity. *American Journal of Obstetrics and Gynecology, 187*(6), S93. Abstract No. 115.

235. Scheller, J. M., & Nelson, K. B. (April 1994). Does cesarean delivery prevent cerebral palsy or other neurologic problems of childhood? *Obstetrics and Gynecology, 83*(4), 624-630.

236. MacLennan, A. (October 1999). A template for defining a causal relation between acute intrapartum events and cerebral palsy: International consensus statement. *British Medical Journal, 319*, 1054-1059.

237. Wilson, R. W., & Schifrin, B. S. (May 1980). Is any pregnancy low risk? *Obstetrics and Gynecology, 55*(5), 653-656.

238. Helfand, H., Marton, K., & Ueland, K. (March 15, 1985). Factors involved in the interpretation of fetal monitor tracings. *American Journal of Obstetrics and Gynecology, 151*(6), 737-744.

239. Low, J. A., Simpson, L. L., Tonni, G., & Chamberlain, S. (March 1995). Limitations in the clinical prediction of intrapartum fetal asphyxia. *American Journal of Obstetrics and Gynecology, 172*(3), 801-804.

240. Nurse's Association of the American College of Obstetricians and Gynecologists. (1991). *Standards for the nursing care of women and newborns (4th ed.).* (1991). Washington, DC: author.

241. Yeh, S. Y., Forsythe, A., Lowensohn, R. I., & Hon, E. H. (January 1, 1977). A study of the relationship between Goodwin's high-risk score and fetal outcome. *American Journal of Obstetrics and Gynecology, 127*(1), 50-55.

242. Sheffer-Mimouni, G., Littner, Y., Mandel, D., Deutsch, V., Dollberg, S., & Mimouni, F. (December 2002). Nucleated red blood cells in infants of asthmatic mothers. *American Journal of Obstetrics and Gynecology, 187*(6), S203. Abstract No. 528.

243. Hon, E. H., Zannini, D., & Quilligan, E. H. (1975). The neonatal value of fetal monitoring. *Transactions of the Pacific Coast Obstetrical and Gynecological Society, 42*, 115-126.

244. Herbst, A., & Ingemarsson, I. (August 1994). Intermittent versus continuous electronic monitoring in labour: A randomised study. *British Journal of Obstetrics and Gynaecology, 101*(8), 663-668.

245. Intrapartum fetal monitoring. (January 1977). *Technical bulletin number 44.* Washington, DC: ACOG.

246. Wilson, R. W., & Schifrin, B. S. (1980). Is any pregnancy low risk? *Obstetrics & Gynecology, 55,* 653.

247. Hobel, C. J., Hyvarinen, M. A., Okada, D. M., & Oh, W. (September 1, 1973). Prenatal and intrapartum high-risk screening. I. Prediction of the high-risk neonate. *American Journal of Obstetrics and Gynecology, 117*(1), 1-9.

248. Low, J. A., Pickersgill, H., Killen, H., & Derrick, E. J. (March 2001). The prediction and prevention of intrapartum fetal asphyxia in term pregnancies. *American Journal of Obstetrics and Gynecology, 184*(4), 724-730.

249. Amini, S. B., Catalano, P. M., & Mann, L. I. (May-June 1996). Effect of prenatal care on obstetrical outcome. *The Journal of Maternal-Fetal Medicine, 5*(3), 142-150.

250. Vintzileos, A. M., Ananth, C. V., Smulian, J. C., Scorza, W. E., & Knuppel, R. A. (May 2002). The impact of prenatal care on neonatal deaths in the presence and absence of antenatal high-risk conditions. *American Journal of Obstetrics and Gynecology, 186*(5), 1011-1016.

251. Low, J. A. (December 1999). Intrapartum fetal surveillance. Is it worthwhile? *Obstetrics and Gynecology Clinics of North America, 26*(4), 725-739.

252. Higgins, S. D., & Garite, T. J. (March 1984). Late abruption placenta in trauma patients: Implications for monitoring. *Obstetrics & Gynecology, 63*(3, Suppl.), 10s-12s.

253. Trauma during pregnancy. (November 1991). Technical bulletin number 161. *International Journal of Gynecology and Obstetrics, 40,*165-170.

254. Dahmus, M. A., & Sibai, B. H. (October 1993). Blunt abdominal trauma: Are there any predictive factors for abruption placentae or maternal-fetal distress? *American Journal of Obstetrics and Gynecology, 169*(4), 1054-1059.

255. Towery, R., English, T. P., & Wisner, D. (November 1993). Evaluation of pregnant women after blunt injury. *The Journal of Trauma, 35*(5), 731-736.

256. Westgate, J. A., Gunn, A. J., & Gunn, T. R. (August 1999). Antecedents of neonatal encephalopathy with fetal acidaemia at term. *British Journal of Obstetrics and Gynaecology, 106*(8), 774-782.

257. Natale, R., Nimrod, C., Liston, R., Lalonde, A., & Hanvey, L. (September 1995). Fetal health surveillance in labour. *Journal of the Society of Obstetricians and Gynecologists of Canada. SOGN Policy Statement.* Retrieved from http://www.sogc.org/sogcnet/sogc%5Fdocs/common/guide/pdfs/ps41.pdf.

258. Poland, R. L., & Freeman, R. K. (Eds.). *Guidelines for perinatal care (3rd ed.).* Elk Grove Village, IL: American Academy of Pediatrics and Washington, DC: ACOG.

259. Gilstrap, L. C., Oh, W., Greene, M. F., & Lemons, J. A. (Eds.). *Guidelines for perinatal care (5th ed.).* Elk Grove Village, IL: American Academy of Pediatrics and Washington, DC: ACOG.

260. American College of Obstetricians and Gynecologists. (September 1989). Intrapartum fetal heart rate monitoring. *Technical bulletin number 132.* Washington, DC: author.

261. Nurse's Association of the American College of Obstetricians and Gynecologists. (February 1992). Nursing responsibilities in implementing intrapartum fetal heart rate monitoring. *NAACOG Position Statement.* Washington, DC: author.

262. EFM, intermittent auscultation found comparable. (1988, November). *ACOG Newsletter, 32*(11), 4-5.

263. Vintzileos, A. M., Nochimson, D. J., Guzman, E. R., Knuppel, R. A., Lake, M., & Schifrin, B. S. (January 1995). Intrapartum electronic fetal heart rate monitoring versus intermittent auscultation: A meta-analysis. *Obstetrics & Gynecology, 85*(1), 149-155.

264. Ingemarrson, I., Arulkumaran, S., Ingemarrson, E., Tambyraja, R. L., & Ratnam, S. S. (December 1986). Admission test: A screening test for fetal distress in labor. *Obstetrics and Gynecology, 68*(6), 800-806.

265. Goodlin, R. C. (1980). Low-risk obstetric care for low-risk mothers. *Lancet, 1,* 1017-1019.

266. Rommal, C. (December 1996). Risk management issues in the perinatal setting. *Journal of Perinatal and Neonatal Nursing, 10*(3), 1-31.

267. Pello, L. C., Dawes, G. S., Smith, J., & Redman, C. W. G. (November 1988). Screening of the fetal heart rate in early labour. *British Journal of Obstetrics and Gynaecology, 95,* 1128-1136.

268. Mires, G., Williams, F., & Howie, P. (June 2001). Randomised controlled trial of cardiotocography versus Doppler auscultation of fetal heart at admission in labour in low risk obstetric population. *British Medical Journal, 322,* 1457-1462.

269. Phelan, J. P. (February 15, 1991). Was it intrapartum fetal distress? *Contemporary OB/GYN, 36,* 26-34.

270. Warenski, J. C., & Kochenour, N. K. (December 1989). Intrapartum management of twin gestation. *Clinics in Perinatology, 16*(4), 889-897.

271. Ducey, J., Guzman, E., Schulman, H., Farmakedis, G., & Karmin, I. (1990). Value of a screening fetal heart rate tracing in the latent phase of labor. *Journal of Reproductive Medicine, 35,* 899-900.

272. Dai, M-S, & Fox, H. (February 1991). Electronic monitoring of fetal heart rate and determination of fetal scalp blood pH in prediction of intrapartum fetal distress. *Chinese Medical Journal, 104*(2), 132-137.

273. Umstad, M. P. (1993). The predictive value of abnormal fetal heart rate patterns in early labour. *Austrialian and New Zealand Journal of Obstetrics and Gynaecology, 33*(2), 145-149.

274. Nieto, A., Matorras, R., Serra, M., & Valenzuela, P. (1996). Fluctuation of cardiotocographic tracings during labor in fetal growth retardation. *Zentralblatt für Gynäkologie, 118*(12), 655-658.

275. Kulkarni, A. A., & Shrotri, A. N. (August 1998). Admission test: A predictive test for fetal distress in high risk labour. *Journal of Obstetric and Gynaecologic Research, 24*(4), 2555-259.

276. Elimian, A., Lawlor, P., Figueroa, R., Wiencek, V., Garry, D., Ogburn, P., et al. (December 2002). Non reassuring fetal admission test and labor outcomes. *American Journal of Obstetrics and Gynecology, 187*(6), S147. Abstract No. 319.

277. Mahomed, K., Nyoni, R., Mlambo, T., Jacobus, E., & Kasule, J. (1992). Intrapartum foetal heart rate monitoring-continuous electronic versus intermittent doppler-a randomised controlled trial. *Central African Journal of Medicine, 38*(12), 458-462.

278. Daddario, J. B. (December 1992). Fetal surveillance in the intensive care unit. *Critical Care Nursing Clinics of North America, 4*(4), 711 -719.

279. Ducey, J., Guzman, E., Schulman, H., Farmakedis, G., & Karmin, I. (September 1990). Value of a screening fetal heart rate tracing in the latent phase of labor. *The Journal of Reproductive Medicine, 35*(9), 899-900.

280. Gray, J. H. (December 1978). Nursing care of monitored women in labor. *American Journal of Nursing,* 2104-2105.

281. Morrison, J. C., Chez, B. F., Davis, I. D., Martin, R. W., Roberts, W. E., Martin, Jr., J. N., & Floyd, R. C. (January 1993). Intrapartum fetal heart rate assessment: Monitoring by auscultation or electronic means. *American Journal of Obstetrics and Gynecology, 168*(1, Pt. 1), 63-66.

282. Hankins, G. D., Leicht, T., Anderson, G. D., & Rowe, T. F. (May 1999). Electronic fetal monitoring. Are we meeting documentation standards? *Journal of Reproductive Medicine, 44*(5), 441-444.

283. Association of Women's Health, Obstetrics, and Neonatal Nurses. (April 2000). Fetal assessment. *Clinical Position Statement.* Washington, DC: author.

284. Banta, H. D., & Thacker, S. B. (2001). Historical controversy in health technology assessment: The case of electronic fetal monitoring. *Obstetrical and Gynecological Survey, 56*(11), 707-719.

285. Schifrin, B. S. (June 1990). Polemics in perinatology: The electronic fetal monitoring guidelines. *Journal of Perinatology, 10*(2), 188-192.

286. Thacker, S. B., Stroup, D. F., & Peterson, H. B. (October 1995). Efficacy and safety of intrapartum electronic fetal monitoring: An update. *Obstetrics and Gynecology, 86*(4, Pt. 1), 613-620.

287. Shenker, L., Post, R. C., & Sellers, J. S. (August 1975). Routine electronic monitoring of fetal heart rate and uterine activity during labor. *Obstetrics and Gynecology, 46*(2), 185-189.

288. Feinstein, N. F., Sprague, A., & Trepanier, M. J. (June/July 2000). Fetal heart rate auscultation. *AWHONN Lifelines, 4*(3), 35-44.

289. Vintzileos, A. M., Nochimson, D. J., Antsaklis, A., Varvarigos, I., Guzman, E. R., & Knuppel, R. A. (October 1995). Comparison of intrapartum electronic fetal heart rate monitoring versus intermittent auscultation in detecting fetal acidemia at birth. *American Journal of Obstetrics and Gynecology, 173*(4), 1021-1024.

290. Mahomed, K., Gupta, B. K., Matikiti, L., & Murape, T. S. (December 1992). A simplified form of cardiotocography for antenatal fetal assessment. *Midwifery, 8*(4), 191-194.

291. Nelson, K. B., & Ellenberg, J. H. (October 1985). Antecedents of cerebral palsy. I. Univariate analysis of risks. *American Journal of Diseases of Children, 139*(10), 1031-1038.

292. Schifrin, B. S. (December 1995). Medicolegal ramifications of electronic fetal monitoring during labor. *Clinics in Perinatology, 22*(4), 837-854.

293. Murray, G. (April 11, 1984). Fetal distress. *Nursing Times, 80*(15), 33-35.

294. Schifrin, B. S., Amsel, J., & Burdorf, G. (February 1992). The accuracy of auscultatory detection of fetal cardiac decelerations: A computer simulation. *American Journal of Obstetrics and Gynecology, 166*(2), 566-576.

295. Miller, F., Pearse, K., & Paul, R. (September 1984). Fetal heart rate pattern recognition by the method of auscultation. *Obstetrics and Gynecology, 64*(3), 332-336.

296. Syndal, S. H. (January/February 1988). Methods of fetal heart rate monitoring during labor. A selective review of the literature. *Journal of Nurse-Midwifery, 33*(1), 4-14.

297. Ellison, P. H., Foster, M., Sheridan-Pereira, M., & MacDonald, D. (May 1991). Electronic fetal heart monitoring, auscultation, and neonatal outcome. *American Journal of Obstetrics and Gynecology, 164*(5, Pt. 1), 1281-1288.

298. Benson, R. C., Shubeck, F., Deutschberger, J., Weiss, W., & Berendes, H. (August 1968). Fetal heart rate as a predictor of fetal distress. *Obstetrics and Gynecology, 32*(2), 259-266.

299. Siemens, R. L. (March 1994). A place for electronic fetal monitoring during labor. *American Family Physician, 49*(4), 749.

300. Hansen, P. K., Smith, S. F., Nim, J., Neldam, S., & Osler, M. (1985). Maternal attitudes to fetal monitoring. *European Journal of Obstetrics & Gynecology, 20,* 43-51.

301. Prentice, A., & Lind, T. (December 12, 1987). Fetal heart rate monitoring during labour-too frequent intervention, too little benefit? *The Lancet, 2*(8572), 1375-1377.

302. Freeman, R. (March 1, 1990). Intrapartum fetal monitoring- A disappointing story. *The New England Journal of Medicine, 322*(9), 624-626.

303. Fields, L. M. (1987). Electronic fetal monitoring: Practices and protocols for the intrapartum patient. *Journal of Perinatal and Neonatal Nursing, 1*(1), 5-12.

304. Steer, P. J. (March 1993). Standards in fetal monitoring-practical requirements for uterine activity measurement and recording. *British Journal of Obstetrics and Gynaecology, 100*(Suppl. 9), 32-36.

305. Turfwar pits midwives vs. physicians. (1995, July 30, Sunday). *The Gazette,* Montreal, pp. Al-A2.

306. Miller, F. C., Pearse, K. E., & Paul, R. H. (September 1984). Fetal heart rate pattern recognition by the method of auscultation. *Obstetrics & Gynecology, 64*(3), 332-336.

307. Strong, Jr., T. H., & Jarles, D. L. (March 1993). Intrapartum auscultation of the fetal heart rate. *American Journal of Obstetrics and Gynecology, 168*(3, Pt. 1), 935-936.

308. Davis, L., & Riedmann, G. (1991). Recommendations for the management of low risk obstetric patients. *International Journal of Gynecology and Obstetrics, 35,* 107-115.

309. Hutson, J. M., & Petrie, R. H. (March 1986). Possible limitations of fetal monitoring. *Clinical Obstetrics and Gynecology, 29*(1), 104-113.

310. Nurse's Association of the American College of Obstetricians and Gynecologists. (March 1990). Fetal heart rate auscultation. *NAACOG OGN Nursing Practice Resource.* Washington, DC: author.

311. Goldstein, K. M., Caputo, D. V., & Taub, H. B. (September 1976). The effects of prenatal and perinatal complications on development at one year of age. *Child Development, 47*(3), 613-621.

312. Kubheka, J., Lephadi, M., Majola, V., Mbawa, E., Mokoena, A., Monaheng, C., Mulaudzi, F., Ngetu, Z., Nomtuli, G., & Peters, E. (September 1985). Intrapartum foetal distress. *Curationis, 8*(3), 49-51.

313. Sykes, G. S., Molloy, P. M., Johnson, P., Gu, W., Ashworth, F., Stirrat, G. M., & Turnbull, A. C. (February 27, 1982). Do Apgar scores indicate asphyxia? *The Lancet,* 494-496.

314. Curzen, P., Bekir, J. S., McLintock, D. G., & Patel, M. (November 7, 1984). Reliability of cardiotocography in predicting baby's condition at birth. *British Medical Journal, 289*(6455), 1345-1347.

315. Emory, E. K., & Noonan, J. R. (1984). Fetal cardiac responding: A correlate of birth weight and neonatal behavior. *Child Development, 55,*1651-1657.

316. Krebs, H. B., Petres, R. E., Dunn, L. J., & Smith, P. J. (May 15, 1982). Intrapartum fetal heart rate monitoring. VII. The impact of mode of delivery on fetal outcome. *American Journal of Obstetrics and Gynecology, 143*(2), 190-194.

317. Lissauer, T. J., & Steer, P. J. (October 1986). The relation between the need for intubation at birth, abnormal cardiotocograms in labour and cord artery blood gas and pH values. *British Journal of Obstetrics and Gynaecology, 93*(10), 1060-1066.

318. Braithwaite, N. D. J., Milligan, J. E., & Shennan, A. T. (February 1986). Fetal heart rate monitoring and neonatal mortality in the very preterm infant. *American Journal of Obstetrics and Gynecology, 154*(2), 250-254.

319. Larson, E. B., van Belle, G., Shy, K. K., Luthy, D. A., Strickland, D., & Hughes, J. P. (October 1989). Fetal monitoring and predictions by clinicians: Observations during a randomized clinical trial in very low birth weight infants. *Obstetrics & Gynecology, 74*(4), 584-589.

320. Association of Women's Health, Obstetric, and Neonatal Nurses. (February 1997). *Issue: The role of unlicensed assistive personnel in the nursing care for women and newborns.* Washington, DC: author.

321. Liston, R., Crane, J., Hughes, O., Kuling, S., MacKinnon, C., & Milne, K. (April 2002). Fetal health surveillance in labour. *Journal of Obstetric and Gynaecology of Canada, 24*(4), 342-355.

322. Sprague, A., & Trépanier, M-J. (August/September 1999). Charting in record time. *AWHONN Lifelines, 3*(4), 35-40.

323. Cady, R. (January/February 2001). Legal issues surrounding the use of unlicensed assistive personnel. *MCN, 26*(1), 49.

324. Schifrin, B. S. (Ed.). (1993). Fetal surveillance during labor: The role of the expert witness. *Journal of Perinatology, 13*(2), 151-152.

325. Nurse's Association of the American College of Obstetricians and Gynecologists. Electronic fetal monitoring. (1986). *Joint NAACOG/ACOG statement.* Washington, DC: author.

326. Reeves, M. (April/May 2001). Building expertise. Making the case for fetal heart monitoring certification. *AWHONN Lifelines, 5*(2), 71-72.

327. Chagnon, L., & Easterwood, B. (September/October 1986). Managing the risks of obstetrical nursing. *MCN, 11*(5), 303-310.

328. McMullen, P. (Summer 1990). Liability in obstetrical nursing. *Nursing Connections, 3*(2), 61-63.

329. Knox, G., Simpson, K., & Garite, T. (Spring 1999). High reliability perinatal units: An approach to the prevention of patient injury and medical malpractice claims. *Journal of Healthcare Risk Management, 19*(2), 24-32.

330. Simpson, K., & Knox, G. (December 2000). Risk management and electronic fetal monitoring: Decreasing risk of adverse outcomes and liability exposure. *Journal of Perinatal and Neonatal Nursing, 14*(3), 40-52.

331. Murray, M. L. (January-February 1999). Certification in fetal heart monitoring: Is it really worth the additional effort and expense for perinatal nurses? *MCN, 24*(1), 10.

332. Cary, A. H. (January 2001). Certified registered nurses: Results of the study of the certified workforce. *American Journal of Nursing, 101*(1), 44-52.

333. Kinnick, V. L. (1989). Learning fetal monitoring under three conditions of concept learning. *Unpublished doctoral dissertation*, University of Colorado, Boulder.

334. Murray, M. L. (1992). A comparison of fetal monitoring concept learning from a learner-controlled versus teacher-controlled instructional strategy. *Unpublished doctoral dissertation*, University of New Mexico, Albuquerque.

335. Guild, S. D. (January 1994). A comprehensive fetal monitoring program for nursing practice and education. *JOGNN, 23*(1), 34-41.

336. McCartney, P. R. (1995). Fetal heart rate pattern analysis by expert and novice nurses. *Unpublished doctoral dissertation abstract*, University at Buffalo, State University of New York.

337. Schmidt, J. (1987). A second view on polemics in electronic fetal monitoring. *Journal of Perinatology, 7*(3), 229-230.

338. Catanzarite, V. A. (May 1987). FM TUTOR: A computer-aided instructional system for teaching fetal monitor interpretation. *American Journal of Obstetrics and Gynecology, 156*(5), 1045-1048.

339. Trépanier, M-J., Niday, P., Davies, B., Sprague, A., Nimrod, C., Dulberg, C., & Watters, N. (June 26-30, 1994). Development and evaluation of an education program: Fundamentals of intrapartum fetal monitoring [Abstract]. *AWHONN 1994 Annual Meeting*, Cincinnati, OH.

340. Association of Women's Health, Obstetrics, and Neonatal Nurses. *Clinical competencies and education guide: Antepartal and intrapartal fetal surveillance.* Washington, DC: author.

341. Feinstein, N., & McCartney, P. (Eds.). (1997). *Fetal heart monitoring principles and practices (2nd ed.).* Dubuque, Iowa: Kendall/Hunt Publishing Company and washington, DC: Association of Women's Health, Obstetrics, and Neonatal Nurses.

342. Afriat, C. I. (July 1987). Historical perspective on electronic fetal heart rate monitoring: A decade of growth, a decade of conflict. *Journal of Perinatal and Neonatal Nursing, 1*(1), 1-4.

343. Arulkumaran, S., Lilja, H., Lindecrantz, K., Ratnam, S. S., Thavarasah, A. S., & Rosen, K. G. (1990). Fetal ECG waveform analysis should improve fetal surveillance in labour. *Journal of Perinatal Medicine, 18*(1), 13-22.

344. McRae, M. J. (January 1993). Litigation, electronic fetal monitoring, and the obstetric nurse. *JOGNN, 22*(5), 410-419.

345. Fetal monitoring problems during labor associated with most serious OB claims. (1986). *Forum, 7*, 19-20.

346. Donker, D. K., van Geijn, H. P., & Hasman, A. (July 1993). Interobserver variation in the assessment of fetal heart rate recordings. *European Journal of Obstetrics & Gynecology, and Reproductive Biology, 52*(1), 21-28.

347. Simpson, N., Oppenheimer, L. W., Siren, A., Bland, E., McDonald, O., McDonald, D., & Dabrowski, A. (1999). Accuracy of strategies for monitoring fetal heart rate in labor. *American Journal of Perinatology, 16*(4), 167-173.

348. Fisher, C. W., Dombrowski, M. P., Juszczak, S. :E., Cook, C. D., & Sokol, R. J. (June 1995). The expert witness: Real issues and suggestions. *American Journal of Obstetrics and Gynecology, 172*(6), 1792- 1800.

349. Northrop, C. E. (1986). Malpractice and standards of care. *Nursing Outlook, 34*(3), 160.

350. The Health Law Center & Streiff, C. J. (Eds.). (1975). *Nursing and the law (2nd ed.).* Maryland: Aspen Systems Corporation.

351. Lent, M. (April 1999). The medical and legal risks of the electronic fetal monitor. *Stanford Law Review, 51*(4), 807-837.

352. Association of Women's Health, Obstetrics, and Neonatal Nurses. (1998). *Achieving consistent quality care: Using evidence to guide practice.* Washington, DC: author.

353. Rooks, J. P., Weatherby, N. L., & Ernst, E. K. M. (September-October 1992). The national birth center study–Intrapartum and immediate postpartum and neonatal care. *Journal of Nurse-Midwifery, 37*(5), 301-330.

354. Wiley, J. (September/October 1976). The nurse's legal responsibility in obstetric monitoring. *JOGNN Nursing Supplement*, 77s-78s.

355. Cetrulo, C. L., & Cetrulo, L. G. (March 1987). Medicolegal dystocia. *Clinical Obstetrics and Gynecology, 30*(1), 106-113.

356. Nurse's Association of the American College of Obstetricians and Gynecologists. (September 1991). *Issue: Appropriate use of technology in nursing care.* NAACOG Committee Opinion. Washington, DC: author.

357. Pheigaru, J. L. (September/October 1988). Keeping staff up on electronic fetal monitoring. *MCN, 13*, 334-335.

358. Cohen, J. (August/September 2001). Fetal monitoring discrepancies. *Lifelines, 5*(4), 11.

359. McRae, M. J. (May/June 1999). Fetal surveillance and monitoring: Legal issues revisited. *JOGNN, 28*(3), 310-319.

360. Koniak-Griffin, D. (May/June 1999). Strategies for reducing the risk of malpractice litigation in perinatal nursing. *JOGNN, 28*(3), 291-299.

361. $30 million verdict. OB not contacted on poor EFM strips; child has CP. (May 2000). *OB-GYN Malpractice Prevention*, 40.

362. Nurses are persons of superior knowledge. (December 1993). *American Journal of Nursing*, 9.

363. Mahlmeister, L. (September/October 2000). Legal implications of fetal heart assessment. *JOGNN, 29*(5), 517-526.

364. Mahlmeister, L. (May/June 1999). Professional accountability and legal liability for the team leader and charge nurse. *JOGNN, 28*(3), 300-309.

365. Sandmire, H. F. (October 1993) Auscultation of the fetal heart: How to do it [Letter to the editor]. *American Journal of Obstetrics and Gynecology, 169*(4), 1078-1079.

366. Avery, J. K. (December 1987). Fundamentals Fundamental. *Journal of the Tennessee Medical Association, 80*(12), 738.

367. Tammello, A. (Ed.). (July 1986). Misuse of fetal monitor: Brain damage results. *The Regan Report on Nursing Law, 27*(2), 4.

368. American College of Obstetricians and Gynecologists. (1989). *Standards for obstetric-gynecologic services (7th ed.).* (1989). Washington, DC: author.

369. National Institute of Child Health and Human Development Research Planning Workshop. (1997). Electronic fetal heart monitoring: Research guidelines for interpretation. *American Journal of Obstetrics and Gynecology, 177,* 1385-1390.

370. National Institute of Child Health and Human Development Research Planning Workshop. (1997). Electronic fetal monitoring: Research guidelines for interpretation. *JOGNN, 26,* 635-640.

371. Devoe, L., Golde, S., Kilman, Y., Morton, D., Shea, K., & Waller, J. (August 2000). A comparison of visual analyses of intrapartum fetal heart rate tracings according to the new National Institute of Child Health and Human Development guidelines with computer analyses by an automated fetal heart rate monitoring system. *American Journal of Obstetrics and Gynecology, 183*(2), 361-366.

372. Mandeville, L. K. (June 4-7, 1995). Legalities in perinatal nursing: Case reviews. In Tune With the Country. *AWHONN 1995 Convention Session Resources,* 84-86. Nashville, TN.

373. Chez, B. F., & Verklan, M. T. (1987). Documentation and electronic fetal monitoring: How, where, and what? *Journal of Perinatal and Neonatal Nursing, 1*(1), 22-28.

374. Pluta, M., Dudenhausen, J. W., Gesche, J., & Saling, E. (1983). Fetal heart rate monitoring on the operating table immediately before delivery by cesarean section. *Journal of Perinatal Medicine, 11*(2), 85-96.

375. Murchison, I., Nichols, T. S., & Hanson, R. (1978). *Legal accountability in the nursing process.* St. Louis: The C. V. Mosby Company.

376. Murray, M. L. (1996). Electronic fetal monitoring: Role of the nurse. In S. M. Donn & C. W. Fisher (Eds.), *Risk management techniques in perinatal and neonatal practice,* pp 213-238. Armonk, NY: Future Publishing Company, Inc.

377. Fall, O., Ek, B., Nilsson, B. A., & Rooth, G. (1979). Time factor in oxygen transfer from mother to fetus. *Gynecology, Obstetrics Investigation, 10*(5), 231-236.

378. Baxi, L. V. (June 1982). Current status of fetal oxygen monitoring. *Clinical Perinatology, 9*(2), 423-431.

379. Tammelleo, A. D. (Ed.). (December 1992). Failure to monitor FHR: Catastrophic results. *The Regan Report on Nursing Law, 33*(7).

380. Tammelleo, A. D. (Ed.). (December 1992). Fetal distress: "Failure to call for help." Case in point: Fairfax Hosp. System, Inc. v. McCarty (419 S.E. 2d 621 - VA [1992]). *The Regan Report on Nursing Law, 33*(7).

381. Nurse's Association of the American College of Obstetricians and Gynecologists. (1991). *Nursing practice competencies and educational guidelines. Antepartum fetal surveillance and intrapartum fetal heart monitoring (2nd ed).* Washington, DC: author.

382. Nurse's Association of the American College of Obstetricians and Gynecologists. (October 1988). *Nursing responsibilities in implementing intrapartum fetal heart rate monitoring.* NAACOG Position Statement. Washington, DC: author.

383. Tauer, C. A. (1993). When pregnant patients refuse interventions. *AWHONN's Clinical Issues 4*(4), 596-605.

384. Miller-Slade, D. (July 1994). What is "informed consent" and what is the nurse's role in the informed consent process? *AWHONN Voice 2*(7), 4.

385. Oxford, A. (Personal communication, April 20, 1995).

386. Symonds, E. M. (March 1993). Litigation and the cardiotocogram. *British Journal of Obstetrics and Gynaecology, 100*(Suppl. 9), 8-9.

387. Hirsch, C. S., Morris, R. C., & Moritz, A. R. (1979). *Handbook of Legal Medicine (5th ed.)* (pp. 315-318). St. Louis: The C. V. Mosby Company.

388. Cohn, S. D. (October 1987). Trends in perinatal nursing professional liability. *Journal of Perinatal and Neonatal Nursing, 1*(2), 19-27.

389. Schmidt, J. (1987). Documenting EFM events. *Perinatal Press, 10*(6), 79-81.

390. Feather, H., & Morgan, N. (November 1991). Risk management: Role of the medical record department. *Top Health Record Management, 12*(2), 40-48.

391. Patient Discharge. Fraudulent charting. (July 1990). *Nursing90,* 18.

392. Specht, J. (June 4-7, 1995). Bedside computerization in an LDRP setting. In Tune With The Country. *AWHONN 1995 Convention Session Resources,* Nashville, TN.

393. Skiba, D. (Spring 1993). Collaborative tools. *Reflections,* 10-12.

394. Boyd, W. (August 1989). Transmission of cardiotocograph material by facsimile for expert interpretation. *Australian & New Zealand Journal of Obstetrics & Gynaecology, 29*(3, Pt. 2), 368-369.

395. Perlow, J. H., & Garite, T. J. (1991). Update on electronic fetal monitoring systems. *Contemporary OB/GYN, 36*, 44-55.

396. Devoe, L. D. (April 1990). Computerized analysis of fetal heart rate. *The Female Patient, 15*, 41-47.

397. Wolman, W-L., Chalmers, B., Hofmeyr, J., & Nikodem, V. C. (May 1993). Postpartum depression and companionship in the clinical birth environment: A randomized, controlled study. *American Journal Obstetrics and Gynecology, 168*(5), 1388-1393.

398. Kennell, J., Klaus, M., McGrath, S ., Robertson, S., & Hinkley, C. (May 1, 1991). Continuous emotional support during labor in a US hospital. *The Journal of the American Medical Association, 265*(17), 2197-2201.

399. Kardong-Edgren, S . (October 1994). Labor assistants [Letter to the editor] . *JOGNN, 23*(8), 637.

7

Hemodynamic and Biochemical Fetal Monitoring

INTRODUCTION

Fetal acid-base information has been indirectly obtained by tissue pH sampling, transcutaneous oxygen pressure monitoring, electrocardiography, electroencephalography, reflectance pulse oximetry, mass spectrophotometry, near infrared spectroscopy, real-time ultrasound, and Doppler blood flow studies (1-3). A direct measure of fetal acid-base status requires a sample of fetal scalp capillary blood, umbilical artery blood, or blood from a fetal artery on the placental chorionic plate. Analysis of fetal hemodynamics and acid-base status supplements information obtained from the electronic fetal monitor. This chapter presents techniques that have been used to assess fetal hemodynamic and acid-base status and maternal interventions to resuscitate the fetus in utero.

ANTENATAL HEMODYNAMIC ANALYSIS AND BIOCHEMICAL TESTS
DOPPLER BLOOD FLOW STUDIES

Placental pathology and fetal compromise are indirectly assessed by Doppler-derived blood flow information. Abnormal Doppler blood flow waveforms are associated with fetal acidemia. Doppler study data influences the decision to deliver the baby versus maintain the pregnancy. In some cases, asphyxia will be suspected and the baby will be delivered prior to heart failure or death (4-5).

Placental status is indirectly reflected by umbilical artery Doppler blood flow information. Divon (5) believes women with a high-risk pregnancy need umbilical artery Doppler blood flow studies to prevent fetal death. Doppler imaging

significantly decreased perinatal mortality compared to pregnancies where Doppler tests were not done (12.2 deaths/1000 births versus 27.1 deaths/1000 births) (5). A meta-analysis of 20 randomized controlled trials of umbilical artery Doppler ultrasonography confirmed definite benefits of Doppler blood flow information in high-risk pregnancies. There were fewer cases of :
- intrapartum "fetal distress"
- cesarean sections for "fetal distress"
- perinatal deaths and
- hypoxic-ischemic encephalopathy (6).

In addition to analysis of blood flow through the umbilical arteries, blood flow may be measured in maternal or fetal vessels during diastole. Diastolic blood flow is passive. Using Doppler technology, the systolic to diastolic (S/D) ratio, the pulsatility index (PI), and the resistance index (RI) may be determined.

Pulsatility Index

The PI quantifies blood flow waveforms (7). Normally, umbilical artery PI is 0.5 to 1.5 at 20 w (8). PI increases when placental circulation resistance increases (9). Abnormally elevated umbilical vein adenosine was associated with abnormally elevated *uterine artery* PI, even if the fetus had normal *umbilical artery* blood gases (10). These findings reflect diminished uterine blood flow, anaerobic metabolism of adenosine triphosphate, and compensation for chronic hypoxia.

Resistance Index (RI)

Preterm fetuses have a higher umbilical artery RI than term fetuses because their placental capillary walls are thicker. As gestation advances, placental tertiary stem villi capillary walls become thinner and RI decreases (11). Umbilical artery pH may be predicted from the RI. A *low* umbilical artery RI (less than the 10th percentile for that gestational age) is associated with hyperdynamic fetal circulation and an increased risk of antepartal hemorrhage, preterm premature rupture of membranes, preterm labor, high umbilical venous blood flow, and increased days in the neonatal intensive care unit (NICU). Fetuses with hyperdynamic blood flow were less mature than those with a normal RI (12).

The Brain

Cerebral and umbilical artery PI decreases from 26 weeks' gestation to term (13). Cerebral blood flow and blood vessel diameter are related to fetal PO_2 and base excess (BE). The PI of the fetal *internal carotid artery* was related to fetal PO_2 and BE but not pH or PCO_2 (14). As a fetus becomes acidemic, *middle cerebral artery* perfusion of the basal ganglia decreases. Cocaine exposed neonates had basal ganglia lesions (15). An abnormal middle cerebral artery S/D ratio (≤ 3.1) was found in intrauterine growth restricted (IUGR) fetuses who were 26 to 37 weeks' gestation with a preacidotic (7.20 to 7.25) umbilical artery pH (16).

The Cardiovascular System

As the risk of cardiac failure increases in IUGR fetuses and twins who had twin-twin transfusion syndrome, *jugular vein* diastolic velocity decreases or blood flow reverses during atrial contraction of the heart (17). Fetuses who had cardiac failure were also bradycardic (18).

Doppler blood flow studies in the *ductus venosus and inferior vena cava* may suggest impending fetal heart failure. Normally there is high flow through the ductus venosus during the cardiac cycle. Hypoxemia and acidemia decrease the velocity of blood flow during an atrial contraction (9). If there is no flow or reversal of flow, the fetus may be acidotic or asphyxiated. For example, reversed end diastolic blood flow in the *ductus venosus* is abnormal and has been associated with increased fetal atrial pressure and impending fetal heart failure (9, 19). Decreased aortic and pulmonic valve outflow during peak velocity times is also indicative of cardiac function deterioration (20).

These studies suggest that if the fetus is compromised blood does not move normally through the inferior vena cava. The S/D ratio may be abnormally high or low. A high S/D ratio reflects decreased central venous pressure. A decrease in inferior vena cava flow increases the PI and suggests failure of compensatory mechanisms with hypoxic myocardial failure. Fetal afterload may increase due to high umbilical artery resistance and/or impending cardiac failure. High afterload decreases blood flow through the *inferior vena cava* to the point where blood flow may be reversed during diastole, suggesting tricuspid valve regurgitation (4, 21). The inferior vena cava diameter of *compromised* fetuses is greater at the end of diastole than early in diastole and there is a low pulsatile waveform (22).

Umbilical Artery Blood Flow

Abnormal umbilical artery blood flow reflects placental pathology and fetal compromise. The Doppler waveform will be affected by cardiac contractility, the fetal heart rate (FHR), fetal breathing movements, preload, vessel elasticity, and blood viscosity (5, 21). The fetus may be compromised due to deranged afterload and/or cardiac contractility. Or, there may be increased intravascular resistance in the placenta, i.e., downstream resistance, which causes umbilical artery-placental insufficiency. An abnormal umbilical artery Doppler waveform, e.g., a notched waveform, was related to placental infarction, decidual vessel muscular thickening, placental fibrinoid necrosis, fetal stem vessel obliteration, hemorrhagic endovasculitis, and avascular terminal villi (23-24).

Downstream placental resistance is inversely related to umbilical artery end-diastolic blood velocity. If the placenta has increased blood flow impedance, diastolic flow decreases or becomes absent or reversed. *Absent umbilical artery end-diastolic velocity in preterm pregnancies* was associated with IUGR, operative delivery, necrotizing enterocolitis, and perinatal death (25). Gestational age of fetuses with abnormal umbilical artery blood flow was related to their survival. *Only 25% of fetuses with abnormal umbilical artery blood flow who were less than 26 weeks' gestation survived.* If they were 26 to 28 weeks' gestation, 53.85% lived. The majority of fetuses greater than 28 weeks' gestation (92.86%), who had abnormal umbilical artery blood flow, lived (26).

When the number of placental blood vessels decrease to fewer than 50% of normal, umbilical artery PI increases (5). Elevated PI indicates high placental vascular resistance. PI increases and the FHR changes when the fetus is becoming hypoxic or acidotic (27). Visser, Bekedam, and Ribbert (28) found umbilical artery *PI increased nine days to three weeks prior to the onset of decelerations.* They identified a continuum in fetal deterioration (see Figure 7.1).

Figure 7.1: Continuum of fetal deterioration during the antenatal period

Abnormal Doppler waveform pattern precedes decelerations by 1 to 3 weeks

▼

Maternal perception: more weak fetal movements, fewer strong, rolling movements
Ultrasound: slow, monotonous movements

▼

Disturbed transition from behavior state to state, e.g., change from 1F to 2F

▼

Decelerations (may be late, variable, or prolonged)
Hypoxemia

▼

Decreased long-term variation (to 30 milliseconds (msec), the lower range of normality)
Hypoxemia

▼

Fewer accelerations, loss of accelerations
Acidemia

▼

Decreased overall variability (< 5 beats per minute (bpm))

▼

Decreased fetal movement
Hypoxia and acidemia

▼

Absent fetal movement +
Terminal FHR patterns, e.g., sinusoidal pattern or absent variability with subtle late decelerations or spontaneous decelerations
pH < 7.15 in 70% of cases

▼

Death within 1 week of terminal FHR pattern

Thus, abnormal umbilical artery blood flow is an earlier sign of impending fetal decompensation than an abnormal FHR pattern. Abnormal umbilical artery blood flow occurs days before hypoxemia affects the FHR. Decelerations are often an earlier warning sign of fetal hypoxia than the loss of variability, loss of accelerations, or loss of fetal movement. When Doppler blood flow study results are evaluated with FHR changes, physicians may decide that delivery is warranted to prevent fetal injury from asphyxia.

Doppler Blood Flow Studies of the IUGR Fetus

Preeclamptic women have an increased risk of abnormal *uterine artery* blood flow (7). Sixty-six percent of hypertensive women had fetuses with abnormal Doppler blood flow and 61% of fetuses with abnormal blood flow were IUGR (26). Many IUGR fetuses are already hypoxemic and acidemic before labor (29). They have redistributed their blood flow and *increased* impedance in their descending thoracic aorta with *decreased* impedance in their cerebral circulation. Flow across their mitral and tricuspid valves decreases in response to decreased venous return to their heart (9). IUGR fetuses with an abnormal umbilical artery PI had a normal size cerebellum, illustrating the brainsparing effect that occurs during chronic hypoxia (7). Abnormal umbilical artery PI was associated with an increased risk of long-term neurologic impairment and death (5).

Decreased variability, the lack of accelerations, and abnormal umbilical artery blood flow predict acidemia. If the *uterine artery* PI was abnormal, umbilical vein adenosine was higher than normal. The elevated adenosine level was even found when IUGR fetuses had normal blood gases (10). Adenosine inhibits the SA node and sympathetic nerves to decrease variability. Low variation of the FHR baseline was a better predictor of fetal acidemia than the umbilical artery S/D ratio, PI or RI (30).

Acidemic fetuses have reduced variability, no accelerations, and decelerations (29). Low variation for more than 50 minutes was associated with a pH less than 7.20 in 67% of IUGR fetuses. Fetal pH was always less than 7.20 if short-term variation (STV) was less than 3.5 msec and there were no accelerations (31). *One hour of STV less than 2.5 msec, and long-term variation less than 12.5 msec, increased the risk of impending fetal death (32). Therefore, after 50 minutes of monitoring the IUGR fetus, if STV is less than 3.5 msec, there are no accelerations, and there is abnormal umbilical artery blood flow, fetal acidemia is highly probable* creating a high risk for acidosis, asphyxia, and death. Women should be advised of the fetal risk and the fetus should be delivered to avoid asphyxia and its sequelae.

Cordocentesis

As a reflection of placental function, umbilical vein blood gases may be obtained during the antenatal period by cordocentesis or percutaneous umbilical blood sampling (PUBS). To obtain umbilical venous blood, a 21 gauge long (spinal) needle is inserted through the maternal abdomen and uterus and into the umbilical vein under real-time ultrasound sector scanner guidance. Blood is collected in a heparinized syringe (33-34). The common complications of PUBS include:

- umbilical cord bleeding
- cord hematoma
- a prolonged deceleration or
- bradycardia.

Bleeding depends on the size of the needle and the puncture site. Bradycardia may be transient (a prolonged deceleration) or profound and may be a response to hypoxia related to development of a cord hematoma or umbilical vessel spasm. Two of nine fetuses, less than 32 weeks' gestation, had a prolonged deceleration for five to seven minutes following PUBS (33). Profound bradycardia is more common if the fetus is IUGR or severely anemic (35). PUBS may precede preterm labor, a fetomaternal hemorrhage (in as many as 40% of cases), abruption, and 1% of fetuses die from exsanguination. Exsanguination has been associated with Glanzmann's thrombasthenia or alloimmune thrombocytopenia (33, 35). In this disease, maternal antiplatelet antibodies transfer through the placenta into the fetus causing alloimmune thrombocytopenia (36-37).

Umbilical blood gases have been obtained prior to elective cesarean section (cordocentesis) and may be obtained immediately following delivery (umbilical cord sampling). There are differences in umbilical venous values before and after the hypoxic stress of labor and delivery. These norms reflect findings from several studies and include values for fetuses 18 to 38 weeks' gestation (38-40).

Table 1: Umbilical Vein Blood Gases Obtained by Cordocentesis Prior to Labor and Following Elective Cesarean Section

	Cordocentesis	After Elective Cesarean
pH	7.33 - 7.45	7.27 - 7.35
SO$_2$	58.39 - 97.09%	
PO$_2$	24.38 - 52.77 mm Hg	22.54 - 31.4
PCO$_2$	25.16 - 47.12 mm Hg	40.58 - 52
Bicarbonate	19.71 - 23.81 mEq/L	
Base Excess	-3.45 to 1.64 mEq/L	-3.84 to 0.88

INTRAPARTAL BIOCHEMICAL TESTS

During labor, nurses monitor the physical condition of the mother and fetus. At times, the FHR pattern suggests fetal compromise. Noninvasive tests that *rule in well-being* and rule out metabolic acidosis include acoustic stimulation, scalp stimulation, or the scalp electrode stimulation test. The physician may sample scalp capillary blood for pH and/or fetal blood gases. An acceleration that peaks 15 bpm above the baseline and lasts 15 seconds at its base following any of these tests rules out metabolic acidosis (41).

Fetal Acoustic Stimulation Test (FAST)

The fetus responds to sound, not vibration (42). The fetal cochlea, the organ of hearing, is fully developed by 20 weeks' gestation (43). However, neonates do not respond to sound until 25 to 28 weeks' gestation (42, 44). Usually, the fetus responds to external sounds at about 26 weeks' gestation (45). In one study, a 3 second sound stimulus elicited NO response in fetuses 28 or fewer weeks' gestation, but did elicit an acceleration in fetuses greater than 28 weeks' gestation (46). Therefore, *the best time to use FAST is when the fetus is 28 or more weeks' gestation*. The device is used when the FHR baseline is evident and not during a deceleration. The goal is to elicit an acceleration in the FHR.

Acoustic stimulation is used when the cervix is not dilated enough to apply firm digital pressure to the fetal scalp (scalp stimulation), when baseline variability is minimal or absent and accelerations have not appeared for 50 or more minutes, or when confirmation is needed that the fetus is not metabolically acidotic (47). Depending on hospital protocol, the midwife or physician may be notified of the FHR pattern prior to use of the acoustic stimulator. In some cases, the acoustic stimulator is used and then the midwife or physician are notified of the FHR pattern before and after stimulation. Prior to device application on the maternal thigh or abdomen, the woman should see it and hear it. She should be asked to acknowledge fetal movement following sound stimulation. The clinician may also palpate the maternal abdomen to detect fetal movement following stimulation.

Sound Intensity

The fetus is constantly surrounded by sound from maternal breathing, vascular pulsations, the heartbeat, intestinal peristalsis, placental sounds, and external noises such as music and voices (43, 48-51). This background noise has been measured at 60 to 95 decibels (dB) (42, 48, 52).

There is no evidence that use of the acoustic stimulator impairs fetal hearing. Eighty-two 4 year olds were tested using pediatric audiometry techniques. There was no difference in the hearing between children whose had a FAST and those who did not (53).

External sound is attenuated by the abdominal wall and intensified after passing through fluid (54). Acoustic stimulation devices are usually 75 or more megahertz (MHZ) and 72 or more dB (55-56). An artificial larynx can produce sounds of 91 to 111 dB (42, 55). At 80 dB, a deceleration following acoustic stimulation was more common than an acceleration in low-risk fetuses who were 37 to 40 weeks' gestation. At a sound intensity of 90 or more dB, an acceleration was more common (57). Therefore, a device that provides 90 or more dB would be best to rule out metabolic acidosis.

Sound is loudest when the device is placed over the fetal ear. An 103 dB artificial larynx on the ewe's abdomen and over the fetal lamb's ear created 134.9 dB of sound at the ear. Three inches from the ear, it was 114.3 dB. Six inches from the ear it was 101.4 dB (58). A pneumatic jack hammer or severe thunder produce 120 dB. 125 dB is close to the sound of a jet upon takeoff as heard on the runway (59). Since 90 or more dB is all that is needed to produce a fetal acceleration, it might be best to start at the maternal thigh, near the fetal ear and repeat the stimulus one or two times as the device is moved closer to the fetal ear.

Sound Duration

Usually, a three second stimulation is applied near or over the fetal vertex (47). Best results will be obtained if the device is applied 30 seconds *after a contraction has ended*, when the fetus has replenished most of its oxygen (O_2) reserves (60).

Fetal Response

In a study of low-risk women, 75% of the fetuses accelerated and 19% had a variable deceleration or prolonged deceleration following acoustic stimulation. Decelerations were innocuous (60). When an *acceleration was immediately followed by a deceleration*, a nuchal cord was present 39.2% of the time. Perhaps when the fetus moved after stimulation, the nuchal cord was tightened which caused the variable deceleration. A nuchal cord was present in 15% of fetuses who accelerated and 11% of fetuses that had no FHR change in response to acoustic stimulation (55).

A nonacidotic fetus *"awakens" and urinates* after being startled by acoustic stimulation (54, 61). Blood flow to the brain increases and the FHR accelerates an average of 13 bpm (46). If the acceleration peaked 15 bpm above the baseline, the fetal scalp pH was greater than 7.19 (62). The number of fetal movements, the baseline rate, and baseline variability often increase following acoustic stimulation (63). In fact, *the fetus may remain in a 4F state for one hour after acoustic stimulation* (64).

Narcotics and the fetal response. Narcotics reduce fetal movement but do not prevent a fetal response to acoustic stimulation (65-66). When Stadol, a narcotic agonist-antagonist, was administered, 78% of fetuses responded to acoustic stimulation. One hour after drug administration, the other fetuses responded (67). Narcotics change the fetal wake state and put the fetus into a quiescent (1F) state. If the fetus is stimulated with sound, the sympathetic response may last only 10 minutes and the fetus will return to "sleep" (66). Although *it is best to let women sleep or rest after narcotic administration*, if concern heightens for the fetus, use of acoustic

stimulation to elicit an acceleration will shorten the period of nonreactivity.

Rupture of membranes and the fetal response. The FHR response decreases as labor progresses, possibly due to the loss of amniotic fluid which diminishes sound intensity, or fetal hypoxia which diminishes the response to sound (60). Therefore, *when membranes are ruptured, the well fetus may be unresponsive to acoustic stimulation*. During the second stage of labor, there may be a decline in the fetal O_2 supply which will diminish the fetal response due to a sensori-neural hearing loss. Maternal inhalation of O_2 by mask increases the near-term fetus' response to acoustic stimulation (42, 55, 60).

Scalp Stimulation

Fetal scalp stimulation may be an intermediate diagnostic step before fetal scalp blood sampling or operative delivery (68). A protocol should be written so that staff nurses can use this technique at their discretion when they are unable to assess STV and they wish to elicit an acceleration to rule out metabolic acidosis or they are concerned because they observe an abnormal pattern that is associated with acidosis, e.g.,

- late decelerations with baseline STV
- severe variable decelerations
- absent variability
- tachycardia
- no accelerations for at least 40 minutes of monitoring (the end of state 1F)
- no fetal movement for 45 to 60 minutes
- the clinician is unsure of the fetal status
- a sinusoidal pattern exists on admission, it could be a benign sinusoidal pattern
- the baseline changed to a tachycardic or bradycardic rate and variability decreased
- an abnormal FHR pattern has not resolved following interventions
- an arrhythmia is suspected (62, 69-70).

When and How To Do Fetal Scalp Stimulation

Scalp stimulation has been accomplished by grasping the fetal skin with an atraumatic allis clamp, firm digital pressure, traction on the spiral electrode, and puncture (scalp capillary pH sampling). Scalp stimulation is most commonly done by firm digital pressure. The clinician dons a sterile glove. Using two fingers, the fetal scalp over a parietal bone is vigorously rubbed between contractions and decelerations when a baseline FHR has been established. It is NOT appropriate to rub the fetal scalp during a deceleration as it serves absolutely no purpose. The deceleration usually reflects a vagal response which prevents any sympathetic nerve response during scalp stimulation. The goal is to elicit a sympathetic nerve response. An acceleration in the FHR after stimulation is associated with a scalp blood pH of greater than 7.19 (62).

346

Fetal Response

If the FHR accelerates after scalp stimulation, it is highly unlikely that the fetus is acidotic (69). *An acceleration is a good predictor of a nonacidemic fetus. The lack of an acceleration is a poor predictor of an acidemic fetus* (68-69, 71-73). Fetuses, who had FHR patterns associated with acidemia, i.e., tachycardia, severe variable decelerations, late decelerations, or absent variability, where tested by scalp stimulation. If the FHR accelerated 15 bpm and lasted 15 seconds (15 x 15), fetal scalp pH was greater than or equal to 7.25. Almost half (47%) of the fetuses that did not accelerate were not acidemic (69). An acceleration greater than 15 bpm lasting greater than 15 seconds in response to scalp puncture reflected a scalp pH greater than 7.20 (71). In both of these studies, researchers did not say whether or not the acceleration was sustained for 15 seconds at 15 bpm above the baseline nor did they identify which part of the baseline (top, middle, or bottom) they used to measure the 15 bpm rise in the FHR.

Scalp Electrode Stimulation Test

An easy test of fetal well-being is to elicit fetal pain by pulling on the spiral electrode. In nonacidotic fetuses, following *5 short consecutive tractions over a 5 second period* during a fetal 2F active state, every fetus moved and accelerated and 95.8% accelerated and moved within 1 minute following stimulation. Twelve of 15 fetuses in a quiescent (1F) state moved immediately, 14 of 15 moved within 10 seconds of stimulation, 10 of 14 resumed their 1F state after stimulation, and 13 of 15 accelerated within 1 minute of stimulation (74).

FETAL SCALP BLOOD SAMPLING (FSBS)

In 1962, prior to the development of the first commercial electronic fetal heart monitor, Erich Saling developed the technique of fetal scalp capillary blood sampling for acid-base studies during labor (75-76). Although the use of FSBS is waning, it is still being used in many centers in the United States and Europe.

Indications

A normal FHR pattern predicts a healthy fetus and newborn with 99% accuracy (77-78). It is harder to predict the depressed newborn based only on the FHR pattern. FSBS, in conjunction with the FHR pattern, increases the physician's ability to predict outcome (78). *However, FSBS is not indicated when FHR patterns are clearly indicative of fetal well-being or decompensation (79).*

FSBS verifies fetal status when there is an abnormal FHR pattern, such as tachycardia with absent variability (80). Other FHR patterns which may precede FSBS include:
- unexplained absent STV
- sinusoidal pattern
- cardiac arrhythmia patterns
- mixed deceleration patterns (two or more types of decelerations)
- contradictory patterns, such as absent variability with accelerations (81-82).

Contraindications

Because the fetus can bleed from the scalp and possibly exsanguinate, contraindications to FSBS include:
- a suspected blood dyscrasia, such as alloimmune thrombocytopenia, hemophilia, or von Willebrand's disease
- when undesirable rupture of membranes would be required
- when there is vaginal bleeding (maternal blood could contaminate the sample)
- when several previous scalp punctures have been made
- when maternal herpes simplex or human immunodeficiency virus is confirmed and/or
- when there is a confirmed genital tract infection such as gonorrhea or β-hemolytic streptococcus (83).

Limitations

The feasibility of performing intermittent FSBS is influenced by fetal presentation, position, station, and the degree of cervical dilatation and effacement. Presence of thick fetal hair may hinder collection of the blood sample. Marked scalp swelling (caput succedaneum) is accompanied by venous stasis, which may produce an erroneously low pH (79).

It has been recommended that more than one sample of scalp capillary blood be analyzed prior to deciding if delivery should be by cesarean section (84-85). Therefore, once FSBS is initiated, it is usually repeated. The collection of multiple samples may precede scalp abscess or hemorrhage or may unnecessarily prolong labor and increase the risk of fetal hypoxia and acidosis. On the other hand, the fetus with an abnormal FHR pattern may have a congenital defect which would not warrant an immediate cesarean delivery. Bossart (86) describes this situation as a "treatment paradox," i.e., whether scalp sampling or a cesarean delivery would be an excessive intervention or preventive medicine. Because there is no characteristic abnormal FHR that is associated with major congenital malformations, in the absence of ultrasound studies that indicate an anomaly, FSBS would be beneficial to assist the clinician in decision making when the possibility exists that an infant will be unnecessarily operatively delivered (87-88).

Even if conditions for FSBS are ideal, FSBS may not be done or may yield erroneous information because of:
- an unskilled physician
- unavailable pH analysis equipment
- misinterpretation of results
- a need to repeat FSBS prior to a final diagnosis and/or
- insufficient training or opportunities to practice FSBS and maintain proficiency.

The financial considerations of having 24 hour laboratory equipment and assistance, with the degree of skill and experience required to properly perform blood analysis, are the most frequent limiting factors of FSBS (79).

ANTEPARTAL AND INTRAPARTAL FETAL MONITORING

Requirements Prior To Sampling

Once the need for FSBS has been determined, the woman should be given as much information as is reasonable about the circumstances for testing and about how the procedure will be performed. This usually is a process shared by the physician and nurse. Many facilities require a signed consent prior to FSBS. In addition, the following must exist:

- an experienced physician who knows the correct technique for blood acquisition
- a "low enough" fetal presenting part
- "adequate" dilatation
- fetal head in the pelvis or use of fundal pressure to bring the head down into the pelvis and
- appropriate equipment with a prewarmed, calibrated blood analyzer (89-90).

The physician cannot perform this procedure without assistants. At least two nurses or a nurse and a technician are needed to assist with maternal positioning, blood sample handling, and sample analysis. The nurse provides emotional support and assists the physician. The other nurse or the technician is responsible for the rapid transport of the specimen to the analyzer site. A physician, nurse, or skilled technician should run the analyzer.

The woman is positioned on her side or her back with the head of the bed slightly elevated and/or a wedge under her right side. Supine positioning is avoided as hypotension and blood flow reduction may cause a lower pH which would not reflect the true fetal condition. A knee-chest position may be used as it facilitates uterine blood flow while allowing adequate access to the fetus (91). If a lateral position is used, the woman's leg may be supported on the side rail or may be held by the nurse.

Sampling Technique

Sterile disposable kits are available for FSBS. FSBS equipment includes:
- endoscope with a light source
- sponges on a long holder
- silicone gel to facilitate beading of blood droplets
- 2 x 2 mm lancet at the end of a long holder
- long capillary tubes for blood collection and
- a prewarmed and calibrated blood gas analyzer.

The physician inserts the lighted endoscope into the vagina then dries the fetal scalp with swabs. Silicone gel is applied. The scalp is punctured but not over a fontanel (89). Capillary glass tubes, used to collect the specimen, have a maximum length of 15 centimeters (cm), and usually no more than 10.7 cm are needed to supply 85 to 125 microliters (μl) of blood. Between 25 and 125 μl of blood is needed, depending on analyzer requirements (90).

Blood gas analyzers must be warmed prior to use. Analysis of scalp blood pH should take less than three minutes. *If the analyzer has a paper printout, it should be retained in*

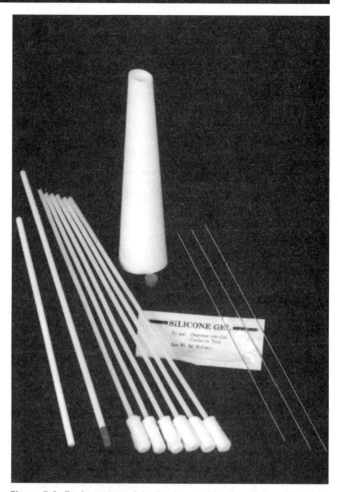

Figure 7.2: Equipment used for fetal scalp blood sampling. The light source and blood analyzer are not in this picture. (Photograph by Pam Barncastle, Castle Studios, Albuquerque, NM).

the medical record as evidence of results. The physician should write a progress note discussing the procedure and results with a plan of care. The nurse may record maternal position during FSBS, maternal and fetal tolerance of the procedure, pH results, and the FHR response to scalp puncture, e.g., the height and duration of the acceleration.

Complications

The lancet may break (85). Bleeding is the most serious complication following FSBS. Sites may bleed during vacuum extraction. A laceration may require suturing. Fetal death has occurred from exsanguination. A sinusoidal pattern suggests fetal anemia. Some babies have developed a scalp infection (83).

Acidemia and Acidosis

pH values determine the presence or absence of acidemia. Blood gases determine the presence or absence of acidosis. Fetuses who had *no decelerations* or *only early decelerations* (head compression) in the 20 minutes prior to FSBS consistently had pH values above 7.25. Scalp capillary blood *pH values dropped with the appearance of tachycardia, variable decelerations, and late decelerations. pH values became lower as decelerations became deeper and longer* and were higher when accelerations in the FHR were present within the 20 minute period prior to FSBS (82). Fetuses with an acidotic pH (< 7.20) had a lower average FHR prior to FSBS than fetuses with preacidotic or normal pH values (92). Norms for fetal scalp blood gases reflect the findings of multiple studies (14, 93-95).

Table 2: Scalp Capillary Blood Gases

Scalp Capillary pH

normal	> 7.25
preacidemic	7.20 to 7.25
acidemic	< 7.20

Scalp Capillary Blood Gases

pH	7.25 - 7.43
PO$_2$	20 - 48 mm Hg
PCO$_2$	30 - 53 mm Hg
Base Excess	-6.9 to 4.2 mEq/L

Scalp Capillary Blood Gases of Low Risk Women at 5 or More Centimeters Dilatation

pH	≥ 7.25
PO$_2$	> 10.48 mm Hg
PCO$_2$	> 38.7 mm Hg
Bicarbonate	> 21.05 mEq/L

Scalp Capillary Blood with Respiratory Acidosis

pH	**< 7.20**
PO$_2$	> 10 mm Hg
PCO$_2$	**> 60 mm Hg**
Base Excess	> -10 mEq/L

Scalp Capillary Blood with Metabolic Acidosis

pH	**< 7.20**
PO$_2$	**usually < 20 mm Hg**
PCO$_2$	45-55 mm Hg
Base Excess	**< -10 mEq/L**

Fetal scalp pH values depend upon maternal acid-base status and the temporal relationship of sampling to uterine contractions and decelerations.

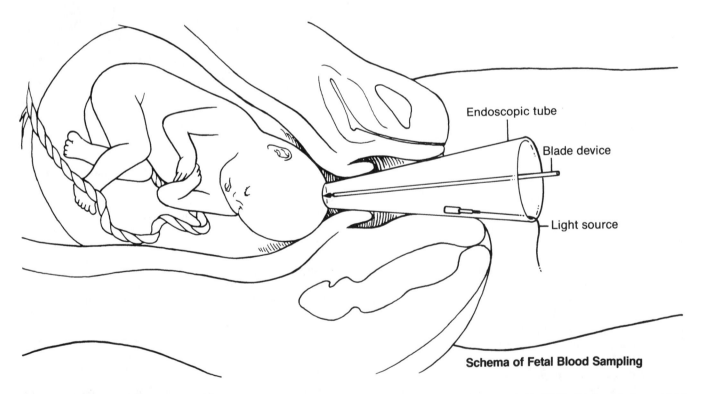

Schema of Fetal Blood Sampling

Figure 7.3: Schema of fetal blood sampling (Reproduced with permission of The C. V. Mosby Company from Tucker, S. M. (1978). *Fetal monitoring and fetal assessment in high-risk pregnancy*).

Maternal pH influences fetal pH. There is a strong relationship between maternal and fetal pH. Maternal venous pH is usually no more than 0.17 units higher than fetal scalp pH. Maternal artery pH is usually no more than 0.20 units higher than fetal pH. If the woman is alkalotic or acidemic, fetal scalp blood pH may not reflect the true fetal pH (78). Maternal metabolic acidosis can *falsely lower fetal pH* due to the transplacental transfer of maternal hydrogen ions or infusion acidosis (96-97). Catecholamine release, in response to pain, and the lack of food during labor can create a mild maternal metabolic acidosis. The accumulated hydrogen (H+) ions decrease maternal and fetal pH, especially if labor is prolonged. *Maternal respiratory or metabolic diseases* may also decrease fetal pH, e.g., maternal ketoacidosis.

To clarify the maternal influence on fetal pH values, it has been recommended that maternal venous (from the antecubital vein) or capillary pH (from a finger stick) be obtained at the time the fetal scalp blood sample is collected (78, 85). Maternal blood should not be collected from the arm which has the intravenous (IV) infusion. If maternal blood is collected, prolonged constriction of the mother's arm with a tourniquet should be avoided.

Temporal relationship of sampling to uterine contractions. *Blood should be collected between contractions.* A biological oscillation of fetal pH occurs with uterine activity. pH decreases during contractions, followed by a gradual increase from the onset of the intercontractile pause (the interval) to the peak of the following contraction. These changes may cause pH to vary by as much as 0.05 units (84).

Fetal scalp pH was lower in nulliparous women than in women who had at least one prior delivery (average 7.276 versus 7.304). The difference in fetal pH may be a reflection of the fact that nulliparous women may suffer more pain, catecholamine release, and relative starvation due to their longer labors. Fetal lactate increases as labor progresses. The rise in lactate increases the H+ ion concentration and lowers pH. Scalp blood pH decreased from 7.34 to 7.4 in early labor to 7.29 to 7.37 by the end of the first stage of labor (95). These are all normal scalp blood pH values.

Prediction of Neonatal Status

Fetal scalp pH should predict Apgar scores. If the fetal scalp pH was greater than 7.25 during the second stage of labor, 92% of neonates had an Apgar score of 8 to 10 at 2 minutes of age. If the pH was less than 7.15, 80% had an Apgar score at 2 minutes less than 6. A pH between 7.15 and 7.25 did not predict the Apgar score (98-99).

Errors in interpretation and prediction of neonatal status may result from sampling technique, improper analyzer calibration, or maternal or fetal factors (85). The pH may be normal, but the neonate is depressed. Or, the pH may be low, and the neonate is fine (see Table 3).

Table 3: Maternal and Fetal Factors That Influence Fetal pH and Neonatal Outcome (83)

pH ≥ 7.25 but Depressed Newborn
Maternal factors:
maternal alkalosis (pH > 7.45), e.g., with hyperventilation

Neonatal factors:
upper airway obstruction
meconium aspiration
respiratory depression due to maternal narcotics
birth trauma
congenital anomalies affecting brain, heart, and/or lungs
infection, sepsis
prematurity

Other:
slow collection of sample
contamination of sample with amniotic fluid
asphyxia between sampling time and delivery

pH < 7.25 with Normal Newborn
Maternal factors:
maternal acidosis (pH ≤ 7.35), e.g., after a prolonged lack of food, vomiting, dehydration, and/or ketoacidosis

Fetal factors:
small amount of scalp bleeding
caput succedaneum
fetal respiratory acidosis and positive pressure ventilation

Other:
sample collected during a uterine contraction rather than between contractions
delay in sample analysis

Slow blood flow from the scalp increases the pH because blood combines with O_2 in the atmosphere. A time lapse of as little as 10 seconds causes pH to increase by 0.18 to 0.22 units (88, 100). The rate of blood flow into the capillary tube can be increased by decreasing the internal tube diameter (101).

Decreased Use of Fetal Scalp Blood Sampling

Drs. Goodwin, Milner-Masterson, and Paul (41) questioned the role of FSBS in current clinical practice. They found FSBS was rarely used outside of teaching centers and there was no consensus regarding its role in contemporary obstetric practice. They also discovered that the lack of FSBS did not increase their cesarean section rate, incidence of five minute Apgar scores less than five, nor the diagnoses of perinatal asphyxia or meconium aspiration syndrome. In their large university facility, FSBS was only done in 0.03 to 2% of all labors depending on the year they reviewed. Yet, it appears that FSBS will be a part of obstetric practice until it is replaced with a reliable technique that determines fetal acid-base status.

BIOCHEMICAL TESTS AFTER BIRTH
UMBILICAL CORD AND PLACENTAL BLOOD SAMPLING
Benefits of Fetal Blood Gas Analysis
Umbilical cord gases provide an objective assessment of the placenta (venous gases) and fetus (arterial gases) at the time of birth (18). The majority of academic medical centers in the Unites States and Canada obtain fetal blood gases from the umbilical cord routinely after certain situations. More than 50% of centers collect separate umbilical artery and umbilical vein specimens. Approximately one third only analyze blood from the umbilical artery. Ten percent collect a mixed arterial-venous sample. All determine pH. Most determine PO_2, PCO_2, bicarbonate and BE. Fewer than 50% analyze O_2 saturation, O_2 content, and hemoglobin (Hb) concentration (102). Blood gases provide immediate feedback on the adequacy of antepartal and intrapartal surveillance and may be used as an objective marker of the quality of intrapartal care. Gases can rule out intrapartal asphyxia as a cause of fetal neurologic damage and can be used in the management of the depressed neonate, i.e., to determine if sodium bicarbonate is needed to treat metabolic acidosis (103-107). Fetal gases may assist the physician in determining the etiology of neonatal complications. For example, in the presence of low Apgar scores and normal blood gases, neonatal compromise may be related to a congenital defect or resuscitative measures rather than an intrapartum asphyxial event.

Indications
The FHR pattern may suggest hypoxia, acidosis, or asphyxia. However, abnormal patterns do not always precede an adverse outcome. In addition, Apgar scores may not reflect fetal acid-base status (108). Therefore, collection of fetal blood after birth of the depressed neonate may shed light on the cause of neonatal depression.

Proponents of fetal blood gas studies believe routine blood gas assessment is clinically helpful and could lead to a better understanding of the frequency and severity of fetal acidosis (18). However, collection of blood gases on all fetuses may not be cost-effective. Therefore, it was recommended that if the one minute Apgar score is less than 7, umbilical artery gases should be collected to detect the presence or absence of acidosis and to differentiate between respiratory and metabolic acidosis (109). Other indications for blood gas analysis include thick meconium-stained amniotic fluid, delivery of a very premature infant, or a nonreassuring FHR pattern prior to delivery (94).

Syrinage Preparation
Syringe Preparation
Blood gas analysis requires unclotted blood. A heparinized syringe must be used for blood collection. Prepackaged, pre-heparinized syringes may be used or syringes may be prepared with heparin. To heparinize a syringe, 1000 U/ml heparin is aspirated into a syringe then expelled, leaving *less than* 0.2 ml of solution in the syringe. When 0.2 ml of 1000 U/ml heparin was mixed with 0.8 ml of blood, pH was unchanged but there was a significant drop in PCO_2, bicarbonate, and BE and an increase in PO_2 (110-111).

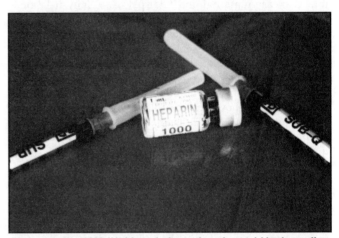

Figure 7.4: Use 1000 U/ml heparin for cord or placental blood sampling. Less than 0.2 ml should remain in the syringe prior to mixing with blood. More than 0.2 ml per 0.8 ml of blood causes a dilutional error. (Permission to photograph provided by Lovelace Medical Center, Albuquerque, NM. Photograph by Pam Barncastle, Castle Studios, Albuquerque, NM).

Use of 10,000 U/ml heparin caused erroneously low bicarbonate and BE. Greater than 0.2 ml of 10,000 U/ml heparin in the syringe lowers pH because sodium heparin is an acid mucopolysaccharide (111).

Mixed Venous-Arterial Samples
A heparinized Vacutainer® tube (green top) may be used to collect mixed venous-arterial blood samples (112). However, a mixed sample neither reflects placental function nor fetal acid-base status because mixing the two blends the values. Therefore, it is best to use two syringes and draw a sample of blood from a fetal vein and artery.

Collection Technique
Accurate umbilical vessel blood gases can only be obtained if the cord is clamped prior to the neonate's first respiration. Blood gases in the unclamped cord change very rapidly. Within one minute after birth in an unclamped umbilical cord, umbilical artery pH and BE fell and PCO_2 increased. pH dropped an average of 0.043 units, BE fell an average of 1.3 mEq/L, and PCO_2 rose an average of 5 mm Hg (113).

The following is a list of supplies needed to collect blood from the umbilical cord or placenta:

- 4 to 8 inches of umbilical cord clamped on either end or
- a placenta
- two 1 or 3 ml plastic syringes with needles and
- a vial of 1000 U/ml heparin (89).

To avoid puncture of the posterior wall of the umbilical cord vessel, it may be helpful to use a tangential approach (approximately 45 degree angle) with the bevel of the needle facing down.

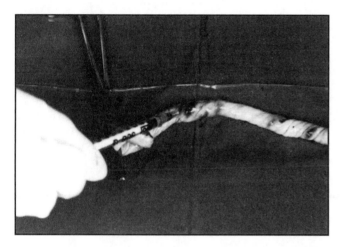

Figure 7.5: Collect blood first from the vessel inside the umbilical cord. It looks like a blue streak. Then, collect blood in a new syringe from an outer vessel. Use a tangential approach with the bevel facing down. After collecting blood, air is removed and the syringe is capped prior to transport to the laboratory. (Permission to photograph by Lovelace Medical Center, Albuquerque, NM. Photograph by Pam Barncastle, Castle Studios, Albuquerque, NM).

Umbilical vein blood reflects placental function or the respiratory status of the placenta. It has a higher O_2 content than arterial blood and *will be pinker in color than arterial blood*. Umbilical *artery values reflect fetal acid-base status*. Umbilical artery blood is deoxygenated and *darker than venous blood. Without collecting two samples, there is <u>absolutely no way</u> one can distinguish which blood sample is venous and which is arterial.* The only way to tell which vessel has been punctured and which blood has been removed is to compare the color of the blood in the two syringes. The pinker blood is venous, the darker is arterial. The difference between the blood gases of each sample will confirm the clinical observation of color that was used to differentiate the samples. The syringes should be labeled with the last name of the neonate, the date and time of collection, and the words "fetal venous blood" and "fetal arterial blood." If venous values are not desired, the person collecting fetal blood samples should document two samples were collected and the pinker (venous) sample was discarded while the darker sample was sent for analysis. This validates the blood gases are arterial in origin.

Transportation of Blood Samples

If fetal blood samples are drawn and analyzed within the first hour after birth, there is no clinical advantage to icing the syringes because very little change occurs in pH or PCO_2 (114). However, blood gases must be analyzed as soon as possible because National Committee for Clinical Laboratory Standards state that *blood gas samples not analyzed within 60 minutes of collection must be discarded* (110).

At room temperature, a clamped umbilical cord segment has minimal pH changes up to 20 minutes after birth (94). Others reported insignificant changes in blood gases if the cord segment was clamped and at room temperature for up to one hour after birth (89, 110, 115). *After 60 minutes, significant changes occur in blood gases* due to metabolically active leukocytes that release CO_2 and consume O_2. The pH and PO_2 fall and PCO_2 rises (110, 115). pH may fall as much as 0.05 units and PCO_2 may increase as much as 9 mm Hg (110).

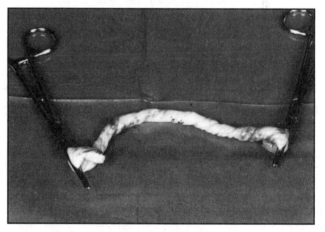

Figure 7.6: Cord blood gases do not significantly change if a clamped segment of cord is at room temperature up for up to 60 minutes after the birth. (Permission to photograph by Lovelace Medical Center, Albuquerque, NM. Photograph by Pam Barncastle, Castle Studios, Albuquerque, NM).

Sampling Fetal Blood From Placental Vessels

The chorionic membrane on the placenta contains fetal blood vessels. Usually arteries cross over veins, but can only be differentiated by looking at the color differences in the blood drawn from vessels (116). If placental arterial and venous blood was drawn immediately after delivery, pH, pO_2, bicarbonate, and BE were higher and PCO_2 was lower than blood drawn at 30 and 60 minutes after delivery (117). Therefore, it is best to draw placental blood samples within a half hour of delivery.

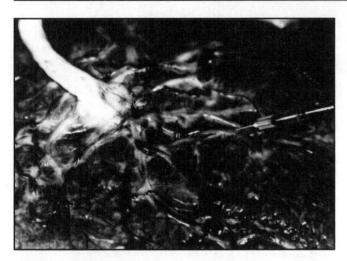

Figure 7.7: Arteries tend to traverse over larger veins but may be difficult to differentiate from veins. Use a tangential approach and obtain two syringes. The pinker sample is venous. The darker sample is arterial. (Permission to photograph by Lovelace Medical Center, Albuquerque, NM. Photograph by Pam Barncastle, Castle Studios, Albuquerque, NM).

Normal Blood Gases After Birth

Maternal blood flow, gestational age, blood O_2 content, maternal position, sedation, and anesthesia management, such as preoxygenation and IV fluid administration, affect acid-base values. As the fetus ages, changes in the umbilical vein include a fall in PO_2 and a rise in Hb, PCO_2, bicarbonate, BE, and lactate. Changes in the umbilical artery include a fall in pH and PO_2 and a rise in PCO_2. Blood gases in the umbilical artery were better when women delivered in a sitting versus a supine position. Umbilical artery PO_2 was 22.5 to 23.3 mm Hg (sitting) versus 19.1 to 21.1 mm Hg (supine) (118). These values are all within a normal range.

In spite of these maturational changes, there is no significant difference between term and preterm umbilical cord gases (34). The values listed are at least two standard deviations from the mean (18, 34, 89, 94, 108, 110, 117, 119-124).

Traditionally, an umbilical cord vessel pH of 7.20 was the cut off between normal and low, although the vessel sampled was not necessarily known. Umbilical artery pH is always lower than umbilical vein pH. An arterial pH of 7.10 or more, and an umbilical vein pH of at least 7.25, has been considered "normal" by some researchers (101). However, numerous studies suggest normal umbilical artery pH is higher (7.15 to

Table 4: Preterm and Term Fetal Blood Gas Norms for Samples Collected After Birth

Umbilical Vein (Placental Function)

pH	7.26 - 7.49
O_2 sat	29.4 - 66.3%
PO_2	15.4 - 48.2 mm Hg
O_2 content	5.6 - 13.1 mmol/L
PCO_2	23.2 - 51.7 mm Hg
Bicarbonate	16.3 - 24.9 mEq/L
Buffer Base	40.9 - 46.5 mEq/L
Base Excess	-5.1 to 0.1

Umbilical Artery (Fetal Blood)		**Placental Artery** (117)
pH	7.15 - 7.43	7.23 - 7.33
O_2 sat	7.1 - 42.1%	
PO_2	10 - 33.8 mm Hg*	11.2 - 25.6
PCO_2	31.1 - 74.3 mm Hg**	43.7 - 55.9
Bicarbonate	13.3 - 27.5 mEq/L**	22.6 - 25.4
Buffer Base	38.6 - 45.4 mEq/L	
Base Excess	-6.1 to -3.9 mEq/L***	-5 to - 1.2
Lactate	2.7 - 3.2 mEq/L***	

* Goldaber and Gilstrap III (18) reported a low PO_2 of 3.8 mm Hg following uncomplicated vaginal delivery.

** ACOG suggested an abnormally high umbilical artery PCO_2 is a value greater than 65 torr and a low bicarbonate is 17 mEq/L or less (89).

*** Ruth and Raivio (125) reported a BE of -3.5 to -1.5 and a lactate of 1.7 to 2.3 mEq/L after elective cesarean birth versus vaginal delivery.

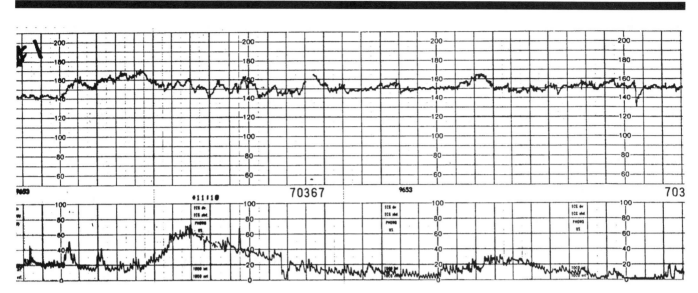

Figure 7.8: Tracing during induction attempt two days prior to delivery (#1).

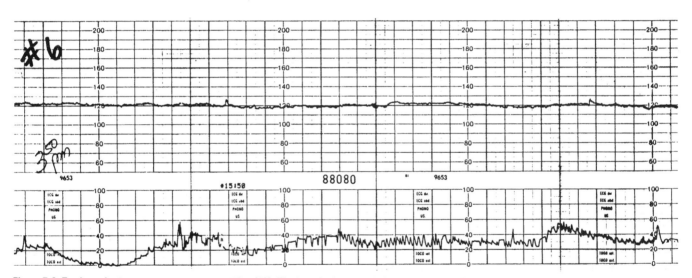

Figure 7.9: Tracing prior to emergency cesarean section (#6). The fetus had a nonreactive tracing on admission with a FHR near 135 bpm. The rate gradually fell from 135 to 120 bpm then to 105 bpm over a period of 3 hours. Then the FHR dropped to 90 bpm just prior to surgery. The Apgar scores were 0, 0, 1, and 3 at 1, 5, 10, and 15 minutes. The umbilical vein gases were: pH 7.14, PO$_2$ 17.11 mm Hg, PCO$_2$ 46.7 mm Hg, BE -11 mEq/L. The umbilical artery gases were pH 6.87, pO$_2$ 16.4 mm Hg, PCO$_2$ 89.5 mm Hg, BE -20 mEq/L. There was thick meconium in the amniotic fluid. Based on umbilical vein results, placental tissue was metabolically acidotic. The fetus was asphyxiated.

7.43). In spite of this research, there remains a lack of consensus in obstetrics regarding normal and abnormal pH values. Abnormally low pH has been defined as a pH less than 7.00, 7.05, 7.10, and 7.20 (104). Some believe the normal range is 7.09 to 7.25 (124). A pH of 7.19 was only 1 standard deviation below the mean for more than 4500 fetuses (108, 125). An umbilical artery PO$_2$ of 14 mm Hg or less was considered low, and bicarbonate was considered low if it was less than 17 mEq/L. PCO$_2$ was high if it was greater than 65 torr (122).

Acidosis and Asphyxia

Respiratory acidosis is defined by a *low umbilical artery pH, high PCO$_2$, and a normal BE*. A PCO$_2$ of 60 to 65 mm Hg or more and a BE of -8 to -9 mEq/L or less (e.g., -11 mEq/L) in umbilical cord samples has been considered abnormal (109, 126). Usually, PCO$_2$ higher than 65 mm Hg is associated with respiratory acidosis. Metabolic acidosis is reflected by a *low pH, normal PO$_2$, normal PCO$_2$, and a low BE (high base deficit)*. ACOG (89) suggested these values to define acidosis:

Table 5: Umbilical Artery Values: Acidosis and Asphyxia

Respiratory Acidosis

pH	< 7.20
PO$_2$	≥ 18 mm Hg
PCO$_2$	> 65 mm Hg
Base Excess	< - 8.3 mEq/L
Bicarbonate	≥ 22 mEq/L

Metabolic Acidosis

pH	< 7.20
PO$_2$	≤ 18 mm Hg*
PCO$_2$	< 65 mm Hg
Base Excess	< -18.7 mEq/L
Bicarbonate	≤ 17 mEq/L

* Based on other norms, if the PO$_2$ is less than 10 torr, the fetus is hypoxic with metabolic acidosis prior to birth.

Mixed Respiratory and Metabolic Acidosis

pH	< 7.20
PO$_2$	≤ 18 mm Hg
PCO$_2$	≥ 65 mm Hg
Base Excess	< -12.1 mEq/L
Bicarbonate	≤ 17 mEq/L

Asphyxia (108, 120)

pH	6.76 - 7.08
PO$_2$	4.8 - 17 mm Hg
PCO$_2$	57.5 - 118.3 mm Hg
Buffer Base	17.5 - 30.7 mEq/L
Buffer Base	< 34 mEq/L

Interpretation of Umbilical/Placental Blood Gases

Oxytocin, epidural anesthesia, labor lasting 12 or more hours, meconium-stained amniotic fluid, and cord compression are all associated with lower umbilical artery pH values (124). The use of some analgesic and anesthetic drugs, combined with a supine position or infection, cardiac disease, dehydration, vomiting or hyperventilation, may enhance mild maternal acid-base aberrations and produce misleading fetal blood gas values. Epidural versus spinal anesthesia prior to cesarean delivery is associated with higher umbilical artery pH and BE values (127). There may have been more maternal hypotension following spinal anesthesia, which would limit uteroplacental blood flow and fetal O$_2$ delivery, increasing lactate levels and decreasing pH. Fetal sepsis and lower Apgar scores at one and five minutes were associated with an umbilical artery pH less than 7.20 (125). Twins differ in their umbilical vein PO$_2$. The second twin, who was delivered by cesarean section, had a lower PO$_2$ than the first twin who was vaginally delivered (24.3 ± 3.1 mm Hg versus 29.8 ± 6.8

mm Hg). Umbilical artery bicarbonate was lower if they were both delivered vaginally (23 ± 2.2 (first twin) versus 21.2 ± 3.1 mEq/L (second twin)). However, these differences were not clinically significant (128).

Knowledge of maternal pH is helpful in interpreting fetal cord or placental blood gas findings. It is also helpful to know the time blood was collected. For example, if blood was collected from placental vessels 30 or 60 minutes after the time it was delivered, pH dropped from a mean of 7.28 at birth to 7.20 at 30 minutes and 7.10 at 60 minutes. PO$_2$ fell from an average of 18.4 mm Hg just after birth to 15.8 torr by 30 minutes and 13.8 torr by 60 minutes after birth. PCO$_2$ rose from an average of 49.8 mm Hg just after birth to 55.2 torr at 30 minutes and 70.6 torr at 60 minutes. Bicarbonate fell from 24 mEq/L just after birth to an average of 22.4 mEq/L at 30 minutes and 20.8 mEq/L at 60 minutes. Lastly, the BE fell from an average of -3.1 mEq/L to -6.6 mEq/L by 30 minutes and -9.9 mEq/L by 60 minutes (117).

Calculation of the Degree of Asphyxial Insult

Blood gases reflect the accumulation of acids and enzymes as a result of damage. Calculation of the difference between the umbilical vein and artery buffer base quantifies the severity of the asphyxial insult just prior to birth. Terminal asphyxia, just before delivery, will create an arteriovenous difference greater than 6 mEq/L (mmol/L). But, asphyxia of long duration will result in an arteriovenous buffer base difference less than or equal to 6 mEq/L (120).

Lactate

The concentration of lactate increases prior to the onset of metabolic acidosis (27). Thus, the level of fetal lactate provides indirect information on cellular respiration and metabolism. Transient or short-term respiratory acidosis is harmless to the fetus, whereas metabolic acidosis, with the production and metabolism of lactate, is associated with a risk of organ damage (129). Knowledge of an abnormal fetal lactate level may prompt actions to treat metabolic acidosis while preparing for delivery.

Lactate is an alternative energy substrate to glucose. The placenta produces lactate, contributing to the fetal lactate load (130). The fetus produces lactate anaerobically from glycogen and glucose (131). Lactic dehydrogenase (LDH) catalyzes pyruvate to create lactate. Lactic acid begins to accumulate in fetal lambs whose SaO$_2$ is less than 60%. Normally, only 15% of lactate is transferred across the placenta to maternal circulation. If fetal O$_2$ delivery is reestablished following tissue hypoxia and the production of lactic acid, and SaO$_2$ exceeds 60%, *approximately 14 minutes is needed to remove excess lactic acid from fetal circulation* (132).

Several factors other than tissue hypoxia influence the concentration of fetal lactate. For example, maternal hyperventilation, *glucose* or β-mimetic administration, and the time interval between sampling and analysis *may increase fetal lactate*. When the fetus produces lactate during anaerobic metabolism, adenosine triphosphate (ATP) is consumed, adenosine increases, bicarbonate ions are consumed, BE drops, and the metabolic rate decreases to only 20% of the aerobic, oxidative metabolic rate (132). During the second stage of labor, an abnormal lactate level was related to placental vessel dilation, decreased variability, decelerations, and/or bradycardia (3, 133). Adenosine most likley caused placental vessel vasodilation and decreased variability. Cardiac depletion of glucose probably caused decelerations and bradycardia.

Umbilical artery lactate is significantly related to pH, PCO_2, Hb, and BE and an elevation in the ST segment of the fetal ECG (134-135). Lactate can be measured from a fetal scalp capillary blood sample or the umbilical artery (134-136). Until recently, fetal lactic acid analysis during labor was impractical because of the relatively large amount of scalp capillary blood required (150 μl). Using a test strip sampling device requires only 5 to 20 μl of blood for lactate analysis (129, 137). Results are available within 60 seconds.

Fetal lactate above 1.5 mmol/L is considered abnormal (131). Moderate lactic acidosis is 1.6 to 2.2 mmol/L (27). A "high lactate level" was considered to be greater than 3.2 mmol/L (134). Lactate levels were highest in fetuses delivered by cesarean section for "fetal distress" and lowest in fetuses delivered by elective cesarean section (134-135).

Lactate may be less predictive of outcome than pH and BE. When lactate increases, pH decreases. The umbilical artery pH was a better predictor of the one minute Apgar score than lactate or the BE. BE was a better predictor of the five minute Apgar score than lactate (134). Lactate was not predictive of neonatal outcome (138). Research has yet to identify a lactate "cut-off" level which requires operative intervention (137).

INVESTIGATIONS OF FETAL ACID-BASE STATUS

Investigations of fetal acid-base status during the intrapartal period have included fetal pulse oximetry, near infrared spectroscopy, tissue pH sampling, transcutaneous tissue PO_2 and PCO_2 ($tcPO_2$ and $tcPCO_2$), and mass spectroscopy. Currently, fetal pulse oximetry has the greatest potential for clinical adaptation.

FETAL SpO_2 ($FSpO_2$) MONITORING

Fetal pulse oximetry was believed to be a possible adjunct to electronic FHR monitoring (139-142). When the fetal pulse oximeter was used, the $FSpO_2$ level could be printed on the tracing along with the FHR and uterine activity.

Benefits of Fetal Pulse Oximetry

$FSpO_2$ is related to the FHR pattern during the first stage of labor (139-152). Nonreassuring FHR patterns are associated with decreasing $FSpO_2$ (143-145, 147, 149, 151). Fluctuations in $FSpO_2$ occur during compensatory FHR changes (146, 151). $FSpO_2$ decreases during decelerations due to hypoxia but not early decelerations due to fetal head compression (153). Therefore, $FSpO_2$ changes may be helpful in differentiating the truly hypoxic fetus from the well, quiescent fetus or the

well fetus with an abnormal FHR pattern (140, 143-149, 154). Evaluation of the FHR pattern and $FSpO_2$ identifies well and compromised fetuses better than evaluation of the FHR pattern alone (139, 141). Clinician confidence about fetal well-being may increase when $FSpO_2$ is determined as an adjunct to electronic FHR monitoring (148). Normal $FSpO_2$ may prevent unnecessary interventions when a nonreassuring FHR pattern is identified (155). *$FSpO_2$ values greater than 50% have been associated with normal fetal outcomes regardless of nonreassuring FHR patterns when the oximeter employed the red wavelength of 660 nanometers (nm).* As fetal saturation decreased towards 40%, the strength of the relationship between a nonreassuring FHR pattern and poor fetal outcome increased (140-141, 144-145, 152). The nearly continuous printout of $FSpO_2$ allows prompt recognition of desaturation (156-160). In addition, $FSpO_2$ provides data to evaluate the effectiveness of interventions to improve fetal oxygenation.

Sometimes there is a need to clarify fetal acid-base status because the FHR pattern is unclear, e.g., during a dysrhythmia (144-145, 161-164). In the case of heart block, the persistence of a normal $FSpO_2$, even with a FHR below 60 bpm, may encourage physicians to perform a vaginal delivery rather than a cesarean section.

$FSpO_2$ determinations may become an alternative to fetal scalp sampling (165). $FSpO_2$ monitoring is available in Europe. However, in the United States in 1996, fetal pulse oximetry was considered investigational. Additional research is ongoing to establish clinically significant normal and abnormal $FSpO_2$ values.

Pulse Oximetry: Hemoglobin and Oxyhemoglobin Light Absorption

Tissue and the heme portion, not the globin portion, of red blood cells (RBCs) absorb light. Although fetal hemoglobin and adult hemoglobin have structurally different globin chains, they are optically equivalent at the wavelengths of light used in pulse oximetry. Fetal hemoglobin (HbF) absorbs as much light as adult hemoglobin (HbA). The pulse oximeter "sees" a hemoglobin molecule, whether HbF or HbA, as either saturated with oxygen or reduced (165).

Reduced hemoglobin (Hb) and oxyhemoglobin (HbO_2) absorb different amounts of red and infrared light. *Hb absorbs more red light than HbO_2. HbO_2 absorbs more infrared light than Hb* (161). Pulse oximeters use red light in the wavelength range of 660 to 735 nm. Pulse oxim2eters also use infrared light in the wavelength range of 890-935 nm. A nanometer is one billionth of a meter (166).

The absorption of red and infrared light during each arterial pulse is calculated to determine $FSpO_2$. A weak relationship was found between $FSpO_2$ and umbilical vein SO_2 when the sensor emitted a red wavelength of 660 nm and an infrared wavelength of 920 nm (r = 0.47) (167). A sensor that emits red and infrared light at 735 and 890 nm respectively performed better than the 660/920 sensor (168). The Nellcor FS 14® sensor emits light at 735 (red) and 890 (infrared) nm wavelengths (169). Computer mathematical modeling and

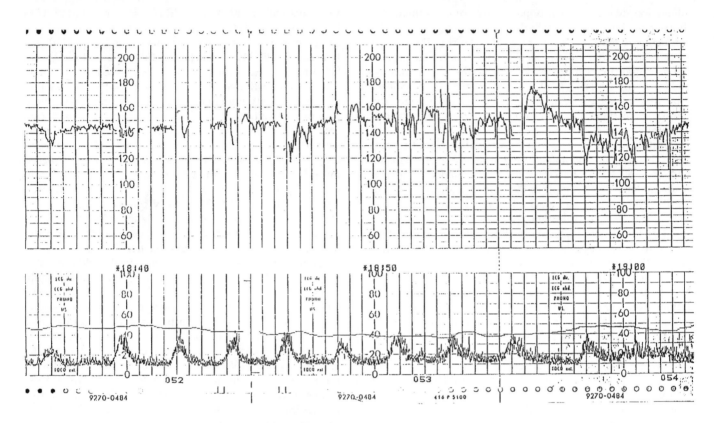

Figure 7.10: Fetal heart rate tracing with fetal SpO₂ data recorded on the same scale as uterine activity. Note the strip speed is 1 cm/min and the fetal heart rate paper is in 5 bpm increments. (Tracing courtesy of Nellcor Puritan Bennett, Pleasanton, CA.).

animal testing confirm this wavelength combination (735 nm and 890 nm) provides more accurate readings at low saturations than the conventional pulse oximetry wavelength combination of 660 nm and 890 nm (168, 170).

Determination of FSpO₂

Saturation can be determined in three ways: non-invasively by pulse oximetry and invasively by blood sampling with either a laboratory hemoximeter (co-oximeter) or blood gas analyzer. Pulse oximeters, including fetal oxygen saturation monitoring systems, determine *functional* hemoglobin oxygen saturation which is expressed as $HbO_2/(HbO_2 + Hb)$. This is the amount of oxyhemoglobin over the total hemoglobin concentration available to bind with oxygen. The saturation reported by pulse oximeters is determined differently than that reported by a laboratory hemoximeter and by a blood gas analyzer. The laboratory hemoximeter, like the pulse oximeter, *measures* saturation, but includes the dysfunctional hemoglobins carboxyhemoglobin (HbCO) and methemoglobin (MetHb) in its determination when they are present in blood (156). The hemoximeter reports chemical or *fractional* saturation and is expressed by the equation $HbO_2/(HbO_2 + Hb + HbCO + MetHb)$. Functional and fractional saturation are often equal, but differ when HbCO and MetHb are present. MetHb contains ferric iron rather than ferrous iron and is incapable of reversibly binding with oxygen (171).

A blood gas analyzer measures PO_2, PCO_2 and pH, but *calculates* saturation based on oxygen's affinity for hemoglobin and the oxyhemoglobin dissociation curve. Often the reported saturation is different than the pulse oximeter saturation at the time the blood gas was obtained. This is the result of the blood gas analyzer's inability to correct for certain shifts in the oxyhemoglobin dissociation curve.

Reflectance Pulse Oximetry

The two types of sensors, *transmission* and *reflectance*, are used in adult, pediatric, and neonatal pulse oximetry. Transmission sensors are impractical for fetal use because they require opposition of the sensor's light emitting diodes and photodetector across a pulsatile vascular bed (such as a finger or earlobe) (172).

Given the limited accessible sites for fetal sensor application, reflectance sensors, where the optical components lie side by side, are best for fetal saturation monitoring. Adult reflectance pulse oximeters are not suitable for fetal use because the red wavelength of 660 nanometers (nm) is less accurate at the normally low FSpO$_2$ values encountered in labor (173). At SaO$_2$ levels below 80%, adult pulse oximeters are not as accurate as at higher saturations. They overestimate the true FSpO$_2$ value (174-176). Therefore, reflectance pulse oximeters had to be modified for FSpO$_2$ monitoring (172). The electronics have been optimized to reliably obtain a signal despite the small size of the fetal vascular bed and low intensity peripheral pulses generated in the fetal scalp (173). FSpO$_2$ has been measured with three different types of devices.

The Knitza System (Oxycardiotocography). Dr. Reinhold Knitza and his group from Munich, Germany, have incorporated light emitting diodes and a photodetector into a spiral electrode (SE). With this system, the simultaneous acquisition of FHR data and FSpO$_2$ is possible. The sensor is invasive and is applied to the fetal scalp. Although concerns exist about the accuracy of signal transmission in the presence of fetal hair or caput, researchers contend these had no effect on FSpO$_2$ in more than 250 fetuses (172, 177). The Knitza system was not calibrated for fetal use and emitted red light at 660 nm, possibly creating erroneous FSpO$_2$ readings. Additional testing and development of this system is needed prior to its clinical application (178).

The Balloon Probe. A multi-parameter balloon probe has been developed by Dr. Jason Gardosi of Nottingham, England. This system combines pulse oximetry, contact electrodes for FHR data acquisition, an intrauterine pressure transducer, and an amnioinfusion port in one sensor. The probe is inserted like an intrauterine pressure catheter (IUPC), but it is not placed as high as an IUPC in the uterine cavity. It is a flat probe that is placed between the fetal biparietal bone and the uterine wall. A 50 ml balloon is inflated with sterile saline or water to hold the device in place. It measures intrauterine pressure while a gold plated contact sensor determines the fetal electrocardiogram (FECG). Complications of probe application may include bradycardia related to nuchal cord compression. The balloon probe also uses a 660 nm red wavelength, has not been calibrated for fetal use, and needs additional testing prior to clinical use (179, 180).

The Nellcor Puritan Bennett (NPB) N-400® Fetal Oxygen Saturation Monitoring System. The NPB system was calibrated specifically for low FSpO$_2$ levels. This system reliably obtains a signal despite the small size of the fetal vascular bed and low peripheral pulses generated by the fetus (173). Versions of the NPB system, prior to October 1993, utilized a red wavelength of 660 nm. The sensor now uses a 735 nm red wavelength and was calibrated and verified in animal and human studies (168).

Pulse Oximetry Assumptions

Fetal reflectance technology measures light absorption on the same side of the skin and is based on the following assumptions:

- all pulsations are arterial and not from motion or venous blood
- all light reaching the photodetector passes through vascularized tissue
- the hemoglobin concentration is adequate
- oxyhemoglobin (HbO$_2$) and deoxyhemoglobin or reduced hemoglobin (Hb) are the only significant light absorbers in arterial blood
- dysfunctional hemoglobins, such as carboxyhemoglobin and methemoglobin, are not present and
- no extraneous dyes are present in the vascular system or on the skin (156, 172).

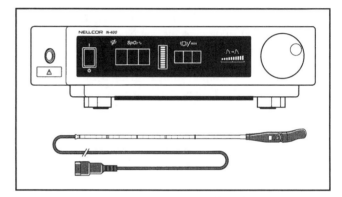

Figure 7.11: Nellcor Puritan Bennett N-400® fetal oxygen saturation monitoring system® (Reprinted by permission of Nellcor Puritan Bennett, Pleasanton, CA).

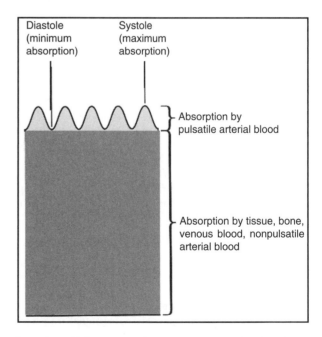

Figure 7.12: Light absorption by various tissue components during the cardiac cycle. Plethysmographic waveforms fluctuate during the cardiac cycle. (Reprinted by permission of Nellcor Puritan Bennett, Pleasanton, CA).

The Reflectance Sensor or Probe

Light-emitting diodes. All pulse oximetry sensors contain light-emitting diodes and a photodetector. The NPB sensor® also uses contact electrodes. Two light-emitting diodes (LEDs) are on the surface of the sensor that is applied to the fetus. LEDs emit red and infrared light (164-165). Infrared light is invisible to the human eye. Light moves through fetal tissue and enters the pulsating capillary bed (162, 183).

Photodetector. Most light not absorbed by Hb and HbO_2 is reflected back to a spectrophotometer or photodetector on the probe's surface (140, 156, 165). This information is transmitted back to the pulse oximeter.

Contact-electrodes that measure impedance. In addition to the LEDs and photodetector, the Nellcor Puritan Bennett sensor® has three contact electrodes that measure electrical impedance across the sensor's surface. Impedance varies between skin, hair, amniotic fluid, and air. Because of this difference, it is possible to determine when the sensor is in good contact with the underlying tissue of the fetal face.

The Pulse Oximeter

Pulse oximetry is based on the principles of plethysmography and spectrophotometry.

Optical plethysmography. *Optical plethysmography* is a technology that produces a waveform from pulsatile blood. Some oximeters display this waveform on a digital screen. Light transmission and light absorption differences during the cardiac cycle are calculated by the microprocessor in the pulse oximeter (see Figure 7.12). The pulse oximeter also displays the optical pulse rate and $FSpO_2$ (156).

Spectrophotometry. Spectrophotometry is the measurement of the amount of absorbed light. Absorption of light by a substance is dependent upon the light's wavelength, the concentration of the absorbing substance, and the distance light traveled (172, 184). The microprocessor in the pulse oximeter calculates the difference between light transmission and absorption, determines the percentage of HbO_2 and Hb, analyzes the arterial pulse waveform (plethysmograph) and signal quality against algorithms, then calculates $FSpO_2$. Signal quality is graded for amplitude, purity, and synchronicity with the FHR (165, 185-186).

Fetal signal quality may be affected by:
- sensor placement
- light shunting artifact
- maternal pulses
- perfusion at the sensor site
- hair or vernix which might decrease signal transmission (181, 185).

Automatic gain control in some oximeters strengthens the weak fetal signal and increases background noise which increases the risk of artifact (185). Electronic background noise may be filtered prior to analysis of the fetal signal (181).

Sensor or Probe Insertion

Application of the sensor on the amniotic membranes in front of the fetal head is likely to yield inaccurate $FSpO_2$ calculations. Meconium in amniotic fluid artificially lowers $FSpO_2$ because it is a red filter similar to tissue (187). Therefore, prior to application of the probe, membranes must be ruptured. The most reliable, consistent reading of $FSpO_2$ is obtained when the sensor has good contact with the skin. Poor sensor-to-skin apposition causes light shunting artifact, violating the second assumption on page 17 (181).

Prior to NPB sensor® insertion, the pulse oximeter is plugged in, turned on, and the LEDs are inspected. A red light should be visible. Sensor insertion does not appear to increase the postpartal infection rate, although cleansing of the woman's vulva prior to insertion may be done. When Savlon, a disinfectant, was used there was no increase in the infection rate in women whose fetuses were monitored by pulse oximetry and those who were not monitored (188). The maximal postpartal temperature of women whose fetuses were monitored by pulse oximetry was 0.2° F higher than the temperature of women whose fetuses were not monitored (189).

Insertion of the sterile, disposable Nellcor Puritan Bennett FS-14 oxisensor® is similar to insertion of an IUPC. The sensor is inserted to the level of the fetal cheek of a fetus in a cephalic presentation. The introducer is stiff enough to insert between the fetal head and the uterine wall, yet it bends to follow the contour of the fetal head (139). The NPB system® indicates when a contact is achieved and a good signal is and *is not* obtained.

Limitations of $FSpO_2$ Monitoring [Artifact]

Membranes must be ruptured to apply to probe. Therefore, use of this technology is an invasive maternal procedure but not necessarily an invasive fetal procedure. Signal error limits information continuity and arises from incomplete sensor-skin contact, the presence of caput succedaneum, nonarterial pulsatile signals, and meconium (185, 187, 190). In most circumstances meconium, blood and vernix do not affect the signal quality after rupture of membranes, however, thick or tenacious meconium or vernix has the potential to obstruct light transmission (187). Meconium-stained skin has an insignificant effect on $FSpO_2$ readings (191).

Artifact or signal errors are due to interference by maternal pulsations, motion, optical shunting of light passing over the skin surface or through nonvascular layers of the skin (172). A significant increase in deoxygenated hemoglobin, changes in blood optical properties due to fetal hemolysis, a high HbF level, maternal carbon monoxide exposure with an increase in fetal HbCO, or the presence of methemoglobin do not affect fetal pulse oximetry readings. However, they may affect hemoximetry determination of SaO_2 (192). Signal errors may prevent a continuous $FSpO_2$ reading during labor. In one study, $FSpO_2$ was detected an average of 58% of the

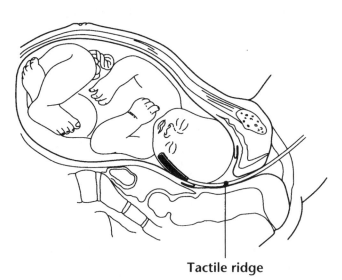

Tactile ridge

Figure 7.13: Illustration of reflectance Nellcor Puritan Bennett (NPB) fetal oxisensor® in contact with tissue. The sensor is inserted until the 15 cm tactile ridge is felt at the midpoint of the presenting part. It is held in place by pressure from the uterine wall. (Reprinted by permission of Nellcor Puritan Bennett, Pleasanton, CA).

monitoring time. Signal transmission improved as labor progressed. Even if $FSpO_2$ did not significantly change during labor, pH sometimes changed (193). The fetal signal was often lost during variable decelerations (194).

The type of equipment and their calibration algorithms used to determine $FSpO_2$ affects the meaning of results. For example, the Ohmeda Biox 3700® $FSpO_2$ correlated best with *fractional* SaO_2 whereas the early NPB prototypes correlated best with *functional* SaO_2 (195). Manufacturers of fetal pulse oximetry systems should provide a list of references documenting the norms for $FSpO_2$ during labor using their equipment.

Although fetal hair or caput were found to have no effect on $FSpO_2$ with the Knitza system, others have determined that their presence may affect $FSpO_2$ readings (177). Hair can affect oximetry readings several ways. First, hair, if present in sufficient quantity, may prevent the sensor from making adequate contact with the fetal skin and, consequently cause light shunts. Dark hair absorbs a significant amount of red light, thereby greatly reducing signal amplitude. Placement of the oximetry sensor beyond the hairline reduces the likelihood of these artifacts occurring. Caput, with blood stasis, may cause inaccurate information to be transmitted due to light shunting through the edematous area (172, 196).

What is Normal $FSpO_2$?

$FSpO_2$ determined with fetal pulse oximeter sensors that emitted a red wavelength of 660 nm found the "normal" range of $FSpO_2$ was:

- 25.2 to 87.5% (197)
- 30.0 to 65% (172)

- 48.0 to 67% (198) and
- 70 to 90% (199).

Researchers have even suggested the normal $FSpO_2$ range is 40 to 100% (139, 200-201). It now appears that at a red wavelength of 660 nm, true $FSpO_2$ may be overestimated when SaO_2 is below 80%. *At a red wavelength of 735 nm, "normal" $FSpO_2$ during labor is between 30 and 70% (196).*

Researchers are investigating the critical SaO_2 or $FSpO_2$ values in human fetuses where metabolic acidosis begins and O_2 consumption depends entirely on O_2 supply (202). In comparison to extrauterine values, a $FSpO_2$ of 30% is incredibly low, but fetal lamb research suggests otherwise. In lambs, there is little change in pH *until SaO_2 is between 30 and 40%. At that point, lactic acid accumulates and metabolic acidosis becomes apparent* (203-204). Furthermore, fetal cerebral O_2 uptake, and redistribution of blood flow to maintain cerebral O_2 delivery, was not significantly decreased until SaO_2 was less than 30%. At that time, pH and BE decreased (204-205). *The critical $FSpO_2$ where metabolic acidosis becomes apparent appears to be 30%* (197). In one case of a tight nucal cord, the human fetus had a SpO_2 of 20 to 30% prior to birth, the pH was 7.09 and the umbilical artery SaO_2 was 23.9% (139). Multicenter human studies conducted by a consortium of French researchers revealed a $FSpO_2$ greater than 30% predicted a scalp pH above 7.20 (unpublished data on file at Nellcor Puritan Bennett).

$FSpO_2$ does not change when there is chorioamnionitis evidenced by a maternal temperature above 38° C, a C reactive protein above 2 mg/dl, or a white blood cell count greater than 16,000/μl (169). Eventually, an elevation of maternal and fetal temperature decreases O_2 binding to Hb and causes Hb desaturation and tissue hypoxia (206).

As determined by pulse oximetry, $FSpO_2$ decreases during contractions (199). Transient cerebral blood desaturation occurred during contractions as measured by near infrared spectroscopy (207). When a pulse oximetry sensor with a 660 nm red wavelength was used, a decreasing trend in $FSpO_2$ was found as labor progressed (208-210). $FSpO_2$ ranged from 62 to 68% during early labor and from 53 to 58% during late first stage and second stage labor (211).

Table 6: Fetal SpO2 During Labor Using the 660 nm Red Wavelength (144, 193, 198, 211)

Dilatation (cm)	FSpO2 (%)
0 to 4	52 - 71.1
4	40 - 80
5 to 7	48.9 - 71.1
8 to 10	47.2 - 67.8

A statistically significant decrease in fetal SpO_2 was observed as labor progressed in women with normal neonatal outcomes. Normal and abnormal outcome groups had significantly different FSpO$_2$ values (211). FSpO$_2$ significantly decreased prior to the birth of a depressed neonate (141, 212).

Average readings from the fetal buttocks of a breech fetus were lower than readings from the fetal face or head of a vertex fetus (213-214). Norms for IUGR and preterm fetuses may be different than norms for term fetuses. For example, FSpO$_2$ values were higher in preterm gestations and lower in IUGR fetuses than in term fetuses (199, 214).

FSpO$_2$ may change following maternal O$_2$ administration or withdrawal (163, 211, 215-217). Individual fetal responses to maternal hyperoxygenation during labor vary. However, in 2 studies, there was a significant increase in FSpO$_2$ in response to maternal administration of 100 percent O$_2$ (with an anesthesia face mask) compared with the fetal response to breathing room air (F^{I}O$_2$ 21%), 27%, or 40% O$_2$ (163, 211, 215-216). When O$_2$ was delivered with an anesthesia mask at a F^{I}O$_2$ of 100%, FSpO$_2$ increased an average of 14% (216). Discontinuation of maternal O$_2$ decreased FSpO$_2$ to below the baseline level (163, 211, 215-217).

Maternal hyperoxygenation may increase fetal FSpO$_2$. For example, O$_2$ was administered to 8 healthy women in normal labor at concentrations of 27% and 100% alternating with 10 minutes of room air. At 27%, FSpO$_2$ increased an average 7.5%. At 100% FSpO$_2$ increased an average of 11% (215). A tight-fitting simple face mask, commonly used in labor and delivery, provides more than 40% but less than 100% F^{I}O$_2$, and should therefore increase FSpO$_2$.

NEAR INFRARED SPECTROSCOPY (NIRS)

Near infrared spectroscopy (NIRS) detects fetal blood O$_2$ content. Two interoptrodes are applied 6 cm apart on the fetal head. Infrared light, at a wavelength of 700 to 900 nm, is emitted every 0.2 microseconds at a speed of 0.5 kHz from 4 laser diodes. Light returns to a photodetector and HbO$_2$, Hb, and total hemoglobin are measured (218). The first study using NIRS was published in 1992. SaO$_2$ in 6 of 8 human fetuses was 33 to 53% during "normal" contractions. Problems encountered included determination of the optical path length, restricted access to the fetal head, and probe movement (207).

TISSUE pH (TpH)

Although TpH was once thought to be a promising area of fetal research, TpH is no longer being investigated. Tissue pH was measured with a special spiral electrode imbedded in fetal scalp subcutaneous tissue. There was no relationship between TpH, Apgar scores, umbilical artery pH, and umbilical vein pH (219). The FHR changed two to three minutes prior to a change in the TpH (220). TpH values and scalp pH values differed by 0.002 to 0.351 units. A TpH less than 7.09 was the lower limit the machine could reliably measure, and there were technical problems with probe application, calibration, and removal. Technical requirements for TpH included the need for membranes to be ruptured, a 3 to 4 cm dilatation, and a supine maternal position. The procedure for application of the device was awkward for personnel and time-consuming (219).

TRANSCUTANEOUS PO$_2$ and PCO$_2$ (tcPO$_2$ and tcPCO$_2$)

To assess tcPO$_2$ and tcPCO$_2$, an electrochemical sensor with two electrodes is attached to the fetal scalp with tissue adhesive or a vacuum. Electrodes are calibrated to CO$_2$ gas and O$_2$ in the atmosphere prior to application. An amnioscope is inserted into the woman's vagina, the fetal scalp is cleansed of vernix and blood. Sometimes the fetal head must be shaved prior to electrode application. After electrodes are secured to the scalp, they are heated to 43 to 45° C. The warmth of the electrodes causes hyperemia in the subepidermal capillaries. Oxygen and CO$_2$ diffuse through the skin through a Teflon® membrane which overlies electrodes that are covered with an electrolyte solution (221-222). Transcutaneous gases must be monitored for more than 11 minutes prior to interpretation. After an average of 11.4 minutes, tcPO$_2$ reaches a steady state. After an average of 18.4 minutes, tcPCO$_2$ reaches a steady state. A multichannel recorder prints uterine contractions, the FHR, tcPO$_2$, and tcPCO$_2$ (222). Researchers found a strong relationship between tcPO$_2$ and scalp capillary PO$_2$ (r = 0.93) but tcPO$_2$ was lower than scalp PO$_2$. There was also a strong relationship between tcPCO$_2$ and scalp capillary PCO$_2$ (r = 0.95) (222-223). There was no relationship between tcPO$_2$ and umbilical artery PO$_2$. tcPO$_2$ reflects O$_2$ levels under a heated transcutaneous sensor but not PaO$_2$ in fetal arteries (222). Others found tcPO$_2$ during the active phase of labor had a "good" correlation with umbilical artery PO$_2$. They believed tcPO$_2$ better reflected the fetal condition than tissue pH (224).

Transcutaneous *PO$_2$ fell to 19 mm Hg during variable decelerations* (222). Transcutaneous PO$_2$ may decrease during contractions (224). Even if tcPO$_2$ decreased, there might be no change in tissue pH or the FHR (222, 224).

Transcutaneous *PCO$_2$ increased during variable decelerations and contractions stronger than 30 mm Hg (at their peak)* (222, 224). A sitting position did not alter the FHR, but there was a change in tcPCO$_2$ and tcPO2. Transcutaneous PCO$_2$ slightly increased and tcPO$_2$ slightly decreased when women sat up during labor. The reason for the change is these blood gases is not clear. In a left lateral position tcPO$_2$ increased and tcPCO$_2$ returned to a normal level (222). Therefore, *when variable decelerations are observed, a lateral position may be better than a sitting up position to normalize fetal PCO$_2$.*

Transcutaneous PO$_2$ decreased and tcPCO$_2$ increased during fetal descent, but did not change during pushing efforts or between contractions during the second stage of labor when the FHR pattern only had "small" variable decelerations (222). Transcutaneous PO$_2$ may appear to decrease, even though it may be normal, when there is caput succedaneum, compression of the electrode, or a rise in fetal catecholamines resulting in scalp vessel vasoconstriction (221). Due to the difficulty with electrode application and the errors in data acquisition, transcutaneous blood gas analysis was never adopted for clinical use.

SUBCUTANEOUS (TISSUE) PO$_2$

Subcutaneous scalp PO$_2$ was measured by a special electrode in the fetal scalp. Subcutaneous PO$_2$ was found to increase during the ascending limb of a contraction then decrease no more than 5 mm Hg below the level recorded prior to the contraction. Tissue PO$_2$ fell more than 5 mm Hg during the contraction in conjunction with moderate to severe variable decelerations, bradycardia less than 100 bpm, tachycardia greater than 180 bpm, or late decelerations. At times, PO$_2$ was zero. *Late decelerations were only seen when subcutaneous PO$_2$ was less than 20 torr (225).* It is probable that the fetus was hypoxic during late decelerations.

MASS SPECTROMETRY (PsO$_2$, PsCO$_2$)

Mass spectrometry is a noninvasive technique that measures gas molecules that diffuse through and out of the skin. Fetal scalp O$_2$ tension measured by mass spectrometry (PsO$_2$) was 4 to 27 mm Hg and CO$_2$ tension (PsCO$_2$) was 49 to 85 mm Hg. PsO$_2$ dropped and PsCO$_2$ rose during decelerations (see Table 7) (226).

Table 7: Scalp O$_2$ and CO$_2$ Tension Changes During Contractions and Decelerations

Deceleration	PsO$_2$ Decrease (%)	PsCO$_2$ Increase (%)
Early	0 to 20	less than 20
Variable	40 to 80	45 to 75
Late	60 to 90	30 to 85

Head compression was not related to a change in fetal blood gases. The changes recorded may be due to the contraction's compression of intramural vessels more so than compression of the fetal head. *Cord compression (variable decelerations) and uteroplacental insufficiency (late decelerations) were related to hypoxia and hypercapnia.* Researchers did not quantify the duration or depth of decelerations.

Hyperoxygenation increases PsO$_2$. The driving force for O$_2$ transfer across the placenta is the O$_2$ pressure gradient between maternal veins and fetal tertiary stem villi capillaries (96). When O$_2$ was administered by face mask at 7 liters per minute (LPM), maternal PaO$_2$ increased to greater than 170 mm Hg and fetal PsO$_2$ increased in 7 of 8 fetuses by 9 to 21 mm Hg. *Fetal PsO$_2$ increased within two minutes after O$_2$ therapy was initiated (226).* Therefore, *within 2 minutes of administrating O$_2$, O$_2$ should reach the fetus, including fetal cerebral vessels. The clinician should expect an improvement in the FHR pattern.*

MONITORING THE FETUS, EVALUATING THE FETAL BRAIN, AND NEUROPROTECTIVE THERAPY

PEP/VET Ratio, Noninvasive Monitoring of the FHR and Maternal and Fetal Temperature

Researchers are interested in how the fetal electrocardiogram (ECG) changes as acid-base balance changes. The ratio between the preejection period (PEP) and the ventricular ejection time (VET) may predict fetal acid-base status. PEP is the time from the onset of the QRS complex to opening of the aortic valve or systole (S$_1$). VET is the time from opening of the aortic valve to its closure or diastole (S$_2$). The ratio, PEP/VET, indicates left ventricular function and is a sensitive indicator of fetal status. PEP is prolonged when the fetus is hypoxic and acidemic. PEP increases more than 10 msec when the fetus is asphyxiated. Additional research is needed prior to use of the PEP/VET ratio in clinical practice (227).

Researchers in the United Kingdom developed a noninvasive polyurethane probe with sensors that measure intrauterine maternal and fetal temperature. The probe is inserted into the uterus and placed against the fetal skin next to the lower uterine segment. The average initial uterine wall temperature was 36.87º C. The average initial fetal temperature was 37.10º C. Maternal temperature sometimes fluctuated with contractions, fetal temperature was stable. After epidural anesthesia, maternal temperature increased an average of 0.37º C and the FHR increased an average of 7.5 bpm. The FHR was weakly related to fetal (r = 0.532) and maternal (r = 0.567) temperatures (228).

1H MR Spectroscopy of the Human Fetal Brain

Proton magnetic resonance spectroscopy (^{1}H MRS) is a noninvasive tool that may be able to predict brain damage and detect signs of insufficient cerebral O$_2$ supply. ^{1}H MRS detects brain metabolites such as choline and creatine (229). If fetal brain damage is detected in the antenatal period, women can be counseled regarding their birth options and neonatal prognosis.

Transvaginal Ultrasound (TVU)

The fetal brain may be visualized by abdominal ultrasound or transvaginal ultrasound. Brain damage during the antenatal period was suspected following ultrasonographic imaging of the fetal brain at 36 weeks' gestation. The diagnosis of a massive cerebellar hemorrhage was confirmed by a computerized tomography (CT) scan. The FHR baseline was flat at 150 bpm (230).

TVU creates images of the cortical surface of the fetal brain (231). Fetal brain anatomy was clearly seen 92% of the time (232). TVU predicted intraventricular hemorrhage or periventricular leukomalacia in 97% of the neonates that had

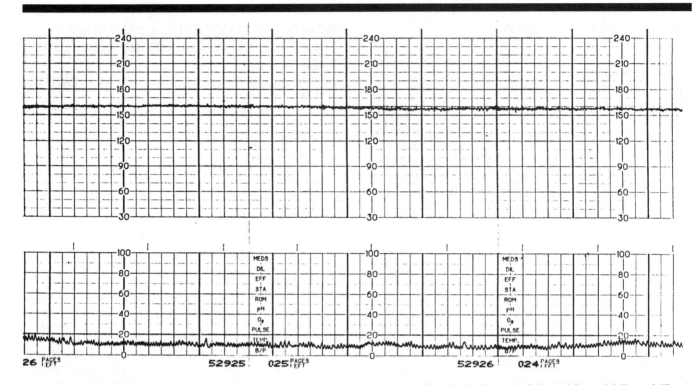

Figure 7.14: FHR pattern of a fetus with an intraventricular hemorrhage and periventricular leukomalacia prior to admission to labor and delivery. A 17 year old married primigravida with a history of barbiturate, amphetamine, alcohol, and benzodiazepam use was admitted at 37 weeks' gestation not in labor. The cervix was 1 cm dilated, thick, and long. The fetus was ballottable and vertex. Her temperature was 99.1º F, other vital signs were normal. An intravenous bolus and hyperoxygenation were initiated. Note absent variability. A primary cesarean section was performed. Apgar scores were 1, 1, and 0 at 1, 5, and 10 minutes. The 8 lb 8 ounce baby had hydrocephalus, bilateral intracranial hemorrhages, an obstructive left side intraventricular bleed, and periventricular leukomalacia on the right side. A 23 minute resuscitation attempt ended with demise of the neonate.

evidence of IVH or PVL (233). If TVU failed to identify fetal brain anatomy, magnetic resonance imaging (MRI) was done. Prior to the MRI, the fetus had to be immobilized by a percutaneous umbilical vein injection of atracurium or pancuronium (234). Detection of IVH or PVL prior to birth may influence the physician's decision for early delivery versus conservative management of preterm labor.

Glutamate Antagonist to Prevent Brain Damage

Since glutamate has been implicated in brain injury, a glutamate antagonist may prevent brain injury. In 1995, researchers reported the intravenous administration of the glutamate antagonist MK-801 that created a biphasic response in fetal lambs. First there was global inhibition with decreased fetal breathing movements, decreased heart rate variability, and there was a drop in O_2 consumption and cerebral blood flow. Then, there was arousal, an increase in low voltage electrocortical activity, continuous fetal breathing movements, normal O_2 consumption and normal cerebral blood flow (235). Of course, more research is needed before this drug is used in humans.

Healing the Damaged Brain: Monosialogangliosides (GM₁)

Some day a drug may be developed to give to asphyxiated fetuses to heal damaged cells and minimize or prevent permanent brain damage. Preliminary experiments with fetal lambs who had bilateral carotid occlusion and suffered hypoxic-ischemic brain damage has suggested ganglioside GM_1, a sialylated glycospingolipid, may stabilize brain nerve cells and improve outcome. Cell walls are composed of lipids and proteins (236). Researchers believe this lipid, ganglioside GM_1, is incorporated into the damaged nerve cell wall which repairs it. Treated lambs had better electroencephalograms (EEGs) and less neuronal loss in the striatum, hippocampus, and cortex of the brain. Their EEGs were normal 72 hours after the asphyxial episode (237).

INTRAUTERINE RESUSCITATION

Over the last four decades, intrauterine fetal resuscitation techniques have evolved. For example, in the 1960s, women were given sodium bicarbonate, 66 to 125 mEq via an IV drip over 1 to 3 hours, in the hopes of correcting fetal metabolic acidosis. Fetal BE and pH increased but so did maternal and fetal PCO_2 (238-239).

In the 1970s, fetal resuscitative actions included Nikolaev's Triad, which included 50 ml of 40% glucose in water IV followed by 300 mg of ascorbic acid IV and inhalation of O_2. Sometimes intramuscular (IM) or IV estradiol dipropionate was administered. If the woman was acidotic, 150 to 200 ml of 5% sodium bicarbonate was administered IV followed by 100 ml of 10 to 20% glucose (1).

Today, is is known that IV glucose is contraindicated for intrauterine resuscitation because it may worsen fetal acidemia. Glucose is aerobically metabolized by the fetus to produce CO_2 and anaerobically metabolized to produce lactic acid (240). Therefore, *when an IV bolus is given in response to a nonreassuring FHR pattern, a nondextrose containing solution should be used* (241). If the woman is bolused with glucose or dextrose shortly before birth, the placenta will transfer a large amount of glucose to the fetus. The fetus will produce insulin. When the umbilical cord is cut after birth, the neonate may experience rebound *hypoglycemia*.

O_2 delivery is dependent upon uteroplacental and umbilical cord blood flow and blood O_2 content (240). Actions to improve fetal oxygenation focus on *increasing blood flow* to the uterus, placenta, and fetus and *increasing blood O_2 content* (242). Without uterine blood flow, any increase in maternal arterial O_2 will not reach the fetus. Therefore, *actions are first directed at blood flow to the uterus and umbilical cord blood flow improvement, followed by actions to increase blood O_2 content.* Uteroplacental blood flow (Q_{ut}) is dependent upon maternal:
- cardiac contractility
- cardiac output
- intravascular volume
- systemic vascular resistance
- blood viscosity
- uterine vessel diameter and
- placental vessel diameter (243).

Hb oxygen affinity differs in maternal and fetal blood due to differences in:
- Hb type
- RBC glycolytic metabolism
- RBC 2,3-diphosphoglycerate (DPG)
- pH
- PCO_2 and
- temperature (244).

Health care providers can act to improve blood flow to the uterus, placenta, and fetus, to improve blood flow through the umbilical cord, and to increase fetal blood O_2 content. Possible intrauterine resuscitation actions are listed in Table 8.

Table 8: Intrauterine Resuscitation: Assess, Act, Communicate, Evaluate

ASSESS: IDENTIFY THE PROBABLE CAUSE OF HYPOXIA
- Maternal? Assess blood pressure (BP), pulse, temperature, hemoglobin, hematocrit, medications
- Uterine? Assess uterine activity, hyperstimulation or hypertonus?
- Placental? Assess maternal behavior, e.g., restless?, pain, and vaginal bleeding

- Fetal? Assess FHR, amniotic fluid, and perform vaginal examination to rule out cord prolapse.

ACT TO DIMINISH OR REMOVE THE HYPOXIC INSULT:
INCREASE RED BLOOD CELL VOLUME
- Maternal blood transfusion to maintain Hb above 10 grams/deciliter (gm/dl)
- Fetal blood transfusion needed if hemolysis (pathological sinusoidal pattern?)

ENHANCE BLOOD FLOW
Treat Maternal Disease Processes
- Antihypertensive needed?
- Magnesium sulfate needed?

Increase Maternal Cardiac Output and Uterine Perfusion
- Change maternal position (avoid supine and Trendelenburg positions)
- Hydrate: Intravenous bolus of nonglucose solution (241, 245)
- Correct hypotension: ephedrine may be needed
- Decrease anxiety and fear, explain procedures

Increase Placental Perfusion
- Decrease or discontinue pitocin depending on fetal status and uterine activity
- Administer tocolytic unless abruption is diagnosed

Improve Umbilical Cord Blood Flow
- Change maternal position, knee-chest or Trendelenburg with right wedge if cord prolapse
- Fill bladder (for cord prolapse) (246-248)
- Amnioinfusion (for oligohydramnios, variable decelerations, thick meconium)

INCREASE BLOOD OXYGEN CONTENT
Increase Maternal P_vO_2 to Increase Umbilical vein PO_2
- Hyperoxygenate with a tight fitting face mask and O_2 at 8 to 10 LPM (249)

COMMUNICATE URGENCY AS NEEDED
- Notify charge nurse or supervisor
- Notify midwife and/or physician

EVALUATE
- Maternal response
- Fetal response

DELIVER if
- Placental abruption
- Cord prolapse
- Uterine rupture
- Maternal or fetal hemorrhage
- Ominous FHR pattern

Act First, Call Second

After intrauterine resuscitation measures are initiated, the charge nurse or supervisor may be called and the midwife or physician are informed of the previous and current FHR patterns, clinical findings prior to interventions, actions taken, and the maternal and fetal response to actions. When the fetus is hypoxic, it is best to avoid narcotic administration because narcotics diminish the fetal compensatory response and heighten the risk of acidosis. If oligohydramnios has been diagnosed and the fetus isn't in immediate jeopardy, an amnioinfusion may be ordered. Prior to amnioinfusion, cord prolapse should be ruled out, membranes must be ruptured, and an IUPC must be inserted (83).

If the fetus reestablishes homeostatic balance following interventions, intrauterine resuscitation was successful. If, on the other hand, intrauterine resuscitative measures fail to improve the FHR pattern and scalp blood pH or blood gases are not available, expeditious delivery must be considered the next option.

UTEROPLACENTAL BLOOD FLOW
Placental Blood Flow

Oxygen and nutrient delivery is dependent upon maternal and fetal circulation (250-251). The delivery of O_2 via the placenta, rather than the condition that might adversely affect the rate of delivery, is a primary predictor of fetal growth and oxygenation (250). A secondary predictor of fetal growth is acid-base balance. Quadriceps and left ventricular myocardium growth were delayed in fetal lambs who had tissue hypoxia (252).

An increase in placental blood flow increases placental O_2 consumption (253). A decrease in fetal umbilical artery flow decreases placental O_2 consumption (250). Increasing uterine blood flow increases fetal SaO_2 and umbilical vein and artery BE (254). A decrease in maternal cardiac output by 60% or more (in the ewe) decreases placental blood flow and produces fetal acidemia (255).

Reduce Anxiety, Fear, and Pain

A reduction in anxiety, fear, and pain should diminish maternal catecholamine levels. The reduction in norepinephrine and epinephrine should dilate blood vessels and improve uteroplacental blood flow and fetal O_2 delivery.

Recognize cultural differences. It is possible that the current healthcare system creates anxiety, fear, or access barriers in some women who are not part of the majority culture. For example, women who only spoke Spanish were more likely to have HELLP syndrome, cerebral bleeds, blindness, liver rupture, dialysis, transfusions, and admission to an intensive care unit. Some even died. Although women of all ethnic groups had equal access to care and translation services, Spanish-speaking women were more likely to develop pregnancy complications and become critically ill than English speaking women (256). Hispanic women were also less likely to receive epidural anesthesia during labor than women from other ethnic groups (257). Reasons for these differences need to be investigated.

Meet expectations. *Culturally-relevant care* meets the woman's expectations and needs, and not necessarily the health care providers needs. This type of care may be more effective than routine or ritualistic behavior in reducing anxiety, fear, and pain during labor. Married women, who attended a Lamaze childbirth preparation class, expected to receive pain relief during labor. In their opinion, the ideal labor nurse was calm, compassionate, concerned, understanding, accepting of feelings, able to offer praise, and was interested in the woman as a person. They also felt supportive nursing activities included the following:

- provided comfort measures and reassurance
- used conversation as a diversion
- provided encouragement
- offered praise for the woman's efforts during labor and delivery
- provided feedback for doing well
- demonstrated friendly behaviors
- demonstrated knowledge
- was a patient advocate
- listened
- respected opinions and
- accepted the woman's behavior.

Women from other ethnic backgrounds may have other or additional expectations for the nurse's behavior, but these have yet to be elucidated.

If a woman's expectations are not met, anxiety may heighten, and dissatisfaction with care may occur. Health care providers would be wise to assess each woman's unique needs and expectations. Some women may desire less intense nursing care than others (258).

Be empathetic. Empathy is the capacity for participation in another person's feelings or ideas (259). Nurses are usually empathetic and the first to respond to a woman's pain and distress. Communication is required to express empathy. The quality of the communication can decrease the woman's pain and anxiety or heighten it (260).

Touch is essential. Touch is an essential nursing strategy that has meaning and intent. Touch should be sincere and reciprocal. Labor nurses touch laboring women when they cry, moan, beseech, scream, reach out, or have a facial expression of fear, pain, or panic (261). Nurses who are present at the bedside and are sensitive to these behaviors will more likely be able to allay fear and reduce pain better than nurses who are out of the room.

Music is a distraction. Music can alter pain perception by providing a distraction (43). By therapeutic manipulation of the environment, e.g., turn off the television, dim the lights, and turn on soft music, women may be able to derive increased relaxation during the early phase of labor.

Biofeedback didn't work. Devices that provide information about finger temperature and other bodily responses to stress have not been helpful in decreasing maternal anxiety during labor, partly because women don't use them even when they have been instructed in their use. Instead, women found the most helpful labor coping strategies included ASPO/Lamaze breathing and coaching (262).

Hydrotherapy is therapeutic. Even if membranes are ruptured, women can soak in warm water to alleviate the pain of labor without increasing their risk of infection. Women, 34 or more weeks pregnant who soaked after spontaneous prelabor rupture of membranes, needed more pitocin but had *fewer cesarean sections* (2.4% versus 5.1%) than women who were not ruptured but took a bath during labor (263).

ANALGESIA AND ANESTHESIA

Analgesia has been defined as a *lack of pain* without the loss of consciousness (166). Women in labor, who only receive IV or intramuscular (IM) narcotics, never receive total analgesia. Narcotics act on the brain and alter pain perception. Analgesia during labor has been achieved by epidural drug administration.

In 1979, *anesthesia* was defined as the *loss of all sensation* with or without the loss of consciousness (259). Thus, *analgesia (loss of pain) differs from anesthesia (loss of sensation).* An anesthetic is a drug that is capable of producing a complete or partial loss of sensation or feeling. Anesthetic drugs, such as bupivacaine (Marcaine), can also provide analgesia if they are delivered in very small doses. Anesthetic drugs block the passage of pain impulses along nerve fibers to the brain (171).

Administration of Anesthesics for Analgesia

All too often, especially in rural hospitals, staff nurses, who are not certified registered nurse anesthetists (CRNAs), are asked to administer epidural medications when the CRNA or anesthesiologist is off the unit or out of the building. This practice, i.e., *management of epidurals by nonanesthesia providers, has been viewed as suboptimal care* (J. Stem, CRNA, personal communication, February 1996). Obstetric staff nurses should not reinject an epidural catheter. Instead, the nurse needs to work closely with anesthesia providers who will need to manage the epidural infusion. Anesthesiologists administer anesthetics and provide respiratory and cardiovascular support during anesthetic procedures. A nurse anesthetist is qualified by advanced training in an accredited program in the speciality of nurse anesthesia to manage the anesthetic care of a patient in certain surgical situations (166). Based on their training and experience, shouldn't anesthesiologists or CRNAs be present at the bedside when medication is injected into an epidural? Hospital administrators need to promote the proper policies and personnel mix so that women in labor may have their pain managed by an appropriately educated health care professional. Management of epidural analgesia in the laboring women is not the same as giving other forms of analgesic medications.

American CRNAs believe the appropriate training to manage a complicated technique like epidural analgesia lasts 24 to 30 months in an accredited school of nurse anesthesia or occurs in medical school and anesthesia residency. Skills that are required for management of complications of epidural analgesia include airway management, advanced cardiac life support (ACLS), recognition of impending difficulties, knowledge of when to call for assistance and when to terminate an injection or a continuous epidural infusion (J. Stem, CRNA, personal communication, February 1996).

Even though most women do not suffer complications of epidural analgesia, *complications have unexpectedly occurred.* The injection of local anesthetics, regardless of concentration, significantly increase the risk of life threatening complications. Annoying side effects, such as numb lips and a metallic taste can occur. Or, there can be life threatening complications, including seizures and cardiovascular collapse (J. Stem, CRNA, personal communication, February, 1996). Women in labor may have ketoacidosis. Miller (264) believes the pregnant woman may be more susceptible to the cardiotoxic effects of anesthetic drugs. Bupivacaine (Marcaine), in the presence of hypoxia and acidosis, becomes extremely cardiotoxic and may cause dysrhythmias or asystole *which may be irreversible.*

Even if the epidural catheter was initially placed in the epidural space, it may still migrate into the spinal column (J. Stem, CRNA, personal communication, February 1996). When the epidural catheter is initially inserted, unintentional intravascular placement occurs two to three percent of the time (265). However, there are no statistics on the number of times epidural catheters migrate during the labor and delivery process.

The American Association of Nurse Anesthetists (AANA) has specific guidelines for the management of pain via continuous epidural, intrathecal, intrapleural, peripheral catheters and other pain relief devices (266). Their position statement 2.8, part II, section B, states:

> *"Obstetrical laboring patients receiving epidural analgesia may be MONITORED (emphasis added) by an obstetrical nurse, appropriately trained...reinjection or continuous infusion of epidural catheters for anesthesia or analgesia for the obstetrical patient in labor may ONLY (emphasis in the original text) be performed by a qualified/credentialed anesthesia provider."*

Guidelines for obstetrical anesthesia and conduction analgesia for the certified registered nurse anesthetist, found in the AANA Practice Manual (266) state: "Conduction analgesia (via epidural or intrathecal single dose or via catheter) should be...*managed by a CRNA or other qualified anesthesia provider.*"

Unintentional subarachnoid (intraspinal) injection of anesthetic drugs, such as bupivacaine (Marcaine) or opiates may lead to total spinal anesthesia, cardiovascular collapse, and respiratory arrest. In general, *obstetrical nurses are not adequately trained to manage these complications*, nor can they manage these complications, call a code blue, intubate and resuscitate the pregnant woman all at the same time. Obstetric nurses do not practice maternal intubation enough to be competent in this procedure. Massive hypotension, loss of airway reflexes, and regurgitation with aspiration are life threatening, especially if these complications are inappropriately managed. Ostheimer (265) believes poor maternal and neonatal outcome during obstetrical anesthesia occurs as a result of ignoring the basic principles of anesthesia (J. Stem, CRNA, personal communication, February 1996). If these complications challenge educated, professional anesthesia providers, how can one expect nonanesthesia providers, such as obstetric staff nurses, to properly manage this technique even with "education beyond licensure?" If the obstetric nurse believes her actions may endanger the laboring woman, she should refuse to perform the procedure. It may be necessary to follow the hospital conflict resolution protocol should pressure be exerted on the obstetric nurse to perform a task that is outside of the scope of practice.

BLOOD PRESSURE ASSESSMENT
What is Hypotension?
Hypotension is a systolic blood pressure (BP) of 90 mm Hg or a systolic drop of more than 30 mm Hg (267-268). The risk of hypotension increases when a β-mimetic tocolytic is given in conjunction with epidural anesthesia or following injection of an anesthetic drug for epidural or spinal anesthesia (268-269). Hypotension diminishes placental perfusion and fetal O_2 delivery (270).

Treatment for Hypotension: Maternal Plasma Volume Expansion and Ephedrine
A prolonged deceleration or a series of late decelerations may occur as a result of maternal hypotension. If either of these fetal responses occur after epidural or spinal anesthesia, maternal BP should be assessed. The first response to maternal hypotension is to change maternal position. Women are positioned on their side or a wedge is placed under their right side, especially prior to and after regional anesthesia (267). Relieving mechanical compression of the aorta, inferior vena cava, and iliac vessels by a knee-chest or lateral position should decrease intrapulmonary shunting, maintain maternal PaO_2, increase cardiac output, and increase O_2 delivery to the fetus. If hypotension is severe, the legs may be raised. If the woman is able to turn around in the bed, the head of the bed could be raised which easily raises her legs.

As the woman changes her position, an IV bolus of an isotonic solution, such as lactated Ringer's solution or normal saline, is initiated. An increase in maternal plasma volume should increase venous return to the heart, cardiac output, and fetal O_2 delivery (271). The woman's midwife, physician, CRNA, or anesthesiologist should be notified as soon as possible of maternal hypotension. They may order ephedrine to be administered or they may administer it themselves.

Ephedrine, 2.5 to 10 mg IV push or IM, is the preferred vasoconstrictor for the laboring hypotensive woman because it has little vasoconstrictive effect on uterine vessels (20). Ephedrine is an α and β-adrenergic agonist that activates cardiac β-receptors and blood vessel α-receptors. It restores uteroplacental blood flow by increasing maternal heart rate and cardiac output (269). Ephedrine crosses the placenta, increases fetal norepinephrine, and may increase the FHR (272).

Antenatal Hydration By Mouth (PO)
The amniotic fluid index (AFI) is determined by ultrasound evaluation of the four quadrants of the uterus. The largest pocket of fluid in each quadrant is measured in centimeters and the pockets are added. An AFI of 5 cm or less is considered to be oligohydramnios. Fetuses with oligohydramnios have sig-nificantly lower birth weights than those with a normal AFI and are more vulnerable to acidosis than normal fetuses (273). Oligohydramnios increases the risk of umbilical cord compression, hypoxia, and acidosis. There is an association between oligohydramnios, IUGR, and chronic abruption (274). Prior to PO hydration, placental abruption should be ruled out by clinical asssessment of maternal vital signs, pain, and behavior, uterine activity, vaginal bleeding, the FHR pattern, and ultrasound evaluation of the placenta.

Ingestion of a large amount of water may increase the AFI. For example, ingestion of one liter of water in one hour increased the AFI and significantly decreased maternal urine specific gravity. The AFI increased an average of 1.8 cm in women who consumed one liter of water and only 0.87 cm in the group that ingested 150 ml of water. AFI increased most in women whose original AFI was less than 8 cm. In some of these women, the AFI increased 60% (275). Although ingestion of water may increase the AFI, an AFI increase does NOT diminish concern for the fetus because *an increase in the AFI does not reverse the factors that created IUGR or oligohydramnios.* However, increasing amniotic fluid volume may be beneficial when it aides the ultrasonographer's identification of the fetus.

The mechanisms by which amniotic fluid increases following water ingestion are most likely bulk flow and increased uteroplacental perfusion which improves fetal O_2 delivery, renal perfusion, and urine output (276). Water crosses the chorionic and amniotic membranes based on an osmotic or hydrostatic gradient (277). In sheep, intake of 20 ml per kilogram (kg) of water over an 8 hour period decreased maternal and fetal plasma osmolality and increased maternal and fetal urine production (278). Women with oligohydramnios who said they drank two liters of water over a two to four hour period increased their AFI an average of 1.5 cm. Women who did not increase their fluid intake had an average AFI increase of 0.31 cm (279). After two liters of water were ingested over a two hour period, the AFI increased an average of 3.2 cm. Also, uterine artery blood flow increased. Fewer than one third of the fetuses increased their urine output. However, umbilical artery velocity and fetal blood flow did improve.

Table 9: Ingestion of More than 1 Liter of Water Increases Amniotic Fluid Volume in Women who Have Oligohydramnios

Primary Researcher	Amount of Water Ingested/Time	Increase in AFI
Ross (278)	20 ml/kg titrated over 8 hrs (sheep/lamb study)	3.3-5.1 AFI increased to 5.5-9.3 at 8 hours and 6.9-10.1 at 24 hours
Kerr (275)	1000 ml vs. 150 ml over 1 hr	Nonsignificant increase in AFI (average increase 1.8 cm vs. 0.87 cm)
Flack (276)	2000 ml over 2 hours	Average AFI increase 3.2 cm if there was an AFI less than 7 cm. Significant decrease in plasma and urine osmolality
Kilpatrick (279)	2000 ml over 2 to 4 hours	Average AFI increase 1.5 vs. 0.31 cm

Intrapartal Intravenous Hydration

A bolus is a large amount of fluid, often 400 ml or more. Twelve of 14 term women with oligohydramnios who received an IV *bolus of 500 ml* increased their AFI. Seven of the 12 increased their AFI by 50% or more, and 3 of 12 increased their AFI by 100% or more. *The increase in AFI was greater with IV fluid administration than PO fluid administration* (280). In some cases, an IV bolus did not improve fetal oxygenation as there was no improvement in end-diastolic umbilical artery blood flow (276).

Some pregnant women should not receive a bolus of IV fluid, even when their fetus appears compromised. The physician should specify the desired flow rate when the woman has any condition that would be exacerbated by a bolus of IV fluid or that would increase her risk of complications. For example, preeclamptic women who received *only one liter* of normal saline reduced their colloid osmotic pressure (COP) an average of 12%. The decrease in COP lasted 2 to 5 days and increased their risk of pulmonary edema (281).

Women in labor need glucose. Women in labor consume approximately 1200 kcal of glucose in an 8 to 10 hour labor. They need 2.55 mg of glucose per kg of body weight per minute to avoid hypoglycemia (282-283). Therefore, a standard IV solution given to laboring women is 5% dextrose in lactated Ringer's solution (D_5LR). Provision of dextrose during labor prevents maternal hypoglycemia and its sequelae, i.e., maternal seizures. In addition to glucose consumption during labor, women increase their O_2 consumption from an average of 281 ml/minute to 703 ml/minute (283).

There is *a misconception* that glucose administered to a pregnant woman will help resuscitate her acidotic fetus. Maternal hyperglycemia has no effect on fetal body movements, however, fetuses *moved more when their mother had a hypoglycemic blood glucose level of less than 60 mg/dl* (284). Supplemental oral or IV glucose of 25 gms increased the incidence of fetal *breathing movement* as well as the amplitude of breathing movements, and the frequency of breathing movements within 10 minutes after glucose administration. Maternal glucose levels peaked 45 to 75 minutes after IV administration. The infusion of 5% dextrose in water (D_5W) dilutes maternal blood and *lowers the sodium concentration* resulting in a net transfer of water to the fetus (285). *Maternal and fetal hyponatremia* can occur if IV solutions that do not contain sodium are continuously administered over a long period of time. When 3000 ml of D_5W was infused over a 3 hour period in women who had preterm premature rupture of membranes, there was no change in their urine specific gravity, serum osmolality, or AFI. Fetal effects of the bolus were not studied (286).

Avoid a bolus of dextrose or glucose. There is an increase in fetal insulin production associated with a maternal glucose bolus. Fetal metabolism increases, O_2 consumption increases, CO_2 production increases, and PO_2 decreases (287). Fetal pH may decrease as a result of a maternal glucose bolus. If the fetus was well, a maternal bolus of glucose preceded a rapid fall in fetal plasma pH (244). *If the fetus is acidemic, maternal glucose administration could precede a further decrease in pH and rise in PCO_2 which could potentially worsen the fetal condition and increase the risk of asphyxia.* A liter of IV fluid containing 5% dextrose contains 50 gms of dextrose. Fifteen to 50 grams of dextrose infused over 4 or more hours was related to a significant reduction in neonatal capillary blood sugars (288). Hypoglycemic neonates, following maternal IV dextrose administration, have a greater risk of developing physiologic jaundice. They had high lactate and insulin levels and suppressed glucagon release secondary to anaerobic glucose metabolism (289).

Bolus with a nondextrose containing solution. Laboring women need glucose and IV fluids that contain a balanced electrolyte solution to minimize the incidence of fetal hyperglycemia and neonatal hypoglycemia (290). The woman in

Table 10: Tocolytics

DRUG	ROUTE	ONSET	ACTION
Isoxuprine	5 mg IVP in 20 ml D$_5$W over 30 seconds (298)	10 minutes	Decreases UA from 4.3 ± 1.7 to 3 ± 1.5 contractions in 10 minutes, no fetal tachycardia, an initial fall then rise in maternal diastolic BP, a slight rise in systolic BP, and a slight decrease in maternal heart rate (MHR)
Fenoterol	IV		When given with supplemental maternal O$_2$ significant increase in fetal tcPO$_2$ and maternal PaO$_2$ (305)
Hexoprenoline	IV push over 1 minute 5-10 μg (306)		
Ritodrine	IV 150 to 400 μg (50 mg in 500 ml D$_5$W at 2.5 to 4 ml/min) continuous infusion (248, 306)		No contractions after 5 to 10 minutes (248)
Terbutaline	0.125 to 0.25 mg SQ or IVP over 1 minute (249)	within 1 to 2.5 minutes (292, 307) halves UA in 7 to 24 minutes (297)	12 of 15 fetuses had no further decelerations, 4 of 6 had "improved" variability; increased MHR from an average of 79.5 bpm to 101.8 bpm, with a maximum of 125 bpm (292)
MgSO$_4$	4 gm over 20 minutes or 2 gm IVP slowly	within 2 minutes (308)	Decreases frequency but doesn't stop UA, often maintains contraction amplitude (309)

SQ = subcutaneous injection
IVP = intravenous push

labor should maintain a blood glucose at 120 mg/dl or less. *IV dextrose should be limited to 6 grams per hour or 125 ml/hr of a 1000 ml solution containing 5% dextrose (291). An IV bolus may decrease uterine activity to indirectly increase fetal oxygenation.* Some nurses have found it helpful to use blood tubing when the IV is initiated. They connect D$_5$LR to one side of the Y tubing and LR to the other. If they need to give a fluid bolus, they discontinue the D$_5$LR infusion and begin the LR bolus.

TOCOLYSIS

Tocolysis is a decrease in uterine activity (UA). Uterine activity may be decreased by administration of a tocolytic drug or discontinuance of a uterine stimulant such as pitocin. Tocolysis buys time to determine fetal acid-base status or to set up for a cesarean delivery (292). In 1969, Dr. Caldeyro-Barcia used metaproterenol sulfate as a continuous IV infusion or hexoprenaline in an IV push injection to diminish UA (293). In the United Kingdom and Europe, IV salbutamol has been used to diminish or eliminate UA in the presence of hyperstimulation and hypertonicity (283, 294-296). The

physician who orders tocolysis must carefully consider the benefits and risks of drug administration. *Tocolytics are not recommended in cases of abruption where immediate delivery is indicated (297).* In addition, β-mimetic tocolytics may alter fetal hemodynamics, increase myocardial intracellular calcium, resulting in overexcitation and *necrosis of cardiac cells* (3).

Tocolytic medications are more commonly administered when repositioning, an IV bolus, and hyperoxygenation do not improve the FHR pattern and preparations are being made for emergency delivery. Tocolytics have also been administered in response to umbilical cord prolapse or prior to bilateral ultrasonographically guided fetal thoracocentesis, a procedure that decompresses fluid collection around the fetal lungs (247, 296).

Combination Therapy: Tocolysis Plus O$_2$ Is Better than Tocolysis or Hyperoxygenation Alone

Intrauterine resuscitation is more effective if tocolytics are given in conjunction with maternal hyperoxygenation by face mask (221). *When the tocolytic isoxuprine was administered in conjunction with maternal O$_2$ in response to late decelerations* *during the first stage of labor, there was a 95% recovery in the FHR. When O$_2$ was given without tocolysis, there was only an 18% recovery in the FHR (298).*

Tocolytics

Magnesium sulfate (MgSO$_4$) has been used as a tocolytic. It decreases systemic vascular resistance and increases cardiac output in preeclamptic women. However this effect is minimal after the initial bolus (299). In the uterus, β-mimetics, such as salbutamol, terbutaline, ritodrine (Yutopar), isoxsuprine, and metaproterenol (Alupent), bind with β$_2$-receptors. Then, adenylate cyclase within uterine cells is activated which enhances the conversion of ATP to cyclic adenosine 3^1 5^1-monophosphate (cAMP). cAMP *decreases* intracellular calcium which causes uterine smooth muscle relaxation or tocolysis (292, 298, 300-303). Terbutaline (Brethine) binds with β$_1$- and β$_2$-receptors. Cardiac contractility increases, blood vessels dilate, peripheral blood flow increases, and placental perfusion may improve (303).

Contraindications to Use of β-mimetics

β-mimetics should not be given if there is evidence of maternal
- cardiac disease or a history of cardiac surgery, e.g., mitral valve prosthesis, atrial fibrillation
- hyperthyroidism
- uncontrolled hypertension
- pulmonary hypertension
- asthma
- uncontrolled diabetes mellitus or
- chronic hepatic or renal disease (246, 304).

When to Discontinue Uterine Stimulants Such as Pitocin

When there is excessive uterine activity and a nonreassuring FHR pattern, it has been suggested that pitocin be decreased or discontinued (249). Fetal recovery should be faster if pitocin is totally discontinued versus just decreased. It has been recommended that pitocin be discontinued when fetal bradycardia occurs (297).

Modified Pushing During the Second Stage of Labor

Maternal BP increases when women push (310). Rhesus monkeys with intraamniotic pressures of 40 to 50 torr had almost complete cessation of placental blood flow (311). Therefore, women with intrauterine pressures exceeding 80 torr (common with pushing) would be expected to have no placental perfusion during pushing efforts. In spite of the cessation of placental blood flow with pushing, sometimes maternal bearing down using a Valsalva Maneuver had no effect on umbilical artery pH (312). During the second stage, many fetuses have "spikes" or "dips" in their FHR during pushing efforts. The baseline may decrease 20 or more bpm as a vagal response to head and cord compression. Rather than being focused on large decelerations or bradycardia, it is important to identify and record signs of fetal well-being, such as short-term variability or accelerations.

If the fetus decelerates during the second stage to a rate less than 100 bpm and baseline variability is decreased, intrauterine resuscitation actions should be initiated. Fetal blood gases are better when women sit to deliver versus lay down. At delivery both the umbilical vein and artery gases had a higher pH, SO$_2$, PO$_2$, BE and lower PCO$_2$ when women were sitting versus laying down for delivery (118). In as many as 60% of fetuses, decelerations and bradycardia were related to a nuchal cord. Decelerations that continue to increase in depth and duration may precede severe, persistent, progressive bradycardia (307). The increase in deceleration depth and duration suggests additional interventions are necessary. For example, women may be asked to not push with every other contraction, they may be hyperoxygenated, or tocolytics may be given. Assess for the presence of a prolapsed umbilical cord if during maternal pushing variable decelerations continue to become deeper and longer lasting.

It has been recommended that the FHR should be assessed *and recorded* every 15 minutes if women are low-risk and every 5 minutes if women are high-risk during the second stage of labor (241). End-stage bradycardia, with a FHR between 80 and 100 bpm, occurs in 1 to 35% of all labors and is expected (307). But a rate between 60 to 80 bpm (sinus bradycardia) has been associated with severe acidosis and requires swift intervention. In the case of a persistent bradycardia when delivery is not imminent, it may be helpful to administer tocolytics and hyperoxygenate the laboring woman.

MATERNAL HYPEROXYGENATION

Oxygen was discovered by the Swedish chemist Carl Wilhelm Scheele and the English chemist Joseph Priestley in the late 1700s. Today, their discovery is used as part of a two-pronged approach to increase fetal oxygenation: increase blood flow and increase blood O$_2$ content. Hyperoxygenation is a safe, efficient, life-saving, expedient procedure which benefits the hypoxic fetus (313-315).

Hyperoxygenation Concerns

Criticisms that hyperoxygenation might cause vasoconstriction in the placenta are based on laboratory experiments, not in vivo studies. For example, an in vitro study of placental arteries found that a 100 mm Hg O$_2$ bath caused contractions in the umbilical artery, possibly due to increased vessel sensitivity to vasoconstrictors and decreased sensitivity to vasodilators (316). Placentas in a high O$_2$ solution increased thromboxane A$_2$ production, a vasoconstrictor (317). Hyperoxygenation with tocolytic medication administration should reverse any placental vasoconstriction (318).

In vivo studies with pregnant sheep revealed no decrease in placental perfusion when 100% O$_2$ was administered to the ewe. Fears that a high O$_2$ concentration might cause fetal vasoconstriction are unfounded. In fact, maternal hyperoxygenation did not change fetal umbilical vessel blood flow. Hyperoxygenation increased fetal PO$_2$ in both the umbilical vein and arteries. Umbilical vein PO$_2$ averaged 40 mm Hg and umbilical arterial PO_2 averaged 16 mm Hg after maternal hyperoxygenation (319). Indications for maternal hyperoxygenation include

- emergency intervention for fetal indications during labor (320-323)
- as an adjunct to diminish a fetal adverse response in high risk, complicated labors (322)
- in conjunction with induction of anesthesia prior to a cesarean delivery (324-328) or
- as long term antenatal therapy when the fetus is immature and as an attempt to improve fetal status prior to labor and delivery (313, 329-336).

Hyperoxygenation Benefits

Both animal and human studies clearly show evidence of fetal improvement following maternal hyperoxygenation. For example, when rhesus monkeys were given 100% O_2, maternal PaO_2 increased to 349.1 ± 26.2 mm Hg and fetal PaO_2 increased from 29.4 ± 4.6 to 34.2 ± 5.5 mm Hg (337). Fetal and neonatal benefits of maternal hyperoxygenation include:

- increased fetal cerebral oxygenation (320-321)
- improved fetal circulation (329-330, 334-335)
- increased fetal PaO_2 (323, 326, 334, 338)
- increased fetal SaO_2 (215, 327-328, 339)
- increased fetal $tcPO_2$ (313, 322, 333, 340-341)
- increased fetal breathing movements (331-333, 336, 342)
- increased fetal movements (313, 331, 333, 336)
- FHR accelerations (333)
- increased FHR variability (331, 333)
- amelioration of late decelerations (323) and
- a lower incidence of neonatal resuscitation (326).

Maternal PaO_2 Increases Fetal PaO_2

A common *misconception* regarding hyperoxygenation is that the woman's hemoglobin O_2 saturation is normal therefore any attempt to increase it will not help the fetus. However, *SaO_2 or SpO_2 reflects O_2 not available for transfer across the placenta because it is bound to hemoglobin. O_2 must first dissociate from Hb and disolve in plasma before it is available for transfer. Maternal uterine PaO_2 and PvO_2 must increase to increase fetal PaO_2.*

Fetuses with the lowest PaO_2, had the greater improvement in their PaO_2 following maternal hyperoxygenation (338). An increase in maternal PaO_2 from 123 to 440 mm Hg increased fetal PaO_2 from 17.8 to 31.5 mm Hg (314). Although the maternal increase in PaO_2 is much greater than the fetal increase, a review of the fetal oxyhemoglobin dissociation curve indicates a much greater increase in fetal SaO_2 with smaller increases in PaO_2.

By increasing maternal F^IO_2, maternal PaO_2 increases (343). When maternal PaO_2 increases, PvO_2 increases. Maternal uterine vein PO_2 determines the placental-fetal O_2 gradient. The rise in maternal vein PO_2 increases O_2 transfer to fetal circulation. Therefore, increasing maternal PaO_2 increases fetal PO_2 (315).

The concentration of O_2 that reaches the trachea (F^IO_2) depends on the speed O_2 enters the mask. Newman, McKinnon, and Phillips (315) found the most effective way to increase fetal PaO_2 was by administering 100% O_2 by mask versus a nasal cannula. To maximize the concentration of O_2 at the trachea, the mask should be tight and the O_2 flow rate should be high (344). Ten people who had a tracheostomy participated in an experiment to measure intratracheal O_2 content following O_2 delivery by a simple plastic face mask. As the O_2 flow rate increased, the percentage of O_2 reaching the trachea increased (345). Results were:

Table 11: Simple O_2 Mask and Intratracheal O_2 Content

LPM	TRACHEAL CONCENTRATION (%)
5	40
10	60
15	70
20	80

When an O_2 sensor was placed within the mask, the following concentrations were obtained (346):

Table 12: O_2 Flow Rate via a Simple Mask and Maternal O_2 Concentration (in the mask)

LPM	CONCENTRATION IN THE MASK (%)
5	64
10	81
15	88

Based on tables 12 and 13, it is obvious that O_2 is lost to the atmosphere prior to the time it reaches the trachea. When a tight fitting face mask is applied and supplied with 100% O_2 (from the flow meter or tank) at a rate of 8 to 10 LPM, there should be a rapid rise in fetal PO_2 and pH and a decline in fetal PCO_2 (315). When the flow rate is less than 10 LPM, the risk of maternal hypercapnia increases. To diminish the risk of maternal CO_2 retention, O_2 masks should have side holes (345). When pregnant primates, who had a fetus with late decelerations, were hyperoxygenated with 100% O_2, fetal PaO_2 increased and late decelerations were temporarily abolished (323).

In instances of maternal hyperoxygenation using a nasal cannula during labor, it may be quite difficult, if not impossible, to obtain an adequate maternal O_2 concentration due to the inability of the mother to breathe solely through her nares in combination with irritation of the nasal mucosa with high flow rates of oxygen (322).

Table 13: Maternal PaO₂ Greater than 300 mm Hg Offers Insignificant Increases in Fetal Umbilical Vein PO₂

O₂ Concentration Before C-section (%)	Maternal F^IO₂ (torr)	Maternal PaO₂ (torr)	Umbilical Vein PO₂ (torr)	Umbilical Artery PO₂ (torr)
28	207 - 211	87.98 - 93.43	24.64 - 37.36	17.28 - 20.88
33	250 - 254	117.3 - 132.7	25.91 - 30.75	15.60 - 20.4
33 1/3		124.32 - 145.68	22.96 - 35.44	11.95 - 24.25
66 2/3		211.99 - 298.01	28.58 - 50.02	18.67 - 36.33
65	**486 - 490**	**272.63 - 292.57**	**33.91 - 36.01**	**22.32 - 23.76**
93-97	714 - 722	375.03 - 399.61	39.61 - 42.79	24.85 - 27.07
100		361.22 - 517.78	28.70 - 44.1	16.15 - 27.85

The Standard of Practice: Hyperoxygenate if the FHR Pattern is Nonreassuring

Maternal O₂ administration is clearly part of fetal resuscitative measures. Oxygen administered at high flow rates for intrauterine fetal resuscitation is a short-term intervention. Therefore, it need not be humidified. For long term use during the antepartal period, humidification is recommended to counteract mucosal irritation and dryness (334).

In 1980, researchers stated, "The generally beneficial effect of maternal oxygen inhalation on the hypoxic fetus can no longer be questioned" (305). In spite of this, some clinicians find it necessary to question the use of supplemental O₂ for suspected fetal hypoxia. *Research over the past 30 years overwhelmingly supports supplemental maternal O₂ administration when the fetus is hypoxic.*

Maternal PaO₂ should be above 100 mm Hg in order to increase PvO₂. The most efficient way to do this is by an anesthesia mask. The next best way to increase maternal PaO₂ is by a mask with an oxygen reservoir (partial rebreathing mask). Lastly, a simple, straight face mask can be used. *A nasal cannula is unreliable and its use during labor for fetal resuscitation was not recommended as early as 1967* (315). Hyperoxygenation with a tight fitting face mask can be expected to promptly increase fetal PaO₂ when there is adequate placental gas exchange and unobstructed umbilical vein circulation (249). The face mask may be a simple mask or partial rebreathing mask with a reservoir. When a partial rebreathing mask is used, an O₂ flow rate of 12 LPM should deliver 100% O₂ to the fetus (211, 216).

Failure to apply maternal O₂ by a *tight fitting face mask* at 8 to 10 LPM, as recommended by ACOG (241) in response to a nonreassuring FHR pattern, is substandard care which may result in fetal harm, neonatal injury, and even cerebral palsy. Of 339 children who had CP, 23 (6.8%) who were term, nonmalformed, singleton babies with hypoxic-ischemic encephalopathy (HIE) had health care providers that failed to respond to a FHR less than 100 bpm for 30 minutes, severe variable decelerations for 90 minutes, late decelerations for 90 minutes, or tachycardia greater than 180 bpm for 90 minutes (347).

The Goal of Hyperoxygenation

The goal of maternal hyperoxygenation is to achieve a maternal PaO₂ greater than 100 but less than 300 mm Hg. A PaO₂ over 300 torr was accompanied by a slight drop in umbilical vein and umbilical artery PO₂ (315, 348). When maternal PaO₂ exceeds 100 torr, fetal PaO₂ and SaO₂ increase (314, 323, 326-327, 334, 338). A maternal PaO₂ greater than 300 torr did not offer any extra benefit to the fetus (see Table 14) (348-349).

After reviewing this table, it should be clear that to attain a normal umbilical vein PO₂ (between 22 to 53 torr), O₂ delivered to the mask should be close to 65%. Apgar scores and umbilical vein and artery PO₂ were higher when 66 2/3% O₂ was administered versus 33 1/3%. (348). The administration of 100% O₂ may require use of an anesthesia mask, used commonly in the operating room but not the labor room. When an anesthesia mask was used to provide 100% O₂ to the woman, a maternal PaO₂ of 78 to 133 mm Hg was related to an increase in umbilical vein PO₂. But, when maternal PaO₂ exceeded 200 mm Hg, there was no relation to umbilical vein PO₂ (350). Just as there is a positive linear correlation between maternal and fetal PCO₂, *there is a positive correlation between maternal and fetal PO₂ as long as maternal PaO₂ is not greater than 300 mm Hg* (351).

Nasal Prongs (Cannula) Versus A Mask

Nasal prongs provide a low-flow O₂ delivery system and are unreliable and less effective than an O₂ mask in increasing maternal PaO₂ (315, 352). An O₂ concentration of 21 to 90% can be delivered by a nasal cannula depending on the O₂ flow rate. Inspiration of room air dilutes O₂ so inspired O₂ levels will vary from breath to breath. A nasal cannula works best with normal respiratory rates and breathing depths (352).

If an emergency cesarean section is undertaken, maternal administration of 100% O₂ via a face mask results in higher umbilical artery PO₂ and less need for neonatal resuscitation than those infants who were delivered under similar circumstances to women who received 50% O₂ (326).

If the cesarean section is elective, i.e., planned and not an emergency, a nasal cannula would be appropriate for O₂ delivery following epidural anesthesia. Nasal prongs with an O_2 flow rate of 4 LPM or a simple face mask with an O_2 flow rate of 8 LPM preceded the cesarean birth of well neonates (353). There was also no statistical difference in fetal PO_2 or neonatal outcome when O_2 was administered by mask at a 50% versus 100% concentration from the time of hysterotomy to birth (average duration 3 minutes) in 20 normal, healthy patients undergoing elective cesarean delivery (325).

Fetal acidemia may be prevented prior to cesarean birth if supplemental O_2 is provided. Concentrations of O_2 between 28 and 97% administered to women prior to their elective cesarean section caused no significant change in maternal pH, $PaCO_2$, or BE. Maternal PaO_2 increased to greater than 300 mm Hg faster at higher concentrations of O_2. At an O_2 concentration of 90%, maternal PaO_2 exceeded 300 mm Hg in 12 seconds (349).

When anesthesia was administered with supplemental O_2 and the induction to delivery time was greater than 10 minutes, fetal PaO_2 increased (354). Fetal pH decreased as the time increased from regional anesthesia to delivery or the time from uterine incision to delivery increased. *In a nonemergency cesarean delivery with a known healthy fetus where the time from uterine incision to birth averages three minutes, O_2 may be delivered by nasal prongs or a simple face mask without any adverse effect on the neonate* (355-356)

If a face mask is applied in response to a nonreassuring FHR pattern, and the women pulls it off even though she is instructed more than once to leave it on, it is necessary to document her behavior and quote her words, detail explanations about the need for the O_2 mask, then apply the nasal cannula at 5 LPM if she refuses to wear the mask.

Duration of O_2 Therapy

From initial administration of O_2 to the mother until placental transfer to the fetus requires a minimum of *50 to 60 seconds* (341). Fetal scalp PO_2 reached normal levels in 5 minutes when 100% O_2 is administered by anesthesia mask (315). Maximum fetal SaO_2 occurs by *nine minutes* (215, 328). In normal, non-stressed fetuses during the second stage of labor, maternal O_2 therapy was associated with an increase in fetal cord arterial pH and an improvement in venous BE when the duration was *10 minutes* or less (346). To summarize:

> In 1 minute: O_2 reaches the fetus
> In 5 minutes: scalp blood PO_2 returned to normal
> In 9 minutes: maximum SaO_2 levels are reached
> In 10 minutes: umbilical artery pH increased, umbilical vein BE improved.

A continuation of maternal O_2 therapy during the *second stage of labor* beyond 10 minutes in *normal* fetuses was accompanied by a decrease in cord arterial pH and a decrease in venous BE (346). Therefore, if after maternal hyperoxygenation a normal FHR pattern has been established, consider discontinuing O_2 after 10 minutes of a reassuring or compensatory pattern and continue fetal surveillance until delivery.

INTERVENTIONS FOR UMBILICAL CORD PROLAPSE

Cord prolapse may be *occult*, with the umbilical cord alongside the fetal head, or *overt*, with the cord palpated in front of the fetal presenting part. Umbilical cord prolapse occurred in as few as 0.08% of all women who delivered at one medical center (357). The presentation of the umbilical cord ahead of the fetus usually requires immediate delivery to prevent fetal anoxia and its sequelae. Fetal mortality due to cord prolapse was as high as 51.6% prior to hospital admission, but as low as 2.2 to 18.6% after hospital admission (358-359). Fetuses are delivered primarily by cesarean section (85%) versus vaginally (15%) after cord prolapse is diagnosed.

The risk of cord prolapse increases when there is a poor fit of the presenting part in the pelvis (246). Risk factors for umbilical cord prolapse are listed in Table 15 (246-247, 357-362).

Table 14: Risk Factors for Umbilical Cord Prolapse

- malpresentation:
  breech
  transverse lie
  oblique lie
  face
  brow
  compound presentation, e.g., hand and head are presenting
- prematurity
- low birth weight, especially less than 2500 grams
- twins, especially the second twin
- lack of prenatal care
- low socioeconomic class
- maternal age greater than 30 years
- hydramnios
- spontaneous rupture of membranes
- a floating station (unengaged head) with artificial rupture of membranes
- cephalopelvic disproportion (CPD)
- cord length > 50 cm
- low lying placenta.

At a hospital in India, the incidence of cord prolapse was only 0.011%. Artificial rupture of the membranes (AROM) was only associated with 6.41% of the cord prolapses, suggesting the lack of a relationship between cord prolapse and AROM. AROM was related to cord prolapse when the fetus was not in the pelvic inlet or was at a -3 station (with the tip of the fetal skull or presenting part 3 or more cm above the ischial spines) or higher (357).

Traditionally, the knee-chest or Trendelenburg position have been used to shift the baby off of its umbilical cord (246-

247, 360). However, a Trendelenburg (head down, feet up) position is also a supine position, which may *decrease* maternal cardiac output and uterine, placental, and fetal O_2 delivery. If a Trendelenburg position is required, e.g., following sensory blockade by epidural anesthesia, a wedge should be placed under the right hip so that the uterus is tilted to the left off the major vessels. Use of a wedge should be documented as well as all actions related to umbilical cord prolapse and the FHR. In addition to a position change when cord prolapse is diagnosed, all or part of the following actions may be taken:

• pitocin is discontinued
• a foley catheter is inserted, the catheter balloon is inflated, the bladder is filled with sterile saline or water, and the foley is clamped until just before incision of the peritoneum during the cesarean section
• hyperoxygenation with O_2 at 8 to 10 LPM by tight fitting face mask
• an IV bolus of a solution free of dextrose
• electronic FHR monitoring
• elevation of the presenting part by two gloved fingers (a full bladder can accomplish this)
• saturation of 4 x 4 gauze with warm normal saline to wrap the exposed umbilical cord and prevent spasm of umbilical vessels from cooling
• tocolysis
• an ultrasound to confirm cord prolapse and
• preparation for emergency cesarean section (247, 360).

Interventions for cord prolapse depend on whether or not the cord is pulsating and the fetus is alive, the presentation of the fetus, cervical dilatation, and time required to set up for and accomplish a cesarean section (362).

Digital Decompression of the Cord and Funic Reduction

Digital decompression of the cord is the application of two fingers of a sterile gloved hand on the presenting part with pressure to lift the fetus off the umbilical cord (246).This practice has been considered the "best treatment" if delivery by cesarean section is imminent (363). However, bladder inflation may be an even better treatment than digital decompression. Head displacement may be more effective in occult versus overt prolapse (361). However, overaggressive displacement of the head did not usually affect outcome and *tocolysis with bladder infusion or filling* was recommended as an alternative to digital decompression (358).

Funic reduction, with replacement of the cord into the uterus, has been accomplished when the fetus could be elevated above 0 station (the level of the ischial spines) and four or more cm of umbilical cord was in front of the fetal head. However, this procedure was not recommended if more than 25 cm of cord was presenting or there were signs of "fetal distress." With gentle simultaneous suprapubic pres-

sure, the cord is digitally elevated above the widest part of the fetal head to place it in the nuchal area. At the same time, preparations are being made for a cesarean section. In a report of 5 cases, delivery occurred 14 to 512 minutes after funic reduction. All five babies had a five minute Apgar score of seven or higher (364).

Knee-chest Position

Trendelenburg with a tilt or the knee-chest position *are common positions* women are placed in upon discovering a prolapsed umbilical cord (357). Unfortunately, a *misconception* about the knee-chest position has been created by statements such as, "Some states, e.g., California, prohibit knee-chest position in the presence of ruptured membranes" (365). No legal, medical, or nursing reference was given for this statement. When talking to California nurses, it appears many of them were told in a seminar that there was an association between air embolism and a knee-chest position. This, of course, is a *gross* misconception which is not based on facts, statute, or statistics. Thousands of women have been placed in a knee-chest position when a cord prolapse was discovered or suspected, even in the state of California, without any adverse outcome. There is absolutely no risk that a woman positioned on elbows and knees, with her head down and her bottom raised, will have open blood vessels and develop an embolism.

Bladder Filling for Umbilical Cord Prolapse

Bladder inflation buys time. A full bladder may stop uterine contractions or decrease uterine activity and is easier and less awkward than digital elevation of the presenting part. By filling the bladder to lift the fetus off its cord, the empty vagina can accommodate the cord to prevent its exposure to air and possible clotting (246). Care should be taken to NOT touch the umbilical cord. If the cord is exposed, it should be wrapped with sterile gauze that has been soaked in warm sterile normal saline. In conjunction with filling the bladder, a tocolytic may be administered (248, 366). *After five years of using normal saline for bladder filling and IV ritodrine, all fetuses survived with an average five minute Apgar score of 9.5 (248).*

Supplies for bladder inflation. To fill the bladder, the following supplies are needed:

Prolapse Kit
• sterile no. 16 foley catheter, drainage tubing and bag
• hemostat
• 1000 ml bottle of sterile water or sterile bladder irrigation fluid or 1000 ml of normal saline with IV tubing
• large syringe with pointed tip, preferably 60 ml

These supplies should be immediately available at the bedside. If the cord prolapse is found during a vaginal examination, and the nurse is not alone, the other clinician should obtain supplies for bladder inflation and notify the physician.

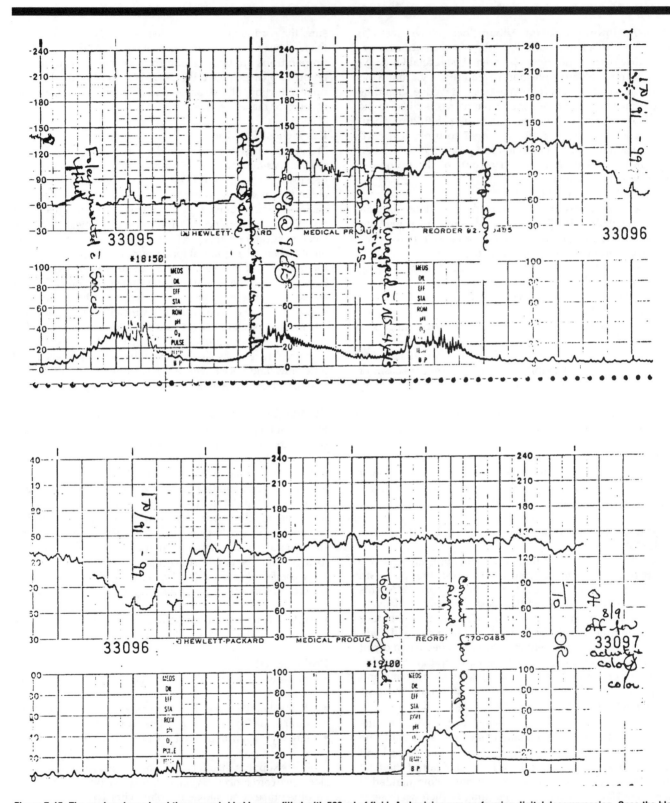

Figure 7.15: The cord prolapsed and the woman's bladder was filled with 500 ml of fluid. A physician was performing digital decompression. Once the bladder was filled, digital elevation of the presenting part was not necessary. Oxygen was applied at 9 1/2 LPM, the exposed cord was wrapped in wet 4 x 4s, and the woman was prepared for surgery. Note the improvement in the FHR pattern. There wasn't even a deceleration with the last contraction! Apgar scores were 8 and 9 at 1 and 5 minutes.

Technique. After insertion of the foley catheter and catheter balloon inflation, the catheter is clamped with a hemostat and the drainage tubing is removed. If an IV line is in place, the woman should be bolused (unless contraindicated) with a non-dextrose containing solution during this procedure.

To inflate the bladder a dextrose-free IV solution, usually a 1000 ml bag of normal saline, should be hung on an IV pole with IV tubing. The IV tubing is inserted into the end of the foley catheter and the hemostat is removed. Infuse 400 to 750 ml into the end of the catheter and reclamp the foley. Reattach the drainage tubing. Leave the clamp in place. The hemostat is removed just before the physician incises the peritoneum during the cesarean section.

An alternative and more cumbersome technique of bladder filling requires a large cath-tip (pointed) syringe to instill water into the foley catheter (246, 367). A foley catheter is inserted and the foley balloon is inflated. The foley is clamped. The drainage tubing is removed. The water bottle is opened and 60 ml of fluid is aspirated using the large syringe. The syringe is inserted into the end of the foley catheter. The clamp is removed and fluid is instilled into the foley. The foley is clamped again and the process is repeated until a minimum of 400 ml has been instilled.

Bladder inflation causes pain. The woman will be scared. Therefore, during foley catheter insertion and bladder filling it is imperative that the clinician stay calm and speak slowly saying such things as, "Your baby is on top of the umbilical cord, so I need to fill your bladder with sterile water. Your full bladder will lift your baby off of its cord. I need your help. While I'm doing this I know it will hurt, but you need to keep thinking I'm helping my baby. Send positive thoughts to your baby. Now, breathe deeply and slowly. Take deep breaths for me now." After the bladder is filled, the fetus should regain a normal baseline rate, and should reestablish normal blood gases.

Act First, Call Second, Communicate Urgency
If the clinician is alone, the bladder is filled then the physician who can perform a cesarean section, an anesthesia provider, and the operating room team are called (247). After

filling the bladder, the woman should be placed in a knee-chest position. If this is awkward for her, a modified Trendelenburg position (with a wedge) should be used. A tocolytic may be ordered and administered while the physician is on the way to the hospital.

CONCLUSION
Doppler blood flow provides hemodynamic information about the fetus prior to labor. During labor, scalp stimulation, acoustic stimulation, and fetal blood sampling provide information about the presence or absence of possible fetal metabolic acidosis. After birth, the umbilical cord or placental blood gases provide additional information about fetal acid-base status near the time of birth. Fetal lactate assessment may provide additional information about fetal well-being. Fetal oxygen saturation monitoring by pulse oximetry may replace fetal scalp blood sampling or become an adjunct to intrapartum FHR assessment. The decade of the 1990s reflects maturation of fetal assessment and interventions to improve fetal acid-base status. The future holds the promise of new techniques that will diagnose and possibly cure fetal brain injuries.

Currently, fetal resuscitation requires unimpeded maternal and umbilical cord blood flow and high blood oxygen content. Fetuses, who are hypoxic with a risk of metabolic acidosis, have nonreassuring FHR patterns. There might be unrelenting bradycardia, late decelerations or severe variable decelerations with a lack of accelerations, or a lack of FHR baseline variability. Successful intrauterine resuscitation requires maternal PaO_2 increase to 100 to 300 mm Hg. This is best accomplished by hyperoxygenation with 100% oxygen delivered by a tight fitting face mask at a flow rate of 8 to 10 liters per minute. The FHR pattern should improve in 1 to 9 minutes. If the fetus recovers, oxygen is usually discontinued. Scalp pH sampling, scalp stimulation, or acoustic stimulation may be used to evaluate fetal well-being following intrauterine resuscitative measures. If the cord prolapses, interventions such as digital decompression and bladder inflation may be helpful in preventing fetal anoxia. Tocolytics may also be given and are best used with hyperoxygenation.

References

1. Persianinov, L. S. (1973). The effect of normal and abnormal labour on the foetus. A survey. Acta et Obstetricia Gynecologica Scandinavica, 52(1), 29-36.

2. Freeman, J. M. (Ed.). (April 1985). Prenatal and perinatal factors associated with brain disorders. NIH Publication No. 85-1149, 240-250, 288-299.

3. van Geijn, H. P., Copray, F. J. A., Donkers, D. K., & Bos, M. H. (December 1991). Diagnosis and management of intrapartum fetal distress. European Journal of Obstetrics, Gynecology and Reproductive Biology, 42(Suppl.), s63-s72.

4. Trudinger, B. J., Mori, A., & Reed, V. (January 1995). Central venous pressure and flow waveforms of the human fetus in normal and complicated pregnancy. American Journal of Obstetrics and Gynecology, 172(1, Pt. 2), 356. SPO abstracts #349.

5. Divon, M. Y. (January 1996). Umbilical artery doppler velocimetry: Clinical utility in high-risk pregnancies [Clinical Opinion]. American Journal of Obstetrics and Gynecology, 174(1, Pt. 1), 10-14.

6. Alfirevic, Z., & Neilson, J. P. (May 1995). Doppler ultrasonography in high-risk pregnancies: Systematic review with meta-analysis. American Journal of Obstetrics and Gynecology, 172(5), 1379-1387.

7. Uerpairojkit, B., Chan, L., Ludomirski, A., Copel, J. A., Martinez, E., & Reece, E. A. (January 1996). Cerebellar doppler velocimetry in the appropriate and small-for-gestational-age fetus. American Journal of Obstetrics and Gynecology, 174(1, Pt. 2), 460. SPO abstracts #555.

8. Khandelwal, M., Rasanen, J., Ludormirski, A., Addonizio, P., & Reece, E. A. (January 1996). Fetal and uterine hemodynamics during and after maternal cardiopulmonary bypass (CPB). American Journal of Obstetrics and Gynecology, 174(1, Pt. 2), 460. SPO abstracts #554.

9. Hecher, K., Snijders, R., Campbell, S., & Nicolaides, K. (July 1995). Fetal venous, intracardiac, and arterial blood flow measurements in intrauterine growth retardation: Relationship with fetal blood gases [General Obstetrics & Gynecology. Fetus-Placenta-Newborn]. American Journal of Obstetrics and Gynecology, 173(1), 10-15.

10. Yoneyama, Y., Sawa, R., Suzuki, S., Shin, S., Power, G. G., & Araki, T. (January 1996). The relationship between uterine artery doppler velocimetry and umbilical venous adenosine levels in pregnancies complicated by preeclampsia. American Journal of Obstetrics and Gynecology, 174(1, Pt. 1), 267-271.

11. Mitra, S. C., Venkataseshan, V. S., & Gil, J. (January 1995). Morphometric study of human placental vessels: Relationship with umbilical artery doppler flow. American Journal of Obstetrics and Gynecology, 172(1, Pt. 2), 310. SPO abstracts #179.

12. Challis, D. E., Gill, R. W., & Warren, P. S. (January 1996). The significance of a low umbilical artery resistance index in a high risk population. American Journal of Obstetrics and Gynecology, 174(1, Pt. 2), 459. SPO abstracts #551.

13. Luzi, G., Clerici,G., & Di Renzo, G. C. (January 1996). The significance of cerebral doppler velocimetry in normal and growth retarded fetuses. American Journal of Obstetrics and Gynecology, 174(1, Pt. 2), 424. SPO abstracts #420.

14. Simonazzi, E., Wladimiroff, J. W., & van Eyck, J. (May 1989). Flow velocity waveforms in the fetal internal carotid artery relative to fetal blood gas and acid-base measurements in normal pregnancy. Early Human Development, 19(2), 111-115.

15. Smeltzer, J. S., Dogra, V. S., Walentik, C., Menon, P. A., Cai, H., & Poblete, J. (January 1995). Middle cerebral artery blood flow indices in cocaine-exposed appropriate-for-gestational-age neonates. American Journal of Obstetrics and Gynecology, 172(1, Pt. 2), 367. SPO abstracts #393.

16. Guzman, E., Vintzileos, A., & Martins, M. (January 1995). Relationship between middle cerebral artery velocimetry, computer fetal heart rate assessment and degree of acidemia at birth in intrauterine growth restricted fetuses. American Journal of Obstetrics and Gynecology, 172(1, Pt. 2), 337. SPO abstracts #280.

17. Gonzalez, R., Mari, G., Gomez, R., Mondion, M., Insunza, A., & Rojas, I. (January 1996). Flow velocity waveforms of the jugular vein in the appropriate-for-gestational-age fetus and in the fetus at risk for cardiac failure. American Journal of Obstetrics and Gynecology, 174(1, Pt. 2), 459. SPO abstracts #549.

18. Goldaber, K. G., & Gilstrap, III, L. C. (March 1993). Correlations between obstetric clinical events and umbilical cord blood acid-base and blood gas values. Clinical Obstetrics and Gynecology, 36(1), 47-59.

19. Goncalves, L. F., Romero, R., Silva, M., Ghezzi, F., Soto, A., & Munoz, H. (January 1995). Reverse flow in the ductus venosus: An ominous sign. American Journal of Obstetrics and Gynecology, 172(1, Pt. 2), 266. SPO abstracts #33.

20. Weiner, Z., Farmakides, G., Barnhard, Y., Maulik, D., Bar-Hava, I., & Henderson, C. E. (January 1995). Cardiac function in postterm fetuses: A prospective longitudinal study. American Journal of Obstetrics and Gynecology, 172(1, Pt. 2), 386. SPO abstracts #459.

21. Trudinger, B. J., Mori, A., Challis, D., & Turner, A. (January 1995). The influence of cardiac contractility and afterload on central venous pressure and flow waveforms in fetal lambs. American Journal of Obstetrics and Gynecology, 172(1, Pt. 2), 356. SPO abstracts #350.

22. Mori, A., Trudinger, B., Mori, R., Reed, V., & Takeda, Y. (January 1995). The fetal central venous pressure waveform in normal pregnancy and in umbilical placental insufficiency. American Journal of Obstetrics and Gynecology, 172(1, Pt. 1), 51-57.

23. Guzman, E., Shen-Schwarz, S., Vintzileos, A., Chavez, M., Waldron, R., & Walters, C. (January 1995). Correlation between uterine artery doppler velocimetry and histopathology of decidual blood vessels and placental infarction. American Journal of Obstetrics and Gynecology, 172(1, Pt. 2), 387. SPO abstracts #465.

24. Salafia, C., Divon, M., Minior, V., & Pezzullo, J. (January 1996). Correlation of comprehensive placental pathology with umbilical artery doppler studies in growth-retarded fetuses. American Journal of Obstetrics and Gynecology, 174(1, Pt. 2), 459. SPO abstracts #550.

25. Koons, A., & Sengupta, S. (January 1995). Neurodevelopmental outcome of premature fetuses with reversed end diastolic flow of umbilical artery. American Journal of Obstetrics and Gynecology, 172(1, Pt. 2), 367. SPO abstracts #392.

26. Zelop, C. M., Richardson, D. K., & Heffner, L. J. (January 1995). Management implications and outcome of severe abnormal umbilical artery doppler velocimetry. American Journal of Obstetrics and Gynecology, 172(1, Pt. 2), 387. SPO abstracts #464.

27. Pardi, G., Cetin, I., Marconi, A. M., Franchi, A. L., Bozzetti, P., & Ferrazzi, E. (March 11, 1993). Diagnostic value of blood sampling in fetuses with growth retardation. The New England Journal of Medicine, 328(10), 692-696.

28. Visser, G. H., Bekedam, D. J., & Ribbert, L. S. M. (May 1990). Changes in antepartum heart rate patterns with progressive deterioration of the fetal condition. International Journal of Bio-Medical Computing, 25(4), 239-246.

29. Ribbert, L. S. M., Snijders, R. J. M., Nicolaides, K. H., & Visser, G. H. A. (August 1991). Relation of fetal blood gases and data from computer-assisted analysis of fetal heart rate patterns in small for gestation fetuses. British Journal of Obstetrics and Gynaecology, 98,(8), 820-823.

30. Guzman, E., Vintzileos, A., & Martins, M. (January 1995). Prediction of umbilical artery and vein pH in intrauterine growth restricted fetuses based on fetal and maternal doppler velocimetry and computer fetal heart rate parameters. American Journal of Obstetrics and Gynecology, 172(1, Pt. 2), 269. SPO abstracts #41.

31. Guzman, E., Vintzileos, A., & Martins, M. (January 1995). The efficacy of individual computer fetal heart rate parameters in detecting acidemia at birth in intrauterine growth restricted fetuses. American Journal of Obstetrics and Gynecology, 172(1, Pt. 2), 338. SPO abstracts #281.

32. Dawes, G. S., Rosevear, S. K., Pello, L. C., Moulden, M., & Redman, C. W. G. (September 1991). Computerized analysis of episodic changes in fetal heart rate variation in early labor. American Journal of Obstetrics and Gynecology, 165(3), 618-624.

33. Shalev, E., Dan, U., Yanai, N., & Weiner, E. (1991). Sonography-guided fetal blood sampling for pH and blood gases in premature fetuses with abnormal fetal heart rate tracings. Acta Obstetricia et Gynecologica Scandinavica, 70(7-8), 539-542.

34. Gregg, A. R., & Weiner, C. P. (March 1993). "Normal" umbilical arterial and venous acid-base and blood gas values. Clinical Obstetrics and Gynecology, 36(1), 24-32.

35. Ghidini, A., Sepulveda, W., Lockwood, C. J., & Romero, R. (May 1993). Clinical section. Complications of fetal blood sampling. American Journal of Obstetrics and Gynecology, 168(5), 1339-1344.

36. Leonardi, M. R., Berry, S. M., Wolfe, H. M., Dombrowski, M. P., Lanouette, J. M., & Cotton, D. B. (January 1995). Determination of fetal platelet counts in pregnancies complicated by ITP. American Journal of Obstetrics and Gynecology, 172(1, Pt. 2), 281. SPO abstracts #74.

37. Sciscione, A., Bessos, H., Blakemore, K., Callan, N., & Kickler, T. (January 1995). Assessment of glycocalicin levels in the amniotic fluid and cord blood of the thrombocytopenic fetus. American Journal of Obstetrics and Gynecology, 172(1, Pt. 2), 317. SPO abstracts #197.

38. Khoury, A. D., Moretti, M. L., Barton, J. R., Shaver, D. C., & Sibai, B. M. (October 1991). Fetal blood sampling in patients undergoing elective cesarean section: A correlation with cord blood gas values obtained at delivery. American Journal of Obstetrics and Gynecology, 165(4, Pt. 1), 1026-1029.

39. Hsieh, F-J., Chang, F-M., Ko, T-M., Kuo, P-L., Chang, D-Y., & Chen, H-Y. (November 1989). The antenatal blood gas and acid-base status of normal fetuses and hydropic fetuses with Bart hemoglobinopathy. Obstetrics & Gynecology, 74(5), 722-725.

40. Lazarevic, B., Ljubic, A., Stevic, R., Sulovic, V., Rosic, B., & Radunovic, N. (December 1991). Respiratory gases and acid base parameter of the fetus during the second and third trimester. Clinical and Experimental Obstetrics and Gynecology, 8(2), 81-84.

41. Goodwin, T. M., Milner-Masterson, L., & Paul, R. H. (June 1994). Elimination of fetal scalp blood sampling on a large clinical service. Obstetrics & Gynecology, 83(6), 971-974.

42. Sohmer, H., Geal-Dor, M., & Weinstein, D. (May 1994). Human fetal auditory threshold improvement during maternal oxygen respiration. Hearing Research, 75(1-2), 145-150.

43. Spies Pope, D. (Winter 1995). Music, noise, and the human voice in the nurse-patient environment. IMAGE: Journal of Nursing Scholarship, 27(4), 291-295.

44. Blackburn, S. T., & Loper, D. L. (1992). Maternal, fetal, and neonatal physiology. A clinical perspective. Philadelphia, PA: W. B. Saunders Company.

45. Phelan, J. P. (April 1991). Acoustic stimulation during the third trimester. Contemporary OB/GYN, 36, 87-94.

46. Kofinas, A., Cabbad, M., & Kofinas, G. (January 1995). The effect of vibratory acoustic stimulation on fetal middle cerebral artery resistance and instantaneous fetal heart rate from 20 to 42 weeks gestational age. American Journal of Obstetrics and Gynecology, 172(1, Pt. 2), 322. SPO abstracts #220.

47. Edersheim, T. G., Hutson, J. M., Druzin, M. L., & Kogut, E. A. (December 1987). Fetal heart rate response to vibratory acoustic stimulation predicts fetal pH in labor. <u>American Journal of Obstetrics and Gynecology, 157</u>(6), 1557-1560.

48. Walker, D., Grimwade, J., & Wood, C. (1971). Intra-uterine noise: A component of the fetal environment. <u>American Journal of Obstetrics and Gynecology, 109,</u> 91-95.

49. Henshall, W. R. (1972). Intra-uterine sound levels. <u>American Journal of Obstetrics and Gynecology, 112,</u> 576-578.

50. Murooka, H., Koie, Y., & Suda, N. (1976). Analyse des sons intrauterins et leurs effets tranquillisants sur le nouveau-ne. <u>Journal de Gynecolecologie, Obstetrique et Biologie de la Reproduction, 5</u>(3), 367-376.

51. Querleu, D., Renard, X., & Crepin, G. (1981). Perception auditive et reactivite foetale aux stimulations sonores. <u>Journal de Gynecologie, Obstetrique et Biologie de la Reproduction, 10</u>(4), 307-314.

52. Bench, R. J. (1968). Sound transmission to the human fetus through the maternal abdominal wall. <u>Journal of General Psychology, 113,</u> 85-87.

53. Mariona, F., Kelly, R., Saltmarche, P., Nemec, S., Lipshaw, L., & Lower, S. (January 1993). Long-term effects of fetal vibroacoustic stimulation on infant hearing. <u>American Journal of Obstetrics and Gynecology, 168</u>(1, Pt. 2), 337. SPO abstracts #337.

54. Zimmer, E. Z., & Divon, M. Y. (March 1993). Fetal vibroacoustic stimulation. <u>Obstetrics & Gynecology, 81</u>(3), 451-457.

55. Anyaegbunam, A. M., Ditchik, A., Stoessel, R., & Mikhail, M. S. (June 1994). Vibroacoustic stimulation of the fetus entering the second stage of labor. <u>Obstetrics & Gynecology, 83</u>(6), 963-966.

56. Jensen, O. H. (1984). Fetal heart rate response to controlled sound stimuli during the third trimester of normal pregnancy. <u>Acta Obstetricia et Gynecologica Scandinavica, 63,</u> 193-197.

57. Groome, L. J., Mooney, D. M., Holland, S. B., Bentz, L. S., Atterbury, J. L., & Dykman, R. A. (January 1996). Assessing cognitive processing in the human fetus. <u>American Journal of Obstetrics and Gynecology, 174</u>(1, Pt. 2), 381. SPO abstracts #255.

58. Gerhardt, K. J., Abrams, R. M., Kovaz, B. M., Gomez, K. J., & Conlon, M. (July 1988). Intrauterine noise levels produced in pregnant ewes by sound applied to the abdomen. <u>American Journal of Obstetrics and Gynecology, 159</u>(1), 228-232.

59. Romero, R., Mazor, M., & Hobbins, J. C. (May 1988). A critical appraisal of fetal acoustic stimulation as an antenatal test for fetal well-being. <u>Obstetrics & Gynecology, 71</u>(5), 781-786.

60. Richards, D. S., Cefalo, R. C., Thorpe, J. M., Salley, M., & Rose, D. (April 1988). Determinants of fetal heart rate response to vibroacoustic stimulation in labor. <u>Obstetrics & Gynecology, 71</u>(4), 535-540.

61. Thomas, R. L., Johnson, T. R., Besinger, R. E., Rafkin, D., Treanor, C., & Strobino, D. (July 1989). Preterm and term fetal cardiac and movement responses to vibratory acoustic stimulation. <u>American Journal of Obstetrics and Gynecology, 161</u>(1),141-145.

62. Harvey, C. J. (July 1987). Fetal scalp stimulation: Enhancing the interpretation of fetal monitor tracings. <u>Journal of Perinatal Nursing, 1</u>(1), 13-21.

63. Barton, J. R., & Hiett, A. K. (January 1995). The effect of vibroacoustic stimulation on fetal heart rate parameters utilizing computer analysis. <u>American Journal of Obstetrics and Gynecology, 172</u>(1, Pt. 2), 338. SPO abstracts #282.

64. Visser, G. H., Mulder, H. H., Wit, H. P., Mulder, E. J., & Prechtl, H. F. (July 1989). Vibro-acoustic stimulation of the human fetus: Effect on behavioural state organization. <u>Early Human Development, 19</u>(4), 285-296.

65. Rayburn, W. F. (December 15, 1982). Clinical implications from monitoring fetal activity. <u>American Journal of Obstetrics and Gynecology, 144</u>(8), 967-980.

66. Lewinsky, R. M., & Degani, S. (January 1996). Spectral analysis of heart rate variability gives new insight into fetal autonomic response to vibroacoustic stimulation. <u>American Journal of Obstetrics and Gynecology, 174</u>(1, Pt. 2), 380. SPO abstracts #252.

67. Schucker, J. L., Sarno, A. P., Egerman, R. S., & Sibai, B. M. (January 1996). The effect of butorphanol on the fetal heart rate reactivity during labor. <u>American Journal of Obstetrics and Gynecology, 174</u>(1, Pt. 2), 491. SPO abstracts #672.

68. Rice, P. E., & Benedetti, T. J. (October 1986). Fetal heart rate acceleration with fetal blood sampling. <u>Obstetrics & Gynecology, 68</u>(4), 469-472.

69. Smith, C. V., Nguyen, H. N., Phelan, J. P., & Paul, R. H. (October 1986). Intrapartum assessment of fetal well-being: A comparison of fetal acoustic stimulation with acid-base determinations. <u>American Journal of Obstetrics and Gynecology, 155</u>(4), 726-728.

70. Reddy, U. M., Paine, L. L., Gegor, C. L., Johnson, M. J., & Johnson, T. R. B. (October 1991). Fetal movement during labor. <u>American Journal of Obstetrics and Gynecology, 165</u>(4, Pt. 1), 1073-1076.

71. Clark, S. L., Gimovsky, M. L., & Miller, F. C. (November 15, 1982). Fetal heart rate response to scalp blood sampling. <u>American Journal Obstetrics and Gynecology, 144</u>(6), 706-708.

72. Clark, S. L., Gimovsky, M. L., & Miller, F. C. (February 1, 1984). The scalp stimulation test: A clinical alternative to fetal scalp blood sampling. <u>American Journal of Obstetrics and Gynecology, 148</u>(3), 274-277.

73. Spencer, J. A. D. (1991). Predictive value of a fetal heart rate acceleration at the time of fetal blood sampling in labour. <u>Journal of Perinatal Medicine, 19,</u> 207-215.

74. Zimmer, E. Z., & Vadasz, A. (January 1989). Influence of the fetal scalp electrode stimulation test on fetal heart rate and body movements in quiet and active behavioral states during labor. American Journal of Perinatology, 6(1), 24-29.

75. Cohen, W. R., & Schifrin, B. S. (1983). Clinical management of fetal hypoxemia. In W. R. Cohen, & E. A. Friedman (Eds.). Management of labor (pp. 163-188). Baltimore: University Park Press.

76. Mathews, D. D., & Loeffler, F. E. (March 1968). The effect of abdominal decompression on fetal oxygenation during pregnancy and early labour. Journal of Obstetrics, and Gynaecology of the British Commonwealth, 75(3), 268-270.

77. Hon, E. (1967). Detection of fetal distress. In C. Wood (Ed.). Fifth world congress of gynaecology and obstetrics, Sidney, Australia.

78. Bowen, L. W., Kochenour, N. K., Rehm, N. E., & Woolley, F. R. (April 1986). Maternal-fetal pH difference and fetal scalp pH as predictors of neonatal outcome. Obstetrics & Gynecology, 67(4), 487-495.

79. Clark, S. L., & Paul, R. H. (December 1, 1985). Intrapartum fetal surveillance: The role of fetal scalp blood sampling. American Journal of Obstetrics and Gynecology, 153(7), 717-720.

80. Neutra, R., Greenland, S., & Friedman, E. A. (June 15, 1981). The relationship between electronic fetal monitoring and Apgar score. American Journal Obstetrics and Gynecology, 140(4), 440-445.

81. Cabaniss, M. L. (1993). Fetal monitoring interpretation. Philadelphia, PA: J. B. Lippincott Company.

82. Kubli, F. W., Hon, E. H., Khazin, A. F., & Takemura, H. (August 15, 1969). Observations on heart rate and pH in the human fetus during labor. American Journal of Obstetrics and Gynecology, 104(8), 1190-1206.

83. West, J., Chez, B. F., & Miller, F. C. (1993). Fetal heart rate. In R. A. Knuppel, & J. E. Drukker (Eds.), High risk pregnancy a team approach (pp. 316-336). Philadelphia, PA: W. B. Saunders Company.

84. Bretsher, J. (1966). Felhler and irrtum bei pH anf mikroblutproben des feten. (Mistakes and errors in pH analysis of microscopic blood specimens.) Gynaecologia, 162, 369.

85. Fetal blood sampling. (October 1976). Technical bulletin number 42, 1-3.

86. Bossart, H., Jenkins, H. M. L., van Geijn, H. P., & Sureau, C. (February 1987). Fetal monitoring, present and future. European Journal of Obstetrics, Gynecology and Reproductive Biology, 24(2), 105-121.

87. Phillips, W. D. P., & Towell, M. E. (April 1980). Abnormal fetal heart rate associated with congenital abnormalities. British Journal of Obstetrics and Gynaecology, 87(4), 270-274.

88. Zernickow, K. (1966). Der luftkontakt airfulss anf miroblutproben des feten (Effect of air contact on microscopic blood specimens of the fetus). Gynaecologia, 161, 277.

89. Caring for cocaine's mothers and babies. (October 1989). NAACOG Newsletter, 16(10), 1, 4-6.

90. Arulkumaran, S., Talbert, D., MacLachlan, N., & Rodeck, C. H. (August 1990). The selection of capillary tube diameter for fetal scalp blood sampling. British Journal of Obstetrics and Gynaecology, 97, 744-747.

91. Young, D. C., Popat, R., Luther, E. R., Scott, K. E., & Writer, W. D. (February 1, 1980). Influence of maternal oxygen administration on the term fetus before labor. American Journal of Obstetrics and Gynecology, 136(3), 321-324.

92. Lazebnik, N., Neuman, M. R., Lysikiewicz, A., Dierker, L-R., & Mann, L. I. (July 1992). Response of fetal heart rate to scalp stimulation related to fetal acid-base status. American Journal of Perinatology, 9(4), 228-232.

93. Freeman, R. K., & Garite, T. J. (1981). Fetal heart rate monitoring. Baltimore: Williams and Wilkins.

94. Boesel, R. R., Olson, A. E., & Johnson, J. W. C. (November 1986). Umbilical cord blood studies help assess fetal respiratory status. Comtemporary OB-GYN, 63, 2.

95. Ingemarsson, I., & Arulkumaran, S. (July 1986). Fetal acid-base balance in low-risk patients in labor. American Journal of Obstetrics and Gynecology, 155(1), 66-69.

96. Blechner, J. N., Stenger, V. G., Eitzman, D. V., & Prystowsky, H. (September 1, 1970). Oxygenation of the human fetus and newborn infant during maternal metabolic acidosis. American Journal of Obstetrics and Gynecology, 108(1), 47-55.

97. Cowan, D. B. (August 30, 1980). Intrapartum fetal resuscitation. South African Medical Journal, 58(9), 376-379.

98. Bretscher, J., & Saling, S. (April 1, 1967). pH values in the human fetus during labor. American Journal of Obstetrics and Gynecology, 97(7), 906-911.

99. Mendez-Bauer, C., Arnt, I. C., Gulin, L., Escarcena, L., & Caldeyro-Barcia, R. (1967). Relationship between blood pH and heart rate in the human fetus. American Journal of Obstetrics and Gynecology, 97(4), 530.

100. Sherman, D. J., Arieli, S., Raziel, A., Bukovski, I., & Caspi, E. (January 1994). The effect of sampling technique on measurement of fetal blood pH and gases - an in-vitro system. American Journal of Obstetrics and Gynecology, 170(1, Pt. 2), 391. SPO abstracts #421.

101. Miller, Jr., J. M., Bernard, M., Brown, H. L., St. Pierre, J. J., & Gabert, H. A. (April 1990). Umbilical cord blood gases for term healthy newborns. American Journal of Perinatology, 7(2), 157-159.

102. Johnson, J. W. C., & Riley, W. (March 1993). Cord blood gas studies: A survey. Clinical Obstetrics and Gynecology, 36(1), 99-101.

103. Richards, D. S., & Johnson, J. W. C. (March 1993). The practical implications of cord blood acid-base studies. Clinical Obstetrics and Gynecology, 36(1), 91-97.

104. Chauhan, S. P., Cowan, B. D., Meydrech, E. F., Magann, E. F., Morrison, J. C., & Martin, Jr., J. N. (June 1994). Transactions of the sixty-first annual meeting of the central association of obstetrics and gynecologists. Determination of fetal acidemia at birth from a remote umbilical arterial blood gas analysis. American Journal of Obstetrics and Gynecology, 170(6), 1705-1712.

105. Blackstone, J., & Young, B. K. (March 1993). Umbilical cord blood acid-base values and other descriptors of fetal condition. Clinical Obstetrics and Gynecology, 36(1), 33-46.

106. Johnson, J. W. C., Richards, D. S., & Wagaman, R. A. (March 1990). The case for routine umbilical acid-base studies at delivery. American Journal of Obstetrics and Gynecology, 162(3), 621-625.

107. Goldenberg, R. L., Huddleston, J. F., & Nelson, K. G. (July 15, 1984). Apgar scores and umbilical arterial pH in preterm newborn infants. American Journal of Obstetrics and Gynecology, 149(6), 651-654.

108. Low, J. A. (November 1988). The role of blood gas and acid-base assessment in the diagnosis of intrapartum fetal asphyxia. American Journal of Obstetrics and Gynecology, 159(5), 1235-1240.

109. Boehm, F. H., Fields, L. M., Entman, S. S., & Vaugh, W. K. (April 1986). Correlation of the one-minute Apgar score and umbilical cord acid-base status. Southern Medical Journal, 79(4), 429-431.

110. Riley, R. J., & Johnson, J. W. C. (March 1993). Collecting and analyzing cord blood gases. Clinical Obstetrics and Gynecology, 36(1), 13-23.

111. Kirshon, B., & Moise, Jr., K. J. (April 1989). Effect of heparin on umbilical arterial blood gases. The Journal of Reproductive Medicine, 34(4), 267-269.

112. Eggert, J. V., Weidner, W., Eggert, L. D., Woods, R. E., & Mattern, D. (October 1986). A simplified method of obtaining umbilical cord blood for pH using a heparinized vacutainer versus heparinized syringe. American Journal of Perinatology, 3(4), 311-314.

113. Lievaart, M., & de Jong, P. A. (January 1984). Acid-base equilibrium in umbilical cord blood and time of cord clamping. Obstetrics & Gynecology, 63(1), 44-47.

114. Duerbeck, N. B., Chaffin, D. G., & Seeds, J. W. (June 1992). A practical approach to umbilical artery pH and blood gas determinations. Obstetrics & Gynecology, 79(6), 959-962.

115. Strickland, D. M., Gilstrap, III, L. C., Hauth, J. C., & Widmer, K. (1984). Umbilical cord pH and PCO_2 : Effect of interval from delivery to determination. American Journal Obstetrics and Gynecology, 148(2), 191-194.

116. Benirschke, K. (1990). Placental implantation and development. In R. D. Eden, F. H. Boehm, & M. Haire (Eds). Assessment and care of the fetus. Physiological, clinical, and medicolegal principles. Norwalk, CT: Appleton & Lange.

117. Meyer, B. A., Thorpe, J. A., Cohen, G. R., & Yeast, J. D. (January 1994). Umbilical cord blood gases: The effect of smoking on delayed sampling from the placenta. American Journal of Obstetrics and Gynecology, 170(1, Pt. 2), 320. SPO abstracts #158.

118. Koga, S., Koga, Y., & Nagai, H. (1988). Physiological significance of fetal blood gas changes elicited by different delivery postures. Tohoku Journal of Experimental Medicine, 154(4), 357-363.

119. Yeomans, E. R., Hauth, J. C., Gilstrap, III, L. C., & Strickland, D. M. (March 15, 1985). Umbilical cord pH, PCO_2, and bicarbonate following uncomplicated term vaginal deliveries. American Journal of Obstetrics and Gynecology, 151(6), 798-800.

120. Low, J. A., Panagiotopoulos, C., & Derrick, E. J. (March 1995). Newborn complications after intrapartum asphyxia with metabolic acidosis in the preterm fetus. American Journal of Obstetrics and Gynecology, 172(3), 805-810.

121. Porter, K., Williams, M., O'Brien, W., & Casanova, C. (January 1993). Intrapartum pulse oximetry predicts neonatal depression. American Journal of Obstetrics and Gynecology, 168(1, Pt. 2), SPO abstracts #251.

122. Gaudier, F. L., Goldenberg, R. L., Du Bard, M., Nelson, K. G., & Hauth, J. C. (January 1994). Acid-base status at birth in small for gestational age vs appropriate for gestational age $\leq$ 1,000 grams infants. American Journal of Obstetrics and Gynecology, 170(1, Pt. 2), 309. SPO abstracts #112.

123. Dickenson, J. E., Eriksen, N. L., Meyer, B. A., & Parisi, V. M. (April 1992). The effect of preterm birth on umbilical cord blood gases. Obstetrics & Gynecology, 79(4), 575-578.

124. Ruth, V. J., & Raivio, K. O. (July 2, 1988). Perinatal brain damage: Predictive value of metabolic acidosis and the Apgar score. British Medical Journal, 297, 24-27.

125. Terence, T., Lao, M. B., & Ohlsson, A. (February 1993). Effect of fetal sepsis on umbilical cord blood gases [Letters]. American Journal of Obstetrics and Gynecology, 168(2), 738-739.

126. Assessment of fetal and newborn acid-base status. (April 1989). Technical bulletin number 127, 1-4. Washington, DC: ACOG.

127. Caritis, S. N., Abouleish, E., Edelstone, D. I., & Mueller-Heubach, E. (November 1980). Fetal acid-base state following spinal or epidural anesthesia for cesarean section. Obstetrics & Gynecology, 56(5), 610-615.

128. Borgida, A. F., Eng, F., Egan, J. F. X., Rodis, J. F., Smeltzer, J. S., & Turner, G. W. (January 1996). Umbilical cord gas assessment in high risk twin gestations. American Journal of Obstetrics and Gynecology, 174(1, Pt. 2), 383. SPO abstracts #262.

129. Nordstrom, L., & Arulkumaran, S. (July 1993). Lactate in fetal surveillance. Singapore Journal of Obstetrics and Gynecology, 24(2), 87-98.

130. Nicolaides, K. H., Economides, D. L., & Soothill, P. W. (October 1989). Blood gases, pH, and lactate in appropriate- and small-for-gestational-age fetuses. American Journal Obstetrics and Gynecology, 161(4), 996-1001.

131. Pardi, G., Marconi, A. M., Cetin, I., Baggiani, A. M., Lan Franchi, A., & Bozzetti, P. (1991). Fetal oxygenation and acid base balance during pregnancy. Journal of Perinatal Medicine, 19(Suppl. 1), 139-144.

132. Moll, W., & Kastendieck, E. (1985). Kinetics of lactic acid accumulation and removal in the fetus. In W. Kunzel (Ed.), Fetal heart rate monitoring. Clinical practice and pathophysiology (pp. 161-169). Berlin, Germany: Springer-Verlag.

133. Figueroa, R., Martinez, E., Fayngersh, R. P., Jiang, H., Tejani, N., & Wolin, M. S. (January 1995). Gestational diabetes impairs relaxation of human placental veins to H_2O_2 and lactate. American Journal of Obstetrics and Gynecology, 172(1, Pt. 2), 328. SPO abstracts #244.

134. Westgren, M., Divon, M., Horal, M., Ingemarsson, I., Kublickas, M., & Shimojo, N. (November 1995). Routine measurements of umbilical artery lactate levels in the prediction of perinatal outcome. American Journal of Obstetrics and Gynecology, 173(5), 1416-1422.

135. Deans, A. C., & Steer, P. J. (January 1994). The use of the fetal electrocardiogram in labour. British Journal of Obstetrics and Gynaecology, 101, 9-17.

136. Eguiluz, A., Lopez Bernal, A., McPherson, K., Parrilla, J. J., & Abad, L. (December 15, 1983). The use of intrapartum fetal blood lactate measurements for the early diagnosis of fetal distress. American Journal of Obstetrics and Gynecology, 147(8), 949-954.

137. Nordstrom, L., Ingemarsson, I., Persson, B., Shimojo, N., & Westgren, M. (1994). Lactate in fetal scalp blood and umbilical artery blood measured during normal labor with a test strip method. Acta Obstetricia et Gynecologica Scandinavica, 73, 250-254.

138. Gordon, A., & Johnson, J. W. C. (April 1985). Value of umbilical blood acid-base studies in fetal assessment. Journal of Reproductive Medicine, 30(4), 329-336.

139. McNamara, H., & Johnson, N. (1994). Fetal monitoring by pulse oximetry and CTG. Journal of Perinatal Medicine, 21(6), 475-480.

140. Johnson, N., Gupta, G., Johnson, J., McNamara, H., Montague, I. A., & van Oudgaarden, E. D. (1993). Fetal monitoring in labour with pulse oximetry. In J. A. D. Spencer, & R. H. T. Ward (Eds.), Intrapartum fetal surveillance (pp. 317-328). London, England: Royal College of Obstetricians and Gynaecologists.

141. McNamara, H., Johnson, N., & Lilford, R. (July 7-10, 1992). Monitoring the fetus with a pulse oximeter. The 26th British Congress of Obstetrics and Gynaecology, Manchester, England.

142. Knitza, R., Rall, G., Mainz, S., Kleiner, B., Ko, H. K., & Hepp, H. (September 19-24, 1993). Oxycardiotocography: A new tool in monitoring the fetus during delivery. Presented at the 2nd World Congress of Perinatal Medicine. Rome, Italy.

143. Katz, M. (January 1993). Oxygen saturation (SaO_2) monitoring in the presence of non-reassuring fetal heart rate (FHR) patterns. American Journal of Obstetrics and Gynecology,168,(1), 341.

144. Amano, K., Maeda, M., Kurosu, H., Shimada, N., & Nishijima, M. (April 9-12, 1994). Intrapartum fetal pulse oximetry: Relationship between fetal oxygen saturation and fetal heart rate. Unpublished, submitted for presentation at the Congress of the Japanese Society of Obstetrics and Gynecology, Tokyo, Japan.

145. Amano, K., Maeda, M., Kurosu, H., & Nishijima, M. (September 1994). Oxygen saturation and fetal heart rate patterns. International Journal of Gynecology & Obstetrics, 46(Suppl.), 176.

146. Sato, I., Izumi, A., Tamada, T. (September 19-24, 1993). Continuous fetal monitoring with pulse oximeter during labor (168). The 2nd World Congress of Perinatal Medicine, Rome, Italy.

147. Luttkus, A., Fengler, T. W., Friedmann, W., Nimpsch, R., & Dudenhausen, J. W. (March/April 1994). Fetal oxygen saturation in cases with suspected hypoxia and normal cardiotocogram. Zeitschrift fur Geburtshilfe und Perinatologie, 198(2), 62-66.

148. van den Berg, P., Dildy, G. A., Luttkus, A., Mason, G. C., Harvey, C. J., & Nijhuis, J. G. (March 15-18, 1995). The validity of monitoring fetal arterial oxygen saturation with pulse oximetry during labor. Presented at the annual meeting of the Society for Gynecologic Investigation. Chicago, IL.

149. Dildy, G., Clark, S, Loucks C. (January 1995). Intrapartum fetal pulse oximetry: The effects of variable decelerations on fetal arterial oxygen saturation. American Journal of Obstetrics and Gynecology, 172(1, Pt. 2), 366. SPO abstracts #388.

150. Van Hook, J., Harvey, C., Anderson, G., Shailer, T., & Troyer, L. (January 1995). Increases in human fetal hemoglobin oxygen saturation during late fetal heart rate decelerations as a response to intrauterine stress. American Journal of Obstetrics and Gynecology, 172(1, Pt. 2), 365. SPO abstracts #383.

151. Luttkus, A., Fengler, T. W., & Homm-Luttkus, C. (in press). Correlation of fetal oxygen saturation to fetal heart rate patterns: Evaluation of fetal reflectance pulse oximetry with two different oxisensors.

152. Carbonne, B., Langer, B., Dujardin, P., Audibert, F., Boudier, E., & Segard, L. (June 5-8, 1994). Predictive value of fetal pulse oximetry during labor. 14th European Congress of Perinatal Medicine abstract, 512. Helsinki, Finland.

153. Knitza, R., Rall, G., Mainz, S., Kleiner, B., Ko, H., & Hepp, H. (September 19-24, 1993). Oxycardiotocography: A new tool in monitoring the fetus during delivery (169). The 2nd World Congress of Perinatal Medicine, Rome, Italy.

154. Johnson, N., & Johnson, V. (November 1989). Continuous fetal monitoring with a pulse oximeter: A case of cord compression. American Journal of Obstetrics and Gynecology, 161(5), 1295-1296.

155. Katz, M., Petrick, T., Richichi, K., & Belluomini, J. (January 1993). Oxygen saturation (SaO$_2$) monitoring in the presence of non-reassuring fetal heart rate (FHR) patterns. American Journal of Obstetrics and Gynecology, 168(1, Pt. 2), 341. SPO abstracts #153.

156. Letko, M. D. (June 4-7, 1995). Clinical applications of pulse oximetry in the perinatal environment. Symposium conducted at the AWHONN 1995 convention sessions resources. In tune with the country. Nashville, TN.

157. Kulick, R. M. (June 1987). Pulse oximetry. Pediatric Emergency Care, 3(2), 127-130.

158. Pope, L. L., & Hankins, G. D. V. (1991). Pulse oximetry application in the labor and delivery unit of a tertiary care center. Journal of Reproductive Medicine, 853-856.

159. Shailer, T. L., Harvey, C. J., & Guyer, F. (July/September 1992). Principles of oxygen transport in the critically ill obstetric patient. NAACOG's Clinical Issues in Perinatal and Women's Health Nursing, 3(3), 392-398.

160. Severinghaus, J. W., & Kelleher, J. F. (June 1992). Recent developments in pulse oximetry. Anesthesiology, 76(6), 1018-1038.

161. Johnson, N., Johnson, V. A., Bannister, J., & McNamara, H. (1990). The effect of meconium on neonatal and fetal reflectance pulse oximetry. Journal of Perinatal Medicine, 18, 351-355.

162. Audibert, F., Ville, Y., & Fernandez, H. (March 1995). Reflection pulse oximetry in fetal tachyarrythmia. American Journal of Obstetrics and Gynecology, 172(3), 1068-1069.

163. Dildy, G. A., Loucks, C. A., & Clark, S. L. (December 1993). Intrapartum fetal pulse oximetry in the presence of fetal cardiac arrhythmia. American Journal of Obstetrics and Gynecology, 169(6), 1609-1611.

164. van den Berg, P. P., Nijhuis, J. G., & Jongsma, H. W. (January 1993). Intrapartum fetal surveillance with pulse oximetry in complete fetal heart block (CHB)-a case report. American Journal of Obstetrics and Gynecology, 168(1, Pt. 1), 341. SPO abstracts #152.

165. Harris, A. P., Sendak, M. J., Donham, R. T., Thomas, M., & Duncan, D. (July 1988). Absorption characteristics of human fetal hemoglobin at wavelengths used in pulse oximetry. Journal of Clinical Monitoring, 4(3), 175-177.

166. Glanze, W. D., Anderson, K. N., Anderson, L. E. (Eds.). (1990). Mosby's medical, nursing, and allied health dictionary (3rd. ed.). St. Louis, MO: The C. V. Mosby Company.

167. Arikan, G., Haeusler, M. C. H., Kainer, F., & Haas, J. (January 1996). Visual online signal identification and the accuracy of fetal pulse oximetry in second stage of labour. American Journal of Obstetrics and Gynecology, 174(1, Pt. 2), 491. SPO abstracts #671.

168. Nijland, R., Jongsma, H. W., & Nijhuis, J. G. (January 1995). Reflectance pulse oximetry (RPOX): Two sensors compared in piglets. American Journal of Obstetrics and Gynecology, 172(1, Pt. 2), 365. SPO abstracts #386.

169. Luttkus, A., Friedmann, W., & Dudenhausen, J. W. (January 1996). Fetal pulse oximetry for monitoring deliveries with suspected chorionic amnionitis (CA). American Journal of Obstetrics and Gynecology, 174(1, Pt. 2), 492. SPO abstracts #673.

170. Mannheimer, P. D. Wavelength selection for low saturation pulse oximetry. Unpublished - submitted to IEEE Transactions on Biomedical Engineering. Copy on file at Nellcor.

171. Babcock Grove, P. (Ed.). (1976). Webster's third new international dictionary. Springfield, MA: G. & C. Merriam Company.

172. Technical issues of noninvasive fetal oxygen saturation monitoring using the Nellcor N-400. (1994). Reference Note Perinatal Note Number 1, 1-15.

173. Johnson, N., Johnson, V. A., Bannister, J., & Lilford, R. J. (1991). The accuracy of fetal pulse oximetry in the second stage of labour. Journal of Perinatal Medicine, 19, 297-303.

174. Schmitt, H. J., Schuetz, W. H., Proeschel, P. A., & Jaklin, C. (February 1993). Accuracy of pulse oximetry in children with cyanotic congenital heart disease. Journal of Cardiothoracic and Vascular Anesthesia, 7(1), 61-65.

175. Sardesai, S., Durand, M., McEvoy, C., Johnson, C., & Maarek, J-M. (1996). Pulse oximetry in newborn infants with birth weights of 620 to 4285 grams receiving dopamine and dobutamine. Journal of Perinatology, 16(1), 31-34.

176. Chapman, K. R., Liu, F. L.W., Watson, R. M., & Rebuck, A. S. (1989). Range of accuracy of two wavelength oximetry. Chest, 89(4), 540-542.

177. Knitza, R., Pahl, C., Schaffer, I., Schlamp, K., Mainz, S., & Rall, G. (January 1995). Influence of caput succedaneum and hair on fetal O$_2$-saturation measured by pulse oximetry. American Journal of Obstetrics and Gynecology, 172(1, Pt. 2), 366. SPO abstracts #387.

178. Knitza, R. (September 29, 1994). Oxycardiotocography (OCTG) - Fetal surveillance sub partu by CTG and pulse oximetry. Presentation at XIV FIGO World Congress, Montreal, Canada.

179. Gardosi, J. (September 29, 1994). Fetal pulse oximetry. Presentation at XIV FIGO World Congress, Montreal, Canada.

180. Gardosi, J., Reed, N., Sahota, D., & Vanner, T. (January 1995). A minimally invasive method for electronic fetal heart rate monitoring during labor. American Journal of Obstetrics and Gynecology, 172(1, Pt. 2), 366. SPO abstracts #389.

181. Davies, M. G., Curnow, J., & Greene, K. (March 1995). Fetal pulse oximetry: Skin contact and quality-checking algorithms in modern sensor design [Letters]. American Journal of Obstetrics and Gynecology, 172(3), 1062-1063.

182. Harvey, C. J. (June 26-30, 1994). Fetal pulse oximetry: New concepts in fetal surveillance. Paper presented at the annual meeting session resources. AWHONN 1994, Bridge to the future, Cinicinnati, OH.

183. Technology overview: Reflectance sensors for pulse oximetry. (1992). Nellcor Pulse Oximetry Note No. 7, 1-4.

184. Harris, A. P., Sendak, M. J., Chung, D. C., & Richardson, C. A. (May 1993). Validation of arterial oxygen saturation measurements in utero using pulse oximetry. <u>American Journal of Perinatology, 10</u>(3), 250-254.

185. Schram, C. M. H., & Gardosi, J. O. (April 1994). Artifacts in fetal pulse oximetry: Nonarterial pulsatile signals. <u>American Journal of Obstetrics and Gynecology, 170</u>(4), 1174-1177.

186. McNamara, H., & Johnson, N. Can fetal pulse oximetry predict fetal distress? Unpublished.

187. Johnson, N., Johnson, V. A., Bannister, J., & Lilford, R. J. (June 1990). The effect of caput succedaneum on oxygen saturation measurements. <u>British Journal of Obstetrics and Gynaecology, 97,</u> 493-498.

188. Johnson, N., Barker, M., Kelly, M., McNamara, H., Lilford, R., & Montague, I. (1994). The effect of monitoring the fetus with a pulse oximeter on puerperal morbidity. <u>Journal of Obstetrics and Gynaecology, 14</u>(1), 11-13.

189. Dildy, G. A., Loucks, C. A., & Clark, S. L. (January 1996). Intrapartum fetal pulse oximetry: Puerperal morbidity. <u>American Journal of Obstetrics and Gynecology, 174</u>(1, Pt. 2), 491. SPO abstracts #670.

190. Gardosi, J. O., Damianou, D., & Scram, C. M. H. (April 1994). Artifacts in fetal pulse oximetry: Incomplete sensor-to-skin contact [Basic Science Section]. <u>American Journal of Obstetrics and Gynecology, 170</u>(4), 1169-1173.

191. Nellcor, Inc. (May 11, 1995). <u>Questions and answers about Nellcor's N-400 fetal oxygen saturation monitoring system.</u> Pleasanton, CA: Author.

192. Wimberley, P. D., Siggaard-Andersen, O., & Fogh-Andersen, N. (1990). Accurate measurement of hemoglobin oxygen saturation, and fractions of carboxyhemoglobin and methemoglobin in fetal blood using Radiometer OSM3: Corrections for fetal hemoglobin fraction and pH. <u>Scandinavian Journal of Clincal and Laboratory Investigation, 203</u>(Suppl., 50), 235-239.

193. Anderson, G. D., Harvey, C. J., Van Hook, J., Tabb, T. N., & Shailer, T. L. (January 1994). Fetal pulse oximetry: Technical performance and intrapartum values. <u>American Journal of Obstetrics and Gynecology, 170</u>(1, Pt. 2), 313. SPO abstracts #129.

194. Dildy, G. A., Clark, S. L., & Loucks, C. A. (January 1995). Intrapartum fetal pulse oximetry: The effects of variable decelerations on fetal arterial oxygen saturation. <u>American Journal of Obstetrics and Gynecology, 172</u>(1, Pt. 2), 366. SPO abstracts #388.

195. Thilo, E. H., Anderson, D., Wasserstein, M. L., Schmidt, J., & Luckey, D. (1993). Saturation by pulse oximetry: Comparison of the results obtained by instruments of different brands. <u>Journal of Pediatrics, 122</u>(4), 620-626.

196. Introduction to fetal oxygen saturation monitoring. (1995). Nellcor, Inc.

197. Jongsma, H. W., van den Berg, P. P., Menssen, J. J. M., Nijhuis, J. G. (January 1996). The validity of intrapartum pulse oximetry: A quantitative analysis. <u>American Journal of Obstetrics and Gynecology, 174</u>(1, Pt. 2), 492. SPO abstracts #674.

198. Dildy, G., van den Berg, P., Katz, M., Clark, S. L., Jongsma, H. W., & Nijhuis, J. G. (September 30, 1994). Intrapartum fetal pulse oximetry: Fetal oxygen saturation trends during labor and relation to delivery outcome. <u>American Journal of Obstetrics and Gynecology, 171</u>(3), 679-684.

199. Gardosi, J., & Schram, C. Detection of fetal acidosis with intrapartum pulse oximetry. Unpublished.

200. Peat, S., Booker, M., Lanigan, C., & Ponte, J. (July 23, 1988). Continuous intrapartum measurement of fetal oxygen saturation [Letters]. <u>The Lancet,</u> 213.

201. Seelbach-Gobel, B. (September 19-24, 1993). Reflectance pulse oximetry in fetal surveillance during labor (167). <u>The 2nd World Congress of Perinatal Medicine,</u> Rome, Italy.

202. Goodlin, R. C. (August 1993). Preliminary experience with intrapartum fetal pulse oximetry in humans [Letters]. <u>Obstetrics & Gynecology, 82</u>(2), 314-315.

203. Richardson, B., Carmichael, L., Homan, J., & Patrick, J. (March 15-18, 1989). <u>Cerebral oxidative metabolism in fetal sheep with prolonged, graded hypoxaemia</u> (106). 36th Meeting of the Society for Gynecologic Investigation, San Diego, CA.

204. Oeseburg, B., Biny, E. M., Ringnalda, M., Crevels, J. H. W., Jongsma, P., & Mannheimer, J. (May 1992). Fetal oxygenation in chronic maternal hypoxia: What's critical? In W. Erdmann, & D. F. Bruley (Eds.), <u>Advances in experimental medicine & biology, vol. 317. Oxygen transport to tissue XIV</u> (pp. 499-502). New York, NY: Plenum Press.

205. Nijland, R., Jongsma, H. W., Verbruggen, I. M., Menssen, D. J. M., Nijhuis, J. G., & van den Berg, P. P. (May 16-19, 1993). <u>Is there a different adaptation in fetal lambs to low levels of oxygen saturation?</u> 20th Annual Meeting- The Society for the Study of Fetal Physiology, Plymouth, England.

206. Gilbert, R. D., Lis, L., & Longo, L. D. (October 1985). Temperature effects on oxygen affinity of human fetal blood. <u>Journal of Developmental Physiology, 7</u>(5), 299-304.

207. Peebles, D. M., Edwards, A. D., Wyatt, J. S., Bishop, A. P., Cope, M., & Delpy, D. T. (May 1992). Changes in human fetal cerebral hemoglobin concentration and oxygenation during labor measured by near-infrared spectroscopy. <u>American Journal of Obstetrics and Gynecology, 166</u>(5), 1369-1373.

208. McNamara, H.,& Johnson, N. (September 29, 1994). <u>The effect of uterine contractions on fetal oxygen saturation as measured by fetal pulse oximetry.</u> Presentations given at XIV FIGO World Congress, Montreal, Canada.

209. Van Oodgaarden, E., McNamara, H., & Johnson, N. (March 14-15, 1993). Effect of uterine tachysystole on the fetus. Presented at the meeting of the Blair Bell Research Society. London, England.

210. Johnson, N., van Oudgaarden, E., Montague, I., & McNamara, H. (September 1994). Effect of oxytocin-induced hyperstimulation on fetal oxygen. British Journal of Obstetrics and Gynaecology, 101, 805-807.

211. Dildy, G. A., Clark, S. L., & Loucks, C. A. (January 1994). Intrapartum fetal pulse oximetry: The effects of 40% maternal oxygen administration on fetal arterial oxygen saturation. American Journal of Obstetrics and Gynecology, 170(1, Pt. 2), 392. SPO abstracts #424.

212. McNamara, H., Chung, D. C., Lilford, R., & Johnson, N. (September 1992). Do fetal pulse oximetry readings at delivery correlate with cord blood oxygenation and acidaemia? British Journal of Obstetrics and Gynaecology, 99(9), 735-738.

213. Montague, I., & Johnson, N. (March 14-15, 1993). Comparing the oxygen saturation of the breech with cephalic presentation. Blair Bell Research Society, London, England.

214. Gardosi, J. O., Schram, C. M., & Symonds, E. M. (May 25, 1991). Adaptation of pulse oximetry for fetal monitoring during labour. The Lancet, 337, 1265-1267.

215. McNamara, H., Johnson, N., & Lilford, R. (May 1993). The effect on fetal arteriolar oxygen saturation resulting from giving oxygen to the mother measured by pulse oximetry. British Journal of Obstetrics and Gynaecology, 100(5), 446-449.

216. Dildy, G. A., Clark, S. L., & Loucks, C. A. (October 1994). Intrapartum fetal pulse oximetry: The effects of maternal hyperoxia on fetal arterial oxygen saturation. American Journal of Obstetrics and Gynecology, 171(4), 1120-1124.

217. Anderson, G., Harvey, C., Van Hook, J., Shailer, T., & Troyer, L. (January 1995). The effects of maternally-administered oxygen on human fetal SPO_2 values during labor. American Journal of Obstetrics and Gynecology, 172(1, Pt. 2), 365. SPO abstracts #384.

218. Faris, F., Rolfe, P., Thorniley, M., Wickramasinghe, Y., Houston, R., & Doyle, M. (May/June 1993). Non-invasive optical monitoring of cerebral blood oxygenation in the fetus and newborn: Preliminary investigation. Neonatal Intensive Care, 6(3), 40, 42-43.

219. Small, M. L., Beall, M., Platt, L. D., Dirks, D., & Hochberg, H. (August 1989). Continuous tissue pH monitoring in the term fetus. American Journal of Obstetrics and Gynecology, 161(2), 323-329.

220. Young, B. K., Katz, M., & Klein, S. A. (July 15, 1979). The relationship of heart rate patterns and tissue pH in the human fetus. American Journal of Obstetrics and Gynecology, 134(6), 685-690.

221. Baxi, L. V. (June 1982). Symposium on fetal monitoring. Current status of fetal oxygen monitoring. Clinics in Perinatology, 9(2), 423-431.

222. Schmidt, S., Langner, K., Dudenhausen, J. W., & Saling, E. (1985). Measurement of transcutaneous PCO_2 and PO_2 in the fetus during labor. Archives of Gynecology, 236, 145-151.

223. Schmidt, S., Langner, K., Dudenhausen, J. W., & Saling, E. (1985). Reliability of transcutaneous measurement of oxygen and carbon dioxide partial pressure with a combined PO_2-PCO_2 electrochemical sensor in the fetus during labor. Journal of Perinatal Medicine, 13, 127-133.

224. Antoine, C., Young, B. K., & Silverman, F. (1984). Simultaneous measurement of fetal tissue pH and transcutaneous PO_2 during labor. European Journal of Obstetrics, Gynecology and Reproductive Biology, 17, 69-76.

225. Aarnoudse, J. G., Huisjes, H. J., Gordon, H., Oeseburg, B., & Zijlstra, W. G. (November 1, 1985). Fetal subcutaneous scalp PO_2 and abnormal heart rate during labor. American Journal of Obstetrics and Gynecology, 153(5), 565-566.

226. Sykes, G. S., Molloy, P. M., Wollner, J. C., Burton, P. J., Wolton, B., & Rolfe, P. (December 1, 1984). Continuous, noninvasive measurement of fetal oxygen and carbon dioxide levels in labor by use of mass spectrometry. American Journal of Obstetrics and Gynecology, 150(7), 847-858.

227. Lewinsky, R. M. (September 1994). Cardiac systolic time intervals and other parameters of myocardial contractility as indices of fetal acid-base status. Baillieres Clinical Obstetrics and Gynaecology, 8(3), 663-681.

228. Macaulay, J. H., Randall, N. R., Bond, K., & Steer, P. J. (March 1992). Continuous monitoring of fetal temperature by noninvasive probe and its relationship to maternal temperature fetal heart rate, and cord arterial oxygen and pH. Obstetrics & Gynecology, 79(3), 469-474.

229. van den Berg, P. P., & Heerschap, A. (January 1996). Quantitative aspects of in vivo ^{1}H MR spectroscopy of human fetal brain. American Journal of Obstetrics and Gynecology, 174(1, Pt. 2), 381. SPO abstracts #253.

230. Hadi, H. A., Finley, J., Mallette, J. Q., & Strickland, D. (May 1994). Prenatal diagnosis of cerebellar hemorrhage: Medicolegal implications. American Journal of Obstetrics and Gynecology, 170(5, Pt. 1), 1392-1395.

231. Monteagudo, A., & Timor-Tritsch, I. E. (January 1996). Development of fetal gyri, sulci and fissures: An ultrasonographic study. American Journal of Obstetrics and Gynecology, 174(1, Pt. 2), 417. SPO abstracts #392.

232. Mays, J., Lysikiewicz, A., Bracero, L., Evans, R., & Tejani, N. (January 1995). Transvaginal fetal neurosonography-a feasibility study. American Journal of Obstetrics and Gynecology, 172(1, Pt. 2), 348. SPO abstracts #315.

233. Lysikiewicz, A., Mays, J., Klein, S., Verma, U., & Tejani, N. (January 1995). Transvaginal fetal neurosonography for intrauterine diagnosis of periventricular leukomalacia (PVL) and intraventricular hemorrhage (IVH). American Journal of Obstetrics and Gynecology, 172(1, Pt. 2), 347. SPO abstracts #314.

234. Wilkins, I. A., Kramer, L., Slopis, J., Andres, R., & Crino, J. (January 1995). Magnetic resonance imaging in fetal brain abnormalities. American Journal of Obstetrics and Gynecology, 172(1, Pt. 2), 358. SPO abstracts #355.

235. Cedars, L. A., Chao, C. P., & Merita, S. (January 1995). Fetal cerebral metabolic and behavioral effects of glutamate antagonism with MK-801. American Journal of Obstetrics and Gynecology, 172(1, Pt. 2), 315. SPO abstracts #189.

236. Perry, Jr., K. G., & Morrison, J. C. (April 1990). The diagnosis and management of hemoglobinopathies during pregnancy. Seminars in Perinatology, 14(2), 90-102.

237. Tan, W. K. M., Williams, C. E., Mallard, C. E., & Gluckman, P. D. (February 1994). Monosialoganglioside GM_1 treatment after a hypoxic-ischemic episode reduces the vulnerability of the fetal sheep brain to subsequent injuries. American Journal of Obstetrics and Gynecology, 170(2), 663-670.

238. Jauniaux, E., Jurkovic, D., Gulibis, B., Collins, W. P., Zaidi, J., & Campbell, S. (May 1994). Investigation of the acid-base balance of coelomic and amniotic fluids in early human pregnancy. American Journal of Obstetrics and Gynecology, 170(5, Pt. 1), 1365-1369.

239. Newman, W., Mitchell, P., & Wood, C. (January 1, 1967). Fetal acid-base status II. Relationship between maternal and fetal blood bicarbonate concentrations. American Journal of Obstetrics and Gynecology, 97(1), 52-57.

240. Edelstone, D. I., Peticca, B. B., & Goldblum, L. J. (June 1, 1985). Effects of maternal oxygen administration on fetal oxygenation during reductions in umbilical blood flow in fetal lambs. American Journal of Obstetrics and Gynecology, 152(3), 351-358.

241. Standards for obstetric-gynecologic services (7th ed.). (1989). Washington, DC: The American College of Obstetricians and Gynecologists.

242. Salafia, C. M., Minior, V. K., Lopez-Zeno, J. A., Whittington, S. S., Pezzullo, J. C., & Vintzileos, A. M. (October 1995). Relationship between placental histologic features and umbilical cord blood gases in preterm gestations. American Journal of Obstetrics and Gynecology, 173(4), 1058-1064.

243. Meschia, G. (October 1979). Supply of oxygen to the fetus. Journal of Reproductive Medicine, 23(4), 160-165.

244. Madsen, H. (April 1986). Fetal oxygenation in diabetic pregnancy. Danish Medical Bulletin, 33(2), 64-74.

245. Crino, J. P., Harris, A. P., Parisi, V.M., & Johnson, T. R. B. (May 1993). Effect of rapid intravenous crystalloid infusion on uteroplacental blood flow and placental implantation-site oxygen delivery in the pregnant ewe. American Journal of Obstetrics and Gynecology, 168(5), 1603-1609.

246. Barnett, W. M. (March/April 1989). Umbilical cord prolapse: A true obstetrical emergency. The Journal of Emergency Medicine, 7(2), 149-152.

247. Griese, M. E., & Prickett, S. A. (July/August 1993). Nursing management of umbilical cord prolapse. JOGNN, 22(4), 311-315.

248. Katz, Z., Shoham (Schwartz), Z., Lancet, M., Blickstein, I., Mogilner, B. M., & Zalel, Y. (August 1988). Management of labor with umbilical cord prolapse: A 5-year study. Obstetrics & Gynecology, 72(2), 278-281.

249. Fetal heart rate patterns: Monitoring interpretation, and management (July 1995). Technical bulletin number 207, 1-11. Washington, DC: ACOG.

250. Edelstone, D. I. (July 1984). Fetal compensatory responses to reduced oxygen delivery. Seminars in Perinatology, 8(3), 184-191.

251. Schneider, H. (1991). Placental transport function. Reproductive Fertility Development, 3, 345-353.

252. Gagnon, R., Rundle, H., Johnston, L., & Han, V. K. M. (May 1995). Alterations in fetal and placental deoxyribonucleic acid synthesis rates after chronic fetal placental embolization. American Journal of Obstetrics and Gynecology, 172(5), 1451-1458.

253. Maguire, D. J., Cannell,G. R., & Addison, R. S. (1994). Oxygen supply and placental oxygen metabolism. In P. Vaupel, R. Zander, & D. F. Bruly (Eds.), Oxygen transport to tissue XV (pp. 709-715). New York, NY: Plenum Press.

254. Meschia, G. (April 1985). Safety margin of fetal oxygenation. Journal of Reproductive Medicine, 30(4), 308-311.

255. Evans, W., Capelle, S. C., & Edelstone, D. I. (January 1995). Maternal oxygen transport, hemodynamic and metabolic variables as predictors of fetal acidemia in the unanesthetized pregnant sheep. American Journal of Obstetrics and Gynecology, 172(1, Pt. 2), 315. SPO abstracts #191.

256. Harvey, C., Van Hook, J., & Anderson, G. (January 1995). Pregnancy outcomes of pregnancy-induced hypertension in non-English speaking compared to English speaking hispanic women. American Journal of Obstetrics and Gynecology, 172(1, Pt. 2), 381. SPO abstracts #438.

257. Benito, C. W., Thayer, C. F., Lake, M. F., Knuppel, R. A., & Vintzileos, A. M. (January 1996). The effect of hispanic ethnicity on intrapartum management of labor, delivery and analgesia. American Journal of Obstetrics and Gynecology, 174(1, Pt. 2), 485. SPO abstracts #646.

258. Mackey, M. C., & Lock, S. E. (November/December 1989). Women's expectations of the labor and delivery nurse. JOGNN, 18(6), 505-512.

259. Woolf, H. B. et al (Ed.). (1979). Webster's new collegiate dictionary. Springfield, MA: G. & C. Merriam Company.

260. Olson, J. K. (Winter 1995). Relationships between nurse-expressed empathy, patient-perceived empathy and patient-distress. IMAGE: Journal of Nursing Scholarship, 27(4), 317-321.

261. Weaver, D. F. (March/April 1989). Nurses' views on the meaning of touch in obstetrical nursing practice. JOGNN, 19(2), 157-161.

262. Bernat, S. H., Wooldridge, P. J., Marecki, M., & Snell, L. (July/August 1992). Biofeedback-assisted relaxation to reduce stress in labor. JOGNN, 21(4), 295-303.

263. Ladfors, L., Mattsson, L. A., Eriksson, M., & Fall, O. (January 1996). Warm tub bath during labor in women with prelabor rupture of the membranes after 34 weeks of gestation. American Journal of Obstetrics and Gynecology, 174(1, Pt. 2), 345. SPO abstracts #118.

264. Miller, R. D. (1986). Anesthesia (2nd ed.). New York, NY: Churchill Livingstone.

265. Ostheimer, G. W. (1984). Manual of obstetric anesthesia. New York, NY: Churchill Livingstone.

266. Professional practice manual for the certified registered nurse anesthetist (1993). Park Ridge, IL. American Association of Nurse Anesthetists.

267. Fong, J., Gurewitsch, E., Gomillion, M., Press, R., & Volpe, L. (January 1995). Prevention of maternal hypotension by epidural administration of ephedrine sulfate during lumbar epidural anesthesia for cesarean section. American Journal of Obstetrics and Gynecology, 172(1, Pt. 2), 431. SPO abstracts #439.

268. Datta, S., Ostheimer, G. W., Weiss, J. B., Brown, Jr., W. U., & Alper, M. H. (September 1981). Neonatal effect of prolonged anesthetic induction for cesarean section. Obstetrics & Gynecology, 58(3), 331-335.

269. McGrath, J. M., Chestnut, D. H., Vincent, R. D., DeBruyn, C. S., Atkins, B. L., & Poduska, D. J. (May 1994). Ephedrine remains the vasopressor of choice for treatment of hypotension during ritodrine infusion and epidural anesthesia. Anesthesiology, 80(5), 1073-1081.

270. Binder, N. D., & Laird, M. R. (February 1994). Changes in total uterine blood flow do not always reflect changes in maternal placental blood flow [Letters]. American Journal of Obstetrics and Gynecology, 170(2), 701-702.

271. Kitanaka, T., Alonso, J. G., Gilbert, R. D., Siu, B. L., Clemons, G. K., & Long, L. D. (June 1989). Fetal responses to long-term hypoxemia in sheep. American Journal of Physiology, 256(6, Pt. 2), R1348-R1354.

272. Bader, A. M., Datta, S., Arthur, G. R., Benvenuti, E., Courtney, M., & Hauch, M. (April 1990). Maternal and fetal catecholamines and uterine incision-to-delivery interval during elective cesarean. Obstetrics & Gynecology, 75(4), 600-606.

273. Barnhard, Y., Bar-Hava, I., Weiner, Z., & Divon, M. Y. (January 1995). Is oligohydramnios in postdates gestation a function of fetal weight? American Journal of Obstetrics and Gynecology, 172(1, Pt. 2), 294. SPO abstracts #113.

274. Elliott, J., Gilpin, B., & Strong, T. (January 1995). Chronic abruption oligohydramnios sequence (CAOS) a complication of abruptio placentae. American Journal of Obstetrics and Gynecology, 172(1, Pt. 2), 294. SPO abstracts #116.

275. Kerr, J., Borgida, A. F., Hardardottir, H., Calhoun, S., Galetta, J., & Egan, J. F. X. (January 1996). Maternal hydration and its effect on the amniotic fluid index. American Journal of Obstetrics and Gynecology, 174(1, Pt. 2), 416. SPO abstracts #385.

276. Flack, N. J., Sepulveda, W., Bower, S., & Fisk, N. M. (October 1995). Acute maternal hydration in third-trimester oligohydramnios: Effects on amniotic fluid volume, uteroplacental perfusion, and fetal blood flow and urine output. American Journal of Obstetrics and Gynecology, 173(4), 1186-1191.

277. Seeds, A. E. (November 1, 1981). Current concepts in amniotic fluid dynamics [Current Developments]. American Journal of Obstetrics and Gynecology, 138(5), 575-586.

278. Ross, M. G., Cedars, L. A., & Nijland, M. J. M. (January 1995). Treatment of human oligohydramnios with maternal dDAVP-induced plasma hypo-osmolality. American Journal of Obstetrics and Gynecology, 172(1, Pt. 2), 427. SPO abstracts #614.

279. Kilpatrick, S. J., Safford, K. L., Pomeroy, T., Hoedt, L., Scheerer, L., & Laros, R. K. (December 1991). Maternal hydration increases amniotic fluid index. Obstetrics & Gynecology, 78(6), 1098-1102.

280. Bush, J., Minkoff, H., McCalla, S., Moy, S., & Chung, H. (January 1996). The effect of intravenous fluid load on amniotic fluid index in patients with oligohydramnios. American Journal of Obstetrics and Gynecology, 174(1, Pt. 2), 380. SPO abstracts #249.

281. Burke, M. E. (October 1989). Hypertensive crisis and the perinatal period. Journal of Perinatal and Neonatal Nursing, 3(2), 33-47.

282. Jovanovic, L., & Peterson, C. M. (October 1983). Insulin and glucose requirements during the first stage of labor in insulin-dependent diabetic women. The American Journal of Medicine, 75, 607-612.

283. Turner, E. S., Greenberger, P. A., & Patterson, R. (December 1980). Management of the pregnant asthmatic patient. Annals of Internal Medicine, 93(6), 905-918.

284. Bocking, A., Adamson, L., Cousin, A., Campbell, K., Carmichael, L., & Natale, R. (March 15, 1982). Effects of intravenous glucose injections on human fetal breathing movements and gross fetal body movements at 38 to 40 weeks' gestational age. American Journal of Obstetrics and Gynecology, 142(6, Pt. 1), 606-611.

285. Dahlenburg, G. W., Burnell, R. H., & Braybrook, R. (June 1980). The relation between cord serum sodium levels in newborn infants and maternal intravenous therapy during labour. British Journal of Obstetrics and Gynaecology, 87(6), 519-522.

286. Boyle, J., Iams, J., & Gabbe, S. (January 1996). Maternal hydration in patients with preterm premature rupture of membranes. American Journal of Obstetrics and Gynecology, 174(1, Pt. 2), 464. SPO abstracts #562.

287. Yancey, M. K., & Harlass, F. E. (March 1993). Extraneous factors and their influences on fetal acid-base status. Clinical Obstetrics and Gynecology, 36(1), 60-72.

288. Carmen, S. (July/August 1986). Neonatal hypoglycemia in response to maternal glucose infusion before delivery. JOGNN, 15(4), 319-323.

289. Kenepp, N. B., Shelley, W. C., Gabbe, S. G., Kumar, S., Stanley, C. A., & Gutsche, B. B. (May 22, 1982). Fetal and neonatal hazards of maternal hydration with 5% dextrose before cesarean section. The Lancet, 1(8282), 1150-1152.

290. Grylack, L., Chu, S. S., & Scanlon, J. W. (May 1984). Use of intravenous fluids before cesarean section: Effects on perinatal glucose, insulin, & sodium homeostasis. Obstetrics & Gynecology, 63(5), 654-658.

291. Grylack, M. J., & Scanlon, J. W. (January 1982). Effects of intrapartum maternal glucose infusion on the normal fetus and newborn. Anesthesia Analgesia, 61(1), 32-35.

292. Arias, F. (May 1978). Intrauterine resuscitation with terbutaline: A method for the management of acute intrapartum fetal distress. American Journal of Obstetrics and Gynecology, 131(1), 39-43.

293. Patriarco, M. S., Viechnicki, B. M., Hutchinson, T. A., Klasko, S. K., & Yeh, S-Y. (August 1987). A study on intrauterine fetal resuscitation with terbutaline. American Journal of Obstetrics and Gynecology, 157(2), 384-387.

294. Maresh, M. (November 1987). Management of the second stage of labour. Midwife, Health Visitor & Community Nurse, 23(11), 498, 502-506.

295. Parer, J. T., Court, D. J., Block, B. S. B., & Llanos, A. J. (1984). Review. Variability of basal oxygenation of the fetus-causes and associations. European Journal of Obstetrics, Gynecology and Reproductive Biology, 18, 1-9.

296. Mandelbrot, L., Dommergues, M., Aubry, M-C., Mussat, P., & Dumez, Y. (November 1992). Reversal of fetal distress by emergency in utero decompression of hydrothorax. American Journal of Obstetrics and Gynecology, 167(5), 1278-1283.

297. Ingemarsson, I., Arulkumaran, S., & Ratnam, S. S. (December 15, 1985). Single injection of terbutaline in term labor. I. Effect on fetal pH in cases with prolonged bradycardia. American Journal of Obstetrics and Gynecology, 153(8), 859-864.

298. Hidaka, A., Komatani, M., Ikeda, H., Kitanaka, T., Okada, K., & Sugawa, T. (1987). A comparative study of intrauterine fetal resuscitation by β-stimulant and O_2 inhalation. Asia-Oceania Journal of Obstetrics and Gynaecology, 13(2), 195-200.

299. Scardo, J. A., Hogg, B. B., & Newman, R. B. (October 1995). Favorable hemodynamic effects of magnesium sulfate in preeclampsia. American Journal of Obstetrics and Gynecology, 173(4), 1249-1253.

300. Collins, P. L., Zink, E., Moore, R. M., Roberts, J. M., Maguire, M. E., & Moore, J. J. (January 1993). Ritodrine: β-adrenergic receptor antagonist in human amnion. American Journal of Obstetrics and Gynecology, 168(1, Pt. 1), 143-151.

301. Sala, D. J., & Moise, Jr., K. J. (March/April 1990). The treatment of preterm labor using a portable subcutaneous terbutaline pump. JOGNN, 19(2), 108-115.

302. Shortridge, L. A. (January/February 1983). Using ritodrine hydrochloride to inhibit preterm labor. MCN, 8, 58-61.

303. Milner, R. D. G., & De Gasparo, M. (1981). The autonomic nervous system and perinatal metabolism (291-309). The development of the autonomic nervous system. CIBA Foundation Symposium, 83. Pitman Medical, London.

304. Sipes, S. Z., & Weiner, C. P. (April 1990). Venous thromboembolic disease in pregnancy. Seminars in Perinatology, 14(2), 103-118.

305. Schneider, H., Strang, F., Huch, R., & Huch, A. (August 1980). Suppression of uterine contractions with fenoterol and its effect on fetal $tcPO_2$ in human term labour. British Journal of Obstetrics and Gynaecology, 87(8), 657-665.

306. Daddario, J. (June 4-7, 1995). Intrauterine resuscitation. In tune with the country. AWHONN 1995 convention session resources (p. 46). Nashville, TN.

307. Roberts, J. E. (November/December 1989). Managing fetal bradycardia during second stage of labor. The American Journal of Maternal Child Nursing, 14, 394-398.

308. Reece, E. A., Chervenak, F.A., Romero, R., & Hobbins, J. C. (1984). Magnesium sulfate in the management of acute intrapartum fetal distress. American Journal of Obstetrics and Gynecology, 148(1), 104-107.

309. Valenzuela, G. J., & Foster, T, C-S. (May 1990). Use of magnesium sulfate to treat hyperstimulation in term labor. Obstetrics & Gynecology, 75(5), 762-764.

310. Williams, K., & Wilson, S. (January 1996). The effect of labour on maternal cerebral blood flow hemodynamics. American Journal of Obstetrics and Gynecology, 174(1, Pt. 2), 484. SPO abstracts #643.

311. Novy, M. J., Thomas, C. L., & Lees, M. H. (June 15, 1975). Uterine contractility and regional blood flow responses to oxytocin and prostaglandin E_2 in pregnant rhesus monkeys. American Journal of Obstetrics and Gynecology, 122(4), 419-433.

312. Paine, L. L., & Tinker, D. D. (January/February 1992). The effect of maternal bearing-down efforts on arterial umbilical cord pH and length of the second stage of labor. Journal of Nurse-Midwifery, 37(1), 61-63.

313. Bartnicki, J., & Saling, E. (May 1994). The influence of maternal oxygen administration on the fetus. International Federation of Gynecology and Obstetrics, 45, 87-95.

314. Lumley, J., & Wood, C. (1974). Effect of changes in maternal oxygen and carbon dioxide tensions on the fetus. Clinical Anesthesia, 10(2), 121-137.

315. Newman, W., Mc Kinnon, L., Phillips, L., Paterson, P., & Wood, C. (September 1, 1967). Oxygen transfer from mother to fetus during labor. American Journal of Obstetrics and Gynecology, 99(1), 61-70.

316. McCarthy, A. L., Woolfson, R. G., Evans, B. J., Davies, D. R., Raju, S. K., & Poston, L. (March 1994). Functional characteristics of small placental arteries. American Journal of Obstetrics and Gynecology, 170(3), 945-951.

317. Shellhaas, C., Coffman, T., Killam, A., & Kay, H. (January 1995). Effects of different oxygen tensions on placental eicosanoid secretion. American Journal of Obstetrics and Gynecology, 172(1, Pt. 2), 309. SPO abstracts #176.

318. Tervila, L., Vartiainen, E., Finnila, M-J., Kivalo, I., & Vayrynen, M. (1971). The effect of variations in the oxygen content of maternal blood on the perfusion of the uterus and on the oxygen and astrup values of the fetus. Acta Obstetricia et Gynecologica Scandinavica, 9(Suppl. 9), 73.

319. Breathnach, C. S. (July 1991). The stability of the fetal oxygen environment. Irish Journal of Medical Science, 160(7), 189-191.

320. Aldrich, C. J., Wyatt, J. S., Spencer, J. A., Reynolds, E. O., & Delpy, D. T. (June 1994). The effect of maternal oxygen administration on human fetal cerebral oxygenation measured during labour by near infrared spectroscopy. British Journal of Obstetrics and Gynaecology, 101(6), 509-513.

321. Aldrich, C. J., D'Antona, D., Wyatt, J. S., Spencer, J. A. D., Peebles, D. M., & Reynolds, E. O. R. (November 1994). Fetal cerebral oxygenation measured by near-infrared spectroscopy shortly before birth and acid-base status at birth. Obstetrics & Gynecology, 84(5), 861-866.

322. Willcourt, R. J., King, J. C., & Queenan, J. T. (July 15, 1983). Maternal oxygenation administration and the fetal transcutaneous PO_2. American Journal of Obstetrics and Gynecology, 146(6), 714-715.

323. Morishima, H. O., Daniel, S. S., Richards, R. T., & James, L. S. (October 1, 1975). The effect of increased maternal PaO_2 upon the fetus during labor. American Journal of Obstetrics and Gynecology, 123(3), 257-264.

324. Perreault, C., Blaise, G. A., & Meloche, R. (May 1990). Another look at maternal inspired oxygen concentration during cesarean section. Canadian Journal of Anaesthesia, 37(4, Pt. 2), S118.

325. Perreault, C., Blaise, G.A., & Meloche, R. (February 1992). Maternal inspired oxygen concentration and fetal oxygenation during caesarean section. Canadian Journal of Anaesthesia, 39(2), 155-157.

326. Piggott, S. E., Bogod, D. G., Rosen, M., Rees, G. A., & Harmer, M. (September 1990). Isoflurane with either 100% oxygen or 50% nitrous oxide in oxygen for caesarean section. British Journal of Anaesthesia, 65(3), 325-329.

327. Ramanathan, S., Gandhi, S., Arismendy, J., Chalon, J., & Turndorf, H. (July 1982). Oxygen transfer from mother to fetus during cesarean section under epidural anesthesia. Anesthesia & Analgesia, 61(7), 576-581.

328. Young, D. C., Gray, T. H., Luther, E. R., & Peddle, L. T. (February 1, 1980). Fetal scalp blood pH sampling: Its value in an active obstetric unit. American Journal of Obstetrics and Gynecology, 136(3), 276-281.

329. Arduini, D., Rizzo, G., Romanini, C., & Mancuso, S. (April 1989). Hemodynamic changes in growth retarded fetuses during maternal oxygen administration as predictors of fetal outcome. Journal of Ultrasound in Medicine, 8(4), 193-196.

330. Battaglia, C., Artini, P. G., D'Ambrogio, G., Galli, P. A., Segre, A., & Genazzani, A. R. (August 1992). Maternal hyperoxygenation in the treatment of intrauterine growth retardation. American Journal of Obstetrics and Gynecology, 167(2), 430-435.

331. Bekedam, D. J., Mulder, E. J., Snijders, R. J., & Visser, G. H. (December 1991). The effects of maternal hyperoxia on fetal breathing movements, body movements and heart rate variation in growth retarded fetuses. Early Human Development, 27(3), 223-232.

332. Dornan, J. C., & Ritchie, J. W. (March 1983). Fetal breathing movements and maternal hyperoxia in the growth retarded fetus. British Journal of Obstetrics & Gynaecology, 90(3), 210-213.

333. Gagnon, R., Hunse, C., & Vijan, S. (December 1990). The effect of maternal hyperoxia on behavioral activity in growth-retarded human fetuses. American Journal of Obstetrics and Gynecology, 163(6, Pt. 1), 1894-1899.

334. Nicolaides, K. H., Campbell, S., Bradley, R. J., Bilardo, C. M., Soothill, P. W., & Gibb, D. (April 25, 1987). Maternal oxygen therapy for intrauterine growth retardation. The Lancet, 1(8539), 942-945.

335. Rizzo, G., Arduini, D., Romanini, C., & Mancuso, S. (1990). Effects of maternal hyperoxygenation on atrioventricular velocity waveforms in healthy and growth-retarded fetuses. Biology of the Neonate, 58(3), 127-132.

336. Ruedrich, D. A., Devoe, L. D., & Searle, N. (July 1989). Effects of maternal hyperoxia on the biophysical assessment of fetuses with suspected intrauterine growth retardation. American Journal of Obstetrics and Gynecology, 161(1), 188-192.

337. Jackson, B. T., & Piasecki, G. J. (1983). Fetal oxygenation. In W. R. Cohen, & E. A. Friedman (Eds.). Management of labor (pp. 117-142). Baltimore: University Park Press.

338. Gare, D. J., Shime, J., Paul, W. M., & Hoskins, M. (November 15, 1969). Oxygen administration during labor. American Journal of Obstetrics and Gynecology, 105(6), 954-961.

339. Paulick, R. P., Meyers, R. L., & Rudolph, A. M. (July 1992). Effect of maternal oxygen administration on fetal oxygenation during graded reduction of umbilical or uterine blood flow in fetal sheep. American Journal of Obstetrics & Gynecology, 167(1), 233-239.

340. Bartnicki, J., Langner, K., Harnack, H., & Meyenburg, M. (1990). The influence of oxygen administration to the mother during labor on the fetal transcutaneously measured carbon-dioxide partial pressure. Journal of Perinatal Medicine, 18(5), 397-402.

341. Fall, O., Ek, B., Nilsson, B. A., & Rooth, G. (1979). Time factor in oxygen transfer from mother to fetus. Gynecologic and Obstetric Investigation, 10(5), 231-236.

342. Ritchie, J. W., & Lakhani, K. (December 1980). Fetal breathing movements and maternal hyperoxia. British Journal of Obstetrics and Gynaecology, 87(12), 1084-1086.

343. Fruchter, O. (December 1993). Does maternal hyperoxygenation result in fetal oxygenation? <u>American Journal of Obstetrics and Gynecology,</u> <u>169</u>(6), 1657-1658.

344. Jones, H. A., Turner, S. I., & Hughes, J. M. B. (June 30, 1984). Performance of the large-reservoir oxygen mask (ventimask). <u>The Lancet,</u> <u>1</u>(8392), 1427-1431.

345. Wexler, H. R., Aberman, A., Scott, A. A., & Cooper, J. D. (July 1975). Measurement of intratracheal oxygen concentrations during face mask administration of oxygen: A modification for improved control. <u>Canadian Anesthesia Society Journal, 22</u>(4), 417-431.

346. Thorpe, J. A., Trobough, T., Evans, R., Hedrick, J., & Yeast, J. D. (February 1995). The effect of maternal oxygen administration during the second stage of labor on umbilical cord blood gas values: A randomized controlled prospective trial. <u>American Journal of Obstetrics and</u> <u>Gynecology, 172</u>(1, Pt. 2), 465-474.

347. Gaffney, G., Sellers, S., Flavell, V., Squier, M., & Johnson, A. (March 19, 1994). Case-control study of intrapartum care, cerebral palsy, and perinatal death. <u>British Medical Journal, 308,</u> 743-750.

348. Rorke, M. J., Davey, D. A., & Du Toit, H. J. (October 1968). Foetal oxygenation during caesarean section. <u>Anaesthesia, 23</u>(4), 585-596.

349. Marx, G. F., & Mateo, C. V. (November 1971). Effects of different oxygen concentrations during general anaesthesia for elective caesarean section. <u>Canadian Anaesthetists Society Journal, 18</u>(6), 587-593.

350. Baraka, A. (May 1970). Correlation between maternal and foetal PO_2 during caesarean section. <u>British Journal of Anaesthesia, 42</u>(5), 434-438.

351. Newman, W., Braid, D., & Wood, C. (January 1, 1967). Fetal acid-base status. I. Relationship between maternal and fetal PCO_2. <u>American</u> <u>Journal of Obstetrics and Gynecology, 97</u>(1), 43-51.

352. Mathewson, M. (September/October 1983). A nasal cannula guarantees a low oxygen concentration to the patient. <u>Critical Care Nurse,</u> 30.

353. Crosby, E. T., & Halpern, S. H. (April 1992). Supplement maternal oxygen therapy during caesarean section under epidural anaesthesia: A comparison of nasal prongs and face mask. <u>Canadian Journal of Anaesthesia, 39</u>(4), 313-316.

354. Adams, T. J., & Douglas, J. (September 1995). Maternal oxygen administration and fetal well-being [Letters]. <u>American Journal of Obstetrics</u> <u>and Gynecology, 173</u>(3, Pt. 1), 974.

355. Robinson, C. A., & Malee, M. P. (January 1995). Fetal pH - effect of time interval from skin incision to delivery: Under regional anesthesia. <u>American Journal of Obstetrics and Gynecology, 172</u>(1, Pt. 2), 362. SPO abstracts #372.

356. Smith, J. H., Anand, K. J. S., Cotes, P. M., Dawes, G. S., Harkness, R. A., & Howlett, T. A. (October 1988). Antenatal fetal heart rate variation in relation to the respiratory and metabolic status of the compromised human fetus. <u>British Journal of Obstetrics and Gynaecology, 95,</u> 980-989.

357. Isranguranaayudhya, N., & Herabutya, Y. (1988). Prolapse of the umbilical cord: A 5 year review in Ramathibodi hospital. <u>Journal of the</u> <u>Medical Association of Thailand, 71</u>(Suppl. 2), 21-25.

358. Koonings, P. P., Paul, R. H., & Campbell, K. (July 1990). Umbilical cord prolapse. A contemporary look. <u>Journal of Reproductive Medicine,</u> <u>35</u>(7), 690-692.

359. Critchlow, C. W., Leet, T. L., Benedetti, T. J., & Daling, J. R. (February 1994). Risk factors and infant outcomes associated with umbilical cord prolapse: A population-based case-control study among births in Washington State. <u>American Journal of Obstetrics and Gynecology, 170</u>(2), 613-618.

360. Tchabo, J. G. (January/March 1988). The use of the contact hysteroscope in the diagnosis of cord prolapse. <u>International Surgery, 73</u>(1), 57-58.

361. Brown, Jr., R. D., Trupin, S. R., & Brown, M. L. (June 1991). Umbilical cord prolapse: A contemporary look [Letter]. <u>The Journal of</u> <u>Reproductive Medicine, 36</u>(6), 13-14.

362. Nandi, A. K., Saha, S., Sinha, S., & Dutta, S. (August 1988). Cord prolapse: A challenge to the obstetrician. <u>Journal of the Indian Medical</u> <u>Association, 86</u>(8), 206-208.

363. Jacobsen, T., & Madsen, H. (1990). Case report. Unexpected survival after conservative management of cord prolapse in two very preterm babies. <u>Acta Obstetricia et Gynecologica Scandinavica, 69</u>(7-8), 663-664.

364. Barrett, J. M. (September 1991). Funic reduction for the management of umbilical cord prolapse. <u>American Journal of Obstetrics and</u> <u>Gynecology, 165</u>(3), 654-657.

365. Malinowski, J. S., Pedigo, C.G., & Phillips, C. R. (1983). <u>Nursing care during the labor process</u> (3rd ed.). Philadelphia, PA: F. A. Davis Company.

366. Anderson, Jr., G. V., & Anderson, Sr., G. V. (March/April 1989). Umbilical cord prolapse in the emergency department [Editorial]. <u>Journal of</u> <u>Emergency Medicine, 7</u>(2), 207.

367. Vago, T. (May 1994). The management of prolapse of the umbilical cord. <u>American Journal of Obstetrics and Gynecology, 170</u>(5, Pt. 1), 1476-1479.

Notes

Variations of the Fetal Heart Rate

INTRODUCTION

This chapter presents normal and abnormal cardiac electromechanical physiology and changes in the fetal heart rate in response to maternal and fetal conditions, medications, and actions. Since a fetal electrocardiogram is rarely available in the antepartal or intrapartal setting, fetal arrhythmias can only be suspected due to an auscultated irregular fetal heart rate (FHR), or a stable FHR above 180 beats per minute (bpm) or below 90 bpm (1). Knowledge of the effect of conditions, actions, and medications on the FHR may prevent inappropriate antenatal tests or operative delivery.

CARDIAC PHYSIOLOGY

The fetal cardiac conduction system is "functionally mature" at 16 weeks gestation (2-3). Electrical cells, not mechanical cells, of the myocardium are responsible for impulse formation. Electrical cells discharge spontaneous rhythmic impulses (automaticity), react and respond to an electrical impulse (excitability), and transmit impulses serially (conductivity) (4). A change in automaticity, excitability, or conductivity causes a disturbance in the normal conduction of the electrical impulse. An arrhythmia occurs in response to a disturbance in conduction which may have no precipitating cause or may be due to such factors as an electrolyte imbalance, infection and myocarditis, or a heart defect (5). The fetal electrocardiogram (FECG) or a sophisticated ultrasound (echocardiology) are required to diagnose the arrhythmia.

The electrical conduction path in the heart includes the:
1. Sinoatrial (SA) or sinus node
2. Internodal tracts

3. Atrioventricular (AV) node
4. Bundle branch system
5. Purkinje system
6. Ventricular myocardium.

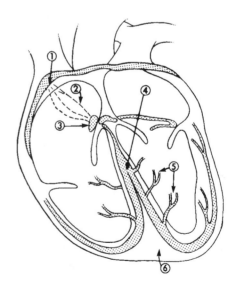

Figure 8.1: Electrical conduction components of the human heart. The sinus node (1) is discernible by the 6th week of gestation. The AV node (3) is discernible by the 10th week. The SA nodal impulse travels via internodal tracts (2) to the AV node, to the His bundle or bundle branch system (4) to the Purkinje fibers (5) and then the ventricles (6) contract. The total system of cardiac conduction is functionally mature by the 16th week of gestation.

Electrical events that cause the heart to beat include depolarization and repolarization. *Depolarization* causes the cardiac cell membrane to become electrically stimulated to form an impulse. When electrical cells depolarize, the difference between sodium and potassium within the cells decreases. *Repolarization* occurs when the cell returns to its resting state. The *refractory period* is the time between depolarization and repolarization.

The SA Node

The normal electrical impulse originates in the SA node, the pacemaker of the heart. The SA node spontaneously depolarizes (6). Potassium (K^+) inhibits SA node function. Acetylcholine, secreted by vagal nerves, increases SA node membrane conductance of K^+ which decreases the duration of the action potential or impulse created by the SA node. Atrial membrane repolarization is accelerated, which slows the FHR (7).

Internodal Tracts

After leaving the SA node, the impulse travels via the three internodal tracts in the right atrium to the AV node. However, both atria are affected by the electrical current generated in tissue fluids. The AV junction is located just below the AV node and it sometimes functions as a "backup" pacemaker. The "junctional" FHR is 40 to 60 bpm.

Bundle Branch System

The impulse travels from the AV node down the Bundle of His and its two branches, the right bundle branch and the left bundle branch. These branches supply the right and left ventricles. Both eventually terminate in smaller branches, known as Purkinje fibers.

Purkinje System

The Purkinje system also serves as a "back-up" pacemaker, but the rate is less than 40 beats per minute. *Any one cell in this conduction pathway can generate and transmit an electrical impulse, create premature depolarizations, and ectopic beats.* Ectopy may originate in the atria or ventricles (8).

The P Wave

The heartbeat recorded on an FECG is composed of a sequence of deflections. The initial deflection is called a P wave. The P wave occurs when the atria depolarize. Normally, the fetal P wave may be inverted for short periods of time, occasionally notched, and/or tall (9). Since the electrical current generated in the body fluids by the SA node is slight, the P wave is small. The atria are thin-walled and the muscle tissue is less than the ventricles.

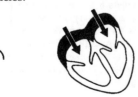

Figure 8.2: The P wave reflects atrial depolarization.

The PR Interval or PR Segment

The PR segment on the FECG is the distance from the end of the P wave to the beginning of the R wave (see page 109). The PR interval represents the amount of time it takes for the impulse to travel from the SA node to the Bundle of His. Normally, the fetal PR interval is less than 0.12 seconds. The PR interval doesn't exceed 0.12 seconds until approximately 17 years of age. In the fetus, the PR segment is often depressed or below the isoelectric line. The PR interval decreases as the level of norepinephrine increases, increasing the FHR. During decelerations, the PR interval decreases but the R-R interval increases, which decreases the FHR (9). Umbilical cord occlusion was associated with a gradual shortening of the PR interval. With prolonged, complete umbilical vessel occlusion, the P wave disappeared and the FHR dropped to 60 bpm (10).

The QRS Complex

The QRS complex or R wave is caused by the depolarization of the ventricles. The ventricles have thicker walls than the atria, and produce a larger deflection on the ECG. The shape of the QRS complex varies depending on the position of the spiral electrode. Sometimes the R wave is notched, or the configuration may be QS with no R or RS with no Q (9).

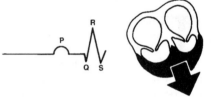

Figure 8.3: The QRS complex or R wave reflects depolarization of the ventricles.

The ST Segment and ST Analysis

Atrial repolarization occurs during ventricular depolarization. Repolarization of the ventricles generates a current in body fluids which produces the T wave. The T wave follows the QRS complex and repolarization is usually not seen on the FECG due to the fast conduction of the impulse through the AV node and Bundle of His and the large QRS complex which follows.

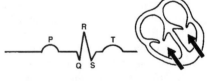

Figure 8.4: Repolarization of the ventricles generates a current in the body fluids and produces the T wave.

The fetal ST segment may be above on or below the isoelectric line (9). Review of the ST segment with the FHR reduced "acute" operative deliveries without an increase in perinatal morbidity and mortality (11-12). To determine the ST waveform, a spiral electrode must be on the fetus or an abdominal ECG must be obtained (12). The FECG waveform is in a sea of electrical noise and must be enhanced prior to interpretation (13-14). Hypoxia and metabolic acidosis elevates the ST segment and T waves (15). In adults, ischemia of the heart creates a negative ST segment, i.e., it is below the isoelectric line (16).

During early decelerations the FECG is unchanged. During severe variable decelerations (lasting longer than 60 seconds with a nadir at or below 70 bpm), the P wave was biphasic. A biphasic P wave suggests a pacemaker other than the SA node exists with bidirectional activation of the atria and ventricles. In some cases, the P wave disappeared, the ST segment became depressed, and the T wave height increased. ST segment depression suggests subepicardiac and endocardiac hypoxia. The T wave amplitude reflects generalized myocardial hypoxia. During *late decelerations that dropped 20 or less bpm*, the PQ interval increased due to depressed atrioventricular conduction and a *mild vagal stimulus*. When late decelerations were *deeper than 20 bpm* below the baseline, the PQ interval decreased suggesting a *stronger vagal stimulus*. SA nodal activity was depressed and there was a wandering pacemaker, i.e., the pacemaker was not the SA node. With late decelerations that dropped to 70 bpm or less, the P wave was absent or biphasic and there was a prolonged or shortened PQ interval (17).

T/QRS Ratio

The normal fetal T wave may be upright or inverted (9). The fetal T/QRS ratio is determined by a microprocessor after three FECG waveforms are obtained (18). A normal T/QRS ratio, i.e., less than 0.25, predicts normal fetal acid-base status 99.3% of the time. However, it poorly predicts a hypoxic fetus (66% positive predictive value), leading some to believe the FECG does not help distinguish fetal status (9, 15). T/QRS is *sometimes* elevated during asphyxia (19).

An abnormal T/QRS ratio is greater than 0.25 (14). Fetal scalp blood sampling has been advocated when ever the T/QRS ratio is abnormal (20). The T/QRS ratio increases when the T wave is elevated due to anaerobic myocardial metabolism and
- altered ionic currents in the myocardial cell
- depleted glycogen, creatine phosphate, and adenosine triphosphate and
- lactate accumulation (16, 21).

Researchers found the T/QRS ratio was positively related to umbilical vein plasma lactate, i.e., as lactate increased the T/QRS ratio increased. Sometimes FHR patterns with variable or late decelerations were associated with an increased T/QRS ratio (22). However, there was no relationship between the T/QRS ratio and abnormal FHR patterns (21). Reed and colleagues (23) are not convinced that the T/QRS ratio identifies fetuses at risk of intrapartum hypoxia. However, a normal T/QRS provided reassurance that any FHR abnormality was not clinically significant.

The U Wave and QT Interval

Additional waves on the FECG are the U wave and QT interval. A U wave may follow the T wave. The significance of the U wave is unclear (4). The U wave is affected by electrolyte changes such as hypokalemia, and medications such as digitalis.

The QT interval represents the time from ventricular depolarization to repolarization. Acidosis prolongs the QT interval and inverts the T wave. A dying fetus has a decreasing FHR and inverted T wave. In fact, researchers believe the QT segment changed most consistently when the fetus was acidotic. *An anoxic fetus accumulates K^+ which depresses myocardial cells to prolong the QT and PR intervals.* In addition, K^+ and sodium enter cardiac cells and release hydrogen which lowers the pH (24).

Atria and SA node depolarization and impulse generation create the P wave
▼
Impulse travels through right and left atria
▼
Atrial systole or contraction
▼
Impulse travels to AV node
▼
His bundle
▼
Purkinje system
▼
Ventricles depolarize ➤ QRS complex
▼
Ventricular systole
▼
Ventricles repolarize ➤ T wave

Figure 8.5: The cardiac cycle.

NORMAL SINUS RHYTHM

Prior to understanding arrhythmias, it is necessary to understand normal sinus rhythm (NSR) which reflects a normal cardiac cycle. An ECG with normal sinus rhythm has P-P and R-R intervals which are very close in length. There is a P wave before each QRS complex. The P waves are similar in shape, and the QRS complexes are also similar in shape. P waves are upright, and the atria contract at the same rate as the ventricles, i.e., there is 1:1 atrioventricular conduction (25).

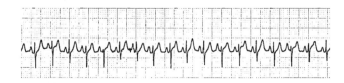

Figure 8.6: Normal sinus rhythm (rate = 150 bpm).

ARRHYTHMIAS OF THE FETAL HEART

An arrhythmia is a malfunction of normal impulse formation which may affect automaticity, excitability, conductivity, or a combination of these, e.g., tachycardia with a heart block (4). Arrhythmias, also referred to as dysrhythmias, may be heard or observed as an irregularity of the FHR or rhythm which has no relationship to uterine activity (26). When there is *a disturbance in the heart cell's ability to form and discharge an impulse independently (automaticity and excitability),* cardiac rhythm may become tachycardic, bradycardic, or irregular with ectopic beats or premature rhythms such as premature atrial contractions. Thus, arrhythmias have been categorized as *fast, slow, and irregular.* Irregular rhythms occur in 1 to 3% of all pregnancies and include:

- premature atrial contractions (PACs)
- premature ventricular contractions (PVCs) (27).

Respiratory sinus arrhythmia is considered an irregular rhythm. Atrial flutter and atrial fibrillation may be irregular depending on the ventricular response, or the FHR may be fixed or flat if there is a one to one atrial-ventricular response (28).

Tachyarrhythmias occur in 0.4 to 0.6% of pregnancies and include:

- sinus tachycardia
- supraventricular tachycardia
- atrial flutter
- atrial fibrillation
- ventricular tachycardia (26-27).

Bradyarrhythmias occur in 0.1 to 0.3% of all pregnancies and represent about 5% of all arrhythmias (27). Brady-arrhythmias include:

- sinus bradycardia
- atrioventricular (AV) block (26).

The most common arrhythmia found during echocardio-graphy was premature atrial contractions (72.2%). Supraven-tricular tachycardia (14.4%) and complete heart block (2.4%) were less frequently encountered. Overall, if the fetus had an arrhythmia, 9.6% had a structural cardiac defect (29).

Irregular rhythms are most common in the last 10 weeks of pregnancy (30). Irregular rhythms, such as isolated extrasystoles caused by PACs, are the most common and represent 85% of all fetal arrhythmias. Tachyarrhythmias are the next most common and represent 10% of fetal arrhythmias (26). Tachyarrhythmias were found in 4 to 26% of referrals to a perinatologist (31-32). The most common fetal tachy-arrhythmia is supraventricular tachycardia (SVT). SVT is usually caused by an impulse that reenters the atria via a reentrant tract. The reentrant tract may be within the AV node or outside of the AV node. The least common cause of SVT is an atrial ectopic pacemaker outside of the SA node (31, 33). Bradyarrhythmias represent 5% of all fetal arrhyth-mias. A rare bradyarrhythmia is complete heart block (CHB). In one report, 234 babies referred to a tertiary center for

diagnosis had the following arrhythmias:

PACs (190 or 81.2%)
PVCs (3 or 0.13%)
SVT (17 or 7.26%)
Atrial Flutter (5 or 2.14%) and
CHB (19 or 8.12%) (34).

Fetal arrhythmias are rare, occurring in only 1 to 5% of all pregnancies (5, 27, 29, 35). Six to 15% of fetuses who have an arrhythmia also have a structural cardiac defect (35). In gen-eral, 8 babies per 1000 live births has a cardiac defect, and the majority have no identifiable risk factors (34, 36-37). Half of the babies with a cardiac defect need surgery (37). One to 6.8% of babies with PACs or PVCs had a structural defect (35, 38). If the fetus had a tachyarrhythmia, the likelihood of a structural defect was 1 to 10% (28, 39). If the fetus had CHB, the risk of a cardiac defect was 40% or higher (26, 28, 35, 39).

Table 1: Arrhythmia Incidence in All Pregnancies, Percent of Occurrence, and Incidence of Structural Heart Defects

Arrhythmia Type	Incidence	Percent	Heart Defect
Overall	1-5%		6-15%
Irregular	1-3%	85%	1 to 6.8%
Tachycardic	0.4-0.6%	10%	1 to 10%
Bradycardic	0.1-0.3%	5%	> 40%

COMPLICATIONS OF ARRHYTHMIAS

A real-time ultrasound scan will only identify 23% of fetuses with a heart defect (40). However, echocardiography which uses sophisticated ultrasound and microprocessor technolo-gy can identify cardiac anatomy, arrhythmias, and their hemodynamic effect on the fetus (23, 41-43). Almost all forms of structural heart defects and arrhythmias, but not necessari-ly their electrophysiologic mechanism, have been identified using echocardiography (35, 40, 44). Most fetal arrhythmias (90%) are hemodynamically harmless (5, 45).

Irregular FHRs caused by PACs or premature ventricular contractions (PVCs) rarely require treatment. If PACs precede the development of SVT, treatment may be required. PACs and PVCs disappear shortly after birth. Complications of tachyarrhythmias include:

- decreased ventricular filling
- decreased cardiac output
- congestive heart failure
- hydrops fetalis
- death (2, 23, 46).

Tachyarrhythmias, with a FHR sustained above 180 bpm, and bradyarrhythmias, with a FHR below 60 bpm, have been associated with fetal cardiac failure and hydrops (39). A FHR less than 50 bpm or greater than 230 bpm significantly decreases cardiac output, increasing the risk of fetal death (47).

Nonimmune Hydrops Fetalis

Hydrops is an abnormal fluid collection in two or more body cavities or edema with an abnormal collection of fluid in one body cavity (48-49). Half of all fetuses with a tachyarrhythmia develop hydrops and *more than 50% of fetuses with hydrops die* (48, 50). Hydrops has been reported as early as 17 weeks' gestation in a fetus with SVT (3). Hydrops is a result of increased right atrial pressure, increased venous blood pressure, and third spacing of intravascular fluid or edema (43). Hydropic fetuses may have:

- scalp edema
- ascites
- placental thickening (more than 6 cm by ultrasound)
- anasarca (generalized, massive edema)
- hepatosplenomegaly
- cardiomegaly
- bilateral pleural effusions
- pericardial effusion
- dilated cardiac chambers
- tricuspid incompetence
- atrioventricular valve regurgitation
- pulmonary valve stenosis
- circulatory collapse
- polyhydramnios (35, 51-53).

Pericardial effusion often is the first sign of fetal hydrops and can be visualized by M-mode echocardiography (personal communication, Dr. G. Joffe, April, 1996). Hydrops fetalis is preterminal, therefore, it demands immediate treatment. Pleural effusions were associated with the death of 38 to 82% of fetuses (35, 53). Dilatation of the right atrium and/or ventricle is due to increased intracardiac volume (that was not normally being pumped out). Tricuspid valve incompetence or dysfunction reflects cardiac compromise and is an early sign of imminent congestive heart failure (43). The placenta may accumulate fluid and be more than 6 centimeters (cm) thick based on ultrasound measurement. Tables have been established for placental thickness versus gestational age (personal communication, Dr. G. Joffe, April 1996). There may be polyhydramnios. The umbilical vein may be dilated more than 1 cm. When the fetus is diagnosed with hydrops, tests may be performed to rule out toxoplasmosis, cytomegalovirus, coxsackie B virus, varicella, or the presence of lupus anticoagulant, anticardiolipin, and/or antinuclear antibodies (26, 39, 42, 48). SS-A and SS-B are more likely to be associated with congenital hydrops and heart block than lupus anticoagulant or anticardiolipin (personal communication, Dr. G. Joffe, April 1996). Prompt treatment is needed to prevent fetal death (52).

More than 80 conditions have been associated with hydrops (54). For example, hydrops may be related to:

- fetal anemia
- fetal hypoproteinuria
- chromosomal anomalies such as trisomy 21
- congenital infection, e.g., coxsackie B virus
- umbilical cord torsion
- a single umbilical artery
- a true knot in the umbilical cord
- cord entanglement
- twin to twin transfusion (in the polycythemic twin)
- chylothorax (the accumulation of liquid products of digestion from the thoracic duct into the pleural space, often due to a tumor that invades the thoracic duct)
- congenital cystic adenomatoid malformation, a cystic lung lesion, and
- cardiac failure (54-57).

Cardiac failure, which preceded hydrops, may be caused by:

- a conduction system defect
- fetal cardiomyopathy, e.g., due to viral myocarditis
- a cardiac tumor
- endocardial fibroelastosis
- a structural defect(s)
- obstructed or diverted cardiac outflow
- inadequate venous return to the heart
- inadequate ventricular filling and/or
- inadequate inotropic force
- tachy- or bradyarrhythmias
- severe fetal anemia related to parvovirus or a fetomaternal blood transfusion
- polycythemia (42, 49).

Hydrops prior to 24 weeks' gestation is usually related to a fetal chromosomal abnormality. Amniotic fluid tests may include a karyotype and viral cultures. Viral titers of the woman's blood may be obtained for cytomegalovirus, toxoplasmosis, parvovirus, and herpes. Other maternal tests may include a complete blood count and Kleihauer-Betke stain, ABO and Rh typing, an indirect Coombs test, a VDRL, and G_6PD deficiency screen. Cordocentesis will be required for assessment of fetal hemoglobin and hematocrit to determine the need for transfusion. In addition, fetal blood can be used for karyotyping, assessment of umbilical vein IgM, and thyroid levels. The fetus may need a paracentesis, thoracentesis, or drug therapy (54). It has been theorized that cord torsion, a tight twist in the cord versus a helix or coil, causes cord compression which causes a myocardial conduction defect or cardiac dysfunction which creates an arrhythmia, heart failure, and hydrops (57).

CLASSIFICATION OF ARRHYTHMIAS

Arrhythmias may be classified by their site of origin. Fetal arrhythmias that will be discussed in this chapter are listed in Table 2.

Table 2: Fetal Arrhythmias

Sinus Arrhythmias (origin = SA node)
- respiratory sinus arrhythmia
- sinus bradycardia
- sinus tachycardia
- sinus block or sinus arrest with and without junctional escape beats
- sick sinus syndrome

Irregular Rhythms
- premature atrial contractions (origin = AV node or atria)
- premature ventricular contractions (origin = ventricles)
- parasystole
- idioventricular rhythm

Ventricular Tachyarrhythmias (origin = ventricles)
- ventricular tachycardia
- ventricular fibrillation

Supraventricur Tachyarrhythmias (origin = atria)
- reentrant supraventricular tachycardia or atrioventricular reentry tachycardia
- atrial or junctional ectopic tachycardia
- atrial flutter
- atrial fibrillation

Bradyarrhythmias (AV node conduction defect)
- blocked atrial premature beat
- first-degree heart block
- second-degree heart block
- complete heart block (27-28)

SINUS NODE DISORDERS

Features of a sinus node disorder include:
- "pacemaker" is within the SA node
- normal impulse conduction.

Respiratory Sinus Arrhythmia

The most common irregular arrhythmia is respiratory sinus arrhythmia with increased SA node firing during inspiratory efforts and decreased firing during exhalation efforts (4). The R-R interval varies and is reflected by small changes in the heart rate and similar upward and downward changes in blood pressure (58). This is an innocuous arrhythmia that requires no treatment (4).

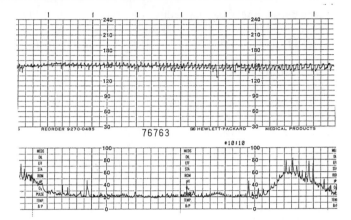

Figure 8.7: Respiratory sinus arrhythmia documented as a sawtooth pattern.

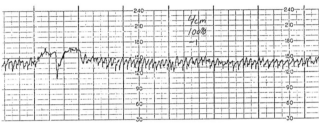

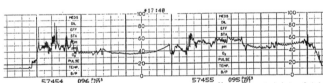

Figure 8.8: Respiratory sinus arrhythmia and spontaneous accelerations with Lambda pattern in a G₂ P₁ woman at 39 weeks' gestation. She delivered vaginally with Apgar scores of 3, 7, and 9 at 1, 5, and 10 minutes. The FHR dropped to 60 bpm prior to birth, 25 minutes after Demerol and Vistaril administration.

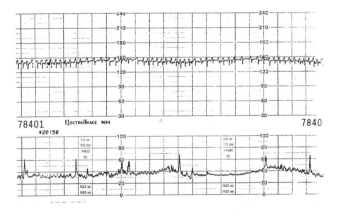

Figure 8.9: Respiratory sinus arrhythmia in a woman who was a G₂ P₁ at 39 weeks' gestation. She is married and does not smoke, drink alcohol, or use "recreational" drugs. She delivered vaginally with Apgar scores of 8 and 9. The neonate had a normal cardiovascular system.

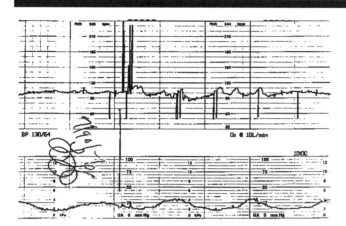

Figure 8.10: Moderate to marked sinus bradycardia. The presence of accelerations and short-term variability confirm the pacemaker is the sinoatrial node. The downward deflections represent blocked premature atrial impulses or artifact. The upward deflections may represent conducted premature atrial beats or artifact. This 19 year old G$_4$ P$_1$ woman at 39 weeks' gestation delivered a 9 lb 2 oz baby vaginally. Apgar scores were 7 and 8 at 1 and 5 minutes.

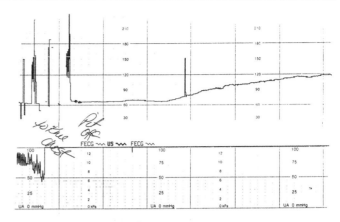

Figure 8.11: Marked sinus bradycardia is usually related to anoxia, metabolic acidosis, or asphyxia and requires immediate action. The woman was G$_2$ P$_0$ with an uncomplicated pregnancy at 41 weeks' gestation. Labor was induced with artificial rupture of membranes and pitocin. Apgar scores were 1, 7, and 9 at 1, 5, and 10 minutes following positive pressure ventilation with 100% oxygen. Note the junctional escape beats in the first, second, and fourth minutes of monitoring.

Sinus Bradycardia (Nodal Rhythm)

Features of sinus bradycardia include:

- SA node is firing at less than its inherent rate (2, 4)
- FHR is less than 100 bpm and has been reported as low as 70 bpm at 14 weeks' gestation (2, 59)
- confirmed during echocardiography
- may be intermittent, e.g., the FHR falls to 50 to 70 bpm for 20 to 30 seconds (which was termed a "carrot") or asystole occurred for 5 to 7 seconds during a 90 second deceleration
- sometimes followed by a compensatory sinus tachycardia for 1 to 2 minutes (60)
- P-P and R-R intervals are similar but not fixed
- atrial and ventricular rates are the same, i.e., 1 to 1 conduction
- causes may be: increased vagal tone, e.g. from chronic hypoxia, hypercapnia, pan-hypopituitary disease, myocardial depression, or a cardiac defect such as ventricular septal defect with situs inversus of the stomach and heart failure (32, 59).

Sinus bradycardia is usually innocuous when it is not related to hypoxia. A FHR between 100 and 120 bpm may be defined as moderate bradycardia in some texts. This rate is associated with a healthy fetus when accelerations and short-term variability are also present (61). Accelerations in the FHR confirm the sinoatrial node (SA node) is the pacemaker. Sinus bradycardia is easy to differentiate from CHB because *there is no short-term variability when there is atrioventricular (AV) block and the FHR is usually less than 90 bpm, flat, and stable during CHB* (62). Some references define marked bradycardia as a FHR less than 100 bpm (61). Marked sinus bradycardia due to anoxia, metabolic acidosis, and/or asphyxia requires

immediate action. Marked sinus bradycardia is not accompanied by accelerations, is not a stable rate, and there are no accelerations and rare to no fetal movements.

Sinus Tachycardia

Features of sinus tachycardia include:

- SA node is firing at greater than its inherent rate
- FHR greater than 160 bpm with short-term variability
- normal conduction of impulse
- may be due to SA node impulse reentry
- P-P and R-R intervals are similar but not fixed
- baseline range or bandwidth is 5 to 15 bpm
- normal P waveform.

The increase in the rate is usually a response to a demand by the body for an increase in cardiac output. Sinus tachycardia may be caused by:

- maternal thyrotoxicosis
- fetal hyperthyroidism
- hypoxia
- drugs, e.g., cocaine (hypoxia response), amphetamines, β-mimetics such as terbutaline (drug response)
- amnionitis, with or without fever
- hypovolemia
- maternal anxiety and increased epinephrine and norepinephrine
- maternal infection and/or fever
- congenital infection, e.g., cytomegalic inclusion disease (2, 4, 27, 31, 52, 63).

A common cause of sinus tachycardia is hypoxia related to intraamniotic infection. Symptoms of chorioamnionitis include at least two of the following: hyperthermia (≥ 38° C), maternal tachycardia (> 100 bpm), fetal tachycardia (> 160 bpm), uterine tenderness, leukocytosis, and/or foul-smelling amniotic fluid (64). Sinus tachycardia may be differentiated from SVT by echocardiography prior to treatment. If the cause is hypoxia, intrauterine resuscitation measures are required. If the cause is SVT, antiarrhythmics may be ordered.

Sinus Block or Sinoatrial (SA) Block with Junctional Escape

Transient asystole is also called sinus block, sinoatrial block, sinus arrest, or vagal cardiac arrest. Sinus arrest (a sinus nodal pause) may occur *at the bottom of a deceleration* (see Figure 8.13) followed by junctional escape beats. Sinus arrest may also occur *during an acceleration*, which creates the appearance of a Lambda pattern (see Figure 8.14, also see Figure 2.12 on page 39). A strong vagal stimulus may suppress the SA node to the point that new impulses are blocked. A nodal rhythm (originating in or near the AV node) with ventricular escape beats will be seen on the fetal ECG (65). The result is transient or reflex asystole, particularly at the bottom or nadir of a variable deceleration (2, 65). Prolonged asystole is "quite unusual and death is rare" (65).

Asphyxial sinus block may also occur in "seriously asphyxiated" fetuses who have myocardial depression. They have a bradycardic rate with absent variability. The bradycardia reflects a sinus rhythm (65). Hypoxia and acidosis alter the sensitivity of the heart's impulse conduction system to autonomic nervous system stimuli (66). When the fetus is asphyxiated, vagal cardiac arrest may precede complete cardiac arrest and death. When cord compression is relieved, the vagal stimulus ceases, and the heart should beat again. If the SA node is completely inhibited from releasing an impulse, escape beats may originate along the atrial internodal tracts, and persist until the sinus node functions again. At heart rates below 60 bpm, the impulse for the heartbeat originates in the AV node. The generation of the cardiac impulse from the AV node, and the resultant ECG, is referred to as an AV rhythm. The FECG will show P waves of decreased amplitude, which will disappear or change their shape as the inhibition of the sinus node progresses (2).

A Lambda pattern is an acceleration preceded or followed by a reflex drop in the FHR. Lambda patterns, including those reflective of sinus arrest, are rarely documented because they are not clinically significant. When the FHR drops to below half the baseline FHR, the heart essentially stopped beating. The heart begins to beat after this sinus pause with a junctional depolarization. A junctional depolarization appears on an FECG as a QRS complex which is *not* preceded by a P wave. In the healthy fetus, this pause, a transient cardiac asystole or a vagal cardiac arrest, is harmless (2, 67).

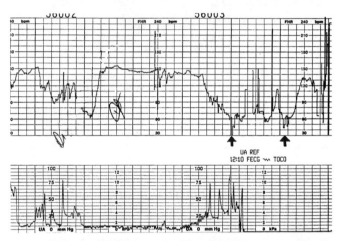

Figure 8.13: Transient asystole or vagal cardiac arrest at the nadir of a prolonged deceleration (see rate above arrows). Note upward excursions of the FHR from the base of the deceleration which reflect junctional escape beats that originate in the AV node.

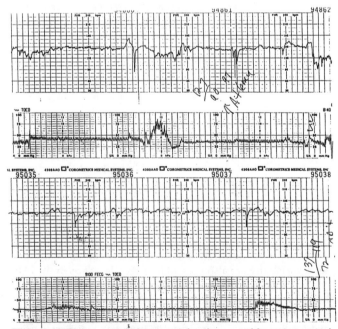

Figure 8.14: Sinus arrest during an acceleration caused by a strong vagal stimulus. Also note dropped beat (sinus arrest) above the hand-written words "Pit 6 mU." The woman is $G_2 P_1$ at 39 weeks' gestation, 6 cm, +1 station. The baby was delivered following a vacuum-assist with Apgar scores of 9 and 9 at 1 and 5 minutes. The transient sinus arrest is innocuous.

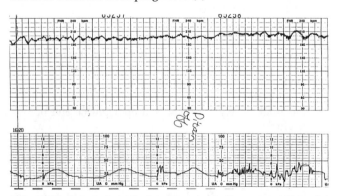

Figure 8.12: Sinus tachycardia in a fetus of a $G_1 P_0$ woman at 42 weeks' gestation at 4 cm, 0 station with a vertex presentation. Apgar scores were 9 and 9 at 1 and 5 minutes.

Sick Sinus Syndrome

An unusual cause of sinus arrest is a bradycardia/tachycardia syndrome known as sick sinus syndrome or sinus node dysfunction. One case report of sick sinus syndrome diagnosed at 27 weeks' gestation was identified in the literature. In that case, the fetus was eventually delivered at 37 weeks' gestation. The FHR due to sick sinus syndrome included persistent, unexplained bradycardia that never exceeded 70 bpm. The FECG demonstrated a 1 to 1 atrial-ventricular rate. Each QRS complex was preceded by a P wave. Atropine was administered to the woman with no effect on the FHR. There were no anti-DNA, antinuclear, or cardiac tissue (SS-A/Ro or SS-B/La) antibodies found in the maternal circulation (68).

IRREGULAR RHYTHMS

Irregular FHR rhythm features are:
- the most common type of fetal arrhythmia
- PACs and PVCs have an unknown cause
- the atrial and ventricular rate is between 120 and 160 bpm during normal cardiac conduction
- are usually benign
- have no treatment.

PREMATURE ATRIAL CONTRACTIONS (PACs)

Premature atrial contractions are also called premature supraventricular systoles or premature atrial depolarizations (PAD). If one were to evaluate the FECG, the PAC would be diagnosed by a P wave that precedes a normal, but premature, QRS complex (6). PACs in adults may be caused by atrial distention or various drugs (69). They may also be followed by an abnormal QRS complex due to aberrant impulse conduction. Features of PACs include:
- the most common arrhythmia and the most common irregular rhythm (43 to 84% of all arrhythmias diagnosed by echocardiography) (32)
- diagnosed as early as 13 weeks' gestation (70).
- usually ectopic focus causes PAC (33)
- primary cause of ectopy is an aneurysmal atrial septum which bulges into the left atrium causing mechanical irritation of myocardial fibers (76% of fetuses with PACs) (39, 70-72)
- secondary causes may be related to cardiac malformations, diaphragmatic hernia, and illicit drug use, caffeine or alcohol use, or cigarette smoking (31, 67, 73-74)
- may occur with sinus node reentry of impulse within atrium, but there are no accessory conduction pathways (33)
- if sinus node reentry, P waves all have similar morphology, vagal stimulus will slow the rate (33)
- may be bigeminal or trigeminal, i.e., occur as two or three PACs in a row (70)
- following a PAC, cardiac contractility is enhanced and fractional shortening increases 49 to 64% (8)
- Frank-Starling Mechanism has been confirmed by Doppler ultrasound valvular flow (8)
- 1% of PACs precede SVT (32, 70)
- PAC may not be conducted resulting in a heart rate at 60 or 70 bpm creating downward deflections on the FHR pattern (dropped beats) (32, 70)
- not clinically significant (33)
- usually resolve spontaneously after birth (70).

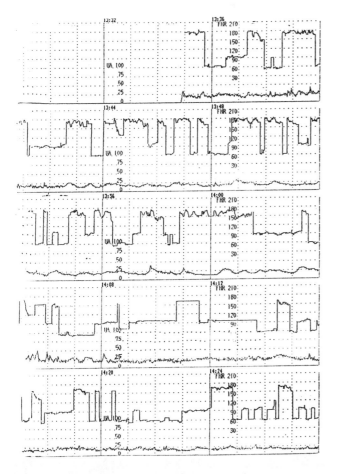

Figure 8.15: Sick sinus syndrome might be suspected with this unusual FHR pattern that includes tachycardia, bradycardia, and a normal fetal heart rate. After birth, the neonate was found to have two sinoatrial nodes, an extremely rare and unusual anomaly. Ablation of one SA node was attempted but failed.

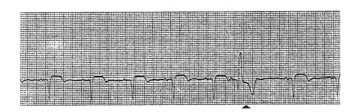

Figure 8.16: Adult ECG illustrating PAC with aberrant conduction.

Fractional shortening is determined by an ultrasound measurement of heart size at the end of diastole and systole. Fractional shortening is the percent change in the dimension of cardiac size at the level of the atrioventricular valves and is calculated by the following formula:

$$\text{end-diastolic dimension - end-systolic dimension} \div \text{end-diastolic dimension} \times 100 \quad (75)$$

Fractional shortening was decreased and end-diastolic dimensions were larger in fetuses who were 26 to 30 weeks' gestation with SVT. These findings suggested cardiomyopathy. With the very fast rate, it would have been expected to find smaller end-diastolic dimensions (76).

An atrial septal aneurysm can be visualized by two-dimensional, cross-sectional echocardiography as a bulge into the left atrium or it appears as mobile, redundant atrial septal tissue. This is thought to be a form of a prematurely obstructed foramen ovale. Some aneurysms are restrictive and others are not (71, 77). The septum primum (the normal septum) creates a flap that postnatally closes the foramen ovale (77). It moves with biphasic oscillations during atrial contraction (78). When there is an atrial septal aneurysm, this septum extends at least half way across the left atrium and even strikes the left atrial free wall or mitral valve annulus. It has even prolapsed into the mitral valve (77). The septal wall may be weak which causes it to move across the left atrium (72). Atrial septal aneurysms are also associated with SVT (20%) and atrial flutter with or without 2:1 AV conduction (4%) (71-72). Atrial septal aneurysms spontaneously resolve after birth due to the change in blood flow in which the right to left shunt (through the foramen ovale) is no longer present (72). In fact, almost all PACs resolve by 12 weeks of age (32).

Since PACs may precede SVT, careful evaluation of the FHR at each prenatal visit is required (32). The woman should be instructed to report a decrease in fetal movement. She may be asked to return to the obstetrician's office for FHR assessment every one to two weeks or she may have a home health nurse assess the FHR.

Less than one percent of fetuses with atrial arrhythmias have a structural cardiac defect (77). PACs may appear as little upward deflections followed immediately by downward deflections on the FHR tracing (see Figure 8.17) (79). PACs are clinically nonsignificant and commonly disappear before or shortly after birth, e.g., within 30 minutes (2, 67, 79).

PACs and Supraventricular Tachycardia

PACs may also include a premature P wave with a different configuration from the sinus P wave (2). This premature P wave may not be conducted due to the absolute refractory

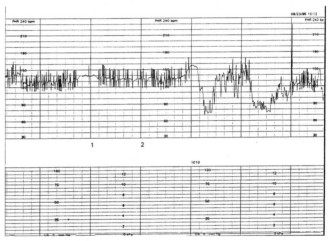

Figure 8.18: Premature atrial depolarizations produce upward and downward deflections in the FHR pattern. Note the upward deflection (the conducted PAC) precedes the downward deflection (the compensatory pause). The 41 week fetus had Apgar scores of 9 and 9 at 1 and 5 minutes.

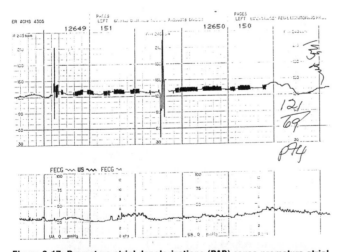

Figure 8.17: Premature atrial depolarizations (PAD) cause premature atrial contractions. Dropped beats occur when the PAD is not conducted. The upward excursion of the fetal heart rate reflects conducted PACs. The little upward and downward deflections probably reflect PACs in a bigeminal pattern, although the exact arrhythmia would need to be confirmed by echocardiography. The woman was $G_2 P_1$ and 39 5/7 weeks' gestation who "quit smoking during her pregnancy." Smoking has been implicated in the occurrence of fetal PACs.

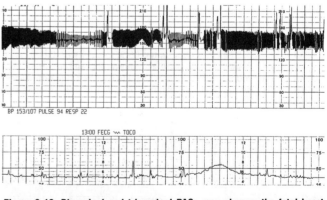

Figure 8.19: Bigeminal and trigeminal PACs may obscure the fetal heart rate baseline. This 40 week fetus had Apgar scores of 8 and 9 at 1 and 5 minutes. By turning logic on these lines would disappear. If an ultrasound transducer were in place, the atrial rate would be printed. When the spiral electrode is used, the rate calculated between consecutive R waves is printed.

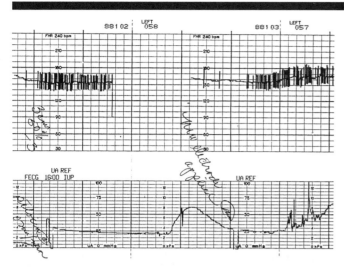

Figure 8.20: Premature atrial depolarizations persist, even when a new spiral electrode is applied. Apgar scores were 9 and 9 at 1 and 5 minutes. The baby was 36 6/7 weeks' gestation and macrosomic (8 lbs 11½ ounces). There was oligohydramnios and the woman had gestational diabetes.

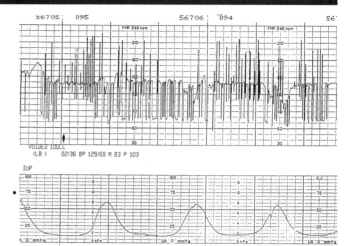

Figure 8.22: Dropped beats reflect blocked premature atrial depolarizations in a 38 week fetus whose Apgar scores were 8 and 9 at 1 and 5 minutes. Note the occasional 2:1 AV block, particularly at the end of the second minute in frame 56706.

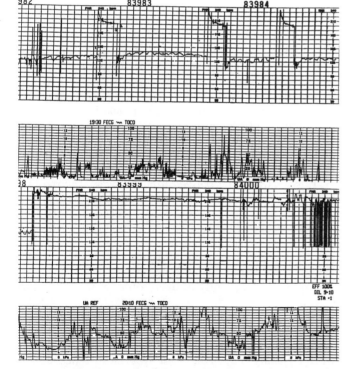

Figure 8.21: Formerly called paroxysmal atrial tachycardia, supraventricular tachycardia is triggered by a premature atrial depolarization in a 39 week fetus born to a $G_2 P_1$ woman with a normal pregnancy. Apgar scores were 9 and 9 at 1 and 5 minutes. Supraventricular tachycardia recurred during the neonatal period. The baby received two doses of digoxin and two of adenosine and was later diagnosed with Wolff-Parkinson-White syndrome. The neonate was discharged home on digoxin.

period in the AV node. If it is conducted, SVT may occur (see Figure 8.21) (80). In only 1% of cases, PACs precede SVT (39). In some cases, SVT may be associated with a structural cardiac abnormality (62, 81-82). SVT has an abrupt onset and termination, i.e., the rate becomes tachycardic or returns to a normal baseline with only one heartbeat (1). However, sometimes SVT begins after a bigeminal or coupled supraventricular rhythm (two fast beats occur together) (30, 83).

PACs and Dropped Beats
Features of FHR patterns reflective of premature atrial depolarizations followed by a nonconducted impulses include:
* atrial rate faster than ventricular rate, e.g. 130-140 bpm versus 60 to 90 bpm (51, 80)
* bradycardic episodes disappear by 2 months of age (80).

A PAC is usually followed by a brief or partial compensatory pause. However, a nonconducted PAC causes the fetal monitor microprocessor to calculate a very slow rate because the R-R interval increases when the PAC is never conducted. The calculated rate is usually between 60 to 90 bpm (see Figure 8.22 and 8.23). *The downward deflections from the FHR baseline are called dropped beats.* The long compensatory pause which creates the dropped beat may follow a retrograde atrial premature impulse that is not conducted due to the refractory period of the SA node (80). In that case, there is no R wave, a dropped beat, and the ventricles do not depolarize. This is similar to the heart "skipping a beat."

Dropped beats may also be artifact due to signal loss (see Figure 8.24). A similar tracing can occur when R waves are absent due to fetal demise. Maternal electrical activity may be transmitted through the fetus to the spiral electrode. The signal will be amplified by the monitor's automatic gain control, counted, and recorded (84). When this type of pattern

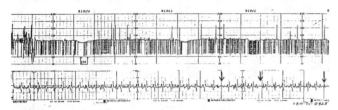

Figure 8.23: This tracing shows a series of downward deflections of the fetal heart rate. The lack of an R wave creates the dropped beats. (Reproduced with permission of Williams and Wilkins, Inc., Baltimore, MD from Freeman, R. K., & Garite, T. (1981). *Fetal heart rate monitoring*).

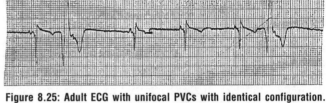

Figure 8.25: Adult ECG with unifocal PVCs with identical configuration. This suggests only one area in the ventricle is irritable.

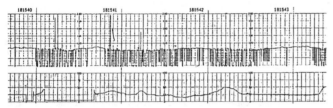

Figure 8.24: This tracing also shows a series of downward reflections. In this instance, the heart rate is maternal conducted through the dead fetus' spiral electrode. The downward deflections represent a weak maternal signal with intermittent noncounted beats. (Paul, R., & Freeman, R. (1971). Selected records of intrapartum fetal monitoring. USC Pub., reproduced with permission of Williams and Wilkins, Inc. from Freeman, R. K., & Garite, T. (1981). *Fetal heart rate monitoring*).

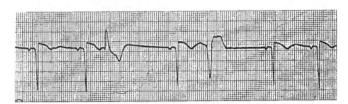

Figure 8.26: Adult ECG with multifocal PVCs that vary in configuration and indicate a widespread problem in the ventricles.

appears, it is important to listen to the FHR with a fetoscope or assess fetal movement. The maternal heart rate should be compared to the rate recorded on the fetal monitor paper. To confirm demise, the physician may scan the fetus using real-time ultrasound technology. Sounds heard with a fetoscope reflect the ventricular, not the atrial, rate. Fetal movement confirms fetal life.

PREMATURE VENTRICULAR CONTRACTIONS (PVCs)

Features of PVCs include:
- they are less common than PACs (70)
- their cause is unknown, but an ectopic focus in the ventricles triggers the premature contraction
- they may be related to cocaine (70)
- there is a wide QRS complex which represents aberrant ventricular conduction (85)
- the atrial and ventricular rate is between 120 and 160 bpm when there is normal cardiac conduction
- after the premature ventricular contraction, there is a compensatory diastolic pause or interval (70)
- PVCs are benign and have no treatment
- PVCs may precede ventricular tachycardia (70)
- echocardiography can identify which ventricle prematurely contracts (70)
- PVCs usually disappear within two weeks after birth (83).

Premature ventricular contractions are also called premature ventricular depolarizations. Their cause is an irritable focus in the ventricles which discharges before the arrival of the next impulse from the SA node. The *PVC is always followed by a compensatory pause* before repolarization and the next normal sinus impulse. The absence of the P wave prior to an abnormal, prolonged, widened, distorted QRS complex is diagnostic of a PVC versus a PAC (6). The ST segment and/or T wave changes (2).

If the FHR tracing derived from an external ultrasound transducer records fast and slow rates, e.g., a rate near 80 bpm and a rate near 140 bpm, it is possible that PVCs exist (86). Anytime there is an unusual rate, it is wise to use a fetoscope or real-time ultrasound to determine the actual ventricular rate. If it sounds irregular, a M-mode echocardiography would be needed to diagnose the actual arrhythmia. PVCs may occur as frequently as every other beat of the heart (bigeminy) or every third beat (trigeminy) (see Figure 8.27). Although PVCs are the most common of all arrhythmias in human beings and are usually associated in adults with acute myocardial infarction, overdoses with digitalis (especially when bigeminy is observed), and hypokalemia, they are less common in the fetus. The cause of fetal PVCs is unknown. They are usually benign, requiring no intervention (2). Fetal PVCs may be unifocal or multifocal in origin. *The upward deflections on the tracing reflect the PVC, the downward deflections*

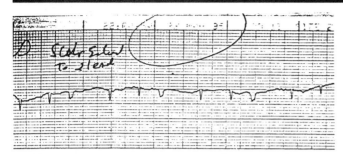

Figure 8.27: Fetal electrocardiogram reflecting trigeminy. Every third heartbeat was a premature ventricular contraction. Note the wider QRS complex.

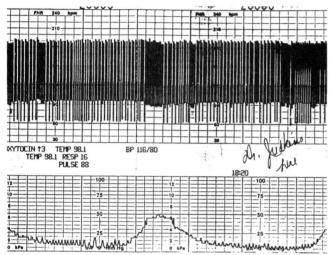

Figure 8.28: The tracing of a 41 week fetus of a G$_3$ P$_2$ nonsmoker with multifocal PVCs. Note the change in color near the middle of these lines. Below the middle, the two distinct lengths of lines are noted. When the compensatory pause lines are of two or more lengths, there are multifocal PVCs. The neonate was born with a loose nuchal cord, trigeminy, and Apgar scores of 2, 8, and 9 at 1, 2, and 5 minutes.

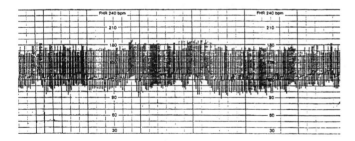

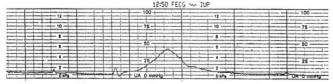

Figure 8.29: Unifocal PVCs include upward and downward deflections of similar lengths. A baseline rate can be discerned near 120 to 130 bpm. If PACs were present, the baseline would be totally obscured.

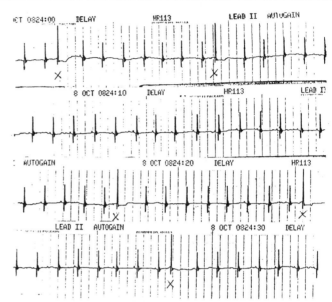

Figure 8.30: Neonatal ECG of baby in Figure 8.29. Premature ventricular contractions are marked with an X.

reflect the compensatory pause. The compensatory pause often equals the time of two normal heartbeats (39, 69). PVCs often resolve during labor or shortly after birth and pharmacologic therapy is not indicated (62, 67).

Parasystole

Features of parasystole include:
- vertical deflections of varying lengths
- automatic focus of ectopic impulse generation in the ventricle
- discharged impulse exits ventricle before or after ventricle is refractory but without any fixed relationship to the normal impulse generated by the SA node
- interectopic intervals are multiples of the shortest interectopic interval
- in adults, it is a benign arrhythmia
- it is rare in the fetus (67).

Idioventricular Rhythm

An irregular ventricular rate which may occur with PVCs is idioventricular rhythm. There is a ectopic focus in the ventricle which spontaneously depolarizes. The impulse does not leave the ventricles until the SA node impulse is less than the rate of the idioventricular cell(s). Idioventricular impulses alternate with normal sinus impulses. Adults, who have had a myocardial infarction with SA and AV node ischemia, may have an idioventricular rhythm. The cause of this arrhythmia in the fetus is unknown (67).

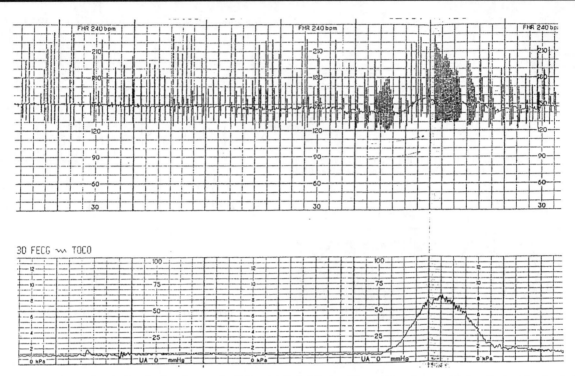

Figure 8.31: Parasystole is suspected when the baseline can be distinguished and there are excursions above and below the baseline level of differing lengths. The interval between the PVC lines is a multiple of the shortest interval between lines, a distinguishing feature of parasystole.

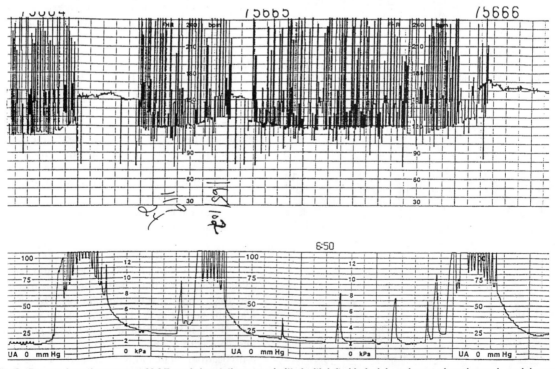

Figure 8.32: The G$_1$ P$_0$ preeclamptic woman at 36 3/7 weeks' gestation was admitted with left side facial weakness, slurred speech, and decreased strength on her left side. Her blood pressure was greater than 160/90, she had 1 gram of protein in her 24 hour urine collection. Artificial rupture of the membranes revealed clear fluid. She is now completely dilated and pushing. Magnesium sulfate is at 2.5 gm/hour. The neonate was delivered by midforceps with Apgar scores of 8 and 9 at 1 and 5 minutes. Although a fetal arrhythmia was confirmed, the exact diagnosis was not available. Therefore, it can only be assumed that this is an example of idioventricular rhythm.

Ventricular Tachycardia

- uncommon
- due to sustained ventricular ectopy
- often related to cardiac tumor, long QT syndrome, e.g., Romano-Ward syndrome
- may be sustained or intermittent
- FHR 140 to 400 bpm
- atrioventricular (AV) dissociation
- possible that ventricular rate is faster than atrial rate
- FHR pattern is indistinguishable from SVT
- diagnose with echocardiography
- do NOT give digoxin (70, 87).

Ventricular tachycardia is defined as three or more consecutive PVCs (2). This arrhythmia is *rarely found in the fetus*. In adults, it has been associated with hypomagnesemia (88). During ventricular tachycardia, there is a total dissociation between the atrial and ventricular rhythms. The atrial rate is slower than the ventricular rate (25). Drugs, such as digoxin or verapamil, used to treat SVT or atrial flutter should NOT be used to treat this dysrhythmia (52). They are inappropriate and ineffective, especially if ventricular tachycardia is due to retrograde conduction of each cardiac impulse (25, 89). Digoxin shortens the refractory period in the atrium and AV node to slow AV conduction and the ventricular rate. This decreases the antegrade (atrial) refractory period but may increase the ventricular response as cardiac impulses sent back into the atrium via retrograde accessory pathway(s) are more likely to be conducted and exacerbate ventricular tachycardia or create ventricular fibrillation (52, 90). Therefore, finding a medication that is effective in the treatment of this arrhythmia is extremely difficult. Agents used to treat ventricular tachycardia in children have included lidocaine, bretylium, procainamide, phenytoin, amiodarone, propranolol, and mexiletine. As many as 43% of children with ventricular tachycardia had a history of myocardial infarction (MI). The presence of sustained ventricular tachycardia plus a MI resulted in an 80% mortality rate (91). In one case, a fetus with ventricular tachycardia was given an umbilical vein injection of lidocaine followed by maternal administration of quinidine and procainamide (87). If the fetus develops signs of congestive heart failure, e.g., hydrops fetalis, delivery and neonatal treatment is advised.

Ventricular Fibrillation

No cases of fetal ventricular fibrillation have been reported, however, a neonate developed ventricular fibrillation on the second day of life. The baby had complete congenital atrioventricular block at 30 weeks' gestation with a structurally normal heart. Due to sudden circulatory failure, an emergency cesarean section was performed. On the second day of life ventricular fibrillation necessitated the surgical insertion of a pacemaker which reestablished normal circulation (92). In another neonatal case of ventricular fibrillation, *digoxin* was administered to a baby who had Wolff-Parkinson-White syndrome (93).

SUPRAVENTRICULAR TACHYCARDIA

Supraventricular tachycardia (SVT) has an atrial or junctional origin and includes atrioventricular reentry tachycardia and ectopic tachycardia. Ectopic supraventricular tachycardia is subdivided into atrial ectopic tachycardia where there is an ectopic atrial focus and junctional ectopic tachycardia with AV dissociation and a ventricular rate higher than the atrial rate (94). Fetal SVT includes

- atrioventricular reentry tachycardia
- atrial ectopic tachycardia
- junctional ectopic tachycardia
- atrial flutter and
- atrial fibrillation (27, 94).

Junctional ectopic tachycardia has also been called accelerated junctional ectopic tachycardia (95). All of these produce a fast FHR greater than 180 bpm. SVT may be initiated by an impulse in or near

- the atria
- the AV node or
- an accessory conduction (reentry) pathway outside the AV node (33).

SVT is the second most frequent fetal tachyarrhythmia. Sinus tachycardia is the most frequent (62). SVT is an umbrella term for a tachyarrhythmias in which extra cardiac impulses are conducted to or from the atria to the AV node. Paroxysmal atrial tachycardia (PAT) and paroxysmal junctional tachycardia are outdated terms for SVT (55). Tachyarrhythmias usually have a FHR greater than 180 bpm. SVT is usually greater than 200 bpm. It starts *abruptly, i.e., with one beat of the heart, either a PAC or PVC*, and is usually initiated and terminated by a PAC (52, 70). Supraventricular tachycardia features include the following:

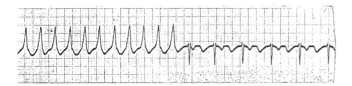

Figure 8.33: An example of ventricular tachycardia (adult ECG).

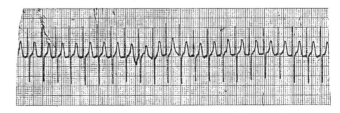

Figure 8.34: Supraventricular tachycardia (adult ECG). Fixed R-R intervals suggest a reentrant mechanism versus an ectopic focus.

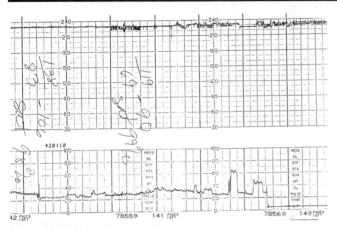

Figure 8.35: Supraventricular reentrant tachycardia is suspected when the FHR is greater than 200 bpm with fixed variability.

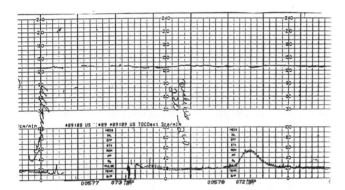

Figure 8.36: Suspect supraventricular tachycardia when a flat line appears near 125 to 130 bpm. Most fetal monitors print half the rate when it exceeds 240 bpm (the top of the FHR channel). In this case, the FHR was near 250 bpm.

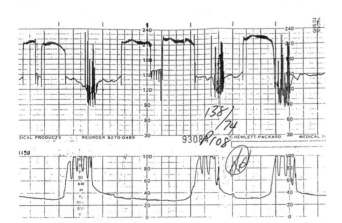

Figure 8.37: Supraventricular tachycardia may be intermittent. Apgar scores were 8 and 9 at 1 and 5 minutes. During pushing, the FHR decelerates and the vertical lines may be artifact or they may reflect premature atrial contractions.

- usually the FHR is greater than 200 bpm (96)
- the FHR may be as high as 300 bpm (97)
- FHR during SVT is lower than the FHR during atrial flutter or fibrillation (79)
- 1 in 4347 fetuses have SVT (98)
- SVT has occurred as early as 17 weeks' gestation (3)
- SVT may be associated with a structural cardiac anomaly in as many as 10% of cases (98-99)
- SVT is found in 95% of cases with a tachyarrhythmia (5% are atrial flutter or fibrilllation) (99)
- reentrant SVT (the most common) has fixed R-R intervals, P waves precede each narrow QRS complex
- P waves may be difficult to discern on a FECG
- P wave configuration is similar unless the impulse is generated in an accessory pathway (33).
- due to the fixed R-R intervals, there is absent variability (2, 62)
- junctional ectopic tachycardia, triggered by an ectopic focus, has variability, accelerations, and decelerations
- SVT may be intermittent or continuous lasting a few seconds to hours (6)
- there is 1:1 AV conduction (2, 6, 70, 97)
- SVT is more common in male fetuses (2.7:1 male-female ratio) (98)
- Doppler aortic blood flow studies predict the onset of hydrops in fetuses with SVT (97)
- suspect halving of the FHR if the rate is greater than 240 bpm, there will be a flat line printed between 125 and 150 bpm
- auscultate to confirm the ventricular rate or use a real-time ultrasound
- often requires maternal or fetal antiarrhythmic agent to inhibit AV node conduction and prolong the refractory time to prevent risk of heart failure, hydrops, and death (99)
- pharmacologic cardioversion may include maternal medications or medications administered directly to the fetus
- cardioversion by compression of the fetal head or cord have been unsuccessful
- cardioversion using ice applied directly to the fetal vertex or ice water (injected through the outer guide of a spiral electrode with the guide placed firmly on the fetal head) have been attempted but are not documented in the literature
- 20% persist into the neonatal period (99).

A Word About Ice

Ice or ice water is a safe and effective treatment for neonatal SVT (100). The application of an ice-cold washcloth to a neonate's face may cause a diving reflex or vagal response which would cardiovert SVT to a NSR. The diving reflex is oxygen-conserving. Cold water on the afferent nerve endings near the mouth and nose increases sympathetic stimulation of peripheral blood vessels and vagal stimulation of the heart. Peripheral vasoconstriction increases blood flow to the brain and heart. Bradycardia will be seen. Ice water to the face is rapid, effective, easy, safe, noninvasive, painless, and has no side effects (101).

Ice may be placed in a plastic bag and gently applied to the neonate's face avoiding pressure on the eyes and nose (95, 102). Neonates with SVT have been treated with ice water on their face for five seconds which was followed with digitalis therapy. The combination of ice and digoxin restored normal sinus rhythm on 27 of 28 occasions (101). Ice water alone was effective in all 16 children on 53 of 59 occasions (100). In neonates with junctional ectopic tachycardia and a heart rate greater than 200 bpm, ice to the face was unsuccessful in controlling the heart rate, but hypothermia using cooling blankets slowed the rate to a more acceptable level until the neonates eventually cardioverted (95).

Although no report of ice or ice water on the fetal vertex was found in the literature, it has been tried during labor to cardiovert fetal SVT. For example, the outer guide of the spiral electrode is applied to the fetal head over a parietal bone. Ice water has been injected into the guide. Ice may be inserted in the vaginal (in a sterile glove) and pressed on the fetal head. Nurses have filled condoms with water and frozen them to be used against the episiotomy to reduce swelling. It would be interesting to see if this tube of ice could be applied against the fetal vertex for the purpose of cardioversion. If the woman is allergic to latex, this procedure should not be attempted. A curious physician is needed to undertake this experiment to see if ice applied to the fetal head will cardiovert a SVT rate during labor.

Reentry Supraventricular Tachycardia

Atrioventricular reentry tachycardia is also called reentrant supraventricular tachycardia. Atrial reentry tachycardia is another form of SVT. In atrioventricular tachycardia, there is retrograde conduction of the cardiac impulse within the AV node. In atrial reentrant SVT, there is retrograde conduction via a concealed accessory pathway outside the AV node (94, 103). Neonatal treatment of atrial reentry tachycardia may include a combination of an antiarrhythmic agent, such as sotalol, antitachycardia pacemaker or radiofrequency ablation, especially with complex congenital heart disease (103).

When one SA nodal impulse is conducted by multiple paths or reenters the right atrium through a reentry circulating excitation wave, SVT or atrial flutter can occur (90). When the AV node receives the additional reentrant impulse the ventricles contract again. The impulse can travel via one of two types of circuits: antidromic and orthodromic (104). These circuits create a "circus-movement" tachycardia (105).

Antidromic Circuit

When there is an antidromic reentry circuit, the SA nodal impulse is transmitted via more than one anterograde accessory tract to the AV node. There is a normal retrograde pathway after ventricular contraction or the impulse travels back through AV node (104-105).

Orthodromic Circuit

When there is an orthodromic circuit, the impulse travels as follows:
SA node ⇒ AV node ⇒ His bundle ⇒ Purkinje fibers ⇒ ventricles contract ⇒ impulse reenters the AV node through a retrograde accessory pathway ⇒ His bundle ⇒ Purkinje fibers, ventricles contract, etc. (104-105).

Reentrant circuit(s) with abnormal excitability and normal conduction. SVT due to reentry of the impulse through the AV node or a bypass tract outside the AV node is the most common form of SVT (52). If the reentry pathway is outside the AV node, preexcitation of the atrium occurs when the His bundle is refractory. A PAC or PVC may initiate or terminate SVT. There may be evidence of heart block, in which the impulse slows or stops. If the reentry pathway is within the AV node, there is usually a retrograde pathway that activates the AV node and the normal antegrade pathway through the AV node. One pathway (retrograde) is fast and one (antegrade) is slow (see Figure 8.38) (31).

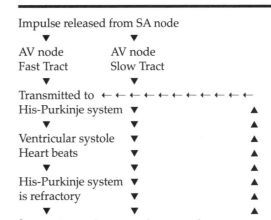

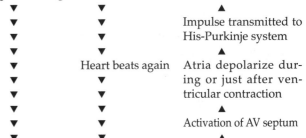

Figure 8.38: AV nodal reentrant tachycardia may be caused by fast and slow tracts that exist within the AV node. When an early atrial beat enters the AV node it travels down the slow pathway since the fast pathway has not yet repolarized from the preceding normal impulse. Then, the impulse in the slow pathway simulates the ventricles (antegrade) and goes up the fast pathway (retrograde) to reexcite the atria (105).

Because two tracts can stimulate atrial depolarization, *P waves differ in their shape*. To treat AV nodal reentry tachycardia, medications are needed to stop the slow tract, antegrade conduction. *Concealed accessory pathways, outside the AV node, may create premature atrial stimuli or rapid atrial pacing.* The SA nodal impulse enters the AV node and even the His bundle but then travels back (retrograde) into the atrium, back over the AV node, and into the His bundle again. During this arrhythmia, *the P wave may be seen within the ST segment or there may be an early T wave. Often, the RP interval is less than the PR interval* (33).

A structural defect may coexist with reentrant SVT (33). Congenital cardiac anomalies associated with SVT include cardiac tumors and Ebstein's anomaly of the tricuspid valve (27-28, 70). Ebstein's anomaly may be detected during a two-dimensional ultrasound. This anomaly includes a dilated right atrium with tricuspid valve leaflets extending into the right ventricular outflow tract. The newborn will have high right atrial pressure and right-to-left atrial shunting due to difficulty or inability of blood to cross the tricuspid valve into the pulmonary artery. Drugs, such as tolazoline (Priscoline), may be needed to lower pulmonary vascular resistance until the child is large enough for surgery to repair this defect (106).

Wolff-Parkinson-White (WPW) Syndrome

WPW syndrome is a preexcitation syndrome caused by accessory antegrade impulse conduction paths outside the AV node, between the SA node and the AV node (31, 33, 107-108). WPW syndrome is impossible to diagnose in the fetus and is only diagnosed after birth (109). Accessory pathways often disappear in utero or shortly after birth (90, 109). If SVT persists, the neonate may be given digoxin. For example, at 30 weeks' gestation, the fetus had intermittent paroxysmal bigeminal and trigeminal tachycardia, i.e., two beats and a pause and three beats and a pause. At 32 weeks' gestation, PVCs were also noted with a pericardial effusion and a hydropic placenta. The FHR tracing generated by an external ultrasound transducer was unusual in that different rates (at 50, 80, and 160 bpm) were recorded intermittently. *The FHR recorded at 50 or 80 bpm was not the true ventricular rate, but reflected the rate calculated between the premature heart beat and the heartbeat after a compensatory pause following the bigeminal and trigeminal beats.* The compensatory pause after the bigeminal tachycardic rhythm or trigeminal rhythm caused dropped beats (downward deflections) when the spiral electrode was in place. *When an unusual or inconsistent FHR pattern is seen with an ultrasound in place, the FHR should be auscultated with a fetoscope or Pinard stethoscope or cardiac motion should be visualized by ultrasound to confirm the true ventricular rate and rhythm.* For example, a FHR was auscultated with a Pinard stethoscope at greater than 200 bpm. Echocardiography revealed a 1:1 relationship between the atrial and ventricular rates with a structurally normal heart. The woman was treated with digoxin and flecainide. Ten days later, fetal pericardial effusion and ascites resolved (110).

If the fetus has WPW syndrome, digoxin *may* increase the ventricular rate, producing atrial flutter or fibrillation and necessitating another drug such as procainamide or quinidine (43, 109). The benefits of digoxin seem to outweigh the risks (109). It seems reasonable, that when digoxin is administered, continuous FHR monitoring should be used to identify its effect on the fetus. Continuous maternal cardiac monitoring may also be used. Digoxin may not be effective in cardioverting the baby. In one case, a woman was given digoxin and after birth the neonate was diagnosed with WPW syndrome and required digoxin for 6 months (107).

Ectopic Tachycardia (Automatic Focus)

Junctional ectopic tachycardia is a rare disorder of automaticity or triggering with atrioventricular dissociation when there is 1:1 retrograde conduction. For example, the atrial rate may be 136 bpm when the ventricular rate is faster (33, 95). The neonate will have a heart rate greater than 200 bpm (95). However, the FHR is usually between 180 and 190 bpm, slower than reentry SVT rates which are usually greater than 200 bpm (33). There will be a narrow QRS complex and P

Table 3: Ectopic Versus Supraventricular Tachycardia

CHARACTERISTIC	ECTOPIC	REENTRANT
Abnormality	Automaticity	Conduction
Fetal Heart Rate	Fluctuates	Monotonous
Onset	"Warm up"	Abrupt
Offset	"Cool down"	Abrupt
P Wave Morphology	May Vary	Similar
R-P to P-R interval	Longer	Shorter or Similar
QRS complex	Narrow	Narrow
Response to Vagal Stimulus	None	Possible cardioversion
Response to Antiarrhythmics	None	Common
Response to Acoustic Stimulation	Acceleration	No response

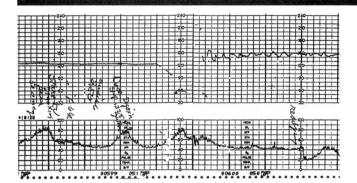

Figure 8.39: Digoxin 0.5 mg (500 mcg) IV push over 2 minutes successfully cardioverted fetal SVT (with a rate of 250 bpm printed at half the rate on the tracing) to a normal sinus rhythm in less than 3 minutes.

waves are difficult to discern. Junctional ectopic tachycardia is often resistant to medications such as lidocaine (Xylocaine) and digoxin (95). It may be present without a known cause. During ectopic tachycardia, an irritable cell in the atrium or AV junction sends an impulse to the AV node. Ectopic SVT, unlike reentrant SVT, is not induced by PACs or stimuli (33). The impulse for the heartbeat comes from a cell above the His bundle that discharges at a faster rate than the SA node. This ectopic cell replaces the SA node as the heart's pacemaker (62, 87). Junctional ectopic tachycardia is also an

- uncommon form of SVT (5% of all tachyarrhythmias)
- with no reentrant circuit
- the ectopic trigger may be intra-atrial or automatic atrial tachycardia with accelerated automaticity

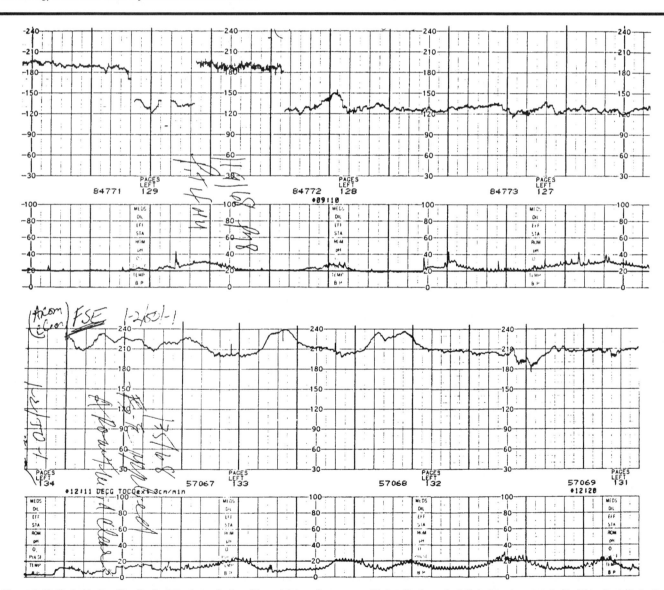

Figure 8.40: Probable junctional ectopic tachycardia in a 37 week fetus of a woman with insulin-dependent diabetes who was admitted for pitocin induction and who had clear amniotic fluid. The FHR at 0905 (top strip) was intermittently in the 180s and 190s. Three hours later (bottom strip), the rate was between 200 and 210 bpm with accelerations. Reentrant SVT does not accelerate.

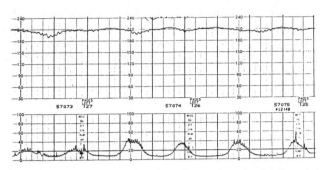

Figure 8.41: Junctional ectopic tachycardia may have decelerations. Late decelerations are evident. The baby was delivered at 8:45 pm. Apgar scores were 9 and 9 and 1 and 5 minutes.

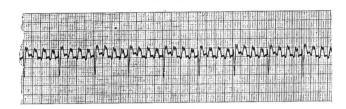

Figure 8.42: Atrial flutter (adult ECG). Note slower ventricular rate and "sawtooth" atrial activity which replaces the P wave.

- the AV node is not part of the tachycardia circuit, and the AV node is not required to maintain it
- the baseline FHR slowly increases to a tachycardic rate greater than 200 bpm
- the R-P interval is longer than the P-R interval
- there may have 1:1 atrioventricular conduction with normal P wave morphology
- conduction from the AV node is not affected, and the QRS complex appears normal
- there may be accelerations and/or decelerations, e.g., early decelerations with pushing during the second stage of labor
- has occurred with digoxin toxicity, ischemic heart disease, and myocarditis
- risk of congestive heart failure
- is associated with high Apgar scores if no cardiac failure (33, 111).

Reentrant SVT and junctional ectopic tachycardia are examples of SVT with distinct differences. Reentrant tachycardia has a constant, monotonous rate. Ectopic tachycardia has a changing FHR. Reentrant tachycardia has an onset after one beat of the heart, e.g., a PAC or PVC triggers it. Ectopic tachycardia has a "warm up" and "cool down" period. Reentrant tachycardia P waves have the same morphology. Ectopic tachycardia P waves may vary depending on the location of the ectopic pacemaker. The R-P interval is longer than the P-R interval in ectopic but

not reentrant tachycardia. Ectopic tachycardia is unresponsive to a vagal stimulus or drugs. If an acceleration follows acoustic stimulation, ectopic tachycardia can be strongly suspected (33, 111).

In a case report of junctional ectopic tachycardia, a fetus at 21 weeks gestation, was diagnosed with atrioventricular dissociation, edema, ascites, and an enlarged liver. The atrial rate was 140 bpm, the ventricular rate was 180 bpm. At one month of age the rate converted to a normal sinus rhythm. In some cases, the tachyarrhythmia is intractable, the prognosis is grave as drugs seldom work, and ablation of the atrioventricular junction is considered. After delivery, the neonate may need surgical ablation or radiofrequency ablation of the ectopic focus if medications, such as propafenone, fail to create a normal sinus rhythm (52, 111-112).

Atrial Flutter

Features of atrial flutter, an unstable supraventricular arrhythmia, include:
- it is a rare disorder of impulse formation and conduction (2, 62)
- atrial rate of 300-500 bpm (2, 25, 52, 62, 70, 90, 113-114)
- atrioventricular (AV) block is usually fixed or variable with periods of 1:1 AV conduction
- there is usually AV block with a ventricular rate between 60 to 300 bpm (2, 25, 62, 90, 99)
- often a 2:1 second-degree heart block with only half of the impulses being conducted, may look like dropped beats with downward deflections from baseline, e.g., atrial rate 492 to 500 bpm, ventricular rate 130 to 194 (113, 115)
- there is usually a macroreentrant electric depolarization circuit (outside the AV node) and
- microreentrant electrical depolarization circuit (within the AV node) (31, 114)
- atrial flutter may also be due to an ectopic focus with increased automaticity (115)
- causes include myocarditis from a viral infection, e.g., coxsackie B, cytomegalovirus or maternal thyrotoxicosis
- 8% of fetuses with atrial flutter also have anomalies such as hypoplastic left ventricle and dilatation of the left atrium (25, 99, 114)
- when the FHR exceeds the paper scale, it will be half-counted, e.g., a flat baseline at 155 bpm (99)
- antenatal pharmacologic treatment is more difficult than treatment of SVT (116)
- can degenerate into atrial fibrillation (115)
- risks: right atrium and ventricle enlargement, mild tricuspid valve regurgitation, decreased cardiac output, heart failure, hydrops fetalis, death (43, 109)
- difficult to control (52)
- treatment goal: slow the ventricular rate by transplacental or direct fetal antiarrhythmic drugs, e.g., digoxin, verapamil, amiodarone, quinidine, procainamide, flecainide acetate, lignocaine, or direct fetal administration of adenosine (50, 52, 62, 90, 96, 109, 116)

- neonatal electrical cardioversion, e.g., with 2 to 5 watt second (joules), may be necessary (90)
- ECG may have sawtooth or undulating baseline appearance with no normal P waves with narrow QRS complexes (on FECG) (6).

Atrial flutter has been associated with biatrial cardiac enlargement and pericardial effusion but a normal biophysical profile. It was treated by the combination of digoxin and flecainide. The neonate required electrocardioversion and oral digoxin due to mild congestive heart failure and a continuation of the tachyarrhythmia (113). Babies with Wolff-Parkinson-White syndrome or fetomaternal hemorrhage may develop atrial flutter (62, 117). Atrial flutter and/or fibrillation are potentially serious arrhythmias which can be diagnosed by M-mode echocardiography. Twenty percent of babies with atrial flutter or fibrillation have congenital heart disease (2, 62).

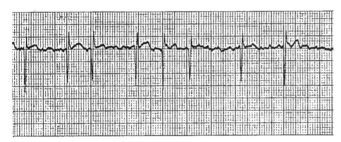

Figure 8.43: Atrial fibrillation (adult ECG). Note low amplitude irregular atrial activity with QRS complexes of various sizes (2, 6).

Atrial Fibrillation
- rarely identified in the fetus
- atrial rate 480 to 520 bpm, ventricular rate 200 to 240 bpm (43)
- identified by echocardiography or FECG
- may be preceded by atrial flutter
- real-time ultrasound reveals quivering atrial wall (43)
- may be related to Wolff-Parkinson-White syndrome or other congenital heart disease (2, 62).
- digoxin is first line drug of choice to decrease ventricular rate or convert rate to normal sinus rhythm (43)

In 1982, Belhassen and his colleagues reported a case of fetal atrial fibrillation at 32 weeks' gestation. There was no structural cardiac defect. Digoxin was administered to the pregnant woman, but the fetal ventricular rate and cardiac size continued to increase. At 34 weeks' gestation the baby was delivered by cesarean section. Recurrent episodes of nonsustained atrial fibrillation occurred in the first hours of life. Wolff-Parkinson-White was ruled out. There was an accessory conduction pathway (118).

Table 4: Suspect the Type of Arrhythmia Based on the Fetal Heart Rate

Fetal Heart Rate (bpm)	Probable Arrhythmia
180-190	Sinus Tachycardia
	Junctional Ectopic Tachycardia
> 200	Supraventricular Tachycardia (atrial rate > 200)
	Atrial Flutter (atrial rate > 300)*
	Atrial Fibrillation (atrial rate > 450)*

*Often accompanied by a second-degree AV block

MANAGEMENT OF FETAL SVT, ATRIAL FLUTTER, AND ATRIAL FIBRILLATION

The hemodynamic effect of tachyarrhythmias on the fetus depends upon myocardial fatigue and cardiac output. If cardiac output is compromised, the fetus may not grow normally or may suffer from congestive heart failure. Medical management varies depending on gestational age, response to medications given to the mother, evidence of worsening hydrops, and evidence of intrauterine growth restriction (IUGR) (6). Once the arrhythmia is defined, the fetus is evaluated for evidence of cardiac anomalies, hydrops, and IUGR. Then, it will be decided if an antiarrhythmic drug will be given to the woman or directly to the fetus.

ANTIARRHYTHMIC MEDICATIONS

Fetal tachyarrhythmias such as SVT, atrial flutter, and atrial fibrillation, may precede heart failure evidenced by hydrops fetalis. The decision to use an antiarrhythmic agent versus deliver the fetus is influenced by the gestational age, lung maturity, and presence or absence of hydrops. If antiarrhythmics are needed, they may be delivered:
- to the pregnant woman either intravenously or by mouth (transplacental route) or
- to the fetus by an intramuscular (IM), an intravenous (IV) or an intraperitoneal injection (39, 50, 119-120).

Antiarrhythmic agents for SVT include:
- digoxin
- sotalol (26, 31)
- verapamil
- propranolol (6)
- procainamide (121)
- quinidine (115)
- flecainide acetate (30, 122)
- amiodarone (52, 123)
- propafenone (45, 52)
- adenosine (26) or a combination such as
- digoxin and quinidine (52, 124)
- digoxin and verapamil (52)
- digoxin and propranolol (52)
- quinidine and procainamide (52).

Antiarrhythmic Classifications

Antiarrhythmic drugs may be classified by their actions (see Table 5) (33, 85)

Table 5: Antiarrhythmic Agents and Their Actions

Drugs that Affect Retrograde Pathways (in and outside the AV node) and Decrease Impulse Speed and Strength (Decreasing Automaticity and Conduction)
- procainamide (class IA-fast sodium channel blocker/local anesthetic)
- quinidine (class IA-fast sodium channel blocker/local anesthetic)
- disopyramide

Drugs that Affect Both Antegrade and Retrograde Accessory Pathways
- flecainide (class IC)
- amiodarone (class III)
- propafenone (class IC)

Drugs that Decrease AV Nodal Conduction
- digitalis (digoxin) (class V cardiac glycoside)
- beta-blockers (class II)
- sotalol (beta-blocker with class III properties)
- edrophonium
- verapamil (class IV calcium-channel blocker)

Class III drugs act on the cardiac cell membrane to prolong the refractory period. This disturbs the reentrant circuit in the AV node or an accessory pathway (45). Sotalol has class III properties (85). Adenosine is also being administered directly to the fetus to convert SVT to a NSR (26).

Digoxin

Digoxin remains the first line drug of choice for treatment of SVT and atrial flutter due to its wide margin of safety. Poor placental transfer may limit its effectiveness (99, 119). Digoxin slows AV conduction and increases the AV nodal refractory period. It also depresses the ventricular response. As a result, the PR interval is prolonged. Digoxin works at the intracellular level to change sodium-potassium and sodium-calcium exchanges (the sodium pump) that occur after systole. The effect is to increase intracellular calcium levels, which produces a positive inotropic effect (125).Thus, digoxin augments cardiac output by increasing cardiac contractility and stroke volume. The QT interval decreases. The ST segment may slope downward, the so-called "digoxin effect" (43, 125). Digoxin is the only antiarrhythmic drug with a positive inotropic effect shown to be safe in patients with heart failure (89, 109). Digoxin is not recommended for use if the fetus is suspected to have Wolff-Parkinson-White syndrome, however, it is not possible to diagnose WPW syndrome until the baby is born (115).

Unfortunately, placental transfer of digoxin is neither quick nor adequate at times (89). Placental transfer decreases when the placenta is hydropic, and ranges from a low of 10 to 40% to a high of 70 to 90% (26, 39, 52). Fetal and maternal serum digoxin levels should be similar within 30 minutes of the initial dose (96).

Standard digoxin doses may be suboptimal during pregnancy due to the normal increase in blood volume, glomerular filtration rate, decreased gastric emptying, and increased fetal metabolism of digoxin (121). When digoxin is given with other antiarrhythmics, its excretion decreases which increases the risk of toxicity. Table 6 illustrates the increase in serum digoxin with the interacting drug (52).

Table 6: Digoxin Excretion Decreases and Serum Concentration Increases When Other Antiarrhythmics are Also Administered

Interacting Drug	Serum Digoxin Concentration Increase(%)
Flecainide	10 to 20
Verapamil	20 to 60
Propafenone	50 to 100
Amiodarone	50 to 100
Quinidine	100 to 200

As a loading dose, digoxin IV in given in a concentration of 10 μg/kg every 12 hours for a total of 1.5 mg in the first 24 hours. The loading dose by mouth (PO) is often an initial dose of 0.5 mg, followed three hours later by 0.5 mg, then another 0.5 mg dose three hours later for a total of 1.5 mg (52, 96, 126). The maintenance dose of digoxin may be 0.25 to 0.5 mg every 12 hours IV or 0.25 to 1 mg PO (5 to 10 μg/kg) 2 to 3 times a day (26, 43, 96). Digoxin has also been given IM to the woman or fetus. The fetal IM dose was 88 μg/kg every 12 to 24 hours for a maximum of 3 doses. With this regimen, fetuses cardioverted in 1.4 to 9.4 hours. By 36 hours 90% of the fetuses had 2 straight hours of NSR. Hydrops was totally resolved within 24 hours (127). *The therapeutic range of maternal serum digoxin is 0.5 to 2 nanograms per milliliter (ng/ml) and fetal serum digoxin is 0.9 to 2 ng/ml (25, 125, 128).* Serum levels are usually drawn 6 hours after the first IV dose and 10 hours after the first PO dose (125). Digoxin has a 36 hour elimination half-life and may require as long as 1 week to reach a steady-state of a therapeutic serum concentration (52). Others found maternal plasma clearance of digoxin occurred in 8.7 to 13.9 hours (109). The plasma elimination half-life of digoxin given directly to the fetus is 15.9 hours (52).

A steady-state need not be achieved for the fetus to cardiovert. For example, 14 hours after a total oral dose of 1.5 mg, fetal movement increased and the FHR dropped to 125 to 130 bpm. The woman continued on a daily digoxin dose of 0.25 mg until delivery (126). Direct administration of digoxin is reserved for the preterm fetus in cardiac failure that has not responded to transplacental therapy (119). In utero therapy is preferable to preterm delivery of a hydropic infant due to the poor prognosis (116).

Symptoms of digoxin toxicity include:
- nausea
- vomiting
- intracellular electrical instability with aberrant action potentials which produce
  - SVT
  - atrial tachycardia
  - accelerated junctional rhythm
  - atrial fibrillation
  - ventricular tachycardia
  - ventricular fibrillation
  - bradycardia
  - AV block
- chest discomfort
- shortness of breath
- a change in color perception, visual acuity, mentation
- decreased sensation
- decreased strength and
- abdominal pain (125).

While digoxin is being administered IV, a cardiac monitor with a continuous ECG should be in place (110). Toxicity is more common if there is a potassium deficiency (hypokalemia) because this increases the sensitivity of cardiac tissue to digoxin. Therefore, maternal electrolytes should be examined prior to digoxin administration. Magnesium and calcium levels may affect the effect of digoxin on the heart. *If the maternal heart rate is bradycardic (less than 60 bpm), the drug is withheld and the physician is notified. If toxic effects occur, the drug is withheld and a 12-lead ECG should be immediately obtained.* If a life-threatening arrhythmia occurs, digoxin immune fab (Digibind) may be given IV. Toxic effects should subside within 20 to 40 minutes after drug administration. Cholestyramine or colestipol may be ordered to increase digoxin clearance. If unstable or pulseless ventricular tachycardia or ventricular fibrillation is noted, the woman may need electrical defibrillation (125).

Sotalol

In the mid-1990s, sotalol was gaining popularity as treatment for SVT in pediatric patients (26, 103). Sotalol is a β-blocker with type III antiarrhythmic properties. It is used to treat arrhythmias with multiple mechanisms, such as Wolff-Parkinson-White syndrome, ectopic atrial tachycardia, atrial reentry tachycardia, and ventricular tachycardia (103). The drug depresses AV nodal conduction, increases the duration of the action potential, increases the refractory period, and prevents atrial fibrillation (31). Drug adverse effects include headache, dizziness, abdominal pain, fatigue, depression, bradycardia, ventricular dysfunction, and it is proarrhythmia (103). It is given by mouth (80 mg twice a day) (26). Sotalol (120 mg) was given with digoxin on the fourth day of digox-

in therapy (0.25 mg every 6 hours following a loading dose of 0.5 mg) when the fetus developed ascites (31).

Flecainide Acetate

Flecainide is a second line drug used to treat atrial, junctional, and ventricular arrhythmias (52). It is a sodium channel blocker that decreases the FHR by depressing abnormal automaticity and slowing conduction in the His-Purkinje system and AV node accessory bypass tracts. This prolongs the PR and QRS intervals (52, 89, 96). Allan and Chita (89) discourage the use of flecainide for atrial flutter because it can actually increase the ventricular response to SA nodal impulses. Flecainide should not be given in cases of atrial flutter or where there is a structural cardiac defect or cardiomyopathy (122).

The effect on the heart is a negative inotropic effect which increases the risk of death in fetuses with cardiac compromise (97). Because flecainide has been associated with death in adults who had a history of myocardial infarction, its use, even during pregnancy with healthy women, is usually reserved for cases of fetal SVT with hydrops (89). In one case, hydrops resolved 11 days after flecainide therapy was started (97).

Flecainide is eliminated by the kidneys (40%) and liver (60%). Renal elimination is decreased if urine is alkaline (52). Fifty to 83% is transplacentally delivered to the fetus (52, 89, 96, 122, 128). It is 73 to 100% effective in cases of SVT. A NSR will be established in one to five days after initiation of drug therapy (89, 97, 122).

The initial maternal dose is 2 mg/kg delivered over 30 minutes IV or 150 mg by mouth twice a day. The maintenance dose will vary and may be:
- 300 to 600 mg/day in 2 to 3 divided doses, e.g., 150 mg every 12 hours, or 1.4 mg/kg/5 minutes IV or 2 mg/kg/30 minutes IV (52, 89)
- 100 to 150 mg by mouth 2 times a day (25)
- 100 mg by mouth 2 to 3 times a day (26, 39, 96-97, 128).

The neonatal dose is 0.5 to 2 mg/kg delivered IV over 2 to 10 minutes (122).

The maternal serum therapeutic level of flecainide is 0.2 to 1 µg/ml (128). Others have suggested the therapeutic level is 0.4 to 0.8 µg/ml (52). It has an elimination half-life of 11 hours, and requires 14 hours to reach a plasma steady state (52, 96). Flecainide will convert SVT to a NSR in two to seven days (52). In one case, it only took 12 hours until there was a NSR (97). In another case, NSR was noted 48 hours after therapy began. Hydrops resolved in one to two weeks after the FHR normalized (89). In a case of atrial flutter, with an atrial rate as high as 500 bpm, the FHR decreased to 180 bpm in 2½ days. The atrial rate was 169 to 319 bpm and the ventricular rate varied between 155 and 175 bpm. A fetal pulse oximeter was applied during labor. The fetal SpO$_2$ ranged from 50 to 85%, a normoxic level (113).

Flecainide interacts with cimetidine which inhibits its metabolism in the liver. In addition, there will be a 20 to 60%

increase in digoxin concentration when flecainide is also administered (52). Side effects of flecainide include blurred vision and dizziness (25). Toxic maternal effects include:

- paresthesia
- visual disturbances
- cardiac failure (if there was a history of left ventricular dysfunction) (52).

Flecainide toxicity, in less than 1% of babies or children that received the drug, reflects it "proarrhythmia" properties. Flecainide "aggravates" ventricular tachycardia. A toxic response to flecainide included SVT but at a slower rate, ventricular fibrillation, atrial flutter, atrial fibrillation, and cardiac arrest (in children) (52, 122). *Women and babies should not be given this drug with milk products because they inhibit oral absorption of flecainide.* Toxic levels of the drug were found when milk was eliminated from the child's diet without changing the drug dosage (122).

Verapamil

Verapamil is a calcium channel blocker which blocks calcium-dependent excitation (115, 129). Since the SA and AV nodes are activated by calcium, use of verapamil will inhibit impulse generation in these nodes (85). Verapamil also has negative inotropic properties, i.e., it decreases cardiac contractility (26, 115). *Verapamil is not recommended for use in adults or fetuses who have a high risk of heart failure or Wolff-Parkinson-White syndrome.* If there is a risk of heart failure and the rate slows due to decreased contractility, heart failure is more likely. *In the case of WPW syndrome, when the ventricular response slows, the risk of reentry tachycardia and atrial fibrillation increases* (115, 129). *Verapamil is also a potent vasodilator, therefore, maternal blood pressure should be assessed prior to and after verapamil administration* (115).

Verapamil may initially be given IV as 10 mg in 10 ml of normal saline at a rate of 1 mg per minute. Then, it may be given by mouth as 120 mg every 8 to 12 hours or 160 mg by mouth every 8 hours (96, 129). The therapeutic serum level of verapamil is 50 to 100 ng/ml (42).

Propranolol (Inderal)

Propranolol blocks the effect of epinephrine on β-receptors (130). Potential adverse reactions of this agent are weighed against the risk of nonintervention. For example, propranolol has been associated with exacerbation of asthma and heart failure (52). Propranolol is rarely used during pregnancy because it is associated with IUGR and neonatal hypoglycemia, bradycardia, and low Apgar scores (126, 128). Due to its β-blocking properties, propranolol *can cause cardiac standstill if it is given too rapidly IV.* The usual IV dose is 1 to 3 mg at less than 1 mg per minute. This may be repeated after 2 to 5 minutes (52). Propranolol is at a "satisfactory" fetal blood level within 30 minutes of maternal administration (121). This drug slows the ventricular response (115).

Procainamide

Procainamide is a sodium channel blocker which may augment other anticholinergic (antivagal) actions. It is metabolized by the liver to create N-acetyl procainamide (NAPA). NAPA is excreted in the urine. Metabolism is enhanced in "fast acetylators." Half of all Caucasians and 90% of orientals are fast acetylators. Procainamide-induced lupus, with a positive antinuclear antibody titer, has been noted in "slow acetylators" (52).

Maternal and fetal procainamide levels are nearly identical following transplacental transfer from maternal to fetal circulation. Procainamide reaches the fetus within 30 to 40 minutes of administration, and has a maximal effect within 120 minutes, and no effect 9 hours after administration (131). *Therefore, to maintain therapeutic serum levels, procainamide should be administered at least every eight hours.* Fetal concentration may be 30% to 130% of maternal concentration. The concentration of NAPA in the fetus is 90% to 120% of the maternal concentration (52).

Procainamide is usually given IV. It may be given to the woman or injected into the fetus' umbilical vein (25). Procainamide, 340 mg, was given slowly (30 mg/minute) IV on 2 occasions to treat fetal SVT that was resistant to digoxin and propranolol. The procainamide maintenance dose was 1 mg/minute and was increased to 3 mg/minute. Eventually, the woman was given sustained-release oral procainamide (Procan SR), 1 gram every 6 hours by mouth, which was later reduced to 740 mg every 4 hours. The neonate required digoxin, propranolol, and procainamide (121).

Maternal toxic side effects have been reported, and are often due to agranulocytosis, a deficiency of basophils, eosinophils, and neutrophils. Toxic effects include:
- hypotension with QRS and QT prolongation, especially if IV doses exceeded 600 mg
- nausea
- vomiting
- malaise
- fever during the first days of treatment
- agranulocytosis.

Agranulocytosis occurred in 0.2% of women, and is related to fever, prostration, and bleeding ulcers of the rectum, mouth, and vagina (25-26, 52, 55). Prior to and after procainamide administration, maternal blood pressure should be recorded. If procainamide is given with aminoglycosides (such as digoxin) or antihypertensives, there is a heightened risk of hypotension. Excretion is decreased 44% if it is given with cimetidine and decreased 18% if it is given with ranitidiine. If toxic effects occur, a complete blood count with differential may be ordered to rule out agranulocytosis. Side effects, such as nausea and vomiting, should be reported to the physician and may be treated symptomatically.

Quinidine

Quinidine is a vagolytic, α-adrenergic blocking drug for treatment of atrial flutter (52, 114). Quinidine is also a β-adrenergic stimulant (52). Therefore, this drug can slow the atrial rate but may increase AV conduction and the ventricular rate (52, 115). To prevent ventricular tachycardia, quinidine is often given with digoxin, a β-blocker, or verapamil. Eighty percent of this drug is metabolized in the liver and 20% is excreted by the kidneys.

The usual dose of quinidine is 200 to 300 mg by mouth 3 or 4 times a day. A plasma steady-state is achieved in one to two days. The therapeutic plasma concentration is 2 to 5 μg/ml. Twenty-four to 94% is transported to the fetus and higher unbound drug levels were found in the fetus and neonate than the woman, suggesting the fetal concentration should be interpreted with caution. Metabolism of quinidine increases if it is given in conjunction with barbiturates, phenytoin, or rifampin (52). Maternal toxic side effects have been reported and include:

- cinchonism or
    deafness
    headache
    ringing in the ears (tinnitus)
    nausea
    disturbed vision
- ventricular tachycardia
    diagnosed as Torsades de Pointes with prolonged QT
    intervals
- uterine contractions
- neonatal thrombocytopenia
- a rise in serum digoxin levels (quinidine decreases renal and biliary secretion/excretion of digoxin) and
- in high doses, eighth cranial nerve damage (52, 124).

Toxicity is more common if quinidine is given with cimetidine, amiodarone, and verapamil, partly due to decreased hepatic metabolism of the drug (52).

Amiodarone

Amiodarone is a class III drug with class I, II, IV, and α-adrenergic and β-adrenergic blocking properties. It prolongs the PR, QRS, and QT intervals and is metabolized in the liver and excreted in biliary and fecal routes. The plasma elimination half-life is 50 to 60 days! Fetal levels are 10 to 50% of maternal levels. Adverse effects include hypothyroidism (5 to 8%) and hyperthyroidism (2 to 5%) usually 2 weeks after drug therapy has begun. If the fetus develops hypothyroidism, the neonate may need L-thyroxine. Use of amiodarone increases the plasma digoxin concentration, most likely by inhibition of renal excretion of digoxin (52). Amiodarone is usually a very effective, but potentially toxic, drug therefore its use is reserved for drug-refractory, symptomatic, and potentially life-threatening tachyarrhythmias such as SVT or ventricular tachycardia (52, 132). The IV dose of amiodarone is 7.5 mg/kg. It may cause hypotension, therefore, maternal blood pressure should be assessed before and after drug administration.

If amiodarone is given in conjunction with epidural anesthesia, severe refractory vasodilatation and atropine-resistant

bradycardia can occur requiring potent vasopressors such as ephedrine, phenylephrine, and isoprenaline. If amiodarone is given in conjunction with general anesthesia, there is a risk of myocardial depression and sinus arrest, heart block, and severe hypotension. Therefore *amiodarone should not be given close to the time of delivery*. If a woman needs amiodarone to treat her dysrhythmia, vasopressors, external pacing backup, a cardiologist, and a perinatologist should be available at the time of labor and birth (133).

Amiodarone has been used to treat fetal SVT as early as 25 weeks' gestation, particularly after other drugs have failed to cardiovert the fetus and there was evidence of hydrops (132). A 27 week fetus with severe hydrops with a right pleural effusion and scalp edema had a 1:1 atrial-ventricular rate of 240 bpm which changed to atrial flutter with a 2:1 AV block within 48 hours during sotalol and flecainide therapy. The atrial rate was 480 bpm and the ventricular rate was 240 bpm. Since the fetus was becoming more compromised and was unresponsive to sotalol and flecainide, physicians decided to administer amiodarone directly into the umbilical vein. The umbilical vein dose was 15 mg in 15 ml (7 mg/kg plus 25% for the placental circulation). After umbilical vein administration, the needle was moved into the fetal peritoneal cavity and 80 ml of ascites was aspirated. The maternal oral dose was 200 mg every 8 hours which was reduced to 200 mg a day after 2 weeks. Within 24 hours of the umbilical vein dose, the atrial rate dropped to 280 bpm with a 2:1 AV block. At that point, another dose of amiodarone (15 mg in 15 ml) was delivered into the fetal peritoneum (intraperitoneal). The baby was delivered at 37 weeks' gestation and was diagnosed with congenital sinoatrial disease (sick sinus syndrome) with atrial flutter and sinus bradycardia (50).

Concerns exist regarding amiodarone's long half-life and the effect of this drug on fetal, neonatal, and maternal thyroid function (26). Neonatal hypothyroid goiter is a possible complication of maternal amiodarone administration (132). According to Ito and Magee (52) there are 75 mg of iodine in 200 mg of amiodarone. As a result of this high iodine concentration, amiodarone inhibits thyroidal iodine conversion to thyroxine which causes an increase in thyroid stimulating hormone (TSH), increasing the risk of fetal goiter. Fetal and maternal thyroxine (T_4) levels, TSH, and triiodothyronine (T_3) may be assessed during drug therapy (45).

Table 7: Normal Range of Fetal Thyroid Hormones (45)

T_4	5.5 - 13 pmol/l
T_3	9 - 18 pmol/l
TSH	2 - 10 mU/l

The optimal daily dose of iodine is 200 to 800 micrograms (μg) a day. A woman who was given amiodarone to treat her ventricular tachycardia had preterm labor and a baby that

Table 8: Adenosine (52, 105, 108, 134-135)

Indications	Supraventricular tachycardia without SA node involvement, i.e., no Wolff-Parkinson-White Syndrome
Dose	Maternal: 6 or 12 mg IVP, may repeat 12 mg x 2 at 2 minute intervals
	Fetal: 300 μg direct IV (108)
Onset	20 to 30 seconds
Placental transfer	12% reaches the fetus, it is degraded by the placenta
Actions	Depresses SA node, slows conduction through AV node, shortens action potential of the atrial tissue with little to no effect on the ventricles, dilates coronary vessels, may increase potassium and decrease calcium conductance
Metabolized in	Red blood cells and endothelial cells
Biologic half life	10 to 30 seconds (its effect lasts no more than 30 seconds)
Plasma elimination half life	0.6 to 1.5 seconds
Adverse reactions	Chest pain, dyspnea, flushing, transient bradycardia, *transient heart block or asystole, e.g., for 6-10 seconds*, hypotension
Contraindications	sinus node dysfunction, use of dipyridamole
Interactions	Theophylline inhibits receptor binding with adenosine making adenosine ineffective, caffeine decreases adenosine's effectiveness, phenobarbital and valium potentiate the effects of adenosine
Assessments	*Blood pressure before and after administration, ECG during administration.*

was undergrown, although it was not clear how this drug might have interfered with fetal growth. Only 10 to 25% of the drug is transferred to the fetus suggesting the placenta retains a high percentage of the drug, possibly interfering with nutrient transport. Adverse fetal and neonatal effects of amiodarone include bradycardia, systolic murmur, prolonged QT interval, hypothyroidism (9%), small for gestational age (SGA), prematurity, spontaneous abortion, and death. Neonatal thryoid function should be assessed soon after delivery (132).

Propafenone
Propafenone is similar to sotalol because it has β-blocking activity. Propafenone also is a class IC (sodium channel blocker) agent. Propafenone suppresses ventricular discharges and has been used to treat atrioventricular reentry tachycardia, atrial reentry tachycardia, atrial flutter, atrial or junctional ectopic tachycardia, and ventricular arrhythmias (52, 94). Propafenone may be given IV or PO (94). It is metabolized by the liver. However, *1 to 10% of adults are unable to metabolize this drug.* Unbound drug levels are equal in the mother and fetus, however the fetal to maternal ratio of albumin-bound drug is 1 to 0.2. Adverse effects are similar to other β-blockers: aggravation of asthma, hypotension, dizziness, and blurred vision. This drug decreases digoxin clearance, therefore, digoxin doses should be halved when

propafenone is given. (52). Very little has been reported about propafenone as a treatment for fetal SVT. However, it has been used with partial success to treat neonatal SVT (94). The initial dose may be 2 mg/kg delivered IV over 10 minutes followed by 100 to 300 mg PO every 8 hours (45, 52). The serum therapeutic range is 100 to 1000 ng/ml (52). The average neonatal oral dose was 13.5 mg/kg/day. Propafenone was administered 3 to 4 times a day at a dose of 10 to 20 mg/kg body weight. Better results were observed in neonates with normal hearts (80% success rate) (94).

Adenosine
Adenosine (Adenocard) was approved for use by the Food and Drug Administration of the United States in 1990 (105). In 1992, Severson and Meyer (105) wrote "Adenosine is a promising new drug." Adenosine stimulates adenosine receptors to block conduction through the AV node (108). It has a rapid onset, and an extremely short elimination half-life. Therefore it must be given (100 to 200 μg/kg) directly to the fetus via the umbilical vein in cases of SVT, atrial flutter, or atrial fibrillation that were unresponsive to other antiarrhythmics (26, 31, 105). If the woman has SVT and needs adenosine because carotid sinus massage and/or drugs such as digoxin (1 mg IV) or verapamil (12.5 mg IV) failed to cardiovert her SVT, adenosine (6 to 12 mg) may be given IV push, followed by at least 1 ml of normal saline. It has no

Table 9 summarizes antiarrhythmic medications used to treat supraventricular tachycardia, atrial flutter, and atrial fibrillation.

Table 9: Antiarrhythmic Medications (25-26, 39, 42, 52, 89, 96-97, 128, 133)

DRUG	MATERNAL DOSE	THERAPEUTIC SERUM LEVEL
Digoxin	0.25 to 1.0 mg every 8 hr PO 0.25 to 0.75 mg every 8 hrs IV	0.5 to 2 ng/ml
Sotalol	80 mg every 12 hours PO	
Flecainide	0.5 to 2 mg/kg in 30 minutes IV 150 mg PO every 12 hours then 100 mg PO every 8 or 12 hours	0.2 to 1 μg/ml
Verapamil	80 to 100 mg every 6 to 8 hrs IV 120 to 160 mg every 8 hrs PO	50 to 100 ng/ml
Propranolol	1 to 3 mg IV given VERY slow (< 1 mg/minute), may be repeated in 2 to 5 minutes Up to 320 mg/day in divided doses every 6 to 8 hrs IV	20 to 100 ng/ml
Procainamide	6 mg/kg every 4 hrs IV or 100 mg IV over 4 minutes, repeated every 5 minutes until therapeutic goal, toxicity, or 1 gram has been given or 20 mg/minute until 1 gm is given Maintenance dose: 2 to 6 mg/min IV or 7.2 gm/day PO	3 to 14 μg/ml or 8 to 20 μg/ml of NAPA
Quinidine	200 to 300 mg every 6 or 8 hrs PO	2 to 5 μg/ml
Amiodarone	7.5 mg/kg IV or 25 mg/kg/day or 1600 mg/day	
Propafenone	2 mg/kg over 10 minutes IV then 100 to 300 mg every 8 hrs PO	100 to 1000 ng/ml

effect on uterine activity (134). It will not cross the placenta nor affect the FHR (52, 134).

MANAGEMENT OF WOMEN WHO ARE RECEIVING ANTIARRHYTHMICS

Prior to administration of an antiarrhythmic, a maternal ECG should be obtained and the maternal blood pressure and heart rate and rhythm should be assessed and recorded. The FHR should be assessed and recorded. If the maternal rhythm is irregular or abnormally slow, suggesting heart block, the drug should be withheld until the woman is evaluated by a physician. Oral doses of antiarrhythmic medications, such as flecainide, should not be given with milk. Six hours after the first IV dose and 10 hours after the first PO dose of digoxin, serum levels may be drawn (125). Maternal thyroid function may also be assessed if amiodarone is administered.

It may take as many as five or more days for the fetus to establish a NSR (122). During this time, women may need reassurance about their fetus' health. Frequent assessment of the FHR may be necessary to allay maternal fear, or daily ultrasound evaluation may be done to assess signs of cardiac failure (97). If continuous fetal monitoring is ordered, the nurse should request that orders specify it be removed for maternal bathing and/or other activities such as ambulation. Daily maternal ECGs may be ordered (128). Since

hypokalemia predisposes women to digoxin toxicity, daily electrolytes may be drawn (52). If hydrops fetalis was diagnosed, an ultrasound examination may occur daily to evaluate the resolution of hydrops. When the woman goes home from the hospital, she may be instructed to use a Doppler to assess the FHR twice a day (3).

BRADYARRHYTHMIAS: ATRIOVENTRICULAR (HEART) BLOCK

Bradycardia has been defined as a sustained FHR below 100 bpm (39). However, the FHR during heart block is usually 45 to 80 bpm (2, 28, 39, 48, 51, 136). Suspect heart block if the FHR is stable at less than 60 BPM *and the fetus is moving* (2). Features of heart block include:

- occurs in 1 in 20,000 to 25,000 live births (137-139)
- reported as early as 13 weeks' gestation (2:1 block) (140)
- as many as 86% had structural cardiac anomalies, but overall about 47% have anomalies (26, 137-138)
- as many as 50% have mothers with an autoimmune collagen vascular disease related to atrial axis discontinuity with the SA and AV node replaced by fibrous and adipose tissue and calcification along ventricular portions of the conduction system and the SA node (138-139)
- may be a result of a viral infection with myocarditis and heart block (32)

- if there is complete heart block, there is no in utero treatment and almost 50% of neonates need a permanent pacemaker (42, 138)
- delivery is prompted by a FHR less than 50 bpm with hydrops fetalis
- some or all atrial depolarizations do not produce ventricular depolarizations, i.e., dissociation of atrial and ventricular activity (79). For example, Fabbri and Hamner (48) reported a case of a fetus with an atrial rate of 144 bpm and a ventricular rate of 44 bpm who had hydrops
- P waves may not be followed by QRS complexes or there will be no relationship between P waves and QRS complexes
- if an ultrasound transducer is used to detect the FHR, atrial or ventricular or both rates will be printed
- if the spiral electrode is used, the ventricular rate will be printed.

Heart block occurs because the SA nodal impulse is blocked within the SA node, the internodal tracts between the atria and the ventricles, the AV node, or there are disturbances in conduction below the level of the bifurcation of the Bundle of His. An impulse from the His bundle often acts as the ventricles' pacemaker during CHB. The fetus is not in jeopardy until the ventricular rate approaches 50 bpm and the risk of congestive heart failure and hydrops increases.

Causes of Heart Block

In adults, heart block may be caused by increased vagal activity, digitalis toxicity, myocardial infarction with ischemic damage to the AV node, or hypokalemia (141). In the fetus, heart block is associated with cardiac anomalies or maternal connective tissue disease (2, 48, 142).

Structural defect. If there is a structural defect, the connection between the SA and AV nodes may be missing or there may be an abnormal AV node position (48). Nearly half of all fetuses with CHB have a *structural abnormality* (27). Therefore, when heart block is suspected, a two-dimensional "echo" may be done to examine cardiac anatomy. Neonates with a structural defect may not survive. For example, left atrial isomerism with nonimmune hydrops preceded neonatal death (26). If the neonate survives, as many as 95% of survivors live for 20 or more years (48).

Structural anomalies associated with heart block are:
- malalignment of the conduction system such as failure of fusion between the atrial muscle and AV node or AV node and His bundle
- atrial septal defect
- aortopulmonary transposition of the great arteries
- atrial isomerism (left or right) with anatomical discontinuity between the AV node and the conduction system
- complete atrioventricular canal with atrial isomerism
- pulmonary stenosis
- double outlet right ventricle

- double inlet left ventricle
- ventricular septal defect
- absent right atrioventricular connection
- anomalous pulmonary venous connection
- aortic coarctation (constriction or contraction of the vessel walls)
- pulmonary stenosis or atresia (no opening)
- subvalvular aortic stenosis (26-27, 51, 137, 142).

In aortopulmonary transposition, the pulmonary artery arises from the left ventricle instead of the right ventricle and the aorta arises from the right ventricle instead of the left ventricle so there is no communication between the systemic and pulmonary circulations. Life is impossible without septal defects and a patent ductus arteriosus to allow mixing of oxygenated and deoxygenated blood (55). Fox (143) reported a case of transposition of the great vessels with a hypoplastic, fibrotic sinus node. The neonate died. Isomerism is the presence of two left or right sides of the thoracic or abdominal organs due to abnormal embryonic development. Isomerism is associated with a 90% mortality rate (27).

Irreversible fibrotic destruction of the AV node. In the absence of a cardiac defect, heart block is a result of a change in the AV node such as its absence with atrial-axis discontinuity (5%) or AV nodal discontinuity with fibrous and adipose tissue in the area of the AV node (95%) (137). Irreversible fibrotic destruction of the AV node has occurred in fetuses of approximately 4% of women who have connective tissue disorders (26, 144). There is an 8% risk that a sibling of a child who was born with heart block will also develop heart block. Antibodies that pass through the placenta and "attack" the conductive cells of the fetal heart usually appear in the fetus after the 22nd week of gestation (144).

Connective tissue diseases include rheumatoid arthritis, anti-Ro (SS-A) lupus erythematosus, Sjögren's syndrome, Raynaud's syndrome, and scleroderma (137-138, 142). Sjögren's syndrome is characterized by deficient moisture production of the lacrimal, salivary, and other glands resulting in abnormal dryness of the mouth, eyes, and other mucous membranes. Scleroderma is characterized by fibrous degeneration of the connective tissue of the skin, lungs, internal organs, especially the esophagus and kidneys (55). As many as 60% of babies with complete heart block have mothers with *connective tissue disease*, such as rheumatoid arthritis or systemic lupus erythematosus (SLE) (27, 66). Fetuses have heart block due to conduction system fibrosis and calcification (48).

First-degree Heart Block

In first-degree heart block, the only abnormality is a prolonged PR interval. The QRS complex may be slightly widened. The P-P interval is shorter than the R-R interval. The QRS complex may or may not be distorted depending on the site of origin of the ventricular signal. To date, there are no reports in the literature of fetal first-degree heart block (2, 67).

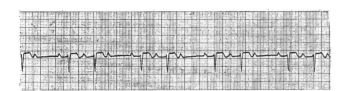

Figure 8.44: Second-degree heart block (adult ECG). Wenckebach or Type I or Mobitz I type heart block.

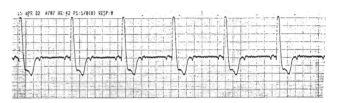

Figure 8.46: A 2:1 second-degree heart block (adult ECG).

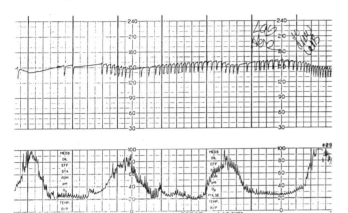

Figure 8.45: Probable Wenckebach (Mobitz I) heart block in a 39 week fetus with a normal karyotype. A fetal ECG is needed to confirm the diagnosis. The woman passed a blood clot approximately 6 cm in diameter. Light meconium stained fluid was evident as the spiral electrode was applied. This FHR persisted until delivery by emergency cesarean section. The neonatal hemoglobin was 5 gm/dl and the hematocrit was 16%. The baby received a transfusion of packed red blood cells in the operating room, but died within 24 hours of birth as a complication of acidosis and disseminated intravascular coagulopathy (DIC). There was a 10% placental abruption. The downward deflections suggest the nonconduction of the SA nodal impulse (absent QRS) followed by progressive shortening of the PR interval and an increase in the FHR.

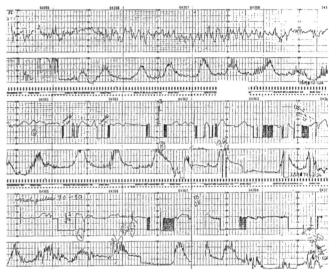

Figure 8.47: The top panel is the FHR detected by the ultrasound transducer. The middle and bottom panels are recorded by the spiral electrode. The intermittent abrupt drops to 60 bpm from 120 bpm reflect 2:1 AV block. (Reproduced with permission of Williams and Wilkins, Baltimore, MD from Freeman, R. K., & Garite, T. (1981). *Fetal heart rate monitoring*).

Second-degree Heart Block

Features of second-degree AV block include:

- commonly due to blocked PACs alternating with normal sinus beats (70)
- may be due to atrial flutter with AV block and ventricular bradycardia (70).

Mobitz I heart block or Wenckebach heart block is a form of second-degree atrioventricular block with:

- a progressive beat-to-beat prolongation
- caused by an increase in the PR interval
- which finally results in a nonconducted P wave
- then there is no ventricular beat or no QRS complex (a pause occurs) after which there is
- progressive shortening of the PR interval and the cycle repeats itself (55)

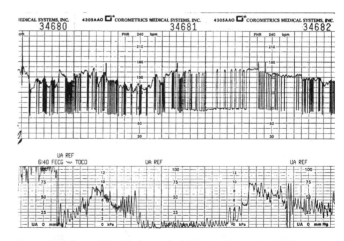

Figure 8.48: Second-degree heart block (Mobitz II) in a 41 week fetus who was delivered vaginally with Apgar scores of 7 and 9 at 1 and 5 minutes. Note short-term variability is present in the baseline between dropped beats.

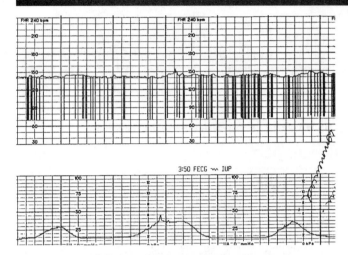

Figure 8.49: 2:1 AV block. Note the baseline near 140 bpm and the bottom of the dropped beats (ventricular rate during the block) near 70 bpm in a 37 2/7 week male delivered vaginally with Apgar scores of 9 and 10 at 1 and 5 minutes. There were two loops of nuchal cord. This tracing could be documented as "BL 140 - 145, STV +, LTV absent to minimal, with dropped beats. Suspect 2:1 AV block." Because the baseline is in the normal range, fetal myocarditis may be related to AV block. Had the baseline been tachycardic, nonconducted impulses would have been suspected.

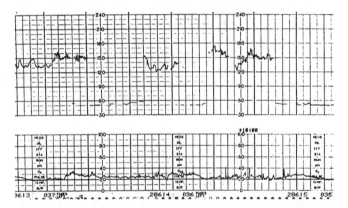

Figure 8.50: Intermittent heart block diagnosed at 33 weeks' gestation, probably due to immaturity. Cardiac anatomy was normal. Wolff (79) reported a similar case that spontaneously converted to a normal sinus rhythm after one week. No cause of the heart block was ever found.

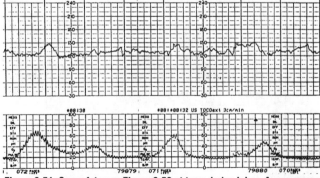

Figure 8.51: Same fetus as Figure 8.50 at term during labor. Apgar scores were 9 and 9 at 1 and 5 minutes.

Features of Mobitz II heart block include:
- second-degree or partial AV block
- a sudden nonconduction of an atrial impulse and a periodic dropped beat without prior lengthening of the PR interval
- may progress to complete heart block (55).

A 2 to 1 atrioventricular block is a type of Mobitz II heart block. During 2 to 1 AV block, the atrial rate is twice as fast as the ventricular rate. The tracing will contain dropped beats when there is no QRS complex, and the baseline will have variability (see Figure 8.47 and 8.49) (145).

Causes of Second-degree Heart Block

The fetus, who has SVT with atrial flutter or fibrillation, may also have second-degree AV block due to nonconducted impulses through the AV node (2). Heart block may occur due to an immature conductive system (see Figures 8.50 and 8.51) (48). Second-degree heart block may also be caused by myocarditis and impaired conduction in the bundle branches. Copel and Buyon (146) reported a case of 2:1 Mobitz II second-degree AV block where the atrial rate was 140 bpm and the ventricular rate was 70 bpm. After two weeks of maternal dexamethasone (6 mg/day), the arrhythmia changed to Wenckebach or Mobitz type I heart block. Within four weeks the rate converted to a NSR. If myocarditis is suspected during the antenatal period, corticosteroids that decrease cardiac inflammation to improve impulse conduction may be ordered.

Second-degree AV block is usually a temporary disorder of conduction, but it may lead to third-degree or complete heart block and rarely to ventricular standstill and sudden death. Based on the causes of second-degree heart block it is more probable than not that the fetus would be admitted to labor and delivery with the block and it would not occur "out of the blue." Health care providers should be skeptical if the FHR abruptly changes from a normal rate to a sustained bradycardic rate. For example, Wright (147) reported that during surgery to remove the gallbladder, the FHR changed from 140 bpm to 70 bpm. The woman was given lidocaine which "abolished the fetal bradycardia." However, an external monitor was used, and the report did not mention the maternal heart rate, which could have been 70 bpm. Therefore, this case report causes the reader to be skeptical about the effect of lidocaine given to a woman as a treatment for fetal heart block with an abrupt onset.

When ever the atrial and/or ventricular rate is unclear or there appears to be a wide variation in the baseline when the ultrasound is used (see Figure 8.47 top panel), the FHR should be confirmed by auscultation or real-time ultrasound (86). Fetoscopes may be nonexistent in some labor and delivery units, making it impossible to hear the ventricular rate. Even if a fetoscope is available, some arrhythmias are transient and will be missed by auscultation. Any FHR less than 100 bpm or greater than 180 bpm on admission should be investigated. If there is an irregular rhythm, and delivery is not imminent, the physician may choose to evaluate the fetus by real-time ultrasound or echocardiography. The nurse should notify the physician of

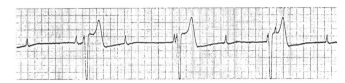

Figure 8.52: Complete heart block produces a bradycardic rate (adult ECG).

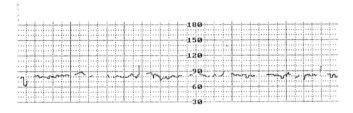

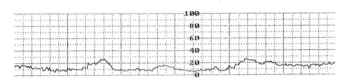

Figure 8.53: Complete heart block. An ultrasound transducer-derived FHR near 80 bpm in a term fetus with Apgar scores of 7 and 7 at 1 and 5 minutes. The FHR remained near 80 bpm and differed from the maternal heart rate. After birth, the neonate had blocked premature atrial depolarizations, but was discharged with essentially a normal sinus rhythm and occasional premature atrial contractions. There were no structural cardiac defects and "no unusual maternal labs."

any auscultated irregular rhythm. While it may seem that the irregular rhythm is heard on the audio output of the fetal monitor, this is an unreliable method to assess an arrhythmia because it is a machine-generated sound (2).

Thus, to confirm the ventricular rate, a fetoscope or real-time ultrasound must be used. If the hand-held Doppler records a faster rate (most likely the atrial rate) than the rate heard with a fetoscope or Pinard stethoscope, and the fetoscope rate is below 90 bpm and differs from the maternal heart rate, heart block should be suspected. If there is a 2 to 1 heart block, the FHR head with the fetoscope may be half of the rate printed when an external ultrasound device is used. The external ultrasound may detect the atrial rate and/or the ventricular rate (67). If the FHR baseline abruptly changes to a bradycardic or tachycardic rate, maternal heart rate should be assessed and the FHR may be confirmed by auscultation. If the spiral electrode is used, the recorded rate should reflect the fetal ventricular rate.

Third-degree Heart Block

Third-degree heart block is the same as congenital heart block, congenital complete heart block (CCHB), and complete heart block (CHB). During CHB, there is an absence of SA node impulse conduction to the ventricles. Instead, the ventricular pacemaker is located below the AV node producing an atrioventricular junctional rhythm. The atria and ventricles beat independently, each controlled by a separate pacemaker. CHB is more common than first- or second-degree

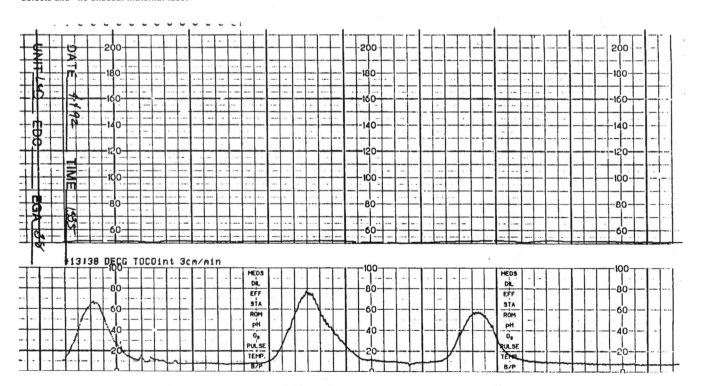

Figure 8.54: Complete heart block. This spiral-electrode derived tracing printed on European-scaled paper (5 bpm increments) demonstrates a stable FHR near 52 bpm. Usually these fetuses are delivered at a level III center with a pediatric surgeon available to provide a temporary pacemaker if necessary.

block when a congenital defect exists (70, 145). If the fetus has a cardiac structural defect, CHB may be caused by abnormal connections at the atrioventricular junction due to atrial isomerism, a discordant AV connection, or an abnormal AV junction (146). In adults, third-degree heart block is usually a result of injury to the AV junctional area, the conduction system below it, or digitalis toxicity (145). Complete heart block, detected with a spiral electrode, produces a smooth, stable baseline, often between 45 and 60 bpm. CHB has been found as early as 16 weeks' gestation (48).

Frank-Starling Mechanism. The Frank-Starling Mechanism was operational, but limited, during CHB in an 18 week fetus (76, 142). The Frank-Starling Mechanism compensates for the slow heart rate and increases systolic performance and stroke volume (8). Although the FHR is slow, the heart pumps out more blood than it would at a normal FHR. The increase in stroke volume is due to:
- increased ventricular size and wall thickness
- increased ventricular filling (volume)
- increased fractional shortening
- increased ventricular output (75-76).

Even with a bradycardic FHR below 80 bpm, the fetus is able to increase stroke volume by increasing fractional shortening or the index of ventricular function which correlates with stroke volume. The fetal heart can pump 11.4 to 12.6 ml per cardiac contraction (148). Circulatory efficiency is seldom affected in cases of heart block, and infants have been delivered vaginally, especially when fetal SpO_2 or pH have been monitored during labor. Neonates with complete heart block should be delivered at a medical center with neonatology services, as the neonate may require a pacemaker after birth. In rare cases, the condition improves or disappears spontaneously after birth without treatment (79). A pacemaker is most likely needed if the ventricular rate is less than 50 bpm. Therefore, a pediatric cardiologist should be in attendance at delivery (48).

ANTIPHOSPHOLIPID ANTIBODY SYNDROME (APAS)

Antiphospholipid antibody syndrome is a disorder of the maternal immune system. The presence of *IgG and/or IgM antiphosphatidylserine and/or antiphosphatidylinositol antibodies* confirm the diagnosis. Other autoantibodies found in women with APAS include:
- lupus anticoagulant antibodies
- IgG anticardiolipin
- immunoglobulin M (IgM) anticardiolipin
- antinuclear or anti-double-stranded deoxyribonucleic acid antibodies (anti-DNA), including
  • IgG anti-Ro (anti-SS-A) and/or
  • anti-La (anti-SS-B)
- rheumatoid factor.

Antiphospholipid antibodies damage blood vessels and activate platelets to liberate thromboxane which causes vasoconstriction and platelet agglutination (149). Phosphatidylserine, phosphatidylethanolamine, and phosphatidylcholine are principal components of cell plasma membranes. Phosphatidylserine is on the outer surface of cells and therefore reacts with antibodies. *Lupus anticoagulant, anticardiolipin, and antiphosphatidylserine antibodies* appear to be from the same family of autoantibodies, however, their relationship was unclear in 1996 (150).

Autoantibodies may be detected by an enzyme linked immunoassay (ELISA), an immunoblot technique that uses recombinant SS-A/Ro antigen, and/or an immunodiffusion test (144, 146, 151-152). *Rheumatoid factor* is normally less than 60 units/ml (138).

Lupus anticoagulant (LAC) antibodies. Lupus anticoagulant antibodies are antiphospholipid antibodies that disrupt endothelial and platelet cells and decrease prostacyclin (PGI_2) production in some women (149, 153). Prostacyclin is a vasodilator that also decreases platelet adhesiveness. Lupus anticoagulant is a "double misnomer" according to Gilson (149) because most women who are positive for this antibody do not have systemic lupus erythematosus; and, the antibody is an anticoagulant in vitro but a thrombotic agent in vivo.

Anticardiolipin antibody. Ten to 30% of people with lupus anticoagulant antibodies also have anticardiolipin antibodies. Anticardiolipin antibodies are antiphospholipid antibodies that have anticoagulant properties in vitro but thrombotic properties in vivo (149). Anticardiolipin antibody syndrome is now called antiphospholipid antibody syndrome. Cardiolipin is a phospholipid and part of the mitochondrial membrane within cells (150, 154). *Anticardiolipin antibodies* may be measured with a cofactor-dependent ELISA (155). β_2-glycoprotein I is the plasma cofactor that binds anticardiolipin antibodies to cardiolipin phospholipids (154). Aoki (151) reported that β_2-glycoprotein I-dependent anticardiolipin antibodies were a more specific marker of autoimmune disease and thrombotic risk than cofactor-independent anticardiolipin antibodies. In addition, he noted autoimmune diseases often involve more than one autoantibody type. Women, who were positive for both anticardiolipin and lupus anticoagulant antibodies, had a higher rate of spontaneous abortion, fetal death, arterial and venous thrombosis, and thrombocytopenia.

Anti-SS-A(Ro) antibody. Anti-SS-A is a IgG antinuclear autoantibody which is directed against saline-soluble tissue composed of ribonucleic protein antigens. Cytoplasmic antibodies are *anti-Ro* antibodies (137). Anti-SS-A and anti-Ro are thought of as one in the same. Antibodies to SS-A (Ro) particles react with monocytes and cause myocarditis. Myocarditis alters the action potential required for repolarization because there is a perturbance in transmembrane signaling and calcium fluxes. When the concentration of anti-SS-A/Ro is greater than 1:64, Sjögren's syndrome may be present. The *SS-B (La)* antigen is on the surface of fetal myocardial fibers. Anti-SS-B antibodies will react with myocardial fibers and cause myocarditis (146).

Placental Damage by Autoantibodies
The placenta and the fetal heart are the primary target of maternal antiphospholipid antibodies. IgM antiphosphatidylserine or IgM anticardiolipin antibodies are in maternal blood that bathes the placental syncytiotrophoblast. These antibodies cause direct damage to placental villi (the syncytiotrophoblast and cytotrophoblast cells) and are related to decidual thrombosis and placental dysfunction (150, 156). Thromboses and increased syncytial knots occur and increase the risk of IUGR, abruption, prematurity, and early and severe preeclampsia (150).

Cardiac Damage by Autoantibodies
Maternal immunoglobulin G (IgG) antibodies appear to be transported across the placenta at or after 18 weeks' gestation (146). IgG antibodies readily cross the placenta and inflame fetal cardiac conductive fibers resulting in endocardial fibroelastosis or damage (48). When CHB is caused by transplacental transfer of maternal autoantibodies, the following occurs:
Antiphospholipid antibodies cross the placenta

Immune inflammatory response of villi and/or

Antibodies bind to cardiac conduction cells

Myocyte immune response ➤ Myocarditis

SA and AV nodes replaced by fibrous and adipose tissue
+
Calcification along ventricular portions of conducting system and the SA node

▼

Complete heart block

Figure 8.55: Autoantibody damage of fetal myocardial conduction cells creates heart block.

Endothelial Damage and Pregnancy Complications
More than 50% of antiphospholipid antibodies react with endothelial cell (blood vessel cell) surface antigens and are related to the development of venous thromboses, thromboemboli, arterial occlusion, placental ischemia, thrombocytopenia, spontaneous abortion, recurrent miscarriage, pregnancy loss (50% of pregnancy losses occur in the second trimester), IUGR, oligohydramnios, and stillbirth (151, 157). The reason they have an increased risk for spontaneous abortion may be inflammation of spiral arteries due to direct injury by antiphospholipid antibodies and decidual thrombosis, infarcts, and chronic intervillositis (156, 158-159). Women with anticardiolipin antibodies are at increased risk for

thrombosis, pregnancy losses, and an autoimmune syndrome (160). Thromboses form due to inappropriate and increased platelet activation which is stimulated by radyl-platelet activating factor. In addition, there is an increase in thromboxane production (a vasoconstrictor), decrease in prostacyclin production (a vasodilator), and inhibition of the anticoagulant mediators antithrombin III and protein C (161). If the woman with APAS remains pregnant, there is a 50% chance she will develop pregnancy-induced hypertension and a 20 to 30% chance she will have an IUGR fetus (156). If she also has a connective tissue disease, such as systemic lupus erythematosus, there is an increased risk her baby will have CHB (162). Mothers who appeared healthy at the time of delivery of an infant with CHB, have been found to later develop systemic lupus erythematosus, often within 5 or more months postpartum (163). *Therefore, any woman who delivers a baby with CHB should be screened for APAS.*

Systemic Lupus Erythematosus
Women who have systemic lupus erythematosus (SLE), an autoimmune connective tissue disease, have been shown to have a higher incidence of infants with CHB than women who do not have SLE (66). Women with SLE may also have the following:
- malar rash (on the cheeks)
- discoid rash
- photosensitivity
- oral ulcers
- arthritis
- serositis
- renal disorder
- neurologic disorder
- hematologic disorder
- immunologic disorder
- positive (> 1:80) antinuclear antibody titer
- positive anti-DNA
- positive anti-Ro
- positive anti-Sm (149).

SLE is associated with an increased level of nitric oxide or endothelium-derived relaxing factor (164). The pathophysiologic mechanism behind the increase in this vasodilator is unknown. Antibodies to tissue ribonucleoprotein antigen, the Ro antigen or sicca syndrome antigen (SS-A), and lupus anticoagulant antibodies, have been found in the sera of women with SLE (27, 165). SS-A autoantibodies cause immune-mediated cardiac conduction tissue injury. Women with SLE have an increased risk for cesarean section, hypertension, and a neonate who will be admitted to the neonatal intensive care unit. Fetuses may demonstrate absent end-diastolic velocity as a result of cardiac cell injury. They may also be IUGR and be born preterm (166). *One in 20 (5%) women with a high titer of the SS-A antibody (anti-SS-A), i.e., greater than or equal to 1:16, had a fetus with CHB.* The SS-A antigen has been identified in human fetal myocardial tissue from 10 to 20 weeks' gestation (66). Initially, CHB is related to myocarditis. As time passes, degenerative changes occur in the conduction system (167). The SA and AV nodes of infants who had CHB and died were found to be replaced with granulation tissue (168). Fibrosis in the His bundle has also been reported (169). To minimize the cardiac inflammatory process and to ameliorate signs of congestive heart failure, women with SLE may be given corticosteroids (148, 170). Antibody-mediated CHB *is irreversible*, therefore, treatment is aimed at prevention or amelioration of myocarditis once heart block is diagnosed (139).

Sjögren's Syndrome
The baby of a woman who had Sjögren's syndrome and anti-SS-A/Ro antibodies had CHB and needed a transvenous temporary pacing bipolar pacemaker electrode. This type of pacemaker is introduced into the right femoral vein and progressed until it reaches the apex of the right ventricle. It may be fixed to the skin with sutures. Sometimes the pacemaker electrode perforates the neonate's myocardium which can cause a hemopericardium (blood collection) and cardiac tamponade or pressure which stops the flow of blood. A permanent pacemaker must be inserted surgically for epicardial pacing (51). In another case report, the baby of a woman with Sjögren's syndrome had CHB with a FHR of 60 bpm at 22 weeks' gestation that dropped to 48 bpm with an atrial rate of 110 to 112 bpm at 28 weeks' gestation. By 31 weeks' gestation the atrial rate was 102 bpm with a ventricular rate of 42 bpm. The fetus had ascites, hepatosplenomegaly, pericardial effusion, an enlarged ventricular size, including enlarged wall thickness, increased fractional shortening, and increased stroke volume. Following a cesarean section, the neonate received IV isoproterenol and a temporary pacemaker was placed until one week of age when a permanent pacemaker was implanted (75).

Anti-SS-A, Anti-SS-B, and the HLA DR3 Gene
The majority of women who are positive for anti-SS-A (Ro) and anti-SS-B (La) antibodies have normal fetuses. Therefore, it is believed that another factor may be responsible for the cardiac damage that results in CHB. Olah and Gee (139) proposed that a virus may initiate immune damage, for example, the cytomegalovirus. Another interesting finding related to neonatal lupus syndrome and CHB is the HLA DR3 antigen.

HLA DR3, imbalanced cytokine production, and heart block. Autoimmune diseases have a genetic basis (171). For example, Sjögren's syndrome was associated with the presence of the HLA DR3 antigen (172). The genes that are responsible for the production of the HLA DR3 antigen are DRB1*03, DRB3*01, and DRB2 which are arranged as DRB1, DRB2, and DRB3 on chromosome 6. Vincek and his colleagues (173) at the University of Miami School of Medicine believe these genes evolved from a common ancestor which existed before the separation of the human, gorilla, and chimpanzee lineages. They believe these genes are more than

six million years old. These genes are recessively inherited, however heterozygous people, e.g., they have the DR2/DR3 genes or DR2/DR7 genes, have been diagnosed with systemic lupus erythematosus (174-175).

The HLA DR3 antigen is a human leukocyte antigen produced by HLA genes (176-178). HLA-B8, DR3 is "over represented" in people who have autoimmune diseases, subacute cutaneous lupus erythematosus, the neonatal lupus syndrome (with heart block), Sjögren's syndrome, and rheumatoid arthritis. The HLA DR3 antigen is also found in insulin-dependent diabetics (179-193). In fact, HLA DR3 and HLA DR4 are markers for diabetes susceptibility (194). HLA DR3 was associated with autoantibodies to types I, II, III, and IV collagen (195). Blood antiphospholipid antibody levels are significantly higher in young females who were HLA-B8, DR3 positive (196). Human B-LCL. 174 (DR3) cells express transgene-encoded HLA-DR3 (197). People with the HLA-B8, DR3 chromosome may have impaired T cells that have a low immune response (198-199). They have an impaired ability to produce the cytokines interleukin 1 (IL-1) and interleukin 2 (IL-2) and the receptor of IL-2, i.e., sIL-2R (198, 200). People with rheumatoid arthritis had a significantly increased level of HLA DR3 than their relatives who did not have rheumatoid arthritis (180).

Women who had children with neonatal lupus erythematosus and CHB had the HLA DR3 antigen. A woman who had a child with neonatal lupus and CHB also had autoimmune hepatitis. She was positive for lupus anticoagulant and anti-nuclear antibodies and was in remission due to immunosuppressive therapy (152). Women who had the HLA DR2 gene did not have a baby with heart block (139).

Testing for Antiphospholipid Antibody Syndrome
Women who have APAS usually have a history of recurrent pregnancy loss, i.e., three or more first trimester spontaneous abortions, an unexplained second or third trimester intrauterine fetal demise, unexplained thromboses, unexplained thrombocytopenia, recurrent and/or early onset of preeclampsia (prior to 34 weeks' gestation), IUGR, and the presence of lupus anticoagulant or anticardiolipin antibody. In women who had three or more spontaneous abortions, 5 to 10% were positive for lupus anticoagulant antibodies and 5 to 15% were positive for anticardiolipin antibodies. As many as 4% of "normal" pregnant women will be positive for these antibodies (149).

Management of Women Who Have Antiphospholipid Antibody Syndrome
In September 1995, Silver and Mullen wrote that there was no consensus on the best medical regimen for women with antiphospholipid antibody syndrome. However, treatment to prevent preeclampsia, placental thrombosis and infarction, IUGR, and fetal death has included low-dose aspirin and heparin to prevent thrombosis formation, and intravenous gamma globulin and prednisone for immunosuppression.

Low-dose aspirin. Low-dose aspirin (80 mg per day reduced to 20 mg per day) significantly decreases thromboxane production which inhibits platelet aggregation but does not decrease antibody titers (149, 153). Aspirin acts to block lipid peroxide (endoperoxide) stimulation of cyclooxygenase which converts platelet wall arachidonic acid to thromboxane. By permanently inactivating some of the existing platelets' cyclooxygenase, both thromboxane A_2 and B_2 production decreases (201-202). Since thromboxane also stimulates platelet aggregation, clot formation is decreased when thromboxane decreases.

Immunoglobulin. Intravenous immunoglobulin (0.4 to 0.6 mg/kg/day) may be given for 5 days to women who had a history of spontaneous abortion (149, 203). Immunoglob-ulins inhibit antibody formation and block placental antibody transport. Unfortunately, the cost of treatment may be $5,000 or more (149). Immunoglobulin injections were administered every 3 weeks until 25 weeks' gestation. In spite of this regimen, there was no difference in pregnancy outcome between women who received the immunoglobulin and women who did not receive injections (203). Immuno-suppressive drugs, such as Azathioprine, have been used to treat active lupus during pregnancy (139).

Corticosteroids. Women who were positive for anti-SS-A and anti-SS-B antibodies have been given corticosteroids to diminish the fetal cardiac inflammatory response (204). Unfortunately, corticosteroids increase the woman's risk of developing diabetes mellitus, infection, and poor healing should she need surgery for placement of a *fetal* pacemaker (a rare procedure) (205). Dexamethasone (four IM doses of 12 mg every 12 hours) and prednisone (30 mg/day) followed by dexamethasone (6 mg/day reduced to 2 mg/day) was initially administered to a woman at 28 weeks' gestation whose fetus had hydrops. Eventually following dexamethasone administration, the FHR increased from 48 to 60 bpm. At 35 weeks' gestation, the fetus had a heart rate of 27 bpm and was delivered by emergency cesarean section. The umbilical artery pH was 6.710 with a -21.2 mEq/L base excess. The neonate received a temporary pacemaker but died 18 days after birth (170).

Prednisone is largely inactivated by the placenta and has serious side effects, e.g., osteoporosis, osteonecrosis, adrenal insufficiency, and preterm labor and birth (146, 149). Therefore, *dexamethasone is the better steroid because it is not metabolized by the placenta and it reaches the fetus in active form.* Dexamethasone may be given IM, 4 to 6 mg per day. In another case following 6 mg per day of dexamethasone, the FHR increased to 65 to 70 bpm within a week from a rate of 50 to 55 bpm (146).

Heparin. Heparin, 12,000 to 30,000 units, may be given by subcutaneous injection every 12 hours instead of low-dose aspirin to increase the partial thromboplastin time (PTT) and prevent intervillous thromboses (149, 157). Unfortunately, heparin has serious side effects such as bleeding, osteoporosis, and thrombocytopenia (149). Women who are taking aspirin or heparin may receive a weekly partial thromboplastin time (PTT) (157). Heparin decreased the rate of fetal demise, IUGR, and placental infarction, but aspirin and prednisone offered no added benefit to 72 women diagnosed with APAS (206).

β-mimetics. In addition to corticosteroids, women were given β-mimetics (fenoterol or terbutaline 5 mg PO every 6 hours) in an attempt to elevate the FHR. From a FHR of 56 bpm, the rate increased to 87 bpm and hydrops improved in 4 of 6 fetuses who were 25 to 32 weeks' gestation (204). In another case, following 5 mg of terbutaline every 4 hours, the FHR increased from the 40s to the 50s (146).

Plasmapheresis. Plasmapheresis before 20 weeks' gestation, when transplacental passage of antibodies is more likely, has been performed without improvement in fetal outcome (170). Plasmapheresis does not reverse CHB, is a time-consuming risky procedure, and most cases of CHB are found *after 22 weeks' gestation when damage and autoantibody transfer has already occurred* (139).

Follow-up during pregnancy. Women who are diagnosed with APAS may be seen every two weeks during their pregnancy. They may have an ultrasound for fetal growth every four weeks. Nonstress testing will occur on a regular basis. The woman will be tested for maternal serum alpha feto protein (MSAFP) and platelets and partial thromboplastin times (149). Nurses may be involved in teaching women about signs and symptoms of thromboses or excessive bleeding. Counseling may be an important option for these women because of their history of pregnancy loss.

Prevention of CHB During a Future Pregnancy

One out of four women (25%) with a collagen vascular disease who delivered a baby with CHB had another child with heart block. To prevent autoantibody fetal cardiac damage during her second pregnancy, a woman with Sjögren's Syndrome who had a baby with CHB received 1 gram per kilogram of IV gamma globulin plus prednisone, 40 mg/day, which was decreased to 10 mg/day over 4 weeks. Drug therapy was initiated at 14 weeks' gestation. IgG was given IV again at 18 weeks' gestation at which time no anti-Ro antibodies were detected (144). Women with a history of APAS, i.e., they were positive for autoimmune antibodies and suffered a pregnancy loss, preterm birth, or had a baby with CHB, may also have a weekly fetal ultrasound (150, 156, 161).

DIAGNOSIS OF FETAL ARRHYTHMIAS

Figure 8.56 illustrates the diagnostic and treatment process of fetal arrhythmias.

Gaps or very fast or slow stable rate noted on external ultrasound tracing

▼

Auscultate using a fetoscope or Pinard stethoscope

▼

Irregular Rate
- suspect PVCs
- suspect PACs with heart block

Regular rate, stable
- fast (> 180 bpm): suspect SVT
- slow (< 90 bpm): suspect heart block

▼

Notify physician

▼

Physician may order tests for autoimmune antibodies if fetal heart block is diagnosed

Real-time ultrasound or echocardiography may be done to confirm cardiac motion and diagnose arrhythmia

▼

Echocardiography identifies cardiac anatomy, rules out cardiac anomalies, diagnoses arrhythmia, rules out hydrops fetalis ‰ if a cardiac defect, amniocentesis and karyotype determination may be done (137)

▼

Physician establishes treatment plan

Figure 8.56: Team approach to diagnosis and management of fetal arrhythmias.

Once the physician has identified the fetal arrhythmia and fetal hemodynamic status, the following may occur:

No Drug Therapy, Deliver
- If term with SVT and no hydrops: deliver by vaginal or abdominal route depending on FHR response to labor
- If term with SVT and hydrops: cesarean section and cardioversion of the neonate
- If term with CHB and no hydrops: monitor by fetal scalp blood sampling and/or fetal pulse oximetry to deliver vaginally or deliver by cesarean section. Pediatric cardiologist with temporary pacemaker should be present at delivery. Delivery should occur in a tertiary center with neonatal services
- If term with CHB and hydrops: deliver by cesarean section in a tertiary center.

Expectant Management (Watch and Wait)
- If lethal cardiac defect counsel parents
- If preterm with SVT or CHB: follow-up with ultrasounds at least every two weeks to rule out hydrops (39).

Active Management/Drug Therapy
- If preterm with SVT: consult with perinatologist,

administer antiarrhythmic medications, follow-up with ultrasounds, lab tests such as electrolytes, maternal ECGs
- If amiodarone is administered, fetal thyroid function should be evaluated (50).
- If preterm with SVT and hydrops: consult with perinatologist, administer antiarrhythmic medications, consider delivery if fetal condition deteriorates
- If preterm with SVT and "severe" hydrops: direct fetal medications and/or delivery (26)
- If preterm with a maternal history of autoimmune, connective tissue disease: consider use of IV immunoglobulin and/or dexamethasone to minimize cardiac conductive tissue damage.

When a normal sinus rhythm is established, weekly ultrasound follow-up will be scheduled until the baby is delivered. The neonate may need antiarrhythmics or cardioversion if SVT persists. If the neonate has CHB and evidence of compromise, e.g., cyanosis, a temporary may be inserted until a permanent pacemaker can be placed.

The physician should counsel the woman and her family about the significance of the arrhythmia and the treatment plan, including the possibility of pregnancy termination with a lethal defect, cesarean section versus a vaginal birth, the healthcare facility best suited for delivery, e.g., a tertiary center for CHB, personnel who might be present at delivery, risks such as congestive heart failure, and the neonatal follow-up such as medications or a pacemaker (34). The nurse is responsible for implementing the physician's plan, which may include administration of antiarrhythmic medications, scheduling future ultrasound examinations, and teaching women about fetal movement and kick counts or the use of a hand-held Doppler. The woman should be instructed to call the physician's office or labor and delivery if she believes fetal movement is decreased. She may be enrolled in home care and be asked to monitor the FHR with a fetal monitor or Doppler device. During labor, the fetus may be monitored by a fetal pulse oximeter, particularly if CHB was diagnosed and there is no sign of congestive heart failure such as hydrops fetalis (136).

ECHOCARDIOGRAPHY

Fetal arrhythmias are rarely diagnosed by FECG. Instead, heart *anatomy* is diagnosed by *two-dimensional echocardiography*. They *type of arrhythmia* is diagnosed by *M-mode (motion mode) echocardiography, and Doppler flow and color flow mapping* are used to evaluate the *hemodynamics* of the arrhythmia (48). Echocardiography is a sophisticated ultrasound which uses a 4 or 5 MHz continuous, linear or phased array Doppler device, a 3 to 5 MHz sector scanner, and a 2.2 MHz pulsed Doppler (38, 107, 207). If the woman was obese, best results were obtained by using a 3.5 MHz transducer (38). In spite of its "sophistication," the quality of the data obtained during echocardiography is diminished by maternal obesity, fetal movement, fetal position or lie, and polyhydramnios (32).

Who Needs Echocardiography?

Electronic fetal monitoring of the FHR raises the suspicion of a fetal arrhythmia but cannot diagnose an arrhythmia. If the FHR is sustained at a rate less than 90 bpm or greater than 180 bpm, or during auscultation there appear to be repetitive, irregular heartbeats, echocardiography is needed. A routine ultrasound might raise suspicion of a chromosomal anomaly, e.g., when there is unexplained hydrops, or might suggest a cardiac anomaly exists (70). However, routine ultrasound often misses an anomaly, for example, a targeted ultrasound picked up only 54.5% of fetuses who had a structural cardiac defect (36, 208-211). Since the ultrasound cannot detect the majority of structural defects, when an arrhythmia or cardiac anomaly is suspected, an "echo" should be done to diagnose the anomaly, arrhythmia, and/or hemodynamics resulting from these abnormalities (211). If an echo, FSpO$_2$, or fetal scalp blood sampling are not available, a cesarean section may be needlessly performed for a nonhypoxic fetus who also has a conduction defect (139). Other indications for an echo include:

- a family history of structural cardiac abnormalities
- any noncardiac anomaly or abnormal four chamber cardiac image noted on ultrasound examination
- the presence of nonimmune hydrops fetalis, i.e., hydrops is not related to Rh isoimmunization
- decreased fetal movement
- an abnormal karyotype
- a fetal arrhythmia is suspected due to an ausculated fast, slow, or irregular rhythm
- the presence of polyhydramnios
- an IUGR fetus
- at-risk women, such as women who
  - are obese
  - are insulin-dependent (type II) diabetics
  - have been exposed to teratogens, such as rubella, which might cause a chromosomal defect (38, 88, 212-217).

Obesity is related to a structural cardiac defect, but 20% of babies with a cardiac defect were missed due to maternal obesity and difficulty in obtaining a clear ultrasound image (218). Insulin-dependent diabetics are at risk for having a fetus with global cardiac enlargement or cardiac hypertrophy (214-215). In one report, 3.1% of insulin-dependent diabetic women had a baby with a structural heart defect. If a structural defect is found, fetal chromosomal analysis should be done. From 5 to 40% of fetuses with a structural cardiac defect also had a chromosomal defect (219).

Two-dimensional, Cross-sectional Echocardiography

Two-dimensional imaging is a *qualitatiave* technique (70). It can identify
- fetal lie
- the heart's position in the chest
- measurements of the four chambers of the heart
- the flap of the foramen ovale

- aneurysmal bulging into the left atrium
- inferior vena cava entering the right atrium
- valves
- septum
- aorta
- the pulmonary artery and aortic root (outflow tracts)
- pulmonary veins
- structures such as tumors, the cisterna magna (a lymph reservoir) and the anterior (ventral) wall of the heart (36, 56, 70, 207, 218, 220-223).

Cardiac dimensions are measured using multiple calipers and a trigonometric formula (224). The cardiac axis is the angle between a line drawn from the spine to the anterior chest wall and a line drawn through the interventricular (cardiac) septum. The cardiac axis alone identifies 63% of fetuses with a structural defect and is abnormal 100% of the time in fetuses with clinically significant structural defects (225-226). The heart occupies 1/3rd of the thorax. The atria are equal in size. The ventricles are equal in size and thickness. Two atrio-ventricular valves, i.e., the tricuspid valve on the right and the mitral valve on the left side of the heart, are near the atrial and ventricular septa at the center of the heart. The aorta arises from the left ventricle to the aortic arch with the head and neck arteries arising from it. The pulmonary artery is slightly larger than the aorta, arises from the right ventricle and branches into the pulmonary arteries. The aorta crosses over the pulmonary artery (30). Ultrasound machines capable of a two-dimensional scan also have a motion-mode (M-mode) capability (60).

Real-time Directed M-mode Ultrasound

M-mode echocardiography provides a real-time, *quantitative* measurement of cardiac activity. Using two cursors over the heart, motion of two distinct structures may be simultaneously measured. For example, atrial and ventricular events can be recorded to measure cardiac cycle durations, premature beat intervals, compensatory pauses, cardiac chamber activities and relationships (70). M-mode "echo" can
- identify ventricular size and function
- identify the aorta and atrial and ventricular movements to
- identify cardiac rhythm and diagnose the arrhythmia
- detect artial and ventricular wall motion and thickness
- detect atrioventricular (semilunar) valve motion
- identify the end-diastolic and end-systolic dimensions of the right and left ventricles
- quantify left ventricular systolic function and stroke volume
- quantify pulmonary artery systolic pressure
- measure cardiac dimensions and wall thickness and
- measure the size of the pulmonary artery and descending aorta
- measure the diameter of atrioventricular valves and
- quantify the ejection fraction (also known as the shortening fraction or fractional shortening) (32, 43, 70, 75, 207, 220-221, 227-228).

Fractional shortening is determined after 10 cardiac cycles (76). Normally with heart block, ventricular fractional shortening increases. However, it will be decreased and right atrial pressures will be increased when there is hydrops fetalis (75).

The P wave corresponds with atrial wall motion. Systole corresponds with the R wave and the closing of the atrioventricular (tricuspid and mitral) valves or ventricular wall thickening (32). Therefore, even though there is no FECG available, physicians are able to identify cardiac events that correspond with FECG events.

The atria and ventricles are observed simultaneously (48, 76). A linear-array ultrasound transducer is used and a cursor is aligned perpendicular to the ventricular septum at the level of the atrioventricular valves. Real-time ultrasound measurements of cardiac motion are recorded on a strip chart that is moving at 50 millimeters per second (76).

Doppler Blood Flow and Color Blood Flow Mapping

Pulsed Doppler can be used to record blood flow patterns and is a *quantitative* technique. Color flow mapping is used to examine valve function or dysfunction, e.g., regurgitation, to determine the severity and hemodynamic compromise experienced by the fetus (70). These blood flow analysis techniques

- measure hemodynamics of the chambers and vessels
- measure the volume and speed of blood flowing through the cardiac chambers, valves, and vessels, e.g., transpulmonary and transaortic blood flow
- pulsed-echo Doppler flow identifies the direction of blood flow in vessels and across valves
- identify flow disturbances such as regurgitation (8, 34, 43, 229).

A pulsed Doppler can be used to estimate ventricular output across the pulmonic and aortic valves. Peak flow velocity can be estimated as well (75). Color flow mapping is helpful in diagnosing structural defects, especially if the atrioventicular valves are insufficient or there is an intracardiac shunt with ventricular or atrial septal defect(s). Hypoplasia and atrioventricular valve obstructions can also be diagnosed (219). A microprocessor analyzes data obtained from the ultrasound images to calculate the cardiothoracic index, aortic peak velocity, ejection time, acceleration time, shortening fraction, left ventricular output, and left ventricular output indexed to fetal weight (220-221).

Transvaginal two-dimensional and Doppler echocardiography has been performed as early as 11 weeks' gestation and was used to diagnose hydrops fetalis, complete AV block, and valvular insufficiency (219). In 14 fetuses, a 5 MHz sector vaginal probe was used to diagnose complete heart block (4/14), atrial flutter (1/14), and PACs (1/14) (230). Usually transabdominal echocardiography is performed from 16 to 36 weeks' gestation (207).

Echocardiography is easiest between 18 and 22 weeks' gestation as the cardiac valves are well developed and the fetal size and position are easily identified (34). Often, the first scan is at 18 weeks' gestation and there is a follow up scan at 24 weeks' gestation (30).

Image Quality

Echocardiography uses ultrasound technology to visualize the fetus. Therefore, any factor that diminishes fetal imaging will decrease image quality. These factors include:

- obesity
- oligohydramnios
- polyhydramnios
- fetal position
- operator skill
- ultrasound equipment (30).

Anomalies Identified by Echocardiography

The following is a list of most of the anomalies that have been identified by echocardiography:

Vessels
- coronary artery anomalies
- coarctation of the aorta (constricture)
- aortic stenosis
- Tetralogy of Fallot with absent pulmonary valve
- Tetralogy of Fallot
- transposition of the great vessels

Valves
- Ebstein's anomaly of the tricuspid valve
- pulmonary valve atresia, stenosis, or dysplasia
- tricuspid valve atresia or dysplasia
- mitral valve atresia
- aortic stenosis
- restrictive foramen ovale or ductus arteriosus

Atria
- atrial isomerism (right or left)

Septum
- atrial septal defect
- secundum atrial septal defect
- ventricular septal defect
- obstructive foramen ovale

Ventricles
- one ventricle
- hypoplastic left ventricle with aorta atresia
- hypoplastic right venticle
- double-outlet right ventricle

Other
- hypoplastic left heart
- intracardiac tumor

- atrioventricular canal defect
  - this defect includes a large common inflow tract
  - if the tricuspid and mitral valve orifices are separated, there is a partial AV canal malformation
  - a single atrioventricular orifice with five leaflets is a complete AV canal malformation (230)
- asymmetrical septal hypertrophy
- endocardial fibroelastosis
- dextrocardia (the heart is on the right side of the chest)
- visceral situs inversus (the organs are on the opposite side of where they should be)
- ectopia cordis (the heart lies outside of the chest)
- bilateral renal agenesis
- polydactyly (extra fingers and/or toes)
- diaphragmatic hernia
- Web neck due to resolution of a cystic hygroma with lympathetic obstruction and flow-related cardiac defects; 60% of fetuses with web neck had a congenital heart defect (34-35, 37-38, 229-231).

Echocardiography is not perfect and one to four percent of fetuses with anomalies have been missed (37, 229). Additionally, a ventricular septal defect may be misdiagnosed when there is no defect (38).

VARIATIONS OF THE FETAL HEART RATE AND MURRAY'S GUIDE© 1996

Murray's Guide© 1996 is a two-sided card with a grid on both sides that includes conditions of the mother or fetus and interventions that may cause variations in the FHR pattern or fetal behavior. This Guide© was developed because it is impossible to memorize all of the factors that affect the FHR. It may be used as a job aide to assist the caregiver during pattern interpretation. After a systematic review of the tracing, it may be consulted as to the possible causes of the observed pattern. For example, tachycardia may be related to maternal anxiety, arrhythmias, hypoxia, etc.

The role of the caregiver is to determine possible causes of the pattern and the need to intervene. The choice of interventions will be based on the perceived cause of the pattern and the fetal and/or maternal response to treatment. For example, if the woman's temperature is normal and she is being treated with terbutaline for preterm labor, no intervention is required for fetal tachycardia as long as the FHR is less than 170 bpm. On the other hand, if the woman is hyperthyroid, one would expect fetal tachycardia from the transplacental transfer of thyroid hormone. Thus, Murray's Guide© is used to determine the possible cause for the pattern to aid decision-making. The darkened square denotes the change(s) in the FHR pattern associated with the maternal or fetal condition or intervention.

MATERNAL CONDITION OR INTERVENTION WITH EFFECT ON THE FHR AND/OR UTERINE ACTIVITY

CONDITION/ACTION	EFFECT
1. **Abdominal palpation**	Fetal stimulation rarely occurs. External manipulation of the fetus or the uterus does not alter the FHR, fetal activity, or baseline variability (232).
2. **Alcohol**	Decreased number and duration of fetal movements (233). There is no difference in the FHR between fetuses with fetal alcohol syndrome (FAS) and those who do not have FAS (234). Lower birth weight was related to paternal alcohol intake (235). Birth weight was inversely related to the amount consumed (236).
3. **Amnioinfusion**	Given in cases of oligohydramnios, meconium stained amniotic fluid, variable and prolonged decelerations (237-240). Uterine rupture may occur due to overdistention (241). The umbilical cord could prolapse due to iatrogenic polyhydramnios.
4. **Amnionitis**	Maternal infection reduces placental efficiency (169). Villous edema increases the distance between fetal capillaries and maternal oxygen in the intervillous space (145). Hypoxia stimulates chemoreceptors and cardioacceleratory nerves to produce tachycardia.
5. **Amniotomy**	Amniotomy increases the likelihood of umbilical cord compression and variable decelerations in labor (242).
6. **Amphetamines**	Cause the release of norepinephrine from sympathetic nerve endings. Expect fetal tachycardia (see Stress) (243). Sympathetic nerve stimulus. Increases maternal catecholamines, decreases fetal pH, increases fetal glucose, insulin, and lactate (244). Tachycardia may be a response to decreased uteroplacental perfusion and hypoxia (245).

7. Analgesics	Transient decrease (for up to 30 minutes) in FHR variability (246-248). Decreased number and duration of fetal movements (233). Analgesics are respiratory and central nervous system (CNS) depressants that cross the placental barrier rapidly (249-251). The *decrease in variability* is dose related (252-253). Nalbuphine (Nubain) may be associated with fetal bradycardia (254). Narcotics may increase oxygen delivery to the fetus due to a decrease in maternal sympathetic nervous system activity and decreased epinephrine levels. Epinephrine inhibits uterine activity. A reduction in epinephrine should improve uterine contraction strength, duration, and frequency (255). As a result of catecholamine reduction, there should be increased uterine blood flow, increased oxygen transfer to the fetus, and moderate to large increases appear in both maternal and fetal serum glucose (256). Analgesics may produce an undulating benign sinusoidal pattern, formerly called a *"pseudosinusoidal" pattern* within 5 to 10 minutes after IV administration due possibly to a direct effect on the autonomic nervous system or the fetal heart (257-259). *Decreased STV and LTV* with 50mg IV Demerol for 10-30 minutes (253). To decrease drug transfer to the fetus, IV injections should begin just after the peak of contractions (take 4 to 5 minutes to complete IV push) (250, 255, 260).
Intrathecal	Subarachnoid opioid administration was associated with *bradycardia* in 7 of 30 fetuses *within 30 minutes* after 50 µg of fentanyl was given. Uterine hyperactivity preceded bradycardia. The mechanism for hyperactivity was unclear, but may be related to hypoperfusion and cytokine release with prostaglandin production (261-262).
8. Anemia	Anemia decreases tissue oxygen delivery (263). To compensate for maternal anemia, the placenta responds by decreasing villous membrane thickness and increasing the number of villous capillaries, increasing the size of the intervillous space, and increasing maternal blood contact with villi. Placental weight may increase or not change (264). Reduction of red blood cells or hemoglobin decreases the amount of bound oxygen available for transfer to the fetus (249). Sickle cell crisis involves episodic capillary occlusion, decreased organ blood flow, and uteroplacental hypoxia, acidosis, and ischemia (265-266). The chronically hypoxic fetus may develop left ventricular hypertrophy without a change in left ventricular systolic function but with lower diastolic function due to a decrease in ventricular relaxation. Stroke volume and cardiac output increase as a hemodynamic adjustment (267). The fetus will not compensate as well if the maternal hemoglobin drops below 10 grams/dl. There was *decreased variability and recurrent late decelerations* when maternal hemoglobin was 7 grams/dl. The FHR should improve after maternal blood transfusion (268).
9. Anesthesia **Epidural or spinal**	Sympathetic nerve blockade, decreased uteroplacental S/D ratios, decreased umbilical artery S/D ratios, decreased uterine and umbilical vessel resistance, uteroplacental hypoperfusion, decreased intervillous blood flow, decreased oxygen delivery commonly precedes fetal respiratory acidosis (72% of fetuses), rarely precedes fetal metabolic acidosis (1 in 231 fetuses) (269-270). The fetal response depends on the dose of anesthetic agents and maternal blood pressure prior to anesthetic administration (270).
Epidural	Continuous electronic fetal monitor has been recommended during epidural anesthesia (271). Lumbar *epidural* block is most effective and least depressant to the woman (272). It causes a sympathetic blockade, vasodilation, and increases the risk of uterine hypoperfusion, which can be minimized by right hip elevation (left tilt) and fluid preloading with 1500 to 2000 ml of Lactated Ringer's solution (LR) prior to drug administration (269, 273). During epidural anesthesia, a decrease in systolic blood pressure of more than 20 mm Hg or to less than 100 mm Hg was associated with *increased variability (when Marcaine was used) and late decelerations* (274-275). Maternal temperature increases and increases the FHR (276). *Decreased variability* may be due to hypotension and uterine hypoperfusion (247). *Bradycardia* may develop due to a reflex mechanism or as a result of maternal hypotension produced by the drug (249). Maternal hypotension reduces blood flow to the uterus and placenta (252). Supine hypotension results from vena caval compression and decreased cardiac output (277-278).

Continuous epidural	There should be no difference in the FHR if a continuous epidural has fentanyl or does not have fentanyl in it. The FHR did *not* change when 0.125% Marcaine plus 50 to 75 µg of fentanyl were administered at 10 to 12 ml per hour (248, 279). If Marcaine and fentanyl were used, there was *a significant decrease in diastolic BP*, no change in fetal movement, *fewer accelerations, more late decelerations, and more mild variable decelerations* (280).
Paracervical block	Vasoconstriction of the uterine arteries may occur leading to fetal hypoxia with subsequent *bradycardia* (247, 281-283). Uterine hypertonus may occur due to uterine artery vaso constriction and hypoxia and have a direct effect on the fetal heart and/or brain (282, 284). Consider the pattern before the block, i.e., if there were decelerations, there was a 39.1% chance of bradycardia after the block (285).
General anesthesia	Expect high fetal umbilical artery PaO_2, especially if women receive 100% oxygen during the procedure (269, 286). Succinylcholine chloride (Scoline), pancuronium bromide (Parvillon), and diazepam (Valium) given during cardiac surgery *decreased FHR variability*. The effect was transient (287). Vigorous hyperventilation is not hazardous to the fetus (288-289). If induction with general anesthesia to delivery (cesarean section) took *longer than 8 minutes*, umbilical artery pH, PO_2, base excess and Apgar scores significantly decreased (290).
10. **Antiarrhythmics**	Adenosine (6 to 12 mg IV) had no effect on the FHR (135, 291). Other drugs cross the placental barrier (246). Propranolol blocks the effect of catecholamines, such as epinephrine, on β-receptors (130). Hypotension may occur and cause uterine hypoperfusion and bradycardia. See Hypoxia.
11. **Antihistamines**	Pseudoephedrine and ephedrine precede fetal *tachycardia* (292-293).
12. **Antihypertensives**	Methyldopa HCl (**Aldomet**) causes a net reduction in the tissue concentration of serotonin, dopamine, norepinephrine, and epinephrine. *Bradycardia* is an adverse reaction.
	Hydralazine (**Apresoline**) side effect is *tachycardia*. Atenolol (**Tenormin**) is a β-blocker or sympathetic nerve blocker that decreases the baseline rate from 143 ± 7 bpm to 133 ± 8 bpm, *decreases LTV 13.1%* to a minimal to average range, and *decreases the amplitude of accelerations* from 23 ± 6 bpm to 18 ± 4 bpm (294). Expect a nonreactive nonstress test (NST) even though the fetus is well-oxygenated. Atenolol may increase uteroplacental and fetus peripheral vascular resistance (295)
	Trandate (**Labetalol**) is a β-blocker that slows the heart rate by blocking epinephrine receptor sites in the myocardium, permitting unopposed vagal tone (141, 169). Propranolol (**Inderal**) has been associated with *decreased FHR variability* (246, 296).
13. **Anxiety**	Expect anxiety in women who have had a bad experience during a previous pregnancy or a history of a long labor (297). Small amounts of maternal epinephrine cross the placental barrier and may *increase FHR variability and create tachycardia* by directly affecting the heart muscle (145, 249). Epinephrine may decrease the intensity of uterine contractions, cause dysfunctional labor, increase or decrease contraction frequency and resting tone resulting in incoordinate or asynchronous uterine activity. Incoordinate uterine activity appears as small contractions alternating with larger ones (298-299). Anxiety reduction decreases the number of cesarean sections and pitocin augmentation, neonatal intensive care unit admissions, and labor duration (7.7 hours vs.15.5 hours) (300). Maternal stress and vasoconstriction may precede fetal *bradycardia* or *a prolonged deceleration* (301).
14. **Barbiturates**	Decrease in fetal movement number and duration (233). Sympathetic nerve blocker causing vasodilation and increased uteroplacental blood flow (301). Depresses fetal central nervous system mechanisms responsible for cardiac control, i.e., cardioaccelerator nerves (249). Accelerations may not appear until the drug is excreted. *Variability decreases* (145).
15. **Betamethasone**	Transient *reduction in FHR variability* and fetal activity after glucocorticoid administration with return to normal after treatment is discontinued. Effects may be mediated by glucocorticoid receptors (302).
16. **Caffeine**	A mild stimulant due to catecholamine release. Antagonist of adenosine receptors. Increases blood pressure. Decreases uterine blood flow (in sheep) 5%, increases mean arterial pressure 7%, but there is no change in fetal oxygen delivery with 8 to 24 mg/kg. An average of 2 cups of coffee (200 mg) had a similar effect, i.e., decreased uterine blood flow, increased mean

arterial pressure with no change in fetal oxygenation (303-304). Caffeine serum level peaks 30 minutes after a cup of coffee. The *FHR dropped* an average of 12 bpm one hour after caffeinated coffee was ingested, but not decaffeinated coffee. Fetal breathing movements increased 3 hours after coffee was ingested. Maternal glucose increased. The elimination half life of two cups of coffee is 4.6 hours (304). The half life of caffeine triples during pregnancy due to decreased clearance speed. Ingestion of more than *8* cups/day was associated with an increased risk of spontaneous abortion, stillbirth, and preterm birth (236).

17. Cardiac arrhythmias

Arrhythmias may be fast, slow, or irregular. The fetus may respond to maternal arrhythmias with an increased heart rate to increase cardiac output as a result of the need for greater oxygenation due to inefficient pumping of maternal blood to the uterus (249).

18. Cardiac disease

Conditions that decrease the pumping of blood reduce blood flow and oxygen delivery to the fetus. See Hypoxia.

19. Cephalopelvic disproportion (fetopelvic disproportion)

Fetal head compression in a tight or small pelvis compresses blood vessels of the head and neck to reduce cerebral blood flow, which activates the central vagus nerve, and decreases the heart rate until the pressure is relieved. Vagal responses due to dural stimulation result in *early decelerations*, often between 4 and 7 cm dilatation, and/or *variable decelerations* (usually during the second stage) (67, 305).

20. Closed glottis pushing

Prolonged breathholding with a Valsalva Maneuver is closed glottis pushing (306). If done in a recumbent, lithotomy position it is related to hypotension and an increased risk of an episiotomy or perineal laceration (307). Breath holding for 10 to 25 seconds decreases maternal SaO_2, fetal PO_2, and increases fetal PCO_2, increases intrathoracic pressure, and decreases cardiac output (308-309). See Hypotension. See Hypoxia.

21. Cocaine

Cocaine is metabolized by placental cholinesterase and converted to norcocaine in the placenta. Norcocaine is 500 to 900% more active physiologically than cocaine, and can be transferred back to maternal circulation or to the fetal circulation. The greatest morbidity of women and their fetus occurs in women who have decreased cholinesterase activity (310). It causes maternal and fetal vasoconstriction, especially in the middle cerebral artery, renal arteries, and internal carotid arteries (311-312). Cocaine-exposed fetuses decrease their urine output, increasing the risk of oligohydramnios (313). The cocaine-addicted woman was at increased risk for syphilis, gonorrhea, hepatitis B antigenemia, vaginal bleeding, abruption, preterm rupture of the membranes, and meconium staining (314). Within about 15 minutes after maternal cocaine use, its metabolite benzoylecgonine affects the fetus' brain structure, mental ability, and behavior and is related to microcephaly and brain lesions (316). The neonate will be unable to habituate to stimuli. The baby has an increased risk of IUGR, morbidity such as seizures, and more hospital days (315, 317). *Decreased variability* seen during antepartum NSTs may be a manifestation of the negative effect on fetal state regulation (318). *Late decelerations*, may be result of decreased uterine blood flow after maternal cocaine administration or abruption (314, 319-320). In cases of intrauterine hypoxia, the fetus does not dilate cerebral vessels, an expected compensatory response (321). *Decreased variability and increased uterine activity* are associated with preterm labor and abruption. Vasoconstriction may lead to fetal hypoxia and an exaggerated fetal cardiac response to hypoxemia, e.g., *marked LTV* (320, 322-323). Crack cocaine is 10 times more potent than pure cocaine. Addiction can occur in two weeks of use versus an average of four years with pure cocaine. *Increased fetal activity* is related to cocaine use. Newborns have an increased risk for microcephaly, anemia, hypocalcemia, low Apgar scores, tremors, irritability, and hypersensitivity to stimuli (324).

22. Contractions

Hypoxia due to decreased placental perfusion (325-327). No change in the FHR is expected unless oxygen reserves are low prior to the contraction. An abnormal labor was associated with a *higher FHR baseline*, especially *tachycardia and absent to minimum LTV with variable decelerations* (328).

23. Chorionic villus sampling

No effect on the FHR baseline but large fluctuations in LTV (329).

24. Cigarettes

See Smoking.

25. Diabetes mellitus

If diabetes is well-controlled there should be no difference in the FHR between the diabetic, the prediabetic, and the nondiabetic (330). Maternal vascular involvement and sclerotic arterial changes reduce uteroplacental perfusion (249). Placental growth may be reduced and placental villi may be edematous, which decreases the intervillous space size and increases the distance between fetal capillaries and maternal oxygen in the intervillous space (145). See Hypoxia.

26. **Eclampsia**

Immediately after maternal breathing ceases during the seizure, fetal bradycardia with decreased variability then rebound tachycardia occurs (331). Uterine hyperactivity occurs immediately after a seizure (332). *Late decelerations* may be present as well (326). Evaluate for abruption if late decelerations appear.

27. **Epidural**

See Anesthesia.

28. **Exercise**

FHR may not change, may increase, or may decrease (333). Exercise poses little to no risk to the fetus, but it may induce hyperthermia, decrease carbohydrate stores, and redistribute blood flow away from the uterus and other organs to the muscle and skin resulting in a *transient decrease in the FHR* during intermediate to moderate intensity bicycling (327, 334). The fetal effect depends on the change in maternal cardiac output, temperature, and uterine blood flow (333, 335-339). If membranes were ruptured, a cycle ergometer used in the bed increased uterine activity, but had no effect on the FHR or fetal movement. Some women thought their baby moved less during exercise (340). There was no change in cardiac output with isometric lower limb extensor exercises, even though maternal heart rate, systemic vascular resistance, and mean arterial pressure increased (341). There was no change in the FHR with 10 minutes of "maximal" aerobic exercise, but 16 of 45 fetuses had *bradycardia to less than 110 bpm for 10 or more minutes* within 3 minutes after exercise ended. The *deceleration or bradycardia* lasted 31 to 180 seconds and ranged from 43 to 102 bpm at its nadir. Decelerations were probably a result of an abrupt decrease in maternal stroke volume coupled with decreased uterine perfusion during exercise (342).

29. **Fever**

Accelerates metabolism of the fetal myocardium, increases sympathetic activity (249). Increase in maternal temperature *increases the FHR and decreases variability* (343).

30. **Heat stress**

Twenty minutes of 70º C (170º F) temperature in a sauna (which increased the skin temperature 5º C and rectal temperature 0.3º C) during 36 to 37 weeks' gestation increased fetal movement slowly and increased the FHR an average of 11 bpm 10 minutes after heat stress ceased. There were a few contractions in 5 of 23 women (344).

31. **Fetal vibroacoustic stimulation**

May cause fetal stimulation as a result of sound produced by an artificial larynx which is placed on the maternal thigh or abdomen near the fetal head. Increase in number of *accelerations* and *increase in variability* seen in healthy fetus (345). Acceleration followed by deceleration after vibroacoustic stimulation suggests the presence of a nuchal cord (232, 346-347).

32. **Hyperoxygenation**

Maternal PaO_2 between 172.8 and 343.2 mm Hg increased fetal PaO_2 (348). Fetal oxygen tension (PO_2) appears to be associated with variability. *Variability increases* with maternal hyperoxygenation (349). Accelerations and an increase in fetal movement frequency reflect improved fetal oxygenation.

33. **Hypertension**

May decrease uterine blood flow and fetal oxygen delivery. FHR pattern depends on fetal oxygen reserves (350). See Hypoxia.

34. **Hyperthyroidism**

Long-acting thyroid stimulating (LATS) hormones cross the placenta in varying quantities (249, 351-352). Uncontrolled maternal hyperthyroidism is a possible cause of fetal *tachycardia* (145)

35. **Hypoglycemia**

Maternal hypoglycemia may cause an increase in maternal secretion of epinephrine and a subsequent decrease in uterine perfusion evidenced by fetal *bradycardia* (353).

36. **Hypotension**

Maternal supine hypotension syndrome decreases venous return to the heart, maternal cardiac output and blood pressure (249, 277, 327). This limits blood flow to the uterus and the delivery of oxygen to the fetus. Decrease in cardiac index (21%), stroke volume index (21%), increase in mean arterial pressure (19%) and systemic vascular resistance (50%) (354). Lack of blood flow to the uterus may precede an increase in uterine activity (278). Uterine hyperstimulation and mechanical pressure on the aorta, vena cava, and iliac vessels result in uterine hypoperfusion, decreased umbilical vein PO_2, decreased fetal cerebral oxygenation, and in some cases *late decelerations or bradycardia* (277-278, 326, 355-358). Ephedrine causes the release of norepinephrine (243).

37. **Hypothermia**	See Surgery, also see Preeclampsia with magesium sulfate.
38. **Hypoxia**	A lack of oxygen in maternal blood may cause fetal hypoxia (246, 359). The fetal response will depend upon the duration of maternal hypoxia, but often includes *late decelerations or bradycardia*.
39. **Magnesium sulfate**	See Preeclampsia with magnesium sulfate.
40. **Marijuana**	Associated with preterm labor and birth (320).
41. **Narcotics**	See Analgesics.
42. **Oxytocin with hyperstimulation**	Hyperstimulation of the myometrium with compression of spiral arteries and reduction of blood flow can cause fetal hypoxia (249). The fetal response will vary based on fetal status before the hyperstimulation. Initially, *LTV may be marked and/or tachycardia may occur*. This pattern may progress to *late decelerations or bradycardia* (246, 360).
43. **Phenergan**	Depresses the central nervous system mechanism responsible for cardiac control, *reducing variability* (249). When given with narcotics has been associated with a *benign sinusoidal pattern and temporary loss of accelerations* (252, 258).
44. **Placental abruption**	Premature separation of the placenta may be accompanied by uterine hyperstimulation, hemorrhage, and hypovolemic shock (141, 249). Decreased fetal oxygen precedes *late decelerations, prolonged decelerations, and bradycardia.*
45. **Placenta previa**	Placental attachment to the lower uterine segment may cause early separation and hemorrhage (249). See placental abruption.
46. **Preeclampsia with magnesium sulfate (MgSO$_4$)**	Hypertensive vascular disease with arterial constriction reduces blood flow to the fetus producing fetal hypoxia (249). See Hypoxia. MgSO$_4$ crosses the placental barrier, and similar maternal and cord blood levels have been found (361). Maternal and fetal levels are closely related *within one hour* of initial IV administration (r = 0.89) (362). MgSO$_4$ may enter the brain (363). It is a CNS depressant with the potential to *decrease variability and frequency of accelerations.* The decrease in variability is not clinically significant, however, confirmation of fetal well-being may not be made based on accelerations or variability (364-367). MgSO$_4$ may increase the duration of the quiet sleep state in the fetus (368). MgSO$_4$ precedes significant maternal hypothermia, perhaps due to the inhibition of skeletal muscle activity which blocks shivering. It also causes vasodilation with heat loss into the environment. The low temperature *may mask an infection* such as chorioamnionitis (369). For example, 12 hours after MgSO$_4$ was initiated for preterm labor, maternal temperature dropped from 97° F to 95.8° F, maternal heart rate dropped from 94 bpm to 64 bpm, blood pressure dropped from 120/80 to 90/50, and respirations were 18/minute. After discontinuing the drug, temperature slowly rose to 98° F (370).
47. **Propranolol (Inderal)**	See Antiarrhythmics.
48. **Ritodrine**	See Tocolytics.
49. **Smoking**	Decreased number and duration of fetal movements (233). Tobacco is the most commonly abused drug during pregnancy (320). *Decrease in FHR variability, fetal movements, and transient increase in FHR* after smoking may be due to acute effect of nicotine causing catecholamine release, peripheral, and placental vasoconstriction plus stimulation of cholinergic postgang-lionic cells and nerves to release acetylcholine which inhibits SA node automaticity (7, 236, 371-372). Fetuses of smokers moved two times as much as fetuses of nonsmokers, which may be related to their increased catecholamine levels (373). When women smoked, there was an immediate decrease in fetal movment and *more nonreactive fetal activity acceleration determination (FAD) tests* (372-373). Smoking may *increase the FHR baseline* but does not result in fetal blood flow velocity and diameter changes (374). Vasoconstriction decreases fetal oxygen delivery and fetal breathing movements (375). Prenatal morbidity includes low birth weight, lower Apgar scores, inguinal hernia and strabismus if more than 1 pack per day (20 cigarettes) are smoked, hyperactivity, attention deficit disorder, decreased reading scores, and an increased risk of leukemia, lymphoma, and Wilm's tumor (236, 320).
50. **Stress**	*Norepinephrine* increases uterine tonus and contraction frequency and intensity. Blood pressure increases, maternal heart rate slightly decreases, and incoordinate uterine activity is possible. *Epinephrine* decreases uterine activity (it is a β$_2$-adrenergic depressor), acts to decrease blood pressure and increase the heart rate (243).

51. **Supine position**	See Hypotension.
52. **Surgery**	Sympathetic nerves are stimulated (see Anxiety). During surgery, shunting of blood away from the uterus occurs (301). The type of surgery may affect the FHR. For example, during mitral valve replacement, the woman was on heart-lung bypass and became *hypothermic*. *There were two decelerations to 60 bpm for 10 minutes* and *late decelerations* after bypass surgery ended. The uterus became "hyperirritable" during cautery (287).
53. **Terbutaline**	See Tocolytics.
54. **Tocolytics**	β-sympathomimetic drugs control excessive uterine activity and improve FHR patterns that reflect fetal compromise (376). They are given to stop preterm labor and have a cardiac stimulant effect similar to epinephrine which can produce fetal *tachycardia* (249). Decreasing uterine activity can possibly correct late decelerations, prolonged decelerations, and improve variability (246, 277).
55. **Tranquilizers**	Depress central nervous system mechanisms responsible for cardiac control with possible *loss of variability and accelerations* which resolves in 90 minutes after the drug has been excreted in 80% of patients (246, 377).
56. **Vaginal examination**	May cause fetal stimulation with increased variability and accelerations if the fetal scalp is vigorously rubbed (scalp stimulation) or may cause a vagal response if a fontanel is pressed. Variable decelerations indicate a vagal response.

FETAL CONDITION OR INTERVENTION WITH EFFECT ON THE FHR

CONDITION/ACTION	EFFECT
1. **Acidosis**	The fall in the FHR is usually proportional to the degree of hypoxia. In the decompensating fetus, the heart may be directly depressed and decelerations may be very subtle or nonexistent (277, 378). *Late decelerations* associated with fetal acidosis (326). Adenosine accumulation will cause a *loss of variability* (379-381).
2. **Acoustic stimulation**	Acoustic stimulation followed by a FHR *acceleration* is indicative of a nonacidotic fetus (382-383). An acceleration followed by a deceleration suggests the presence of a nuchal cord (346).
3. **Age**	See Prematurity. Maturation of central and autonomic nervous systems impact the basal FHR, the amplitude of accelerations, LTV, and the number of decelerations (384-385). See Chapter 3.
4. **Altitude**	Lower PCO_2, higher pH in umbilical vein and artery may be found (386). Clinically insignificant.
5. **Anemia**	Since there are fewer red blood cells to carry oxygen, *tachycardia* occurs as an attempt to provide adequate oxygenation to fetal tissues. When anemia is severe with possible tissue hypoxia, e.g., in cases of erythroblastosis fetalis or fetomaternal transfusion, a *pathologic sinus-oidal* pattern may be seen (259, 387-390). The decrease in STV and LTV depends on the hematocrit (391). *Loss of variability and decelerations* are associated with severe fetal anemia in cases of Rh isoimmunization (390, 392). As hypoxia worsens, the fetus releases epinephrine from the adrenal medulla and arginine vasopressin (AVP) (stress response) (296). *AVP is associated with a pathologic sinusoidal pattern. Pathologic sinusoidal patterns* have been associated with hypoxia (387). Oxygen consumption decreases (393).
6. **Anencephaly**	No specific FHR for defects, although a persistent flat FHR was associated with anencephaly (394).
7. **Antiarrhythmic agents**	Adenosine depresses the SA node's automaticity and slows AV conduction time. It has a biological half life of 10 to 30 seconds (135). However, maternal adenosine does not affect the fetus. There may be a transient vagal arrest after adenosine administration directly to the fetus.

8. **Arrhythmias**	Risk of structural cardiac anomaly (395). Antidepressants may increase the baseline FHR and produce a tachyarrhythmia (396). The rate may be *tachycardic, bradycardic, or irregular* depending on the type of arrhythmia.
9. **Asphyxia**	Decreased fetal body and breathing movements as pH drops (397). Terminal asphyxia is associated with unrelenting *bradycardia* (398).
10. **Breathing movements**	*Increased variability* (respiratory sinus arrhythmia) has been reported in association with fetal sucking (67, 399). A *benign sinusoidal pattern* was associated with clusters of fetal breathing movements (392).
11. **Breech presentation**	Uterine contractions may cause fetal scalp stimulation, which may stimulate the brainstem vagal or sympathetic nerve centers (326, 388). More likely, however, is the umbilical cord is more vulnerable to compression. If just the umbilical vein is compressed (mild cord compression) there will be chemoreceptor and baroreceptor stimulation and a *uniform acceleration*.
12. **Cardiac anomalies**	If there are multiple malformations, the FHR pattern was likely to have *bradycardia, variable decelerations, tachycardia, and/or decreased variability* 83.3% of the time. Chromosomal defects were associated with an "abnormal" FHR pattern 81.8% of the time. CNS lesions were associated with an abnormal pattern 71.4% of the time (400). Early hypoxia, amnionitis with or without fever, drugs, hypovolemia, congestive heart failure, maternal anxiety, maternal fever, and cytomegalic inclusion disease have all been suggested as causes of a change in the normal automaticity and conductivity of fetal cardiac impulses (2, 6, 63).
13. **Cardiac failure**	Hydrops may be detected by real-time ultrasound. There may be a tachy- or bradyarrhythmia.
14. **Electrode placement**	May stimulate fetus and cause movement, *increased variability,* and/or an *acceleration*.
15. **Heart block**	Third-degree heart block is reflected by a *stable bradycardic baseline usually less than 80 bpm with absent variability* (75, 139, 401).
16. **Hemorrhage**	Fetomaternal hemorrhage can result in *profound bradycardia, absent variability and/or a sinus-oidal pattern* (402-403).
17. **Hydrops**	Decreased fetal movement due to hemodynamic compromise (233). Usually associated with a tachy- or bradyarrhythmia.
18. **Hyperparathyroidism**	Congenital hyperparathyroidism and rickets causes severe hypocalcemia and a vitamin B deficiency. There will be *absent variability* and no decelerations with a normal pH. Probably the decrease in variability is related to the lack of calcium which depresses cardiac activity (404).
19. **Hypothermia**	Reduces myocardial metabolism, decreasing oxygen requirements (249). Oxygen transfer across the placenta is unaffected (405). *FHR decreases* as a result of maternal cooling and increases with maternal warming, e.g., during brain aneurysm surgery (406-407). Hypothermia may occur during $MgSO_4$ administration due to less skeletal muscle activity from the inhibition of acetylcholine release at the neuromuscular junction, and/or by a direct effect on the muscles (369-370).
20. **Hypovolemia**	See Hemorrhage.
21. **Hypoxia**	A fetal condition which is a result of decreased delivery of oxygen, prolonged hypoxia may directly depress myocardial electrical activity (249, 296). With mild hypoxia, e.g., with umbilical vein compression, the fetus initially attempts to compensate for the reduced oxygen delivery by an increase in sympathetic activity. There may be *marked LTV or uniform accelerations. Late decelerations* reflect hypoxia (145, 281). A *loss of variability and loss of accelerations* has been associated with adenosine accumulation following hypoxia and anaerobic metabolism (379-381).
22. **Infection**	*Tachycardia or a rising baseline* may be the first sign of a developing intrauterine infection, e.g., following prolonged rupture of membranes, even without a maternal temperature elevation. Tachycardia may reflect fetal sepsis (145, 249).
23. **Intrauterine growth restriction (IUGR)**	Due to chronic hypoxia and adenosine accumulation, the FHR pattern may include *late decelerations or variable decelerations with a slow recovery, and/or fewer, smaller accelerations and absent to minimum LTV* (408).

24. **Movement**	Fetal movement is associated with but not a cause of *increased variability* and *accelerations.*
25. **Occiput posterior (OP) position**	*A low FHR,* not less than 100 bpm, is associated with vagal activity as a result of continuous head compression in the OP or OT position. *Prolonged decelerations* have been observed in some cases (377). In addition, *variable decelerations* have been associated with the OP position due to a fetal vagal response (409).
26. **Occiput transverse (OT) position**	Pressure on the fetal head in a protracted or tight pelvis can increase intracranial pressure to create a vagal response. See Occiput posterior.
27. **Oligohydramnios**	Decreased fetal movement (233). See Umbilical cord compression, Umbilical cord prolapse. Loss of protection of the umbilical cord by the amniotic fluid may occur. Degree of oligohydramnios is positively correlated with unfavorable pregnancy outcome (410-413). *Uniform accelerations and variable or prolonged decelerations* may be seen due to cord compression.
28. **Pancuronium bromide**	A neuromuscular blocking agent that *decreases variability, abolishes accelerations, creates a benign sinusoidal pattern* that is 15 to 30 bpm wide. This drug has vagolytic effects and there is no fetal movement. Used prior to intrauterine transfusions. Fetal movement and accelerations were present 25 to 210 minutes after the procedure (414).
29. **pH sampling**	See Stimulation and activity. Clinically, prolonged decelerations have been observed in some cases (377). However, response to pH sampling depends upon the fetal condition. *Acceleration* at the time of pH sampling indicates a nonacidemic fetus (pH > 7.20). The absence of an acceleration does not always indicate acidosis (415).
30. **Prematurity**	The baseline is above 120 bpm and not expected to be higher than 160 bpm. LTV is present. Accelerations are present even at 16 weeks' gestation. Accelerations increase in size as gestation advances. As the vagus matures, the baseline FHR drops 1 beat per week and stabilizes at approximately 35 weeks' gestation. Dips, not decelerations, are more common in preterm than term fetuses.
31. **Postmaturity**	FHR pattern will depend upon placental function (47). Increased incidence of *variable decelerations* may be due to relative oligohydramnios (416). *Marked variability* and decreased amniotic fluid may be evident (296, 347). *Late decelerations* may be seen (326). *Decreased variability* suggests chronic hypoxia from uteroplacental insufficiency.
32. **Scalp stimulation**	Rubbing the fetal head with the gloved finger is a stimulus, which, in the healthy fetus should cause fetal movement and *accelerations* (145). Pinching the fetal scalp with an allis clamp will cause accelerations in the FHR if the fetus is not obtunded.
33. **Seizures (fetal)**	Seizures in utero may be evidenced by an unusual fetal heart rate pattern with blunted small recurrent nonperiodic variable decelerations and absent accelerations (a *checkmark pattern*). See Chapter 2.
34. **Small for Gestational Age (SGA)**	Reduced placental oxygen reserves, due to decreased perfusion of nutrients and oxygen to the placenta and fetus, may affect the fetal parasympathetic nervous system resulting in *decreased frequency of accelerations and loss of variability* (417-418).
35. **Sleep (fetal)**	Periods of quiesent fetal activity usually last an average of 40 minutes and no longer than 100 for minutes and are associated with *minimal to absent LTV* (249). The 28 to 30 week fetus is active an average of 10.3 minutes and quiet an average of 9.9 minutes. The 38 to 40 week fetus is active an average of 35 minutes and quiet an average of 18.3 minutes (419-420). In the term fetus with an otherwise normal FHR, a *prolonged deceleration* may be associated with a change in behavioral state and is usually not clinically significant (421). Fetal sleep transition states affect FHR variability (232).
36. **Stimulation and activity**	Fetal movement stimulates the nerve centers in the medulla oblongata to produce a transient *acceleration* of the FHR. *Variability will also increase.* Repetitive fetal movement for a prolonged period may produce a merging of accelerations to cause an acceleration which lasts several minutes (249). Fetal movement alters the configuration of the abdomen, putting pressure on the tocotransducer which creates spikes in the uterine activity pattern. Decreased activity may be due to an anomaly, anemia, hydrops, anoxia, or medications with CNS depressant properties (233).

37. **Temperature**	See Hypothermia. The fetus is normally warmer than its mother and body temperature influences the FHR. Epidural anesthesia has been associated with an increase in maternal temperature and the FHR (343, 422).
38. **Umbilical cord compression (vein only)**	Uniform accelerations or shoulders (primary and/or secondary acceleratory phases of the variable deceleration pattern) may be observed.
39. **Umbilical cord compression (vein and arteries)**	Atypical variable decelerations, prolonged decelerations, or bradycardia may be seen. In some cases, there is an agonal, bradycardic pattern.
40. **Umbilical cord prolapse**	Compression of the cord causes fetal hypertension and hypoxia which activates baroreceptors and chemoreceptors which stimulate a vagal reflex and *bradycardia* or repetitive *prolonged decelerations* (249).
41. **Vacuum extractor**	Application of the suction cup to the fetal scalp causes an *increase in LTV* (sympathetic stimulus) or fetal bradycardia (vagal stimulus) due to increased intracranial pressure (423).

CONCLUSION

Nurses may be the first to recognize an abnormal fetal heart rate or uterine activity pattern. This chapter presented arrhythmias and other maternal and fetal conditions that influence the fetal heart rate. Most fetal arrhythmias are innocuous. Tachycardiac rates of 200 bpm or more, and bradycardia rates due to heart block, will usually be detected during the admission assessment. Heart block usually has been present for a long time prior to labor, particularly if the fetus has a congenital heart defect. Complete heart block does not occur spontaneously during labor because it is usually related to a structural cardiac defect or myocarditis. Therefore, if a newly established fetal heart rate is noted during labor, the fetal heart rate should be confirmed by auscultation. In order to accurately assess the ventricular fetal heart rate, a fetoscope must be used or cardiac motion may be assessed by real-time ultrasound. The maternal heart rate should also be assessed and compared with the fetal heart rate. Both should be recorded. When a hand-held Doppler is used to confirm the fetal heart rate, it may pick up maternal aortic movement instead of fetal heart movement.

Cardiac arrhythmias need to be distinguished from artifact. Potential fetal complications of supraventricular tachycardia, atrial flutter, atrial fibrillation, and complete heart block are nonimmune hydrops and congestive heart failure. In some cases, medication may be administered to the pregnant woman to correct fetal tachyarrhythmias. The fetus with complete heart block may require insertion of a pacemaker after birth. Women with collagen vascular disease, such as lupus erythematosus and rheumatoid arthritis, are followed closely during pregnancy, as there is a 5% risk of fetal heart block (2). Echocardiography is used to assess cardiac anatomy, to diagnose the arrhythmia, and to assess the hemodynamic consequences of the arrhythmia.

Electronic fetal heart rate monitoring involves three complex entities: the monitor, the fetus, and the pregnant woman. An understanding of the physiologic mechanisms which affect the FHR rate is essential for accurate monitor tracing interpretation. When the maternal or fetal condition changes, or when multiple interventions take place during labor, the chance of FHR changes increases.

REFERENCES

1. Dunnigan, A. (October 1989). Signs and symptoms associated with cardiac rhythm disorders in the fetus, infant, and child. Comprehensive Therapy, 15(10), 27-37.

2. Shenker, L. (1979). Review: Fetal cardiac arrhythmias. Obstetrical and Gynecological Survey, 34(8), 561-572.

3. Battiste, C. E., Newf., T. W., Evans, J. F., & Cline, B. W. (July 1992). In utero conversion of supraventricular tachycardia with digoxin and procainamide at 17 weeks' gestation. American Journal of Perinatology, 9(4), 302-303.

4. Kolyer, C. (September 1985). CNE 7516 Basic dysrhythmia interpretation [Video course]. (Available from The Hospital Satellite Network and American Journal of Nursing Company) Nurses Continuing Education Program.

5. Young, B. K., Katz, M., & Klein, S. A. (October 1979). Intrapartum fetal cardiac arrhythmias. Obstetrics & Gynecology, 54(4), 427-432.

6. DeVore, G. R., Siassi, B., & Platt, L. D. (August 1, 1983). Fetal echocardiography. III. The diagnosis of cardiac arrhythmias using real-time-directed M-mode ultrasound. American Journal of Obstetrics and Gynecology, 146(7), 792-799.

7. Pappano, A. J. (March 1977). Ontogenetic development of autonomic neuroeffector transmission and transmitter reactivity in embryonic and fetal hearts. Pharmacological Reviews, 29(1), 3-33.

8. Reed, K. L. (August 1989). Fetal arrhythmias: Etiology, diagnosis, pathophysiology, and treatment. Seminars in Perinatology, 13(4), 294-304.

9. Murray, H. G. (1986). The fetal electrocardiogram: Current developments in Nottingham. Journal of Perinatal Medicine, 14, 399-404.

10. Yeh, M-N., Morishima, H. O., Niemann, W. E., & James, L. S. (1975). Myocardial conduction defects in association with compression of the umbilical cord. Experimental observations on fetal baboons. American Journal of Obstetrics and Gynecology, 121(7), 951-957.

11. Eriksen, B. C., Hausken, J., & Eikeland, T. (November 28, 1992). Cardiotocography with ST-waveform analysis for fetal monitoring. The Lancet, 340(8831), 1349.

12. Westgate, J., Harris, M., Curnow, J. S. H., & Greene, K. R. (July 25, 1992). Randomised trial of cardiotocography alone or with ST waveform analysis for intrapartum monitoring. The Lancet, 340, 194, 196, 198.

13. Jenkins, H. M. L. (February 1987). Fetal monitoring - present and future. European Journal of Obstetrics, Gynecology, and Reproductive Biology, 24(2), 110-117.

14. Murphy, K. W., Russell, V., Johnson, P., & Valente, J. (January 1992). Clinical assessment of fetal electrocardiogram monitoring in labour. British Journal of Obstetrics and Gynaecology, 99(1), 32-27.

15. Johanson, R. B., Rice, C., Shokr, A., Doyle, M., Chenoy, R., & O'Brien, P. M. S. (February 1992). ST-waveform analysis of the fetal electrocardiogram could reduce fetal blood sampling. British Journal of Obstetrics and Gynaecology, 99, 167-168.

16. Westgate, J., Harris, M., Curnow, J. S. H., & Greene, K. R. (November 1993). Plymouth randomized trial of cardiotocogram only versus ST waveform plus cardiotocogram for intrapartum monitoring in 2400 cases. American Journal of Obstetrics and Gynecology, 169(5), 1151-1160.

17. Pardi, G., Tucci, E., Uderzo, A., & Zanini, D. (January 1974). Fetal electrocardiogram changes in relation to fetal heart rate patterns during labour. American Journal of Obstetrics and Gynecology, 118(2), 243-250.

18. Newbold, S., Wheeler, T., Clewlow, F., & Soul, F. (February 1989). Variation in the T/QRS ratio of fetal electrocardiograms recorded during labour in normal subjects. British Journal of Obstetrics and Gynaecology, 96, 144-150.

19. Rosen, K. G., & Westgate, J. (February 1996). The T/QRS ratio of the fetal electrocardiogram—How to (in)validate experimental data. American Journal of Obstetrics and Gynecology, 174(2), 802-803.

20. Cockburn, J. (September 1992). ST-waveform analysis of the fetal electrocardiogram could reduce fetal blood sampling [Letters]. British Journal of Obstetrics and Gynaecology, 99(9), 783.

21. Newbold, S., Wheeler, T., & Clewlow, F. (February 1991). Comparison of the T/QRS ratio of the fetal electrocardiogram and the fetal heart rate during labour and the relation of these variables to condition at delivery. British Journal of Obstetrics and Gynaecology, 98, 173-178.

22. Lilja, H., Greene, K. R., Karlsson, K., & Rosen, K. G. (June 1985). ST waveform changes of the fetal electrocardiogram during labour-A clinical study. British Journal of Obstetrics and Gynaecology, 92, 611-617.

23. Reed, N. N., Mohajer, M. P., & James, D. K. (September 1994). Plymouth randomized control trial of cardiotocogram only versus ST waveform plus cardiotocogram for intrapartum monitoring in 2400 cases. American Journal of Obstetrics and Gynecology, 171(3), 867-868.

24. Symonds, E. M. (November 1971). Configuration of the fetal electrocardiogram in relation to fetal acid-base balance and plasma electrolytes. Journal of Obstetrics and Gynaecology of the British Commonwealth, 78(11), 957-970.

25. van Engelen, A. D., Weijtens, O., Brenner, J. I., Kleinman, C. S., Copel, J. A., & Stoutenbeek, P. (November 1, 1994). Management outcome and follow-up of fetal tachycardia. Journal of the American College of Cardiology, 24(5), 1371-1375.

26. Meijboom, E. J., van Engelen, A. D., van de Beek, E. W., Weijtens, O., Lautenschutz, J. M., & Benatar, A. A. (1994). Fetal arrhythmias. Current Opinion in Cardiology, 9, 97-102.

27. Cullen, T. (December 1992). Evaluation of fetal arrhythmias. American Family Physician, 46(6), 1745-1749.

28. Beall, M. H., & Paul, R. H. (March 1986). Artifacts, blocks, and arrhythmias: Confusing nonclassical heart rate tracings. Clinical Obstetrics and Gynecology, 29(1), 83-94.

29. Browne, P., Hamner, III, L., & Molina, R. (January 1996). Auscultated fetal arrhythmia: Analysis by echocardiogram. American Journal of Obstetrics and Gynecology, 174(1, Pt. 2), 420. SPO abstracts #402.

30. Allan, L. D. (March 1988). Fetal echocardiography. Clinical Obstetrics and Gynecology, 31(1), 61-79.

31. Joffe, G. M., Izquerdo, L., & Brown, A. (1994). Supraventricular tachycardia. The fetus, 4(3), 1-4.

32. Respondek, A., Huhta, J. C., Wood, D., & Respondek, M. (February 1990). Echocardiographic evaluation of fetal arrhythmias. Kardiologia Polska, 33(2), 136-149.

33. Miles, W. M., & Prystowsky, E. N. (August 1986). Supraventricular tachycardia in patients without overt preexcitation. Cardiology Clinics, 4(3), 429-446.

34. Brook, M. M., Silverman, N. H., & Villegas, M. (September 1993). Cardiac ultrasonography in structural abnormalities and arrhythmias. Recognition and treatment. Western Journal of Medicine, 159(3), 286-300.

35. Snider, A. R. (July/August 1994). Diagnostic procedures: Fetal echocardiography: Indications and limitations. Heart Disease and Stroke, 3(4), 201-204.

36. Ott, W. J. (June 1995). The accuracy of antenatal fetal echocardiography screening in high- and low-risk patients. American Journal of Obstetrics and Gynecology, 172(6), 1741-1749.

37. Wilson, N. J., Allen, B. C., Clarkson, P. M., Knight, D. B., Roberts, A. B., & Calder, A. L. (July 13, 1994). One year audit of a referral fetal echocardiography service. New Zealand Medical Journal, 107(981), 258-260.

38. Martin, G. R., & Ruckman, R. N. (January/February 1990). Fetal echocardiography: A large clinical experience and follow-up. Journal of the American Society of Echocardiography, 3(1), 4-8.

39. Allan, L. D. (1994). Fetal arrhythmias. In D. K. James, P. J. Steer, C. P. Weiner, & B. Gonik (Eds.), High risk pregnancy. management options (pp. 819-826). Philadelphia, PA: W. B. Saunders Company.

40. Brown, C. L., Colden, K. A., Hume, R. F., Johnson, M. P., Treadwell, M. C., & Drugan, A. (January 1996). Positive or faint amniotic fluid acetylcholinesterase band with normal ultrasound. American Journal of Obstetrics and Gynecology, 174(1, Pt. 2), 439. SPO abstracts #439.

41. Fernandez, C. O., Twickler, D. M., & Martin, L. B. (January 1995). Antenatal ultrasound and its sensitivity in detecting congenital heart defects. American Journal of Obstetrics and Gynecology, 172(1, Pt. 2), 261. SPO abstracts #23.

42. Pinsky, W. W., Rayburn, W. F., & Evans, M. I. (June 1991). Pharmacologic therapy for fetal arrhythmias. Clinical Obstetrics & Gynecology, 34(2), 304-309.

43. Chao, R. C., Ho, E. S., & Hsieh, K. S. (October 1992). Fetal atrial flutter and fibrillation: Prenatal echocardiographic detection and management. American Heart Journal, 124(4), 1095-1098.

44. Knudson, J. M., Kleinman, C. S., Copel, J. A., & Rosenfelf, L. E. (October 1994). Ectopic atrial tachycardia in utero. Obstetrics & Gynecology, 84(4, Pt. 2), 686-689.

45. De Catte, L., De Wolf, D., Smitz, J., Bougatef, A., De Schepper, J., & Foulon, W. (August 1994). Fetal hypothyroidism as a complication of amiodarone treatment for persistent fetal supraventricular tachycardia. Prenatal Diagnosis, 14(8), 762-765.

46. Reed, K. L., Sahn, D. J., Marx, G. R., Anderson, C. F. & Shenker, L. (July 1987). Cardiac doppler flows during fetal arrhythmias: Physiologic consequences. Obstetric & Gynecology, 70(1), 1-6.

47. Tonge, H. M., Wladimiroff, J. W., Noordam, M. J., & Stewart, P. A. (October 1986). Fetal cardiac arrythmias and their effect on volume blood flow in descending aorta of human fetus. Journal of Clinical Ultrasound, 14(8), 607-611.

48. Fabbri, E. L., & Hamner, III, L. H. (September 1992). Congenital complete heart block associated with maternal anti-Ro antibody: A case report. Journal of Perinatology, 12(3), 225-228.

49. Weiner, C. P. (March 1993). Umbilical pressure measurement in the evaluation of nonimmune hydrops fetalis. American Journal of Obstetrics and Gynecology, 168(3, Pt. 1), 817-823.

50. Flack, N. J., Zosmer, N., Bennett, P. R., Vaughan, J., & Fisk, N. M. (October 1993). Amiodarone given by three routes to terminate fetal atrial flutter associated with severe hydrops. Obstetrics & Gynecology, 82(4, Pt. 2), 714-716.

51. So, L. Y., Sung, R.Y., Ho, J. K., Fok, T. F., Chan, Y. L., & Aun, C. (June 1990). Management of a hydropic infant with congenital heart block. Journal of Paediatrics and Child Health, 26(3), 158-159.

52. Ito, S., Magee, L., & Smallhorn, J. (September 1994). Drug therapy for fetal arrhythmias. Clinics in Perinatology, 21(3), 543-572.

53. Chueh, J., Goldberg, J., & Golbus, M. (January 1995). Thoraco-amniotic shunting in fetal pleural effusions. American Journal of Obstetrics and Gynecology, 172(1, Pt. 2), 420. SPO abstracts #620.

54. McCoy, M. C., Katz, V. L., Gould, N., & Kuller, J. A. (1995). Non-immune hydrops after 20 weeks' gestation: Review of 10 years' experience with suggestions for management. Capsules & Comments in Perinatal and Women's Health Nursing, 85, 578-579.

55. Glanze, W. D., Anderson, K. N., & Anderson, L. E. (Eds.). (1990). Mosby's medical, nursing, and allied health dictionary (3rd. ed.). St. Louis, MO: The C. V. Mosby Company.

56. Kato, H., Rikitake, N., & Toyoda, O. (June 1988). Fetal echocardiography: New insight into fetal cardiology—A review. Journal of Cardiology, 18(2), 507-522.

57. Collins, J. H. (March 1995). Prenatal observation of umbilical cord torsion with subsequent premature labor and delivery of a 31-week infant with mild nonimmune hydrops. American Journal of Obstetrics and Gynecology, 172(3), 1048-1049.

58. de Boer, R. W., Karemaker, J. M., & Strackee, J. (July 1985). Relationships between short-term blood-pressure fluctuations and heart-rate variability in resting subjects I: A spectral analysis approach. Medical & Biological Engineering & Computing, 23, 352-358.

59. DeVore, G. R., Steiger, R. M., & Larson, E. J. (March 1987). Fetal echocadiography: The prenatal diagnosis of a ventricular septal defect in a 14-week fetus with pulmonary artery hypoplasia. Obstetrics & Gynecology, 69(3, Pt. 2), 494-497.

60. Mendoza, G. J., Almeida, O., & Steinfeld, L. (May 1989). Intermittent fetal bradycardia induced by midpregnancy fetal ultrasonographic study. American Journal of Obstetrics and Gynecology, 160(5, Pt. 1), 1038-1040.

61. Tournaire, M., Sturbois, G., Zorn, J., Breart, G., & Sureau, C. (1980). Fetal monitoring before and during labor. In S. Aladjem, A. K. Brown, & C. Sureau (Eds.). Clinical perinatology (pp. 331-361). St. Louis, MO: The C. V. Mosby Company.

62. Clement, D., & Schifrin, B. S. (March/April 1987). Diagnosis and management of fetal arrhythmias. Perinatology-Neonatology, 11(2), 9-10, 12, 17-19.

63. Bergmans, M. G. M., Jonker, G. J., & Kock, H.C.L.V. (February 1985). Fetal supraventricular tachycardia. Review of the literature. Obstetrical and Gynecological Survey, 40(2), 61-68.

64. Newton, E. R., Piper, J., & Peairs, W. (January 1995). Does the presence of bacterial vaginosis intrapartum increase the likelihood of intra-amniotic infection? American Journal of Obstetrics and Gynecology, 172(1, Pt. 2), 302. SPO abstracts #147.

65. Kates, R. B., & Schifrin, B. S. (April 1986). Fetal cardiac asystole during labor. Obstetrics & Gynecology, 67(4), 549-555.

66. Ramsey-Goldman, R., Hom, D., Deng, J-S., Ziegler, G. C., Kahl, L. E., Steen, V. D., & La Porte, R. E. (October 1986). Anti-SS-A antibodies and fetal outcome in maternal systemic lupus erythematosus. Arthritis and Rheumatism, 29(10), 1269-1273.

67. Cabaniss, M. L. (1993). Fetal monitoring interpretation. Philadelphia, PA: J. B. Lippincott Company.

68. Degani, S., Abinader, E. G., Shapiro, I., Lewinsky, R., & Sharf, M. (1988). Fetal arrhythmia associated with sinus node dysfunction - A case report. Journal of Perinatal Medicine, 16, 153-155.

69. Meltzer, L. E., et al. (1983). Intensive coronary care. A manual for nurses (4th ed.). Maryland: Robert J. Brady Co.

70. Fyfe, D. A., Meyer, K. B., & Case, C. L. (August 1993). Sonographic assessment of fetal cardiac arrhythmias. Seminars in Ultrasound, CT, and MRI, 14(4), 286-297.

71. Stewart, P. A., & Waldimiroff, J. W. (November/December 1988). Fetal atrial arrhythmias associated with redundancy/aneurysm of the foramen ovale. Journal of Clinical Ultrasound, 16(9), 643-650.

72. Toro, L., Weintraub, R. G., Shiota, T., Sahn, D. J., McDonald, R. W. & Rice, M. J. (April 1, 1994). Relation between persistent atrial arrhythmias and redundant septum primum flap (atrial septal aneurysm) in fetuses. American Journal of Cardiology, 73(9), 711-713.

73. DeVore, G. R. (June 1984). Fetal echocardiography—A new frontier. Clinical Obstetrics and Gynecology, 27(2), 359-377.

74. Oei, S. G., Vosters, R. P. L., & van der Hagen, N. L. J. (March 4, 1989). Fetal arrhythmia caused by excessive intake of caffeine by pregnant women. British Medical Journal, 298, 568.

75. Veille, J-C., & Covitz, W. (May 1994). Fetal cardiovascular hemodynamics in the presence of complete atrioventricular block. American Journal of Obstetrics and Gynecology, 170(5, Pt. 1), 1258-1262.

76. Koyanagi, T., Hara, K., Satoh, S., Yoshizato, T., & Nakano, H. (August 1990). Relationship between heart rate and rhythm, and cardiac performance assessed in the human fetus in utero. International Journal of Cardiology, 28(2), 163-171.

77. Rice, M. J., McDonald, R. W., & Reller, M. D. (November 1988). Fetal atrial septal aneurysm: A cause of fetal atrial arrhythmias. Journal of the American College of Cardiology, 12(5), 1292-1297.

78. Baker, E., Romero, B., D'Alton, M., & Marx, G. (January 1993). Diagnosis of fetal atrial arrhythmia by motion of septum primum. American Journal of Obstetrics and Gynecology, 168(1, Pt. 2), 349. SPO abstracts #178.

79. Wolff, F., Breuker, K. H., Schlensker, K. H., & Bolte, A. (1980). Prenatal diagnosis and therapy of fetal heart rate anomalies: With a contribution on the placental transfer of verapamil. Journal of Perinatal Medicine, 8, 203-208.

80. Todros, T., Presbitero, P., Gaglioti, P., & Demarie, D. (March 1990). Conservative management of fetal bigeminy arrhythmia leading to persistent bradycardia. European Journal of Obstetrics, Gynecology, and Reproductive Biology, 34(3), 211-215.

81. Silverman, N. H., Enderlein, M. A., Stanger, P., Teitel, D. F., Heymann, M. A., & Golbus, M. S. (May 1985). Symposium article: Recognition of fetal arrhythmias by echocardiography. Journal of Clinical Ultrasound, 13, 255-263.

82. Lingman, G., Lundstrom, N. R., & Marsal, K. (1986). Clinical outcome and circulatory effects of fetal cardiac arrhythmia. Acta Paediatrica Scandinavica, 329(Suppl.), 120-126.

83. van den Berg, P., Gembruch, U., Schmidt, S., Hansmann, M., & Krebs, D. (1989). Continuous fetal intrapartum monitoring in supraventricular tachycardia by atraumatic measurement of transcutaneous carbon dioxide tension. Journal of Perinatal Medicine, 17, 371-374.

84. Timor-Tritsch, I., Gergely, Z., Abramovici, H., & Brandes, J. M. (May 1974). Misleading information from fetal monitoring in a case of intrapartum fetal death. Obstetrics & Gynecology, 43(5), 713-717.

85. Harkin, A. H., Honigman, B., & Van Way, III, C. W. (1987). Cardiac dysrhythmias in the acute setting: Recognition and treatment or anyone can treat cardiac dysrhythmias. Journal of Emergency Medicine, 5(2), 129-134.

86. Gray, J. (August 1989). A case of intrapartum fetal arrhythmia creating difficulties in cardiotocograph interpretation. Australian and New Zealand Journal of Obstetrics and Gynaecology, 29(3, Pt. 1), 265-267.

87. Friedman, A. H., Copel, J. A., & Kleinman, C. S. (April 1993). Fetal echocardiography: Indications, diagnosis and management. Seminars in Perinatology, 17(2), 76-88.

88. Varon, M. E., Sherer, D. M., Abramowicz, J. S., & Akiyama, T. (November 1992). Maternal ventricular tachycardia associated with hypomagnesemia. American Journal of Obstetrics and Gynecology, 167(5), 1352-1363.

89. Allan, L. D., Chita, S. K., Sharland, G. K., Maxwell, D., & Priestley, K. (January 1991). Flecainide in the treatment of fetal tachycardias. British Heart Journal, 65(1), 46-48.

90. Till, J., & Wren, C. (January 1992). Atrial flutter in the fetus and young infant: An association with accessory connections. British Heart Journal, 67(1), 80-83.

91. Johnsrude, C. L., Towbin, J. A., Cecchin, F., & Perry, J. C. (June 1995). Postinfarction ventricular arrhythmias in children. American Heart Journal, 129(6), 1171-1177.

92. Yamada, M., Sakakibara, S., Utsu, M., & Chiba, Y. (May 1983). Management of fetal complete atrioventricular block. Australian & New Zealand Journal of Obstetrics & Gynaecology, 23(2), 110-113.

93. Byrum, C. J., Wahl, R. A., Behrendt, D. M., & Macdonald, D. (September 1982). Ventricular fibrillation associated with use of digitalis in a newborn infant with Wolff-Parkinson-White syndrome. Journal of Pediatrics, 101(3), 400-403.

94. Heusch, A., Kramer, H. H., Krogmann, O. N., Rammos, S., & Bourgeois, M. (August 1994). Clinical experience with propafenone for cardiac arrhythmias in the young. European Heart Journal, 15(8), 1050-156.

95. Bash, S. E., Shah, J. J., Albers, W. H., & Geiss, D. M. (November 1987). Hypothermia for the treatment of post surgical greatly accelerated junctional ectopic tachycardia. Journal of the American College of Cardiology, 10(5), 1095-1099.

96. Perry, J. C., Ayres, N. A., & Carpenter, Jr., R. J. (February 1991). Fetal supraventricular tachycardia treated with flecainide acetate. Journal of Pediatrics, 118(2), 303-305.

97. Smoleniec, J. S., Martin, R., & James, D. K. (October 1991). Intermittent fetal tachycardia and fetal hydrops. Archives of Disease in Childhood, 66, 1160-1161.

98. Smith, M. B. H., Colford, D., & Human, D. G. (July/August 1992). Perinatal supraventricular tachycardia. Canadian Journal of Cardiology, 8(6), 565-568.

99. Smoleniec, J. S., James, D. K., & Martin, R. (October 1992). Unreactive fetal heart rate pattern and atrial flutter. British Journal of Obstetrics and Gynaecology, 99(10), 856-857.

100. Sreeram, N., & Wren, C. (January 1990). Supraventricular tachycardia in infants: Response to initial treatment. Archives of Disease in Childhood, 65(1), 127-129.

101. Aydin, M., Baysal, K., Kucukoduk, S., Cetinkaya, F., & Yaman, S. (January/March 1995). Application of ice water to the face in initial treatment of supraventricular tachycardia. Turkish Journal of Pediatrics, 37(1), 15-17.

102. Bisset, III, G. S., Gaum, W., & Kaplan, S. (October 1980). The ice bag: A new technique for interruption of supraventricular tachycardia. Journal of Pediatrics, 97(4), 593-595.

103. Tanel, R. E., Walsh, E. P., Lulu, J. A., & Saul, J. P. (June 1995). Sotalol for refractory arrhythmias in pediatric and young adult patients: Initial efficacy and long-term outcome. American Heart Journal, 129(6), 1171-1177.

104. Akhtar, M., Tchou, P. J., & Jazayeri, M. (January 15, 1988). Mechanisms of clinical tachycardias. American Journal of Cardiology, 61(2), 9A-19A.

105. Severson, A. L., & Meyer, L. T. (July/August 1992). New cardiovascular interventions: Treatment of paroxysmal supraventricular tachycardia with adenosine: Implications for nursing. Heart Lung, 21(4), 350-356.

106. Fanaroff, A. A., & Martin, R. J. (Eds.). (1987). Neonatal-perinatal medicine. Diseases of the fetus and infant (4th ed.). St. Louis, MO: The C. V. Mosby Company.

107. Gonser, M., Dietl, J., Pfeiffer, K., & Clees, J. P. (1989). Evaluation of fetal heart rate artifacts, hemodynamics and digoxin treatment in fetal tachyarrhythmia by doppler measurement of fetal blood flow—case report of a pre-excitation syndrome. Journal of Perinatal Medicine, 17(6), 411-416.

108. Blanch, G., Walkinshaw, S. A., & Walsh, K. (December 10, 1994). Cardioversion of fetal tachyarrhythmia with adenosine [Letters]. The Lancet, 344(8937), 1646.

109. Azancot-Bernisty, A., Jacqz-Aigrain, E., Guirgis, N. M., Decrepy, A., Oury, J. F., & Blot, P. (October 1992). Clinical and pharmacologic study of fetal supraventricular tachyarrhythmias. Journal of Pediatrics, 121(4), 608-613.

110. Mills, M. (June 1992). Treatment of fetal supraventricular tachycardia with flecainide acetate after digoxin failure. American Journal of Obstetrics and Gynecology, 166(6, Pt. 1), 1863.

111. Knudson, J. M. (October 1994). Ectopic atrial tachycardia in utero. Obstetrics & Gynecology, 84(4, Pt. 2), 686-689.

112. Wu, J-M., Young, M-L., Wu, M-H., Wang, T-K., & Lue, H-C. (1991). Junctional ectopic tachycardia in infancy: Report of two cases. Journal of Formosan Medical Association, 90(5), 517-519.

113. Dildy, G. A., Loucks, C. A., & Clark, S. L. (December 1993). Intrapartum fetal pulse oximetry in the presence of fetal cardiac arrhythmia. American Journal of Obstetrics & Gynecology, 169(6), 1609-1611.

114. Chang, J. S., Chen, Y. C., Tsai, C. H., & Tsai, H. D. (May/June 1994). Successful conversion of fetal atrial flutter with digoxin: Report of one case. Acta Paediatrica Sinica, 35(3), 229-234.

115. Olshaker, J. S. (January/February 1988). Atrial flutter. The Journal of Emergency Medicine, 6(1), 55-59.

116. Kleinman, C. S. (1986). Prenatal diagnosis and management of intrauterine arrhythmias. Fetal Therapy, 1, 92-95.

117. Bacevice, Jr., A. E., Dierker, L. J. & Wolfson, R. N. (September 1,1985). Intrauterine atrial fibrillation associated with fetomaternal hemorrhage. American Journal of Obstetrics and Gynecology, 153(1), 81-82.

118. Belhassen, B., Pauzner, D., Blieden, L., Sherez, J., Zinger, A., & David, M. (November 1982). Intrauterine and postnatal atrial fibrillation in the Wolff-Parkinson-White syndrome. Circulation, 66(5), 1124-1128.

119. Weiner, C. P., & Thompson, M. I. B. (March 1988). Direct treatment of fetal supraventricular tachycardia after failed transplacental therapy. American Journal of Obstetrics and Gynecology, 158(3, Pt. 1), 570-573.

120. Hallak, M., Neerhof, M. G., Perry, R., Nazir, M., & Huhta, J. C. (September 1991). Fetal supraventricular tachycardia and hydrops fetalis: Combined intensive, direct, and transplacental therapy. Obstetrics & Gynecology, 78(3, Pt. 2), 523-525.

121. Dumestic, D. A., Silverman, N. H., Tobias, S., & Golbus, M. (October 28, 1982). Transplacental cardioversion of fetal supraventricular tachycardia with procainamide. The New England Journal of Medicine, 307(18), 1128-1131.

122. Perry, J. C., & Garson, Jr., A. (December 1992). Flecainide acetate for treatment of tachyarrhythmias in children: Review of world literature on efficacy, safety, and dosing. American Heart Journal, 124(6), 1614-1621.

123. Rey, E., Duperron, L., Gauthier, R., Lemay, M., Grignon, A., & LeLorier, J. (October 1, 1985). Transplacental treatment of tachycardia-induced fetal heart failure with verapamil and amiodarone: A case report. American Journal of Obstetrics and Gynecology, 153(3), 311-312.

124. Spinnato, J. A., Shaver, D. C., Flinn, G. S., Sibai, B. M., Watson, D. L., & Marin-Garcia, J. (1984). Fetal supraventricular tachycardia: In utero therapy with digoxin and quinidine. Obstetrics & Gynecology, 64(5), 730-735.

125. Murphy, T. G. (December 1993). Digoxin toxicity. Ventricular dysrhythmias to watch for. American Journal of Nursing, 37-41.

126. Harrigan, J. T., Kangos, J. J., Sikka, A., Spisso, K. R., Natarajan, N., & Rosenfeld, D. (1981). Successful treatment of fetal congestive heart failure secondary to tachycardia. The New England Journal of Medicine, 304(25), 1527-1529.

127. Parilla, B. V., Socol, M. L., & Strasburger, J. F. (January 1995). Intramuscular digoxin for fetal supraventricular tachycardia with hydrops fetalis. American Journal of Obstetrics and Gynecology, 172(1, Pt. 2), 426. SPO abstracts #609.

128. Kofinas, A. D., Simon, N. V., Sagel, H., Lyttle, E., Smith, N., & King, K. (September 1991). Treatment of fetal supraventricular tachycardia with flecainide acetate after digoxin failure. American Journal of Obstetrics and Gynecology, 165(3), 630-631.

129. Krikler, D. M. (1986). Verapamil in arrhythmia. British Journal of Clinical Pharmacology, 21(Suppl., 2), 183s-189s.

130. Dalton, K. J., Dawes, G. S., & Patrick, J. E. (June 15, 1983). The autonomic nervous system and fetal heart rate variability. American Journal of Obstetrics and Gynecology, 146(4), 456-462.

131. Kanzaki, T., Murakami, M., Kobayashi, H., Takahashi, S., & Chiba, Y. (January/February 1993). Hemodynamic changes during cardioversion in utero: A case report of supraventricular tachycardia and atrial flutter. Fetal Diagnosis and Therapy, 8(1), 137-144.

132. Widerhorn, J., Bhandari, A. K., Bughi, S., Rahimtoola, S. H., & Elkayam, U. (October 1991). Fetal and neonatal adverse effects profile of amiodarone treatment during pregnancy. American Heart Journal, 122(4, Pt. 1), 1162-1166.

133. Fulgencio, J. P., & Hamza, J. (May 1994). Anaesthesia for caesarean section in a patient receiving high dose amiodarone for fetal supraventricular tachycardia. Anaesthesia, 49(5), 405-408.

134. Harrison, J. K., Greenfield, R. A., Wharton, J. M. (May 1992). Acute termination of supraventricular tachycardia by adenosine during pregnancy. American Heart Journal, 123(5), 1386-1388.

135. Leffler, S., & Johnson, D. R. (November 1992). Adenosine use in pregnancy: Lack of effect on fetal heart rate. American Journal of Emergency Medicine, 10(6), 548-549.

136. van den Berg, P. P., van den Brand, S. F. J. J., Nijland, R., Nijhuis, J. G., Jongsma, H. W., & Eskes, T. K. A. B. (October 1994). Intrapartum fetal surveillance of congenital complete heart block (CCHB) with pulse oximetry. Obstetrics and Gynecology, 84(4, Pt. 2), 683-686.

137. Gembruch, U., Hansmann, M., Redel, D. A., Bald, R., & Knopfle, G. (April 1989). Fetal complete heart block: Antenatal diagnosis, significance and management. European Journal of Obstetrics, Gynecology, and Reproductive Biology, 31(1), 9-22.

138. Davison, M. B., & Radford, D. J. (February 20, 1989). Fetal and neonatal congenital complete heart block. Medical Journal of Australia,150(4), 192-198.

139. Olah, K. S. J., & Gee, H. (September 1993). Antibody mediated complete congenital heart block in the fetus. PACE, 16(9), 1872-1879.

140. Chan, F. Y., Woo, S. K., Ghosh, A., Tang, M., & Lam, C. (August 1990). Prenatal velocimetry of the fetal abdominal aorta and inferior vena cava. Obstetrics & Gynecology, 76(2), 200-205.

141. Reed, B. R., Lee, L. A., Harmon, C., Wolfe, R., Wiggins, J., & Peebles, C. (December 1983). Autoantibodies to SS-A/Ro in infants with congenital heart block. The Journal of Pediatrics, 103(6), 889-891.

142. Schmidt, K. G., Ulmer, H. E., Silverman, N. H., Kleinman, C. S., & Copel, J. A. (May 1991). Perinatal outcome of fetal complete atrioventricular block: A multicenter experience. Journal of the American College of Cardiology, 17(6), 1360-1366.

143. Fox, K. M., Anderson, R. H., & Hallide-Smith, K. A. (May 1980). Hypoplastic and fibrotic sinus node associated with intractable tachycardia in a neonate. Circulation, 61(5), 1048-1052.

144. Kaaja, R., Julkunen, H., Ammala, P., Teppo, A-M., & Kurki, P. (November 1991). Congenital heart block: Successful prophylactic treatment with intravenous gamma globulin and corticosteroid therapy. American Journal of Obstetrics and Gynecology, 165(5, Pt. 1), 1333-1334.

145. Martin, C. B., & Gingerich, B. (September/October 1976). Factors affecting the fetal heart rate: Genesis of FHR patterns. JOGNN, 5(Suppl., 5), 16s-25s, 30s-40s.

146. Copel, J. A., Buyon, J. P., & Kleinman, C. S. (November 1995). Successful in utero therapy of fetal heart block. American Journal of Obstetrics and Gynecology, 173(5), 1384-1390.

147. Wright, A. J. (April 1989). Fetal arrhythmia masquerading as fetal distress. A case report. Journal of Reproductive Medicine, 34(4), 301-302.

148. Alexander, M., Wenstrom, K. D., & Johnson, W. (January 1994). Increased stroke volume in fetuses with heart block. American Journal of Obstetrics and Gynecology, 170(1, Pt. 2), 309. SPO abstract #111.

149. Gilson, G. J. (April 15, 1996). Antiphospholipid syndromes: Obstetrical perspectives. Paper presented at the meeting of the New Mexico Section AWHONN (Association of Women's Health, Obstetrics and Neonatal Nursing) The Best of the West, Albuquerque, NM.

150. Vogt, E., Ng, A-K., & Rote, N. S. (February 1996). A model for the antiphospholipid antibody syndrome: Monoclonal antiphosphatidylserine antibody induces intrauterine growth restriction in mice. American Journal of Obstetrics and Gynecology, 174(2), 700-707.

151. Aoki, K., Dudkiewicz, A. B., Matsuura, E., Novotny, M., Kaberlein, G., & Gleicher, N. (March 1995). Clinical significance of β_2-glycoprotein I-dependent anticardiolipin antibodies in the reproductive autoimmune failure syndrome: Correlation with conventional antiphospholipid antibody detection systems. American Journal of Obstetrics and Gynecology, 172(3), 926-931.

152. Knolle, P., Mayet, W., Lohse, A. W., Treichel, U., Meyer Zum Buschenfelde, K. H., & Gerken, G. (August 1994). Complete congenital heart block in autoimmune hepatitis (SLA-positive). Journal of Hepatology, 21(2), 224-226.

153. Peaceman, A. M., & Rehnberg, K. A. (November 1995). The effect of aspirin and indomethacin on prostacyclin and thromboxane production by placental tissue incubated with immunoglobulin G fractions from patients with lupus anticoagulant. American Journal of Obstetrics and Gynecology, 173(5), 1391-1396.

154. Silver, R. M., Pierangeli, S. S., Gharavi, A. E., Harris, E. N., Edwin, S. S., & Salafia, C. M. (November 1995). Induction of high levels of anticardiolipin antibodies in mice by immunization with β_2-glycoprotein I does not cause fetal death. American Journal of Obstetrics and Gynecology, 173(5), 1410-1415.

155. Julkunen, H., Kaaja, R., Wallgren, E., & Teramo, K. (July 1993). Isolated congenital heart block: Fetal and infant outcome and familial incidence of heart block. Obstetrics & Gynecology, 82(1), 11-16.

156. Katsuragawa, H., Rote, N. S., Inoue, T., Narukawa, S., Kanzaki, H., & Mori, T. (May 1995). Monoclonal antiphosphatidylserine antibody reactivity against human first-trimester placental trophoblasts. American Journal of Obstetrics and Gynecology, 172(5), 1592-1597.

157. Gollin, Y., Howard, C., Bahado-Singh, R., Garofalo, J., Arici, A., & Copel, J. (January 1995). Heparin therapy for the antiphospholipid antibody syndrome: Is full anticoagulation necessary? American Journal of Obstetrics and Gynecology, 172(1, Pt. 2), 335. SPO abstracts #271.

158. Salafia, C. M., & Cowchock, F. S. (January 1995). Placental pathology in treated and untreated women with antiphospholipid antibodies. American Journal of Obstetrics and Gynecology, 172(1, Pt. 2), 335. SPO abstracts #272.

159. Salafia, C. M., & Parke, A. (January 1995). Placental pathology in the phospholipid antibody syndrome and systemic lupus erythematosus. American Journal of Obstetrics and Gynecology, 172(1, Pt. 2), 336. SPO abstracts #273.

160. Scott, J. R., Silver, R. M., & Branch, D. W. (January 1996). Is there an antiphospholipid antibody negative antiphospholipid-like syndrome. American Journal of Obstetrics and Gynecology, 174(1, Pt. 2), 391. SPO abstracts #296.

161. Silver, R. K., Mullen, T. A., Caplan, M. S., O'Connell, P. D., & Ragin, A. (September 1995). Inducible platelet adherence to human umbilical vein endothelium by anticardiolipin antibody—positive sera. American Journal of Obstetrics and Gynecology, 173(3, Pt. 1), 702-707.

162. Gross, K. R., Petty, R. E., Lum, V. L., & Allen, R. C. (1989). Maternal autoantibodies and fetal disease. Clinical and Experimental Rheumatology, 7, 651-657.

163. Reid, R. L., Pancham, S. R., Kean, W. F., & Ford, P. M. (October 1979). Maternal and neonatal implications of congenital complete heart block in the fetus. Obstetrics & Gynecology, 54(4), 470-474.

164. Seligman, S. P., Clancy, R. M., Belmont, H. M., Abramson, S. B., Young, B. K., & Buyon, J. P. (January 1995). Increased serum nitrite levels in lupus pregnancies. American Journal of Obstetrics and Gynecology, 172(1, Pt. 2), 334. SPO abstracts #268.

165. Silver, R. M., Umar, F., Pierangeli, S. S., Harris, E. N., Greenhall, A., & Branch, D. W. (January 1995). Pathogenic antibodies in women with features of antiphospholipid syndrome (APS) who test negative for LA and aCL. American Journal of Obstetrics and Gynecology, 172(1, Pt. 2), 336. SPO abstracts #274.

166. Farine, D., Granovsky-Grisaru, S., Teoh, T. G., Ryan, G., Seaward, G., & Ritchie, J. W. K. (January 1996). The value of umbilical artery blood flow velocity in pregnancies complicated by systemic lupus erythematosus (SLE). American Journal of Obstetrics and Gynecology, 174(1, Pt. 2), 459. SPO abstracts #552.

167. Buyon, J. & Szer, I. (1986). Passively acquired autoimmunity and the maternal fetal dyad in systemic lupus erythematosus. Springer Seminars in Immunopathology, 9, 283-304.

168. Stephensen, O., Cleland, W. P., & Hallidie-Smith, K. (July 1981). Congenital complete heart block and persistent ductus arteriosus associated with maternal systemic lupus erythematosus. British Heart Journal, 46(1), 104-106.

169. Singsen, B. H., Akhter, J. E., Weinstein, M. M., & Sharp, G. C. (July 15, 1985). Congenital complete heart block and SS-A antibodies: Obstetric implications. American Journal of Obstetrics and Gynecology, 152(6, Pt. 1), 655-658.

170. Chua, S., Ostman-Smith, I., Sellers, S., & Redman, C. W. (November 26, 1991). Congenital heart block with hydrops fetalis treated with high-dose dexamethasone. A case report. European Journal of Obstetrics, Gynecology, and Reproductive Biology, 42(2), 155-158.

171. Caruso, C., Candore, G., Colucci, A. T., Cigna, D., Modica, M. A., & Tantillo, G. (November 1993). Natural killer and lymphokine-activated killer activity in HLA-B8, DR3-positive subjects. Human Immunology, 38(3), 226-230.

172. Foster, H., Walker, D., Charles, P., Kelly, C., Cavanagh, G., & Griffiths, I. (May 1992). Association of DR3 with susceptibility to and severity of primary Sjögren's syndrome in a family study. British Journal of Rheumatology, 31(5), 309-314.

173. Vincek, V., Klein, D., Figueroa, F., Hauptfeld, V., Kasahara, M., O'hUigin, C. (1992). The evolutionary origin of the HLA-DR3 haplotype. Immunogenetics, 35(4), 263-271.

174. Jenkins, D., Fletcher, J., Penny, M. A., Mijovic, C. H., Jacobs, K. H., & Bradwell, A. R. (July 1991). DRB genotyping supports recessive inheritance of DR3-associated susceptibility to insulin-dependent diabetes mellitus. American Journal of Human Genetics, 49(1), 49-53.

175. Kukmar, A., Kumar, P., & Schur, P. H. (July 1991). Abundance of DR2/DR3 and DR2/DR7 heterozygotes in Caucasian patients with systemic lupus erythematosus from USA. Tissue Antigens, 38(1), 52.

176. Czaja, A. J., Carpenter, H. A., Santrach, P. J., & Moore, S. B. (October 1995). Significance of human leukocyte antigens DR3 and DR4 in chronic viral hepatitis. Digestive Diseases & Sciences, 40(10), 2098-2106.

177. Cavan, D. A., Kelly, M. A., Jacobs, K. H., Penny, M. A., Jenkins, D., & Mijovic, C. (1994). The BgI II RFLP associated with type I diabetes in DR3-positive subjects is not due to a DQA1 promoter region polymorphism. Autoimmunity, 17(2), 123-125.

178. Bishof, N. A., Welch, T. R., Beischel, L. S., Carson, D., & Donnelly, P. A. (June 1993). DP polymorphism in HLA-A1, -B8, -DR3 extended haplotypes associated with membranoproliferative glomerulonephritis and systemic lupus erythematosus. Pediatric Nephrology, 7(3), 243-246.

179. Candore, G., Cigna, D., Todaro, M., De Maria, R., Stassi, G., & Giordano, C. (April 1995). T-cell activation in HLA-B8, DR3-positive individuals. Early antigen expression defect in vitro. Human Immunology, 42(4), 289-294.

180. Avila-Portillo, L. M., Vargas-Alarcon, G., Andrade, F., Alarcon-Segovia, D., & Granados, J. (September/October 1994). Linkage disequilibrium of HLA-DR3 and HLA-DR4 with HLA-B alleles in Mexican patients with rheumatoid arthritis. Clinical & Experimental Rheumatology, 12(5), 497-502.

181. Cox, A., Gonzalez, A. M., Wilson, A. G., Wilson, R. M., Ward, J. D., & Artlett, C. M. (May 1994). Comparative analysis of the genetic associations of HLA-DR3 and tumour necrosis factor alpha with human IDDM. Diabetologia, 37(5), 500-503.

182. Banerji, M. A., Chaiken, R. L., Huey, H., Tuomi, T., Norin, A. J., & Mackay, I. R. (June 1994). GAD antibody negative NIDDM in adult black subjects with diabetic ketoacidosis and increased frequency of human leukocyte antigen DR3 and DR4. Flatbush diabetes. Diabetes, 43(6), 741-745.

183. Malcherek, G., Falk, K., Rotzschke, O., Rammensee, H. G., Stevanovic, S., & Gnau, V. (October 1993). Natural peptide ligand motifs of two HLA molecules associated with myasthenia gravis. International Immunology, 5(10), 1229-1237.

184. Robinson, W. P., Barbosa, J., Rich, S. S., & Thomson, G. (1993). Homozygous parent affected sib pair method for detecting disease predisposing variants: Application to insulin dependent diabetes mellitus. Genetic Epidemiology, 10(5), 273-288.

185. Regueiro, J. R., Arnaiz-Villena, A., Vicario, J. L., Martinez-Laso, J., Pacheco, A., & Rivera-Guzman, J. M. (July 5, 1993). Experientia, 49(6-7), 553-556.

186. Ivarsson, S. A., Eriksson, S., Kockum, I., Lernmark, A., Lindgren, S., & Nilsson, K. O. (March 1993). HLA-DR3, DQ2 homozygosity in two patients with insulin-dependent diabetes mellitus superimposed with ulcerative colitis and primary sclerosing cholangitis. Journal of Internal Medicine, 233(3), 281-286.

187. Provost, T. T., & Watson, R. (January 1993). Anti-Ro (SS-A) HLA-DR3-positive women: The interrelationship between some ANA negative, SS, SCLE, and NLE mothers and SS/LE overlap female patients. Journal of Investigative Dermatology, 100(1), 14S-20S.

188. Bognetti, E., Meschi, F., Malavasi, C., Pastore, M. R., Sergi, A., & Illeni, M. T. (1992). HLA-antigens in Italian type 1 diabetic patients: Role of DR3/DR4 antigens and breast feeding in the onset of the disease. Acta Diabetologica, 28(3-4), 229-232.

189. Maenpaa, A., Koskimies, S., Scheinin, T., Schlenzka, A., Akerblom, H. K., & Maenpaa, J. (April 1991). Frequencies of HLA-DR3, -DR4, -B8 and -Bw62 in diabetic children diagnosed between 1960 and 1990. Diabetes Research, 16(4), 159-163.

190. Deschamps, I., Beressi, J. P., Khalil, I., Robert, J. J., & Hors, J. (October 1991). The role of genetic predisposition to type I (insulin-dependent) diabetes mellitus. Annals of Medicine, 23(4), 427-435.

191. Modica, M. A., Zambito, A. M., Candore, G., & Caruso, C. (November 1990). Markers of T lymphocyte activation in HLA-B8, DR3 positive individuals. Immunobiology, 181(4-5), 257-266.

192. Modica, M. A., Cammarata, G., & Caruso, C. (February/April 1990). HLA-B8, DR3 phenotype and lymphocyte responses to phytohaemagglutinin. Journal of Immunogenetics, 17(1-2), 101-107.

193. Singal, D. P., Reid, B., Green, D., D'Souza, M., Bensen, W. G., & Buchanan, W. W. (August 1990). Polymorphism of major histocompatibility complex extended haplotypes bearing HLA-DR3 in patients with rheumatoid arthritis with gold induced thrombocytopenia or proteinuria. Annals of the Rheumatic Diseases, 49(8), 582-586.

194. MacMillan, D. R., Foster, M. B., & Key, M. P. (January 1991). HLA type and the genetic risk for type 1 diabetes mellitus. Journal of the Kentucky Medical Association, 89(1), 19-21.

195. Neumuller, J., Menzel, J., & Millesi, H. (May 1994). Prevalence of HLA-DR3 and autoantibodies to connective tissue components in Dupuytren's contracture. Clinical Immunology & Immunopathology, 71(2), 142-148.

196. Colucci, A. T., Di Lorenzo, G., Ingrassia, A., Crescimanno, G., Modica, M. A., & Candore, G. (1992). Blood antiphosolipid antibody levels are influenced by age, sex and HLA-B8, DR3 phenotype. Experimental & Clinical Immunogenetics, 9(2), 72-79.

197. Ceman, S., Rudersdorf, R. A., Petersen, J. M., & DeMars, R. (March 15, 1995). DMA and DMB are the only genes in the class II region of the human MHC needed for class II-associated antigen processing. Journal of Immunology, 154(6), 2545-2456.

198. Candore, G., Cigna, D., Gervasi, F., Colucci, A. T., Modica, M. A., & Caruso, C. (1994). In vitro cytokine production by HLA-B8, DR3 positive subjects. Autoimmunity, 18(2), 121-132.

199. Candore, G., Colucci, A. T., Modica, M. A., & Caruso, C. (1991). HLA-B8, DR3 T cell impairment is completely restored by in vitro treatment with interleukin-2. Immunopharmacology & Immunotoxicology, 13(4), 551-561.

200. Hashimoto, S., Michalski, J. P., Berman, M. A., & McCombs, C. (February 1990). Mechanism of a lymphocyte abnormality associated with HLA-B8/DR3: Role of interleukin-1. Clinical & Experimental Immunology, 79(2), 227-232.

201. Benigni, A., Gregorini, G., Frusca, T., Chiabrando, C., Ballerini, S., & Valcamonico, A. (August 10, 1989). Effect of low-dose aspirin on fetal and maternal generation of thromboxane by platelets in women at risk for pregnancy-induced hypertension. New England Journal of Medicine, 321(6), 357-362.

202. Sibai, B. M., Mirro, R., Chesney, C. M., & Leffler, C. (October 1989). Low-dose aspirin in pregnancy. Obstetrics & Gynecology, 74(4), 551-557.

203. Grandone, E., Margaglione, M., & Pavone, G. (March 1996). Use of intravenous immunoglobulin to prevent recurrent spontaneous abortion. American Journal of Obstetrics and Gynecology, 174(3), 1080.

204. Hare, J. Y., Huhta, J. C., Weil-Chalker, S., Stauffer, N., Cuneo, B. F., & Respondek, M. (January 1995). Beta agonist therapy of fetal complete heart block. American Journal of Obstetrics and Gynecology, 172(1, Pt. 2), 426. SPO abstracts #611.

205. Harrison, M. R. (April 1996). Fetal surgery. American Journal of Obstetrics and Gynecology, 174(4), 1255-1264.

206. Cekleniak, N., Hirshberg, J., Leiva, M. C., Librizzi, R., & Tolosa, J. E. (January 1996). Heparin therapy reduces the risk of fetal death and IUGR and is effective in the treatment of the antiphospholipid antibody syndrome and of repeated pregnancy losses. American Journal of Obstetrics and Gynecology, 174(1, Pt. 2), 392. SPO abstracts #297.

207. Rane, H. S., & Purandare, H. (July 1990). Fetal echocardiography in normal pregnancies—a basis for prenatal detection of cardiac malformations. Indian Pediatrics, 27(7), 729-735.

208. Edwards, M. S., Ellings, J. M., Menard, M. K., & Newman, R. B. (January 1993). Sonographic evaluation for anomalies in twin gestations. American Journal of Obstetrics and Gynecology, 168(1, Pt. 2), 349. SPO abstracts #179.

209. Berghella, V., Pagotto, L., Kaufman, M., Huhta, J., & Wapner, R. (January 1996). Accuracy of prenatal diagnosis of congenital heart defects. American Journal of Obstetrics and Gynecology, 174(1, Pt. 2), 419. SPO abstracts #397.

210. Bork, M. D., Egan, J. F. X., Borgida, A. F., Hardardottir, H., Fabbri, E. L., & Feeney, L. D. (January 1996). Sonographically measured fetal cardiac axis as a marker for congenital heart disease. American Journal of Obstetrics and Gynecology, 174(1, Pt. 2), 418. SPO abstracts #394.

211. Simpson, L. L., Marx, G. R., & D'Alton, M. E. (January 1995). The detection of congenital heart disease in a tertiary care ultrasound practice. American Journal of Obstetrics and Gynecology, 172(1, Pt. 2), 354. SPO abstracts #342.

212. Kirk, J. S., Comstock, C. H., Lee, W., Smith, R. S., Riggs, T. W., & Weinhouse, E. (January 1996). A five-year experience with 111 abnormal fetal hearts: Detected versus undetected. American Journal of Obstetrics and Gynecology, 174(1, Pt. 2), 419. SPO abstracts #400.

213. Mikhail, L. N., Mittendorf, R., & Walker, C. K. (January 1996). The association of maternal obesity and isolated major fetal congenital cardiac anomalies in African-American women. American Journal of Obstetrics and Gynecology, 174(1, Pt. 2), 446. SPO abstracts #497.

214. Gandhi, J., & Yang, X. (January 1995). Fetal cardiac hypetrophy and function in diabetic pregnancies. American Journal of Obstetrics and Gynecology, 172(1, Pt. 2), 355. SPO abstracts #346.

215. Gandhi, J., & Yang, X. (January 1995). Fetal cardiac growth in diabetic pregnancies. American Journal of Obstetrics and Gynecology, 172(1, Pt. 2), 355. SPO abstracts #347.

216. Towner, D., Kjos, S., & Buchanan, T. A. (January 1995). Great vessel and complex cardiac anomalies are the predominant heart defects in infants born to type II diabetics. American Journal of Obstetrics and Gynecology, 172(1, Pt. 2), 282. SPO abstracts #76.

217. Zimmer, E. Z., Avraham, Z., Sujov, P., Goldstein, I., & Bronshtein, M. (January 1996). Impact of ultrasound screening on the prevalence of congenital anomalies at birth. American Journal of Obstetrics and Gynecology, 174(1, Pt. 2), 427. SPO abstracts #431.

218. Smith, R. S., Comstock, C. H., Lorenz, R. P., Kirk, J. S., & Lee, W. (January 1996). Maternal diabetes mellitus: Is fetal echocardiography necessary? American Journal of Obstetrics and Gynecology, 174(1, Pt. 2), 418. SPO abstracts #396.

219. Callan, N. A. (April 1991). Fetal echocardiography. Current Opinion in Obstetrics and Gynecology, 3(2), 255-258.

220. Rokey, R., Belfort, M. A., & Saade, G. R. (October 1995). Quantitative echocardiographic assessment of left ventricular function in critically ill obstetric patients: A comparative study. American Journal of Obstetrics and Gynecology, 173(4), 1148-1152.

221. Lachapelle, M-F., Cote, J-M., Leduc, L., Grignon, A., & Fouron, J-C. (January 1995). Value of fetal echocardiography in the diagnosis of twin-twin transfusion syndrome in presence of polyhydramnios-oligohydramnios. American Journal of Obstetrics and Gynecology, 172(1, Pt. 2), 388. SPO abstracts #467.

222. Kirk, J. S., Comstock, C. H., Lee, W., Smith, R. S., Riggs, T. W., & Weinhouse, E. (January 1996). The prospective evaluation of fetal cardiac anatomy: Addition of the pulmonary artery view does not increase detection rate. American Journal of Obstetrics and Gynecology, 174(1, Pt. 2), 418. SPO abstracts #395.

223. Kirk, J. S., Comstock, C. H., & Lee, W. (January 1993). Optimal gestational ages for the visualization of anatomic structures in the normal fetus. American Journal of Obstetrics and Gynecology, 168(1, Pt. 2), 350. SPO abstracts #185.

224. Bork, M. D., Egan, J. F. X., Diana, D. J., Scorza, W. E., Fabbri, E. L., & Feeney, L. D. (January 1995). A new method to ultrasonically determine fetal cardiac axis. American Journal of Obstetrics and Gynecology, 172(1, Pt. 2), 357. SPO abstracts #351.

225. Bork, M. D., Egan, J. F.X., Campbell, W. A., Diana, D. J., Scorza, W. E., & McLean, D. M. (January 1995). Fetal cardiac axis-a useful screening tool for congenital heart disease? American Journal of Obstetrics and Gynecology, 172(1, Pt. 2), 355. SPO abstracts #344.

226. Fink, N., Ash, K., & Desjardins, C. (January 1996). Fetal cardiac axis in twin pregnancy: A marker for functional and structural cardiac compromise. American Journal of Obstetrics and Gynecology, 174(1, Pt. 2), 419. SPO abstracts #399.

227. Lanouette, J. M., Wolfe, H. M., De Vries, K. L., Puder, K. S., & Gurczynski, J. (January 1996). Adjusted positive predictive value of routine views for the detection of congenital heart disease (CHD). American Journal of Obstetrics and Gynecology, 174(1, Pt. 2), 420. SPO abstracts #401.

228. Veille, J. C., Tatum, K., Steele, L., & McNeil, S. (January 1996). Longitudinal M-mode echocardiography (Ec) of the end diastolic (EDD) and end systolic (ESD) dimension of the right (RV) and left (LV) ventricles from early fetal life to year one. American Journal of Obstetrics and Gynecology, 174(1, Pt. 2), 377. SPO abstracts #239.

229. Hata, T., Takamori, H., Hata, K., Takamiya, O., Murao, F., & Kitao, M. (1988). Antenatal diagnosis of congenital heart disease and fetal arrhythmia by ultrasound: Prospective study. Gynecologic and Obstetric Investigation, (2692), 118-125.

230. Gembruch, U., Knopfle, G., Chatterjee, M., Bald, R., Redel, D. A., Fodisch, H-J., & Hansmann, M. (May 1991). Prenatal diagnosis of atrioventricular canal malformations with up-to-date echocardiographic technology: Report of 14 cases. American Heart Journal, 121(5), 1489-1497.

231. Berdahl, L. D., Wenstrom, K. D., & Hanson, J. W. (January 1995). The relationship of web neck anomaly and congeital heart disease. American Journal of Obstetrics and Gynecology, 172(1, Pt. 2), 394. SPO abstracts #493.

232. Johnson, T. R. B., Besinger, R. E., & Thomas, R. L. (May 1988). New clues to fetal behavior and well being. Contemporary OB/GYN, 108-123.

233. Rayburn, W. F. (December 1987). Monitoring fetal body movement. Clinical Obstetrics and Gynecology, 3(4), 899-911.

234. Sorokin, Y., Chik, L., Brown, C., Martier, S., & Sokol, R. (January 1996). Heart rate patterns in fetuses with fetal alcohol syndrome. American Journal of Obstetrics and Gynecology, 174(1, Pt. 2), 491. SPO abstracts #669.

235. Sokol, R. J., Martier, S. S., Ager, J. W., Abel, E. L., Jacobson, S., & Jacobson, J. (January 1993). Paternal drinking may affect intrauterine growth. American Journal of Obstetrics and Gynecology, 168(1, Pt. 2), 307. SPO abstracts #48.

236. Aaronson, L. S., & Macnee, C. L. (July/August 1989). Tobacco, alcohol, and caffeine use during pregnancy. JOGNN, 18(4), 279-287.

237. Wallerstedt, C., Higgins, P., Kasnic, T., & Curet, L. (1994). Amnioinfusion: An Update. JOGNN 23(7), 573-578.

238. Nageotte, M. P. (1992). Safeguarding the fetus with amnioinfusion. Contemporary OB/GYN, 95-100.

239. Galvan, B., Van Mullem, C., & Broekhuizen, F. (May/June 1989). Using amnioinfusion for the relief of repetitive variable decelerations during labor. JOGNN, 222-229.

240. Sivan, E., Seidman, D. S., Barkai, G., Atlas, M., Dulitzky, M., & Mashiach, S. (1992). Review: The role of amnioinfusion in current obstetric care. Obstetrical and Gynecological Survey, 47(2), 80-87.

241. Ouzounian, J. G., Miller, D. A., & Paul, R. H. (January 1995). Amnioinfusion in women with previous cesarean births. American Journal of Obstetrics and Gynecology, 172(1, Pt. 2), SPO abstracts #88.

242. Garite, T. J., Porto, M., Carlson, N. J., Rumney, P. J., & Reimbold, P. A. (June 1993). The influence of elective amniotomy on fetal heart rate patterns and the course of labor in term patients: A randomized study. American Journal of Obstetrics and Gynecology, 168(6, Pt. 1), 1827-1832.

243. Zuspan, F. P., Cibils, L. A., & Pose, S. V. (October 1, 1962). Myometrial and cardiovascular response to alterations in plasma epinephine and norepinephine. American Journal of Obstetrics and Gynecology, 84(7), 841-851.

244. Ramirez, M. M., Andres, R. L., & Parisi, V. (January 1994). The sympathoadrenal response of the ovine fetus to the direct intravascular administration of methamphetamine. American Journal of Obstetrics and Gynecology, 170(1, Pt. 2), 270. SPO abstracts #18.

245. Stek, A., Fisher, B., Baker, S., & Clark, K. (January 1994). Cardiovascular responses to methamphetamine in fetal sheep. American Journal of Obstetrics and Gynecology, 170(1, Pt. 2), 270.

246. Petrie, R. (October 1980). How intrapartum drugs affect FHR. Contemporary OB/GYN, 1-7.

247. Petrie, R., Yeh, S., Murato, Y., Paul, R., & Hon, E. (February 1978). The effect of drugs on fetal heart rate varibility. American Journal of Obstetrics and Gynecology, 130(3), 294-299.

248. Viscomi, C. M., Hood, D. D., Melone, P. J., & Eisenach, J. C. (December 1990). Fetal heart rate variability after epidural fentanyl during labor. Anesthesia and Analgesia, 71(6), 679-683.

249. Tucker, S. M. (1978). Fetal monitoring and fetal assessment in high-risk pregnancy. St. Louis, MO: The C. V. Mosby Company.

250. McMorland, G. H., & Douglas, M. J. (January 1986). Systemic medication in labour and delivery. Clinics in Anaesthesiology, 4(1), 81-91.

251. Krins, A. J., Mitchells, W. R., & Wood, C. (April 1969). Effect of morphine upon maternal capillary blood oxygen and carbon dioxide tension. Journal of Obstetrics and Gynaecology of the British Commonwealth, 76, 359-361.

252. Barnett, J. M., & Boehm, F. H. (December 1983). Fetal heart rate responses to meperidine alone and in combination with propiomazine. Southern Medical Journal, 76(12), 1480-1483.

253. Baxi, L.V., Petrie, R. H., & James, L. S. (1988). Human Fetal Oxygentation (tcPO$_2$), heart rate variability and uterine activity following maternal administration of meperidine. Journal of Perinatal Medicine 16(1) 23-30.

254. Roumen, F. J. M. E., Aardenburg, R., da Costa, A. J., & Maertzdorf, W. J. (1994). Fetal bradycardia following administration of nalbuphine during labor. The Journal of Maternal-Fetal Medicine, 3, 27-30.

255. Fishburne, J. I. (February 1982). Systemic analgesia during labor. Clinics in Perinatology, 9(1), 29-49.

256. Myers, E., & Myers, S. E. (January 1, 1979). Use of sedative analgesic and anesthetic drugs during labor and delivery: Bane or boon? American Journal of Obstetrics and Gynecology, 133(1), 83-104.

257. Veren, D., Boehm, F. H., & Killam, A. P. (July 1982). The clinical significance of a sinusoidal fetal heart rate pattern associated with alphaprodine administration. Journal of Reproductive Medicine, 27(7), 411-414.

258. Busacca, M., Gementi, P., Ciralli, I., & Vagnali, M. (1982). Sinusoidal fetal heart rate associated with maternal administration of meperidine and promethazine in labor. Journal of Perinatal Medicine, 10, 215-218.

259. Epstein, H., Waxman, A., Gleicher, N., & Lauersen, N. H. (June 1982). Meperidine-induced sinusoidal fetal heart rate pattern and reversal with naloxone. Obstetrics & Gynecology, 59(Suppl., 6), 22s-25s.

260. Spielman, F. J. (September 1987). Systemic analgesics during labor. Clinical Obstetrics and Gynecology, 30(3), 495-503.

261. Clarke, V. T., Smiley, R. M., & Finster, M. (October 1994). Uterine hyperactivity after intrathecal injection of fentanyl for analgesia during labor: A cause of fetal bradycardia [Letter]? Anesthesiology, 81(4), 1083.

262. Valenzuela, G. J., Norburg, M., & Ducsay, C. A. (November 1992). Acute intrauterine hypoxia increases amniotic fluid prostaglandin F metabolites in the pregnant sheep. American Journal of Obstetrics and Gynecology, 167(5), 1459-1464.

263. Paulone, M. E., Edelstone, D. I., & Shedd, A. (January 1987). Effects of maternal anemia on uteroplacental and fetal oxidative metabolism in sheep. American Journal of Obstetrics and Gynecology, 156(1), 230-236.

264. Reshetnikova, O. S., Burton, G. J., & Teleshova, O. V. (September 1995). Placental histomorphometry and morphometric diffusing capacity of the villous membrane in pregnancies complicated by maternal iron-deficiency anemia. American Journal of Obstetrics and Gynecology, 173(3, Pt. 1), 724-727.

265. Olmos, L., Wasserstrum, N., Mombouli, J. V., & Vanhoutte, P. M. (January 1994). Scavenging of EDRF by erythrocytes is altered in pregnancy complicated by sickle cell anemia. American Journal of Obstetrics and Gynecology, 170(1, Pt. 2), 265. SPO abstracts #8.

266. Perry, Jr., K. G., & Morrison, J. C. (April 1990). The diagnosis and management of hemoglobinopathies during pregnancy. Seminars in Perinatology, 14(2), 90-102.

267. Veille, J-C., & Hanson, R. (January 1994). Left ventricular systolic and diastolic function in pregnant patients with sickle cell disease. American Journal of Obstetrics and Gynecology, 170(1, Pt. 1), 107-110.

268. Gimovsky, M. L. (1990). Perinatal/neonatal casebooks. Fetal heart rate monitoring casebook. Journal of Perinatology, 10(2), 198-201.

269. Roberts, S. W., Leveno, K. J., Sidawi, J. E., Lucas, M. J., & Kelly, M. A. (January 1995). Fetal acidemia associated with regional anesthesia for elective cesarean delivery. Obstetrics & Gynecology, 85(1), 79-83.

270. Giles, W. B., Lah, F. X., & Trudinger, B. J. (January 1987). The effect of epidural anaesthesia for caesarean section on maternal uterine and fetal umbilical artery blood velocity waveforms. British Journal of Obstetrics and Gynaecology, 94(1), 55-59.

271. McGlashan, H. E. (August 1994). Elective fetal heart monitoring with epidural analgesia. Australian & New Zealand Journal of Obstetrics and Gynaecology, 34(4), 499-500.

272. Pain relief during labor. (January 1993). ACOG committee opinion number 118. Washington, DC: ACOG.

273. Umstad, M. P., Ross, A., Rushford, D. D., & Permezel, M. (August 1993). Epidural analgesia and fetal heart rate abnormalities. Australian & New Zealand Journal of Obstetrics and Gynaecology, 33(3), 269-272.

274. Lavin, J. P., Samuels, S. V., Miodovnik, M., Holroyde, J., Loon, M., & Joyce, T. (November 15, 1981). The effects of bupivacaine as local anesthetics for epidural anesthesia of fetal heart rate monitoring parameters. American Journal of Obstetrics and Gynecology, 141(6), 717-722.

275. Schifrin, B. S. (April 1972). Fetal heart rate patterns following epidural anaesthesia and oxytocin infusion during labour. Journal of Obstetrics and Gynaecology of the British Commonwealth, 79, 332-339.

276. Fusi, L., Maresh, M. J. A., Steer, P. J., & Beard, R. W. (June 1989). Maternal pyrexia associated with the use of epidural analgesia in labour. The Lancet, i, 1250-1252.

277. Cowan, D. B. (August 30, 1980). Intrapartum fetal resuscitation. South African Medical Journal, 58(9), 376-379.

278. Aldrich, C. J., D'Antona, D., Spencer, J. A., Wyatt, J. S., Peebles, D. M., & Delpy, D. T. (January 1995). The effect of maternal posture on fetal cerebral oxygenation during labour. British Journal of Obstetrics & Gynaecology, 102(1), 14-19.

279. Hoffman, III, C., Guzman, E., Richardson, M., Vintzileos, A., Houlihan, C., & Benito, C. (January 1996). The effects of narcotic and non-narcotic continuous epidural anesthesia on intrapartum fetal heart rate tracings as measured by computer analysis. American Journal of Obstetrics and Gynecology, 174(1, Pt. 2), 431. SPO abstracts #438.

280. Sciscione, A., Boersma, M., Narayan, H., Costigan, K., Gorman, R., & Reddy, U. (January 1995). The effect of epidural anesthesia on intrapartum fetal behavior. American Journal of Obstetrics and Gynecology, 172(1, Pt. 2), 362. SPO abstracts #373.

281. Hon, H. (1967). Detection of fetal distress. In C. Wood (Ed.), Fifth world congress of gynecology and obstetrics. Sydney, Australia.

282. Puolakka, J., Jouppila, R., Jouppila, P., & Puukka, M. (1984). Maternal and fetal effects of low-dosage bupivacaine paracervical block. Journal of Perinatal Medicine, 12, 75-84.

283. Carlsson, B-M., Johansson, M., & Westin, B. (1987). Fetal heart rate pattern before and after paracervical anaesthesia. Acta Obstetricia et Gynecologica Scandinavica, 66, 391-395.

284. Achiron, R., Rojansky, N., & Zakut, H. (1987). Fetal heart rate and uterine activity following paracervical block. Clinical Experiments in Obstetrics and Gynecology, 14(1), 52-56.

285. LeFevre, M. L. (September 1984). Fetal heart rate pattern and postparacervical fetal bradycardia. Obstetrics & Gynecology, 64(3), 343-346.

286. Marx, G. F., & Mateo, C. V. (November 1971). Effects of different oxygen concentrations during general anaesthesia for elective caesarean section. Canadian Anaesthetists Society Journal, 18(6), 587-593.

287. Bahary, C. M., Ninio, A., Gorodesky, I. G., & Neri, A. (May 1980). Tococardiography in pregnancy during extracorporeal bypass for mitral valve replacement. Israel Journal of Medical Science, 16(5), 395-397.

288. Miller, F. C., Petrie, R. H., Arcs, J. J., Paul, R. H., & Hon, E. H. (October 15, 1974). Hyperventilation during labor. American Journal of Obstetrics and Gynecology, 120(4), 489-495.

289. Lumley, J., Renou, P., Newman, W., & Wood, C. (March 15, 1969). Hyperventilation in obstetrics. American Journal of Obstetrics and Gynecology, 103(6), 847-855.

290. Datta, S., Ostheimer, G. W., Weiss, J. B., Brown, Jr., W. U., & Alper, M. H. (September 1981). Neonatal effect of prolonged anesthetic induction for cesarean section. Obstetrics & Gynecology, 58(3), 331-335.

291. Adair, R. F. (December 1993). Fetal monitoring with adenosine administration [Letters]. Annals of Emergency Medicine, 22(12), 1925.

292. Anastasio, G. D., & Harston, P. (September/October 1992). Fetal tachycardia associated with maternal use of pseudoephedrine, an over-the counter oral decongestant. Journal of the American Board of Family Practice 5(5) 527-528.

293. Fetal Distress from something mother ate (April 15, 1985). Emergency Medicine, 57.

294. Montan, S., Solum, T., & Sjoberg, N-O. (1984). Influence of the β_1-adrenoceptor blocker atenolol on antenatal cardiotocography. Acta Obstetricia et Gynecologica Scandinavica, 5118, 99-102.

295. Montan, S., Ingemarsson, I., Marsal, K., & Sjoberg, N-O. (1992). Randomised controlled trial of atenolol and pindolol in human pregnancy. British Medical Journal, 304, 946-949.

296. Bistoletti, P., Lagercrantz, H., & Lunell, N. O. (January 1983). Fetal plasma catecholamine concentrations and fetal heart-rate variability during first stage of labour. British Journal of Obstetrics and Gynaecology, 90(1), 11-15.

297. Cassidy, J. E., & Linthicum, L. (November/December 1987). The effect of anxiety on childbearing. JOGNN, 16(6), 439.

298. Caldeyro-Barcia, R., & Poseiro, J. J. (June 1960). Physiology of the uterine contraction. Clinics in Obstetrics and Gynecology, 3(2), 386-408.

299. Wilcox, D. E. (July 1985). Emergency aspects of complicated labor and delivery: Fetal distress. Topics in Emergency Medicine, 7(2), 33-42.

300. Klaus, M. H., Kennell, J. H., Robertson, S. S., & Sosa, R. (September 6, 1986). Effects of social support during infant morbidity. British Medical Journal, 293, 595-597.

301. Myers, R. E. (May 1, 1975). Maternal psychological stress and fetal asphyxia: A study in the monkey. American Journal of Obstetrics and Gynecology, 122(1), 47-59.

302. Mulder, E. J. H., Derks, J. B., Zonneveld, M. F., Bruinse, H. W., & Visser, G. H. A. (1994). Transient reduction in fetal activity and heart rate variation after maternal betamethasone administration. Early Human Development, 36, 49-60.

303. Conover, W. B., Key, T. C., & Resnik, R. (March 1, 1983). Maternal cardovascular response to caffeine infusion in the pregnant ewe. American Journal of Obstetrics and Gynecology, 145(5), 534-538.

304. Salvador, H. S., & Koos, B. J. (May 1989). Effects of regular and decaffeinated coffee on fetal breathing and heart rate. [published erratum appears in American Journal of Obstetrics and Gynecology, (September 1989), 161(3), 669.] American Journal of Obstetrics and Gynecology, 160(5, Pt. 1), 1043-1047.

305. Ball, R. H. & Parer, J. T. (June 1992). The physiologic mechanisms of variable decelerations. American Journal of Obstetrics and Gynecology, 166(6, Pt. 1), 1683-1689.

306. Barnett, R., & Phillips, C. R. (1988). Physiologic approach to childbirth (pp. 3-16). Batesville, IN: Hill-Rom.

307. Mayberry, L. (February 1994). Intrapartum nursing care: Research into practice. JOGNN, 23(2), 170-174.

308. Strohl, K. P., & Altrose, M. D. (February 1984). Oxygen saturation during breath-holding and during apneas in sleep. Chest, 85(2), 181-186.

309. Caldeyro-Barcia, R., Giussi, G., Storch, E., Poseiro, J. J., Lafaurie, N., & Kettenhuber, K. (1981). The bearing-down efforts and their effects on fetal heart rate, oxygenation and acid base balance. Journal of Perinatal Medicine, 9(Suppl. 1), 63-67.

310. Little, B. B., Roe, D. A., Stettler, R. W., Bohman, V. R., Westfall, K. L., & Sobhi, S. (May 1995). A new placental enzyme in the metabolism of cocaine: An in vitro animal model. American Journal of Obstetrics and Gynecology, 172(5), 1441-1445.

311. Ogunyemi, D., Cook, R., Beverly, S., Brown, P., & Fukushima, T. (January 1993). Effect of positive cocaine toxicology on uterine artery doppler velocimetry. American Journal of Obstetrics and Gynecology, 168(1, Pt. 2), 354. SPO abstracts #201.

312. Shlossman, P., Colmorgen, G., Sciscione, A., Neerhof, M., Craparo, F., & Weiner, S. (January 1993). Effects of cocaine use on fetal blood in appropriately grown fetuses. American Journal of Obstetrics and Gynecology, 168(1, Pt. 2), 355. SPO abstracts #203.

313. Mitra, S. C., Taylor, U. B., Ganesh, V., & Apuzzio, J. J. (January 1993). Effect of maternal cocaine abuse on renal arterial flow and urine output of the fetus. American Journal of Obstetrics and Gynecology, 168(1, Pt. 2), 355. SPO abstracts #202.

314. Miller, Jr., J. M., Boudreaux, M. C., & Regan, F. A. (January 1995). A case-control study of cocaine use in pregnancy. American Journal of Obstetrics and Gynecology, 172(1, Pt. 1), 180-185.

315. Simone, C., Derewlany, L. O., Oskamp, M., Knie, B., & Koren, G. (May 1994). Transfer of cocaine and benzoylecgonine across the perfused human placental cotyledon. American Journal of Obstetrics and Gynecology, 170(5, Pt. 1), 1404-1410.

316. Beck, J. (August 12, 1992). Warn pregnant women about cocaine. Chicago Tribune, A8.

317. Nevils, B., Barada, C., Gilson, G., & Curet, L. (January 1994). Neonatal morbidity and mortality in the pregnant drug abuser. American Journal of Obstetrics and Gynecology, 170(1, Pt. 2), 373. SPO abstracts #351.

318. Tabor, B. L., Soffici, A. R., Smith-Wallace, T., & Yonekura, M. L. (November 1991). The effect of maternal cocaine use on the fetus: Changes in antepartum fetal heart rate tracings. American Journal of Obstetrics and Gynecology, 165(5, Pt. 1), 1278-1281.

319. Perlow, J. H., Schlossberg, D. L., & Strassner, H. T. (October 1990). Intrapartum cocaine use. A case report. Journal of Reproductive Medicine, 35(10), 978-980.

320. Shiono, P. H., Klehanoff, M. A., Nugent, R. P., Cotch, M. F., Wilkins, D. G., & Rollins, D. E. (January 1995). The impact of cocaine and marijuana use on low birth weight and preterm birth: A multicenter study. American Journal of Obstetrics and Gynecology, 172(1, Pt. 1), 19-27.

321. Shlossman, P., Colmorgen, G., Sciscione, A., Neerhof, M., Craparo, F., & Weiner, S. (January 1993). Effects of cocaine exposure on fetal blood flow in small for gestational age fetuses. American Journal of Obstetrics and Gynecology, 168(1, Pt. 2), 355. SPO abstracts #204.

322. Chazotte, C., Forman, L., & Gandhi, J. (September 1991). Heart rate patterns in fetuses exposed to cocaine. Obstetrics & Gynecology, 78(3, Pt.1), 323-325.

323. Peters, H., & Theorell, C. (March/April 1991). Fetal and neonatal effects of maternal cocaine use. JOGNN,20(2), 121-125.

324. Caring for cocaine's mothers and babies. (October 1989). Newsletter. Washington, DC, NAACOG, 1, 4-6.

325. Divon, M. Y., Muskat, Y., Platt, L. D., & Paldi, E. (August 15, 1984). Increased beat-to-beat variability during uterine contractions: A common association in uncomplicated labor. American Journal of Obstetrics and Gynecology, 149(8), 893-896.

326. Hon, E. H., & Quilligan, E. J. (1968). Electronic evaluation of fetal heart rate. IX. Further observations on "pathologic" fetal bradycardia. Clinical Obstetrics, 11, 145-167.

327. Carter, A. M. (1989). Factors affecting gas transfer across the placenta and the oxygen supply to the fetus. Journal of Developmental Physiology, 12(6), 305-322.

328. Low, J. A., Cox, M. J., Karchmar, M. J., McGrath, M. J., Pancham, S. R., & Piercy, W. N. (February 1, 1981). The prediction of intrapartum fetal metabolic acidosis by fetal heart rate monitoring. American Journal of Obstetrics and Gynecology, 139(3), 299-305.

329. Zoppini, C., Donnenfeld, A., Godmilow, L., Ludomirsky, A., & Weiner, S. (January 1993). Immediate effects of chorionic villus sampling on fetal heart rate. American Journal of Obstetrics and Gynecology, 168(1, Pt. 2), 399. SPO abstracts #367.

330. Weiner, Z., Farmakides, G., Barnhard, Y., Maulik, D., Bar-Hava, I., & Divon, M. Y. (January 1995). Fetal heart rate pattern in pregnancies complicated by maternal diabetes. American Journal of Obstetrics and Gynecology, 172(1, Pt. 2), 339. SPO abstracts #285.

331. Conley, N. J., & Olshansky, E. (September/October 1987). Current controversies in pregnancy and epilepsy: A unique chanllenge to nursing. JOGNN, 16(5), 321-328.

332. Paul, R. H., Koh, K. S., & Bernstein, S. G. (January 15, 1978). Changes in fetal heart rate-uterine contraction patterns associated with eclampsia. American Journal of Obstetrics and Gynecology, 130(2), 165-169.

333. Clapp, III, J. F., Little, K. D., & Capeless, E. L. (January 1993). Fetal heart rate response to sustained recreational exercise. American Journal of Obstetrics and Gynecology, 168(1, Pt. 1), 198-205.

334. Clapp, III, J. F., & Little, K. D. (July 1995). The interaction between regular exercise and selected aspects of women's health [Primary Care]. American Journal of Obstetrics and Gynecology, 173(1), 2-9.

335. Bung, P., Huch, R., & Huch, A. (1991). Maternal and fetal heart rate patterns: A pregnant athlete during training and laboratory exercise tests: A case report. European Journal of Obstetrics, Gynecology and Reproductive Biology, 39, 59-62.

336. Collings, C., & Curet, L. B. (February 1985). Fetal heart rate response to maternal exercise. American Journal of Obstetrics and Gynecology, 151(4), 498-501.

337. Watson, W. J., Katz, V. L., Hackney, A. C., Gall, M. M., & McMurray, R. G. (March 1991). Fetal responses to maximal swimming and cycling exercise during pregnancy. Obstetrics & Gynecology, 77(3), 382-386.

338. Fishbein, E., & Phillips, M. (January/February 1990). How safe is exercise during pregnancy? JOGNN,19(1)45-49.

339. Newhall, Jr., J. F. (August 15, 1981). Scuba diving during pregnancy: A brief review. American Journal of Obstetrics and Gynecology, 140, 893-894.

340. Spinnewijn, W. E. M., Lotgering, F. K., Struijk, P. C., & Wallenburg, H. C. S. (January 1996). Fetal heart rate and uterine contractility during maternal exercise at term. American Journal of Obstetrics and Gynecology, 174(1, Pt. 1), 43-48.

341. Van Hook, J., Easterling, T., Schmucker, B., Braeteng, D., Carlson, K., & DeLateur, B. (January 1993). American Journal of Obstetrics and Gynecology, 168(1, Pt. 2), 330. SPO abstracts #107.

342. Carpenter, M. W., Sady, S. P., Hoegsberg, B., Sady, M. A., Haydon, B., & Cullinane, E. M. (May 27, 1988). Fetal heart rate response to maternal exertion. JAMA, 259(20), 3006-3009.

343. Cefalo, R.C., & Hellegers, A. E. (1978). The effects of maternal hyperthermia on maternal and fetal cardiovascular and respiratory function. American Journal of Obstetrics and Gynecology, 131(6), 687-694.

344. Vaha-Eskeli, K., & Erkkola, R. (January 1990). The effects of short term heat stress on uterine contractility fetal heart rate and fetal movements at late pregnancy. European Journal of Obstetrics, Gynecology, and Reproductive Biology, 38(1), 9-14.

345. Bartnicki, J., Ratanasiri, T., Meyenburg, M., & Saling, E. (1992). Effect of the vibratory acoustic stimulation on fetal heart rate patterns of premature fetuses. International Journal of Gynecology and Obstetrics, 37, 3-6.

346. Anyaegbunam, A. M., Ditchik, A., Stoessel, R., & Mikhail, M. S. (June 1994). Vibroacoustic stimulation of the fetus entering the second stage of labor. Obstetrics & Gynecology, 83(6), 963-966.

347. Sulik, S., & Greenwald, J. (April 1994). Evaluation and management of the postdate pregnancy. American Family Physician, 49(5), 1177-1185.

348. Rorke, M. J., Davey, D. A., & Du Toit, H. J. (October 1968). Foetal oxygenation during caesarean section. Anaesthesia, 23(4), 585-596.

349. Bekedam, D. J., Mulder, E. J. H., Snijders, R. J. M., & Visser, G. H. A. (1991). The effects of maternal hyperoxia on fetal breathing movements, body movements and heart rate variation in growth retarded fetuses. Early Human Development, 27, 223-232.

350. Burke, M. E. (October 1989). Hypertensive crisis and the perinatal period. Journal of Perinatal and Neonatal Nursing, 3(2), 33-47.

351. Shearman, R. P. (Ed.). (1979). Human reproductive physiology (2nd ed.). Oxford: England: Blackwell Scientific Publications.

352. Maxwell, K. D., Kearney, K. K., Johnson, J. W. C., Eagan, J. W., & Tyson, J. E. (March 1980). Fetal tachycardia associated with intrauterine fetal thyrotoxicosis. Obstetrics & Gynecology, 55(Suppl., 3), 18s-22s.

353. Langer, O., & Cohen, W. R. (July 15, 1984). Persistent fetal bradycardia during maternal hypoglycemia. American Journal of Obstetrics and Gynecology, 149(6), 688-690.

354. Danilenko-Dixon, D. R., Tefft, L., Haydon, B., Cohen, R. A., & Carpenter, M. W. (January 1996). The effect of maternal position on cardiac output with epidural analgesia in labor. American Journal of Obstetrics and Gynecology, 174(1, Pt. 2), 332. SPO abstracts #75.

355. Abitbol, M. M. (April 1985). Supine position in labor and associated fetal heart rate changes. Obstetrics & Gynecology, 65(4), 481-486.

356. Preston, R., Crosby E. T., Kotarba, D., Dudas, H., & Elliott, R. D. (1993). Maternal positioning affects fetal heart rate changes after epidural analgesia for labour. Canadian Journal of Anesthesia, 40(12), 1136-1141.

357. Waldron, K. W., & Wood, C. (May 1971). Cesarean section in the lateral position. Obstetrics & Gynecology, 37(5), 706-710.

358. de Haan, H. H., Ijzermans, A. C. M., de Haan, J., & Hasaart, T. H. M. (January 1995). The T/QRS ratio of the electrocardiogram does not reliably reflect well-being in fetal lambs. American Journal of Obstetrics and Gynecology, 172(1, Pt. 1), 35-43.

359. Eggert, J. V., Weidner, W., Eggert, L. D., Woods, R. E., & Mattern, D. (1986). Simplified method of obtaining umbilical cord blood for pH using a heparinized vacutainer versus heparinized syringe. American Journal of Perinatology, 3(4), 311.

360. O'Brien-Abel, N. E., & Benedetti, T. J. (1992). Saltatory fetal heart rate pattern. Journal of Perinatology, 12(1), 13-17.

361. Mason, B. A., Strandley, C. A., Whitty, J. E., Irtenkauf, S. M., & Cotton, D. B. (January 1995). The effects of magnesium therapy on umbilical cord ionized magnesium levels. American Journal of Obstetrics and Gynecology, 172(1, Pt. 2), 385. SPO abstracts #457.

362. Hallak, M., Berry, S. M., Romero, R., Evans, M. I., & Cotton, D. B. (January 1993). Maternal-fetal transfer of magnesium across the human placenta. American Journal of Obstetrics and Gynecology, 168(1, Pt. 2), 326. SPO abstracts #91.

363. Hallak, M., & Cotton, D. B. (January 1993). Transfer of maternally administered magnesium sulfate into the fetal compartment of the rat: Assessment of amniotic fluid, blood, and brain concentrations. American Journal of Obstetrics and Gynecology, 168(1, Pt. 2), 326. SPO abstracts #92.

364. Atkinson, M. W., Belfort, M. A., Saade, G. R., & Moise, Jr., K. J. (June 1994). The relation between magnesium sulfate therapy and fetal heart rate variability. Obstetrics & Gynecology, 83(6), 967-970.

365. Guzman, E. R., Conley, M., Stewart, R., Ivan, J., Pitter, M. & Kappy, K. (September 1993). Phenytoin and magnesium sulfate effects on fetal heart rate tracings assessed by computer analysis. Obstetrics & Gynecology, 82(3), 375-378.

366. Keeley, M. M., Wade, R. V., Laurent, S. L., & Hamann, V. D. (February 1993). Alterations in maternal-fetal doppler flow velocity waveforms in preterm labor patients undergoing magnesium sulfate tocolysis. Obstetrics & Gynecology, 81(2), 191-194.

367. Canez, M., Reed, K., & Shenler, L. (April 1987). Effect of maternal magnesium sulfate treatment on FHR variability. Amercian Journal of Perinatology, 4(2)167-170.

368. Petrikovsky, B. M., & Vintzileos, A. M. (April 1990). Magnesium sulfate and intrapartum fetal behavior. American Journal of Perinatology, 7(2), 154-156.

369. Parsons, M. T., Owens, C. A., & Spellacy, W. N. (January 1987). Thermic effects of tocolytic agents: Decreased temperature with magnesium sulfate. Obstetrics & Gynecology, 69(1), 88-90.

370. Rodis, J. F., Vintzileos, A. M., Campbell, W. A., Deaton, J. L., & Nochimson, D. J. (February 1987). Maternal hypothermia: An unusual complication of magnesium sulfate therapy. American Journal of Obstetrics and Gynecology, 156(2), 435-436.

371. Graca, L. M., Cardoso, C. G., Clode, N., & Calhaz-Jorge, C. (1991). Acute effects of maternal cigarette smoking on fetal heart rate and fetal body movements felt by the mother. Journal of Perinatology Medicine, 19, 385-390.

372. Phelan, J. P. (January 15, 1980). Diminished fetal reactivity with smoking. American Journal of Obstetrics and Gynecology, 136(2), 230-233.

373. Brost, B., Joseph, M., Stramm, S., & Eller, D. (January 1996). The acute effects of cigarette use during pregnancy on fetal activity. American Journal of Obstetrics and Gynecology, 174(1, Pt. 2), 336. SPO abstracts #81.

374. Pijpers, L., Wladimiroff, J., McGhie, J., & Bom, N. (September 1984). Acute effect of maternal smoking on the maternal and fetal cardiovascular system. Early Human Development, 10(1-2), 95-105.

375. Cigarette Smoking and pregnancy (September 1979). Technical bulletin number 53. Washington, DC: ACOG.

376. Myers, R. E., Joelsson, I., & Adamson, K. (1978). The effects of isoproterenol on fetal oxygenation. Acta Obstetricia et Gynecologica Scandinavica, 57(4), 317-322.

377. Freeman, R. K., & Garite, T. J. (1981). Fetal heart rate monitoring. Baltimore, MD: Williams & Wilkins.

378. Martin, C. B. (April 1978). Regulation of the fetal heart rate and genesis of FHR patterns. Seminars in Perinatology, 2(2), 131-146.

379. Yoneyama, Y., Shin, S. Iwasaki, T., Power, G. G., & Araki, T. (September 1994). Relationship between plasma adenosine concentration and breathing movements in growth-retarded fetuses. American Journal of Obstetrics and Gynecology, 171(3), 701-706.

380. Weiner, C. P., Power, G., & Yoneyama, Y. (January 1993). Adenosine in the human fetus. American Journal of Obstetrics and Gynecology, 168(1, Pt. 2), 328. SPO abstracts #99.

381. Yoneyama, Y., Wakatsuki, M., Sawa, R., Kamoi, S., Takahashi, H., & Shin, S. (February 1994). Plasma adenosine concentration in appropriate- and small-for-gestational-age fetuses. American Journal of Obstetrics and Gynecology, 170(2), 684-688.

382. Smith, C. V., Nguyen, H. N., Phelan, J. P., & Paul, R. H. (October 1986). Intrapartum assessment of fetal well-being: A comparison of fetal acoustic stimulation with acid-base determinations. American Journal of Obstetrics and Gynecology, 155(4), 726-728.

383. Clark, S. L. (May 1990). How a modified NST improves fetal surveillance. Contemporary OB/GYN, 45-48.

384. Gagnon, R., Campbell, K., Hunse, C., & Patrick, J. (September 1987). Patterns of human fetal heart rate accelerations from 26 weeks to term. American Journal of Obstetrics and Gynecology, 157(3), 743-748.

385. Natale, R., Nasello-Paterson, C., & Turliuk, R. (January 15, 1985). Longitudinal measurements of fetal breathing, body movements, heart rate, and heart rate accelerations and decelerations at 24 to 32 weeks of gestation. American Journal of Obstetrics and Gynecology, 151(2), 256-263.

386. Yancey, M. K., Moore, J., Brody, K., Milligan, D., & Strampel, W. (April 1992). The effect attitude on umbilical cord blood gases. Obstetrics & Gynecology, 79(4), 571-574.

387. Baskett, T. F., & Koh, K. S. (September 1974). Sinusoidal fetal heart pattern. A sign of fetal hypoxia. Obstetrics & Gynecology, 44(3), 379-382.

388. Mueller-Heubach, E., Caritis, S. N., & Edelstone, D. I. (July 1978). Sinusoidal fetal heart rate pattern following intrauterine fetal transfusion. Obstetrics & Gynecology, 52(Suppl., 1), 43s-46s.

389. Young, B. K., Katz, M., & Wilson, S. T. (March 1, 1980). Sinusoidal fetal heart rate. American Journal of Obstetrics and Gynecology, 136(5), 587-597.

390. Olofsson, P., Stangenberg, M., Selbing, A., Rahman, F., & Westgren, M. (1990). Fetal heart rate responses to anemia in Rh isoimmunization. Journal of Perinatal Medicine, 18(3), 187-194.

391. Economides, D. L., Selinger, M., Ferguson, J., Bowell, P. J., Dawes, G. S., & Mackenzie, I. Z. (September 1992). Computerized measurement of heart rate variation in fetal anemia caused by rhesus alloimmunization. American Journal of Obstetrics and Gynecology, 167(3), 689-693.

392. Ito,T., Maeda, K., Takahashi, H., Nagata, N., Nakajima, K. & Terakawa, N. (1994). Differentiation between physiologic and pathologic sinusoidal FHR pattern by fetal actocardiogram. Journal of Perinatal Medicine, 22, 39-43.

393. Darby, M. J., Edelstone, D. I., Bass, K., & Miller, K. (January 1991). Effects of fetal anemia on PO_2 difference between uterine venous and umbilical venous blood. American Journal of Physiology, 260(1, Pt. 2), H276-H281.

394. Van der Moer, P., Gerretsen, G., &Visser, G. (1985). Fixed fetal heart rate pattern after intrauterine accidental decerebration. Obstetrics & Gynecology, 65(1), 125-127.

395. Bork, M. D., Egan, J. F. X., Diana, D. J., Campbell, W. A., Scorza, W. E., & McLean, D. M. (January 1995). Analyses of referral indications for fetal echocardiography in a university and community hospital setting. American Journal of Obstetrics and Gynecology, 172(1, Pt. 2), 355. SPO abstracts #345.

396. Prentice, A., & Brown, R. (January 1989). Fetal tachyarrhythmia and maternal antidepressant treatment. British Medical Journal,298(6667), 190.

397. Matsuda, Y., Patrick, J., Carmichael, L., Fraher, L., & Richardson, B. (May 1994). Recovery of the ovine fetus from sustained hypoxia: Effects on endocrine, cardiovascular, and biophysical activity. American Journal of Obstetrics and Gynecology, 170(5, Pt. 1), 1433-1441.

398. Harned, Jr., H. S., Wolkoff, A. S., Pickrell, J., & MacKinney, L. G. (August 1961). Hemodynamic observations during birth of the lamb. Studies of the unanesthetized full-term animal. American Journal of Diseases of Children, 102, 58-67.

399. Berestka, J. S., Johnson, T. R. B., & Hrushesky, W. J. M. (March 1989). Sinusoidal fetal heart rate pattern during breathing is related to the respiratory sinus arrhythmia: A case report. American Journal of Obstetrics and Gynecology, 160(3), 690-692.

400. Biale, Y., Brawer-Ostrovsky, Y., & Insler, V. (January 1985). Fetal heart rate tracings in fetuses with congenital malformations. The Journal of Reproductive Medicine, 30(1), 43-47.

401. Legun, L. (July 1990). Systemic lupus erythematosus during pregnancy. JOGNN, 19(4),304-310.

402. Goodlin, R. C. (February 1987). The capricious fetal heart rate response to acute blood loss. A report of three cases. The Journal of Reproductive Medicine, 32(2), 126-128.

403. Kosasa, T. S., Ebusugawa, J., Nakayama, R. T., & Hale, R. W. (October 1993). Massive fetomaternal hemorrhage preceded by decreased fetal movement and a nonreactive fetal heart rate pattern. Obstetrics & Gynecology, 82(4, Pt. 2), 711-714.

404. Hagay, Z. J., Mazor, M., Leiberman, J. R., & Piura, B. (1986). The effect of maternal hypocalcemia on fetal heart rate baseline variability. Acta Obstetricia et Gynecologica Scandinavica, 65(5), 513-515.

405. Jadhon, M. E., & Main, E. K. (September 1988). Fetal bradycardia associated with maternal hypothermia. Obstetrics & Gynecology, 72(3, Pt. 2), 496-497.

407. Stange, K., & Haldin, M. (May 1983). Clinical reports: Hypothermia in pregnancy. Anesthesiology, 58(5), 460-461.

408. Odendaal, H. (August 1976). Fetal heart rate patterns in patients with intrauterine growth retardation. Obstetrics & Gynecology, 48(2), 187-190.

409. Ingemarsson, E., Ingemarsson, I., Solum, T., & Westgren, M. (March 1980). Influence of occiput posterior position on the fetal heart rate pattern. Obstetrics & Gynecology, 55(3), 301-304.

410. Vintzileos, A. M., Campbell, W. A., Nochimson, D. J., & Weinbaum, P. J. (August 1985). Degree of oligohydramnios and pregnancy outcome in patients with premature rupture of the membranes. Obstetrics & Gynecology, 66(2), 162-167.

411. Moberg, L. J., Garite, T. J., & Freeman, R. K. (July 1984). Fetal heart rate patterns and fetal distress in patients with preterm premature rupture of membranes. Obstetrics & Gynecology, 64(1), 60-64.

412. Hoskins, I. A., Frieden, F. J., & Young, B. K. (October 1991). Variable decelerations in reactive nonstress tests with decreased amniotic fluid index predict fetal compromise. American Journal of Obstetrics and Gynecology, 165(4, Pt. 1), 1094-1098.

413. Harding, J. A., Jackson, D. M., Lewis, D. F., Major, C. A., Nageotte, M. P., & Asrat, T. (October 1991). Correlation of amniotic fluid index and nonstress test in patients with preterm premature rupture of membranes. American Journal of Obstetrics and Gynecology, 165(4, Pt. 1), 1088-1094.

414. Pielet, B. W., Socol, M. L., MacGregor, S. N., Dooley, S. L., & Minogue, J. (September 1988). Fetal heart rate changes after fetal intravascular treatment with pancuronium bromide. American Journal of Obstetrics and Gynecology, 159(3), 640-643.

415. Spencer, J. A. D. (1991). Predictive value of a fetal heart rate acceleration at the time of fetal blood sampling in labour. Journal of Perinatal Medicine, 19, 207-215.

416. Cibils, L. A., & Votta, R. (1993). Clinical significance of fetal heart rate patterns during labor IX: Prolonged pregnancy. Journal of Perinatal Medicine, 21, 107-116.

417. Ribbert, L. S. M., Visser, G. H. A., Mulder, E. J. H., Zonneveld, M. F., & Morssink, L. P. (1993). Changes with time in fetal heart rate variation, movement incidences and haemodynamics in intrauterine growth retarded fetuses: A longitudinal approach to the assessment of fetal well being. Early Human Development, 31, 195-208.

418. D'Hooghe, T. M., & Odendaal, H. L. (1991). Fewer accelerations and decreased long term variability in the heart rate of small for gestational age fetuses. International Journal of Gynecology and Obstetrics, 35, 133-138.

419. Dierker Jr., L. J., Pillay, S. K., Sorokin, Y., & Rosen, M. G. (July 1982). Active and quiet periods in the preterm and term fetus. Obstetrics & Gynecology, 60(1), 65-70.

420. Dierker, Jr., L. J., Pillay, S., Sorokin, Y., & Rosen, M. G. (May 15, 1982). The change in fetal activity periods in diabetic and nondiabetic pregnancies. American Journal of Obstetrics and Gynecology, 143(2), 181-185.

421. Dawes, G. S., Lobb, M. O., Mandruzzato, G., Moulden, M., Redman, C. W. G., & Wheeler, T. (January 1993). Large fetal heart rate decelerations at term associated with changes in fetal heart rate variation. American Journal of Obstetrics and Gynecology, 168(1, Pt. 1), 105-111.

422. Macaulay, J. H., Randall, N. R., & Steer, P. J. (March 1992). Continuous monitoring of fetal temperature by noninvasive probe and its relationship to maternal temperature, fetal heart rate, and cord arterial oxygen and pH. Obstetrics & Gynecology, 79(3), 469-474.

423. Apuzzio, J. J., Pelosi, M. A., & Ganesh, V. V. (July 1984). Fetal heart bradycardia associated with the vacuum extractor. A case report. The Journal of Reproductive Medicine, 29(7), 496-497.

9

Antepartal Fetal Monitoring

INTRODUCTION

The purpose of antepartal electronic fetal monitoring is to prevent morbidity and mortality of fetuses who have a high risk of hypoxia due to uteroplacental insufficiency (1). The tracing of the fetus before labor is evaluated using the same systematic review as the tracing of the fetus during labor (2). However, antepartal fetal heart rate pattern classifications differ from intrapartal classifications. For example, intrapartal patterns may be classified as reassuring, compensatory, nonreassuring, and ominous. Antepartal patterns may be classified as reactive, nonreactive, negative, reactive/negative, nonreactive/negative, equivocal or suspicious, positive, reactive/positive, nonreactive/positive, hyperstimulation, and inconclusive or unsatisfactory.

Classifications of intrapartal patterns determine intervention choices and the route and timing of delivery. Classifications of antepartal patterns affect pregnancy management decisions (3-6). Just like intrapartal patterns, antepartal patterns predict a normal outcome well and a poor outcome poorly (7).

Antepartal fetal monitoring indirectly assesses fetal brain, cardiac, and placenta function. Antepartal tests include the nonstress test, the fetal activity acceleration determination test, the fetal acoustic stimulation test, and contraction stress tests. This chapter reviews these antepartal tests and the maternal assessment of fetal movement or kick counts.

HISTORY OF ANTEPARTAL TESTS
Oxytocin Challenge Test (OCT)
The first description of a contraction stress test (CST), written by Dr. Hammacher, appeared in 1966 in a German medical journal. The first American report of an OCT was published in 1972 (8). OCT results indirectly reflect *placental function* and fetal oxygen reserves (6, 8-10). Intravenous (IV) oxytocin is administered to produce three 40 to 60 second contractions in a 10 minute period (11). If late decelerations (decels) appear, the fetus may have inadequate oxygen reserves to cope with labor. The popularity of the OCT waned during the 1980s as the use of the biophysical profile (BPP) increased (1, 9).

Nonstress Test (NST)
In 1976, Drs. Rochard, Schifrin, and Goupil described the nonstress test (NST) (6, 12). The NST reflects fetal brainstem, autonomic nervous system, and cardiac function in the absence of contractions. The size and number of accelerations (accels) during a maximum of 40 minutes of monitoring is evaluated to determine fetal well-being (11). In 1984, Dr. Huddleston wrote, "...the nonstress test has generally supplanted the contraction stress test as the primary test for assessment of fetal well-being" (1).

Fetal Acoustic Stimulation Test (FAST)
In 1977, Drs. Read and Miller published a preliminary report on the use of a 5 second 105 to 120 decibel (dB) pure-tone auditory stimulus for "nonstress" testing. They compared test results with the OCT. If the fetus accelerated after acoustic stimulation and the accel was at least 15 bpm above the BL, the subsequent OCT was always negative (13). In 1986, the use of acoustic stimulation was still considered investigational (14). By June 30, 1987, there were 8 papers published on fetal acoustic stimulation as a test of fetal well-

being. Sound intensity in these prospective studies ranged from 80 to 126 dB (measured 10 cm to 1 meter from the sound producing device) at a frequency of 20 to 9000 Hz for 1 to 10 seconds. One to seven stimuli were given one second to three minutes apart (15). By 1989, the FAST was more commonly used and was considered a "modified NST with sound stimulation." If the fetus did not respond to the first 1 to 2 seconds of sound, another sound stimulus was applied to the lower maternal abdomen no more than 10 minutes after the first sound stimulus. An artificial larynx was used to produce the loud sound. Seventeen percent of fetuses who did not accel following 2 sound stimuli had positive OCTs or a BPP score less than or equal to 4 out of 10 (16). Today, acoustic stimulation is used in the antepartal and intrapartal settings as a test of fetal well-being. Acoustic stimulation has also been used as an adjunct to external cephalic version to move the fetus from a midline spine presentation to a lateral spine presentation (17).

Fetal Activity Acceleration Determination Test (FAD)

In 1976, Drs. Lee, DiLoreto, and Logrand added the evaluation of fetal movement (FM) to the NST and called their test the fetal activity acceleration determination test (FAD) (18). In addition to evaluation of accel amplitude and duration, FM was counted and the relationship between FM and accels was evaluated. FM may be recorded by the monitor, e.g., the Toitu actocardiograph®, or the woman may be asked to push a "mark" button when she feels the fetus kick, or the nurse may palpate FM and record "FM" on the tracing. It is less accurate to rely on the "spike" in the uterine activity tracing when a tocotransducer is used as evidence of FM.

Nipple stimulation Contraction Stress Test (NS-CST)

In 1982, an anecdotal report of nipple stimulation for the induction of contractions was published. However, results of prospective studies were not published until 1983 and 1984. When women used nipple stimulation to induce contractions, there was a 57 to 100% success rate (1, 19). Serum oxytocin levels rose in women who successfully completed the NS-CST and women who did not attain 3 contractions in 10 minutes. There was no statistical difference in oxytocin levels between these two groups (20). Just as the use of the OCT waned in the 1990s, the use of this test also diminished as the popularity of the NST and BPP increased.

ANTEPARTAL TEST INDICATIONS

Any fetus who has an increased risk of hypoxia should be evaluated during the last trimester. Women are usually placed in a reclining position, a semi-Fowler's position, or on their side (3). Some high-risk factors associated with an increased risk of hypoxia include
- intrauterine growth restriction (IUGR) (5)
- gestational diabetes (5, 10, 21)
- insulin-dependent diabetes (5-6, 21)
- hypertension (5-6)
- preeclampsia (5-6, 10, 21)

- antiphospholipid antibody syndrome (5-6, 21)
- sickle cell disease (21)
- twin gestation (5-6, 21-22)
- previous fetal loss (5, 23)
- maternal Rh isoimmunization (21, 23)
- decreased FM (6, 21, 24-31).
- postdate pregnancy (3, 6, 10, 21, 32-37).
- antepartal procedures that increase the risk of umbilical cord entanglement or blood loss and
- maternal abdominal trauma.

Discussion

IUGR occurs in 3 to 7% of pregnancies (5). Usually a CST is performed once a week when IUGR is first detected. The CST may be followed by an amniotic fluid volume (AFV) assessment (see Chapter 9). Although CSTs often result in higher intervention rates than BPPs, they predict adverse neonatal outcomes better than BPPs when they are used following a nonreactive NST of an IUGR fetus (38).

Diabetes mellitus increases the risk of polyhydramnios and congenital defects. Weekly antepartal tests may be done if diabetes is diet-controlled (21). However, the insulin-dependent diabetic is usually tested twice a week with a NST and once a week with a BPP beginning at 28 weeks of gestation (5-6, 21).

The hypertensive woman, whose fetus is normal in size, may have a NST each week beginning at 34 weeks of gestation. If the fetus is smaller than expected and/or IUGR, testing usually includes two or more NSTs a week with a weekly BPP (5-6, 21).

If a woman has preeclampsia she is usually followed with NSTs two times a week. Weekly testing may also include a BPP or AFV assessment (5-6, 10, 21). If concern about the fetus heightens, the woman may be evaluated daily.

Antiphospholipid antibody syndrome is associated with IUGR and fetal demise. Therefore, heightened fetal surveillance is recommended. Twice a week NSTs and a weekly BPP may begin as early as 28 weeks of gestation (5-6, 21).

Women with sickle cell disease are anemic. The risk of fetal asphyxia increases during sickle cell crisis. During a crisis, the fetus should be continuously monitored. During the third trimester of pregnancy, a NST is usually performed twice a week (21).

When twin fetuses are growing normally, the likelihood of inadequate oxygenation is low. In that case, a weekly NST and BPP are often initiated at 34 to 36 weeks of gestation. As long as both fetuses are well and their growth and AFV remain normal, no further testing is required. If there is discordance, the risk of fetal demise increases and test frequency increases to two NSTs a week and a weekly BPP (5-6, 21-22). For triplets and higher order multiples, the NST is often *not* done due to the difficulty in finding and monitoring all of the fetuses. Instead, an ultrasound evaluation of fetal breathing movements, body movements, tone, and AFV is the most useful means of evaluating fetal well-being (see Chapter 9) (39).

When a woman has a history of fetal demise due to an unknown etiology, there is a slightly higher than normal risk for another fetal loss. Women with a previous stillbirth become more anxious as they approach their due date. They need reassurance that their fetus is well. Therefore, these women usually begin fetal surveillance at 34 to 36 weeks of gestation (5, 23). In addition to weekly NSTs, they may be instructed to keep a daily record of FM (kick counts) (see procedure in appendix).

Maternal Rh isoimmunization places the fetus at high risk for severe anemia, hypoxia, hydrops, cardiac failure, and death. Antepartal testing often includes NSTs twice a week and a BPP once a week. If the fetus demonstrates an abnormal FHR pattern, e.g., a sinusoidal pattern, or decreased FM, daily NSTs or BPPs may be done until the fetus receives an intrauterine transfusion or is delivered (21, 23).

Fetuses who have decreased movement may be dying. Death of the chronically hypoxic fetus was preceded by decreased FM for 12 hours to 7 days (24-28). *When women report an absence of FM, abnormal FM, an increase in FM, or a decrease in FM, the fetus should be evaluated as soon as possible to distinguish the fetus whose movement is abnormal due to hypoxia or seizures versus the lack of maternal perception of FM* (6, 21, 25, 27-30).

Women who report abnormal or decreased FM should be asked questions such as, "when did your baby move last?" or "what does it feel like when your baby moves?" or "how does movement now differ from movement last week?" The content of the conversation between the nurse and the woman should be recorded as *telephone progress notes* in the prenatal record or in a communication book. If the woman is instructed to come to the clinic or hospital, the time and content of the instructions should be documented. Ask her how long it will take to arrive and record her response. Notify the appropriate health care providers of her future arrival and her concerns. Once she arrives, do *not* feed her until fetal well-being has been confirmed. Palpate her abdomen for FM. If the NST is nonreactive or the fetus is seizing, the physician's presence at the bedside should be requested. While awaiting the physician's arrival, assess

- the woman's last oral intake
- vital signs
- drugs the woman may have taken within two hours prior to arrival at the hospital
- the time the last cigarette was smoked and
- other information that might be needed prior to a cesarean section.

Anticipate the physician's request for an ultrasound examination of the fetus and AFV if the FHR pattern is nonreactive due to a β-blocker such as atenolol (Tenormin®).

If the NST is reactive, provide and/or reinforce kick count instructions and reassure her that her call was appropriate (31). After at least two nurses or a nurse and a physician evaluate the tracing, the woman is usually discharged from the hospital.

Pregnancy that lasts more than 40 weeks and up to 42 weeks is called a *postdate* pregnancy. A *postterm* pregnancy lasts more than 42 weeks. AFV rapidly diminishes after 40 weeks of gestation (32-34). A postterm fetus has an increased risk of meconium aspiration syndrome, "fetal distress" during labor, and an Apgar score less than 7 at 5 minutes (3, 6, 32-33, 35-36). Therefore, after the 40th week of pregnancy the physician may schedule a NST twice a week. During the 41st week, two NSTs will be scheduled plus a BPP (6, 10, 33, 35, 37). If the pregnancy continues to the 42nd week, the physician may choose to induce labor or perform NSTs twice a week plus a weekly BPP. *If a term or postterm fetus has a positive test result, i.e., there is a lack of fetal well-being, no additional tests are needed to justify the decision to induce labor and/or deliver the fetus* (3, 37, 21). In some cases, a preterm fetus will be delivered based on the results of the BPP (which includes the NST).

A NST is usually done prior to and after procedures such as an external cephalic version (turning the breech to a cephalic presentation), an amniocentesis, or a cordocentesis. When pregnant women sustain direct abdominal trauma, e.g., in a motor vehicle accident, during an attack, or by accident, it is necessary to apply the fetal monitor and observe uterine activity for signs of an abruption, e.g., hyperstimulation, and to confirm fetal well-being. A reactive NST indicates the lack of fetal trauma and/or hypoxia. If the fetus sustains a skull fracture, a checkmark pattern representing fetal seizures may be observed (see Chapter 5).

POSSIBLE INDICATIONS FOR ANTEPARTAL TESTS

It may or may not be beneficial to test fetuses on a weekly basis when there is

- placenta previa (40)
- premature rupture of the membranes (PROM) (41-43).
- "advanced" maternal age (≥ 35 years of age)
- preterm labor
- maternal anemia or
- infection with the human immunodeficiency virus (HIV).

Discussion

When the placenta is over the cervical os, there is a placenta previa, and placental perfusion may be diminished as the cervix is less vascular than the uterus. Decreased perfusion increases the risk of fetal hypoxia. Therefore, some physicians advocate weekly NSTs for women who have placenta previa (40). Others advocate initiation of NSTs only after IUGR is diagnosed or there is vaginal bleeding (5).

If membranes rupture prior to labor (PROM), the risk of infection increases. A nonreactive NST was associated with chorioamnionitis in women who had PROM (41-43). In fact, a reactive NST became nonreactive in 90% of women who developed chorioamnionitis after PROM (42). Some physicians do not consider PROM an indication for a NST because the lack of "reactive" accels was not a specific marker for infection or fetal compromise (44-45).

Pregnant women, who are 35 years of age or older, have been labeled as women of "advanced maternal age." Women in this age group have an increased risk of hypertension and gestational diabetes. If they develop any condition that poses a threat to fetal oxygenation, antepartal testing is indicated. However, age, in and of itself, does not warrant fetal testing.

Preterm labor may be related to placental vasculopathy, therefore the fetus should be monitored when a woman presents in preterm labor or threatened preterm labor. Once preterm labor ceases and the FHR is determined to be appropriate for gestational age, FHR monitoring is no longer needed. However, to detect the onset of preterm labor, home uterine activity monitoring may be arranged. In addition, the women may be given "kick count" instructions for daily FM assessment.

The fetus of a chronically anemic woman is at risk for IUGR. If the woman is anemic but the fetus is growing normally, weekly NSTs may be initiated at 34 weeks of gestation. Serial ultrasounds for fetal growth are usually obtained. Additional tests, e.g., the BPP, or more frequent NSTs, are added if fetal growth is less than expected or IUGR is diagnosed.

Many HIV-infected women have complex medical problems which include malnutrition, anemia, and/or opportunistic infections. Some HIV-infected women are also addicted to drugs such as cocaine or heroin. Comprehensive prenatal care of the immunocompromised woman and/or woman who abuses drugs may include serial ultrasounds to evaluate fetal growth. If the fetus is found to be smaller than expected or IUGR, a NST or BPP may be performed twice a week.

THE NONSTRESS TEST (NST)

The NST is the most frequently performed antepartal test (3, 5-6, 21, 35, 46-47).

Definition: an evaluation of the FHR pattern in the absence of regular uterine contractions to determine fetal oxygenation, neurologic, and cardiac function.

Benefits
- noninvasive
- takes less time to complete than a contraction stress test
- no contraindications (6, 21, 48)
- may be performed safely in a home, clinic, or hospital setting (49).

When Testing Begins
Some physicians begin testing as early as the 26th week of gestation.

Test Frequency
If the pregnancy was high-risk, a weekly NST during the third trimester was associated with a stillbirth rate of 6.1 per 1000 births. When there were two NSTs a week, the stillbirth rate dropped to 1.9 per 1000 births (50). The perinatal mortality rate drops even more when the NST is combined with an ultrasound evaluation of the fetus and AFV.

NST Protocol
Prior to application of the fetal monitor, confirm fetal life by palpation of FM or auscultation of the FHR. Assess maternal vital signs and her understanding of the test to be performed and its purpose. Ascertain the woman's last oral intake, including any medications and street drugs. Assess when she smoked last and what she smoked. Obtain a fetal movement history and assess her concerns.

The woman should be positioned off of her back to optimize uterine perfusion and to prevent false positive results. Begin fetal monitoring by applying the ultrasound transducer and tocotransducer. If the fetus is preterm, it is best to apply the tocotransducer at or below the umbilicus. In near term, term, or postterm gestations, the tocotransducer should be placed above the umbilicus for the best recording of uterine activity.

The relationship of any decel to contractions is very important. When a decel is observed, the abdomen should be palpated to assess and confirm uterine activity. By monitoring both the FHR and uterine activity, subtle decels are less likely to be overlooked and the decel type will be more accurately identified.

Establish a NST protocol and follow it. Each institution should establish a protocol for the NST (see sample procedure in appendix). Antepartal test procedures should be compulsively followed to prevent a needlessly prolonged test, misinterpretation of the FHR pattern, or inappropriate discharge of the woman who has a compromised fetus (51).

Do not feed women during antepartal tests. *Although it was once thought that juice or glucose would cause accels, this is a myth that is not supported by research.* Maternal glucose ingestion and blood glucose levels are not related to NST results (30). Even if 50 grams of glucose in 240 ml of water was ingested, and there was a significant increase in maternal whole blood glucose, there was no difference in the average time it took for a fetus to become reactive versus the time it took the fetus to become reactive in women who drank plain water (52). Theoretically, the splash of liquid in the stomach may create an acoustic stimulation which might precede FM and accels. However, until a hydrophone is placed in the uterus and sound is measured before and after women drink, this theory cannot be supported.

Orange juice, or any other kind of liquid, does not cause a reactive NST (5, 21, 52-53). *Glucose does not alter a nonreactive FHR pattern* (54). In a study by Phelan, Kester, and Labudovich (30), the *nonreactive* NST group had slightly *higher* serum glucose levels than the reactive NST group (71.6 ± 17.3 mg/dl versus 70.9 ± 17.3 mg/dl).

Nurses and physicians should base their practice on research not rituals (55). In addition, antepartal tests are used to determine fetal well-being. Women should not be fed until fetal well-being has been confirmed because the acidotic or asphyxiated fetus may be delivered by cesarean section. Eating or drinking prior to surgery is contraindicated.

CLASSIFICATIONS OF NSTS

There are two categories for classifying FHR patterns obtained during a NST: reactive and nonreactive. If the FHR pattern is unclear, the test is classified as inconclusive or unsatisfactory (see Figure 9.5).

A need for standardized categories and classification criteria. Different categories and criteria have been used to classify NST tracings. For example, categories such as reactive, nonreactive, inconclusive, unsatisfactory, and minimally reactive have been used (3, 5-6, 10-11, 21, 31, 35, 56-57). In 1994, the American College of Obstetricians and Gynecologists (ACOG) recommended the following criteria:

Classification: Reactive NST
Recognition Criteria:
- 2 or more accels that
- *peak* at least 15 bpm above the baseline (BL) and
- last 15 seconds from BL to BL (at their base) within
- a 20 minute period
- *with or without FM* discernible by the woman (11).

ACOG (11) did not specify the minimum time required for a reactive NST. However, if two spontaneous "reactive" accels occur within less than 20 minutes of monitoring, the BL level, stability, and variability are "normal," and there are no decels, the fetus is well. It would be reasonable at that point to remove the fetal monitor, schedule the next NST, and send the woman home. Protocol should be written to reflect the minimal time for a reactive NST.

The Accel Need Not be Sustained for 15 Seconds at the Top
It used to be believed that a fetus needed to sustain an accel at a level 15 or more bpm above the BL for 15 or more seconds to be classified as a "reactive" accel (5). In 1990, this belief changed as researchers found no difference in the number of cesarean sections for "fetal distress" if NSTs included accels that were sustained 15 or more seconds at 15 or more bpm above the BL versus accels that only peaked 15 or more bpm above the BL (56).

Two Accels in 20 Minutes are Required for a Reactive NST
If the fetus is oxygenated and moves for 3 or more seconds, an accel should appear 99.8% of the time (59). The number of accels and the minimal testing time for these accels to occur has varied in different studies, but only 2 "reactive" accels are needed in a 20 minute period. For example, physicians have considered a NST reactive if there were 4 accels in 20 minutes (60-61), 3 in 30 minutes (62), 2 in 20 minutes (63-67), or 2 in 10 minutes (68). Waiting for additional "reactive" accels or expecting the fetus to respond in a short period of time will either delay the completion of the test or increase interventions, such as use of the acoustic stimulator.

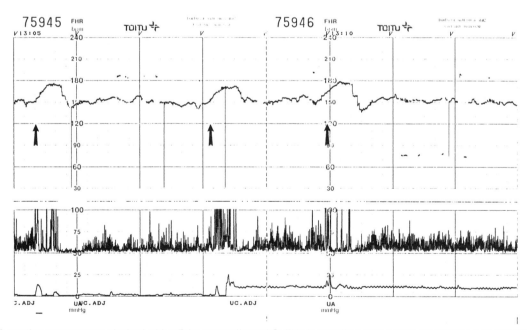

Figure 9.1: A reactive nonstress test obtained with a Toitu actocardiograph®. This is actually a fetal activity acceleration determination test because fetal movement is recorded as spikes. Fetal movement is intensified during accelerations. The third acceleration appears to be a Lambda pattern rather than a combination acceleration/deceleration. A combination acceleration/deceleration suggests the presence of a nuchal cord. (Tracing contributed by Carolyn L. Gegor, CNM, MS, RDMS).

The NST False Negative Rate

A reactive NST and a reactive/negative CST are equally good predictors of fetal status and "good outcomes." A reactive NST is highly unlikely to be associated with a positive CST (69). *False negative* refers to the incidence of stillbirths occurring within one week of a reactive test. When statistics were corrected for congenital anomalies, the *false negative* rate for the NST was 1.4 per 1000 births. The false negative rate for the CST was 0 per 1000 births (46). In other words, if the CST indicates fetal well-being, all fetuses should live another week (if nothing changes in terms of fetal or maternal status). However, if there is a reactive NST, 1 in 1000 fetuses will die prior to the end of the week. Therefore, it is important to remember, *"the NST is only good at the time of the test."* No test can prevent fetal death that is unanticipated or unexpected.

Classification: Nonreactive NST

Recognition Criteria:
- no accels or
- only one accel that meets the 15 x 15 criteria or
- two or more accels that do not meet the 15 x 15 criteria in any 20 minute period of time during a total monitoring period of 40 minutes (11). *The physician should be notified of a nonreactive test as soon as possible.*

NONHYPOXIC CAUSES OF A NONREACTIVE NST

While a reactive NST is predictive of a well-oxygenated fetus *at the time of the test*, a nonreactive NST has a high false positive rate (6, 21, 35). In other words, a nonreactive test may be interpreted to mean the fetus is hypoxic, metabolically acidotic, or asphyxiated due to the lack of "reactive" accels, and will not tolerate labor. However, a false positive test means the fetus is actually well-oxygenated. A false positive nonreactive NST may be caused by one or more of the following factors:
- fetal quiescence (1F state)
- preterm gestation
- smoking prior to the test (59, 70)
- central nervous system (CNS) depressant drugs ingested by or administered to the woman
- a β-blocker, such as atenolol (Tenormin®) (71) and/or
- congenital cardiac or central nervous system anomalies.

Fetal Quiescence

A change in fetal behavioral states reflects an oxygenated brain (47, 72-73). Prior to 34 weeks of gestation, fetal behavioral cycles, breathing movements, eye movements, and changes in BL variability occur irregularly, with little relationship to each other. Near 34 weeks of gestation, behavioral states are more clearly visualized (see Chapter 2) (47, 72). Knowing that a term or near term fetus may normally spend about 40 minutes in a 1F, quiescent state with a nonreactive FHR pattern, may prevent an overreaction to an otherwise normal tracing (59). It may be helpful to obtain a FM history by inquiring about fetal activity prior to fetal monitoring. The physician may request an extension of the NST testing time. If the fetus becomes reactive during the second 40-minute monitoring period, the test is classified as reactive and the woman is discharged.

Extension of NST Testing Time

ACOG (11) has recommended the NST be classified as nonreactive if after 40 minutes 2 accels do not meet reactive criteria within 20 minutes of time. To reduce the false positive rate and to decrease additional unnecessary testing, e.g., with a CST or BPP, the physician may extend testing time. Vigorous shaking of the fetus (after 40 minutes and a nonreactive NST) is no longer recommended because 90% of fetuses do not respond (70, 74). Shaking the fetus did *not* change the fetal behavioral state (74). In fact, vigorous shaking of an asphyxiated fetus is no different than the "shake and shout" in basic life support, i.e., "Annie, Annie are you O.K.?"

60 total test minutes. Oxygenated fetuses, whose FHR pattern became reactive after 60 total minutes of monitoring, were at no higher risk for perinatal complications than those whose tests became reactive in the first 30 minutes of monitoring (75).

80 total test minutes. If the fetus is anatomically normal and there are no drugs in the fetus that prevent accels, *a nonreactive NST after 80 minutes of testing suggests the fetus may be significantly compromised* (64, 76-77). The lack of accels that meet "reactive" criteria may also be related to fetal hypothyroidism.

120 total test minutes. Some researchers have advocated a maximum NST time of 120 minutes in order to increase the positive predictive value of a nonreactive NST and increase the negative predictive value of a reactive NST (78). They have found *if the NST lasts 2 hours, all possible reactive tests should be identified* (62). However, it might be better to provide an acoustic stimulation within the first hour of monitoring rather than to delay evaluation of fetal status until the end of two hours of monitoring.

Preterm Gestation

The predictability of a nonreactive NST of a preterm fetus is lower than a nonreactive NST of a term or postterm fetus because fetuses less than 30 to 32 weeks of gestation are more likely to not meet criteria for a reactive NST (79-81). Therefore, when the preterm fetus is monitored, consideration should be given to the effect of gestational age on the size of accels (6, 21, 35). Once the fetus has a reactive FHR pattern, future antepartal tracings should be reactive. A nonreactive NST of a fetus who was previously reactive should be followed by further testing.

Table 1: Number of Nonreactive Nonstress Tests at Different Gestational Ages (81)

GESTATION (Weeks)	NONREACTIVE NSTs (%)
20 - 24	73
24 - 28	45
28 - 30	24
30 - 32	14
32 - 36	5
36 - 40	1

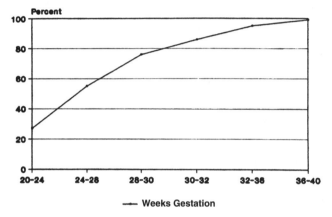

Figure 9.2: Percentage of fetuses that are reactive by gestational age. (Reproduced with permission of Gegor, C. L., Paine, L. L., & Johnson, T. R. B. (1991). Antepartum fetal assessment. A nurse-midwifery perspective. *Journal of Nurse Midwifery, 36*(3), 153-167.

In women who had preeclampsia and a *preterm* pregnancy, the incidence of nonreactive NSTs increased as gestational age and/or fetal weight decreased. Fetuses with nonreactive NSTs had "poor" variability, lower gestational ages, and lower birth weights. They had lower 5 minute Apgar scores, more cesarean sections for "fetal distress," and a lower neonatal blood glucose level than fetuses who were reactive. The lack of long-term variability was predictive of fetal acidemia based on umbilical artery pH analysis. *The presence of long-term variability (LTV) in these preterm fetuses, even without reactive accels, was associated with a normal pH (73). Therefore, a flat or nearly flat BL was associated with a lower pH than a BL with LTV in preterm fetuses of women who had preeclampsia.*

Smoking Prior to the Test
Nicotine depresses the central nervous system and decreases FM (59). The FHR may remain nonreactive for as long as 90 minutes after smoking 2 cigarettes (82).

CNS Depressants, Muscle Relaxants, and Betamethasone
Alcohol significantly decreases the number of FMs. Fetal breathing movements were almost completely arrested after alcohol ingestion (83). *Muscle relaxants and sedatives are usually not prescribed during pregnancy.* Therefore, when a woman reports, "I am taking this drug for my nerves," it is important to document the source of the prescription and/or pills. She should be asked to stop taking the drug because it is harmful to the fetus or neonate. However, at that point, she may be addicted and need a referral to a program or clinic that works with pregnant women addicted to drugs. Diazepam (Valium®) depresses FMs and interferes with the reliability of kick counts as well as FAD results (84). *Betamethasone* is associated with decreased FM, breathing movements, and FHR variation for up to 4 days (85-87).

Drugs That Block Sympathetic Nerves
β-blockers may prevent accels when the fetus is well-oxygenated (see Chapter 8). Therefore, the NST is an unreliable test of fetal well-being if women are being treated with a β-blocker for hypertension or migraine headaches. Fetal evaluation by a BPP should yield a score of 8 out of 10 (0 points for the nonreactive NST) if the fetus is well-oxygenated.

Congenital Anomalies of the Heart or Central Nervous System (CNS)
Fetal CNS, cardiac, and structural anomalies may be associated with abnormal FHR patterns (35). However, no anomaly has been associated with a specific FHR pattern. Occasionally the fetus will have an arrhythmia which creates an uninterpretable tracing. In that case, the BPP and/or echocardiography would be better than a NST to predict fetal well-being.

NONREACTIVE NST RELATED TO HYPOXIA
When the FHR pattern was nonreactive after a total monitoring time of 80 minutes, there was an increased risk of
- oligohydramnios
- IUGR
- fetal acidosis
- meconium-stained amniotic fluid and/or
- placental infarction (88).

SIGNS OF OLIGOHYDRAMNIOS
Uniform Accelerations
Uniform accels may be an early warning sign of oligohydramnios and mild umbilical cord compression (see Figure 9.6). When uniform accels are observed, change the maternal position to see if the cord becomes more compressed. If, after 40 minutes of monitoring, there are no variable decels, there is "normal" long-term variability, and the uniform accels meet "reactive" criteria, the test should be considered reactive and the woman is scheduled for a follow-up test. She should be given kick count instructions and asked to call if FM decreases. It would be interesting to evaluate the intrauterine contents to determine AFV. Research is needed

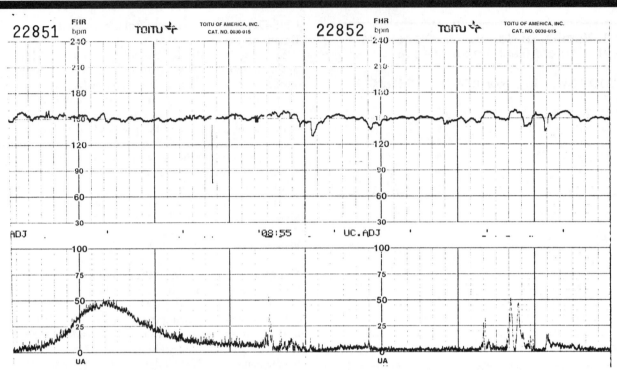

Figure 9.3: A nonreactive nonstress test of a 27 week fetus. Note the normal "dips" in the fetal heart rate. The fetal heart rate is appropriate for gestational age, but the fetus has not yet accelerated to meet the criteria for a reactive nonstress test. (Tracing contributed by Carolyn L. Gegor, CNM, MS, RDMS).

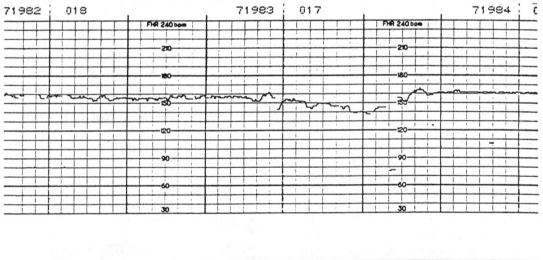

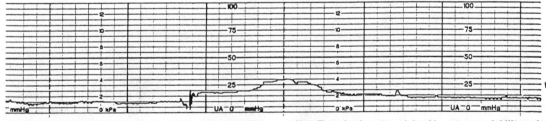

Figure 9.4: Tracing of a fetus who was 39 weeks of gestation with congenital anomalies. There is absent to minimal long-term variability and a late deceleration. No specific fetal heart rate pattern suggests anomalies and this pattern is nonreactive. The woman was a 24 year old G_1P_0 with a history of asthma but no pregnancy complications. The cervix was closed and the fetus was breech. She was delivered by cesarean section. Apgar scores were 1 and 1 at 1 and 5 minutes of age. The fetus had pulmonary hypoplasia, dwarfism, no skull bones, with deformed arms, legs, and ribs.

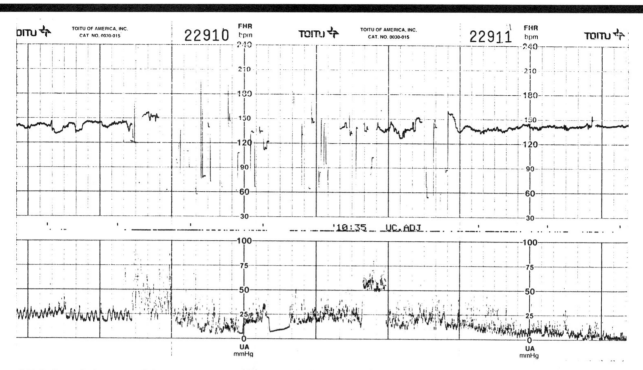

Figure 9.5: An inconclusive or unsatisfactory nonstress test due to gaps in the tracing and artifact. The fetus was very active during that time. The ultrasound should be adjusted, new coupling gel should be applied, and a continuous tracing should be obtained. If an adequate tracing cannot be obtained, an ultrasound scan may be needed to assess the fetus and amniotic fluid volume. (Tracing contributed by Carolyn L. Gegor, CNM, MS, RDMS).

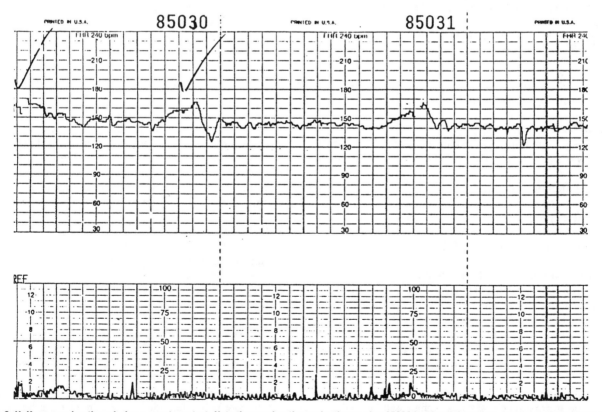

Figure 9.6: Uniform accelerations during a nonstress test. Note the acceleration under the number 85030 is a Lambda pattern, not an acceleration/deceleration combination. The tracing is classified as a reactive nonstress test, but concern should exist regarding the possibility of oligohydramnios.

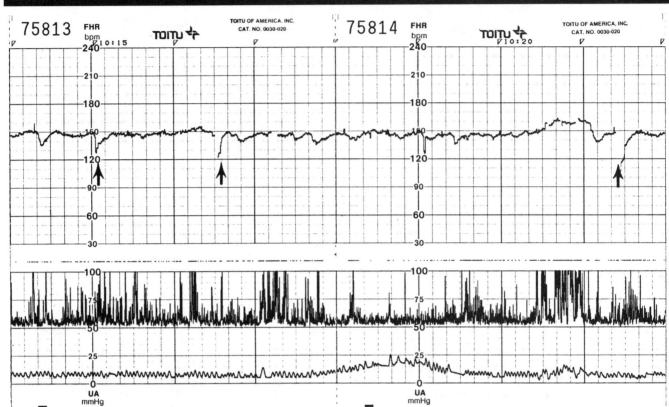

Figure 9.7: A nonreactive nonstress test with multiple small variable decelerations in a term fetus. Oligohydramnios was diagnosed. The amniotic fluid index was only 1.7 cm. This tracing is produced by a Toitu® fetal monitor. The fetus is moving most of the time, but there is only one acceleration. The presence of variable decelerations during antepartal tests should be followed by an ultrasound evaluation of amniotic fluid volume (11). (Tracing contributed by Carolyn L. Gegor, CNM, MS, RDMS).

to determine the strength of the relationship between uniform accels during a NST and AFV.

Variable Decelerations

Decels rarely occur during a NST in the presence of normal AFV (7). Variable decels during a NST or CST may be associated with

- oligohydramnios (11, 61)
- IUGR
- a postterm pregnancy
- PROM (68) and/or
- a short or long umbilical cord (64, 89).

Fetuses who had variable decels during a "minimally" reactive NST were more likely to have a "cord complication," cesarean section, and lower Apgar scores than fetuses who had a reactive NST and no decels (90). *In 1994, ACOG suggested that variable decels, at least 15 seconds in duration, dropping 15 or more bpm below the BL, were evidence of umbilical cord vulnerability and AFV should be evaluated to rule out oligohydramnios or the fetus should be delivered* (11).

The average umbilical cord length was reported to be 56 to 61 cm or approximately 22 to 24 inches, with a minimum "normal" length of 32 cm (12.6 inches) and a maximum

"normal" length of 100 cm (39 inches). Variable decels were more common if the cord was long (75 to 100 cm). When "W" or biphasic variable decels appeared, the cord was 73.07 ± 17.1 cm versus 56.47 ± 11.4 cm in women who did not have biphasic variable decels (89). An abnormal cord position, e.g., a nuchal cord, was present in 55.3% of fetuses whose heart rate decelerated in response to FM (61). Figure 9.7 is an example of a nonreactive NST with variable decels that require "further evaluation or delivery."

Fetal Acidosis and Fetal Deterioration

Signs of fetal deterioration over time include:
- increasing time between accels
- decreasing long-term variability
- decreasing accel amplitude
- decels
- loss of accels
- loss of variability (see Figure 9.9).

Increasing time between accelerations. A subtle indication of deterioration is the increasing time between accels. By comparing past NSTs with the present test, the time between accels may be evaluated. If accels are spacing out, the fetus may have depleted oxygen reserves.

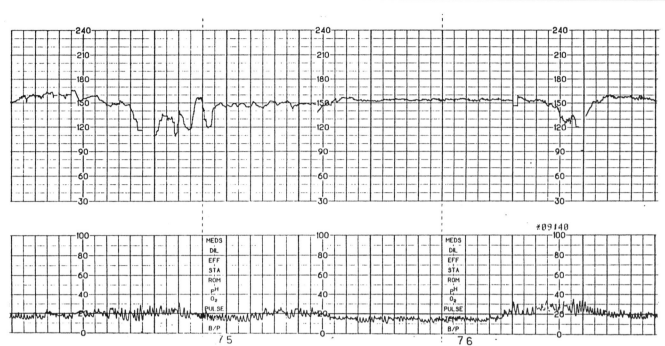

Figure 9.8: A nonreactive nonstress test with variable decelerations in a G_1P_0 woman with an intrauterine growth restricted (IUGR) fetus at 37 weeks of gestation. Note the elevated baseline and absent to minimal long-term variability. The nonstress test was immediately followed by a positive CST and a cesarean section. A 3 lb 8 oz female, 16 inches long, was delivered with Apgar scores of 8 and 9 at 1 and 5 minutes. The placenta was small. It was only 17 cm in diameter. In addition, there were 2 loops of nuchal cord plus the cord was wrapped around the baby's body.

Decelerations. Eden (7) found in postdate pregnancy, *decels* during the NST were associated with:

- a nonreactive NST
- decreased AFV in 90.9% of women
- FHR "abnormalities" and decels during labor
- "low" 5 minute Apgar scores
- meconium passage
- neonatal resuscitation
- congenital anomalies and/or
- perinatal morbidity.

Spontaneous decelerations. Spontaneous decels during a NST were associated with IUGR in 63.6% of women (91). *The fetus who has a nonreactive NST, spontaneous decels, and absent LTV should be delivered* (see Chapter 5 discussion of spontaneous decels). *When spontaneous decels are observed, the physician should be immediately notified.*

Loss of variability. *Absent variability* for at least 80% of the tracing and the presence of decels puts the fetus at high risk for intrapartum death (2). True positive nonreactive NSTs are associated with IUGR, birth by cesarean section, and a fetal scalp blood pH less than 7.25 (75). Therefore, *the absence of variability, particularly in the absence of FM and a history of decreased or absent FM, should prompt immediate notification of the physician.* The nurse should communicate the entire systematic review, including the lack of accels, the BL level, rate, and variability, and the type of decels observed.

TRACING INTERPRETATION: IMPLICATIONS FOR NURSES AND PHYSICIANS

Use a Systematic Review for Tracing Analysis

Contractions are rare or absent during the NST. The lack of uterine activity should be confirmed by palpation and documented. The FHR pattern should be systematically analyzed. Although at least six NST scoring systems have appeared in the literature, they are rarely used to evaluate the tracing (92). The antepartal tracing should be evaluated by nurses or physicians who are aware of the significance of abnormal findings, such as a sinusoidal BL, a flat BL, or variable decels.

The baseline. The BL level should be in a normal range for that gestational age (100 to 160 bpm for term and postterm fetuses, 120 to 160 bpm for preterm fetuses). If it appears high, narrow, or smooth, a previous antepartal test strip should be evaluated to determine the fetus' normal rate and variability.

Accels. The amplitude of each accel should be measured from the middle of the BL on either side of the accel to the top of the accel (51). For example, if the average BL rate is 140 bpm, the accel should peak at 155 bpm to meet height criteria. The duration of the accel is measured from the time the FHR left the BL to the time it returned to the BL. Some nurses use a clear plastic ruler and place it's top edge at the level of the middle of the BL near the accel they are measuring. Then,

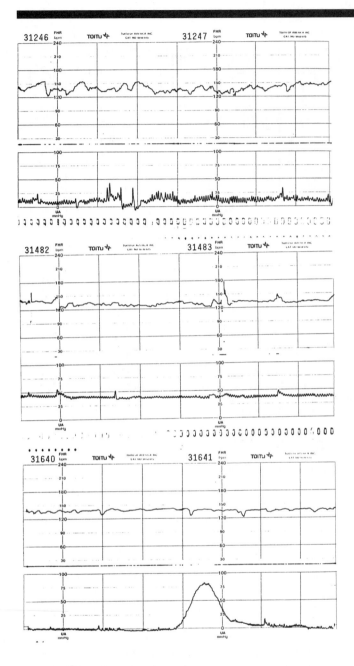

Figure 9.9: Deteriorating fetal status of an intrauterine growth restricted (IUGR) fetus is evident when serial nonstress tests are compared. Top tracing: 35 weeks, reactive nonstress test, amniotic fluid index 12.2 cm. Middle tracing: 36 weeks, increased duration between accelerations, smoothing of accelerations, and decrease in long-term variability. Biophysical profile score 8 out of 10. Amniotic fluid index 7.2 cm. Bottom tracing: 36 3/7 weeks with a nonreactive nonstress test, amniotic fluid index of 3.2 cm, and 4 out of 10 biophysical profile score. Labor was induced, but the fetus did not tolerate labor. The baby weighed 2400 grams and was delivered by cesarean section with Apgar scores were 7 and 8 at 1 and 5 minutes. (Tracing contributed by Carolyn L. Gegor, CNM, MS, RDMS).

they look above the ruler's edge to a level 15 bpm higher than the middle of the BL. If the accel touches or exceeds that level, they place a checkmark above it. They do the same for each accel in a 20 minute period of time. It is also important to examine the shape of accels and classify them as uniform or spontaneous.

Decels. Decels are assessed by looking for transient drops in the FHR that hang below the BL. A variable decel lasts at least 15 seconds (from BL to BL) and the nadir is 15 or more bpm below the BL. The nadir of late decels may be less than 15 bpm, especially if they are subtle late decels.

Document and communicate. The nurse is usually responsible for documenting the systematic review of the tracing. Both nurses and physicians who are skilled in FHR pattern interpretation may classify the tracing as reactive or nonreactive. Nurses and physicians may disagree on the classification of NSTs (6, 21, 35, 93-94). *Therefore, at least two nurses, a nurse and a physician, or two physicians should examine the tracing and agree it is reactive prior to sending the woman home.*

Follow-up Tests After a Nonreactive NST

A nonreactive NST may not be related to fetal jeopardy. Therefore, nonreactive NSTs, especially after only 40 minutes of monitoring, require further fetal evaluation (48). Acoustic stimulation may be used after the first 20 minutes of monitoring. After 40 minutes of monitoring, the physician should be notified of a nonreactive NST. A *nonreactive* NST with or without decels may be followed by an ultrasound to evaluate the fetus, AFV, and umbilical cord position. A nonreactive NST may also be followed by induction of labor or delivery, depending on the perceived fetal status and the physician's plan of care (95). If a follow-up ultrasound or CST indicate fetal well-being, e.g., a BPP score of 8 out of 10 or a reactive/negative CST, there is no increased risk of fetal morbidity (69).

FETAL ACTIVITY ACCELERATION DETERMINATION TEST (FAD)

Definition: the evaluation of fetal movement and accels prior to the onset of labor.

When Testing Begins

Just like the NST, the FAD may begin as early as 26 weeks of gestation.

Test Protocol

Both accels and FM are evaluated during a FAD. *Many clinicians do not distinguish the FAD from the NST, but they are two different tests.* During the NST, FM is not recorded on the tracing. During the FAD however, the woman is asked to push a button on the fetal monitor (the mark button) when she feels the baby move (35). If the fetal monitor records FM, such as the Toitu® monitor, all NSTs automatically become FADs (see Figure 9.11). In spite of these clear cut differences, most clinicians record FADs as NSTs.

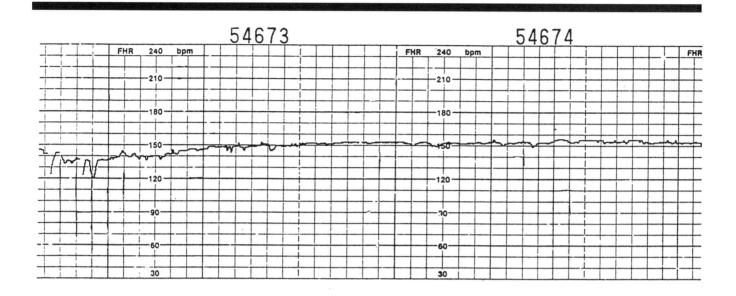

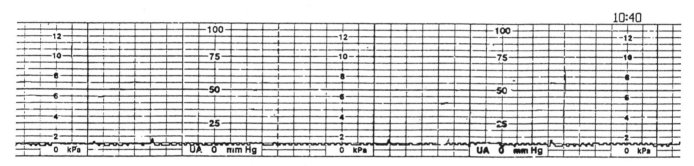

Figure 9.10: Spontaneous deceleration of a 26 week fetus whose G$_5$P$_1$ mother had a history of 3 spontaneous abortions and hypertension and hyperemesis with this pregnancy. When this tracing was obtained, the woman's blood pressure was 140/98. She had 1+ proteinuria and normal reflexes. An anemic, 1 lb 8 ounce fetus was delivered by cesarean section but did not survive. A woman with a history of hypertension and multiple spontaneous abortions should be screened for antiphospholipid antibody syndrome.

Implications of a Reactive FAD

Accels are not a response to fetal movement, accels are associated with fetal movement (79). When motor nerves in the brain and brainstem are activated, the fetus moves. When sympathetic nerves are activated, the FHR accelerates. The stimulus that precedes motor nerve activation also precedes sympathetic nerve activation and spontaneous accels. Spontaneous accels and FM are a response to a sensory stimulus. In a well-oxygenated fetus, spontaneous accels begin near the onset of FM, suggesting coordinated neurologic control of FM and the FHR. The average lag time between FM and the onset of the accel was 1.3 seconds in 23 "low-risk" term women (96).

The relationship between accels and FM increases with gestational age. A *well-oxygenated* term fetus accelerates with 90% of FMs (35, 97). The number of accels in any period of time is related to gestational age. Accels followed FM 65% of the time in term fetuses, but only 20% of the time in fetuses who were 24 weeks of gestation (79). Since the FHR is more

likely to accelerate after FM as gestation advances, several physicians have questioned the validity of the FAD for fetuses who were 32 weeks of gestation or younger (79-80, 98). Natale, Nasello, and Turliuk (98) found that 31% of fetal movements were not associated with accels at 24 to 26 weeks of gestation in "healthy" fetuses. In fetuses who were 30 to 32 weeks of gestation, 15.5% of fetal movements were not followed by an accel, even after 2 hours of testing. Of the 3% of fetuses who were nonreactive at 32 weeks of gestation, 75% had a "normal" neonatal outcome (80). *Thus, the criteria of 15 bpm x 15 seconds is too high to differentiate the truly hypoxic preterm fetus from the oxygenated fetus with immature nerves.*

Implications of a Nonreactive FAD

The association of FM and accels is related to perinatal outcomes. Baser and Johnson found the synchronous onset of FM and FHR accels was strongly predictive of fetal well-being (97). A hypoxic fetus decreases LTV and accel amplitude. In addition, the time between accels lengthens and the

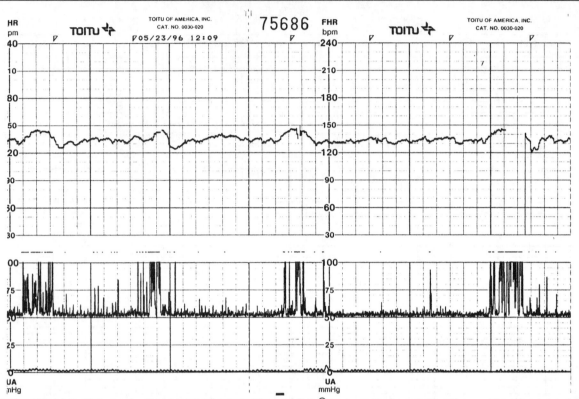

Figure 9.11: Reactive fetal activity acceleration determination test. When the Toitu® fetal monitor is used, the ultrasound transducer detects both fetal movement and cardiac motion. During accelerations, the large spikes in the uterine activity channel denote normal, brisk fetal movements. Rather than documenting "reactive FAD," most clinicians will classify this tracing as a "reactive NST." (Tracing contributed by Carolyn L. Gegor, CNM, MS, RDMS).

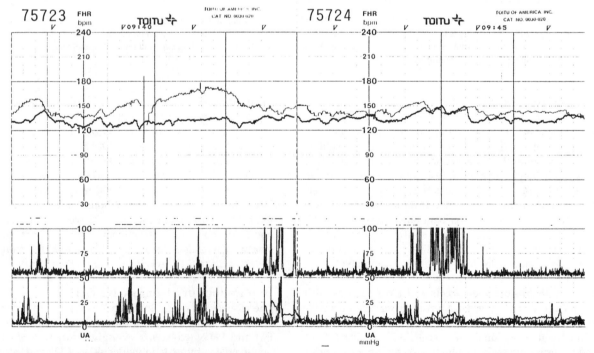

Figure 9.12: Reactive fetal activity acceleration determination test in twins. The Toitu® fetal monitor records the movements of each twin and their heart rates. (Tracing contributed by Carolyn L. Gegor, CNM, MS, RDMS).

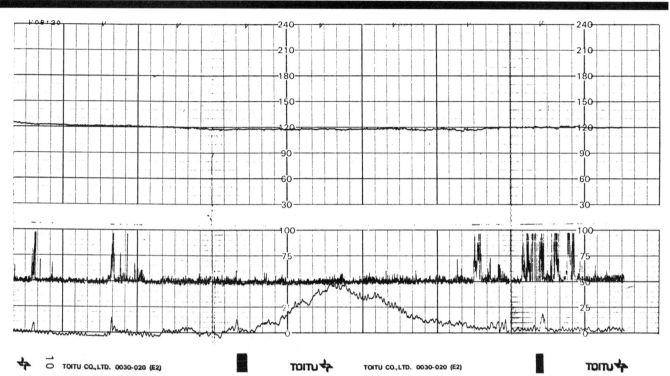

Figure 9.13: Nonreactive fetal activity acceleration determination test in a 34 week fetus. Despite fetal activity, there are no accelerations. If, after 40 minutes, the tracing is still nonreactive, it should be followed by another test such as a biophysical profile. Maternal drug use that might prevent accelerations, e.g., nicotine, narcotics, or β-blockers, should be ruled out. (Tracing contributed by Carolyn L. Gegor, CNM, MS, RDMS).

BL level often increases as FM decreases. As the fetal condition deteriorates, accel frequency decreases and accels and FM dissociate (uncouple) (3, 35, 97, 99). Eventually, accels completely disappear. Thus, a hypoxic fetus has a few small accels or no accels (59, 79, 96).

Sometimes the fetus is well-oxygenated, but FM is never associated with accels. For example, if there are accels but a lack of palpable FM, it is possible the fetus lacks legs or arms and therefore an ultrasound should be done to evaluate fetal anatomy. If there is FM but no accels, a medication with β-blocking properties may be in the fetus.

THE FETAL ACOUSTIC STIMULATION TEST (FAST)
Definition: stimulation of the fetus with a loud sound and identification of the FHR response (100).

Test Purposes
The purposes of fetal acoustic stimulation are to
- evaluate fetal acid-base status and
- reduce antepartal testing time (100).

Benefits
- noninvasive (101)
- low false negative rate, similar to the reactive NST, i.e., if the fetus accels and the tracing is reactive, the fetus is not

metabolically acidotic (102)
- a follow-up test after a nonreactive NST (15, 100, 103-104)
- 70 to 82% of fetuses who had a nonreactive NST had a reactive FHR pattern after acoustic stimulation (105)
- *may* shorten testing time (48, 78, 102, 106)
- a reactive FHR pattern after acoustic stimulation preceded a negative OCT (107)
- has been used to startle a fetus who was holding its umbilical cord
- after acoustic stimulation the hand opened, the cord was released, and severe variable decels disappeared
- has been used to move the fetus during an external cephalic version.

Acoustic stimulation decreased the number of nonreactive NSTs from 14% to 9%, and shortened testing time an average of 4 minutes (100). In another study, acoustic stimulation decreased testing time, decreased the number of nonreactive tests to 2%, and there were no unexpected fetal deaths during a 36 month study of 2,628 women (104).

Limitations
- deaf, oxygenated fetuses will not respond
- fetuses with middle ear infections may not respond
- the response depends on gestational age, e.g., prior to 30 weeks the fetus may accelerate, after 30 weeks of

gestation the fetus may increase the BL rate and accel for up to 1 hour (103, 106)

- some fetuses habituate to repetitive sound stimuli and progressively decrease their response (103)
- high false positive rate, e.g., only 50% of fetuses who did not respond to the sound stimulus were acidotic (100, 107)
- testing time may be lengthened if the accel lasts 15 or more minutes (108)
- variable and/or prolonged decelerations may occur after the sound stimulus (107, 109).

Testing time may be lengthened if the fetus accelerates for a prolonged period after acoustic stimulation. For example, a term fetus may become tachycardic for 1 hour or longer (110-111). The tachycardic fetus must be monitored until the FHR returns to its normal level.

When Testing Begins
The fetus begins to hear at 25 weeks of gestation (112). Therefore, acoustic stimulation is usually initiated after 25 weeks of gestation (106, 113-115).

Equipment
In the past, a model 5C electronic artificial larynx with a sound intensity of 82 decibels (dB) measured in air was used to provide a 5-second stimulus over the fetal head (107-108). Devices have also been sold for the sole purpose of fetal acoustic stimulation. However, nurses and physicians have reported their use of alternative sound-producing devices such as

- a radio
- the TV/radio control on the bed
- the telephone (which is placed on the woman's thigh then the number is called)
- an electric toothbrush
- a pager
- a bedpan pounded by a spoon
- a tambourine
- an electric shaver
- two spoons which were tapped together
- two metal instruments, e.g., two hemostats, which they tapped together and
- their clapping hands.

Researchers have studied the fetal response to the maternal voice (116). Nurses have found the fetus also accels and moves after being spoken to by its father.

Test Protocol
Prior to the sound stimulus, clinicians should express their need to see how the baby responds to a loud sound which will be emitted on the abdomen near the fetal ear (15). Some clinicians prefer to place the sound-producing device on the woman's thigh or some distance away from the fetal ear. With each successive stimulus they place the device closer and closer to the fetal head.

The woman should touch and hear the acoustic stimulator prior to its application. In addition, the fetus should be monitored at least 10 minutes prior to acoustic stimulation, and the room should be as quiet as possible immediately before the sound stimulus (108, 117). If the FHR pattern prior to stimulation is nonreassuring, the physician should be consulted and acoustic stimulation should be withheld until further orders are received from the physician. The number and duration of stimuli and the device used to stimulate the fetus should be documented with the systematic review of the tracing before and after stimulation.

Number and duration of stimuli. A series of 1 to 7 stimuli with a duration of 1 to 10 seconds may be emitted (15). A reasonable protocol would be to have a total of three sound stimuli one minute apart.

Follow-up. Currently, the lack of a fetal accel following acoustic stimulation may be followed by a biophysical profile (ultrasound) or a CST. In the future, the lack of a fetal response may be followed by assessment of fetal brain function using magnetoencephalography. In 1996, magnetoencephalography was investigational, safe, and noninvasive. The magnetic fetal auditory evoked fetal brain response to sound was analyzed after a sound burst of 100 dB for up to 2 seconds. Failure to respond was believed to be related to neurologic immaturity, FM during the sound burst, a low sound intensity reaching the fetus, or unknown causes (118).

FAST Interpretation Criteria
Reactive
- two accels peaking at least 15 bpm above the BL and lasting 15 or more seconds from BL to BL (at their base) within a 20 minute period (11, 15, 119).

Some researchers have proposed other criteria for a reactive FAST.
- two accels peaking at least 15 bpm above the BL and lasting 15 or more seconds (at their base) within 5 minutes of acoustic stimulation (112) or
- 1 accel peaking at least 15 bpm above the BL and lasting 2 or more minutes (100, 112).

Nonreactive
- accels that do not meet reactive criteria within 40 minutes of monitoring (11) or
- after 3 applications of acoustic stimulation at 5 minute intervals, no acceptable accels within 5 minutes of the third stimulus (112).

The Fetal Response to a Sound Stimulus
Acoustic stimulation startles the fetus. Accels after acoustic stimulation are taller and longer than accels during the NST. Some term fetuses increased their BL 11 or more bpm for up to 30 minutes after stimulation and accels lasted an average of 44 seconds with an amplitude of 18 or more bpm (117). In

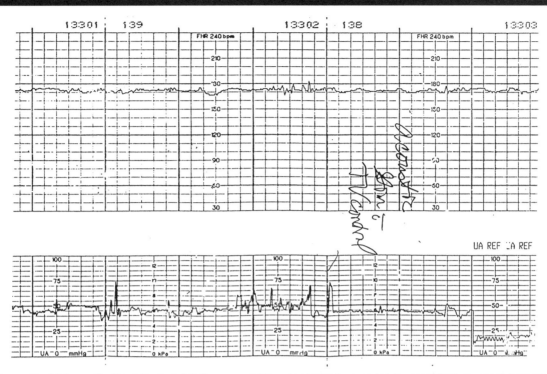

Figure 9.14: Nonreactive fetal acoustic stimulation test. A G_1P_0 woman at 36 weeks of gestation reported decreased fetal movement, headache, and epigastric pain. She was asked to come to the hospital for monitoring. There was a sinusoidal, nonreactive NST. Preeclampsia was ruled out. Monitoring continued for over 6 hours. The baseline rose and eventually became tachycardic and flat. Acoustic stimulation was accomplished using the TV control. A severely anemic baby, who required blood and oxygen, was delivered by cesarean section.

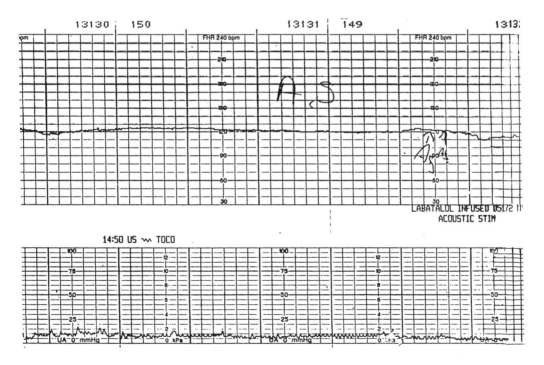

Figure 9.15: A nonreactive fetal acoustic stimulation (A. S.) test of a 36 week fetus of a woman who was severely preeclamptic and who was receiving magnesium sulfate and β-blocker. The fetal heart rate decelerated with two subsequent 3-second sound stimuli that were spaced one minute apart. It would be highly unlikely that a fetus with both magnesium sulfate and a β-blocker "on board" would accelerate. The 4 lb 13 ounce fetus was delivered by cesarean section with Apgar scores of 6 and 7 at 1 and 5 minutes.

other fetuses, accels lasted 10 minutes to 60 minutes or longer.

Even though the fetus was startled, there was no surge of catecholamines as one might have expected (120). Prior to acoustic stimulation, the fetal bladder held 21.7 ± 11.3 milliliters (ml) of urine. After acoustic stimulation, there were only 12.8 ± 9.4 ml in the bladder. In other words, acoustic stimulation caused the fetus to urinate (103)! There are no reports of meconium release following acoustic stimulation.

Acoustic stimulation does *not* impair infant hearing (121). Acoustic stimulation does not identify nuchal cords (46% of fetuses who had a variable decel after acoustic stimulation had a nuchal cord, 64% did not) (122).

CONTRACTION STRESS TESTS (CSTs)

Purpose

The purpose of a contraction stress test is to determine how the fetus responds to decreased oxygen (O_2) delivery during contractions. Since this is a test that may further compromise the fetus, *the woman should not be fed during the procedure* and the test should be performed in a facility with emergency cesarean section capability.

Benefits
- indirectly determines placental function and fetal O_2 reserves.

Limitations
- equivocal/suspicious tests are common (123)
- testing time is longer than the NST, FAD, or FAST
- the OCT is invasive
- more expensive than the NST, FAD, or FAST (6)
- may cost more than the BPP (6)
- women prefer the NST or BPP to the CST, especially when nipple stimulation is required.

Physiology

Contractions that last at least 40 seconds may diminish placental blood flow (124). A hypoxic fetus with borderline O_2 reserves may have late decels as a compensatory response to hypoxia caused by contractions. However, if the fetus is already severely compromised, with an accumulation of adenosine, the BL will be flat or nearly flat, with no accels and no decels. Such a tracing would be classified as nonreactive/negative but the woman should *not* be sent home until fetal well-being has been confirmed either by an ultrasound or a FAST (see Figure 9.18). Some clinicians classify this type of "flat line" pattern as equivocal.

Indications

The CST is mainly used
- as a follow-up test for a nonreactive NST
- when ultrasound evaluation is not available (1, 6, 54)
- in addition to a BPP (9, 21, 23, 125, 153)
- to evaluate a preterm fetus, IUGR fetus, or fetus of a diabetic woman (6, 9-10)

- whenever there is a risk or suspicion of uteroplacental insufficiency and/or
- when other antepartal tests are nonreactive or equivocal, e.g., a BPP score of 6 out of 10 (3, 9, 54).

Contraindications

Initiation of contractions may result in preterm labor. Therefore, if labor is contraindicated for any reason, the CST is contraindicated. Tables 2 and 3 list the absolute and relative contraindications of the CST. The CST may be used despite a relative contraindication. For example, if the preterm fetus has severe IUGR, and life in the newborn nursery may be better than life in the uterus, the CST is an appropriate test. Absolute contraindications mean the CST must never be performed under these circumstances as contractions may compromise the woman or her fetus(es).

Table 2: Contraction Stress Test Absolute Contraindications

- polyhydramnios
- multiple gestation
- a vertical uterine scar
- known placenta previa
- chronic abruptio placentae (46).

Table 3: Contraction Stress Test Relative Contraindications

- threatened preterm labor
- a lack of a desire to initiate preterm labor
- preterm premature rupture of the membranes in the absence of infection.

As many as 7.5% of women had preterm labor within 5 days of a CST, but 7.6% of women who only had a NST had preterm labor. Therefore, there appears to be no increased risk of preterm labor following a CST (126).

False Negative Tests

The CST has an excellent false negative rate. If a CST is reactive and negative, every fetus should be alive 7 days later. If the fetus dies prior to the 7th day, there might have been a cord accident, intrauterine infection, placental abruption, or a congenital anomaly that was incompatible with life (9-10, 54, 123, 127).

False Positive Tests

If a fetus has accels and late decels during the CST, there may be no signs of fetal compromise during labor within 7 days of the test. Therefore, the test was a false positive test. False positive rates have varied from 20 to 70% in different settings (3,

9-10, 128). Maternal hypertension may cause a false positive result. When there are late decels, maternal blood pressure should be assessed to rule out hypotension.

CONTRACTION STRESS TESTS

The Spontaneous Contraction Stress Test

Definition: the presence of 3 or more contractions that last 40 or more seconds in a 10 minute period. The FHR is evaluated during the same 10 minutes.

Protocol:

Uterine activity and the FHR should be recorded at least 10 minutes prior to oxytocin administration or nipple stimulation. If there are 3 or more palpable contractions that last 40 or more seconds in a 10 minute period, the spontaneous CST is complete and the tracing should be systematically reviewed.

The Oxytocin Challenge Test (OCT)

Alternate labels: contraction stress test, exogenous oxytocin contraction stress test (Ex-CST)

Goals

- obtain a continuous FHR pattern and
- stimulate the uterus to create 3 or 4 contractions with a duration of 40 to 60 seconds
- during a 10 minute period of time (11, 124, 129).

Benefits

- assesses fetal oxygen reserve prior to the onset of labor
- may be used as a follow-up test after a nonreactive NST.

Limitations

- invasive
- requires an IV
- risk of a drug allergic reaction
- may take 1 to 3 hours to achieve adequate uterine activity (129).

Protocol

The FHR and uterine activity should be recorded at least 10 minutes prior to the initiation of the oxytocin infusion. Confirm the lack of

- a drug (oxytocin) or latex allergy
- 3 contractions in 10 minutes
- a compromised fetus.

Assess and record maternal vital signs and position the woman to avoid supine hypotension. A main line IV is started, usually with 5% dextrose in lactated Ringer's solution (D_5LR) or 5% dextrose in 20% normal saline (D_5 0.2 NS) at a slow or keep-vein-open (KVO) rate. The oxytocin infusion should not begin if the fetus already has late decels with contractions or if there are 3 contractions within a 10 minute period of time, i.e., there is a spontaneous CST. If the BL is flat or nearly flat, the physician should be consulted prior to initiating the infusion of oxytocin.

To initiate the oxytocin infusion, a secondary IV is attached to an IV pump or IV controller then "piggy-backed" into the main line near the IV site (see procedure in appendix). The secondary solution contains the oxytocic drug. The infusion of oxytocin infusion may begin at a rate as low as 0.5 mU/minute, but is usually begun at 1 mU/minute and increased every 15 minutes by 1 mU/minute until three 40 to 60-second contractions are recorded in a 10 minute period of time (130). At that point, the oxytocin infusion is discontinued and the tracing is analyzed and classified. The woman is usually discharged if

- her fetus has a reactive/negative test and
- her uterine activity is similar to the uterine activity prior to the onset of the oxytocin infusion and/or
- she is not in labor.

During the procedure, the oxytocin infusion is discontinued if

- there are 5 or more contractions in 10 minutes (hyperstimulation) (51)
- there is a tetanic contraction (51)
- there are 2 or more late decels in 10 minutes
- there is a prolonged decel (51)
- if the FHR is nonreactive, with or without decels, after a total monitoring time of 80 minutes. The fetus may be severely compromised (64, 76-77).

If oxytocin is discontinued or concern exists about maternal and/or fetal well-being, the nurse should notify the physician. After discontinuing the oxytocin infusion, additional measures to enhance fetal oxygenation may be needed (see Chapter 6).

The Nipple Stimulation Contraction Stress Test (NS-CST)

Alternative labels: breast stimulation contraction stress test (BS-CST), endogenous oxytocin challenge test

Benefits

- noninvasive
- less maternal pain, time, and expense than the OCT (131)
- assesses fetal oxygen reserves prior to the onset of labor
- may be used as a follow-up test after a nonreactive NST
- can provide useful information during preterm gestations
- 33% of women who applied mineral oil to their breasts (breast massage) had 3 contractions within 10 minutes after beginning massage (129)
- 95% of women who used mineral oil and breast massage had 3 contractions in 10 minutes within 40 minutes of initiating the test (129)
- results from a NS-CST are as predictable as results obtained from an OCT (132).

Physiology

Oxytocin is produced by the hypothalamus and stored in the posterior pituitary gland. During breastfeeding, the level of oxytocin in maternal blood significantly increased within two minutes after sucking began. Researchers believed that manual stimulation of the nipples and breasts could also cause the release of oxytocin and initiate contractions (1, 133-134).

In 1984, Drs. Capeless and Mann (134) suggested contractions caused by nipple stimulation were due to an elevated oxytocin level or heightened sensitivity of the uterus to oxytocin. In 1986, researchers confirmed an increase in plasma oxytocin during nipple stimulation. The difference in oxytocin in women's blood who successfully completed the NS-CST and those that were not successful was not statistically different (133).

Protocol

With any antepartal test, it is important for the nurse to establish rapport with the woman. However, it is even more critical that excellent rapport is established prior to asking a woman to rub her breasts or nipples to stimulate uterine activity. Some women may be reluctant to touch their breasts (51). However, the nurse or another person should not attempt to do this for her as it may produce extreme anxiety which would be counterproductive and result in the lack of contractions. In these situations, it may be better to perform an OCT.

The nurse should ascertain who is in the room prior to the woman's initiation of breast or nipple stimulation. The woman should determine who can remain in the room with her during the test. The nurse should assure the woman's privacy. It is best if one nurse stays with the woman, answers her questions, and explains the test procedure. The fetus and uterine activity should be monitored for at least 10 minutes prior to initiating nipple stimulation.

Stimulation should not begin if the fetus already has late decels with contractions or if there are 3 contractions within a 10 minute period of time, i.e., there is a spontaneous CST. If the BL is flat or nearly flat, the physician should be consulted prior to initiating stimulation. A continuous tracing of the FHR and uterine activity should be obtained throughout the CST. This is more likely if the nurse remains in the room (51, 131). If the nurse must leave, it is best to return at frequent intervals to observe the tracing and to provide verbal reinforcement of the woman's technique. As a courtesy, the nurse should knock on the door prior to entering the room.

Several options for nipple and/or breast stimulation should be discussed. The woman should choose the one she prefers (see sample procedure in the appendix). For example, breast and/or nipple stimulation may be done

- with an electric breast pump which the woman operates for up to 15 minutes at a time

The breast pump should be discontinued during contractions.

- by rubbing a towel on the nipple for approximately 1 minute at a time
- by rolling the nipple for 10 minutes until contractions

begin, then using intermittent nipple stimulation (between contractions)
- by applying warm, moist towels to both breasts then massaging one breast at a time (129).

Nipple stimulation may also be done through the gown using the palmar surfaces of the index and middle fingers. The nipple may be stimulated two minutes and the rest period between stimulation may last as long as five minutes. If the rest period is shorter, e.g., two minutes, the test may be completed in a shorter time. No matter what technique is used, stimulation should be stopped during contractions. If the NS-CST is not completed within 45 minutes, a BPP or OCT should be considered (58, 130, 135).

Complications of the NS-CST
Complications of the NS-CST have included:
- preterm labor within 48 hours of a test in a pregnancy at 32 weeks of gestation (1)
- uterine hyperstimulation (20, 132, 139)
- uterine hypertonus lasting as long as 30 minutes (139)
- a prolonged decel for over 5 minutes (140) and
- fetal bradycardia lasting an average of 12.7 minutes (139).

Intermittent nipple stimulation, without the use of warm compresses, has been recommended to reduce the risk of hyperstimulation which increases the rate of successful test completion (46, 135).

Continuous stimulation increases the risk of uterine hyperstimulation. Uterine hyperstimulation is preventable when intermittent, versus continuous, nipple stimulation is used. It is important to instruct the woman to stop stimulation when contractions begin and to observe her compliance through at least one contraction. She should also be shown a contraction on the fetal monitor paper so that she can see the onset of the contraction even before she feels it. When intermittent stimulation consisted of 2 minutes of stimulation of one nipple alternating with 5 minutes of rest, none of the 345 women hyperstimulated and all successfully completed the NS-CST (1).

Warm compresses increase the risk of hyperstimulation. Some clinicians believe the use of warm, wet compresses on the woman's breast(s) decreases the time between the onset of nipple stimulation and the first contraction (131). However, in one study, only 72% of women who applied hot, moist towels to their breasts achieved adequate contractions in 30 minutes (136). Women who already have some spontaneous contractions are more likely to have their first contraction sooner than women who are not contracting, with or without warm compresses. If warm, wet towels are applied to the woman's breast, the nurse should observe the tracing for hyperstimulation. Hyperstimulation has lasted up to 30 minutes in 4 to 14.28% of women who applied warm compresses to their breasts during a NS-CST (20, 139).

Treatment for hyperstimulation during the OCT or NS-CST. If there is a contraction that lasts longer than 90 seconds or 5 or more contractions within 10 minutes of time, the nurse should

- stop the oxytocin infusion or
- ask the woman to cease nipple stimulation and
- turn to her side.

If late, prolonged, or spontaneous decels occur, O_2 should be administered by a tight-fitting face mask at 8 to 10 liters per minute. If the FHR does not improve, an IV may need to be started (in the case of the NS-CST) to deliver a bolus of fluid. Rarely, a tocolytic will be needed. Interventions should be documented and the physician should be notified of the FHR and uterine activity before and after actions, and actions taken. Terbutaline may not be given by the registered nurse without a physician's order (141).

Following completion of the NS-CST, the woman is usually discharged if

- her fetus has a negative/reactive test and
- her uterine activity is similar to the uterine activity prior to the onset of the oxytocin infusion and/or
- she is not in labor.

CST INTERPRETATION CRITERIA

When there are 3 contractions that last 40 to 60 seconds during a 10 minute period, the CST may be interpreted (11) (see Table 4). If there are 2 contractions in 10 minutes and each is associated with a late decel, the CST can be stopped as this is a positive test result.

Discussion

Unlike the NST, there are no specific guidelines on when the CST should cease. However, if the CST is the first antepartal test, and not a follow-up test for the NST, it would be best to evaluate the tracing in a similar way as a NST. Therefore, after 40 minutes the physician should be notified if the FHR is nonreactive. By 80 minutes, if the fetus remains nonreactive, the physician's presence should be requested as the fetus may be severely compromised (64, 76-77). During the second 40 minutes of an 80 minute test, the woman can also be asked to record FM. Then, the CST actually becomes a combination test: FAD plus CST.

Equivocal CSTs. *Variable decels during a CST have been associated with oligohydramnios, IUGR, and a severely compromised fetus (9, 21, 142). The probable acid-base status of the fetus must be considered when deciding the appropriate*

Table 4: Contraction Stress Test Classifications and Recognition Criteria

CLASSIFICATION	RECOGNITION CRITERIA
Negative	no late decels and
	no variable decels (62) with
	three 40 to 60-second contractions in a 10-minute period
Reactive/negative	meets NST criteria for reactive, no decels
Nonreactive/negative	meets NST criteria for nonreactive, no decels and/or
	absent to minimal long-term variability with no accels and no decels
Equivocal/Suspicious	nonrepetitive or nonpersistent decels, e.g., a spontaneous decel
	one late decel and/or
	variable decels (51, 62)
Equivocal/ Hyperstimulation	decel(s) in conjunction with excessive uterine activity
	Excessive uterine activity is
	• 5 contractions in 10 minutes or
	• 1 or more contractions that last 90 or more seconds (136-138)
Positive	late decels with 2 or more contractions in a 10-minute period
	late decels with at least 50% of contractions, even before there are 3 contractions in 10 minutes (2, 62)
Reactive/positive	meets NST criteria for reactive and CST criteria for positive
Nonreactive/positive	meets NST criteria for nonreactive and CST criteria for positive
Unsatisfactory	fewer than 3 contractions in a 10-minute period (2) or
	a tracing with gaps and artifact that is uninterpretable or
	insufficient contractions after 20 minutes of nipple stimulation (138)

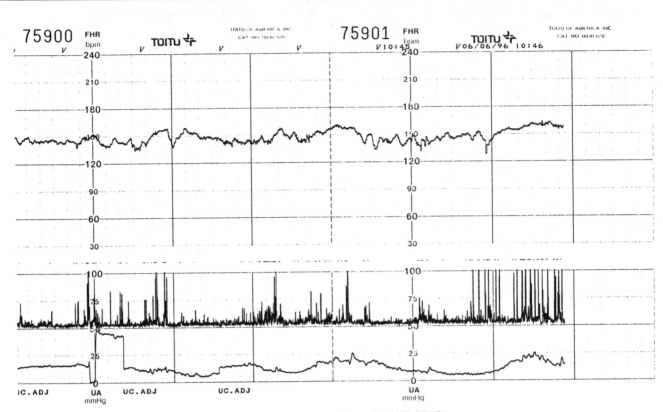

Figure 9.16: Reactive/negative contraction stress test. (Contributed by Carolyn L. Gegor, CNM, MS, RDMS).

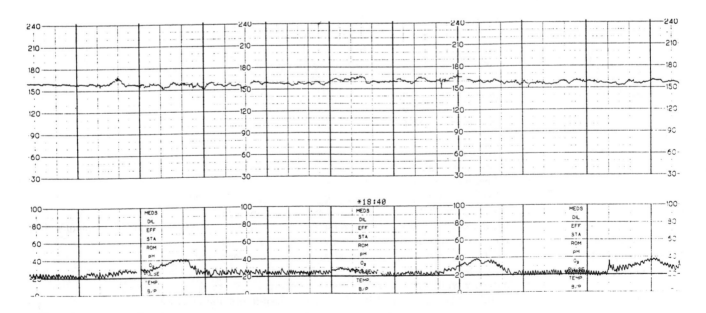

Figure 9.17: Nonreactive/negative contraction stress test (CST). If the tracing is reactive in the minutes preceding or following three 40 to 60 second contractions in a 10 minute period, the fetal heart rate pattern may be classified as "reactive with a negative CST." The presence of "reactive" accels and the lack of decels is evidence of a well-oxygenated fetus. (Contributed by Carolyn L. Gegor, CNM, MS, RDMS).

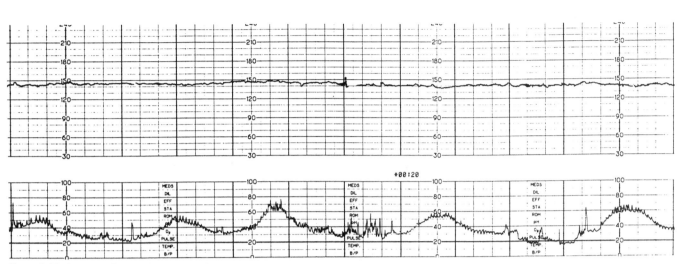

Figure 9.18: A nonreactive/negative contraction stress test with absent to minimal long-term variability, no accels and no decels. Some clinicians have classified this type of tracing as equivocal because it requires follow-up testing. Review previous antepartal tracings to determine the fetus' normal baseline level. Assess fetal movement and maternal drug intake prior to the test, e.g., nicotine, narcotics, or a β-blocker. This test should be followed by a biophysical profile. (Contributed by Carolyn L. Gegor, CNM, MS, RDMS).

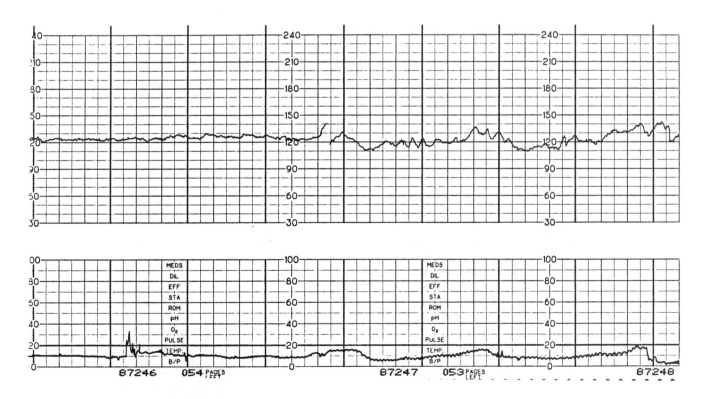

Figure 9.19: This tracing may be interpreted as a reactive/positive contraction stress test. Usually, a reactive/positive test is a false positive test, i.e., there are late decelerations but the fetus tolerates labor that occurs within the next 7 days. (Contributed by Carolyn L. Gegor, CNM, MS, RDMS).

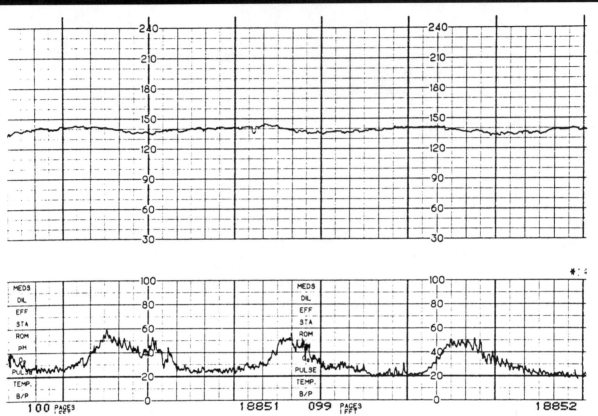

Figure 9.20: Nonreactive/positive contraction stress test (CST). There is absent long-term variability and no accelerations with late decelerations after each contraction. A positive CST also exists if there are late decelerations with two contractions in a ten minute period. (Contributed by Carolyn L. Gegor, CNM, MS, RDMS).

management following an equivocal test result. Some physicians have advocated an equivocal CST should be repeated *the same day*. Others have suggested that an equivocal test should be followed by a BPP. Perhaps, an equivocal test should be followed by delivery as an equivocal test may be worse, in terms of fetal acid-base status, than a positive test. Clinical judgement should supersede "cookbook" recommendations. When variable decels, 15 or more seconds in duration with a nadir 15 or more bpm below the BL, are observed during any antepartal test, the fetus should be "further evaluated" and AFV should be determined *and/or the fetus should be delivered* (11). If an equivocal test is repeated, and subsequent tests are equivocal, NSTs are usually done twice a week (143). A BPP may follow an equivocal CST.

Reactive/Positive CSTs. A reactive FHR pattern is associated with fetal well-being (3, 72). A reactive/positive test was a false positive test in 50% of term fetuses (143). But, 50% of fetuses had a true positive test, suggesting inadequate O_2 reserves to cope with labor. The presence of accels with late decels may be associated with maternal hypotension, therefore blood pressure should be assessed. Schifrin and Clement (3) suggested that late decels occasionally accompany fetal breathing

movements in the normal fetus. They did not explain the physiologic basis of their proposed association between fetal breathing movements and late decels. *If late decels persist, they should be considered an early warning sign of fetal compromise* (127). If the fetus is preterm with a reactive/positive CST, the test is usually repeated within 24 hours, and other tests may be done prior to making a final decision about delivery.

Nonreactive/positive CST. If the woman has occasional spontaneous contractions and each is associated with a late decel, the test is considered positive and no further attempt should be made to stimulate uterine contractions. The physician should be immediately notified of positive CST results and, if applicable, the oxytocin infusion or nipple stimulation are discontinued (2).

The lack of reactive accels and the presence of late decels usually represents fetal deterioration and is associated with IUGR and fetal intolerance of labor (3, 10, 138). *Nonreactive/positive tests have the highest correlation with perinatal mortality* (9-10, 137-138, 144). *A nonreactive/positive CST, even in a preterm fetus, often precedes a poor neonatal outcome and is a strong indication for delivery* (3, 6, 9-10, 35). Prior to a cesarean section, even the term fetus may be observed by ultrasound to rule out a congenital defect that is incompatible with life. In that case, the fetus should be vaginally delivered.

Hyperstimulation. In the case of hyperstimulation, the test cannot be interpreted until the uterus relaxes and there are 3 or 4 contractions in 10 minutes and contractions last less than 90 seconds but are at least 40 seconds in duration.

NURSE AND PHYSICIAN RESPONSIBILITIES DURING ANTEPARTAL TESTING
Know Fetal and Maternal Physiology
Nurses and physicians who perform antepartal tests need a thorough knowledge of high-risk factors, fetal and maternal physiology, and the implications of test results on pregnancy management and fetal outcome.

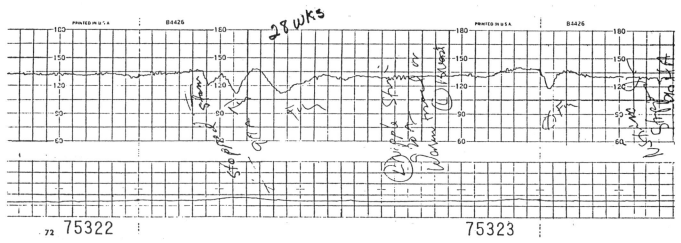

Figure 9.21: Equivocal/suspicious nipple stimulation contraction stress test (NS-CST) that followed a nonreactive nonstress test in a fetus who was only 28 weeks of gestation. The woman presented with decreased fetal movement. There is absent variability, variable decelerations, a spontaneous deceleration which begins in the third minute of monitoring and a late deceleration after the first contraction. The paper is printed in 20 second increments versus 10 second increments, i.e., 3 squares = 1 minute. This preterm fetus has a risk of dying and needs to be delivered as soon as possible (64, 76-77).

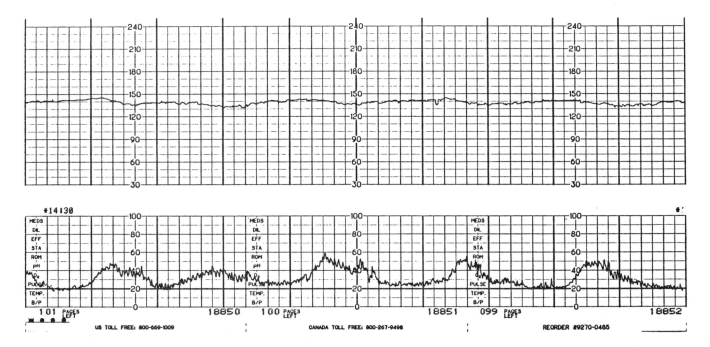

Figure 9.22: Equivocal/hyperstimulation contraction stress test. Note 5 contractions in 10 minutes, each with a late deceleration. Oxytocin or nipple stimulation are discontinued. When there are 3 or 4 contractions in 10 minutes, the test is interpreted. (Contributed by Carolyn L. Gegor, CNM, MS, RDMS).

Follow Protocol
Prior to performing an antepartal test, there should be a procedure in place. The procedure should delineate the scope of nursing practice, including expectations regarding FHR pattern interpretation.

Reduce Anxiety, Assure Privacy, Answer Questions, Provide Instructions, and Reinforce Information Previously Learned
During antepartal tests, the nurse has an opportunity to answer the woman's questions and to teach her about her pregnancy. Women may be anxious and unable to assimilate all of the information they receive during prenatal visits. Therefore, the antepartal testing time may be used to reduce anxiety, explain the FHR and uterine activity patterns and equipment used during testing, the purposes of antepartal tests, and the medical plan of care. Smoking cessation guidelines may also be reinforced, including the request that women not smoke for at least two hours prior to testing.

Obtain a Quality Tracing
Antepartal tests require a continuous or nearly continuous tracing prior to interpretation. The nurse is responsible for the quality of the tracing. Therefore, it is best to stay with the woman as much as possible during antepartal tests.

Analyze the FHR Pattern and Document the Systematic Review
Nurses interpret the tracing and should document their systematic review. Accels and decels should only be measured and documented if the majority of the change in the FHR is observed. When the test is completed, another nurse or physician should confirm the systematic review and agree with the nurse's classification. The names of the nurses and/or physicians who reviewed the tracing should be documented.

Notify the Physician as Soon as Possible if There is a Nonreactive, Equivocal, or Positive Test
If there is a nonreactive, equivocal, or positive test, fetal bradycardia, or spontaneous or prolonged decels, the physician should be contacted after measures have been taken to enhance fetal oxygenation. The time and content of the conversation should be documented in the woman's medical record. Measures should be taken to reduce uterine activity and, if necessary, improve fetal oxygenation. Follow-up tests may be ordered or the woman may be delivered, depending on the perceived fetal condition (see Figure 9.23).

The Physician Establishes the Plan of Care
The nurse and physician should share information which will be used to establish the plan of care. The physician's plan of care will be influenced by the fetus' gestational age, the FHR pattern, uterine activity, condition of the cervix, presentation and station of the fetus, maternal high-risk factors, and ultrasound reports. If the physician decides to perform an "emergency" cesarean section, it is imperative

that someone contact her immediate family and/or significant others *prior to surgery*. There is usually sufficient time to notify the woman's support person of the decision to deliver the fetus and to explain the rationale for the prompt delivery *before* rushing into surgery.

Confirm Fetal Well-Being Prior to Maternal Discharge
Prior to discharge of the woman, the nurse should feel comfortable that fetal well-being has been established. If there is any question about the well-being of the fetus, the physician must see the tracing as soon as possible and prior to the woman's discharge from the antepartal test suite or labor and delivery. Adverse outcomes can be prevented if nurses communicate their entire systematic review to the physician, including findings such as a BL shift (perhaps the BL is rising), absent to minimal LTV, the increased duration between accels, the presence of uniform accels, variable decels, late decels, spontaneous decels, prolonged decels, or bradycardia.

TEST	FOLLOW-UP
NST	
Reactive	→ repeat in 3 to 7 days
Reactive with variable decels	→ ultrasound for AFV or deliver
Inconclusive	→ repeat that day or complete the BPP
Nonreactive	→ increase total test time to 80 minutes (76) or perform a BPP or CST
BPP	
See Chapter 9 for actions according to BPP score	
CST	
Reactive/negative	→ repeat in 3 to 7 days
Equivocal	→ retest ASAP or perform a BPP the fetus should become reactive within 80 minutes of testing (76)
Reactive/positive	→ BPP for further evaluation
Nonreactive/positive	→ transfer woman to labor and delivery enhance fetal oxygenation deliver (may attempt induction or deliver by cesarean section)
Hyperstimulation	→ discontinue stimulation, wait 30 minutes if 3 contractions occur in a 10-minute period, analyze the tracing or begin stimulation again

Figure 9.23: Management of the high-risk woman. This decision tree assumes the absence of a congenital anomaly, medication(s), or a condition that prevents accelerations. NST = nonstress test, AFV = amniotic fluid volume, CST = contraction stress test, BPP = biophysical profile. (modified from Eden (7)).

KICK COUNTS

Nearly one half of all fetal deaths occurred in pregnancies of low-risk women. Therefore, it may be beneficial for all women to be taught to assess FM during the third trimester. In 2519 women who had no formal FM assessment, the fetal mortality rate was 8.7 per 1000 births. When women kept a record of the time it took to feel 10 fetal movements (count-to-ten method), the longest time was 39 minutes and the fetal mortality rate fell to 2.1 per 1000 births. If 2 hours elapsed without 10 movements, women were asked to report to labor and delivery for further testing (145). Although fetal mortality decreased when pregnant women assessed FM, the number of NSTs and other antepartal tests increased 13% and interventions for fetal compromise tripled. The number of fetal movements that women are told they should perceive in an hour is arbitrary. Instead of 10 fetal movements, some protocol require the woman to feel 4 movements within an hour or to call labor and delivery if there have not been 4 movements in 60 minutes (see appendix for sample procedure) (59).

The fetus is more active at night. The fetus is most active in the late evening and early morning hours, i.e., 10:00 p.m. through 2:00 am (27, 72). Therefore, women should be encouraged to count FM in the evening. She should be instructed to lay down with her hand placed on her abdomen over her uterus and, without distractions, feel her baby move. If she has a concern during the day that the fetus is moving less or more than normal, she should be instructed to count FM and to call the physician's office, clinic, or labor and delivery to express her concerns.

CONCLUSION

This chapter presented all of the antepartal tests which require use of the fetal monitor, as well as kick counts. When pregnant women count fetal movements at least once a day, the fetal mortality rate may decrease. In general, antepartal tests are performed on women whose fetus is at risk for hypoxia, metabolic acidosis, and asphyxia. These women may be very anxious about antepartal tests in general, participating in the test, and test results. If the test suggests fetal well-being, women should be reassured that the test is highly reliable as long as the woman and her baby remain physiologically stable. However, since antepartal tests are less accurate in predicting undesirable outcomes, women often need additional tests when criteria are not met for a reactive fetal heart rate pattern (7).

The nurse is usually the first person to evaluate the fetal heart rate and uterine activity patterns. Strict protocol for total testing time and interpretation must be followed. At least two nurses, a nurse and a physician, or two physicians should review the tracing to assure agreement that the fetus is well prior to the woman's departure. The physician should be immediately notified of any nonreactive, equivocal, or positive test results, any actions taken, and the fetal and uterine response to actions.

The physician is responsible for establishing and communicating a plan of care, including follow-up tests and procedures. The teamwork of the woman, her family, nurses and physicians should prevent perinatal morbidity and mortality.

References

1.	Huddleston, J. F., Sutliff, G., & Robinson, D. (May 1984). Contraction stress test by intermittent nipple stimulation. Obstetrics & Gynecology, 63(5), 669-673.

2.	Tournaire, M., Sturbois, G., Zorn, J., Breart, G., & Sureau, C. (1980). Fetal monitoring before and during labor. In S. Aladjem, A. K. Brown, & V. Sureau (Eds.), Clinical perinatology (pp. 331-361). St. Louis, MO: The C. V. Mosby Company.

3.	Schifrin, B. S., & Clement, D. (February 1990). Why fetal monitoring remains a good idea. Comtemporary OB/GYN, 70-86.

4.	Manning, F. A., Morrison, I., Lange, I. R., Harman, C. R., & Chamberlain, P. F. (February 1, 1985). Fetal assessment based on fetal biophysical profile scoring: Experience in 12,620 referred high-risk pregnancies. I. Perinatal mortality by frequency & etiology. American Journal of Obstetrics and Gynecology, 151(3), 343-350.

5.	Freeman, R. K., Garite, T. J., Nageotte, M. P. (1991). Antepartum fetal monitoring. In Fetal heart rate monitoring (pp. 156-178). Baltimore, MD: Williams & Wilkins.

6.	Ware, D. J., & Devoe, L. D. (1994). The nonstress test: Reassessment of the "gold standard." Clinics in Perinatology, 21(4), 779-796.

7.	Eden, R. D., Gergley, R. Z., Schifrin, B. S., & Wade, M. E. (November 15, 1982). Comparison of antepartum testing schemes for the management of the postdate pregnancy. American Journal of Obstetrics and Gynecology, 144(6), 683-692.

8.	Ray, M., Freeman, R., Pine, S., & Hesselgesser, R. (September 1,1972). Clinical experience with the oxytocin challenge test. American Journal of Obstetrics and Gynecology, 114(1), 1-9.

9.	Freeman, R. K., Lagrew, Jr., D. C., (1990). The contraction stress test. In R. D. Eden, & F. H. Boehm (Eds.), Assessment and care of the fetus. Physiological, clinical, and medicolegal principles (pp.351-363). Norwalk, CT: Appleton & Lange.

10.	Gabbe, S. G. (1991). Intrauterine growth retardation. In S. G. Gabbe, J. R. Niebyl, & Simpson (Eds.), Obstetrics: Normal and problem pregnancies (2nd ed). NY: Churchill Livingstone.

11.	Antepartum fetal surveillance. (January 1994). Technical bulletin number 188, Washington, DC: ACOG.

12.	Rochard, F., Schifrin, B. S., Goupil, F., Legrand, H., Blottiere, J., & Sureau, C. (November 15, 1976). Nonstress fetal heart rate monitoring in the antepartum period. American Journal of Obstetrics and Gynecology, 126(6), 699-706.

13.	Read, J. A., & Miller, F. C. (November 1, 1977). Fetal heart rate acceleration in response to acoustic stimulation as a measure of fetal well-being. American Journal of Obstetrics and Gynecology, 129(5), 512-517.

14.	Gagnon, R., Patrick, J., Foreman, J., & West, R. (October 1986). Stimulation of human fetuses with sound and vibration. American Journal of Obstetrics and Gynecology, 155(4), 848-851.

15.	Romero, R., Mazor, M., & Hobbins, J. C. (May 1988). A critical appraisal of fetal acoustic stimulation as an antenatal test for fetal well being. Obstetrics & Gynecology, 71(5), 781-786.

16.	Clark, S. L., Sabey, P., & Jolley, K. (March 1989). Nonstress testing with acoustic stimulation and amniotic fluid volume assessment: 5973 tests without unexpected fetal death. American Journal of Obstetrics and Gynecology, 160(3), 694-697.

17.	Johnson, R. L., & Elliott, J. P. (November 1995). Fetal acoustic stimulation, an adjunct to external cephalic version: A blinded, randomized crossover study. American Journal of Obstetrics and Gynecology, 173(5), 1369-1372.

18.	Lee, C. Y., Di Loreto, P. C., & Logrand, B. (July 1976). Fetal activity acceleration determination for the evaluation of fetal reserve. Obstetrics & Gynecology, 48(1), 19-26.

19.	MacMillan, III, J. B., & Hale, R. W. (April 1984). Contraction stress testing with mammary self-stimulation. Journal of Reproductive Medicine, 29(4), 219-221.

20.	Copel, J. A., Otis, C. S., Stewart, E., Rosetti, C., & Weiner, S. (June 1985). Contraction stress testing with nipple stimulation. Journal of Reproductive Medicine, 30(6), 465-471.

21.	Druzin, M. L. (1992). The nonstress test and contraction stress test. In M. L. Druzin (Ed.), Antepartum fetal assessment (pp. 3-26). Boston, MA: Blackwell Scientific Publications.

22.	Finberg, H. J. (1994). Ultrasound evaluation in multiple gestation. In P. W. Callen (Ed.), Ultrasonography in obstetrics and gynecology (3rd. ed., pp. 102-128). Philadelphia, PA: W B Saunders Company.

23.	Weeks, J. W., Asrat, T., Morgan, M. A., Nageotte, M., Thomas, S. J., & Freeman, R. K. (February 1995). Antepartum surveillance for a history of stillbirth: When to begin? American Journal of Obstetrics and Gynecology, 172(2, Pt. 1), 486-492.

24.	Rayburn, W. F., & McKean, H. E. (August 1980). Maternal perception of fetal movement and perinatal outcome. Obstetrics & Gynecology, 56(2), 161-164.

25. Pearson, J. F., & Weaver, J. B. (1976). Fetal activity and fetal well being: An evaluation. British Medical Journal, 1, 1305-1307.

26. Neldham, S. (June 7, 1980). Fetal movements as an indicator of fetal well being. The Lancet, 1(8180), 1222-1234.

27. Sadovsky, E., & Yaffe, H. (June 1973). Daily fetal movement recording and fetal prognosis. Obstetrics & Gynecology, 41(6), 845-850.

28. Davis, L. (January/February 1987). Daily fetal movement counting: A valuable assessment tool. Journal of Nurse Midwifery, 32(1), 11-19.

29. Gegor, C. L. (1993). Third trimester ultrasound for nurse midwives. Journal of Nurse Midwifery, 38(25), 1-13.

30. Phelan, J. P., Kester, R., & Labudovich, M. L. (October 1982). Nonstress test and maternal serum glucose determinations. Obstetrics & Gynecology, 60(4), 437-439.

31. Gegor, C. L., Paine, L. L., & Johnson, T. R. B. (1991). Antepartum fetal assessment: A nurse-midwifery perspective. Journal of Nurse Midwifery, 36(3), 153-167.

32. Phelan, J. P., Ahn, M. O., Smith, C. V., Rutherford, S. E., & Anderson, E. (August 1987). Amniotic fluid index measurements during pregnancy. Journal of Reproductive Medicine, 32(8), 601-604.

33. Phelan, J. P., Platt, L. D.,Yeh, S. Y., Broussard, P., & Paul, R. H. (February 1, 1985). The role of ultrasound assessment of amniotic fluid volume in the management of postdate pregnancy. American Journal of Obstetrics and Gynecology, 151(3), 304-308.

34. Rutherford, S. E., Phelan, J. P., Smith, C. V., & Jacobs, N. (September 1987). The four-quadrant assessment of amniotic fluid volume: An adjunct to antepartum fetal heart rate testing. Obstetrics & Gynecology, 70(5, Pt. 1), 353-356.

35. Devoe, L. D. (1990). The nonstress test. In R. D. Eden, & F. H. Boehm (Eds.), Assessment and care of the fetus (p. 365). Norwalk, CT: Appleton & Lange.

36. A clinical trial of induction of labor versus expectant management in postterm pregnancy. (March 1994). American Journal of Obstetrics and Gynecology, 170(3), 716-723.

37. Johnson, J. M., Harman, C. R., Lange, I. R., & Manning, F. A. (February 1986). Biophysical profile scoring in the management of the post-term pregnancy: An analysis of 307 patients. American Journal of Obstetrics and Gynecology, 154(2), 269-273.

38. Lien, J. M., Nageotte, M. P., Towers, C. V., de Veciana, M., & Toohey, J. S. (January 1994). Intrauterine growth retardation: Contraction stress test or biophysical profile? American Journal of Obstetrics and Gynecology, 170(1, Pt. 2), 316. SPO abstracts #142.

39. Elliott, J. P., & Finberg, H. J. (February 1995). Biophysical profile testing as an indicator of fetal well-being in higher-order multiple gestations. American Journal Obstetrics and Gynecology, 172(2, Pt. 1), 508-512.

40. Besinger, R. E., & Johnson, T. R. B. (August 1989). Doppler recordings of fetal movement: Clinical correlation with real-time ultrasound. Obstetrics & Gynecology, 74(2), 277-280.

41. Vintzileos, A. M., Campbell, W. A., Nochimson, D. J., Weinbaum, P. J., Mirochnick, M. H., & Escoto, D. T. (October 1986). Fetal biophysical profile versus amniocentesis in predicting infection in preterm premature rupture of the membranes. Obstetrics & Gynecology, 68(4), 488-494.

42. Vintzileos, A. M., Feinstein, S. J., Lodeiro, J. G., Campbell, W. A., Weinbaum, P. J., & Nochimson, D. J. (January 1986). Fetal biophysical profile and the effect of premature rupture of the membranes. Obstetrics & Gynecology, 67(6), 818-823.

43. Vintzileos, A. M., Bors-Koefoed, R., Pelegano, J. F., Campbell, W. A., Rodis, J. F., & Nochimson, D. J. (August 1987). The use of fetal biophysical profile improves pregnancy outcome in premature rupture of the membranes. American Journal of Obstetrics and Gynecology, 157(2), 236-240.

44. Devoe, L. D., Youssef, A. E., Croom, C. S., & Watson, J. (September 1994). Can fetal biophysical observations anticipate outcome in preterm labor or in preterm rupture of membranes? Obstetrics & Gynecology, 84(3), 432-438.

45. Del Valle, G. O., Joffe, G. M., Izquierdo, L. A., Smith, J. F., Gilson, G. J., & Curet, L. B. (July 1992). Poor predictors of chorioamnionitis and fetal nonstress test. Obstetrics & Gynecology, 80(1), 106-110.

46. Antepartum fetal surveillance. (August 1987). Technical bulletin number 107. Washington, DC: ACOG.

47. Pillai, M., & James, D. (1990). Development of human fetal behavior: A review. Fetal Diagnosis Therapy, 5, 15-32.

48. Knuppel, R. A., Lake, M., & Ingram, J. M. (March 1982). A review of the nonstress test. The Journal of Reproductive Medicine, 27(3), 120-126.

49. Naef, III, R. W., Morrison, J. C., Washburne, J. F., McLaughlin, B. N., Perry, Jr., K. G., & Roberts, W. E. (September 1994). Assessment of fetal well-being using the nonstress test in the home setting. Obstetrics & Gynecology, 84(3), 424-426.

50. Boehm, F. H., Salyer, S., Shah, D. M., & Vaughn, W. K. (April 1986). Improved outcome of twice weekly nonstress testing. Obstetrics & Gynecology, 67(4), 566-568.

51. Dauphinee, J. D. (1987). Antepartum testing: A challenge for nursing. Journal of Perinatal and Neonatal Nursing, 1(1), 29-48.

52. Druzin, M. L., & Foodim, J. (March 1986). Effect of maternal glucose ingestion compared with maternal water ingestion on the nonstress test. Obstetrics & Gynecology, 67(3), 425-426.

53. Eglinton, G. S. , Paul, R. H., Broussard, P. M., Walla, C. A., & Platt, L. D. (September 1,1984). Antepartum fetal heart rate testing. XI. Stimulation with orange juice. American Journal of Obstetrics and Gynecology, 150(1), 97-99.

54. Shaw, K. J., & Paul, R. H. (March 1990). Fetal responses to external stimuli. Obstetrics and Gynecology Clinics of North America, 17(1), 235-248.

55. Gegor, C. L., Paine, L. L., Costigan, K., & Johnson, T. R. B. (June 1994). Interpretation of biophysical profiles by nurses and physicians. JOGNN, 23(5), 405-410 .

56. Willis, D. C., Blanco, J. D., Hamblen, K. A., & Stovall, D. W. (September 1990). The nonstress test. Criteria for the duration of fetal heart rate acceleration. Journal of Reproductive Medicine, 35(9), 901-903.

57. Vintzileos, A. M., Campbell, W. A., Ingardia, C. J., & Nochimson, D. J. (1983). The fetal biophysical profile and its predictive value. Obstetrics & Gynecology, 62(3), 271-278.

58. Murray, M. L. (1988). Antepartal and intrapartal fetal monitoring. Washington, DC: Association of Women's Health, Obstetric, and Neonatal Nurses (AWHONN).

59. Rayburn, W. F. (December 15, 1982). Clinical implications from monitoring fetal activity. American Journal of Obstetrics and Gynecology, 144(8), 967-980.

60. Barss, V. A., Frigoletto, Jr., F. D., & Diamond, F. (April 1985). Stillbirth after nonstress testing. Obstetrics & Gynecology, 65(4), 541-544.

61. Phelan, J. P., & Lewis, Jr., P. E. (February 1981). Fetal heart rate decelerations during a nonstress test. Obstetrics & Gynecology, 57(2), 228-232.

62. Devoe, L. D., McKenzie, J., Searle, N. S., & Sherline, D. M. (April 15, 1985). Clinical sequelae of the extended nonstress test. American Journal of Obstetrics and Gynecology, 151(8), 1074-1078.

63. Druzin, M. L., Fox, A., Kogut, E., & Carlson, C. (October 15, 1985). The relationship of the nonstress test to gestational age. American Journal of Obstetrics and Gynecology, 152(2), 386-389.

64. Anyaegbunam, A., Brustman, L., Divon, M., & Langer, O. (October 1986). The significance of antepartum variable decelerations. American Journal of Obstetrics and Gynecology, 155(4), 707-710.

65. Meis, P. J., Ureda, J. R., Swain, M., Kelly, R. T., Penry, M., & Sharp, P. (March 1986). Variable decelerations during nonstress tests are not a sign of fetal compromise. American Journal of Obstetrics and Gynecology, 154(3), 586-590.

66. Keegan Jr., K. A., Paul, R. H., Broussard., P. M., McCart, D., & Smith, M. A. (January 1, 1987). Antepartum fetal heart rate testing. V. The nonstress test—an outpatient approach. American Journal of Obstetrics and Gynecology, 136(1), 81-83.

67. Goldkrand, J. W., & Benjamin, D. S. (January 1984). Antepartum fetal heart testing: A clinical appraisal. Obstetrics & Gynecology, 63(1), 48.

68. Smith, C. V., Greenspoon, J., Phelan, J. P., & Platt, L. D. (1987). Clinical utility of the nonstress test in the conservative management of women with preterm spontaneous premature rupture of membranes. Journal of Reproductive Medicine, 32(1), 1-4.

69. Keane, M. W. D., Horger III, E. O., & Vice, L. (March 1981). Comparative study of stressed and nonstressed antepartum fetal heart rate testing. Obstetrics & Gynecology, 57(3), 320-324.

70. Visser, G. H. A., Zeelenberg, H. J., deVries, J. I. P., & Dawes, G. S. (March 1, 1983). External physical stimulation of the human fetus during episodes of low heart rate variation. American Journal of Obstetrics and Gynecology, 145(5), 579-584.

71. Patrick, J., Carmichael, L., Chess, L., & Staples, C. (January 1, 1984). Accelerations of the human fetal heart rate at 38 to 40 weeks gestational age. American Journal of Obstetrics and Gynecology, 148(4), 386-389.

72. Johnson, T. R. B., Besinger, R. E., & Thomas, R. L. (1988). New clues to fetal behavior and well-being. Contemporary OB/GYN, 108.

73. Odendaal, H. J., Steyn, W., Theron, G. B., Norman, K., & Kirstan, G. F. (May 1994). Does a nonreactive fetal heart rate really mean fetal distress? American Journal of Perinatology, 11(3), 194-198.

74. Issel, E. P. (1983). Fetal response to external mechanical stimuli. The Journal of Perinatal Medicine, 11(5), 232-242.

75. Devoe, L. D., McKenzie, J., Searle, N. S., & Sherline, D. M. (April 15, 1985). Clinical sequelae of the extended nonstress test. American Journal of Obstetrics and Gynecology, 151(8), 1074-1078.

76. Brown, R., & Patrick, J. (November 15, 1981). The nonstress test: How long is enough? American Journal of Obstetrics and Gynecology, 141(6), 646-651.

77. Leveno, K. J., Williams, M. L., DePalma, R. T., & Whalley, P. J. (March 1983). Perinatal outcome in the absence of fetal heart rate auscultation. Obstetrics & Gynecology, 61(3), 347-355.

78. Auyeung, R. M., & Goldkrand, J. W. (May/June 1991). Vibroacoustic stimulation and nursing intervention in the nonstress test. JOGNN, 20(3), 232-238.

79. Navot, D., Yaffe, H., & Sadovsky, E. (May 1, 1984). The ratio of fetal heart rate accelerations to fetal movements according to gestational age. American Journal of Obstetrics and Gynecology, 149(1), 92-94.

80. Lawson, G. W., Dawes, G. S., & Redman, C. (June 1984). Analysis of fetal heart rate on-line at 32 weeks gestation. British Journal of Obstetrics and Gynaecology, 91(6), 542-550.

81. Druzin, M. L., Fox, A., Kogut, E., & Carlson, C. (October 15, 1985). The relationship of the nonstress test to gestational age. American Journal of Obstetrics and Gynecology, 152(4), 386-389.

82. Kelly, J., Mathews, K. A., & O'Conor, M. (February 1984). Smoking in pregnancy: Effects on mother and fetus. British Journal of Obstetrics and Gynaecology, 91(2), 111-117.

83. McLeod, W., Brien, J., Loomis, C., Carmichael, L., Probert, C., & Patrick, J. (January 15, 1983). Effect of maternal ethanol ingestion on fetal breathing movements, gross body movements, and heart rate at 37 to 40 weeks gestational age. American Journal of Obstetrics and Gynecology, 145(2), 251-257.

84. Margulis, E., Binder, D., & Cohen, A. (1984). The effect of propranolol on the nonstress test. American Journal of Obstetrics and Gynecology, 148, 340-341.

85. Katz, M., Meizner, I., Holcberg, G., Mazor, M., Hagay, Z. J., & Insler, V. (1988). Reduction of cessation of fetal movements after administration of steroids for enhancement of lung maturation. I. Clinical evaluation. Israel Journal of Medical Sciences, 24(1), 5-9.

86. Ville, Y., Vincent, Y., Tordjman, N., Hu, M. V., Fernandez, H., & Frydman, R. (1995). Effect of betamethasone on the fetal heart rate pattern assessed by computerized cardiotocography in normal twin pregnancies. Fetal Diagnosis and Therapy, 10, 301-306.

87. Derks, J. B., Mulder, E. J. H., & Visser, G. H. A. (January 1995). The effects of maternal betamethasone administration on the fetus. British Journal of Obstetrics and Gynaecology, 102, 40-46.

88. Leveno, K. J., Williams, M. L., De Palma, R. T., & Whalley, P. J. (March 1983). Perinatal outcome in the absence of antepartum fetal heart rate acceleration. Obstetrics & Gynecology, 61(3), 347-355.

89. Welt, S. I. (March 1984). The fetal heart rate W-sign. Obstetrics & Gynecology, 63(3), 405-408.

90. Tharakan, T., Di Bella, V., & Baxi, L. V. (January 1994). Variable decelerations during nonstress tests-clinical associations. American Journal of Obstetrics and Gynecology, 170(1, Pt. 2), SPO abstracts #317.

91. Pazos, R., Vuolo, K., Aladjem, S., Lueck, J., & Anderson, C. (November 1, 1982). Association of spontaneous fetal heart rate decelerations during antepartum nonstress testing and intrauterine growth retardation. American Journal of Obstetrics and Gynecology, 144(5), 574-577.

92. Flynn, A. M., Kelly, J., Matthews, S. K., O'Conor, M., & Viegas, O. (June 1982). Predictive value of, and observer variability in, several ways of reporting antepartum cardiotocographs. British Journal of Obstetrics and Gynaecology, 89, 434-440.

93. Chez, B. F., Skurnick, J. H., Chez, R. A., Verklan, M. T., Biggs, S., Hage, M. L. (May/June 1990). Interpretations of nonstress tests by obstetric nurses. JOGNN, 19(3), 227-232.

94. Skurnick, J. H., Chez, R. A., & Chez, B. F. (March 1991). Effect of explicit criteria on nonstress test evaluation by obstetric nurses. American Journal of Perinatology, 8(2), 139-143.

95. Smith, C. V., Greenspoon, J., Phelan, J. P., & Platt, L. D. (January 1987). Clinical utility of the nonstress test in the conservative management of women with preterm spontaneous premature rupture of membranes. The Journal of Reproductive Medicine, 32(1), 1-4.

96. Timor-Tritsch, I. E., Dierker, L. J., Zador, I., Hertz, R. H., & Rosen, M. G. (June 1, 1978). Fetal movements associated with fetal heart rate accelerations and decelerations. American Journal of Obstetrics and Gynecology, 131(3), 276-280.

97. Baser, I., Johnson, T. R. B., & Paine, L. L. (July 1992). Coupling of fetal movement and fetal heart rate accelerations as an indicator of fetal health. Obstetrics & Gynecology, 80(1), 62-66.

98. Natale, R., Nasello, C., & Turliuk, R. (March 1, 1984). The relationship between movements and accelerations in fetal heart rate at twenty-four to thirty-two weeks gestation. American Journal of Obstetrics and Gynecology, 91(6), 542-550.

99. Johnson, T. R. B., & Johnson, M. J. (September 1993). Identifying fetal movement and behavior patterns. Contemporary OB/GYN, 11-16.

100. Smith, C. V., Nguyen, H. N., Phelan, J. P., & Paul, R. H. (October 1986). Intrapartum assessment of fetal well being: A comparison of fetal acoustic stimulation with acid-base determinations. American Journal of Obstetrics and Gynecology, 155(4), 726-728.

101. Kisilevsky, B. S., Kilpatrick, K. L., & Low, J. A. (February 1993). Vibroacoustic-induced fetal movement: Two stimuli and two methods of scoring. Obstetrics & Gynecology, 81(2), 174-177.

102. Serafini, P., Lindsay, M. B. J., Nagey, D. A., Pupkin, M. J., Tseng, P., & Crenshaw Jr., C. (January 1, 1984). Antepartum fetal heart rate response to sound stimulation: The acoustic stimulation test. American Journal of Obstetrics and Gynecology, 148(1), 4145.

103. Zimmer, E. Z., Chao, C. R., Guy, G. P., Marks, F., & Fifer, W. P. (February 1993). Vibroacoustic stimulation evokes human fetal micturition. Obstetrics & Gynecology, 81(2)178-180.

104. Clark, S. L., Sabey, P., & Jolley, K. (March 1989). Nonstress testing with acoustic stimulation and amniotic fluid volume assessment: 5973 tests without unexpected fetal death. American Journal of Obstetrics and Gynecology, 160(3), 694-697.

105. Inglis, S. R., Druzin, M. L., Wagner, W. E., & Kogut, E. (September 1993). The use of vibroacoustic stimulation during the abnormal or equivocal biophysical profile. Obstetrics & Gynecology, 82(3), 371-374.

106. Sleutel, M. R. (November/December 1989). An overview of vibroacoustic stimulation. JOGNN, 447-452.

107. Richards, D. S., Cefalo, R. C., Thorpe, J. M., Salley, M., & Rose, D. (April 1988). Determinants of fetal heart rate response to vibroacoustic stimulation in labor. Obstetrics & Gynecology, 71(4), 535-539.

108. Gagnon, R., Patrick, J., Foreman, J., & West, R. (October 1986). Stimulation of human fetuses with sound and vibration. American Journal of Obstetrics and Gynecology, 155(4), 848-851.

109. Sherer, D. M., Menashe, M., & Sadovsky, E. (1988). Severe fetal bradycardia caused by external vibratory acoustic stimulation. American Journal of Obstetrics and Gynecology, 159(2), 334-335.

110. Newnham, J. P., Burns, S. E., & Roberman, B. D. (July 1990). Effect of vibratory acoustic stimulation on the duration of fetal heart rate monitoring tests. American Journal of Perinatology, 7(3), 232-234.

111. Thomas, R. T., Johnson, T. R. B., Besinger, R. E., Rafkin, D., Treanor, C., & Strobino, D. (July 1989). Preterm and term fetal cardiac and movement responses to vibratory acoustic stimulation. American Journal of Obstetrics and Gynecology, 161(1), 141-145.

112. Miller-Slade, D., Gloeb, D. J., Bailey, S. , Bendell, A., Interlandi, E., & Kline-Kaye, V. (March/April 1991). Acoustic stimulation-induced fetal response compared to traditional nonstress testing. JOGNN, 20(2), 160-167.

113. Sohmer, H., Geal-Dor, M., & Weinstein, D. (May 1994). Human fetal auditory threshold improvement during maternal oxygen respiration. Hearing Research, 75(1-2), 145-150.

114. Blackburn, S. T., & Loper, D. L. (1992). Maternal, fetal, and neonatal physiology. A clinical perspective. Philadelphia, PA: W. B. Saunders Company.

115. Phelan, J. P. (April 1991). Acoustic stimulation during the third trimester. Contemporary OB/GYN, 36, 87-94.

116. Abitol, M. M., Udom-Rice, I., Martin, A. K., Toledo, R. B., & Karimi, A. (1992). Fetal sound stimulation using maternal voice. Journal of Maternal-Fetal Investigation, 2, 233-239.

117. Gagnon, R., Hunse, C., Carmichael, L., Fellows, F., & Patrick, J. (February 1987). External vibratory acoustic stimulation near term: Fetal heart rate and heart rate variability responses. American Journal of Obstetrics and Gynecology, 156(2), 323-327.

118. Wakai, R. T., Leuthold, A. C., & Martin, C. B. (May 1996). Fetal auditory evoked responses detected by magnetoencephalography. American Journal of Obstetrics and Gynecology, 174(5), 1484-1486.

119. Tongsong, T., & Piyamongkol, W. (January 1994). Comparison of the acoustic stimulation test with nonstress test. A randomized, controlled clinical trial. Journal of Reproductive Medicine, 39(1), 17-20.

120. Murphy, K. W., Hanretty, K. P., & Inglis, G. C. (December 1993). Fetal catecholamine responses to vibroacoustic stimulation. American Journal of Obstetrics and Gynecology, 169(6), 1571-1577.

121. Mariona, F., Kelly, R., Saltmarche, P., Nemec, S., Lipshaw, L., Lower, S., & Gajda, J. (January 1993). Long-term effects of fetal vibroacoustic stimulation on infant hearing. American Journal of Obstetrics and Gynecology, 168(1, Pt. 2), 337. SPO abstracts #136.

122. Strong, Jr., T. H., Gilpin, M. P., Jordan, D. L., & Sawai, S. K. (January 1993). Fetal acoustic stimulation does not identify nuchal cords. American Journal of Obstetrics and Gynecology, 168(1, Pt. 2), 337. SPO abstracts #135.

123. Freeman, R. K., Anderson, G., & Dorchester, W. (August 1, 1993). A prospective multi-institutional study of antepartum fetal heart rate monitoring. II. Contraction stress test versus nonstress test for primary surveillance. American Journal of Obstetrics and Gynecology, 143(7), 778-781.

124. Freeman, R. K., Garite, T. J., Mondanlou, H., Dorcester, W., Rommal, C., & Devaney, M. (May 15, 1981). Utilization of contraction stress testing for primary fetal surveillance. American Journal of Obstetrics and Gynecology, 140(2), 128-136.

125. Huddleston, J. F., Williams, G. S., & Fabbri, E. L. (1993). Chapter 5. Antepartum assessment of the fetus. In R. A. Knuppel, & J. E. Drukker (Eds.)(2nd ed., pp. 62-77), High-risk pregnancy. A team approach. Philadelphia, PA: WB Saunders Company.

126. Braly, P. S., Freeman, R. K., Garite, T. J., Anderson, G. G, & Dorchester, W. (September 1, 1981). Incidence of premature delivery following the oxytocin challenge test. American Journal of Obstetrics and Gynecology, 141(1), 5-8.

127. Evertson, L. R., Gauthier, R. J., & Collea, J. V. (June 1978). Fetal demise following negative contraction stress tests. Obstetrics & Gynecology, 51(6), 671-673.

128. Goodlin, R. C. (February 1, 1979). History of fetal monitoring. American Journal of Obstetrics and Gynecology, 133(3), 323-352.

129. Gants, M., Kirchhoff, K. T., & Work, Jr., B. A. (November/December 1985). Breast massage to obtain contraction stress test. Nursing Research, 34(6), 338-341.

130. Gegor, C. L., & Paine, L. L. (1992). Antepartum fetal assessment techniques: An update for today's perinatal nurse. Journal of Perinatal and Neonatal Nursing, 5(4), 1-15.

131. Moenning, R. K., & Hill, W. C. (July/August 1987). A randomized study comparing two methods of performing the breast stimulation stress test. JOGNN, 16(4), 253-257.

132. Lenke, R., & Nemes, J. (March 1984). Use of nipple stimulation to obtain contraction stress test. Obstetrics & Gynecology, 63(3), 345-348.

133. Finley, B. E., Amico, J., Castillo, M., & Seitchik, J.(June 1986). Oxytocin and prolactin responses associated with nipple stimulation contraction stress tests. Obstetrics & Gynecology, 67(6), 836-839.

134. Capeless, E. L., & Mann, L. I. (November 1984). Use of breast stimulation for antepartum stress testing. Obstetrics & Gynecology, 64(5), 641-645.

135. Murray, M. L., Harmon, J., & Canfield, S. (September/October 1986). Nipple stimulation-contraction stress test for the high-risk patient. MCN, 11(5), 331-333.

136. Oki, E. Y. (October 1983). A protocol for the nipple-stimulation test. Contemporary OB/GYN, 157-159.

137. Freeman, K., Anderson, G., & Dorchester, W. (August 1, 1982). A prospective multi-institutional study of antepartum fetal heart rate monitoring. I. Risk of perinatal mortality and morbidity according to antepartum fetal heart rate test results. <u>American Journal of Obstetrics and Gynecology, 143</u>(7), 771-777.

138. Druzin, M. L. (1992). Diabetes. In M. L. Druzin (Ed.), <u>Antepartum fetal assessment</u> (pp. 99-110). Boston, MA: Blackwell Scientific Publications.

139. Viegas, O. A., Arulkumaran, S., Gibb, D. M. F., & Ratnam, S. (April 1984). Nipple stimulation in late pregnancy, causing uterine hyperstimulation and profound fetal bradycardia. <u>British Journal of Obstetrics and Gynaecology, 91,</u> 364-366.

140. Viegas, O. A. C., Adaikan, P. G., Singh, K., Arulkumaran, S., Kettegoda, S. R., & Ratnam, S. S. (1986). Intrauterine responses to nipple stimulation in late pregnancy. <u>Gynecologic Obstetric Investigation, 22</u>(3), 128-133.

141. Mayberry, J. L., & Inturrisi-Levy, M. (March/April 1987). Use of breast stimulation for contraction stress tests. <u>JOGNN, 16</u>(2), 121-124.

142. Baskett, T. F., & Sandy, E. A. (September 1979). The oxytocin challenge test: An ominous pattern associated with severe fetal growth retardation. <u>Obstetrics & Gynecology, 54</u>(3), 365-366.

143. Freeman, R. K. (June 1982). Contraction stress testing for primary fetal surveillance in patients at high risk for uteroplacental insufficiency. <u>Clinical Perinatology, 9,</u> 265-270.

144. Slomka, C., & Phelan, J. P. (January 1, 1981). Pregnancy outcome in the patient with a nonreactive nonstress test and a positive contraction stress test. <u>American Journal of Obstetrics and Gynecology, 139</u>(1), 11-15.

145. Moore, T. R., & Piacquadio, K. (May 1989). A prospective evaluation of fetal movement screening to reduce the incidence of antepartum fetal death. <u>American Journal of Obstetrics and Gynecology, 160</u>(5, Pt. 1), 1075-1080.

Notes

10

Biophysical Fetal Assessment

INTRODUCTION

The goals of antepartal fetal surveillance are to prevent and reduce fetal and neonatal morbidity and mortality (1-2). To attain these goals, biophysical assessment by real-time ultrasound may be used for a complete or basic examination, a biophysical profile, a modified biophysical profile, or a limited ultrasound. This chapter presents the history of the biophysical profile, fetal physiology related to biophysical testing, ultrasound equipment, testing indications, biophysical test procedures, scoring criteria, test interpretation, and management based on test results.

History of The Biophysical Profile

Antepartal fetal surveillance in the 1970s used the electronic fetal monitor and included the nonstress test (NST), the fetal activity acceleration determination (FAD) test, and the contraction stress test (CST) or oxytocin challenge test (OCT). In the 1980s, the nipple-stimulation contraction stress test (NS-CST) was developed (3). With refinement of ultrasound technology, a new test was developed for antepartal fetal surveillance. In 1980, Dr. Frank Manning and his colleagues developed the biophysical profile (BPP), which is a NST plus an ultrasound evaluation of the fetus and amniotic fluid. Today, the NST is the most common antepartal surveillance test and is an integral part of the BPP and modified BPP (4-5).

The BPP score is based on five variables: the NST, fetal breathing movements, fetal body movements, fetal tone, and amniotic fluid volume (6). By using a systematic evaluation of the fetus, amniotic fluid volume, and even the placenta, it

was hoped that fetal compromise would be detected early enough to intervene and prevent fetal morbidity (7). In 1983, Dr. Anthony Vintzileos and his colleagues added placental grading to Manning's five variables (7-8). By 1985, the BPP was recognized as an important test of fetal status (6, 8-13). One variable, amniotic fluid volume (AFV), has been extensively investigated (14-23).

Perinatal nurses commonly perform antepartal fetal tests (24-25). The physician or nurse explains test indications to the woman. The nurse usually performs the NST, and many nurses now have the skills to perform the BPP or limited ultrasound examination (24, 26-27). The nurse and physician interpret test results then collaborate on a plan of care that may include ongoing fetal surveillance, labor induction, or delivery by cesarean section.

BIOPHYSICAL FETAL DEVELOPMENT

Development of fetal behavior and organs is predictable and correlates with central nervous system (CNS) development (7, 28). The BPP evaluates *acute and chronic* developmental markers to indirectly evaluate fetal CNS function and oxygenation. Acute markers include the NST, fetal breathing movements, body movements, and tone. Amniotic fluid is assessed as a chronic hypoxia marker (12).

The fetus develops muscle tone, then moves, then develops breathing movements. As early as 7.5 weeks of gestation, muscle tone develops. Fetal movement occurs near 8 weeks of gestation (7). By 10 to 12 weeks of gestation, fetal movement can be detected by real-time ultrasound (29). By 13 to 14 weeks of gestation, there is evidence of expansion and retraction of the thorax and abdomen. By 20 to 21 weeks, the diaphragm contracts and regular fetal breathing movements may be observed (8). By 30 weeks of gestation, the fetal nervous system has matured, and FHR accelerations commonly occur during fetal movements (28, 30).

Table 1: The Progression of Fetal Biophysical Development (modified from Johnson, T. R. B., & Besinger, R. (1989). New clues to fetal behavior. *Contemporary OB/GYN*).

Behavior	Gestational Age (Weeks)
tone, slight movement	7
general movement	8
hiccups	9
limb movements	10
hand to face contact	10
respiratory movements	11
sucking/swallowing	13

Fetuses have a predictable compensatory response to hypoxia (31). Figure 10.1 illustrates the progressive effects of acute fetal hypoxia on biophysical markers and the chronic effects of redistribution of blood, i.e., intrauterine growth restriction (IUGR) and oligohydramnios (32).

Hypoxia → redistribution of cardiac output → increased
▼   blood flow to brain,
                                           heart, adrenal glands,
                                           placenta
Acidosis   decreased blood flow
▼   to kidneys, lungs,
                                           gut, liver, body
Asphyxia   ▼
▼   Oligohydramnios
CNS cellular dysfunction
▼
Nonreactive NST
▼
Absent FBM
▼
Absent FM
▼
Absent tone

Figure 10.1: Fetal response to persistent hypoxia.

THE GRADUAL HYPOXIA CONCEPT

The BPP is based on the Gradual Hypoxia Concept. Depletion of fetal oxygen (O_2) affects brain centers in a specific order (33). Biophysical activities that develop first are the last to disappear (7-8, 12, 31, 34). Accelerations indicate an intact, functioning, nonhypoxic CNS (8, 31-32, 35-36). For example, a reactive FHR pattern and "adequate" AFV is

associated with a umbilical artery pH at or above 7.20 (8, 31, 35). Because a higher O_2 level is required for the fetal brain to regulate fetal breathing movements (FBM), fetal movement (FM), and tone, *the loss of accelerations is a sensitive and early sign of hypoxia*. A nonreactive NST may be the first indicator of fetal hypoxia.

As hypoxia persists, fetal behaviors "disappear" in reverse order of their development. After the loss of accelerations, FBM cease. As the fetus becomes acidotic, FM ceases. Finally, muscle tone disappears, i.e., *tone is the last to go*. When a fetus has no evidence of tone, i.e., the hand is open and limp, the fetus is invariably acidotic and a poor outcome is anticipated (31).

Oligohydramnios is a chronic hypoxia marker. Decreased renal blood flow decreases urine production. Decreased pulmonary blood flow reduces lung fluid production. Therefore, if amniotic fluid volume is normal, the fetus was not *chronically* hypoxic prior to testing, giving AFV long-term significance (7, 20, 37-38).

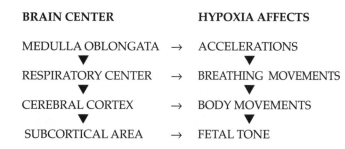

Figure 10.2: The Gradual Hypoxia Concept.

Hypoxemia is associated with a decrease in FBM. *Acidemia, acidosis, and asphyxia are* associated with reduced or absent gross body movements. *Sedatives, analgesics, and anesthetics* may temporarily abolish biophysical activities such as FM. Therefore, prior to the BPP the woman should be asked if she has taken any medications, smoked cigarettes, or ingested CNS depressants such as alcohol. Fetal brain damage secondary to blunt trauma, e.g., domestic violence, resulting in a fetal concussion may also abolish biophysical activities (11). Clearly, many of the same factors that affect the fetal heart rate (FHR) also affect fetal biophysical markers.

ULTRASOUND EQUIPMENT

Intrauterine contents are examined by a real-time ultrasound scanner with a 3.5 MHZ linear array, curved linear array, or sector scanner transducer. For example, a linear array real-time ultrasound scanner can be used to determine:

• fetal presentation and position or lie
• biparietal diameter and serial growth measurements
• FHR and cardiac motion
• placenta location and grade
• AFV

- FBM
- FM
- number of fetuses and
- major fetal organs.

An attached camera may be used to record findings. However, the most common, cost-effective method of image recordation is thermal paper from an attached printer. Printed images kept in a dark, cool environment should remain stable for 25 years. Images may be stored on x-ray film when the ultrasound is performed in the radiology department. Sometimes the BPP is videotaped so that another interpreter may see or clarify images. Storage of videotapes is costly, requires a great deal of space, and videotapes may be difficult to retrieve in the future.

Persons who use the ultrasound machine are responsible for its proper use. The transducer should be cleaned after use. Transducers are fragile. Just like the ultrasound transducer of the fetal monitor, they contain piezoelectric crystals which are easily cracked if the transducer is dropped. Intact crystals are necessary for a quality image. The transducer must always be returned to its proper receptacle on the machine and protected from damage. It is critical that the transducer's cord not be "run over" by the wheels of the machine as some transducer cords contain fragile fiberoptics.

BIOPHYSICAL TEST INDICATIONS

Maternal and fetal risk factors determine the need for a BPP, which is generally initiated at 28 weeks of gestation. If the fetus is IUGR, testing may begin even earlier. A single BPP test may precede and/or follow abdominal trauma, amniocentesis, external cephalic version, or maternal perception of decreased fetal movement. The BPP may also be done during preterm labor or daily following preterm premature rupture of the membranes (PPROM) to rule out infection. Common indications for BPP testing are a significant risk of fetal hypoxia or as follow-up testing for a nonreactive NST or positive CST. The most common indications for the BPP are:
- suspected IUGR
- pregnancy > 40 weeks
- insulin-dependent diabetes
- hypertension
- oligohydramnios
- multiple gestation and
- preterm rupture of the membranes (2, 8, 12, 31-32, 34, 36).

For women at moderate risk for poor perinatal outcomes, weekly BPP assessment beginning at 34 to 36 weeks of gestation is appropriate, e.g., a woman with well-controlled gestational diabetes, well-grown twins, or a history of previous fetal loss.

Duration of the Test
The ultrasound scan is completed within a maximum of 30 minutes. The average length of time for a BPP is 10 minutes (24, 39). Testing time may be affected by the fetal behavioral state, e.g., a fetus who is quiescent may require a longer test time.

Preparation Prior to the Ultrasound Examination
Many practitioners prefer to perform the BPP two hours after a meal with the woman in a semi-Fowler's position and uterine displacement, e.g., a wedge is placed under the right hip (40). Others prefer the woman to sit in an adjustable lounge chair in a semi-recumbent position. Women are instructed to remain sedentary at least one hour prior to the exam and to not smoke for at least 2 hours prior to the exam. They are encouraged to arrive for testing well hydrated. Blood pressure (BP) may be assessed at the initiation of the test, and every 10 minutes during the testing period (13). The woman is asked to remain sedentary prior to the test to promote uterine perfusion. Temporary cessation of smoking should minimize the risk of fetal CNS depression and FBM reduction (41). Assessment of maternal BP documents the lack of hypotension (13).

The NST is usually done prior to the ultrasound examination. After the NST and prior to the ultrasound, women will be asked to drink enough fluid to fill their bladder. As in all procedures, privacy should be maintained and attention to maternal comfort should be provided.

TEST SCORE CRITERIA
The BPP reflects fetal status at the time of the test. If there is a reactive NST, and FBM, FM, and tone are present, it is reasonable to deduce that the CNS is well-oxygenated and functioning normally *at that time* (12). The Manning criteria is the most widely used. Each variable may receive 0 or 2 points, for a total score of 10 (6) (See Table 2).

Table 2: Manning Criteria for the Biophysical Profile Score (36)

The maximal time for the ultrasound is 30 minutes.

Variable	Criteria Score: 2	Criteria Score: 0
NST	2 accelerations 15 bpm x 15 seconds within 20 minutes	Nonreactive NST
Fetal Breathing	30 seconds of continuous FBM	Less than 30 seconds of FBM or absence of FBM (apnea)
Fetal Movement	3 or more gross FM including rolling movement(s)	0 to 2 episodes of FM
Fetal Tone	1 episode of flexion/extension of the fetal spine, limbs, hand or fetal sucking	No evidence of tone
Amniotic Fluid Volume (AFV)	At least 1 cord-free fluid pocket > 2 cms in the vertical diameter	Oligohydramnios (< 2 cm vertical measurement)

If the placenta is graded, a different scoring system is used for the BPP. By adding placental grade, the total possible score is 12 (8).

Table 3: Vintzileos Criteria for Biophysical Profile Scoring (8)

Criteria	Score 2:	Score 1:	Score 0:
NST	5 or more FHR accelerations of at least 15 bpm amplitude and 15 sec. duration during a 20 minute period	2 to 4 FHR accelerations at least 15 bpm amplitude and 15 sec. duration during a 20 min. period	1 or fewer FHR accelerations during a 20 min. period
Fetal Breathing	At least one episode of fetal breathing of at least 60 seconds duration within 30 minutes of observation	At least one episode of fetal breathing lasting 30 to 60 sec. duration within 30 minutes	Absence of fetal breathing or less than 30 second duration within 30 minutes
Fetal Movement	At least 3 episodes of gross (trunk and limbs) FM within 30 minutes. Simultaneous limb and trunk movements are counted as one movement	1 or 2 FM within 30 minutes	Absence of FM within 30 minutes
Fetal Tone	1 episode of extension of extremities with return to flexion, and one episode of extension of spine with return to flexion	At least one episode of extension with return to flexion, or one episode of extension of spine with return to flexion	Extremities in extension. Fetal movements not followed by return to flexion. Opened hand

Criteria	Score 2:	Score 1:	Score 0:
Amniotic Fluid Volume (AFV)	Fluid evident throughout the uterine cavity. A pocket that measures 2 cm or greater in the vertical dimension	A pocket that measures less than 2 cm but more than 1 cm in the vertical dimension	Crowding of small parts. Largest pocket less than 1 cm in vertical dimension
Placental Grade	Placental Grade 0, I, II	Posterior placenta, difficult to grade	Placental Grade III

Fetal Breathing Movements (FBM)

Fetal breathing movements are observed as paradoxical, see-saw movements of the fetal chest and abdomen about the xiphoid (40). On close inspection, and with appropriate ultrasound images, fetal diaphragmatic movement can be seen as well as movement of fetal lung tissue. It is important that the movement seen is actually fetal breathing and is not confused with rhythmic uterine movement due to maternal respirations.

Dr. Geoffrey Dawes (42) was the first physician to record FBM in fetal lambs and humans using the ultrasound. FBM were rapid, irregular, and episodic, particularly during rapid eye movement (REM) sleep (42). FBM episodes are present only 10% of the time at 15 to 19 weeks of gestation and increase in frequency throughout pregnancy. Near term, FBM occurs up to 85% of the time and is more easily visualized (28).

The rate of FBMs in lambs is 60 to 70 per minute (42). In another study, FBM occurred an average of 55 times per minute (43). Fetal tachypnea has been defined as FBM greater than 60 per minute. The incidence of tachypnea in one study was 9% and was *not* associated with fetal compromise (44). Fetal apnea was defined as the absence of FBM for more than 6 seconds (40). The absence of FBM for less than 6 seconds may be included as part of the 30 second evaluation of continuous fetal breathing. Fetal

hiccoughs are considered a normal variant of fetal breathing, and may also be included in the 30 second evaluative period (45).

Episodes of FBM have lasted for 30 seconds or as long as 20 minutes (46). FBM may start and stop spontaneously, especially during nonREM sleep. FBM may be absent up to 108 minutes (36). Usually, the absence of FBM is explained by the behavioral state of the fetus, i.e., the fetus may remain in a 1F, quiescent state for as long as 100 minutes (47).

FBM alone is a poor predictor of outcome. However, fetal hypoxia was related to fetal apnea. Of five women with apneic fetuses, who were delivered within 24 hours, one newborn had low Apgar scores, acidosis, and thick meconium, two had meconium aspiration syndrome, and two were IUGR. Fetal gasping occurred several hours before fetal death (46). In lambs, fetuses died within several days after fetal apnea was detected. Lambs had a terminal episode of gasping and rapid, irregular breathing movements (42).

Fetal Body Movements

The presence of FM is important because it rapidly diminishes or stops 12 to 48 hours before fetal death (48). Fetal movement (FM) is observed as

- the rotation or displacement of the fetal trunk from its initial position (40)

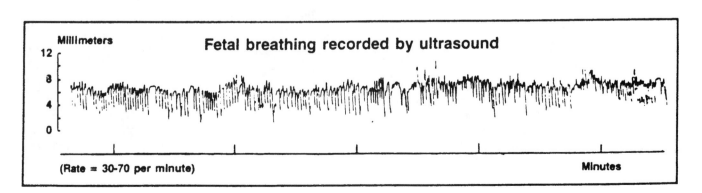

Figure 10.3: Fetal breathing movements from studying breathing movements for clues to fetal health. (42) (Reproduced with permission of Contemporary OB/GYN).

- strong and brisk movement of the whole body (7, 31)
- slow sluggish movements of fetal extremities (7, 31)
- stretching movements and
- rolling movements.

Fetal movement is usually assessed as flexion and extension of an extremity, the whole body, or rolling movements. *When fetal movement is present, fetal tone is also present, as one cannot have purposeful movement without muscle tone.*

Fetal Tone

Fetal tone is the presence of flexion and extension movements (40). Flexion and extension may involve the body, arms, legs, or hands. Tone is evaluated by observing fetal posture, flexion, and extension of the limbs, hand, or spine. An easy way to observe tone is to place the ultrasound transducer over the fetal neck. Even a sleeping or mildly hypoxic fetus should flex its spine. Other observations which can be interpreted as tone include opening or closing of the hand, finger motion, a clenched fist, swallowing, or sucking movements, or thumb sucking (8, 12, 36).

Amniotic Fluid Volume (AFV)

AFV increases as the fetus matures until the 28th week of gestation. At that point, AFV stabilizes until nearly 36 weeks. From 36 to 40 weeks, AFV declines approximately 10% each week. After 40 weeks, there is a dramatic drop in AFV of about 30% per week (14-15). It is important to assess the AFV frequently in a fetus who is suspected to be hypoxic. Just like FM, the AFV can change precipitously within 24 to 48 hours.

Some ultrasonographers make an "eyeball guesstimate" of AFV, i.e., "amniotic fluid appears adequate." A more precise assessment of AFV requires evaluation of each uterine quadrant for the largest cord-free pocket. Its vertical diameter is measured and two points are given if it is 2 or more centimeters (cm) in diameter (20, 45, 49-50). Measurement of the depth of the single largest pocket of fluid correlates well with the actual AFV (21, 23).

This single pocket method can be used to identify oligohydramnios (1, 11-12, 45). Oligohydramnios is diagnosed when there is no fluid pocket measuring 2 or more cm. A pocket greater than 8 cm has been considered polyhydramnios (50).

There is an inverse relationship between the AFV (using a single pocket) and the incidence of a nonreactive NST and decelerations (17). As the size of the pocket decreased, the number of nonreactive NSTs and decelerations increased. This makes sense when one considers how vulnerable the umbilical cord becomes when there is decreased amniotic fluid. A disadvantage of the single pocket measurement is that it does not allow serial AFV evaluation of oligohydramnios, polyhydramnios or comparison of changing quantities of amniotic fluid over time.

Oligohydramnios and polyhydramnios, are associated with poor pregnancy outcomes (7-8, 20, 35, 37-38, 50). Oligohydramnios may indicate chronic uteroplacental insufficiency or a renal anomaly such as agenesis (Potter's syndrome) (36). Postterm and IUGR fetuses with a major congenital anomaly, such as renal agenesis, had a greater incidence of oligohydramnios than a sample of dysmature fetuses with no congenital defects. Perinatal mortality ranged from 4.65/1000 with normal AFV to as high as 187.5/1000 in fetuses with decreased AFV. There were significantly more newborns with congenital anomalies in the group with the higher perinatal mortality rate (37).

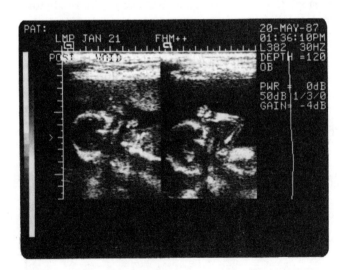

Figure 10.4: Closed fetal hand (fetal tone). (Photograph courtesy of Lovelace Medical Center, Albuquerque, NM).

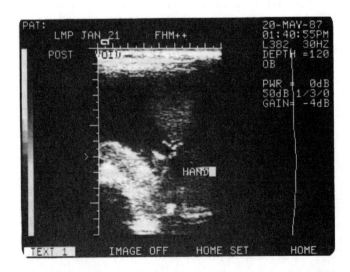

Figure 10.5: Open fetal hand (fetal tone). (Photograph courtesy of Lovelace Medical Center, Albuquerque, NM).

Polyhydramnios is also related to poor perinatal outcome. In a study of 7,562 patients, the perinatal mortality rate was 4.65/1000 when there was normal AFV, but 32.9/1000 in those with polyhydramnios. The rate of congenital defects in the presence of oligohydramnios or polyhydramnios has been reported to be as high as 20% (32). Polyhydramnios was associated with macrosomia, upper gastrointestinal tract obstructions, malformations such as a tracheoesophageal fistula, and hydrops fetalis.

Effect of maternal hydration on AFV. The physiology of the normal decline in AFV is not clear. However, maternal hydration with 1000 ml or more may increase the AFV (22, 51). Conversely, AFV may be decreased when oral fluids are limited (51). The risk of a false positive result, i.e., you observe what you believe to be oligohydramnios but the woman is severely dehydrated, should be avoided if the women reports for testing in a well-hydrated state.

AFV measurement with twins. AFV of each diamniotic twin is very similar to the amount of fluid of a singleton pregnancy (52). The sac separation between the fetuses is identified then the single deepest pocket of fluid which is clearly identifiable as "belonging" to each twin is measured. With monochorionic twins, the single deepest pocket technique or the four quadrant amniotic fluid index (AFI) may be used with serial comparison over the course of the pregnancy.

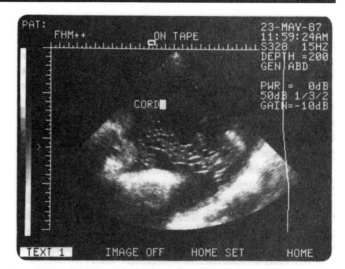

Figure 10.7: Umbilical cord floating in pocket of amniotic fluid. (Photography courtesy of Lovelace Medical Center, Albuquerque, NM).

Placental Grade

The placenta is a fetal organ (53). It matures with other fetal organs and is readily imaged by the 12th to 14th week of pregnancy. It is believed that placentas mature in a predictable way during uncomplicated pregnancies. Immature placentas change their appearance until they look like term placentas (54). Some believed there was a relationship between placental grade and fetal lung maturity and that placental grading would be helpful in evaluating fetal lung maturation prior to preterm birth (53). However, lung maturity is best assessed by analysis of amniotic fluid. Some believe placentas mature faster when women are preeclamptic or the fetus is IUGR (55).

The placental grade is determined after evaluating the ultrasound image of the basal plate (maternal side of the placenta), the chorionic plate (fetal side of the placenta), and the organ substance (See Figure 10.8) (53). As the placenta matures, it becomes grainier, cotyledons become more defined, and the basal plate becomes more heavily calcified. Near term, further changes may be found in the placenta, including calcifications, increasing engorgement of intervillous spaces with maternal blood (venous lakes), and cystic-like changes within the cotyledons secondary to thrombosis (55).

A grade III placenta demonstrates distinct definition of each cotyledon, which may also have a darkened central area of ultrasound "fallout," thought to represent an infarcted area. In 1982, Platt and Petrucha found 95% of all grade III placentas were found in pregnancies beyond 35 weeks of gestation (56). In later research, where a grade III placenta existed *prior to* 35 weeks of gestation, the fetus was found to be IUGR (57). Table 4 summarizes ultrasound evaluation of the placenta, and the relationship between placental grade and fetal lung maturity.

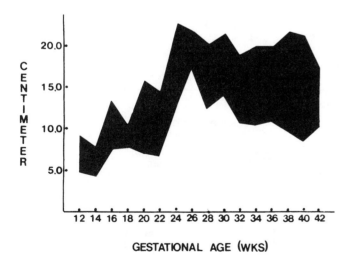

Figure 10.6: Amniotic fluid decline between 12 and 42 weeks' gestation. (Reproduced with permission of Phelan, J. P., Ahn, M. O., Rutherford, S. E., Smith, C. V., & Anderson, E. A. (1987). Amniotic fluid index measurements during pregnancy. *Journal of Reproductive Medicine, 32*(8), 601-604).

Table 4: Placental Grade and Fetal Maturity

GRADE	PLACENTA TEXTURE	LUNG MATURITY	CHARACTERISTICS
0	Smooth chorionic plate	no statistic available	Found prior to 28 weeks
I	Subtle indentations of chorionic plate, echogenic areas which are randomly dispersed	68%	First seen at 14 weeks gestation (56) Expect by 31.5 weeks and 40% of term fetuses (53) Found at 27-36 weeks (55)
II	Basal echogenic densities and comma-like densities	88%	First seen at 26 weeks Expect by 36.6 weeks (53, 56) 45% of term fetuses (53) Found at 28-36 weeks (55)
III	Indentations of chorionic plate, echospared or fallout areas and irregular densities	100%	First seen at 30-31 weeks (55-56) Expect by 38 weeks 15% of term fetuses (53)

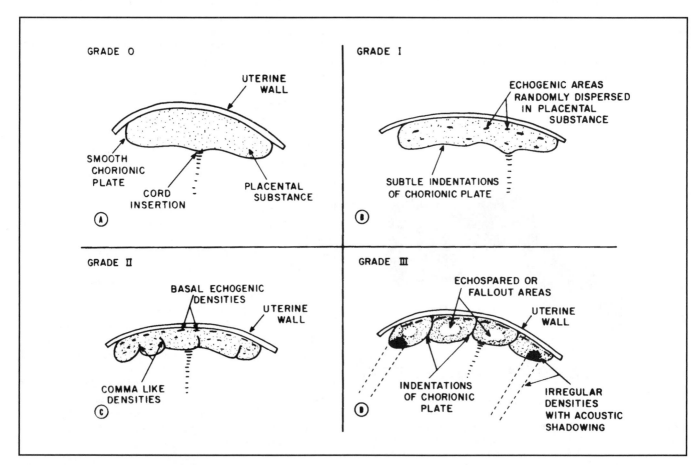

Figure 10.8: Placental maturation changes (53) (Reproduced with permission of the C.V. Mosby Company).

ANTEPARTAL AND INTRAPARTAL FETAL MONITORING

Data is limited on the correlation between fetal lung maturity and placental grade, therefore, this table should be cautiously interpreted. An association between a grade III placenta, an increase in abnormal intrapartal FHR patterns, and placental abruption was reported in 1983 (8). However, a cause and effect relationship between a grade III placenta and later complications of the fetus or placenta has not been proven. For this reason, the placental grade, in and of itself, is not useful in predicting perinatal outcome or in decision-making regarding the time or route of delivery.

BPP INTERPRETATION AND MANAGEMENT GUIDELINES

BPP scores, fetal acid-base status, and perinatal outcome are related. Adequate AFV and a BPP score of 8 or 10 out of 10 was 100% predictive of an umbilical cord artery pH above 7.20. When the BPP score was 4 or 2, the predictive value of a pH less than 7.20 was 69%. When the BPP scores was 0, all fetuses had an umbilical artery pH less than 7.20 (31).

Therefore, if the BPP score is 8 or 10 (out of a possible 10), the woman is discharged and the BPP is usually repeated in 7 days. The BPP may be repeated in less than 7 days if there is a sudden change in the woman's status, if there is a nonreactive NST, or if she perceives a marked decrease in FM.

Individual clinical situations must be carefully evaluated with

a score of 6 out of 10. A BPP scores of 6 out of 10 is *equivocal*. The BPP should be repeated and evaluated by a skilled physician. Platt and his colleagues (13) suggested that if the BPP score was 6 in the morning, the BPP should be repeated that evening. Since BPP scoring is subjective, it might be wise to have another skilled person perform a BPP soon after a score of 6 was obtained.

A BPP score of 4, 2, or 0 suggests fetal acidemia and possibly acidosis and asphyxia. A fetus who is anemic with a sinusoidal pattern may have a score of 2 for AFV only. The severely anemic fetus appears limp. Vintzileos and his colleagues (8) found the incidence of "fetal distress" in labor was 100% when the BPP score was 4 or less using a 12 point scale. Using a 10 point scale, women with a BPP score of 4, 2, or 0 should be admitted to labor and delivery for induction or cesarean section. The route and timing of delivery will depend on the criteria that received zero points. There is a tremendous difference in a BPP score of 8 in a 30 week fetus with a nonreactive NST, and a term fetus with oligohydramnios. Delivery decisions will also be influenced by the FHR pattern following the BPP, the fetus' gestational age, and fetal lung maturity. Table 5 summarizes management guidelines based on a BPP scoring system with a possible 10 points. The perinatal mortality rate within one week of the test is identified for each possible score.

Table 5: Obstetrical Management Based on Biophysical Profile Results With a Maximum of 10 Points (modified from 36)

BPP Score	Assessment	PMR*	Management
8 or 10 normal AFV	Low risk for perinatal asphyxia	<1/1000	• Repeat BPP in 7 days • If high risk for hypoxia: biweekly NST • If postdates, biweekly BPP
8 and abnormal AFV	High risk for perinatal asphyxia	89/1000	• Consider delivery for fetal indications
6 with normal AFV	Equivocal	variable	• If fetus is mature, deliver • If immature, repeat BPP within 24 hours or less
6 with abnormal AFV (and membranes are intact and fetal kidneys are normal)	High risk for perinatal asphyxia	89/1000	• If fetus mature, deliver • If immature, constant observation • Repeat BPP within 24 hours
4	High risk for perinatal asphyxia management	91/1000	• Deliver
2	Perinatal asphyxia almost certain	125/1000	• Deliver
0	Perinatal asphyxia Certain	600/1000	• Delivery recommended • Consult or refer for medical management

* PMR = Perinatal Mortality

The BPP and the Preterm Fetus

A normoxic immature fetus (less than 24 weeks) with a nonreactive NST should attain a score of 8 out of 10 on a BPP. In these immature fetuses, the NST was considered to be "normal" if there was long-term variability and FM was coupled with an acceleration of 5 beats per minute or more above the baseline (31). If decelerations, a positive CST, or a nonreactive NST, preceded a BPP score of 8, *the woman should not be discharged and the fetus should be closely observed with daily BPPs.* When 29 fetuses at less than 32 weeks of gestation with a nonreactive, positive CST were evaluated with continuous fetal monitoring and a daily BPP, there was an average gain of 13.5 days in utero and an increased neonatal survival rate (58).

The BPP and Multiple Gestation

The primary causes of adverse outcome of twins are prematurity and complications related to IUGR (59). Antepartal assessment of fetal well-being is essential during pregnancies with multiple fetuses (59-60). Twins, who are growing normally, are at low risk for hypoxia. Therefore, they may have weekly BPPs beginning at 34 to 36 weeks of gestation. If an ultrasound examination reveals that one or both twins is lagging in size or if oligohydramnios develops, then the pregnancy becomes very high risk, and biweekly BPPs are needed.

Higher order multiples, e.g., triplets and beyond, are at very high risk for poor perinatal outcomes (61). Women often develop preterm labor, hypertension, or gestational diabetes. The fetuses are at risk for IUGR (60). These pregnancies present a fetal monitoring challenge. It is very difficult to find more than two fetuses using an external ultrasound transducer. The potential exists to obtain heart rate information on only two fetuses, missing the third or fourth fetus. In addition, it may take several hours to obtain NST and BPP information on each fetus, which may frustrate the woman and health care providers.

Elliott and Finberg evaluated triplets and quadruplets with a BPP without the NST. The BPP score of 6 or 8 out of 8 was considered normal, 4 out of 8 was equivocal, and 2 or 0 was abnormal. Of the 18 sets of triplets and 6 sets of quadruplets, none were stillborn. Twenty-five percent of the women were delivered for abnormal BPP scores and had good neonatal outcomes (60). The BPP without the NST was found to be a reliable antepartum test of well-being for these higher order multiples (60-61).

Preterm Premature Rupture of the Membranes (PPROM)

Rupture of the amniotic sac does not alter the BPP score of the healthy fetus (62). In fact, the fetal BPP should be 8 or 10 out of 10 between 25 to 44 weeks of gestation (63-64). *Therefore, if there is decreased FM or an absence of FBM, there may be an intraamniotic infection in women who have had PPROM* (62, 65-66). Vintzileos speculated that the causes of decreased or absent FBM may be a reduction in the size of the intrauterine cavity which compresses the thorax. Another possible

cause of decreased FBM may be the effect of prostaglandins released with the rupture of the membranes.

BPP results increase the suspicion of an intrauterine infection (62, 64, 66-67). A BPP score of 7 out of 12 was a good predictor of impending fetal infection in women who had premature rupture of the membranes (62, 67). Dr. Vintzileos and his colleagues (63, 68) used daily BPP testing to predict a developing intrauterine infection in women with PPROM. *The infection rate was 93.75% when the BPP score was 7 or less out of a possible 12 points.* A BPP score of 8 or more out of 12 was associated with a 2.7% infection rate. Several authors have identified a significant decrease in FM and decreased or absent FBM when there was an intraamniotic infection (65-66). The reduction in FM and FBM may be related to the reduction in AFV. Others have found no relationship between decreased FM, FBM, and chorioamnionitis following PPROM (69).

A persistently "low" BPP score with a nonreactive NST and absent FBM was highly predictive of fetal infection. As the infectious process progresses, FBM usually decrease. *Therefore, the presence of FBM strongly predicts the absence of fetal infection.* In fact, when FBM were present within 24 hours prior to delivery, there were no cases of fetal infection. Loss of FM or tone were late signs of infection (62).

THE MODIFIED BIOPHYSICAL PROFILE

The combination of a NST and AFV is referred to as a modified BPP. The modified BPP has the same predictive value as the full BPP when the NST is reactive and the AFV is adequate (36). It is reasonable to assume that a reactive NST is accompanied by FM and tone, especially if FM is palpated during the NST. Therefore, the points that would be given had a full BPP when done would be 6: 2 points for a reactive NST, 2 for FM, and 2 for tone. With the addition of adequate AFV, the score becomes 8. The modified BPP has a perinatal mortality rate of 1.86/1000 when the NST is reactive and AFV is adequate. Biweekly modified BPP testing is suggested for high-risk women (5).

If the NST is nonreactive *or* if the AFV is less than 2 cms, a full BPP must be completed to adequately predict the potential for perinatal asphyxia. In a comparison of the BPP and the CST, both tests were found to have the same ability to predict poor perinatal outcomes, but the CST was associated with a higher rate of operative intervention without an improved outcome (5).

The modified BPP has become very popular as a screening test. It has the advantage of saving time and money, it is easy to perform, it predicts fetal well-being as well as the BPP, and a lower false positive rate than the CST. In other words, the modified BPP has fewer false predictions of a "sick" baby than the CST.

The modified BPP may be used as an admission test to labor and delivery or for weekly or biweekly fetal evaluation (4-5). The individual performing the modified BPP must also have the skills to complete a limited ultrasound scan. When a modified BPP is performed, it is necessary to document the number of fetuses, fetal position, and placental location.

THE AMNIOTIC FLUID INDEX

When serial AFV measurements are desired, a more extensive evaluation of fluid may be desired. Therefore, an amniotic fluid index (AFI) will be obtained. The AFI is performed with the woman supine with uterine displacement to the left (left tilt). The maternal abdomen is visualized as quadrants, using the midline and the umbilicus as landmarks. The transducer is placed in the longitudinal axis, parallel to the maternal midline and directed perpendicular to the floor. The largest pocket of fluid in each quadrant is identified and measured in its vertical dimension. When each measurement is complete, the four values are added together to create the AFI (14-15, 17-19). (Figure 10.9 illustrates fluid pockets measured for the AFI.). The AFI strongly correlated with actual AFV when there were normal amounts of fluid (15, 21).

An advantage of the AFI over the single pocket technique is that the AFI can be followed over time. For example, if an insulin-dependent diabetic has had an AFI of 14 cms for several weeks, and then has a drop to 8 cms in 4 days, this would suggest fetal hypoxia, even though the AFI is still within the normal range.

When the AFI drops, maternal hydration should be investigated. A BPP may be obtained and repeated biweekly. The woman may be encouraged to keep a record of kick counts. The physician may counsel the woman regarding the timing of delivery, e.g., the woman may be scheduled for induction in the near future.

AFI Technique

To increase visualization of each pocket of amniotic fluid, it may be helpful to:

- observe areas near the fetal neck, extremities, or fundus
- be certain that the area being measured is entirely fluid
- carefully evaluate each fluid pocket by angling the transducer in several directions.

It is important to:

- not measure fluid pockets which contain coils of the umbilical cord
- consider FM, as it slightly changes the measurement of the AFI (69)
- accomplish the AFI within a brief period of time to minimize the effect of FM on the total AFI.

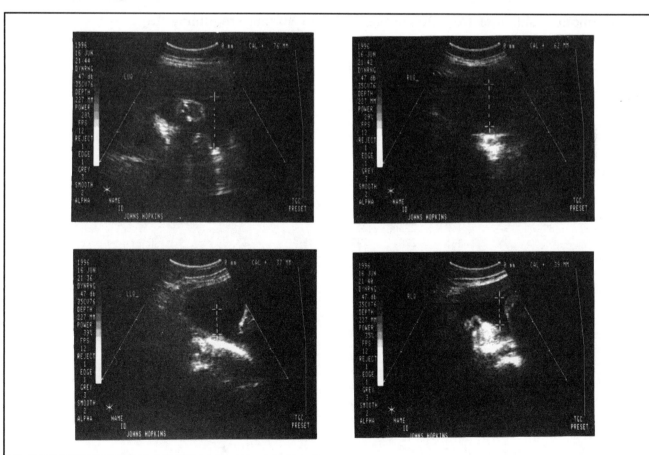

Figure 10.9: Ultasound images of the four quadrant measurements for the Amniotic Fluid Index. Note the absence of the umbilical cord within the measured pockets and the determination of the vertical diameter of each pocket. (Ultrasound images courtesy of C. Gegor, CNM, RDMS, Johns Hopkins University, Baltimore, MD).

It may be necessary to:

- measure a pocket of fluid above or below the cord
- measure fluid that is seen, i.e., at term it is common for the fetus to occupy large amounts of space so that no fluid is seen in one or two quadrants.

Oligohydramnios and Polyhydramnios

At term, the AFI is usually between 8 and 18 cm. AFI values of less than 8 cms have been classified as oligohydramnios, and more than 18 cms has been classified as polyhydramnios (14-15, 19). Oligohydramnios, with an AFI less than 5 cm, was related to meconium staining, cesarean delivery, and Apgar scores less than 7 at 1 and 5 minutes (19).

In women at term with an AFI greater than 8 cms, the incidence of oligohydramnios was 2.3% within 4 days and 2.2% within 1 week of the test. For women with an AFI between 5 and 8 cm, there was a 16.2% risk for oligohydramnios within 4 days of the test, and 16.3% risk within 1 week. Therefore, if the AFI is less than 8 cm, a biweekly AFI has been recommended (71).

When pregnancy lasted 41 weeks or more, women with an AFI greater than 8 cms had a 7.4% chance of developing oligohydramnios within 4 days. If the AFI was 5 to 8 cms, the incidence of oligohydramnios within 4 days was 17.8%. Ideally, women at greater than 41 weeks of gestation should have a biweekly AFI until delivery (71).

There are three methods that have been used to measure AFV using the ultrasound: the single largest vertical pocket, a two-diameter pocket (the vertical and horizontal diameters are multiplied), and the AFI (21). All three strongly correlate with normal amounts of amniotic fluid collected prior to the birth of a fetus being delivered by an elective cesarean section. The AFI was superior to the single pocket measurement in the prediction of both normal and decreased AFV (17). However, the two-diameter measurement had a greater predictive value for identification of *oligohydramnios* than the AFI (23).

AFI nomograms for gestational have been developed for use during the second and third trimesters (See Table 6). Since the AFI changes during pregnancy, age-specific values are more useful than the simplistic and widely varying

Table 6: Amniotic Fluid Index (AFI) Percentile Values in Normal Pregnancy (18)

Week of Gestation	Percentile Values					Number of Women (n)
	2.5th	5th	50th	95th	97.5th	
16	73	79	121	185	201	32
17	77	83	127	194	211	26
18	80	87	133	202	220	17
19	83	90	137	207	225	14
20	86	93	141	212	230	25
21	88	95	143	214	233	14
22	89	97	145	216	235	14
23	90	98	146	218	237	14
24	90	98	147	219	238	23
25	89	97	147	221	240	12
26	89	97	147	223	242	11
27	85	95	146	226	245	17
28	86	94	146	228	249	25
29	84	92	145	231	254	12
30	82	90	145	234	258	17
31	79	88	144	238	263	26
32	77	86	144	242	269	25
33	74	83	143	245	274	30
34	72	81	142	248	278	31
35	70	79	140	249	279	27
36	68	77	138	249	279	39
37	66	75	135	244	275	36
38	65	73	132	239	269	27
39	64	72	127	226	255	12
40	63	71	123	214	240	64
41	63	70	116	194	216	162
42	63	69	110	175	192	30

values of less than 8 cms for oligohydramnios and greater than 18 cms for polyhydramnios. Many believe gestation specific AFI norms offer the most efficient identification of abnormal volumes (17-18). *AFI values that fall below the 2.5th percentile or above the 97.5th percentile are considered to be outside the normal range.*

The Modified BPP and Postterm Pregnancy

Postterm pregnancy is a pregnancy that has lasted more than 42 weeks since the last menstrual period. The ideal management of the uncomplicated pregnancy lasting 41 or more weeks varies based on the woman and fetus' status. It is known that after 41 weeks, there is a greater incidence of meconium, FHR abnormalities, neonatal resuscitation, low 5-minute Apgar scores, and cesarean sections (72). Two approaches to management of the postdate pregnancy include labor induction at 41 weeks of gestation or expectant management, i.e., wait and watch. Labor induction and expectant management, which included biweekly NSTs and amniotic fluid evaluation, produced similar perinatal morbidity, birth weight, and operative delivery statistics (64, 73-74). A rapid decline in the AFV is anticipated after 40 weeks of gestation (5, 15-17, 20-21, 37). The risk of oligohydramnios increases (37). Therefore, AFV should be evaluated twice a week in the postdates woman (37, 72, 74-75). *When oligohydramnios is identified, delivery of the fetus has been recommended* (12, 16-17, 37, 74).

LIMITED THIRD TRIMESTER ULTRASOUND FOR PERINATAL NURSES

The necessity for rapid, on site evaluation of fetal status created a need for a *limited* ultrasound examination. In 1991, the American College of Obstetricians and Gynecologists (ACOG) identified indications for limited, "bedside" ultrasound use:

- antepartal hemorrhage
- determination of fetal lie
- determination of fetal cardiac activity
- determination of fetal number
- guidance for amniocentesis
- guidance for external cephalic version
- guidance for delivery of the second twin
- assessment of fetal well-being
- AFV assessment (76).

The 1991 ACOG committee opinion has been supported by the 1993 ACOG Technical Bulletin, the American Institute of Ultrasound in Medicine, and the American College of Nurse-Midwives (76-79). Prior to publication of the ACOG guidelines, it had been strongly asserted by some ultrasound professionals that each time a scan was performed, a complete or basic scan was required. They were concerned that by looking only for specific data, critical information would be missed. For example, it is unacceptable to determine fetal position by "finding the head," but miss twins, a placenta previa, or a fetal demise. Therefore, a limited scan is

appropriate for women who have had a basic or targeted ultrasound examination during their second or third trimester. If a limited study is performed in an emergency situation, a follow-up basic ultrasound examination should be scheduled if delivery does not occur (76).

Criteria for Limited Ultrasound Examination

To bridge the gap between the comprehensive basic ultrasound examination and the need for specific data, minimal criteria for a limited ultrasound examination must be standardized. Limited scanning primarily assesses fetal wellbeing, often at a time when there is an emergency situation. For example, a woman presents in labor with an uncertain fetal lie, a large amount of vaginal bleeding, and a nonreassuring fetal heart rate pattern. A limited ultrasound may clarify the fetal lie, source of vaginal bleeding, and fetal oxygenation status. A growing number of nurses, nurse-midwives, and nurse practitioners have the skills to perform a BPP, AFI, and limited ultrasound examination.

Nurses who have the appropriate knowledge and skills may perform limited ultrasound studies in the clinic, office or labor and delivery suite (24, 27, 39, 49). Requirements for nurses who perform limited ultrasounds have been recommended by ACOG and the Association of Women's Health, Obstetric and Neonatal Nurses (AWHONN) (25, 76). AWHONN guidelines established the *minimum* criteria for a limited ultrasound examination and detailed knowledge and skill requirements. When nurses have a standardized course of study and develop clinical skills, their performance and interpretation of the BPP, modified BPP, and limited ultrasound examination should be consistent with physicians. Nurses who perform a limited ultrasound may identify:

- the number of fetuses
- their cardiac activity
- their lie or position
- FBM
- FM
- tone
- AFV and
- placental location (25).

Prior to implementation of limited ultrasound scanning by nurses, the following should be exist:

- written policies and procedures, including indications for limited ultrasound by the nurse
- documentation of completed course work and skills validation.

Limited ultrasound is an adjunct to, and never a replacement for, a complete ultrasound examination (25). Ultrasonographers are concerned that the AWHONN guidelines may limit ultrasound information and precede poor decisions. Therefore, only nurses with the educational preparation and skill to collect information on the variables recommended by AWHONN should attempt a limited ultrasound examination. A woman who has had sequential BPP studies should have had a basic or comprehensive scan prior to a limited ultrasound. *This places the responsibility for identification of anomalies and gestational age on the sonographer and/or sonologist* who performed and interpreted the original study. It is critical that those who perform obstetrical ultrasound scans on a limited basis have access to a practitioner who is qualified to perform a complete ultrasound study.

COMPARISON OF ANTEPARTAL TESTS

Many physicians used to prefer the CST as a primary fetal surveillance test, but they now prefer the NST, BPP or modified BPP because they are not invasive and are less time consuming. *The NST and the BPP are equally poor predictors of poor outcomes but good predictors of good outcomes* (13). A normal BPP preceded a normal labor and delivery and neonatal outcome 90 to 95% of the time. On the other hand, the predictive value of an *abnormal* BPP was only 5 to 33% in 132 postterm women (80). Researchers at that time concluded that there was no difference between the use of a NST and the BPP for predicting the postterm fetus at risk for "distress" in labor. In other studies, the BPP had a significantly better predictive value for "fetal distress" during labor than the NST or CST alone (8-9, 32, 37, 50, 81). Advocates of the BPP believe it identifies the hypoxic fetus better than any single test (8). The BPP predicted abnormal outcomes of small for gestational age fetuses better than a CST and provides more information that the NST or CST alone (13). *Decreased amniotic fluid was the best predictor of "fetal distress" in labor and poor perinatal outcomes* (8, 32, 37, 50).

CONCLUSION

The fetus is a unique and complex being, who despite antepartal surveillance, may exhibit an abnormal FHR pattern or be born with an anomaly. For this reason, many antepartal measures are available to assess the fetus, placenta, and amniotic fluid. The biophysical profile is one of several antepartal screening methods which uses ultrasound technology to visualize the intrauterine contents.

Biophysical antepartal fetal assessment techniques are an essential part of prenatal care during high risk pregnancy. Women who had antepartal testing had lower perinatal mortality rates than women at low risk for poor perinatal outcomes who did not have serial testing. In a review of over 170,000 women, Dr. Manning and his colleagues reported a corrected perinatal mortality rate of 1.86/1000 in a high risk group with serial antepartal testing compared with 7.42/1000 in an untested sample (1). This data has raised the question of the value of evaluating *all* fetuses with serial antepartal testing. Over the next decade questions will be asked and answered regarding the cost-effectiveness of prenatal care, including prenatal diagnosis, ultrasound, and antepartal fetal assessment techniques. Undoubtedly, nurses will be involved in the whirlwind of change as researchers strive to determine the true value of technology in improving pregnancy outcomes.

References

1.   Manning, F. A. (1995). Antepartum fetal surveillance. Current Opinion in Obstetrics and Gynecology, 7, 146-149.

2.   Manning, F. A. (1995). Fetal assessment in low-risk pregnancy. Current Opinion in Obstetrics and Gynecology, 7, 461-464.

3.   Murray, M. L., Canfield, S., & Harmon, J. (September/October 1986). Nipple stimulation contraction stress test for the high-risk patient. MCN, 11(5), 331-333.

4.   Nageotte, M. P., Towers, C.V., Asrat, T., Freeman, R. K., & Dorchester, W. (August 1994). The value of a negative antepartum test: Contraction stress test and modified biophysical profile. Obstetrics & Gynecology, 84(2), 231-234.

5.   Nageotte, M. P., Towers, C. V., Asrat, T., & Freeman, R. K. (June 1994). Perinatal outcome with the modified biophysical profile. American Journal of Obstetrics and Gynecology, 170(6), 1672-1676.

6.   Manning, F. A., Platt, L. D., & Sipos, L. (March 15, 1980). Antepartum fetal evaluation: Development of a fetal biophysical profile. American Journal of Obstetrics and Gynecology, 136(6), 787-795.

7.   Vintzileos, A. M., & Knuppel, R. A. (December 1994). Multiple parameter biophysical testing in the prediction of fetal acid-base status. Clinics in Perinatology, 21(4), 823-848.

8.   Vintzileos, A. M., Campbell, W. A., Ingardia, C. J., & Nochimson, D. J. (September 1983). The fetal biophysical profile and its predictive value. Obstetrics & Gynecology, 62(3), 271-278.

9.   Baskett, T. F., Gray, J. H., Prewett, S. J., Young, L. M., & Allen, A. C. (March 1, 1984). Antepartum fetal assessment using a fetal biophysical profile score. American Journal of Obstetrics and Gynecology, 148(5), 630-633.

10.   Finberg, H. J., Kurt, A. B., Johnson, R. L., & Wapner, R. J. (1990). The biophysical profile. A literature review and reassessment of its usefulness in the evaluation of fetal well-being. Journal of Ultrasound in Medicine, 9, 583-591.

11.   Manning, F. A., Baskett, T. F., Morrison, I., & Lange, I. (June 1, 1981). Fetal biophysical profile scoring: A prospective study in 1,184 high-risk patients. American Journal of Obstetrics and Gynecology, 140(3), 289-294.

12.   Manning, F. A., Morrison, I., Lange, I. R., Harman, C. R., & Chamberlain, P. F. (February 1, 1985). Fetal assessment based on fetal biophysical profile scoring: Experience in 12,620 referred high-risk pregnancies. I. Perinatal mortality by frequency and etiology. American Journal of Obstetrics and Gynecology, 151(3), 343-350.

13.   Platt, L. D., Walla, C. A., Paul, R. H., Trujillo, M. E., Loesser, C. V., & Jacobs, N. D. (November 15, 1985). A prospective trial of the fetal biophysical profile versus the nonstress test in the management of high-risk pregnancies. American Journal of Obstetrics and Gynecology, 153(6), 624-633.

14.   Phelan, J. P., Ahn, M. O., Smith, C. V., Rutherford, S. E., & Anderson, E. (August 1987). Amniotic fluid index measurements during pregnancy. Journal of Reproductive Medicine, 32(8), 601-604.

15.   Phelan, J. P., Smith, C. V., Broussard, P. M., & Small, M. (1987). Amniotic fluid volume assessment with the four-quadrant technique at 36-42 weeks gestation. Journal of Reproductive Medicine, 32, 540-542.

16.   Phelan, J. P., Platt, L. D.,Yeh, S. Y., Broussard, P., & Paul, R. H. (February 1, 1985). The role of ultrasound assessment of amniotic fluid volume in the management of the postdate pregnancy. American Journal of Obstetrics and Gynecology, 151(3), 304-308.

17.   Moore, T. R. (September 1990). Superiority of the four-quadrant sum over the single-deepest-pocket technique in ultrasonographic identification of abnormal amniotic fluid volumes. American Journal of Obstetrics and Gynecology, 163(3), 762-767.

18.   Moore, T. R., & Cayle, J. E. (May 1990). The amniotic fluid index in normal human pregnancy. American Journal of Obstetrics and Gynecology, 162(5), 1168-1173.

19.   Rutherford, S. E., Phelan, J. P., Smith, C. V., & Jacobs, D. N. (September 1987). The four-quadrant assessment of amniotic fluid volume: An adjunct to antepartum fetal heart rate testing. Obstetrics & Gynecology, 70(3, Pt. 1), 353-356.

20.   Bastide, A., Manning, F., Harman, C., Lange, I., & Morrison, I. (April 1986). Ultrasound evaluation of amniotic fluid: Outcome of pregnancies with severe oligohydramnios. American Journal of Obstetrics and Gynecology, 154(4), 895-900.

21.   Horsager, R., Nathan, L., & Leveno, K. J. (June 1994). Correlation of measured amniotic fluid volume and sonographic predictions of oligohydramnios. Obstetrics & Gynecology, 83(6), 955-958.

22.   Kilpatrick, S. J., & Safford, K. L. (January 1993). Maternal hydration increases amniotic fluid index in women with normal amniotic fluid. Obstetrics & Gynecology, 81(1), 49-52.

23.   Magann, E. F., Nolan, T. E., Hess, L. W., Martin, R. W., Whitworth, N. S., & Morrison, J. C. (December 1992). Measurement of amniotic fluid volume: Accuracy of ultrasonography techniques. American Journal of Obstetrics and Gynecology, 167(6), 1533-1537.

24. Gegor, C. L., Paine, L. L., Costigan, K., & Johnson, T. R. B. (June 1994). Interpretation of biophysical profiles by nurses and physicians. JOGNN, 23(5), 114-119.

25. Nursing practice competencies and educational guidelines for limited ultrasound examinations in obstetric and gynecologic/infertility settings. (1993). Washington, DC: Association of Women's Health, Obstetric, and Neonatal Nurses, 1-11.

26. Gegor, C. L., Paine, L L., & Johnson, T. R. B. (May/June 1991). Antepartum fetal assessment. A nurse-midwifery perspective. Journal of Nurse-Midwifery, 36(3), 153-167.

27. Gegor, C. L. (1992). Antepartum fetal assessment techniques: An update for today's perinatal nurse. Journal of Perinatal and Neonatal Nursing, 5(4), 115.

28. Johnson, T. R. B., Besinger, R.E., & Thomas, R. L. (May 1988). New clues to fetal behavior and well-being. Contemporary OB/GYN, 31(5), 108-119, 123.

29. Jorgensen, N. P., Marshal, K., & Lindstrom, K. (January 1989). Quantification of fetal motor activity in early pregnancy. European Journal of Obstetrics, Gynecology, & Reproductive Biology, 30(1), 11-18.

30. Gagnon, R., Campbell, K., Hunse, C., & Patrick, J. (September 1987). Patterns of human fetal heart rate accelerations from 26 weeks to term. American Journal of Obstetrics and Gynecology, 157(3), 743-748.

31. Manning, F. A., Snijders, R., Harman, C. R., Nicolaides, K., Menticoglou, S., & Morrison, I. (October 1993). Transactions of the thirteenth annual meeting of the society of perinatal obstetricians. Fetal biophysical profile score. VI. Correlation with antepartum umbilical venous fetal pH. American Journal of Obstetrics and Gynecology, 169(4), 755-763.

32. Manning, F. A., Lange, I. R., Morrison, I., & Harman, C. R. (September 1984). Fetal biophysical profile score and the nonstress test: A comparative trial. Obstetrics & Gynecology, 64(3), 326-331.

33. Lodeiro, J. G., Vintzileos, A. M., Feinstein, S. J., Campbell, W. A., & Nochimson, D. J. (June 1986). Fetal biophysical profile in twin gestations. Obstetrics & Gynecology, 67(6), 824-827.

34. Vintzileos, A. M., Gaffney, S. E., Salinger, L. M., Kontopoulos, V. G., Campbell, W. A., & Nochimson, D. J. (September 1987). Transactions of the seventh annual meeting of the society of perinatal obsetricians. The relationships among the fetal biophysical profile, umbilical cord pH, and Apgar scores. American Journal of Obstetrics and Gynecology, 157(3), 627-631.

35. Manning, F. A. (1995). Fetal biophysical profile scoring: Theoretical considerations and clinical application. In F. A. Manning (Ed.), Fetal medicine: Principles and practice (p. 285). Norwalk, CT: Appleton-Lange.

36. Manning, F. A., Morrison, I., Lange, I. R., & Harman, C. (June 1982). Antepartum determination of fetal health: Composite biophysical profile scoring. Clinics in Perinatology, 9(2), 285-296.

37. Chamberlain, P. F., Manning, F. A., Morrison, I., Harman, C. R., & Lange, I. R. (October 1, 1984). Ultrasound evaluation of amniotic fluid volume. I. The relationship of marginal and decreased amniotic fluid volumes to perinatal outcome. American Journal of Obstetrics and Gynecology, 150(3), 245-249.

38. Johnson, J. M., Harman, C. R., Lange, I. R., & Manning, F. A. (February 1986). Biophysical profile scoring in the management of the post-term pregnancy: An analysis of 307 patients. American Journal of Obstetrics and Gynecology, 154(2), 269-273.

39. Gegor, C. L. (March/April 1993). Third-trimester ultrasound for nurse-midwives. Journal of Nurse-Midwifery, 38(2, Suppl.), 49S-61S.

40. Devoe, L. D., Searle, N., Searle, J., Phillips, M., Castillo, R. A., Saad, S., & Sherline, D. M. (October 1, 1985). Computer-assisted assessment of the fetal biophysical profile. American Journal of Obstetrics and Gynecology, 153(3), 317-321.

41. Goodman, J. D. S., Visser, F. G. A., & Dawes, G. S. (July 1984). Effects of maternal cigarette smoking on fetal trunk movements, fetal breathing movements and the fetal heart rate. British Journal of Obstetrics and Gynaecology, 91(7), 657-661.

42. Dawes, G. S. (October 1978). Studying breathing movements for clues to fetal health. Contemporary OB/GYN, 12, 71-72, 77.

43. Campogrande, M., Alermanno, M. G., Viora, E., & Bussolino, S. (1982). FHR short- and long-term variability associated with fetal breathing. Journal of Perinatal Medicine, 10(4), 203-208.

44. Devoe, L. D., Castillo., R. A., Searle, N., & Searle, J. (February 1987). Clinical significance of fetal tachypnea during antepartum biophysical testing. Obstetrics and Gynecology, 69(2), 187-190.

45. Manning, F. A., & Harman, C. R. (1990). Chapter 28. The fetal biophysical profile. In R. D. Eden, & F. H. Boehm (Eds.), Assessment and care of the fetus (pp. 385-396). Norwalk, CT: Appleton-Lange.

46. Benacerraf, G. R., & Frigoletto Jr., F. D. (April 1986). Fetal respiratory movements: Only part of the biophysical profile. Obstetrics and Gynecology, 67(4), 556-557.

47. Pillai, M., & James, D. (January 1990). Behavioural states in normal mature human fetuses. Archives of Disease in Childhood, 65(1 Spec No.), 39-43.

48. Pearson, J. F., & Weaver, J. B. (May 29, 1976). Fetal activity and fetal well being: An evaluation. British Medical Journal, 1, 1305-1307.

49. Fresquez, M. L., & Collins, D. E. (1992). Advancement of the nursing role in antepartum fetal evaluation. Journal of Perinatal Neonatal Nursing, 5(4), 16-22.

50. Chamberlain, P. F., Manning, F. A., Morrison, I., Harman, C. R., & Lange, I. R. (October 1, 1984). Ultrasound evaluation of amniotic fluid volume. II. The relationship of increased amniotic fluid volume to perinatal outcome. American Journal of Obstetrics and Gynecology, 150(3), 250-254.

51. Kilpatrick, S. J., Safford, K. L., Pomeroy, T., Hoedt, L., Scheerer, L., & Laros, R. K. (December 1991). Maternal hydration increases amniotic fluid index. Obstetrics & Gynecology, 78(6), 1098-1102.

52. Magann, E. F., Whitworth, N. S., Bass, J. D., Chauhan, S. P., Martin, J. N., & Morrison, J. C. (1995). Amniotic fluid volume of third trimester diamniotic twin pregnancies. Obstetrics & Gynecology, 85, 957-960.

53. Grannum, P. A. T., Berkowitz, R. L., & Hobbins, J. C. (April 15, 1979). The ultrasonic changes in the maturing placenta and their relation to fetal pulmonic maturity. American Journal of Obstetrics and Gynecology, 133(8), 915-922.

54. Key, T. C., & Moore, T. R. (1984). Evaluation of high-risk pregnancy using ultrasonography: An overview. Journal of Perinatology, 5(3), 49-53.

55. Hopper, K. D., Komppa, G. H., Bice, P., Williams, M. D., Cotterill, R. W., & Ghaed, N. (June 1984). A reevaluation of placental grading and its clinical significance. Journal of Ultrasound in Medicine, 3, 261-266.

56. Platt, L. D., & Petrucha, R. A. (November 15, 1982). Relationship of placental grade to gestational age. American Journal of Obstetrics and Gynecology, 144(6), 733-735.

57. Petrucha, R. A., & Platt, L. D. (September 15, 1989). Relationship of placental grade to gestational age. American Journal of Obstetrics and Gynecology, 144(6), 733-735.

58. Merrill, P. A., Porto, M., Lovett, S. M., Dorchester, W., Nageotte, M. P., & Garite, T. J. (July 1995). Evaluation of the nonreactive positive contraction stress test prior to 32 weeks: The role of the biophysical profile. American Journal of Perinatology, 12(4), 229-231.

59. Finberg, H. J. (1994). Ultrasound evaluation in multiple gestation. In P. W. Callen (Ed.), Ultrasonography in obstetrics and gynecology (pp. 102-128). Philadelphia, PA: W. B. Saunders Company.

60. Elliott, J. P., & Finberg, H. J. (February 1995). Biophysical profile testing as an indicator of fetal well-being in high-order multiple gestations. American Journal of Obstetrics and Gynecology, 172(2, Pt. 1), 508-512.

61. Alcalay, M., Lipitz, S., Rafael, Z. B., Barkai, G., & Mashiach, S. (June 1994). Fetal biophysical profile score in triplet pregnancies. Journal of Reproductive Medicine, 39(6), 436-440.

62. Vintzileos, A. M., Campbell, W. A., Nochimson, D. J., Connolly, M. E., Fuenfer, M. M., & Hoehn, G. J. (July 1, 1985). The fetal biophysical profile in patients with premature rupture of the membranes--an early predictor of fetal infection. American Journal of Obstetrics and Gynecology, 152(5), 510-516.

63. Vintzileos, A. M., Feinstein, S. J., Lodeiro, J. G., Campbell, W. A., Weinbaum, P. J., & Nochimson, D. J. (June 1986). Fetal biophysical profile and the effect of premature rupture of the membranes. Obstetrics & Gynecology, 67(6), 818-823.

64. Johnson, J. M., Harman, C. R., Lange, I. R., & Manning, F. A. (1986). Biophysical profile scoring in the management of the postterm pregnancy: An analysis of 307 patients. American Journal of Obstetrics and Gynecology, 154(2), 269-273.

65. Roberts, A. B., Goldstein, I., Romero, R., & Hobbins, J. C. (1991). Comparison of total fetal activity measurement with the biophysical profile in predicting intra-amniotic infection in preterm premature rupture of membranes. Ultrasound in Obstetrics and Gynecology, 1, 36-39.

66. Goldstein, I., Romero, R., Merrill, M., Wan, M., O'Connor, T. Z., Mazor, M., & Hobbins, J. C. (August 1988). Fetal body and breathing movements as predictors of intraamniotic infection in preterm premature rupture of membranes. American Journal of Obstetrics and Gynecology, 159(2), 363-368.

67. Vintzileos, A. M., Bors-Koefoed, R., Pelegano, J. F., Campbell, W. A., Rodis, J. F., & Nochimson, D. J. (August 1987). The use of fetal biophysical profile improves pregnancy outcome in premature rupture of the membranes. American Journal of Obstetrics and Gynecology, 157(2), 236-240.

68. Vintzileos, A. M., Campbell, W. A., Nochimson, D. J., Weinbaum, P. J., Mirochnick, M. H., & Escoto, D. T. (October 1986). Fetal biophysical profile versus amniocentesis in predicting infection in preterm premature rupture of membranes. Obstetrics and Gynecology, 68(4), 488-494.

69. Devoe, L. D., Youssef, A. E., Croom, C. S., & Watson, J. (September 1994). Can fetal biophysical observations anticipate outcome in preterm labor or preterm rupture of membranes? Obstetrics & Gynecology, 84(3), 432-438.

70. Wax, J. R., Costigan, K., Callan, N. A., Gegor, C., & Johnson, T. R. B. (January 1993). Effect of fetal movement on the amniotic fluid index. American Journal of Obstetrics and Gynecology, 168(1, Pt. 1), 188-189.

71. Wing, D. A., Fishman, A., Gonzalez, C., & Paul, R. H. (January 1996). How frequently should the amniotic fluid index be performed during the course of antepartum testing? American Journal of Obstetrics and Gynecology, 174(1, Pt. 1), 33-36.

72. Nageotte, M. P., Towers, C. V., Asrat, T., & Freeman, R. K. (1994). Perinatal outcome with the modified biophysical profile. American Journal of Obstetrics and Gynecology, 170, 1672-1676.

73. A clinical trial of induction of labor versus expectant management in postterm pregnancy. The National Institute of Child Health and Human Development network of maternal-fetal medicine units. (March 1994). American Journal of Obstetrics and Gynecology, 170(3), 716-723.

74. Hannah, M. E., Hannah, W. J., Hellmann, J., Hewson, S., Milner, R., & Willan, A. (1992). Induction of labor as compared with serial antenatal monitoring in post-term pregnancy trial group. New England Journal of Medicine, 326, 1587-1592.

75. Shaw, K., & Clark, S. L. (December 1988). Reliability of intrapartum fetal heart rate monitoring in the postterm fetus with meconium passage. <u>Obstetrics & Gynecology, 72(6),</u> 886-889.

76. Ultrasound imaging in pregnancy. (August 1991). <u>Committee Opinion Number 96,</u> 156-157. Washington, DC: ACOG.

77. Ultrasonography in pregnancy. (December 1993). <u>Committee Opinion Number 187,</u> 1-9. Washington, DC: ACOG.

78. American institute of ultrasound in medicine. (1993). <u>Standards and guidelines for the performance of the antepartum obstetrical examination,</u> Bethesda, MD: AIUM.

79. Third trimester limited ultrasound for nurse-midwives. (1996). In <u>Clinical bulletin No. 1,</u> Washington, DC: American College of Nurse-Midwives.

80. Sachs, B. P., Hann, L., McArdle, C., & Acker, D. (February 1985). The use of non-stress test versus biophysical profile for screening postdate pregnancies (Abstract #196). Society of Perinatal Obstetricians Annual Meeting, Las Vegas, Nevada.

81. Platt, L. D., Eglinton, G. S., Sipos, L., Broussard, P. M., & Paul, R. A. (April 1983). Further experience with the fetal biophysical profile. <u>Obstetrics and Gynecology, 61</u>(4), 480-485.

Appendix

Suggested Abbreviations:

A

a	arterial
AB or ab	abortion
Abd	abdomen
ABG	arterial blood gases
accel(s)	acceleration(s)
ACTH	adrenocorticotropic hormone
adm	admission
A/G ratio	albumin/globulin ratio test
AFP	alpha fetoprotein
AGA	appropriate for gestational age
AgNO₃	silver nitrate
alb	albumin
AMA	against medical advice
amb	ambulate or ambulatory
amnio	amniocentesis
amt	amount
ANA	antinuclear antibodies
Angio	angiocath (intravenous catheter brand)
AO	aorta
AP	apical pulse
A-P	anterior/posterior
ARDS	Adult Respiratory Distress Syndrome
AROM	artificial rupture of membranes
ASA	acetylsalicylic acid (aspirin)
ASAP	as soon as possible
AV	Atrioventricular
ax	axilla

B

BBOW	bulging bag of water
b.i.d.	twice a day
BL	baseline

BM	bowel movement
BOW	bag of water
BP	blood pressure
BPM or bpm	beats per minute
BPP	biophysical profile
BR	bathroom
BTL	bottle
BUN	blood urea nitrogen

C

C	Centigrade/celsius
°C	degrees Celcius
CAN	cord around neck (nuchal cord)
CBC	complete blood count
CBG	capillary blood gases
cc	cubic centimeter(s)
cm	centimeter(s)
CO	carbon monoxide
CO₂	carbon dioxide
COHb or HbCO	carboxyhemoglobin
CPAP	continuous positive airway pressure
CPD	cephalopelvic disproportion
CPK	creatinine phosphokinase
CPR	cardiopulmonary resuscitation
CRP	C-reactive protein
C/S, C-Section	cesarean section
CSF	cerebrospinal fluid
CST	contraction stress test
CTX or UCs	contraction(s)/uterine contractions
CV	cardiovascular
CVA	cerebrovascular accident
CVP	central venous pressure
CX, cx	cervix

D

D_5LR	5% dextrose in lactated Ringer's (solution)
2,3-DPG	2, 3-diphosphoglycerate
Δ	delta (Gk) representing change or difference
DAT	diet as tolerated
DC	discontinue
DC'd or dc'd	discontinued
decel(s)	deceleration(s)
del	delivery
decr or ↓	decrease
DFM	decreased fetal movement
DI	diabetes insipidus
DIC	disseminated intravascular coagulation or coagulopathy
Dig	digoxin
dil	dilatation
Disch	discharge
dk	dark
DKA	diabetic ketoacidosis
DM	diabetes mellitus
DNA	do not announce
DOB	date of birth
DR	delivery Room
Dr.	doctor
drsg	dressing(s)
DX or Dx	diagnosis

E

early decel(s)	early deceleration(s)
EBL	estimated blood loss
EBOW	evident bag of water
ECG	electrocardiogram
Echo	echocardiogram
EDC	estimated date of confinement (see EDD)
EDD	estimated date delivery/estimated due date
EDH	epidural hematoma
EEG	electroencephalogram
EENT	eyes, ears, nose and throat
EF	ejection fraction
EFM	electronic fetal monitoring
EFW	estimated fetal weight
EGA	estimated gestational age
ENT	Ears, nose and throat
epis	episiotomy
Eq	equivalent(s)
est	estimate or estimated
ETA	estimated time of arrival
ER	emergency room
ETT	endotracheal tube
exam	examination
Ext	external

F

F	fetal
FBS	fasting blood sugar
FA	fetus active
FAS	fetal accoustic stimulator
FBM	fetal breathing movements
FD	fetal demise (see IUFD for intrauterine fetal demise)
FDP	fibrinogen degradation products
Fe	iron
FECG	fetal electrocardiogram
FF or ff	fundus firm
FFP	fresh frozen plasma
FHR	fetal heart rate
FHT	fetal heart tones
F^IO_2	fractional inspired oxygen
fld	fluid
FM	fetal movement
FOB	father of baby
FP	fundal pressure
FSE	fetal scalp electrode (more appropriately abbreviated SE as it is only applied to the fetus)
FSH	follicle-stimulating hormone
FT	fingertip
F/U	fundus at umbilicus
FUO	fever of undetermined origin
Fx	fracture

G

g or gm	gram(s)
G	gravida
GA	gestational age
GBM	gross body movement(s)
GEST	gestation
G T P A L	gravida, term, preterm, aborta, living children
GTT	glucose tolerance test
gtt	drop(s)
GU	genitourinary
GYN	gynecology

H

h. or hr.	hour(s)
HA	headache
Hb or hgb	hemoglobin
HbA	adult hemoglobin
HbA_{1C}	hemoglobin A_{1C} (glycosylated hemoglobin)
HbF	fetal hemoglobin
HBP or HTN	high blood pressure/hypertension
HB_SA_g	hepatitis B surface antigen
HCT or hct	hematocrit
HCVD	hypertensive cardiovascular disease
HDL	high density lipoprotein
HEENT	Head, eyes, ears, nose and throat
HELLP	hemolysis, elevated liver enzymes, low platelets
HFD	high forceps delivery
H & H	hemoglobin and hematocrit
HL	heparin lock
H_2O	water

HOB	head of bed	LFD	low forcep delivery
Hosp	hospital	lg	large
H & P	history and physical	LGA	large for gestational age
hs	at bedtime	liq	liquid
ht	height	LLQ	left lower quadrant
HTN	hypertension	LMP	last menstrual period
HTVD	hypertensive vascular disease	LPM	liters per minute or liters by mask
HX or Hx	history	L → R	left to right
		L/S	lecithin/sphingomyelin ratio

I

I	iodine	LTV	long-term veriability
IASD	Intra-atrial septal defect	LTV abs/LTV O	long-term variability absent (0-2 bpm BL bandwidth)
IBOW	intact bag of water	LTV min/LTV ↓	long-term variability minimal (3-5 bpm BL bandwidth)
IBW	ideal body weight		
ICA	internal carotid artery	LTV av	long-term variability average (6-10 bpm BL bandwidth)
ICH	intracranial hemorrhage		
ict	icterus	LTV mod/LTV ↑	long-term variability moderate (11-25 bpm BL bandwidth)
ICU	intensive care unit		
I & D	incision and drainage	LTV marked	long-term variability marked or saltatory (> 25 bpm bandwidth)
IDM	infant of diabetic mother		
IG	immune globulin	LOA	Left occiput anterior
incr or ↑	increase	LOP	left occiput posterior
Ind or ind	induction of labor	LR	lactated Ringer's (solution)
inf	infection	L-spine	lumbar spine
inj	inject(ion)	L	left
IU	International Unit (of hormone activity)	LUOQ	left upper outer quadrant
IUFD	intrauterine fetal demise	LUQ	left upper quadrant
IUGR	intrauterine growth restriction, formerly intrauterine growth retardation	lytes	electrolytes
IUPC	intrauterine pressure catheter	**M**	
IV	intravenous	mat	maternal
IVAC	volume infusion pump	max	maximum
IVH	intraventricular hemorrhage	mcg	microgram (also μg)
IVPB	intravenous piggyback	MCH	mean corpuscular hemoglobin
IVSD	intraventricular septal defect	MCHC	mean corpuscular hemoglobin concentration
		MCV	mean corpuscular volume
K		mec	meconium
K	potassium	mEq(s)	milliequivalent(s)
K-B	Kleihauer-Betke test	MFD	midforceps delivery
KCL	potassium chloride	mg	milligram
Kg or kg	kilogram	mg%	milligrams percent
kPa	kilopascal (1 kPa = 7.5 mm Hg)	MgSO$_4$	magnesium sulfate
		MHR	maternal heart rate
L		MI	myocardial infarction
L or l	liter	midnoc	midnight
lab	laboratory	min	minute
lac	laceration	ML	midline
lap	laparotomy	ml	milliliter
lat	lateral	MLE	midline episiotomy
late decel(s)	late deceleration(s)	mm	millimeter
lb.	pound	mm Hg	millimeters of mercury (1 mm Hg = 0.133 kPa)
LBP	low back pain	mmol	millimole
LBW	low birth weight	MO	mineral Oil
LC	living child	MOM	milk of magnesia
LDH	lactic dehydrogenase	mo(s)	month(s)
LDRP	labor, delivery, recovery, post partum	mosm	milliosmole

MPV	mean platelet volume	ROM	rupture of membranes
MSF	meconium-stained fluid	R → L	right to left
mU	milliunits	RR	recovery room
mU/min	milliunits per minute		

N

N	number	**S**	
NB	newborn	S	saturation, as in SaO_2
NICU	neonatal intensive care unit	SE	spiral electrode
NKA	no known allergies	SGA	small for gestational age
NSVD	normal spontaneous vaginal delivery	SIDS	sudden infant death syndrome
NST	nonstress test	SKB	single, keeping baby
NSY	nursery	SNKB	single, not keeping baby
N/V	nausea and vomiting	spont	spontaneous
		SROM	spontaneous rupture of membranes

S

S	saturation, as in SaO_2
SE	spiral electrode
SGA	small for gestational age
SIDS	sudden infant death syndrome
SKB	single, keeping baby
SNKB	single, not keeping baby
spont	spontaneous
SROM	spontaneous rupture of membranes
S/S	signs and symptoms
S → S	side to side
STAT	immediately
STDs	sexually transmitted diseases
STV	short-term variability
STV +	short-term variability present
STV 0	short-term variability absent
STV inter	short-term variability intermittent
SVE	sterile vaginal examination
SVT	supraventricular tachycardia

O

O_2	oxygen
OA	occiput anterior
OB	obstetrics
OBRR	obstetrics recovery room
OCT	oxytocin challenge test
OP	occiput posterior
OT	occiput transverse

T

TAB	therapeutic abortion
ThAB	threatened abortion
T/L	tubal ligation
TOCO or toco	tocodynamometer, tocotransducer
TOL	trial of labor
TOLAC	trial of labor after cesarean

P

p	probability
P	partial pressure, eg. PO_2 is the partial pressure of oxygen
PAC	premature atrial contractions
PP	post partum
P_{50}	point on partial pressure axis on oxyhemoglobin dissociation curve of 50% hemoglobin saturation
PGE_2	prostaglandin E_2
PIGI	pregnancy-induced glucose intolerance
PIH	pregnancy-induced hypertension
PNV	postnatal visit
prolonged decel	prolonged deceleration
PP	post partum
PPROM	preterm premature rupture of membranes
PTL	postpartal tubal ligation
PROM	premature rupture of membranes
pt	patient

U

UAC	umbilical artery catheter
UCs	uterine contractions
US	ultrasound (external monitoring)
UVC	umbilical venous catheter

V

vag	vaginal
var decel(s)	variable decelerations
VBAC	vaginal birth after cesarean section
VE	vaginal examination
VTX or vtx	vertex
VO_2	oxygen delivery (or oxygen consumption)

Q

q	every
Q	blood flow

W, X, Y, Z

WNL	within normal limits
wt	weight
xylo	xylocaine
YOB	year of birth

R

RBCs	red blood cells
R/CS	repeat cesarean section

References

1. Madsen, H. (April 1986). Fetal oxygenation in diabetic pregnancy. Danish Medical Bulletin, 33(2), 64-74.

2. Rose, L. (February 15, 1995). Proposed abbreviation list. Heartland New Beginnings Obstetrics, St. Joseph, MO.

3. Abbreviations and symbols. (March 10, 1995). Eastern New Mexico Medical Center, Roswell, NM.

Glossary of Fetal Heart Monitoring Terms

A

Ab:	number of miscarriages (abortions) and births before 20 weeks' gestation, includes spontaneous (SAB) and therapeutic abortions (TAB).
Abruptio placentae (placental abruption):	premature separation of the placenta prior to delivery of the fetus.
Acceleration:	an increase in the fetal heart rate above the baseline level. There are two types: uniform and spontaneous (see Chapter 5).
Acidemia:	abnormal increase in hydrogen ion concentration due to the accumulation of an acid or a loss of base.
Acidosis:	the abnormal accumulation of carbon dioxide (respiratory acidosis) or lactic acid (metabolic acidosis).
Amnioinfusion:	instillation of an isotonic, glucose-free solution, such as normal saline, into the uterus.
Amnion:	inner membrane of the sac that encloses the fetus.
Amniotomy:	breaking the bag of waters, the artificial rupture of the fetal membranes (AROM) usually performed to stimulate the onset of labor.
Antepartal:	before birth, pertaining to the period spanning conception to the onset of labor.
Anoxia:	absence of oxygen within the tissues.
Apgar score:	system of scoring neonate's physical condition one minute and five minutes after birth. The color or appearance (A), heart rate or pulse (P), response to stimuli or grimace (G), muscle tone or activity (A), and respirations (R) are assessed. Each can receive a maximum of 2 points. The maximum Apgar score is 10.
Arrhythmia:	any variation from the normal rhythm of the heart.
Artifact:	irregularities on the monitor tracing due to poor reception of the fetal heart signal which appears as scattered dots, gaps on the tracing, or lines.
Asphyxia:	a condition due to lack of oxygen resulting in impending or actual cessation of life, from Greek meaning "a stopping of the pulse." Implies a reduction in PO_2 (hypoxia), elevation of PCO_2 (hypercapnia), and lowering of blood pH and bicarbonate or mixed acidosis with respiratory and metabolic components. Asphyxia is preceded by anaerobic metabolism. Asphyxia can precede cell damage and/or death.
Auscultation:	act of listening for sounds within the body; assisted by use of a stethoscope and/or fetoscope.

B

Baseline (BL):	the fetal heart rate over a period of time, not including accelerations or decelerations. The BL may be recorded as a range or an average rate.
Beat-to-beat variability (BTBV):	the fluctuation in milliseconds (msec) between consecutive R to R intervals of fetal QRS complexes (heartbeats).
Bradycardia:	a fetal heart rate less than 100 bpm for 10 or more minutes.

C

Caput succedaneum:	swelling occurring in and under the scalp of the fetus during labor. A localized pitting edema in the scalp of a fetus that may overlie sutures of the skull. It is usually formed during labor as a result of the circular pressure of the cervix on the fetal occiput.
Cervix (Cx):	neck of the uterus which protrudes into the vagina.

Contraction stress test (CST):	antepartum surveillance method using induced or spontaneous contractions to evaluate fetal oxygen reserves and placental function. Induced contractions may be from endogenous or exogenous oxytocin.

D

Deceleration:	a distinct decrease in the FHR with a return to a baseline with a duration of less than 10 minutes. Decelerations are classified by their shape and timing in relation to uterine contractions.
Dilatation:	expansion of the opening of the cervix from 1 to 10 cm.
Doppler ultrasound:	instrument that emits and receives sound waves to determine the fetal heart rate.

E

Early deceleration:	a FHR deceleration which is caused by compression of the fetal head and characterized by a gradual onset at the beginning of a contraction and a slow return, gradual offset, or gradual recovery to the baseline soon after the contraction ends.
EDD/EDC:	expected date of delivery or confinement or due date calculated from the first day of the last menstrual period or estimated by other clinical parameters such as ultrasound measurements of the fetus.
Effacement:	shortening or thinning of the cervical canal, usually during the early phase of dilatation, estimated by a percent. For example, 80% effaced indicates the cervix is approximately 4/5th of its original length. The closed cervix is 2.5 to 3 cm long.
Electronic fetal monitor (EFM):	computer with paper printout used to show graphically and continuously the relationship between maternal uterine activity and the FHR.
Engagement	of the vertex occurs when the biparietal diameter has passed through the pelvic inlet and is clinically diagnosed when the leading bony portion of the fetal head is at or below the level of the ischial spines (station 0 or more) (see ACOG 1989 technical bulletin on Obstetric Forceps).
Epidural:	regional anesthesia administered through the back between L3 and L4 via a thin catheter in the epidural space outside of the spinal canal or the dura mater.

F

Fetal heart rate (FHR):	fetal ventricular rate in beats per minute.
Fetal scalp electrode:	see spiral electrode.
Fundus:	portion of the uterus which lies above the insertion of the fallopian tubes at the top of the uterus. The portion farthest from the mouth of an organ.

G

Gestation:	time from conception to birth.
Gestational age:	age of the embryo or fetus computed from the first day of the last menstrual period to the present, usually expressed in weeks.
Gravida (G):	number of pregnancies.

H

Hematoma:	localized collection of blood, usually clotted, caused by a break in the wall of a blood vessel.
Hypoxemia:	low blood oxygen content.
Hypoxia:	deficiency of oxygen in the cells.

I

Intensity:	when an IUPC is in the uterus, the peak IUP minus the resting tone.

Intrapartal:	the period of time during labor and birth.
Intrauterine pressure catheter (IUPC):	a fluid-filled or solid catheter inserted transvaginally into the uterus. Intrauterine pressure is conducted through the catheter, exerted on a pressure transducer, and transformed to an electronic signal, then printed on the tracing.
Introitus:	entrance to the vagina.
Ischial spines:	the shortest diameter of the pelvis. Two prominent, palpable bony prominences.

L

Late deceleration:	a FHR deceleration caused by uteroplacental insufficiency (low oxygen delivery) and characterized by a gradual, slanted onset after the contraction begins, and *usually* a slow return to baseline. The nadir is always after the contraction peak. Late decelerations tend to be similar in shape. They return to baseline after the contraction ends.
Low forceps:	The application of forceps when the leading point of the skull is at station +2 or more.
Long-term variability (LTV):	the fluctuation of the fetal heart rate above and below an average baseline rate (cycles) evaluated each minute of the baseline.

M

Meconium:	dark-green mucilaginous material in the intestine of the fetus. The normal contents of the baby's intestines, i.e., 80% water, 20% mucoproteins, mucopolysaccharides, and biliverdin.
Membranes:	the sac surrounding the fetus.
Molding:	shaping of the fetal head in adjustment to the size and shape of the pelvis and birth canal.
Midforceps:	The application of forceps when the head is engaged but the leading point of the skull is above station +2. Application of forceps above station +2 may be attempted while simultaneously initiating preparations for a cesarean delivery in the even that the forceps maneuver is unsuccessful (see ACOG, 1989 technical bulletin on Obstetric Forceps).
Montevideo units:	from Uruguay, invented by Dr. Caldeyro-Barcia, the sum of the intensity of contractions in a ten minute period.
Multipara:	a woman who has completed two or more pregnancies to the stage of viability.

N

Nadir:	the lowest possible point of the curve, for example, nadir of the deceleration.
Nonperiodic (pattern):	decelerations not related to contractions.
Nonstress test (NST):	antepartum surveillance method used to evaluate fetal condition by evaluation of the FHR pattern. An oxygenated, nonacidotic term fetus should have at least 2 accelerations in a 20 minute period with each acceleration peaking 15 bpm above the baseline and lasting 15 or more seconds at its base.

O

Outlet forceps:	The application of forceps when a) the scalp is visible at the introitus without separating the labia, b) the fetal skull has reached the pelvic floor, c) the sagittal suture is in the anterior-posterior diameter or in the right or left occiput anterior or posterior position, and d) the fetal head is at or on the perineum (see ACOG, 1989 technical bulletin on Obstetric Forceps).
Occiput:	back part of the head.
Oxytocic:	agent which acts like the naturally occurring hormone oxytocin, and stimulates contractions of the pregnant uterus.

Oxytocin Challenge Test (OCT):	a CST which is conducted by stimulation of uterine contractions with intravenously administered oxytocin. NST criteria also apply to the CST, i.e., a well fetus has a reactive negative test.

P

Para (P):	represents parity or the number of *pregnancies* reaching viability, *rather than the number of fetuses* delivered. Past obstetric history may be summarized in a series of numbers connected by hyphens. For example, pregnancies (gravida), term infants, premature infants, abortions, number of children currently alive may appear on the prenatal record as 3-2-1-0-3.
Paracervical block:	local anesthesia injected around the cervix to relieve the pain of uterine contractions.
Parity:	the condition of having carried pregnancy to the point where the fetus weighs 500 grams or is 20 weeks of gestation regardless of the outcome.
Periodic pattern:	decelerations occurring in relation to contractions.
Pattern:	the fetal heart rate plotted on heat sensitive paper in an electronic fetal heart monitor; including baseline rate, variability, accelerations, and decelerations.
Placenta previa:	placenta lying partially or totally over the cervical os or opening.
Position:	the relation of the presenting part, eg., fetal head or buttocks, to the maternal pelvis.
Presentation:	the part of the baby that is over the birth canal.
Presenting part:	portion of the fetus which is touched by the gloved examining finger(s) during a vaginal examination. The part of the fetus that is first into the birth canal.
Primigravida:	a women pregnant for the first time.
Primipara:	a woman who has delivered a fetus weighing 500 or more grams or who is 20 or more weeks' gestation.
Prolonged deceleration:	a periodic pattern which is characterized by a deceleration of the FHR lasting at least 2 minutes but less than 10 minutes.
Prostaglandins:	hormone-like unsaturated fatty acids that have an effect on blood vessels, smooth muscles, platelets, endocrine glands, the uterus, and the nervous system.

S

Short-term variability (STV):	the consecutive beats per minute (bpm) rates plotted on moving fetal monitor paper, which appears as bumps, squiggles or grass. STV is determined from beat-to-beat variability (BTBV).
Spiral electrode:	usually a stainless steel curved wire which is inserted under the fetal skin of the presenting part. It transmits the fetal heart electric current to the fetal monitor.
Station:	the level (in centimeters) of the presenting part to the ischial spines. (-) is above the spines, "O" is at the spines, and (+) is below the spines. If the fetal head (vertex) is presenting, station is the relationship of the estimated distance, in centimeters, between bony portion of the fetal head and the level of the maternal ischial spines..

T

Tachycardia:	in the fetus, a heart rate above 160 bpm for 10 or more minutes. Maternal tachycardia is a rate above 100 bpm.
Tocodynamometer/tocotransducer (toco):	pressure sensing instrument applied externally to the maternal abdomen to assess uterine contractions.
Tonus or resting tone:	partial contraction of the uterine muscle between contractions, measured in mm Hg by an intrauterine pressure catheter or assessed by palpation.

Tracing:	the paper and pattern of the fetal heart rate and/or contractions produced by an electronic fetal monitor.
Transducer:	a device which senses a signal for conversion to an electronic form.

U

Uterine contractions (UC):	periodic increase in intrauterine pressure. When externally palpated, uterine contractions are classified as: mild, moderate, and strong.
Uterine resting tone:	see tonus or resting tone.
Uteroplacental reserve:	the amount of blood and oxygen available to support the fetus during contractions.
Uteroplacental insufficiency:	an inadequate flow of oxygen from the intervillous space to the fetus, resulting in fetal hypoxemia.

V

Variability (FHRV):	fetal heart rate variability has two components: long-term variability (the slow rhythmic fluctuations above and below an average baseline rate) and short-term or beat-to-beat variability which are instantaneous fluctuations in the FHR. The combination of these two types of variability reflects the interaction between parasympathetic and sympathetic branches of the central nervous system.
Variable deceleration:	a deceleration of the fetal heart rate caused by umbilical cord compression and/or head compression (especially in the second stage of labor with pushing), characterized by a rapid onset and return to baseline, and a variable relationship to the contraction (may occur at any time in the contraction phase). Variable decelerations may be preceded or followed by acceleratory phases or shoulders.
Shoulders:	brief increases in the fetal heart rate (usually 20 seconds in duration) preceding or following a variable deceleration and attached to the variable deceleration in response to umbilical vein compression.
Overshoot:	immediately following a variable deceleration, a high increase (> 20 bpm above the baseline) or a long increase (> 20 seconds in duration). Neither a shoulder or an overshoot is classified as an acceleration. Rather, this acceleratory phase suggests fetal compensation for hypoxia with release of catecholamines.
Variation:	computer-generated analysis of the fetal heart rate over 1/16th of a minute (short-term variation) and each minute (long-term variation). Variation is calculated in milliseconds and is determined with an ultrasound transducer in place or a spiral electrode.
Viable:	a reasonable potential for subsequent survival if the fetus were delivered. In determining parity, viability is considered to be 500 grams or 20 weeks' gestation. A reasonable potential for subsequent survival appears to be delivery at 23 or more weeks' gestation, if neonatal intensive care facilities are available.

References:

Obstetric forceps. (February 1988). Committee opinion, Number 59, 1-2. Washington DC: ACOG.

Janulis, D. M. (1989). A primer on electronic fetal monitoring. Personal Injury Review, 175-214.

Glanze, W. D., Anderson, K. N., & Anderson, L. E. (Eds.). (1990). Mosby's medical, nursing, and allied health dictionary (3rd ed.). St. Louis, MO: The C. V. Mosby Company.

Notes

Index

— A —

Abdominal wall fetal electrocardiogram, 17-19
    electrical noise, 19
    fetal/maternal position, 19
    gestational age, 19
    reliability, 19
Abruption of placenta, 17, 38, 73, 79, 135, 222, 277
Absent baseline variability, 76-77, 140
Absent end-diastolic velocity, 225-226
Absent long-term variability, 85
    cause/physiology of, 85
    response to, 85-86
Absent short-term variability, 258-259
Absent variability response, 76-77
Acceleration, 7, 13-14, 59-60, 62, 66, 71, 83, 95-96
    cause/physiology, 95
    during labor, 96
    lack of, response to, 95
    misconceptions about, 95-96
    prolonged, 168
    recognition, 95
    spontaneous, 65, 80, 96-98, 101
        alternative labels, 96
        cause/physiology of, 96
    uniform, 97-100, 102, 175, 438-440, 463-466
        cause/physiology, 99-100
        recognition, 97-99
Accels. *See* Acceleration
Acetylcholine, 436
Acid-base balance, 241-304, 306, 318-319
Acid-base status, 95
Acidemia, 100, 242-243, 255-257, 310, 345, 349-351
Acidosis, 12, 70-71, 83, 217, 227, 243-244, 349-351, 355-356,
    437, 466-467

Acids, 241
Acoustic stimulation, 90, 311, 346-347, 437, 472
Acoustic stimulation test, 473
Acoustic stimulator, 346
Active transport, placenta, 209
Actocardiograph, 9
Addiction, 434
Adenosine, 181, 224, 226, 246, 418-419, 433, 437
Adenosine accumulation, 106
Adenosine levels, 226-227
Adenosine triphosphate, 246
Adipose tissue, 180-181
Adlomet, 433
Adrenal cortex, 178-179
    aldosterone, 178
    atrial natriuretic peptide factor, 179
    cortisol, 178
    Rh isoimmunization, 179
Adrenal medullae, 179-180
Adrenocorticotropic hormone, 178
Adult respiratory distress syndrome, 268
Advanced maternal age, 122
AFI. *See* Amniotic fluid index
Afterload, 203-205
    left, 205
    right, 204-205
Agonal pattern, 63, 71, 440
    cause/physiology of, 71
    response to, 71
Air embolism, 270-271
Alcohol use, 431, 463
Aldosterone, 178, 184
Alert/alarm function, computer, 12
Alkalosis, 243
Alternative label, 77

Amiodarone, 417-418
Amniocentesis, 222
Amnioinfusion, 100, 105, 117-125, 431
    amount of fluid infused, 117-188
    benefits, 118
    blanket warmer, 123
    complications of, 119
    contraindications, 118
    embolism, 120, 122
        modified response to, 121
        nursing response to, 122
    factors associated with, 121
    IV fluid, temperature, 122-123
    limitations, 118
    meconium, 122
    medical responsibilities, 123-125
    nursing responsibilities, 123-125
    oligohydramnios, 118
    oxytocin, 121-122
    phases of, 121
    for thick meconium, 262-263
    transabdominal amnioinfusion, 118
    transcervical amnioinfusion, 118
    trial of labor after cesarean, 119-120
    type of fluid for, 117
    ultrasound, prior to initial bolus, 118-119
    uterine rupture, 120
Amnionitis, 222, 431
Amniotic fluid, 209
Amniotic fluid-derived humoral substances, 120
Amniotic fluid embolism, 120-121
    modified response to, 121
    nursing response to, 122
Amniotic fluid index, 466, 501-503
Amniotic fluid optical density, 91
Amniotic fluid volume, 179, 496-497
Amniotomy, 431
Amphetamines, 273-275, 431
Amplitude, 64
Amylase, 278
Anaerobic metabolism, 181-182
Analgesics, 282, 367-368, 432
Anatomic shunts, 182-183
Anemia, 89, 201, 218-222, 279-280, 437
Anencephaly, 79, 437
Anesthesia, 270, 367
    epidural, 432-433
    general, 273
    high spinal, 270
    paracervical, 128
    regional, 70
Anoxia, 217, 246
Antepartal fetal monitoring. *See* Fetal monitoring
Anti-Kell antibodies, 219
Anti-SS-A gene, 426
Anti-SS-B gene, 426
Anti-SS-(Ro) antibody, 424-425

Antiarrhythmic agents, 413-419, 433, 437
Anticardiolipin antibodies, 424-425
Antidepressants, 438
Antidromic circuit, 409
Antihistamines, 433
Antihypertensives, 433
Antiphospholipid antibody syndrome, 424-427, 458
Anxiety, 282, 433
Apgar score, 248, 318-319, 352
Apresoline, 276
ARDS. *See* Adult respiratory distress syndrome
Arginine vasopressin, 89, 93, 173, 178, 184, 227
Arrhythmia, 14, 64, 82, 85, 396-398, 428-431, 434, 438
Artery compression, 175
Artifacts, 8, 14, 64
    elimination switch, 5
Artificial larynx, 472
Ascites, 397
Asphyxia, 1, 12, 79, 83, 227, 246-249, 251-253, 259-261, 305-342, 355-356, 438
    Apgar score, 248
    asphyxia, 248-249
    clinical, 248
    hypoxic-ischemic encephalopathy, 249
    intrapartal fetal, 305-342
    metabolic, 248
Aspirin use, 427
Asthma, 266-267
Asynchronous twin fetal heart rates, 137
Atenolol, 95, 433, 459
Atria, 395
Atrial fibrillation, 398, 413-419
Atrial flutter, 398, 412-413
Atrial natriuretic peptide factor, 179, 184
Atrial systole, 395
Atrioventricular block, 419-424
Atropine, 78, 172
Atypical biphasic variable decelerations, 114
Atypical variable deceleration, 114-116, 440
Auscultation, 2, 7, 316-318, 321-322
Autoantibodies, 425
Autocorrelations, 21, 23-25, 29
Automatic gain control, 7-8, 19
Automaticity, 393
Autonomic nervous system, 169
Avascular villi, 214
Average long-term variability, cause/physiology of, 86

— B —

Barbiturates, 433
Baroreceptors, 78, 111, 164, 174-178
Baseline characteristic variability, 80
Baseline fetal heart rate, 10
Baseline stability, 71-73
    falling baseline, 73

rising baseline, 71
wandering baseline, 73
Baseline variability, 68, 73-77
absent, 76-77
cause/physiology, 75
decreased, 76-77
documentation, 76
increased, 76
response to, 76
recognition, 75
visualization, 76
Baselines, 14-15, 59, 63, 65-73, 125, 131
stability, 71-73
unstable, response to, 83
Bases, 241
Behavior, fetal, 14, 226
cycles, 167-169
EEG patterns, association, 169
fetal heart rates, 167-168
Benign sinusoidal pattern, 88-89, 436, 438-439
cause/physiology of, 88-89
response to, 89
Beta blockers, 172-173
Beta-mimetics, 371, 427
Beta-sympathomimetics, 21
Betamethasone, 433
Bigeminal premature atrial contractions, 402
Biochemical fetal monitoring, 343-392
Biofeedback, 367
Biophysical fetal assessment, 491-518
Biophysical profile, 491, 499
Biphasic variable decelerations, 116
Birth canal, rupture of, 121
Birth weight, 274
Bishop's score, 13
Bladder filling, umbilical cord prolapse, 375
Blocked atrial premature beat, 398
Blood flow, 212, 226, 274-275
Blood gas analysis, 352
Blood glucose, 370
Blood sampling, fetal, 13
Blood vessels, 179
Blood viscosity, 279
Body movements, fetal, 495-496
Bradyarrhythmias, 419-424
Bradycardia, 63, 68-71, 119, 127, 227, 258-260, 433, 436, 440
end-stage, 63, 70
classification of, 70-71
response to, 69-70
terminal, 63, 71, 85
cause/physiology of, 71
response to, 71
Brain, 344
Brainstem, 163-169
Braxton Hicks contractions, 216, 281
Breathing movements, 164-165, 259, 438, 495
Breech presentation, 438

Buffers, 241
Bulk flow, placenta, 209
Bundle branch system, 394
Bupivacaine, 269
Butorphanol, 282

— C —

Cable block/leg plate, 30-31
conductive gel, 31
Caffeine, 433-434
Calcium accumulation, 246-247
Cannula, 373-374
Capillary hydrostatic pressure, 199-200
Carbon dioxide, 197
Carbon monoxide, 271
Cardiac arrest, 204
Cardiac contractility, 203-205
decrease in, 205
increase in, 205
Cardiac disease, 434
Cardiac failure, 397, 438
Cardiac glycogen, 259
Cardiac output, 202, 205, 268, 273-274
Cardiotocography, 305
Cardiovascular system, 344
Cardiovert SVT, 408
Catecholamine response, 100
Catecholamines, 76, 78, 282, 433, 436
Central display functions, computer, 10
Central nervous system depressants, 79
fetal sleep, 83
Cephalhematoma, 124
Cephalopelvic disproportion, 434
Cerebral anoxia, 246
Cerebral palsy, 250-251, 313
cerebral palsy, 251
intraventricular hemorrhage, 250
periventricular leukomalacia, 250
Cervix, 214-215
ripening, 215
Cesarean section, 309
with continuous electronic fetal monitoring, 1
rates, 308-309
Charting by exception, 324
Checkmark pattern, 64, 102, 116, 125-127, 137, 439
due to seizures, 127
nonperiodic decelerations, 125-127
response to, 125-127
Chemoreceptors, 78, 164, 174
activation of, 111, 175
Chorioamnionitis, 69, 118-119, 202, 250-251, 255, 257, 263
Chorioangiosis, 209
Chorionic membrane on placenta, 353
Chorionic villus sampling, 434
Circulation, 182

Closed glottis pushing, 434
Clustered FBM, long-term variability, 166
Coagulopathy, 107
Cocaine, 276-277, 434
    intrauterine pressure catheter, 38
    transfer of, 209
Codeine, 280
Coffee, 434
Colloid osmotic pressure, 199
Compensatory fetal heart rate patterns, 139
Compensatory mechanisms, 178-180
Compensatory response, 138
Complete heart block, 398, 423
Computers, 10-12
    accelerations, 10
    alert/alarm function, 12
    analysis with, 14-15
    central display functions, 10
    data retrieval, 10-11
    electronic point-of-care charting, 10
    fetal heart rate, 10, 13-14
    graphical user interface, 10
    hard drive, 10
    long-term variability, 10
    monitoring equipment, 10-12
    optical disk archiving, 10
    peak intrauterine pressure, 10
    point-of-care documentation, 10-11
    purchase of, 11
    remote access, 11
    remote display, 10
    resting tone, 10
    short-term variability, 10
    software, 13
    statistics, 11
    system implementation, 12
    uterine contraction frequency, 10
Conceptual knowledge development, fetal monitoring, 62
Concurrent flow system, 211-212
Concurrent flow/venous equilibrium exchange model, 211-212
Conductivity, 393
Congenital anomalies, 464
Congenital heart block, 219
Congestive heart failure, 396
Continuous electronic fetal monitoring
    benefits of, 1-2
    cesarean section with, 1
    limitations of, 1-2
    post partum endometritis with, 1
Continuum of fetal welfare, 138-140
Contraction stress test, 474-475, 477
Contractions, 63, 281, 434
Coombs test, 91
Cord compression, 125, 176, 217-218
    hiccups, seizures, differentiating, 127
Cord length, 218

Cordocentesis, 135, 346
Corticosteroids, 427
Cortisol, 178, 184
Coupling, 63
Coupling gel, 20
Cross-channel verification, 9
Cultural differences, 366
Cyanotic heart disease, 273
Cytomegalovirus, 90

— D —

Data entry devices, 9
Data retrieval, computer, 10-11
Death, fetal, 1, 7, 29, 89, 222
Deceleration, 13-14, 59, 62, 69, 167, 227, 259
    early, 102-103, 171-172, 395
        cause/physiology of, 104
        significance of, 104
    late, 60, 98, 102, 104-107, 109-110, 134, 140, 176, 257, 259, 263, 306, 313, 395, 433-438
        characteristics of, 110-111
        hypoxic myocardial failure, 107
        late/variable decelerations, 109
        recognition, 106-107
        reflex late decelerations, 107
        response to, 109-111
        subtle late decelerations, 107
        types of, 107-111
    mild variable, 433
    mixed, 125
        recognition, 125
        response to, 125
    nonperiodic, 102-103
        Checkmark pattern, 125-127
        recognition, 102-104
        taxonomy of, 102
    periodic, 102
        taxonomy of, 102
    prolonged, 127-129, 433, 439-440
        bradycardia, 260
        cause/physiology, 127-128
        classification, 127
        response to, 128-129
    reflex late, 108, 139
    severe variable, 113-114, 134, 140, 395
    spontaneous, 129-131, 225-226, 467, 469
        cause/physiology, 130
        classification, 130
        recognition, 129
        response to, 130-131
        significance abnormally, 130
    subtle late, 108
    variable, 102, 109, 111-113, 171-172, 176, 257, 259, 313, 438-439, 466
        cause/physiology, 111-113

classification of, 113-114
documentation of, 117
mild, 113
moderate, 113
overshoots, 111
with overshoots, 112
recognition, 111
response to, 116
shoulders, 111
with shoulders, 112
Decompensation, 70-71
Decrease short-term variability, 78
Decreased fetal monitoring, 458
Decreased variability, 258, 345
response to, 76-77
Deficient placental transfer, 209
Dehydration, 280
Demerol, 89, 280, 282
Depolarization, 394
Dextrose, 369
Diabetes, 213, 225, 278, 434-435
Diazepam, 79, 433, 463
Digital decompression of cord, 375
Digital scalp stimulation, 307
Digoxin, 411, 414-415
Dilantin, 269
Direct/internal monitoring techniques, 30-38
Disagreements, 12
Discontinuance, monitor, 15-16
Discordance, 135
Discordant twins, 214
Disseminated intravascular coagulopathy, 120
Diuresis, 179
Dizygotic twins, 135
Documentation, 323-325
fetal monitoring, 62-64
long-term variability, 87-88
Dopamine, 180
Doppler blood flow, 343-344, 430
Doppler devices, 25
Doppler principles, 6, 20-22
Doppler ultrasonography, 343
Doppler velocimetry, 91, 135
Doppler waveforms, 24, 344
Doubling fetal heart rate, 25-27
Dropped beats, 403

— E —

Echocardiography, 428-431
Eclampsia, 83, 269, 435
Ectopic tachycardia, 410-412
Education, 320
Electrocardiogram, 13, 17, 19, 21
abdominal wall, 17-19
electrical noise, 19

fetal/maternal position, 19
gestational age, 19
reliability, 19
reliability of, 19
direct, 17
indirect, 17
ST analysis, 311-312
Electrode placement, 438
Electroencephalogram, fetal, 169-171
Electromagnetic waves, 10
Electronic fetal monitoring, 1-2, 305-307, 309-310
Electronic point-of-care charting, 10
Embolism, amniotic fluid, 120
Empathy, 366
End-diastolic blood flow, 225
End-diastolic blood velocity, 344
End-stage bradycardia, 63, 70
classification of, 70-71
Endometritis, intrauterine pressure catheter, 38
Endomyometritis, 119
Endorphins, 178, 184
Ephedrine, 86, 128, 433, 435
Epidural, 276, 283, 432, 435
Epilepsy, 269
Epinephrine, 179, 184, 277, 282, 432-433, 436
Equipment for monitoring, 1-58
continuous electronic fetal monitoring, 1-2
direct/internal monitoring techniques, 30-38
external fetal heart rate monitoring devices, 17-20
features of, 3-10
fetal heart rate analysis, 12-15
indirect/external uterine monitoring, 16-17
intrauterine pressure catheter, 34-38
monitor start-up, discontinuance, 15-16
problems with, 38-40
spiral electrode, 30-33
tocotransducer, 16-17
ultrasound transducer, 20-30
uterine activity assessment, 40-47
Equipment problems, 38-40
intrauterine pressure catheter, 39
spiral electrode, 40
ultrasound transducer, 38
Equivocal/hyperstimulation contraction stress test, 481
Erythroblastosis fetalis, 219
Erythropoietin, 222-223
European scaled paper, for monitoring, 3
Excitability, 393
Exercise, 274
External fetal heart rate monitoring, devices for, 17-20
Extrinsic factors
fetal heart rate, 197-233
oxygen delivery, 197-233

— F —

Facilitated diffusion, 209
Falling baseline, 73
FAST. *See* Fetal acoustic stimulation test
Features of fetal monitor, 3-10
Fentanyl, 282, 433
Fetal acoustic stimulation test, 346, 457-458, 471-474
Fetal activity acceleration determination test, 436, 458, 468-471
Fetal demise, 1, 7, 29, 89, 135, 222
Fetal electrode stimulation test, 311
Fetal monitoring, 29, 59-162
    accelerations, 65, 95-96, 130
    acid-base balance, 241-304, 306, 318-319
    acidemia, 255-257
    admission test, 315-316
    amnioinfusion, 117-125
    amniotic fluid index, 501-503
    antepartal, 457-490
    antiphospholipid antibody syndrome, 424-427
    Apgar scores, 318-319
    arrhythmias, 396-397, 428-431
    asphyxia, 247-249, 251-252, 259-261, 305-342
    atrial fibrillation, 413-419
    atrioventricular block, 419-424
    auscultation, 316-317
    baseline, 65-73
        identification of, 65
        variability of, 73-77
    biochemical, 343-392
    biophysical profile, 491-518
    bradyarrhythmias, 419-424
    carbon monoxide, 271
    cardiac output, 273-274
    cerebral palsy, 250-251
    cesarean section, 308-309
    Checkmark pattern, 125-127
    compensatory mechanisms, 178-180
    computer applications, 10-12
    conceptual knowledge development, 62
    continuous electronic fetal monitoring
        benefits of, 1-2
        limitations of, 1-2
    contraction stress tests, 474-475
    cord compression, 127
    decelerations, identification of, 65
    discontinuance, 15-16
    distress, 307
    documentation, 62-64
    electronic, 305-306
    equipment problems, 38-40
    evaluation of learning, 62-64
    external fetal heart rate, 17-20
    extrinsic factors, 197-233
    fetal acoustic stimulation test, 471-474
    fetal activity acceleration determination test, 468-471

    fetal scalp blood sampling, 348-352
    fetal welfare continuum, 138-140
    gradual hypoxia, 492
    heart rate, 12-15, 224-227
        control mechanisms, 163-177
    hemodynamic, 343-392
    hiccups, 127
    hyperoxygenation, 371-374
    hypoxemia, 253-254
    hypoxia, 224-227, 254-255
    instructional design, 61-62
    instructor responsibilities, 61
    intrauterine pressure catheter, 34-38
    intrauterine resuscitation, 364-365
    intrinsic factors, 163-196
    kick counts, 483
    labor, 282-283
    lambda pattern, 100-101
    late decelerations, 104-107
        types of, 107-111
    learner responsibilities, 61
    measurement, 80-84
    meconium, 261-264
    metabolic acidosis, 254-255, 258-259
    misconceptions, 60-61
    mixed deceleration patterns, 125
    nonperiodic changes, 101-104
    nonperiodic decelerations, 125-127
    nonstress test, 460
    normal sinus rhythm, 395
    overview, 59-61
    oxygen delivery, 197-198, 217-224
    oxygenation, 251-252
    pattern components, 59
    pattern identification, 65
    periodic changes, 101-104
    placenta, 207-214
    premature atrial contractions, 401-404
    preterm fetus, 131-135
    procedural knowledge development, 62
    prolonged decelerations, 127-129
    prototype formation, 62
    recognition, 60
    risk categories, 314-315
    seizures, 127
    sensitivity, 306
    sinusoidal patterns, 88-95
    specificity, 306
    spiral electrode, 30-33
    spontaneous accelerations, 96-97
    spontaneous decelerations, 129-131
    start-up, 15-16
    third trimester ultrasound, 503-504
    tocolysis, 370-371
    tocotransducer, 16-17
    twins, 135-138
    ultrasound transducer, 20-30

umbilical cord prolapse, 374-377
uniform accelerations, 97-100
uterine activity, 40-47
uterine rupture, 283-285
uteroplacental blood flow, 366
uterus, 214-217
variability, 77
    long-term, 84-88
    short-term, 77-84
variable decelerations, 111-113
    atypical, 114-117
    classification, 113-114
    typical, 114-117
variations in heart rate, 393-456
visualization, 80-84
Fetal movement, 7, 27, 66, 83, 167, 282, 433. *See also*
    Fetal monitoring
accelerations, 166
betamethasone administration, 131
decelerations, 167
hypoxia and, 169
lack of, 7
multiple gestation, 136
reduction in, 30
representation of, 88
ultrasound transducer, 27-30
Fetal vibroacoustic stimulation, 435
Fetomaternal hemorrhage, 219, 438
Fetomaternal transfusion, 219-220
Fetopelvic disproportion, 434
Fetoscope, 7, 21, 86
Fibrin, 214
Fibronectin, 214
Fibrotic destruction, AV node, 420
Fick Principle, 206
Fifth's disease, 90
First-degree heart block, 398, 420-421
First generation monitors, 1, 23, 25, 28
First stage of labor, 216
Flecainide acetate, 415-416
Fractional shortening, 401-402
Frank Starling Law, 203-204, 424
Fraternal twins. *See* Dizygotic twins
Free fatty acids, 180-181
FSpO$_2$, 360-362
Fundal pressure, 121
Funisitis, 73

— G —

Gamma globulin, 427
General anesthesia, 433
Gestational age, fetal heart rate, 171
Gestational diabetes, 458
Glucagon, 180
Glucocorticoid administration, 433

Glucola, 278
Gluconeogenesis, 180
Glucose, 180, 365, 369
Glutamate, 246, 364
Glycogenolysis, 180
Glycosylated hemoglobin, 278
Gonorrhea, 434
Gradual hypoxia, 492
Graphical user interface, computer, 10
Gross body movements, 164

— H —

Halving fetal heart rate, 25-27
Hand-held Doppler, 7, 20
Hard drive, computer, 10
Head compression, 125, 171-172
Heart block, 420, 438
Heart rate, 12-15, 64, 202-203
    antiphospholipid antibody syndrome, 424-427
    arrhythmias, 396-397, 428-431
    atrial fibrillation, 413-419
    baseline, 13
    bradyarrhythmias, 419-424
    computer analysis, 13-14
    control mechanisms, 163-177
    data analysis, 13
    extrinsic factors, 197-233
    hypoxia, 224-227
    intraventricular hemorrhage prediction, 132
    intrinsic factors, 163-196
    measurement techniques, 18
    normal sinus rhythm, 395
    oxygen delivery, 197-233
    premature atrial contractions, 401-404
    short-term variability, 164-165
    variations, 393-456
Heart rate volume, 6
Heat stress, 435
Hematocrit, 201-202
Hemoconcentration, 280
Hemodynamic fetal monitoring, 343-392
Hemoglobin, 201-202, 218
Hemoglobin affinity, 200-201
Hemoglobin types, 200-201
Hemoglobinopathies, anemia, 279
Hemorrhage, 89, 120-121, 438
Heparin, 427
Hepatitis B, 434
Hiccups, seizures, cord compression, differentiating, 127
High amplitude/low frequency Braxton Hicks, 215
High-risk factors, 264
HIV. *See* Human immunodeficiency virus
HLA DR3 gene, 426
HLA gene, 426
Homeostasis, 178

Hon, Dr. Edward, 30, 307, 310, 321
Human immunodeficiency virus, 32-33
    maternal-fetal transmission, 33, 209
    zidovudine, 33
Human parvovirus, 90
Hydralazine, 276
Hydration, 497
Hydration by mouth, 368
Hydrops, 89, 219, 396-397, 438-439
Hydrotherapy, 367
Hyperbilirubinemic, 278
Hypercapnia, 116, 245, 255
Hyperinsulinemia, 243
Hyperkalemia, 222
Hyperoxygenate, 110, 373
Hyperoxygenation, 76, 363, 371-374, 435
Hyperparathyroidism, 438
Hyperstimulation, 128, 281, 436, 457, 476-477, 481-482
    intrauterine pressure catheter, 38
    with uterine hypertonus, 47
Hypertension, 83, 212-213, 225, 276, 435, 458
Hypertensive vascular disease, 436
Hyperthyroidism, 435
Hypertonic labor, 121
Hypertonus, 63, 281
Hyperventilation, 273
Hypoglycemia, 243, 435
Hypoglycemic, 278
Hypotension, 70, 275-276, 368, 435
Hypothalamic-pituitary-adrenal axis, 178
    adrenocorticotropic hormone, 178
    arginine vasopressin, 178
    endorphins, 178
Hypothermia, 202, 436, 438, 440
Hypothyroid fetus, 96
Hypothyroidism, 202
Hypoventilation, 266
Hypovolemia, 69, 275, 438
Hypovolemic shock, 283
Hypoxemia, 242, 253-254, 282, 310
    without metabolic acidosis, 252
Hypoxia, 2, 12, 70-71, 76, 82-83, 89, 93, 106, 183, 216-217, 224-227, 242, 252, 310, 436, 438
    admission test, 253
    chronic, 224, 491
    fetal movement, 169
    fetal response to, 180-184
    gradual, 492
    intrauterine growth restriction, 253
    with metabolic acidosis, 252
    preterm response to, 132-135
    response to, 76
    with risk of metabolic acidosis, 254-255
Hypoxic-ischemic encephalopathy, 249
Hypoxic myocardial depression, 107
Hypoxic myocardial failure, 64
    late decelerations, 109
    lates, 140

— I —

Iatrogenic hydramnios, 119
Identical twins. See Monozygotic Twins
Idioventricular rhythm, 398, 405-406
Immune reaction, 90
Immunoglobulin, 427
Increased fetal activity, 434
Increased variability, 439
    response to, 76
Inderal, 416, 433, 436
Indirect/external fetal heart rate, 20-30
Indirect/external uterine monitoring, 16-17
Infection with human immunodeficiency virus, 32-33, 459
    maternal-fetal transmission, 33, 209
    zidovudine, 33
Informed consent, 322-323
Infusion acidosis, 242-243
Instructional design, fetal monitoring, 61-62
Instructor responsibilities, fetal monitoring, 61
Insulin, 180
Insulin-dependent diabetes, 458
Interleukin 1, 278
Intermittent heart block, 422
Internodal tracts, 394
Interobserver agreement, 12
Interobserver interpretation, 310
Intraerythrocytic glycolytic metabolism, 201
Intrapartal asphyxia, 1, 12, 79, 83, 227, 246-249, 251-253, 259-261, 305-342, 355-356, 438
Intraperitoneal abscess, intrauterine pressure catheter, 37
Intrapulmonary shunt, 267-268
Intrauterine growth restriction, 1, 77, 86, 95, 99, 131, 135, 179-180, 184, 207, 214, 216-217, 222, 224-227, 243, 271, 345, 438, 458, 491
Intrauterine pressure catheter, 34-38, 104, 109-110, 117
    abruption, 36, 38
    amnioinfusion, 36
    amniotic fluid index, 35
    atmospheric pressure, 35
    cocaine use, 38
    complications, 37
    contractions, 36
    endometritis, 38
    equipment problems, 39
    fluid-filled, solid, pressure differences, 36-37
    hydrostatic pressure, 35-36
    hyperstimulation, 38
    infarction of placenta, 38
    insertion, 34-38
    intraperitoneal abscess, 37
    maternal movement, 36
    offset error, 36
    oxytocin administration, 36
    perforation, 37
    preeclampsia, 38
    resting tone, 36

spiral electrode, 1
uterine perforation, 37
Intrauterine resuscitation, 364-365
Intrauterine transfusion, 91, 220-222
complications of, 91
success of, 91-92
Intravenous hydration, 369
Intraventricular bleed, 364
Intraventricular hemorrhage, 250, 364
Intrinsic factors, fetal heart rate, 163-196
Irregular rhythm, 396
IUGR. *See* Intrauterine growth restriction
IUPC. *See* Intrauterine pressure catheter

— J —

Junctional ectopic tachycardia, 398, 407, 411-412

— K —

Karotype, 91
Ketoacidosis, 243, 278
Kick counts, 483
Kidneys, 179
Kleihauer-Betke reaction, 90-91, 220
Knee-chest position, 268
umbilical cord prolapse, 375

— L —

L-lactic acid, 245
Labetalol, 224, 433
Labor, 282-283
first stage, 216
second stage, 86, 217, 371
Lactate, 181, 211, 273, 356-357
Lactic acid, 181-182, 184
Lacticemia, 242
Lambda pattern, 64, 100-101, 166, 175-178, 400, 465
cause/physiology, 100-101
differentiating, 101
recognition, 100
response to, 101
Learner responsibilities, fetal monitoring, 61
Leg plate, cable block, 30-31
Leopold's maneuvers, 27, 99
Leukotrienes, 120, 122
Limb movement, 226
Lipolysis, 180-181
Liver, 180
Logic off, 4-5
Logic on, 4
Long-acting thyroid stimulating hormones, 435

Long-term variability, 10, 14, 59, 62, 64, 71, 80, 84-88, 95, 125, 131, 173-174
absent, 85-86
cause/physiology of, 85
response to, 85-86
amplitude, 85
average, 86
cause/physiology of, 86
categories of, 85
cause, 84
computer studies, 10
cycles, 84
documentation, 87-88
label
amplitude, 85
cycles, 84
during labor, 84
marked, 70, 86-87, 434, 438
cause/physiology, 86
response to, 86-87
minimal, 86
cause/physiology of, 86
moderate, 86
cause/physiology of, 86
physiology, 84
recognition, 84-86
saltatory pattern, 86
Loss of variability, 259, 261, 437
Loudspeaker, 6-7
Lumbar epidural block, 432
Lupus anticoagulant antibodies, 424

— M —

Macrosomia, 121
Magnesium sulfate, 269, 371, 436
Malformations, 438
Malnutrition, 224-226
Manning, Dr. Frank, 491
Manning criteria, 494
Marcaine, 127, 269-270
Marijuana, 436
Marked long-term variability, 86
cause/physiology, 86
response to, 86-87
Marked variability, 439
Mass spectrometry, 363
Maternal abdominal trauma, 458
Maternal age, 459
Maternal anemia, 459
Maternal blood flow, 212
Maternal brain oxygen delivery/consumption, 206
Maternal cardiac output, 211
Maternal electrocardiogram, 1-58
Maternal-fetal transmission, human immunodeficiency virus, 33, 209

Maternal fever, 122
Maternal heart deceleration, 8
Maternal heart rate, 21-22, 27, 69, 99-100, 110, 202-203
Maternal hypoxemia, 218
Maternal oxygen administration, 13
Maternal oxygen extraction, 206
Maternal pulse, 21
Maternal Rh isoimmunization, 89, 458-459
Maternal risk factors, limiting fetal oxygen delivery, 265
Maternal temperature, 119
Maternal tissue oxygen consumption, 206
Meconium, 86, 117, 122, 124, 222, 261-264, 312-313, 355
    metabolic acidosis, 264
Meconium aspiration syndrome, 244, 262
Meconium-stained amniotic fluid, 261
Medication effects, 76
Medulla oblongata, 79, 93
Membrane, partial pressure of gas, 197-199
Meperidine, 89
Metabolic acidosis, 25, 29, 181, 245, 258-259, 310-311, 351
    hypoxemia without, 252
    hypoxia with, 252
    meconium, 264
Methadone, 280
Methyldopa HCl, 433
Minimal long-term variability, cause/physiology of, 86
Mixed acidosis, 245-246
Mobitz heart block, 421
Modems, 10
Moderate long-term variability, cause/physiology of, 86
Modified biophysical profile, 500
Monitor, 15-16
Monitor clock, 8
Monitor paper, 13
Monitoring equipment, 10-12
Monitoring ports, 8
Monosialogangliosides, 364
Monozygotic twins, 135
Morphine, 280, 282
Mortality, fetal, 1, 7, 29, 89, 135, 222
Multifocal PVCs, 405
Multiple gestation, biophysical profile, 500
Muscle relaxants, 463
Music, 366
Myocardium, 393, 435

— N —

Nalbuphine, 432
Narcotics, 79, 282-283, 366, 436
Nasal prongs, 373-374
National Institute of Neurological and Communicative
    Disorders and Stroke Collaborative Perinatal Project,
    307
Natriuesis, 7, 179
Near infrared spectroscopy, 362

Neonatal death rates, 1
Neonatal EEG, 127
Networking, 11
NICHD Research Planning Workshop, 322
Nicotine, 271
NIH Consensus Development Conference Task Force on
    Cesarean Childbirth, 308
Nipple stimulation contraction stress test, 458, 475
NIRS. *See* Near infrared spectroscopy
Nitric oxide, 271
Non-Rh alloimmunization, 219
Nonimmune hydrops, 91, 219, 397
Nonreactive/negative contraction stress test, 478-479
Nonreactive nonstress tests, 463, 468
Nonreactive/positive contraction stress test, 480-481
Nonstress test, 71, 135, 457, 459-460
    nonreactive, 462
    reactive, 461-462
Norepinephrine, 179, 184, 274, 277, 435-436
Normal fetal behavior, 76
Normal maturation, 76
Normal sinus rhythm, 395
NRBCs. *See* Nucleated red blood cells
NS-CST. *See* Nipple stimulation contraction stress test
Nubain, 88-89, 432
Nuchal cord, 137, 255-256
Nuchal notch, 256
Nucleated red blood cells, 201, 218, 222-223, 252
Nursing education, 320

— O —

Occiput posterior position, 104, 439
Occiput transverse position, 439
Oligohydramnios, 30, 91, 99, 103, 111, 118, 124, 131, 183-184,
    226-227, 259, 434, 439, 463-467, 492, 496, 502-503
Ominous fetal heart rate pattern, 260-261
Ominous patterns, response to, 140
On/off recorder button, 3
Open glottal pushing, 266
Opioids, 432
Optical disk archiving, computer, 10
Optical laser disks, 10
Orange juice, 460
Orthodromic circuit, 409-410
Oscillatory effect, vagus, 171-172
Over monitoring, 2
Overdistention, 119
Overshoot, 114, 139
Oxycardiotocography, 359
Oxygen affinity, 201
Oxygen-carrying capacity, 200-201
Oxygen consumption, 208, 223
Oxygen delivery, 197-233, 282
Oxygen extraction, 224
    ratios, 223-224

Oxygen free radicals, 247
Oxygen reserves, 206, 217, 223, 227
Oxygen therapy, 374
Oxygenation, 66, 227
Oxytocin, 121-122, 282
    with hyperstimulation, 436
Oxytocin challenge test, 457, 475

— P —

P wave, 394
PACs. *See* Premature atrial contractions
Pain, 282-283
Palpation, abdominal, 431
Pancreas, 180
Pancuronium bromide, 433, 439
Paper, for monitoring, 3-5
Paper speed switch, monitor, 5
Paracervical block, 433
Parasympathetic activity, increased, 76
Parasympathetic nervous system, 131, 169-171
Parasympatholytic drugs, 78
Parasystole, 405-406
Parathyroid hormone-related protein receptors, 211
Paroxysmal atrial tachycardia, 403
Parvillon, 433
Passive diffusion, 208-209
Pathologic sinusoidal pattern, 76, 89-90, 166, 437
    cause/physiology, 89-90
    recognition, 89
    response to, 90
Paul, Dr. R.H., 310
Peak detection, 21, 23
    autocorrelation, 23
Peak pressure, 63
Pericardial effusion, 397
Peripheral equipment, 9-10
Periventricular leukomalacia, 250, 364
Persistent nonreactive fetal heart rate, 260-261
Phenergan, 89, 436
Phonocardiography, 17
Picket fence pattern, 63
Piezoelectric crystals, 20, 22
Pinocytosis, 209
Pitocin, 282, 371, 433
Placenta, 212
    oxygen delivery to, 199-203
Placenta previa, 436, 459
Placental abruption, 121, 436
Placental anatomy, 207-214
Placental blood flow, 212
Placental blood gases, 356
Placental gas, 110
Placental grade, 497-499
Placental growth, 435
Placental lesions, 212-214

Placental oxygen consumption, 209-210
Placental resistance, 344
Placental transport mechanisms, 208-211
Placental vasoconstriction, 210-211
Placental vessel vasospasm, 214
Placental villi, 207-208, 435
Plasmapheresis, 427
Plethysmography, 360
Plot, fetal monitoring, 5-6
Pneumonia, 267
Point-of-care documentation, computer, 10-11
Polycythemia, 218-222
Polyhydramnios, 121, 135, 496-497, 502-503
Post partum endometritis with continuous electronic fetal monitoring, 1
Postdate pregnancy, 458
Postmaturity, 439
Postterm pregnancy, 263
    modified biophysical profile, 503
Potassium leakage, 246-247
PR interval, 394
Prednisone, 427
Preeclampsia, 83, 135, 214, 275, 278, 280, 369, 406, 436, 458
Preload, 203-205
    high, 204
    low, 204
    measurement of, 204
Premature atrial contractions, 398, 401-404
    dropped beats, 403-404
Premature atrial depolarizations, 402-403
Premature rupture of membranes, 117, 122, 222, 459
Premature ventricular contractions, 25, 404-407
Premature ventricular contractors, 398
Prematurity, 439
Preterm fetus, 132, 135, 251, 261, 277, 462-463
    accelerations, 132
        vs. decelerations, 132
    baseline changes, 132
    baseline level, 131
    baseline variability, 132
    betamethasone administration, 131
    biophysical profile, 500
    fetal heart rate pattern, 132
    fetal movement, 131
    hypoxia, 132-135
    initiation of monitoring, 132
    intraventricular hemorrhage, 132
    late decelerations, 135
    monitoring, 131-135
    nonstress testing, 132
    variable decelerations, 132-135
    variation, 131
Preterm labor, 222, 277, 459
Preterm premature rupture of membranes, 500
Previous fetal loss, 458
Printer, for monitor, 5
Procainamide, 416

Procedural knowledge development, fetal monitoring, 62
Prolapsed cord, 128
Propafenone, 418
Propranolol, 173, 416, 433, 436
Prostacyclin, 271
Prostaglandin gel, 109
Prostaglandins, 179, 184, 211
Prototypes, 13
Pseudoephedrine, 433
Pseudosinusoidal pattern, 432
Pulmonary edema, 267-268
Pulmonary shunting, 267
Pulmonary volumes, 199
Pulsatility index, 343
Pulse oximeter, 270, 360
Pulse oximetry, 311, 357-360
Pulsed-echo Doppler ultrasound, 22, 29
Pulsing sound, 7
Purchase of computer, 11
Purkinje system, 394-395
Pushing pattern, 63
PVCs. *See* Premature ventricular contractions

— Q —

QRS complex, 394
Quiescence, 462
Quinidine, 416-417

— R —

R waves, 13
Rapid eye movement, 27, 226
Reactive fetal heart rate, 260-261
Reactive/negative contraction stress test, 478
Reactive/positive contraction stress test, 479-480
Reactive tracings, 15
Reactivity, 61
Real-time data, 10
Real-time directed M-mode ultrasound, 429-430
Real-time ultrasound, 7
Reassuring fetal heart rate patterns, 138
Recognition, 13, 139
Red blood cell 2,3 diphosphoglycerate, 201
    decrease in, 201-202
    increase in, 201
Redistribution of blood streaming, 182
Reduced fetal movement, 30
Reentry supraventricular tachycardia, 409, 412
Reflectance pulse oximetry, 358-359
Refractory period, 394
Regional anesthesia, 70
Remote access computer, 11
Remote display computer, 10
Renin, 184

Renin-angiotensin, 179
Repolarization, 394
Resistance index, 344
Respiratory acidosis, 245
Respiratory arrest, 270
Respiratory distress, 278
Respiratory sinus arrhythmia, 63, 83, 165-166, 396, 398
Response to abnormal heart rate, 66-67
Resting tone, 63
    computer, 10
Resting zone, 281-282
Rh D hemolytic disease, 89
Rh incompatibility and, 219
Rising baseline, 71, 438
Ritodrine, 436
Rupture of birth canal, 121
Rupture of membranes, 347

— S —

SA node, 394
Saltatory pattern, 64, 85
Sawtooth pattern, 63, 82, 166
    short-term variability, 83
        response to, 84
Scalp abscess, 30
    spiral electrode, 32
Scalp blood sampling, 348-352
Scalp capillary blood gases, 350
Scalp capillary blood pH, 256
Scalp electrode stimulation test, 346, 348
Scalp pH, 25, 311, 351
Scalp stimulation, 311, 346-348, 437, 439
Scoline, 433
Scopolamine, 172
Second-degree heart block, 398, 421-423
Second generation fetal monitors, 1
Second generation monitors, 23, 25, 27-28
Second stage of labor, 86, 217, 266-267, 371
Seizures, 83, 89, 127, 244, 249, 268-270, 308, 313, 439
    cause/physiology of, 125
    hiccups, cord compression, differentiating, 127
Serotonin, 180
Short-term variability, 13-14, 23, 25, 31, 59, 62, 66, 71, 77-84, 95, 109-110, 125, 131, 172
    absent, 78-79
        response to, 83
    categories, 80
    cause/physiology, 78, 83-84
    documentation, 81
    measurement, 80-81
        vs. visualization, 81
    normal range of, 80
    recognition, 78, 83
    sawtooth pattern, 83
        response to, 84

ultrasound, 25
visualization, 81
Shoulders, 103, 175
Shunting of blood, to vital organs, 183-184
Sick sinus syndrome, 401
Sickle cell disease, 279-280, 458
Signal loss, 14
Signal source, 21
Sinoatrial block, with junctional escape, 400
Sinus arrest, 398
Sinus block, 398
    with junctional escape, 400
Sinus bradycardia, 398-399
Sinus tachycardia, 398-400
Sinusoidal pattern, 64, 87-95, 133, 220, 227
    benign, 88-89, 439
        cause/physiology of, 88-89
        response to, 89
    benign *vs.* pathological, 173-174
    documentation of, 95
    pathologic, 88, 90, 220-221
Sjögren's syndrome, 426
Skewed contractions, 63
Skills validation, 320
Sleep, fetal, central nervous system depressants, 83
Smoking, 271-273, 277, 434, 436, 463
Sotalol, 415
Spectrophotometry, 360
Spiral artery diameter, 214
Spiral electrode, 1-2, 6, 8-9, 13, 15, 17, 30-33, 110, 263, 279
    application, 31
    calculations, 31-32
    complications, 32
    double helix, 30-31
    endometritis, 32
    equipment problems, 40
    preeclampsia, 30
    removal of, 31
    scalp abscess, 30, 32
    short-term variability, 31
    single helix, 30-31
Spontaneous contraction stress test, 475
Stability of baseline, 71-73
    falling baseline, 73
    rising baseline, 71
    wandering baseline, 73
Stadol, 89, 282
Standard of care, 321-322
Start-up, monitor, 15-16
Statistics, 11
Stethoscope, 7
Stress, 436
Stroke volume, 203-204
Sturge-Weber syndrome, 269
Subcutaneous PO_2, 363
Sublimaze, 282
Suboptimal care, 305

Succinylcholine chloride, 433
Supine hypotension, 17, 435
Supine position, 276, 437
Supraventricular reentrant tachycardia, 408
Supraventricular tachyarrhythmias, 398
Supraventricular tachycardia, 27, 219, 398, 402-403, 407-409
Swallowing, 259
Swishing sound, 7
Sympathetic influences, 173
Sympathetic nervous system, 131, 172-174
Sympathoadrenal medullary system, 179
Synchronous twin tracings, 138
Synchrony, twin monitoring, 136-138
Syphilis, 434
Syringe preparation, 352
Systematic review for tracing analysis, 467-468
Systemic lupus erythematosus, 425-426
Systole, 13

— T —

T/QRS ratio, 19-20, 395
    metabolic acidosis, 19
    PR interval, 19
Tachyarrhythmias, 396
Tachycardia, 63, 67-69, 71, 100, 127, 139, 202, 227, 256-257, 261, 433, 437-438
    response to, 67-68
Tachysystole, 63
    with uterine hypertonus, 47
Tachysystole with, uterine hypertonus, 47
Telemetry, 10
Temperature, fetal, 202
Tenormin, 433, 459
Terbutaline, 9, 437
Terminal bradycardia, 63, 71
    cause/physiology of, 71
    response to, 71
Test button, monitor, 6
Tetanic contraction, 63
Thick meconium, 355
Third-degree heart block, 423-424
Third trimester ultrasound, 66, 70, 503-504
    abnormal baseline, 66
    baseline, 66
    bradycardia, 69
    chorioamnionitis, 69
    classifications, 67
    decelerations, 69
    fetal hypovolemia, 69
    recognition, 66-67
    response to abnormal heart rate, 66-67
    tachycardia, 67, 69
        response to, 67-68
Thrombocytopenia, 79
Thromboemboli, 280

Thromboxane, 247, 278
Tissue hypoxia, 252
Tissue oxygen consumption, fetal, 223
Tissue pH, 362
Tissue thromboplastins, 122
Toco. *See* Tocotransducer
Tocodynamometer mechanism, 16
Tocolysis, 370-371
Tocolytics, 371, 437
Tocotransducer, 1, 16-17
Toitu monitor, 29
TOLAC. *See* Trial of labor after cesarean
Tone, fetal, 496
Tonic effects of vagus, 171-172
Trandate, 433
Tranquilizers, 437
Transabdominal amnioinfusion, 118
Transcervical amnioinfusion, 118
Transcutaneous PO$_2$, PCO$_2$, 362
Transcutaneous scalp PO$_2$, 282
Transfusion
    intrauterine, 90-91
        complications of, 91
    twin-twin, 89, 91
Transient tachycardia, 135
Tray, for monitor paper, 3-5
Trendelenburg, 268, 375
Trial of labor after cesarean, 283-285
Trigeminal premature atrial contractions, 402
Triplet monitoring, 2
Twin baseline offset, 9
Twin gestation, 458, 497
Twin monitoring, 2, 135-138
    accelerations, 136-138
    asynchronous accelerations, 138
    baseline, 136
    dizygotic twins, 135
    monozygotic twins, 135
    multiple gestation, 136
    synchrony, 136-138
Twin-twin transfusion, 89, 91

— U —

Ultrasound energy, 22-23
Ultrasound signal reliability, 22
Ultrasound signal transmission, 22
Ultrasound technology, 1
Ultrasound transducer, 1, 20-30
    cleaning, 20
    equipment problems, 38
    fetal movement monitoring using, 27-30
    testing, 20
Umbilical artery, 225, 344
    blood flow, 222
Umbilical artery blood flow, 344-345

Umbilical artery gases, 355
Umbilical artery lactate, 357
Umbilical artery pH, 354
Umbilical artery resistance, decreased, 222
Umbilical artery values, 356
Umbilical cord, 110, 209, 225
Umbilical cord blood flow, 217, 365
Umbilical cord compression, 102, 127, 175, 218, 440
Umbilical cord entanglement, 458
Umbilical cord hematoma, 220
Umbilical cord prolapse, 374-377, 440
    bladder filling, 375
        digital decompression of cord, 375
        knee-chest position, 375
        prolapse kit, 375-377
Umbilical vein blood, 353
Umbilical vein blood gases, 346
Umbilical vein compression, 176
Umbilical vein pH, 354
Umbilical vein thrombosis, 90
Umbilical venous pressure, increased, 222
Uneven placental perfusion pattern, 211-214
Unifocal PVCs, 405
Unsatisfactory nonstress test, 465
Unstable baseline, response to, 83
USA scaled paper, for monitoring, 3
Uterine activity, 3, 40-47, 62, 64, 127
    abnormal, 43-44
    abruption of placenta, 17
    active pressure, 41
    Alexandria units, 41-42
    analysis, 16-17
    baseline at zero, 16
    baseline setting, 16
    catheters, solid, transducer-tipped, 48
    cocaine addiction, 47
    contractions, 42
    coupling, 44
    documentation, 42-43
    doubling, 44
    duration, 41
    fetal heart rate, 48
    fetal hypoxia, 47
    fetal monitors, 48
    fluid-filled intrauterine pressure catheters, 48
    frequency, 41
    hypercontractility, 44-45
    hyperstimulation, 41, 44-47
    hypertonus, 41
    increased contraction frequency, 44-45
    increased peak IUP, 47
    injection, 47
    intensity, 41
    interval, 41
    intrauterine pressure catheter, 48
    kilopascal units, 41
    late decelerations, 17

low amplitude, high frequency waves, 43
maternal position, 17
Montevideo units, 41
oxygen reserves, 44
oxytocin, 47
pattern deviations, 43-47
patterns, 12, 14
peak IUP, 41
persistent occiput posterior, 45
persistent occiput transverse, 45
placenta, 47
quadrupling, 44
recognition, 17
resting tone, 41
skewed contractions, 44
supine hypotension, 17
tachysystole, 44-45, 47
tocotransducer, 16
tripling, 44
ultrasound, 48
uterine activity, 48
uterine reversal pattern, 42
waveform, 17
Uterine activity monitor, 6
Uterine blood flow, 202
Uterine contraction frequency, 10
Uterine contractions, 215-217
Braxton Hicks contractions, 215-216
cocaine, 217
coupling, 105
doubling of, 105
estrogen/progesterone, 216
gap junctions, 216
labor
first stage of, 216
second stage of, 217
oxytocin receptors, 216
prostaglandins, 216
resting tone, 217
Uterine hyperactivity, 269
Uterine hyperstimulation, 108, 436
Uterine hypertonus, 119, 433
Uterine hypoxia, 280
Uterine overdistention, 119
Uterine perforation, intrauterine pressure catheter, 37
Uterine reversal pattern, 63
Uterine rupture, 106, 119-120, 128, 283-285
Uteroplacental blood flow, 365-366, 433
Uteroplacental insufficiency, 102, 125, 176, 183, 206-207, 218, 224
Uteroplacental oxygen, 206-207
delivery, 205
consumption, 206
Uterus, 214-217

— V —

Vacuum extractor, 440
Vagal arrest, 113
Vagal influences, 173
Vagal reflex, 440
Vagal stimulus, 176
Vaginal birth after cesarean, 309
Vaginal examination, 437
Vaginal insufflation syndrome, 270-271
Vagus, 169-171
Valium, 79, 433, 463
Valsalva maneuver, 266, 434
Variability. *See under* type
classification of, 76
Variation, 14
vs. variability, 77
Vascular defects, congenital, 79
Vasculitis, 135
Vasoconstriction, 183, 433
Vein compression, 175
Ventricles, 395
Ventricular fibrillation, 398, 407
Ventricular tachycardia, 398, 407
Verapamil, 416
Villous edema, 213-214
Vintzileos criteria, 494-495
Visual analysis, 12-15

— W —

Wandering baseline, 73
Wedge pressure, increased, 199-200
Wenckebach heart block, 421
Wharton's jelly, 216, 218
Whispered rumble, 7
Whole blood oxygen content, 200
Wolff-Parkinson-White syndrome, 410

— Z —

Zero-crossings, 84
Zidovudine, 33